AF838908

Global Cleft Care in Low-Resource Settings

Jordan W. Swanson
Editor

David W. Low
Illustrator

# Global Cleft Care in Low-Resource Settings

Springer

*Editor*
Jordan W. Swanson
Children's Hospital of Philadelphia
University of Pennsylvania
Philadelphia, PA
USA

*Illustrator*
David W. Low
Children's Hospital of Philadelphia
University of Pennsylvania
Philadelphia, PA
USA

ISBN 978-3-030-59104-5 ISBN 978-3-030-59105-2 (eBook)
https://doi.org/10.1007/978-3-030-59105-2

© Springer Nature Switzerland AG 2021
This work is subject to copyright. All rights are reserved by the Publisher, whether the whole or part of the material is concerned, specifically the rights of translation, reprinting, reuse of illustrations, recitation, broadcasting, reproduction on microfilms or in any other physical way, and transmission or information storage and retrieval, electronic adaptation, computer software, or by similar or dissimilar methodology now known or hereafter developed.
The use of general descriptive names, registered names, trademarks, service marks, etc. in this publication does not imply, even in the absence of a specific statement, that such names are exempt from the relevant protective laws and regulations and therefore free for general use.
The publisher, the authors and the editors are safe to assume that the advice and information in this book are believed to be true and accurate at the date of publication. Neither the publisher nor the authors or the editors give a warranty, expressed or implied, with respect to the material contained herein or for any errors or omissions that may have been made. The publisher remains neutral with regard to jurisdictional claims in published maps and institutional affiliations.

This Springer imprint is published by the registered company Springer Nature Switzerland AG
The registered company address is: Gewerbestrasse 11, 6330 Cham, Switzerland

*This book is dedicated to the memory of Joseph Gruss, Don LaRossa, and Peter Randall – cleft pioneers and our dear mentors, who emphasized excellence above all else in the quest to expand access to cleft care.*

*This book is also dedicated to the memory of Marco Aurelio Gamborgi, an exceptionally talented and inspirational cleft surgeon, and author of Chapter 7 in this book, whose magnetic life was tragically cut short as this book went to press.*

–J.W.S. and D.W.L.

# Foreword

Surgery is the art of changing a life of despair into a better life.

Ten years ago, our island country saw much of this despair. The red island, Madagascar, is one of the poorest countries in the world. Our 30 million people see perhaps a thousand or more children born with clefts each year. The majority of patients are from disadvantaged families and live far from the capital city.

We have made recent strides to improve the treatment of patients with cleft lip and palate in our country. Some of the best examples of this work represent how we have reached out to patients. I am proud to have been among the pioneers of "Operation Smile" in Madagascar, one of several organizations working to improve access to surgical care. Patients tell me that they feel much supported because these healthcare programs are not only limited to surgery and hospitalization. Rather, a whole package of patient care is taken into account, starting from the fieldwork for the diagnosis, following by the explanation of the treatment process, and finally providing psychological support to the parents or the adult patients. Our team accompanies the patient through to the surgery site for screening and care.

Particularly special in caring for children with clefts is the camaraderie of a team that is created. It shows the willingness of all of us to help others. Doctors become friends by working together, by learning from each other. Surgeons from all over the world come together in missions to share ideas as they care for patients. This learning has created energy among our teams in Madagascar, as the exchange of experiences and the contribution of new techniques by renowned surgeons both increases the quality of our care, and motivates young people to become trained in cleft surgery.

This book reflects the close bonds between doctors. One of the things I find wonderful about this book is its internationality. The authors herald from 29 different countries, and many of the chapters are written by a combination of authors from higher- and lower-income countries, or different lower-income countries.

Writing a foreword to this prestigious work is a great honor for me and my beloved country.

The comprehensive writing and clear guidance, from more than 100 authors, including many of the top authorities globally, show all aspects of treatment used in cleft lip and palate cases. Surgeons of different nationalities share their experiences and knowledge focused on how to give patients a better future. And it makes available the most recent techniques for all readers.

Above all, this book reminds us of the importance in showing empathy to our patients (and our colleagues) at all times. Our capacity to heal patients is unfortunately often limited, sometimes by the hours in the day or a week that we can do surgery. We can't usually afford to give satisfaction to all of them. Yet we are always proud of our intervention, as we are there to bring smiles and a new start in their lives. For those patients who we can't take care of today, we hope that we can take care of tomorrow, or soon. And that the care we provide them tomorrow is even better than the care we provide today. I really prefer to use the name "servant" instead of "surgeon" to illustrate the compassion so engrained in this work. It takes a lot of humility and self-sacrifice to be able to contribute to the joy and happiness of others.

I end this foreword with words of thanks to all the authors of this work. All of our collective actions are possible because of the involvement of the whole team. This book helps make the team stronger.

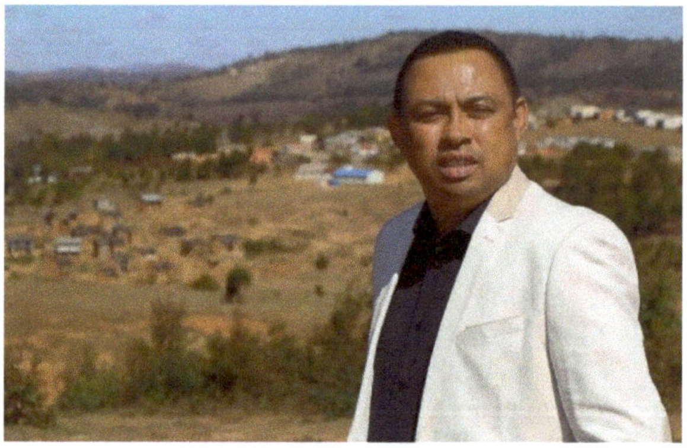

Andriamanarivo Mamy Lalatiana, MD
Plastic Surgeon and Head of Pediatric Surgery Department
CHU-JRA Antananarivo, Former Dean, Medical School of Antananarivo
Former Minister of Public Health
Antananarivo, Madagascar

# Foreword

It is a great honour to write this foreword for *Global Cleft Care for Low Resource Settings*. I look forward to sharing this book with its pearls of wisdom from many wonderful teachers.

We, as cleft surgeons, find commonality in our desire to create a perfect lip and nose, together with a palate that works well and allows the maxilla to grow. We all know the handcuffs of perfectionism, as we torture ourselves with the minute details of tissues, in our quest to relieve ourselves of the burden of not being good enough. We meet each other and we know we have met ourselves.

Once enticed, we devote years in pursuing a surgical art that remunerates modestly, haunts us with the deforming face of time, and then provokes our angst as we confront our shortcomings, long after we can change anything about what we might have done differently.

Ultimately, we married the partner we loved rather than the one who had all the money or the status. And how blessed we are!

I ponder the journey that brought me to cleft surgery. Like many of you, it drew me in with an early experience. I loved it from the first moment I watched a surgeon repair a cleft lip. His hands moved with the help of his assistant, in an orchestra of purposeful motion. He worked, reposed serenely, in concentration and attention. A chess game evolved, as he wrestled the tissues into harmony. In my case, that surgeon was Harold McComb. The result was awesome. The moment contagious. I wanted to be a cleft surgeon too.

I wasn't even sure I would be good at surgery. I still don't know if I am good at surgery. And perhaps it's that notion, the lingering voice in my head that tells me I am not good enough, that drives me to create as close to perfection as I can, reflected on the face that abides in front of me. As I finish each surgical attempt, how the asymmetries of the lip accuse me, how that persisting nasal slump chides me. At least with time and age, the voice grows softer. Maybe it's become more of a friend now.

Other voices also speak to me. Deep from a time past, a quiet promise pulls insistently on my mind. A reminder to never forget what it was like to be a child. A time when, what I wanted for myself didn't seem to matter to adults. Somehow, I kept that oath to myself. I can reach through that fog. And reach that child. And tell him I remember. And I am there to let him know what he feels is important. And now I will look after every child remembering that.

There is also a slightly crueller memory. Fingers pointed at me. A time in my life when I felt the judgement of others based on how I looked. What could I do to change what they said about me? How could they think they knew me just from the way I looked? Somehow as a child, trauma is worn as fault. "I am faulty. That's why this is happening to me." This I also remember. And each time I am given an opportunity to change that for a child, perhaps I am also healing a part of myself.

What a gift we have, friends. To be able to change the way even one life is lived. To do our best to minimise the pain felt by our patients, from the cruelty that potentially resides in the dark side of all of us.

Like many of you, I am thankful that I am in a place in life to give back. And how ideally suited cleft surgery is to enable this, to give away something that was given to us. Devoting our careers, we understand the importance of quality, audit, teamwork and training. We have much to offer as we share what we have with people in other countries that have fewer resources and opportunities.

Sending missions to help in different parts of the world is a wonderful enterprise when they are geared with human connection. Anyone who has participated in a mission can attest to the magic of lives changed, both those who give, as well as those that receive.

However, a shift is beginning to happen. The fact that I volunteer and intend to do good does not justify any action I choose. Cleft care rarely means a single operation. With limited resources, we are faced with increasingly difficult questions. How do we prioritise our surgeries? When there is not enough time, do we help those who haven't been helped yet, or finish the care of someone we have started with? How do we know we did a good job? What happens when we don't do a good job? What is the best way to make lasting difference?

We seem to do better as we listen to the needs of a country, as we work alongside local leaders and medical staff. We are learning to increase our awareness of the effect of our intentions.

A particularly notable change is in our approach to palate surgery. We increasingly understand the impact of a well-executed primary procedure and the importance of providing the environment to ensure it. The emotional impact of a lip repair can distract us from the significance of palate reconstruction. It sometimes seems like palates are treated as the invisible poorer cousins. It is palate surgery that affects a lifetime of being understood and the repercussions of poor surgery can be hard to correct.

Palatoplasty is technically demanding surgery. Operating with limited access, with bleeding obscuring vision while dealing with tissues that are difficult to dissect, can be unforgiving. Adequate time, instrumentation and lighting is required. Education and supervision of younger surgeons is needed, with emphasis on the training and support of local practitioners. It is particularly important to avert creating large fistulas, which then require multiple interventions with difficult surgical solutions in scarred tissues. A palate repair done hastily is more likely to leave a complication than one done carefully and patiently, resulting in many more hours of surgery than the time initially "saved." Sadly, as many of us have seen, the situation can be irretrievable and in those situations it is better if we had done nothing. All are avoided by a primary procedure performed well. The ego and bravado of fast surgery should be thoroughly discouraged. It is better to do well than to be quick.

It is our job to be advocates. To shift the paradigm to prioritising each patient. To remember a name, to acknowledge a life, to greet family members, to perform the surgery we are trained to do, to emphasise the capacity building for local teams, and to recreate the team approach that we know is paramount to the care of each child affected with cleft lip and palate. Who else can understand the significance of all these factors but the cleft surgeon who has devoted their career to marrying this pursuit? For it is about helping others in the way we would have liked to be helped, if fate had found us on the other side of the equation.

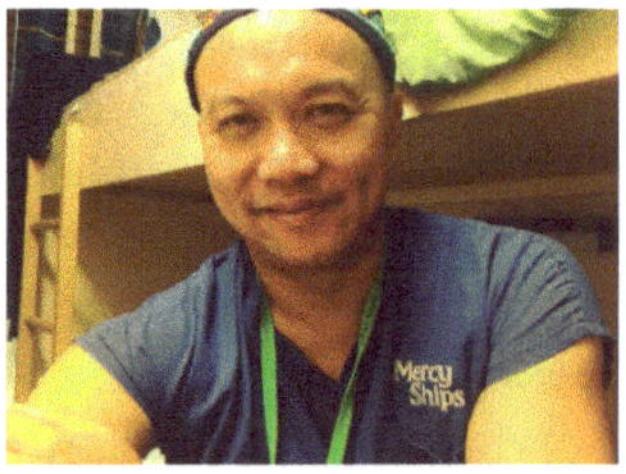


David K. Chong, MBBS, FRACS
Cleft Surgeon, Royal Children's Hospital
President Australasian Cleft Lip and Palate Association
Melbourne, Australia

# Preface

The impetus for this book was, sadly, a surgical complication. Early in my career, practicing in Managua, Nicaragua, I repaired the bilateral cleft lip of a young girl, and all went smoothly. She was slender, with an asymmetry to her cleft pattern, but she passed our screening examinations without concerns and tolerated anesthesia and surgery well. When she left the hospital the next day for her nearby village, her mother beamed with pride.

But when I saw her back in clinic a week later, something wasn't right: the incisions were turning red, with a whitish slough over top. Over the following weeks, the skin and muscle of her upper lip philtrum slowly melted away, despite our best efforts. A hole formed between her upper lip and nose. As it healed, it retracted her upper lip, and she is likely to need further surgical reconstruction of her upper lip when she is older.

I had never seen a lip dehisce like this, and it is considered exceedingly rare in the North American centers in which I had trained. Yet, as I got to know the faces and scars of children with clefts in Nicaragua, I realized that surgical outcomes were far more variable. Why did her cleft lip repair become infected and dehisce? What about the patient, the surgeon or surgical technique, or the post-operative environment may have played a role in the complication occurring?

Seeking the answers to these questions over the last several years has introduced me to a dynamic cadre of emerging leaders in low-resource settings. Surgeons, orthodontists, nurses, pediatricians, anesthesiologists, therapists, engineers, program coordinators, and others, they are passionately and adaptively caring for children with clefts. They are devising novel ways to help families surmount the myriad barriers that stymy access to care in areas of entrenched poverty. They are carefully studying outcomes of cleft treatment and verifying what I observed in Nicaragua: adverse outcomes are occurring more often than suspected, creating an urgency to improve the quality of our care. Because they realize that treatment approaches refined in high-income settings don't often translate well to low-resource settings, they are conducting research efforts to develop practical solution sets that work in these environments. They are developing new and innovative ways to teach, which is so critical to bolstering low numbers of medical and surgical personnel. And they are often teaming up together, forging collaborations across borders to build energy and accountability to sustain these efforts.

This is their book. The 100 contributing authors hail from 29 countries, most of them constituting low-resource settings. Many chapters are co-authored by colleagues in both high and low-resource environments, in which they present contemporary treatment strategies and techniques with guidance for adapting them to different settings. But perhaps more importantly, they illustrate fundamental challenges and mindsets for improvement that are likely to continue to guide our efforts – your efforts – to advance global cleft care well into the future. Finally, we return to the most important people in this process, our patients – past, present, and future. They are for whom, and through whom, we seek to do better.

Philadelphia, PA, USA — Jordan W. Swanson

# Acknowledgments

Surgeons are the products of their mentors, and I have been incredibly fortunate for the many who have guided me. Rick Redett at Johns Hopkins first introduced me to cleft surgery, and set me on my path with inspiration. Craig Birgfeld, Joseph Gruss, Richard Hopper, and Raymond Tse trained me with patience and exacting standards at the University of Washington, and their partnership with surgeons in Africa was a visionary model for international academic collaboration. Scott Bartlett and Jesse Taylor at the Children's Hospital of Philadelphia are extraordinarily versatile cleft and craniofacial surgeons, and greatly expanded my operative intuition. I am lucky indeed to now come to work each day with Oksana Jackson, David Low, and both of them as my partners. Bill Magee (III) at USC was courageous in taking me on as the Tsao Global Surgery fellow and as a junior partner, and I remain deeply grateful for his support and coaching as we together tackled challenges of improving cleft outcomes and training surgeons in austere settings. Finally, much of my favorite learning comes from the remarkable clinical instinct (and sense of humor) of my beloved partner Armando Siu in Nicaragua, who has built much through his resilient career on the front lines.

Operation Smile is a very special organization, and has been forward thinking in taking on big challenges ahead of their time, including establishing local teams, developing comprehensive care centers, building orthognathic and craniofacial programs, strengthening health systems, and empowering its volunteers in program countries. I am grateful to Bill and Kathy Magee, Ruben Ayala, and Jordi Baron for the opportunities to learn alongside them and to help co-develop some of these programs together with them. I am further thankful to Indiana Siu, Tatiana Morales, Jaffa Coen, and Albertina McGregor of Operacion Sonrisa Nicaragua and the countless Ministry of Health staff who relentlessly advocate for children and adults with clefts, and who welcomed our family to what is now a second home.

Alex Campbell is a young plastic surgeon who has not only cared for the most vulnerable in India and Colombia, but brought keen scientific intellect and clever problem-solving to these efforts; he is a pioneer and role model. David Chong, Neema Kaseje, Edwar Alvarez, Gaurav Deshpande, Nicolas Sierra, Nivaldo Alonso, and Marco Swanson are likewise emerged and emerging changemakers in global cleft surgery, and teaming up with each of them continues to be a real privilege. Thanks to Caitlin Prim at Springer who set this book in motion, and to Dhanapal Palanisamy our production manager and Miranda Finch our supervising editor who carried it the distance. Finally, most importantly, thank you to my dear Magda, Lazaro, and Joaquin, whose love gives purpose to the adventure.

*–J.W.S.*

I am incredibly fortunate to be a living extension of Don LaRossa and Peter Randall, having been inspired and mentored by Don to become a plastic surgeon. I had the distinction of being Peter Randall's last chief resident, and I was honored to have been asked to join the Penn faculty by the great craniofacial pioneer Linton Whitaker. Penn Plastic Surgery and The Children's Hospital of Philadelphia have always supported my career as both a surgeon and a medical illustrator.

I am indebted to my colleagues who have encouraged me to participate in and have accompanied me on many cleft missions, beginning with Rotaplast and culminating in Smiles for Guatemala. I have formed many new professional friendships during the creation of this book, and I have learned so many innovative techniques in cleft care from this international group of experts in the field.

I have always dedicated my life to my three children, Jenny, Jamie, and Katie (a Disney animator who introduced me to the drawing app Procreate, which I used exclusively to create every illustration in this book), and I have happily made additional room in my heart for Evelyn and Hudson.

*–D.W.L.*

# Contents

# Case Studies in Cleft Surgery

Edwar Alvarez, David Alvarez, Percy Rossell-Perry, and Vilma Arteaga

# About the Editors

## Editor

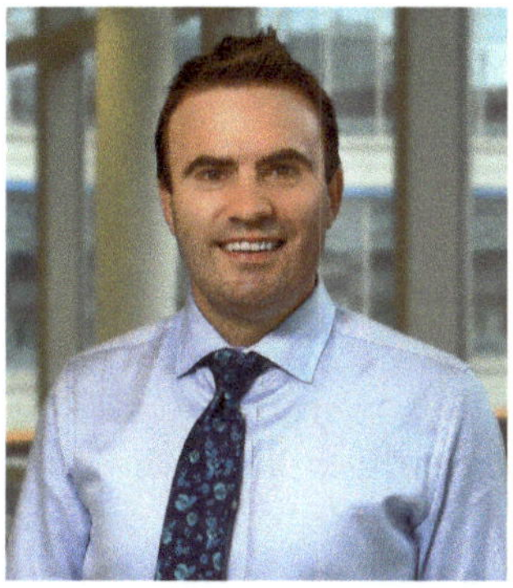

**Jordan W. Swanson, MD, MSc** is a pediatric plastic and craniofacial surgeon at the Children's Hospital of Philadelphia and assistant professor of surgery at the University of Pennsylvania. He trained at the University of Washington and completed his cleft and craniofacial surgery fellowship at Penn. He also holds an MSc in international development management from the London School of Economics and was the Tsao Fellow in Global Surgery. He previously lived and worked in Nicaragua, collaborating with Operation Smile and the Nicaraguan Ministry of Health to help build a joint comprehensive cleft and craniofacial program. He went on to serve as the director of surgical innovation at Operation Smile, working to expand rural access to surgical care through the *Surgery for the People* program in Nicaragua. He partners with cleft teams in several countries to develop adaptive solutions for improving access to care, training, and quality of outcomes.

## Illustrator

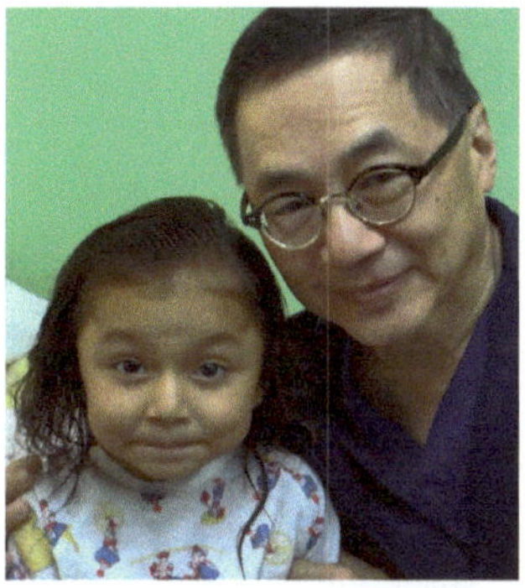

**David W. Low, MD** is professor of surgery at the University of Pennsylvania and an attending physician at The Children's Hospital of Philadelphia where he has more than 30 years' experience in treating patients with cleft lip and palate. A graduate of Harvard College and Harvard Medical School, he completed all of his surgical training at Penn under the guidance of plastic surgery giants Don LaRossa, Linton Whitaker, and Peter Randall. He serves as the medical director for his CHOP-based team, Smiles for Guatemala, which provides multidisciplinary cleft care biannually to the indigent population of Guatemala. A certified medical illustrator, Dr. Low has contributed to many publications through his artwork. His personal experience in cleft care has provided a unique advantage in the creation of the many illustrations in this book.

## Section Editors

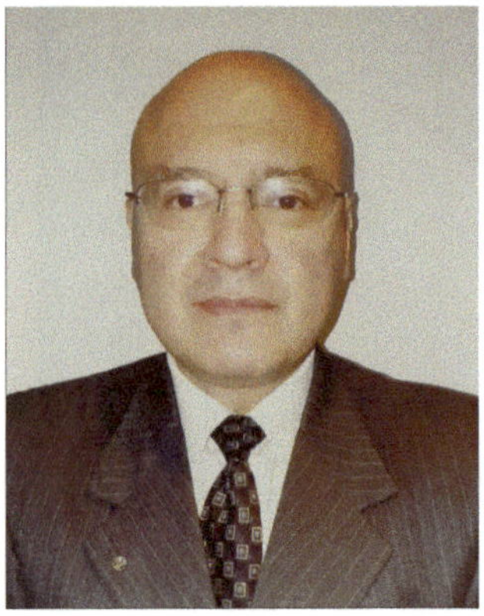

*Case Studies in Cleft Care*

**Edwar Alvarez, MD** is a reconstructive and aesthetic plastic surgeon and serves as medical director of the Plastic Surgery Service at the Hospital Clinic Continental. He has developed several new cleft surgical techniques, particularly aimed at reducing complications and improving outcomes in lower-resource countries. He serves as scientific coordinator of Operation Smile Ecuador and is a sought-out surgeon educator throughout Latin America. He is a Member of the Ecuadorian Society of Reconstructive and Aesthetic Plastic Surgery and FILACP, and recipient of the Arcadio Forereo Colombia Award and Stephen Pratt Award.

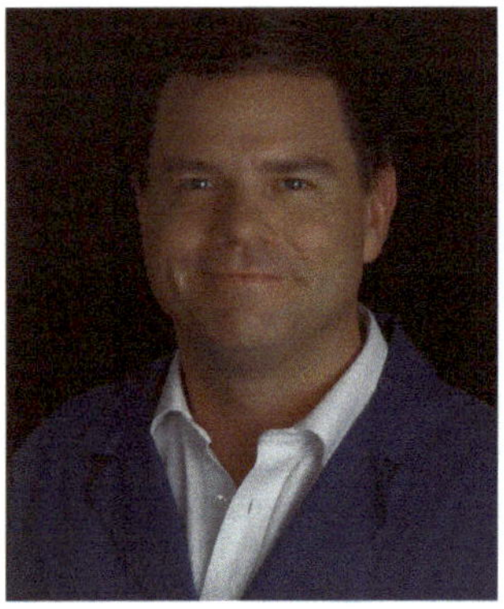

*Complete Surgical Treatment*

**Alex Campbell, MD** is a diplomate of the American Board of Plastic Surgery and Member of the Colombian Society of Plastic Surgery. He is the founding medical director of the Guwahati Comprehensive Cleft Care Center in Assam, India, and served as a senior medical advisor to Operation Smile, where he designed the Cleft Surgery Training Program and the Surgical Outcomes Program. Dr. Campbell is a clinical assistant professor of surgery at Penn State University and serves as chief medical officer for Mobile Surgery International and Medical Advisor to the United States Embassy in Colombia. Dr. Campbell has authored dozens of articles and book chapters and is co-editor of the surgical handbook *Essentials of Cleft Surgery*. He lives with his wife and partner, Dr. Carolina Restrepo, in Cartagena, Colombia.

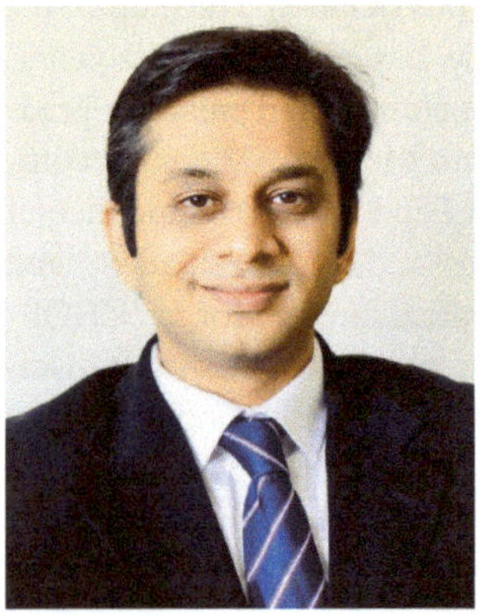

*Care Delivery Models*

**Gaurav Deshpande, MD** is associate professor of maxillofacial surgery and fellowship director for cleft and craniofacial surgery at MGM Dental College and Hospital, Navi Mumbai. He has led pioneering cleft surgery technique and outcomes research in India, and is an invited lecturer internationally. He has participated with numerous cleft care missions with Operation Smile, where he is passionate about teaching and believes in strengthening young surgeons' foundation by emphasizing mastery of basic principles.

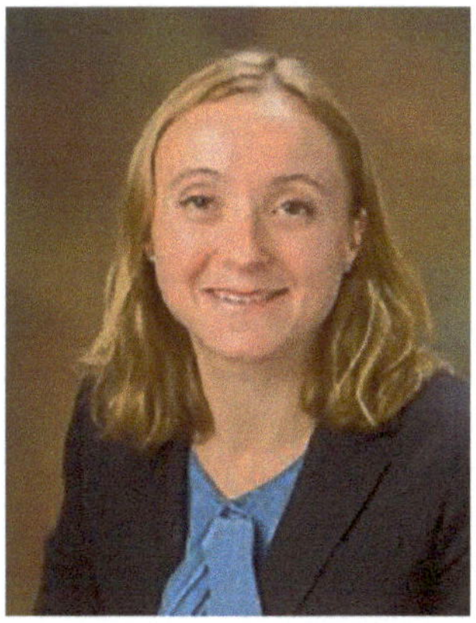

*Comprehensive Cleft Care*

**Oksana A. Jackson, MD** is co-director of the Cleft Lip and Palate Program and director of the Velopharyngeal Dysfunction Program at the Children's Hospital of Philadelphia and associate professor of surgery at the University of Pennsylvania. She is a graduate of the University of Pennsylvania School of Medicine and completed plastic surgery residency and fellowship at the University of Pennsylvania and the Children's Hospital of Philadelphia. Dr. Jackson has been involved in numerous international surgical missions for cleft care over the past 12 years, primarily in South and Central America and Eastern Europe. She also serves on the board of directors for the humanitarian organization SARA (Sharing America's Resources Abroad).

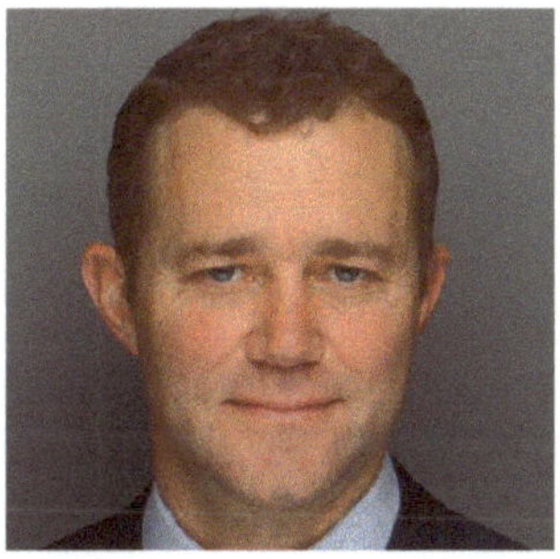

*Introduction to Global Cleft Care*

**William P. Magee III, MD, DDS** is a respected leader and visionary in global surgery who has made significant contributions to this field through his life-long work with Operation Smile transforming pediatric reconstructive surgery in low- and middle-income countries. As founder and director of the Operation Smile Global Surgery Fellowship, he mentors surgical trainees from around the world to become leaders, educators, and innovators within global surgery. In addition, he holds professorships at Children's Hospital Los Angeles and University of Southern California while also serving as chief of plastic and reconstructive surgery at Shriners Hospital for Children – Pasadena where he continues to advance the field of pediatric reconstructive surgery.

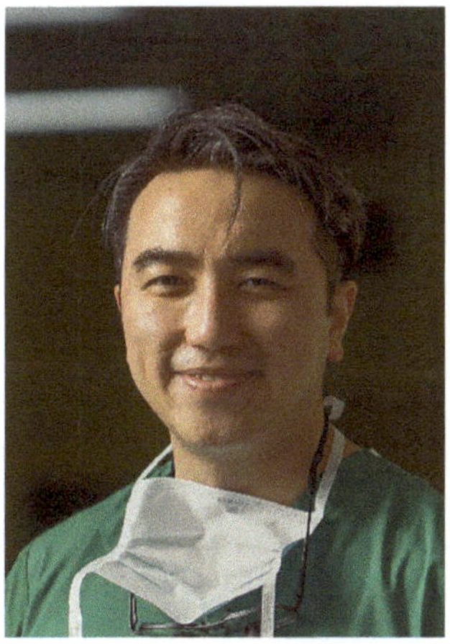

*Educational Innovation*

**Phuong D. Nguyen, MD** is director of craniofacial surgery and assistant professor of surgery in the Division of Plastic and Reconstructive Surgery at the University of Texas Health Sciences Center, McGovern Medical School, and Children's Memorial Hermann Hospital. He has been engaged in international medical outreach and reconstructive surgical missions for over 16 years in 8 countries. Dr. Nguyen is also a first-generation Vietnamese American, born in a refugee camp in Indonesia. He has dedicated his professional career to reconstructive surgery for children and is the co-founder of Nuoy Reconstructive International, a humanitarian organization that seeks to improve access to reconstructive care, education, collaboration, and transparency.

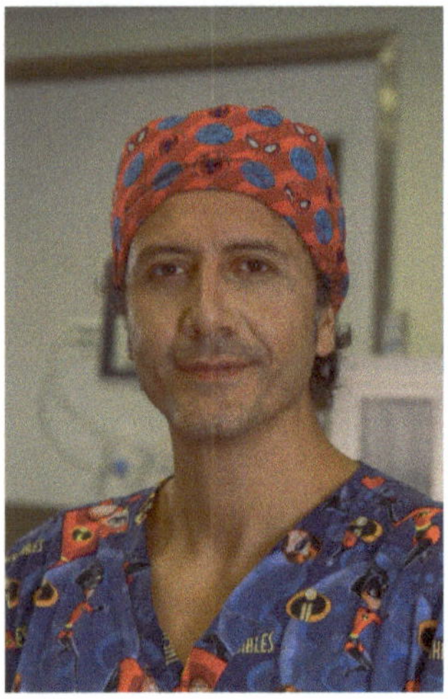

*Cleft Patient Assessment*

**Nicolas E. Sierra, MD** is medical director and chief surgeon for Mobile Surgery International at the Mobile Surgical Center in Oaxaca-México, where a model of comprehensive surgical care for cleft patients is under development with the support of Smile Train. He is also associate surgeon of pediatric oral and maxillofacial surgery at the Vall d'Hebrón University Hospital in Barcelona, Spain, where he has dedicated his career to the management of congenital facial anomalies. He has trained within the Operation Smile's Cleft-Surgery-Training-Program at the Guwahati Comprehensive Cleft Care Center in Assam, India, and completed his cleft-craniofacial fellowship at the Federal University of Paraná in Curitiba, Brazil. He serves as a volunteer for Operation Smile, where has helped develop the global Orthognathic Surgery program.

# Contributors

**Karoon Agrawal, MS, MCh** Smile Train, New Delhi, India

**Adriana Agell-Sogbe, DMD** Orthodontics and Maxillary Orthopedics Unit, Oral and Maxilofacial Surgery Department, Vall d´Hebrón University Hospital, Barcelona, Spain

**Allyson R. Alfonso, BS, BA** New York University Langone Health Hansjörg Wyss, Department of Plastic and Reconstructive Surgery, New York City, NY, USA

**Nivaldo Alonso, MD, PhD** Faculty of Medicine of the University of São Paulo, Hospital das Clinicas at the University of São Paulo, São Paulo, Brazil

**Emmanuella Amoako, MD** Cape Coast Teaching Hospital, Cape Coast, Ghana

**Yader Arce, RN** Operacion Sonrisa Nicaragua, Managua, Nicaragua

**Vilma L. Arteaga, DDS** Maxillofacial Orthodontics and Orthopedics Ortodent, Guatemala City, Guatemala

Juan Pablo II Children Hospital, Operation Smile Guatemala, Guatemala City, Guatemala

**Ruben Ayala, MD** Operation Smile, Virginia Beach, VA, USA

**Keith L. Ballance** Surgical Instruments Maintenance Department, Operation Smile, Virginia Beach, VA, USA

**Patricia Bannister, MBE, MSc, RN, SCM, HV** Pullum House, Beggars Ash, Ledbury, UK

University of Manchester, Manchester, UK

**Jordana Baron, MPH, MBA** Johns Hopkins University Bloomberg School of Public Health (at time of writing), Washington, DC, USA

**Scott P. Bartlett, MD** University of Pennsylvania, Children's Hospital of Philadelphia, Philadelphia, PA, USA

**Craig Birgfeld, MD** Division of Plastic Surgery, Department of Surgery, University of Washington and Seattle Children's Hospital, Seattle, WA, USA

**Diana Bohórquez, MD** Oral and Maxillofacial Surgery Department, Vall d'Hebron University Hospital, Barcelona, Spain

**Adrian Bosenberg, MBChB, FFA(SA)** Department Anesthesiology and Pain Management, Seattle Children's Hospital, University Washington, Seattle, WA, USA

**Alex Campbell, MD** Division of Plastic Surgery, Penn State Hershey College of Medicine, Hershey, PA, USA

Operation Smile, Inc, Virginia Beach, VA, USA

Mobile Surgery International, Mexico City, Mexico

Premium Care Plastic Surgery, Cartagena, Colombia

**James Chang, MD, FACS** Division of Plastic and Reconstructive Surgery, Stanford Medical Center, Stanford, CA, USA

**Philip Kuo-Ting Chen, MD** Craniofacial Center, Taipei Medical University Hospital, Taipei, Taiwan

Department of Surgery, Taipei Medical University, Taipei, Taiwan

**David K. Chong, MBBS** Plastic and Maxillofacial Surgery Department, Royal Children's Hospital, Melbourne, VIC, Australia

**Noreen Clarke, DNP, RN, CNS** Children's Hospital Los Angeles, Los Angeles, CA, USA

Keck Scholl of Medicine of USC, Los Angeles, CA, USA

**D. Scott Corlew, MD, MPH** Program in Global Surgery and Social Change, Harvard Medical School, Boston, MA, USA

**Nicolas S. Dhooghe** Plastic, Reconstuctive and Esthetic Surgery, Ghent University Hospital, Ghent, Oost-Vlaanderen, Belgium

**James M. Drake, MD, MSc** Division of Neurosurgery, The Hospital for Sick Children, Toronto, ON, Canada

**Gaston Echaniz, MD** Department of Pediatric Anesthesia, Sant Joan de Déu Barcelona Children's Hospital, Barcelona, Spain

**Ghulam Qadir Fayyaz, MD** Plastic Surgery Services Institute of Medical Sciences, & CLAPP Hospital, Lahore, Pakistan

**Caleb J. Figge, PhD** Department of Mental Health, Johns Hopkins Bloomberg School of Public Health, Baltimore, MD, USA

**David M. Fisher, MB, BCh, FRCS(C), FACS** Division of Plastic & Reconstructive Surgery, University of Toronto, Toronto, ON, Canada

The Cleft Lip and Palate Program, Division of Plastic & Reconstructive Surgery, The Hospital for Sick Children, Toronto, ON, Canada

**Roberto L. Flores, MD** Hansjörg Wyss Department of Plastic Surgery, NYU Langone Health, New York, NY, USA

**David Aldrete Flores** Division of Biomedical Engineering, Operation Smile, Guadalajara, Jalisco, Mexico

**Christopher R. Forrest, MD, MSc** Division of Plastic & Reconstructive Surgery, University of Toronto, Toronto, ON, Canada

The Cleft Lip and Palate Program, Division of Plastic & Reconstructive Surgery, The Hospital for Sick Children, Toronto, ON, Canada

**Muhammad Ashraf Ganatra** Department of Plastic Surgery, Dow University of Health Sciences, Karachi, Pakistan

**Amanda A. Gosman, MD** University of California San Diego, San Diego, CA, USA

**Usama S. Hamdan, MD, FACS** Global Smile Foundation, Boston, MA, USA

Tufts University School of Medicine, Boston, MA, USA

Harvard Medical School, Boston, MA, USA

Boston University School of Medicine, Boston, MA, USA

**Anne Hing, MD** Seattle Children's Hospital, Seattle, WA, USA

**Oksana A. Jackson, MD** Division of Plastic Surgery, Children's Hospital of Philadelphia and University of Pennsylvania, Philadelphia, PA, USA

**Luv Javia, MD** Children's Hospital of Philadelphia, University of Pennsylvania Perelman School of Medicine, Philadelphia, PA, USA

**Desmond T. Jumbam, MSGH** Program in Global Surgery and Social Change, Harvard Medical School, Boston, MA, USA

Department of Plastic and Oral Surgery, Boston Children's Hospital, Boston, MA, USA

**Melissa Kanack, MD** Department of Aesthetic & Plastic Surgery, UC Irvine School of Medicine, Irvine, CA, USA

**Rami S. Kantar, MD, MPH** New York University Langone Health Hansjörg Wyss, Department of Plastic and Reconstructive Surgery, New York City, NY, USA

The University of Maryland Medical System, Baltimore, MD, USA

**Serena N. Kassam, DMD** Pediatric Dentistry Department, New York University College of Dentistry, New York, NY, USA

Global Smile Foundation, Norwood, MA, USA

**Nima Khavanian, MD** Department of Plastic and Reconstructive Surgery, Johns Hopkins School of Medicine, Baltimore, MD, USA

**Anna Kolentz, MD** Hospital Casa de Saúde Bon Jesus, Caruaru, Pernambuco, Brazil

**Prasetyanugraheni Kreshanti, MD** Cleft and Craniofacial Center Cipto Mangunkusumo Hospital, Plastic Surgery Division, Department of Surgery, Faculty of Medicine Universitas Indonesia, Jakarta, Indonesia

**Ann W. Kummer, PhD, CCC-SLP, FASHA** Division of Speech-Language Pathology, Cincinnati Children's Hospital Medical Center and University of Cincinnati College of Medicine, Cincinnati, OH, USA

**Florence C. Kuyt, MD** Pediatric Clinical Specialty Advisor, Operation Smile's Medical Council, Virginia Beach, VA, USA

**Marco A. Lopes-Gamborgi, MD** Centro de Atendimento Integral aof Fissurado Labiopalatal, Curitiba, Brazil

Núcleo de Pesquisa e Reabilitação de Lesões Lábio Palatais Prefeito Luiz Gomes, Joinville, Brazil

**David W. Low, MD** Division of Plastic Surgery, Children's Hospital of Philadelphia and University of Pennsylvania, Philadelphia, PA, USA

**Anna Luan, MD, MS** Division of Plastic and Reconstructive Surgery, Stanford Medical Center, Stanford, CA, USA

**Fabiola Grigoletto Lupion, MD** Hospital de Clínicas, Federal University of Paraná, Curitiba, Brazil

**Donald R. Mackay, DDS, MD** Division of Plastic Surgery, PennState Hershey College of Medicine, Hershey, PA, USA

**Anil Madaree, MD** Department of Plastic and Reconstructive Surgery, Inkosi Albert Luthuli Central Hospital; University of Kwazulu-Natal, Durban, South Africa

**Leanne Magee, MD, DDS** Division of Plastic and Reconstructive Surgery, Department of Child and Adolescent Psychiatry and Behavioral Sciences, Children's Hospital of Philadelphia and University of Pennsylvania, Philadelphia, PA, USA

**William P. Magee III** Division of Plastic and Reconstructive Surgery, University of Southern California, Los Angeles, CA, USA

Division of Plastic and Maxillofacial Surgery, Children's Hospital Los Angeles, Los Angeles, CA, USA

Shriners Hospital for Children, Pasadena, CA, USA

**Meghan McCullough, MD, MS** Keck School of Medicine, University of Southern California, Los Angeles, CA, USA

**Felicity V. Mehendale, MBBS, MS, FRCS, FRCS** University of Edinburgh, Edinburgh, Scotland, UK

**Naikhoba C. O. Munabi, MD** Division of Plastic and Reconstructive Surgery, Keck School of Medicine of the University of Southern California, Los Angeles, CA, USA

**Eric Nagengast, MD** Division of Plastic and Reconstructive Surgery, University of Southern California, Los Angeles, CA, USA

**Isis Juliane Guarezi Nasser, MD** Assistance Center for Cleft Lip and Palate (CAIF), Hospital do Trabalhador, Curitiba, Paraná, Brazil

**Kusezweni Kevin Nduku, MBChB** Department of Plastic and Reconstructive Surgery, University of Zimbabwe, Harare, Zimbabwe

**Phuong D. Nguyen, MD, FACS, FAAP** Division of Plastic Surgery, Department of Surgery, Children's Memorial Hermann Hospital, University of Texas Health Science Center, Houston, TX, USA

**Solomon Obiri-Yeboah, MD, DMD** Department of Oral and Maxillofacial Sciences, Kwame Nkrumah University of Science and Technology, Kumasi, Ghana

School of Medicine and Dentistry and Komfo Anokye Teaching Hospita, Kumasi, Ghana

**Jorge Pamias, MD, DDS** Orthognatic Surgery Unit, Oral and Maxilofacial Surgery Department, Vall d´Hebrón University Hospital, Barcelona, Spain

**Vikram Pandit, MDS** Pandit Clinic, Pune, India

**Teresita Pannaci, DDS** Vall d' Hebron Institute of Research, Barcelona, Spain

Operation Smile Venezuela, Virginia Beach, VA, USA

Operation Smile Morocco, Casablanca, Morocco

**Eugene Park, MD** Division of Plastic Surgery, Northwestern University Feinberg School of Medicine, Chicago, IL, USA

**Dale J. Podolsky, MD, PhD** Division of Plastic & Reconstructive Surgery, University of Toronto, Toronto, ON, Canada

**Allan Porras, DDS** Oral and Maxillofacial Surgery, Proactive Dental Solutions and Operation Smile Nicaragua, Managua, Nicaragua

**Shankar Man Rai, MD** National Academy of Medical Sciences, Kirtipur Hospital, Kathmandu, Nepal

**Anjaramamy Ramamonjisoa** Operation Smile Madagascar, Washington, DC, USA

**Elie P. Ramly, MD** Global Smile Foundation, Norwood, MA, USA

Hansjörg Wyss Department of Plastic Surgery, NYU Langone Health, New York, NY, USA

**Krishna Shama Rao, MBBS** Consultant Craniomaxillofacial Surgeon, Inga Health Foundation, Bangalore, India

**Sashank K. Reddy, MD, PhD** Department of Plastic and Reconstructive Surgery, Johns Hopkins School of Medicine, Baltimore, MD, USA

**Richard J. Redett III, MD** Department of Plastic and Reconstructive Surgery, Johns Hopkins School of Medicine, Baltimore, MD, USA

**Carolina Restrepo, MD** Operation Smile, Inc, Virginia Beach, VA, USA

**Diógenes L. Rocha, MD, PhD** Plastic and Reconstructive Department, Hospital das Clinicas, Universidade de Sao Paulo, Sao Paulo, Brazil

**Derek J. Rogers, MD** Pediatric Otolaryngology, Madigan Army Medical Center, Tacoma, WA, USA

**Percy Rossell-Perry, MD, PhD, FACS** E. Rebagliati Martins Hospital ESSALUD Lima PERU, Lima, Peru

**Alexis Rothermel, MD** Division of Plastic Surgery, PennState Hershey College of Medicine, Hershey, PA, USA

**Gisela H. Sánchez Sosa, MSc** Division of Biomedical Engineering, Tecnológico de Monterrey, Guadalajara, Jalisco, Mexico

**Michelle Scott, DDS, MBA** Department of Plastic and Reconstructive Surgery, Children's Hospital of Philadelphia, Philadelphia, PA, USA

**Chen Shen, BS** Hansjörg Wyss Department of Plastic Surgery, NYU Langone Health, New York, NY, USA

**Nicolas E. Sierra, MD, FEBOMFS** Mobile Surgery International, Oaxaca, Mexico

Oral and Maxillofacial Surgery Department, Vall d'Hebron University Hospital, Barcelona, Spain

**Plinio Sierra, MD** Department of Pediatric Anesthesia, King Abdullah Specialized Children's Hospital, Riyadh, Saudi Arabia

**Renato da Silva Freitas, MD** Plastic Surgery Unit, Federal University of Parana, Curitiba, Brazil

Assistance Center for Cleft Lip and Palate (CAIF), Hospital do Trabalhador, Curitiba, Paraná, Brazil

**Armando Siu, MD** Operation Smile Nicaragua, Managua, Nicaragua

**Brian C. Sommerlad, MBBS, FRCS** Consultant Plastic Surgeon, Great Ormond Street Hospital for Children, London, UK

**Jordan W. Swanson, MD, MSc** Division of Plastic Surgery, Children's Hospital of Philadelphia and University of Pennsylvania, Philadelphia, PA, USA

**Jesse A. Taylor, MD, FACS, FAAP** Department of Plastic Surgery, The Children's Hospital of Philadelphia, Philadelphia, PA, USA

**Raymond W. Tse, MD, FRCS(C)** Division of Plastic Surgery, Department of Surgery, University of Washington, Seattle, WA, USA

Division of Craniofacial and Plastic Surgery, Department of Surgery, Seattle Children's Hospital, Seattle, WA, USA

**Charanya Vijayakumar, MD** Department of Plastic & Reconstructive Surgery, Sri Ramachandra Institute of Higher Education and Research (SRIHER), Chennai, Tamil Nadu, India

**Aurora G. Vincent, MD** Otolaryngology, Head and Neck Surgery, Madigan Army Medical Center, Tacoma, WA, USA

**Raj M. Vyas, MD, FACS** Department of Aesthetic & Plastic Surgery, UC Irvine School of Medicine, Irvine, CA, USA

Global Smile Foundation, Boston, MA, USA

**Karen W. Y. Wong Riff, MD, PhD** Division of Plastic and Reconstructive Surgery, Hospital for Sick Children, Toronto, ON, Canada

The Cleft Lip and Palate Program, Division of Plastic & Reconstructive Surgery, The Hospital for Sick Children, Toronto, ON, Canada

**Robin Yang, MD, DDS** Department of Plastic Surgery, Johns Hopkins Hospital, Baltimore, MD, USA

**Caroline A. Yao, MD, MS** Program in Global Surgery and Social Change, Harvard Medical School, Boston, MA, USA

Department of Plastic and Oral Surgery, Boston Children's Hospital, Boston, MA, USA

**Carrie Zimmerman, BS** Children's Hospital of Philadelphia, Philadelphia, PA, USA

# Part I

# Introduction to Global Cleft Care

# Introduction: A Paradigm Shift in Global Cleft Care

# 1

Jordan W. Swanson

**Key Points**

- Major evolution in global cleft care is being driven by five exciting—but challenging—forces.
  1. Surgery is increasingly seen as a critical but underdeveloped component of public health delivery in low-resource settings, and cleft surgery is an important potential bellwether to mediate this shift.
  2. Locally delivered cleft care offers many advantages, but creates a systemic transition from the international missions that were prominent in early outreach efforts.
  3. Patient-perceived outcomes of good function and appearance are the ultimate goals of cleft care, and employing outcome measures in these settings is critically important.
  4. Innovation borne out of low-resource settings can be nurtured by bringing voice and tools to emerging leaders in these settings.
  5. The evidence base for cleft surgery needs to be inclusive of low-resource settings, which often yield different findings than high-resource settings.

Lizmarlin was 4 years old when we first met, in the stale, humid air of a clinic room attached to the Esteban Serrano Hospital, in the Caribbean jungle of eastern Nicaragua. Cowering behind a door in the room, tears streamed down her cheeks and onto her pink dress, her nicest one, which had become dusty during the 8-hour walk and bus ride to our clinic. Each half of her full upper lip was splayed widely to the side, and mucous poured from the wide cleft in her lip and palate. Though this was the furthest that she had ever been from home, she was still another 10 hours by bus away from the capital city of Managua, where her cleft could be surgically repaired. The exhausted eyes of her young mother, sitting with us, revealed stoicism and love, but also divulged uncertainty about her daughter's future.

Lizmarlin's story is different from those of the children born with clefts whom I meet at the Children's Hospital of Philadelphia. In Philadelphia, I often meet them for the first time while they are still in the womb, parents tipped off to the pending cleft by a prenatal ultrasound. These parents can count on successful lip and palate repairs to be completed by a year of age, with their child likely to begin to smile, speak, and sing shortly thereafter.

In truth, Lizmarlin's story was graced with some good fortune. She was spotted by a coffee buyer, one of many who logs regular travel through rural agricultural regions and are trained up through an inspired effort of the Nicaraguan government and Operation Smile to identify children with clefts and inform their families of available treatment. And her family surmounted a number of barriers common to low-resource settings; Lizmarlin's mother sought out and managed to reach care for her daughter. In high-resource settings, an orofacial cleft is not thought to be a fatal disease, but Smile Train data from low-resource settings suggest that fewer than half of children with clefts in some regions survive to their fifth birthday—due to a combination of malnutrition, aspiration pneumonia, and purposeful neglect [1]. In these ways, a cleft lip and palate exemplify health inequality in the modern world.

As a young surgeon living and working in Nicaragua, I struggled to understand the pathophysiology of clefts and their optimal care in the setting of poverty and a constrained health system. Was it appropriate to perform a palate repair in an older patient? How had infection led to dehiscence of a bilateral lip

J. W. Swanson (✉)
Division of Plastic Surgery, Children's Hospital of Philadelphia and University of Pennsylvania, Philadelphia, PA, USA
e-mail: swansonj@email.chop.edu

© Springer Nature Switzerland AG 2021

J. W. Swanson, D. W. Low (eds.), *Global Cleft Care in Low-Resource Settings*, https://doi.org/10.1007/978-3-030-59105-2_1

repair, something I had not seen before? Despite being trained by outstanding cleft surgeons at leading programs in the United States, the answers to these questions and others—the widely ranging cleft patterns and severity, and patient ages and comorbidities—exceeded my clinical experience and training.

Most challenging was caring for patients who had been left with poor outcomes from previous surgery. Specifics of the surgery were often unknown to the family or health system. Facing children stigmatized by appearance and function, their faces and mouths severely scarred, often elicited a sense of duty to bring mercy, even as we vowed not to repeat past mistakes that were not always evident. I also saw the consequences of well-intentioned efforts by well-trained surgeons from afar: for instance, the teaching of a Furlow palatoplasty under loupe magnification to young surgeons who did not have loupes, and who then struggled in subsequently emulating the technique. I know there were similar consequences resulting from my own efforts, and even others which I did not fully appreciate.

Fortunately, a growing cadre of specialists who care for children with clefts in these settings are marshaling keen observation, intuition, and problem-solving to significantly improve paradigms of care. Doctor Armando Siu, my senior partner in Nicaragua, has honed a remarkable surgical instinct over three decades of practice, deploying adroit maneuvers so that surgical repairs better stand up to the realities of poor hygiene, sugary diets, and irregular follow-up. Nurse Tatiana Morales, a fierce patient advocate, set up my visit with Lizmarlin in the rural hospital and as a patient coordinator meticulously tracks patients throughout the country and devises creative ways of reaching out to them. Tatiana and other similarly committed doctors and nurses are among a passionate and inspiring band of cleft providers in low-resource settings who are quick to improvise to bring practical help to people in need (Fig. 1.1). They seem to share three common attributes: (1) they have sought out excellent clinical training, (2) they have committed themselves to serving vulnerable and marginalized cleft patient populations, and (3) they work to be data-driven in their decision-making, collecting data where possible and studying outcomes in settings in that are simply not addressed in the vast majority of existing academic literature.

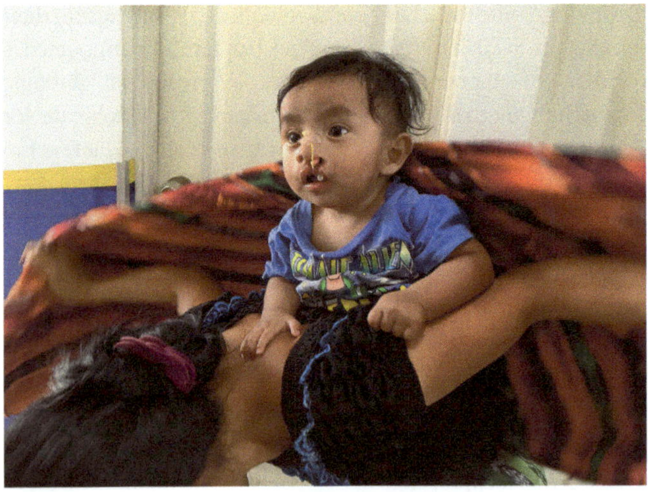

Fig. 1.1 Infant with a cleft lip and nasal deformity is treated with an improvised naso-alveolar molding device by an unknown dentist in a region without known trained cleft providers

These unsung problem-solvers are forming a growing fraternity of cleft providers around the world. Accessible technologies such as WhatsApp give voice to surgeons in remote settings, and cleft organizations and societies help to mobilize disparate providers. These innovators are now becoming thought leaders in their own right, and whose ideas are worth spreading. This book was both inspired and, importantly, authored by these scholar-pragmatists—practitioners who have made it their mission to deliver the best possible cleft care to all people of the world using methods appropriate to their realities and circumstances.

Just as low-resource settings vary dramatically in their unique and specific economic, technological, and cultural constraints and attributes, perspectives on traditional and emerging approaches to cleft treatment at times diverge. The approximately 100 authors who have contributed to this textbook hail from 29 countries, most of them constituting low-resource settings (Fig. 1.2). Great efforts have been taken to present multiple perspectives where they exist, and nurture evolving surgical techniques and approaches by practitioners in low-resource settings even as they contrast with traditional surgical techniques originating in quite dissimilar clinical settings. In identifying, curating, and reviewing these contributions to the academic literature on cleft repair, much credit is due to this book's talented section editors, each of whom possesses a unique depth of experience as medical directors and leaders of cleft centers and outreach programs in these challenging settings.

## Five Forces Shaping Global Cleft Care

We find ourselves amidst an exciting but challenging time of major evolution in the field of global cleft care. This book was conceived and inspired in the hopes of better understanding of how we should address these changes, and it aims to squarely take on each one.

### Surgery as Public Health

First, the potential of surgery to contribute to dramatic improvements in global health looms bright. Not so long ago, surgery was thought to be too expensive or complex to scale effectively in poorer countries—a service peripheral to

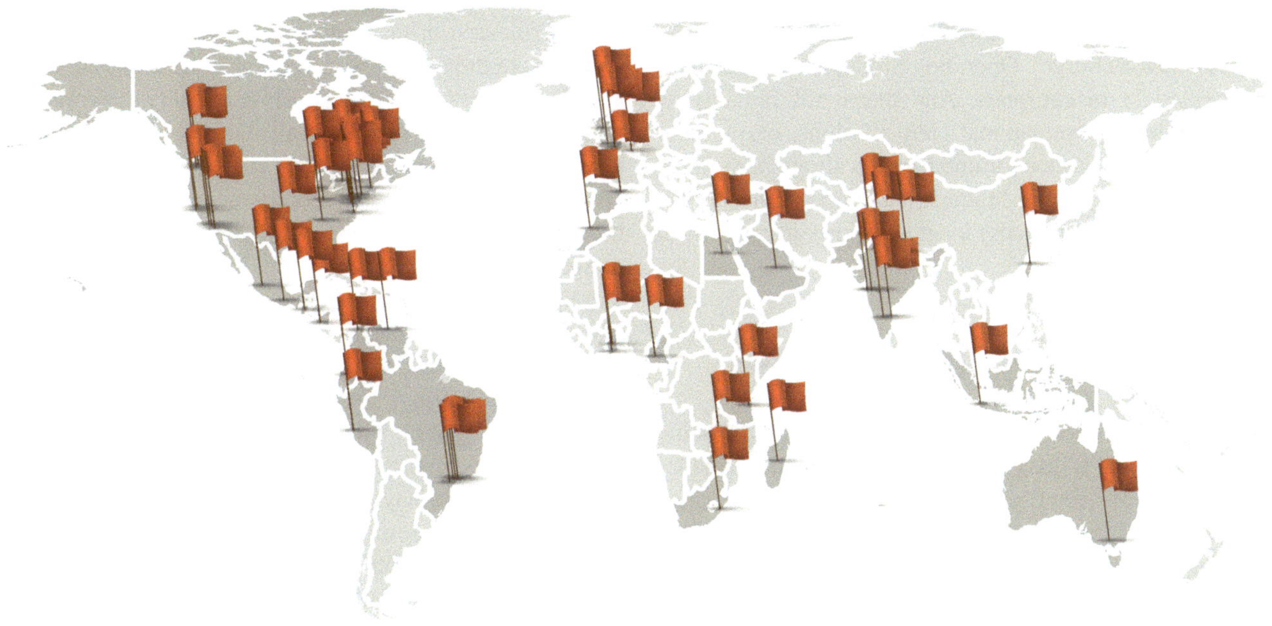

**Fig. 1.2** Authorship of *Global Cleft Care for Low-Resource Settings*. (Map courtesy of Chris Kalmar, MD)

public health. This viewpoint is being challenged by recent findings from the World Health Organization and *The Lancet* that more people die each year from surgically treatable conditions than HIV/AIDS, malaria, and tuberculosis combined [2, 3]. Surgically treatable diseases are among the top causes of disability in the world, particularly in low- and middle-income countries (LMICs).

In fact, surgical treatment of many conditions, including cleft lip and palate, can be highly effective relative to investment costs; it is, for example, more cost-effective than anti-hypertensive medicines for cardiovascular disease or antiretrovirals for HIV/AIDS [2]. Especially in poorer settings, surgical treatment of a laborer's injured hand or a child's congenital deformity is a form of *Surgical Justice*, the concept that surgery imparts freedom even beyond the receiving patient to their family, community, and society [4]. Cleft surgery is well-positioned to be a global bellwether for this shift in thinking about surgery. Cleft care represents the largest sector of philanthropically funded global surgery [5], and a compelling argument can be made for "diagonal development" of a health system by scaling up cleft care [6]. It is a field with leadership potential to strengthen surgical systems in low-resource settings.

## Locally Delivered Cleft Care

Second, a major transition is occurring in how cleft care is delivered in low-resource settings—and by whom. Many of the most visible early cleft outreach efforts were conducted by international volunteer teams who traveled from higher to lower income countries for 1–2-week surgical missions to places that had no cleft care providers. The power of reconstructing major visible congenital deformities through relatively quick, safe procedures is remarkable, bringing hope to communities unfamiliar with cleft treatment. Surgical missions also provide a rare forum for doctors, nurses, and therapists to work side by side, sharing ideas, and learning from each other.

Perhaps inspired by these outreach missions, a growing corpus of local providers have begun to develop local cleft teams and programs. Home-grown teams have important advantages over visiting clinicians, including the possibility of offering year-round care continuity to patients and an intimate familiarity with the nuances of local health system dynamics. Unfortunately, these programs are often challenged by limited financing, and surgeons and clinical teams frequently serve in unpaid volunteer capacities. Moreover, in places where such local efforts have taken root, they have also served to expose some of the downsides of the traditional international surgical mission model: difficulty in offering patient continuity and following outcomes, undermining the reputation of local surgeons and of local cultural and social practices, outsized travel and cargo transport expenses (often exceeding the cost of a local surgeon's full-time salary for up to a year), and limited ability to offer ongoing dental, speech, and other multi-disciplinary care.

In response, many cleft organizations that started out solely as surgical mission providers are working to adapt their programs to this changing landscape. Building and investing in local cleft centers staffed by local teams, embracing an educational focus to clinical efforts, financing local teams, and drawing volunteer providers from other low-resource settings, are several tactics that groups such as Interplast (now ReSurge), Operation Smile, and Smile Train have adopted in recent years. And there still remains an important role for international cleft missions, particularly in locations where properly trained staff is altogether scarce, such as to provide care in Madagascar (population 29 million, with 2 plastic surgeons) even as efforts to train local surgeons are underway.

## Focus on Achieving Great Patient Outcomes

Third, the effectiveness of cleft care is increasingly being judged not by what is done to patients, but by what it enables in them. A simple count of total cleft surgeries performed cannot be the primary yardstick for success. Success might be better defined as a patient who feels socially and functionally integrated into society. In settings where patient follow-up is challenging and provider presence is intermittent, it is particularly important to ensure that impactful outcomes are achieved consistently. Several recent studies have reported that post-surgical complications such as dehiscence and fistula, which typically occur in fewer than 5% of cases in high-income settings, occur in an astonishing 25–56% of cases in LMICs [7–9]. Thus we have to be cautious not to proliferate care that is ineffective, or worse, harmful, in settings where factors of poverty, medical care, nutrition, environment, and culture may influence healing differently.

Moreover, publicizing a high number of procedures or care episodes that an organization performs or a patient receives can be problematic. Increased numbers can indicate reaching more patients with better care, but it can also signify the repetition of care episodes or surgical revisions that reflect inadequate solutions to the underlying problem. Patients and families seek the best possible function and appearance delivered through the fewest possible episodes of treatment. Therefore, quality of care is paramount. Refining and tracking robust outcome metrics—reflecting the breadth of speech, oral health, appearance, and self-confidence—are critical to these efforts, and this is an exciting area of rapidly evolving research discussed in Chap. 37.

## Innovation Borne of Low-Resource Settings

Fourth, innovations in cleft care are increasingly being developed in low-resource settings. "Poverty devises skills," proposed the Greek poet Theocritus. If "necessity is the mother of invention," as his contemporary Plato wrote, it seems logical that new and practical solutions would arise in constrained settings. Further, in many cases, these innovations and improvisations may be well-suited to other low-resource settings.

Historically, factors such as low densities of providers, a lack of research infrastructure, and the high costs of prototyping were thought to pose structural barriers to innovation and sharing in these settings. More recently, however, technological advances in communication, online collaboration, and 3-D printing, among others, are enabling a more conducive ecosystem to emerge. Compared to high-income countries, less complex regulatory environments and health care delivery systems may actually reduce barriers to entry for these innovations, even as the rights and vulnerability of patients involved in these efforts must be respected. In paradoxical and exciting ways, some innovations originating in low-resource settings are spreading to high-resource settings, including nerve blocks, obturator techniques, and cleft severity and outcome tools. Innovations derived from low-resource settings may be particularly timely as healthcare costs soar in high-resource settings, and efficacious lower-cost alternatives are increasingly being sought.

To be sure, there remain many challenges in identifying new innovations and vetting their efficacy, which is particularly important when resources to scale up new innovations are limited. Good ideas and good intentions do not always lead to better outcomes. But when they do, they can dramatically alter our patients' lives for the better, and the desire to find these innovations—regardless of their place of origin—unites us all.

## The Conundrum of Evidence-Based Medicine

Finally, while we all seek to practice "evidence-based" medicine, how that applies to low-resource settings is often far from clear. Much of the "evidence," if defined as scientific literature published in high impact journals, originates from high-income countries. Mounting examples suggest that when these techniques or protocols are re-deployed in low-resource settings, the results can be very different [10]. Where higher quality studies do exist, they can lead to different recommendations than in high-resource settings. For instance, the best US evidence supports no postoperative antibiotic use after palatoplasty [11]. However, a double-blinded, randomized controlled trial in India showed superior outcomes when a 5-day prophylactic oral antibiotic was used postoperatively [12].

In the absence of clear data, practice patterns around the world vary widely; decision-making is often guided by intuition and personal experience, and multiple approaches often seem reasonable. Throughout this textbook, we strive to seek out and present these multiple approaches. With time, it is quite possible that some aspects of cleft care will converge toward a single most optimal technique or protocol, whereas others will continue to see evidence supporting multiple approaches. Further, higher fidelity studies may show us how and why cer-

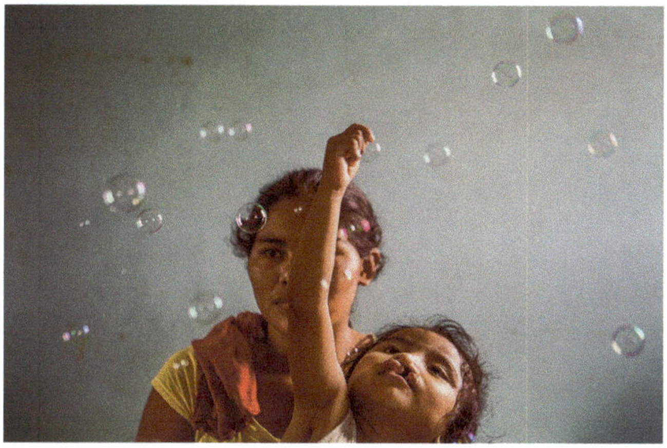

**Fig. 1.3** Lizmarlin, a 4-year-old girl in Nicaragua with unrepaired cleft lip and palate, 1 month after her family's initial visit to a cleft surgeon and shortly before her cleft lip repair. (Photo courtesy of Inti Ocon)

tain approaches are better in certain places, and this may depend on broad socioeconomic factors or specific epigenetic factors in ways that we are now only beginning to understand.

Dr. Bill Magee, the founder of Operation Smile and an early advocate for global cleft surgery, often remarks that the surgeon plays at most 10% of the part in helping to heal a child with a cleft. Indeed, a few moments before I repaired Lizmarlin's cleft lip, a photographer took this photo (Fig. 1.3). Although she had not undergone any surgical care at this point, a transformation was already well underway. A pediatrician found that she was otherwise healthy, with good growth potential; a speech therapist had counseled her family that her speech would improve after surgery; a child life specialist was helping her self-confidence grow through interactive games; and a team of caring specialists was already at her side.

Ingenuity and problem-solving are not unique to cleft repair nor to surgery in general—medical practitioners have always sought out the best possible solutions with the resources at hand. This textbook first seeks to honor that tradition by presenting the techniques of leading experts from around the world, and by doing so and illustrating them in such a way to be accessible by all global providers. But it further seeks to recognize that ingenuity is an innate part of the practice of medicine, and that improvisation and practical adaptation are not necessarily less than ideal or second-rate care. They are often the right care for the setting in which they are being performed, and this textbook seeks to elevate these practices to their rightful place in the literature—or at the very least, validate the ingenuity and pragmatism that their originators were facing in developing them. It finally seeks to pay tribute to the many talented people dedicated to caring for children with clefts in low-resource settings, as we endeavor to learn from each other to do better for our patients.

## References


1. Mossey PA, Modell B. Epidemiology of oral clefts 2012: an international perspective. Front Oral Biol. 2012;16:1–18.
2. Meara JG, Leather AJ, Hagander L, Alkire BC, Alonso N, Ameh EA, Bickler SW, Conteh L, Dare AJ, Davies J, Mérisier ED. Global surgery 2030: evidence and solutions for achieving health, welfare, and economic development. Lancet. 2015;386(9993):569–624.
3. World Health Organization. World health assembly resolution 68.15: strengthening emergency and essential surgical care and anaesthesia as a component of universal health coverage. 68th World Health Assembly. 2015; 27. Available at http://apps.who.int/gb/ebwha/pdf_files/WHA68/A68_R15-en.pdf?ua=1.
4. Morrison SD, Swanson JW. Surgical justice. Plast Reconstr Surg. 2015;136(2):291e–2e.
5. Gutnik L, Dieleman J, Dare AJ, Ramos MS, Riviello R, Meara JG, et al. Funding allocation to surgery in low and middle-income countries: a retrospective analysis of contributions from the USA. BMJ Open. 2015;5(11):e008780. https://doi.org/10.1136/bmjopen-2015-008780.
6. Patel PB, Hoyler M, Maine R, Hughes CD, Hagander L, Meara JG. An opportunity for diagonal development in global surgery: cleft lip and palate care in resource-limited settings. Plast Surg Int. 2012;2012:892437.
7. Maine RG, Hoffman WY, Palacios-Martinez JH, Corlew DS, Gregory GA. Comparison of fistula rates after palatoplasty for international and local surgeons on surgical missions in Ecuador with rates at a craniofacial center in the United States. Plast Reconstr Surg. 2012;129:2. https://doi.org/10.1097/prs.0b013e31823aea7e.
8. Daniels KM, Yu EY, Maine RG, et al. Palatal fistula risk after primary palatoplasty: a retrospective comparison of a humanitarian organization and tertiary hospitals. Cleft Palate Craniofac J. 2016;55:807. https://doi.org/10.1597/16-007.
9. Rossell-Perry P, Segura E, Salas-Bustinza L, Cotrina-Rabanal O. Comparison of two models of surgical care for patients with cleft lip and palate in resource-challenged settings. World J Surg. 2015;39:47–53. https://doi.org/10.1007/s00268-013-2395-9.
10. Deshpande G, Wendby L, Jagtap R, Schönmeyr B. The efficacy of vomer flap for closure of hard palate during primary lip repair. J Plast Reconstr Aesthet Surg. 2015;68(7):940–5.
11. Rottgers SA, Camison L, Mai R, Shakir S, Grunwaldt L, Nowalk AJ, Natali M, Losee JE. Antibiotic use in primary palatoplasty: a survey of practice patterns, assessment of efficacy, and proposed guidelines for use. Plast Reconstr Surg. 2016;137(2):574–82.
12. Aznar ML, Schönmeyr B, Echaniz G, Nebeker L, Wendby L, Campbell A. Role of postoperative antimicrobials in cleft palate surgery: prospective, double-blind, randomized, placebo-controlled clinical study in India. Plast Reconstr Surg. 2015;136:59e–66e.

# Burden of Cleft Disease and Opportunity for Impact

# 2

Naikhoba C. O. Munabi and Nivaldo Alonso

**Key Points**

- Clefts cause both functional limitations on feeding and speech, and aesthetic consequences with profound psychosocial impact due to social stigma, which together lead to poor educational and employment opportunities as well as inability to achieve major life milestones.
- The long-term effects of untreated cleft lip and palate lead to a large social and economic impact, thus cleft repair is considered an essential surgery that should be available to all people everywhere by the 2015 Lancet Commission on Global Surgery.
- Cleft lip and palate can be caused by a genetic mutation, either inherited or spontaneous. Its frequency is also increased by environmental exposures often experienced before a young mother knows that she is pregnant.
- Even in regions where primarily lip and palate repair can be accessed, there is often a large backlog of patients who suffer from untreated or inadequately treated sequelae of cleft lip/palate.
- Cleft conditions disproportionately impact low-resource countries, where many additional social determinants and barriers may impact the ability of individuals to seek and receive appropriate care.
- Increased focus on comprehensive delivery of cleft care in austere settings, and assuring adequate outcomes of care, has the potential to dramatically improve social and economic well-being, and demonstrate the transformative impact of surgical care in these settings.

## Introduction

Cleft lip and/or palate is the most common congenital malformation of the head and neck worldwide with a prevalence of 0.5–1.6 in 1000 live births [1]. Cleft conditions can vary in appearance and severity from small incomplete clefts of the lip to wide bilateral combined cleft lip and palate. Clefts present both functional and aesthetic challenges. Functionally, clefts particularly of the palate can result in challenges with feeding and speech. Aesthetically, an atypical appearance due to cleft can have a profound psychosocial impact due to social stigma and lack of community acceptance, leading to poor educational and employment opportunities as well as inability to achieve major life milestones [2]. These long-term effects of cleft lip and palate can lead to a large economic impact, and it is this combined individual and economic impact that makes cleft repair one of the essential surgeries listed by the 2015 Lancet Commission on Global Surgery that should be available from either in country or visiting skilled providers [3].

In order to create systems that care for cleft conditions globally, we must understand their epidemiology and the impact such conditions have on communities, domestic and international society. Cleft conditions disproportionately impact low-resource countries, where many additional social determinants and barriers may impact the ability of individuals to seek and receive appropriate care. In this

N. C. O. Munabi (✉)
Division of Plastic and Reconstructive Surgery, Keck School of Medicine of the University of Southern California, Los Angeles, CA, USA
e-mail: Naikhoba.munabi@med.usc.edu

N. Alonso
Faculty of Medicine of the University of São Paulo, Hospital das Clinicas at the University of São Paulo, São Paulo, Brazil
e-mail: Nivalonso@usp.br

© Springer Nature Switzerland AG 2021

J. W. Swanson, D. W. Low (eds.), *Global Cleft Care in Low-Resource Settings*, https://doi.org/10.1007/978-3-030-59105-2_2

chapter, we review the nature and burden of cleft disease, and introduce options for cleft care delivery and their potential impact.

## Defining Cleft Conditions

Orofacial clefts originate from a failure of fusion of the frontonasal and lateral processes during development [4, 5] (Fig. 2.1). This failure occurs early in the development process between weeks six and eight of gestation [6]. Therefore, in cases where environmental exposures are the suspected cause of cleft conditions, these exposures may occur prior to awareness of pregnancy, highlighting the need for more preventive global policies and interventions rather than those just targeting expectant mothers.

The degree of disruption of the embryologic fusion process leads to the severity of the cleft condition, which can range from an incomplete unilateral cleft of just the lip to full bilateral cleft of the lip and palate. Studies by Yao et al. and Campbell et al. have graded the severity of cleft lip conditions on a 4-point scale, allowing for more universal language describing cleft lip presentations [7, 8] (Fig. 2.2). Similarly, classifications such as Veau and Kernahan aim to stratify clefts of the palate by either severity or component of the palate involved [9]; classifications are discussed further in Chap. 6.

In addition to clefts occurring as a result of intrinsic impairment in facial process fusion, clefts can also occur when the palatal shelves are otherwise obstructed from fusion by an intervening structure. Such a phenomenon is the case in Pierre Robin Sequence (PRS), where stunted mandibular growth leads to inability of the tongue to descend to the floor of the mouth resulting in the tongue physically obstructing palate fusion [10]. Despite being associated with multiple structural abnormalities, PRS can occur independently of a genetic cause, however is often seen in Stickler syndrome [10].

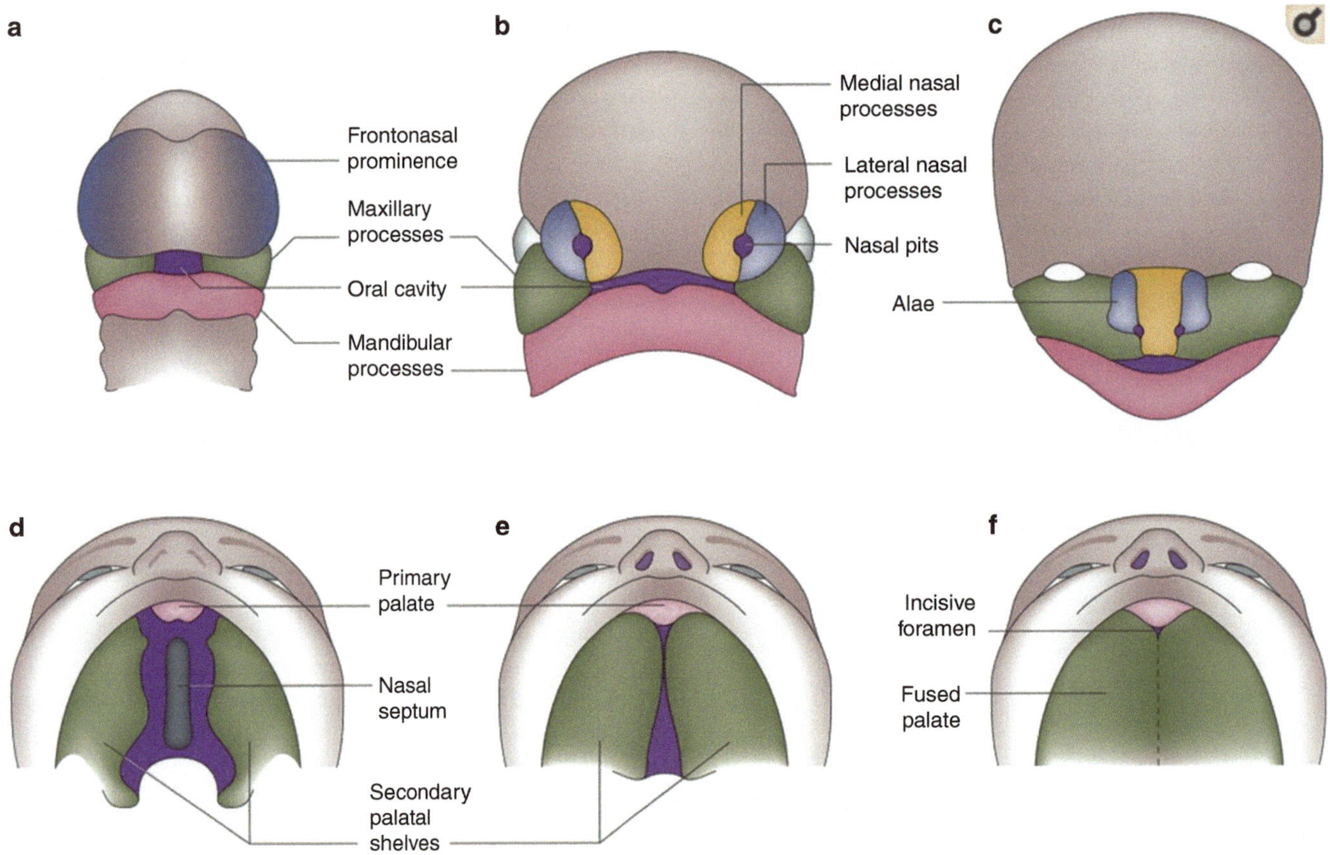


**Fig. 2.1** Embryonic development of the lip and palate in humans at the end of the (**a**) fourth, (**b**) fifth, and (**c**), sixth weeks of gestation. Disruption in movement and fusion of the frontonasal and maxillary processes during this time period can lead to cleft lip development. Primary and secondary palate fusion occur between weeks six and eight of gestation (**d**–**f**), with failures in fusion during this time period contributing to the development of cleft palate. (Reproduced from Dixon and colleagues [6] by permission of Nature Reviews)

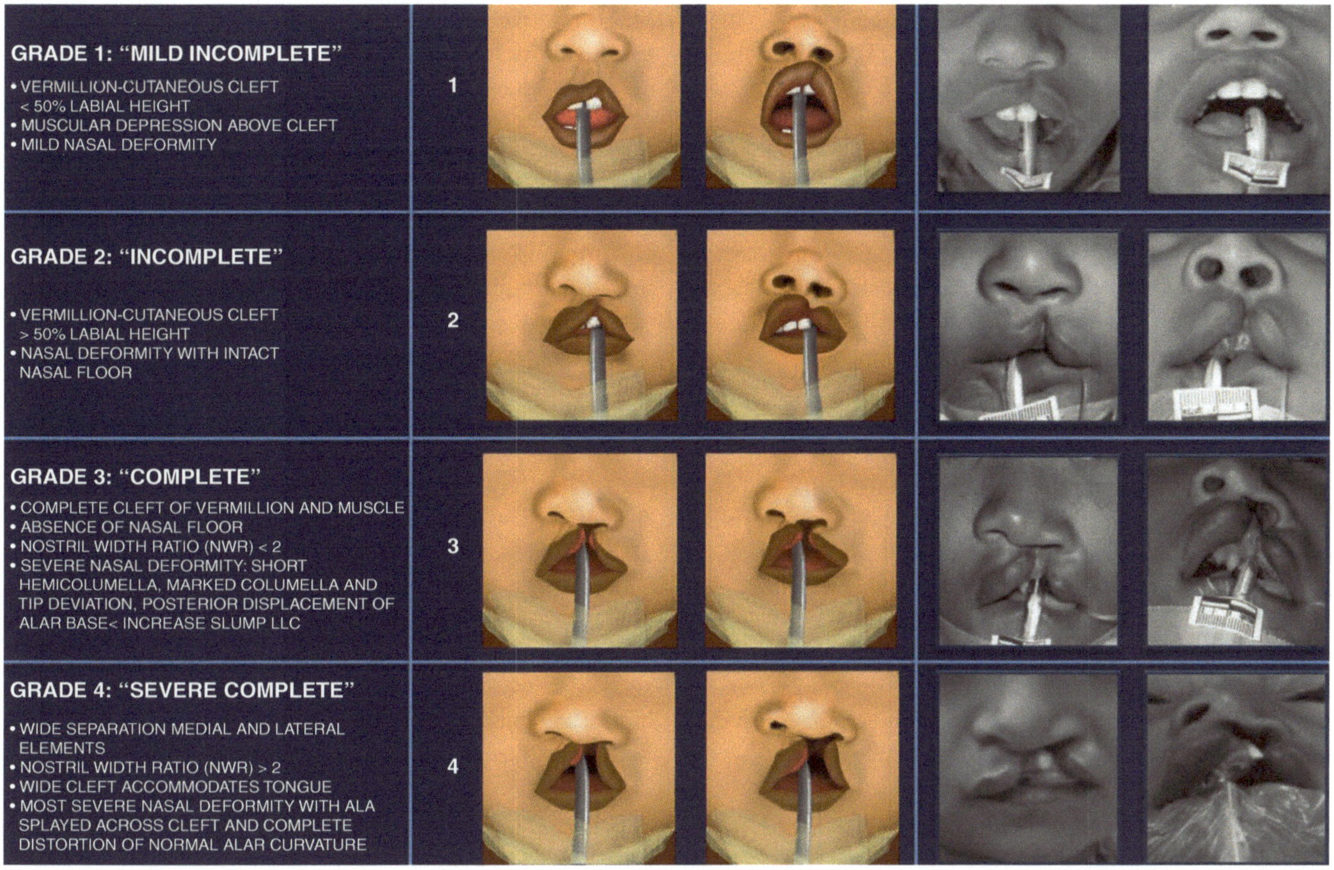


**Fig. 2.2** The Cleft Severity Index. Criteria for each of the 4 grades of the cleft severity and associated examples. (Reproduced from Campbell and colleagues [7] by permission of Plastic and Reconstructive Surgery Global Open)

## The Burden of Cleft Disease

### Epidemiology

Cleft lip and/or palate (CL/P) is one of the four most common congenital defects in children, and is the most common congenital anomaly of the head and neck. It affects between 1 in 500 and 1 in 2500 children born worldwide [11]. In general, Asian and Amerindian populations have the highest reported birth prevalence rates, often as high as 1/500, European-derived populations have intermediate prevalence rates at about 1/1000, and African-derived populations have the lowest prevalence rates at about 1/2500 [6].

Males are affected twice as often as females and for every bilateral cleft, there are three times as many patients affected with a cleft on the right, and six times as many with a cleft on the left [12].

The variability in incidence is due to a combination of genetic predisposition and environmental factors. Approximately 30% of cleft patients have a diagnosed syndrome, suggesting a genetic cause of the cleft. For the 70% of patients who are identified as non-syndromic, factors such as family history, rarer genetic mutations, and environmental exposures likely each play a role in the frequency of cleft development [13, 14]. For example, in Brazil, the familial recurrence rate for CL/P is dependent on the region of the country, with some areas demonstrating a recurrence risk as low as 0.6–0.7% compared to other regions with a three- to four-fold higher risk (2.2–2.8%) [15]. In this population, IRF6 may be one such gene associated with non-syndromic CL/P, as has been seen in other ethnic groups [14, 16]. However, environmental factors may also account for the geographic discrepancy observed.

Folate deficiency is perhaps the most well-known environmental factor associated with CL/P. Due to the effect of folate deficiency on neural tube formation, fortification of grains with folic acid has been mandated in many countries. In the United States, where fortification of grains was mandated in 1998, a 6–12% reduction in cleft palate prevalence was observed over the course of 12 years [16]. Convincing evidence also exists for other environmental factors influencing the rate of CL/P in a population. These factors all relate to maternal health and exposures during pregnancy such as gestational hypertension, seizures, smoking, and indoor cooking over an open fire stove [6, 13]. These factors can also show a geographic distribution due to ethnicity, culture, and socioeconomic status. Altogether, genetic predisposition, in addition to differential regulations and environmental exposures, may account for why some populations appear to be more afflicted by CL/P than others worldwide. Understanding the true nature of this gene by environment interaction may allow for improved pre-natal diagnosis and prevention of cleft conditions.

## Outcomes for Cleft Patients

The effectiveness of cleft care influences the burden of cleft disease, and this depends on the availability and accessibility of cleft care, its timeliness, and quality of outcomes. Ideal timing of primary cleft repair is between 4 and 6 months of age for cleft lip, and 8 and 12 months of age for cleft palate [17]. Delayed repair can be defined as repair occurring at an age over twice the ideal: 1 year for cleft lip and 2 years for cleft palate [18]. These recommendations stem from studies demonstrating the negative psychosocial impact of the response individuals can have to a person with a cleft, as well as the need for a functionally intact palate during the development of speech [2, 17]. The collective of patients who do not have their CL/P repaired, or who have an unsatisfactory outcome of the repair, by the appropriate time points constitute the backlog of cases [11, 18]. This backlog also represents the number of patients who need to be cared for in order to arrive at the lowest rate of cleft surgery required—sustainability for the birth rate.

Studies have estimated the backlog, or unmet need of cleft surgery, is highest in central Africa and southern Asia [19] (Fig. 2.3). However, these estimates focus on the unmet need of primary cleft repair only. Primary cleft lip or palate repair is only a portion of cleft care which can be defined as either complete or comprehensive. Complete cleft care includes all the necessary surgical procedures that should occur over the course of childhood to result in normal oral function, speech, and aesthetics. Complete care differs from comprehensive care which refers to the ability for a cleft patient to receive all necessary services surrounding their cleft condition. For example, in addition to cleft repair, patients with cleft palate may require nutrition consultation, speech therapy, tympanostomy tubes placed by an otolaryngologist, and audiology intervention among other services.

In today's current reality, many parts of the world are unable to deliver complete or comprehensive cleft care. Without access to such services, or even just primary cleft surgery, untreated individuals face considerable risk of morbidity and mortality. Morbidity can stem from functional limitations due to the cleft, including challenges with feeding and speech. However, the psychosocial impact of untreated clefts can also be tremendous due to stigma surrounding the condition in many countries. This stigma leads to limited engagement in educational opportunities, learning difficulties, poor self-esteem, depression, and anxiety, all of which ultimately impact individual potential to participate and achieve major milestones in life [2].

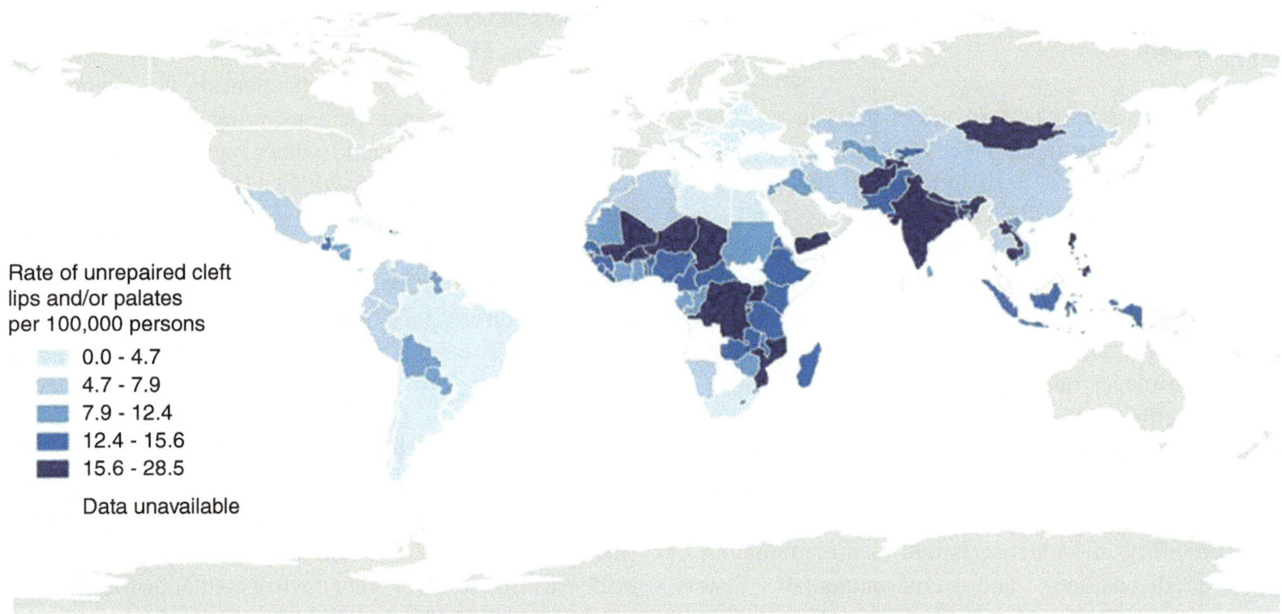


**Fig. 2.3** Map demonstrating the unmet need for cleft lip and cleft palate surgery worldwide. The highest burden of need is observed in low- and middle-income countries. (Reproduced from Carlson and colleagues [19] by permission of World Journal of Surgery)

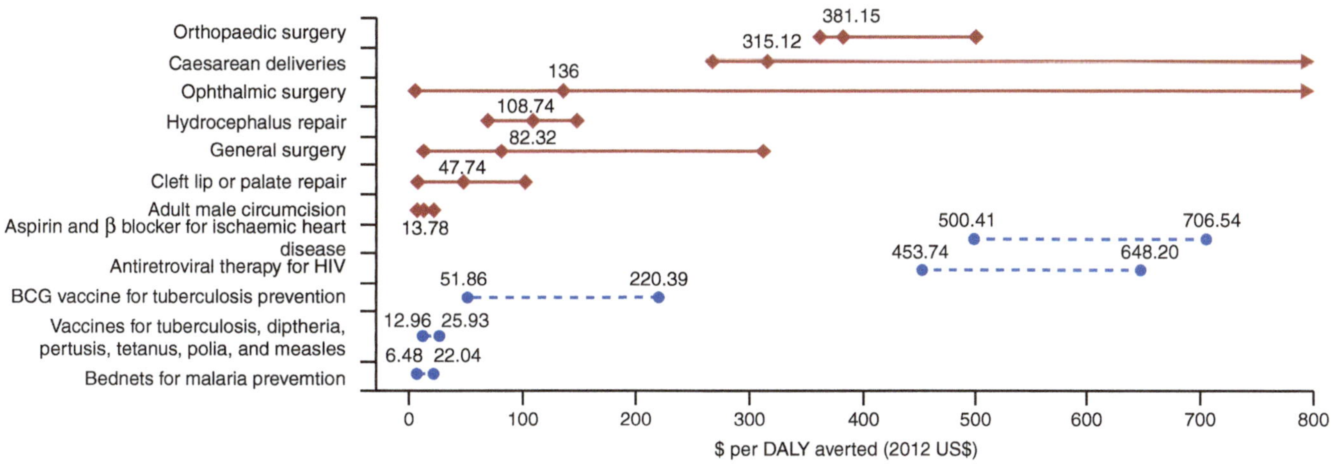


Fig. 2.4 Cost-effective comparison of cleft surgery to other surgeries and public health initiatives. Data points represent median disability-adjusted life years and error bars show range. Surgical interventions appear in red diamonds and solid lines. Public health interventions appear as blue circles with dashed lines. (Reproduced from Meara and colleagues [3] by permission of The Lancet)

Patients with untreated clefts also experience a higher rate of mortality. A 2012 study by Mossey et al. found an exponential decrease in estimated survival to less than 10% by age 20 in cleft patients who did not receive surgery in India. By comparison, cleft patients who did receive surgery had long-term survival estimates similar to the UK population with survival only decreasing below 90% by age 50 [11]. Mortality burden was attributed to two broad categories: nutritional failures and infanticide. In rural areas with limited education and literacy, where lack of understanding exists for feeding options and techniques, mortality from dehydration and starvation can occur frequently in the neonatal period for patients with severe defects [11]. With regard to infanticide, the true incidence remains unknown. However, given the known stigma surrounding cleft conditions, an element of infanticide or neglect can be assumed to be present, especially in areas where the birth rate is either unreported or significantly lower than anticipated [11]. Regardless of mortality cause, an estimated 16.9% of preventable deaths due to lack of surgery could be averted by scaling up access to cleft lip and palate surgical care [20].

## Economics of Cleft Care

The dichotomy of cleft conditions is that they are associated with a high economic burden and yet predominantly affect countries with the lowest income. The lack of subspecialty surgical care in low- and middle-income countries (LMICs) contributes to 38.9 million avertable disability-adjusted life years (DALYs) per year [20]. When looking at a cost-effective profile of surgical and public health interventions, the cost of providing cleft surgery is lower relative to life years (DALYs) saved than both certain vaccine programs and antiretroviral therapy for HIV [3] (Fig. 2.4). This economic burden of cleft conditions is further exacerbated in low-resource environments where limited or often no providers are available who can perform cleft repair. In such instances the backlog exponentially increases, compounding the detrimental economic effects of the condition [21] (Fig. 2.5).

## Approaches to Cleft Care

### Defining Adequate Cleft Care

Ensuring adequate cleft care requires increasing the accessibility of cleft care services for those who receive no interventions, as well as recognizing the need and providing for more complete or comprehensive care for patients who may have received one or two surgical interventions. The prevalence and global distribution of patients who have not received any cleft care has been well studied and reported. However, identifying populations that have received incomplete or non-comprehensive cleft care is more challenging due to the need to perform qualitative and longitudinal assessments of patient care. A 1998 study by the Clinical Standards Advisory Group (CSAG) for cleft lip and palate found that only 63.1% of cleft teams in the UK longitudinally tracked their cleft lip patients and associated outcome [22]. For those that did follow their patients, 37–39% cited "poor" or "very poor" dental outcomes. A follow-up CSAG study found that fewer than 30% of these patients had an associated good cosmetic outcome [23]. Studies of overall cleft care quality have been performed in few countries, and these data are particularly sparse for low-resource settings. Even without granular data, given that the UK is a high-income country, the majority of

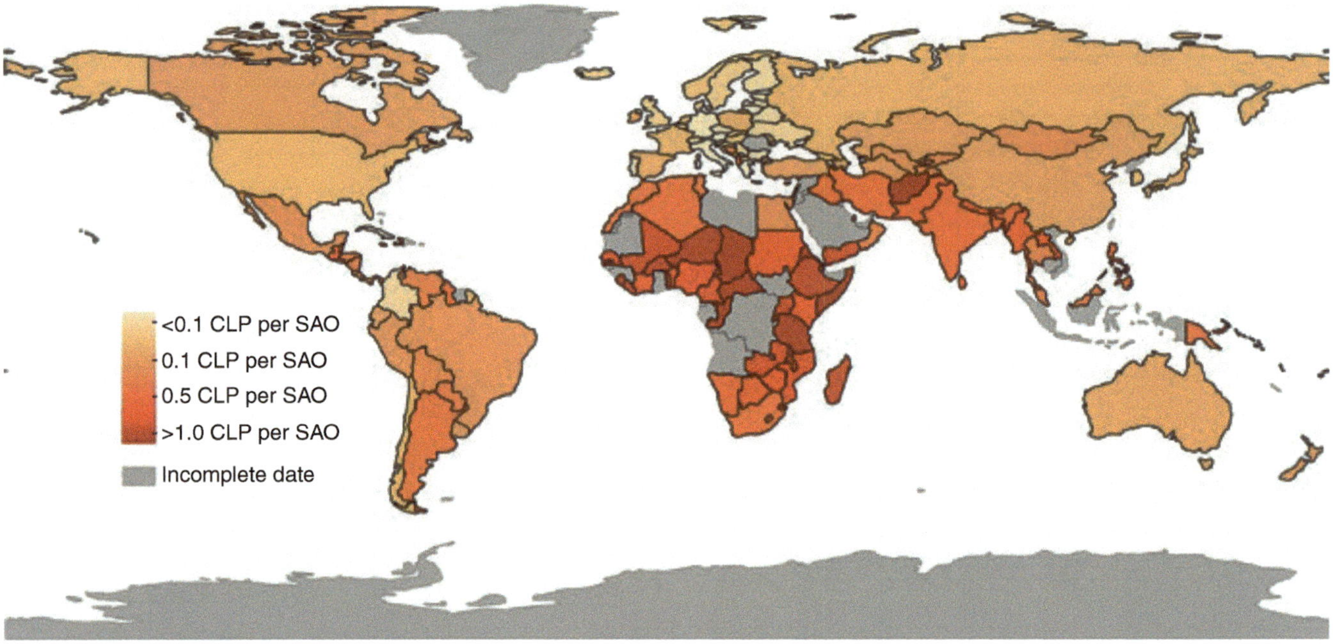


**Fig. 2.5** Map of the incidence of cleft lip and/or palate (CLP) per surgeon, anesthesiologist, and obstetrician (SAO) available in each country. Of note, SAO density does not represent cleft specific providers but is used as a proxy for the density of CLP workforce. (Reproduced from Massenberg and colleagues [21] by permission of Springer Nature)

the world likely lags behind the CSAG outcomes, which in themselves show major opportunity for improvement.

An additional challenge to the provision of adequate cleft care lies in the debate that has existed in the elements required for comprehensive and complete cleft care. The desire for improved quality in cleft outcomes led to the push for more extensive guidelines on comprehensive cleft care. The American Cleft-Palate Craniofacial Association (ACPA) guidelines for cleft palate and craniofacial teams states minimum mandates: the presence of a patient care coordinator; core team members from surgery, orthodontics, and speech-language pathology; and community resources to access psychology, social work, audiology, genetics, general and pediatric dentistry, otolaryngology, and pediatrics/primary care services [24]. Given this list of specialty requirements, comprehensive cleft care is currently only available in middle- and high-income countries.

Providing complete cleft care—the assurance that patients receive the full sequence of necessary procedures for their conditions—requires a varied set of surgical capabilities as well as the ability to longitudinally track a cleft patient throughout their childhood and into adulthood. Per McIntyre et al., patients with CL/P at a tertiary children's hospital in the United States typically undergo an average of 8.6 surgical procedures prior to the age of 21 [25]. These surgeries would include combinations of lip repair, palate repair, alveolar bone grafting, surgery to address velopharyngeal insufficiency, orthognathic surgery, rhinoplasty, and revisions. The ability to provide all of these surgeries as needed over the course of two decades may be feasible with some but not all cleft care delivery models.

## Methods of Reaching Untreated or Undertreated Patients

Multiple methods have been used to try and deliver cleft care to areas with high burden of disease and limited locally available resources. Initiatives for the delivery of cleft care to LMICs first began with the surgical mission, where human resources, equipment, and supplies provided by nongovernmental organizations (NGOs) were temporarily transferred to an area of high burden in order to deliver surgical care to a large volume of patients in a condensed time frame. The introduction of the surgical mission was one of the first ways that many rural and low-resource environments learned of the potential for cleft treatment, the specialized needs of cleft patients, and the ability for cleft patients to lead normal lives when they have the chance to receive appropriate care.

Surgical missions, which have many benefits and performed regularly throughout the world, are a challenging method for delivering ongoing patient follow-up and complete cleft care. Recognizing the deficits in this model, multiple NGOs have created cleft centers with independent facilities or through hospital partnerships, where patients can access ongoing comprehensive care. However, in order to have center activity, countries must have baseline infrastructure to support a facility and enough trained providers for reliable accessibility of services. Therefore, while centers have been valuable in some circumstances, they are not universally applicable or appropriate for all environments.

For countries with a high burden of need, but limited infrastructure and/or providers, the challenge remains for how to deliver ongoing rather than episodic cleft care. In-country education initiatives aimed at increasing the number of skilled providers have been incorporated into the cleft care programs of multiple NGOs through independent and partnership programs [26]. In addition to being able to provide more cleft services on an ongoing basis, education initiatives have served as an economic builder for countries by allowing for expansion of employment opportunities through community health worker, patient advocate, and other outreach care positions.

Additional methods for reaching untreated or undertreated patients exist, which have been employed by various NGOs and governmental bodies. Upcoming chapters will discuss these methods of cleft care delivery in further detail, including history of their use, sustainability of care, their compatibility to run concurrently, and their relative efficacy in different environmental circumstances.

## The Potential Impact of Cleft Care

Patients in LMICs struggle to obtain access to cleft care due to a number of barriers including structural, cultural, financial, and educational factors among other reasons. In a 2016 study of cleft patients in Vietnam, the most reported barriers to obtain cleft care included lack of care continuity (68%), equipment or medication shortage (67%), physician unavailability, unaffordability of food costs when receiving care (66% each), and lack of knowledge of where to obtain care or cost of living expenses while receiving care (64% each) [27]. Barriers to care however can be regionally different. In Brazil, patients reported the greatest barriers to care to be predominantly structural: lack of availability of hospitals able to perform cleft surgery (54%) and doctors capable of performing the surgery (51%) [28]. Provider opinions overlap with patient reports, with the greatest barriers felt to be patient travel costs (60.7%), lack of patient awareness (54.1%), and lack of financial support (52.8%). Similar to patient reports, provider opinions varied depending on country of origin, with over 1997 individuals surveyed worldwide [29].

Developing methods to safely and sustainably deliver cleft care will require minimizing patient barriers to care. These barriers, however, do not uniquely affect cleft patients, and can impair any individual from obtaining surgical services. Addressing cleft care, therefore, has the ability to decrease the overall burden of disease, increase the economic productivity of LMICs, and augment surgical and healthcare capacity in a sustainable way to improve the quality of surgical care for the whole population.

## References


1. Panamonta V, Pradubwong S, Panamonta M, Chowchuen B. Global birth prevalence of orofacial clefts: a systematic review. J Med Assoc Thailand = Chotmaihet thangphaet. 2015;98(Suppl 7):S11–21.
2. Hunt O, Burden D, Hepper P, Johnston C. The psychosocial effects of cleft lip and palate: a systematic review. Eur J Orthod. 2005;27(3):274–85. https://doi.org/10.1093/ejo/cji004.
3. Meara JG, Leather AJM, Hagander L, Alkire BC, Alonso N, Ameh EA, et al. Global surgery 2030: evidence and solutions for achieving health, welfare, and economic development. Lancet. 2015;386(9993):569–624. https://doi.org/10.1016/S0140-6736(15)60160-X.
4. Merritt L. Part 1. Understanding the embryology and genetics of cleft lip and palate. Adv Neonatal Care. 2005;5(2):64–71.
5. Suzuki A, Sangani DR, Ansari A, Iwata J. Molecular mechanisms of midfacial developmental defects. Dev Dyn. 2016;245(3):276–93. https://doi.org/10.1002/dvdy.24368.
6. Dixon MJ, Marazita ML, Beaty TH, Murray JC. Cleft lip and palate: understanding genetic and environmental influences. Nat Rev Genet. 2011;12(3):167–78. https://doi.org/10.1038/nrg2933.
7. Campbell A, Restrepo C, Deshpande G, Bernstein SM, Tredway C, Wendby L, et al. Validation of the unilateral cleft lip severity index for surgeons and laypersons. Plast Reconstr Surg Glob Open. 2017;5(9):e1479. https://doi.org/10.1097/gox.0000000000001479.
8. Yao CA, Imahiyerobo T, Swanson J, Auslander A, De Cardenas D, Figueiredo JC, et al. The smile index: part 1. A large-scale study of phenotypic norms for preoperative and postoperative unilateral cleft lip. Plast Reconstr Surg. 2018;141(1):137–46. https://doi.org/10.1097/prs.0000000000003931.
9. Allori AC, Mulliken JB, Meara JG, Shusterman S, Marcus JR. Classification of cleft lip/palate: then and now. Cleft Palate Craniofac J. 2017;54(2):175–88. https://doi.org/10.1597/14-080.
10. Mackay DR. Controversies in the diagnosis and management of the Robin sequence. J Craniofac Surg. 2011;22(2):415–20. https://doi.org/10.1097/SCS.0b013e3182074799.
11. Mossey PA, Modell B. Epidemiology of oral clefts 2012: an international perspective. Front Oral Biol. 2012;16:1–18. https://doi.org/10.1159/000337464.
12. Matthews JL, Oddone-Paolucci E, Harrop RA. The epidemiology of cleft lip and palate in Canada, 1998 to 2007. Cleft Palate Craniofac J. 2015;52(4):417–24. https://doi.org/10.1597/14-047.
13. Figueiredo JC, Ly S, Magee KS, Ihenacho U, Baurley JW, Sanchez-Lara PA, et al. Parental risk factors for oral clefts among Central Africans, Southeast Asians, and Central Americans. Birth Defects Res A Clin Mol Teratol. 2015;103(10):863–79. https://doi.org/10.1002/bdra.23417.
14. Brito LA, Bassi CF, Masotti C, Malcher C, Rocha KM, Schlesinger D, et al. IRF6 is a risk factor for nonsyndromic cleft lip in the Brazilian population. Am J Med Genet A. 2012;158a(9):2170–5. https://doi.org/10.1002/ajmg.a.35526.
15. Brito LA, Cruz LA, Rocha KM, Barbara LK, Silva CB, Bueno DF, et al. Genetic contribution for non-syndromic cleft lip with or without cleft palate (NS CL/P) in different regions of Brazil and implications for association studies. Am J Med Genet A. 2011;155a(7):1581–7. https://doi.org/10.1002/ajmg.a.34036.
16. Wehby GL, Murray JC. Folic acid and orofacial clefts: a review of the evidence. Oral Dis. 2010;16(1):11–9. https://doi.org/10.1111/j.1601-0825.2009.01587.x.
17. Nahai FR, Williams JK, Burstein FD, Martin J, Thomas J. The management of cleft lip and palate: pathways for treatment and longitudinal assessment. Semin Plast Surg. 2005;19(4):275–85. https://doi.org/10.1055/s-2005-925900.
18. Poenaru D, Ozgediz D, Gosselin RA. Burden, need, or backlog: a call for improved metrics for the global burden of surgical dis-

ease. Int J Surg. 2014;12(5):483–6. https://doi.org/10.1016/j.ijsu.2014.01.021.
19. Carlson LC, Stewart BT, Hatcher KW, Kabetu C, VanderBurg R, Magee WP. A model of the unmet need for cleft lip and palate surgery in low- and middle-income countries. World J Surg. 2016;40(12):2857–67. https://doi.org/10.1007/s00268-016-3637-4.
20. Bickler SW, Weiser TG, Kassebaum N, Higashi H, Chang DC, Barendregt JJ, et al. Global burden of surgical conditions. In: Debas HT, editor. Essential surgery volume I: disease control priorities. Washington, D.C.: The World Bank; 2015. p. 31.
21. Massenburg BB, Riesel JN, Hughes CD, Meara JG. Global cleft lip and palate care: a brief review. In: Alonso N, Raposo-Amaral C, editors. Cleft lip and palate treatment. Cham: Springer; 2018.
22. Sandy J, Williams A, Mildinhall S, Murphy T, Bearn D, Shaw B, et al. The Clinical Standards Advisory Group (CSAG) cleft lip and palate study. Br J Orthod. 1998;25(1):21–30.
23. Williams AC, Bearn D, Mildinhall S, Murphy T, Sell D, Shaw WC, et al. Cleft lip and palate care in the United Kingdom—the Clinical Standards Advisory Group (CSAG) study. Part 2: dentofacial outcomes and patient satisfaction. Cleft Palate Craniofac J. 2001;38(1):24–9. https://doi.org/10.1597/1545-1569_2001_038_0024_clapci_2.0.co_2.
24. American Cleft Palate-Craniofacial Association.Standards for approval of cleft palate and craniofacial teams. 2016. https://acpa-cpf.org/wp-content/uploads/2017/06/standards.pdf. Accessed on 23 Feb 2019.
25. McIntyre JK, Sethi H, Schönbrunner A, Proudfoot J, Jones M, Gosman A. Number of surgical procedures for patients with cleft lip and palate from birth to 21 years old at a single children's. Hospital. 2016;76:S205–S8. https://doi.org/10.1097/sap.0000000000000765.
26. Jenny HE, Massenburg BB, Saluja S, Meara JG, Shrime MG, Alonso N. Efficacy of facilitated capacity building in providing cleft lip and palate care in low- and middle-income countries. J Craniofac Surg. 2017;28(7):1737–41. https://doi.org/10.1097/scs.0000000000003884.
27. Yao CA, Swanson J, Chanson D, Taro TB, Gura B, Figueiredo JC, et al. Barriers to reconstructive surgery in low- and middle-income countries: a cross-sectional study of 453 cleft lip and cleft palate patients in Vietnam. Plast Reconstr Surg. 2016;138(5):887e–95e. https://doi.org/10.1097/prs.0000000000002656.
28. Ise A, Menezes C, Batista Neto J, Saluja S, Amundson JR, Jenny H, et al. Patient-perceived barriers to accessing cleft care at a tertiary referral center in Sao Paulo, Brazil. Cleft Palate Craniofac J. 2018;56:1055665618796018. https://doi.org/10.1177/1055665618796018.
29. Massenburg BB, Jenny HE, Saluja S, Meara JG, Shrime MG, Alonso N. Barriers to cleft lip and palate repair around the world. J Craniofac Surg. 2016;27(7):1741–5. https://doi.org/10.1097/scs.0000000000003038.

# Patient Barriers to Care

3

Caroline A. Yao, Desmond T. Jumbam, and D. Scott Corlew

**Key Points**

- Cleft surgical care must be available, affordable, and acceptable in order for patients to receive it.
- There are many supply and demand-side barriers to obtaining cleft care in the developing world, including those related to infrastructure, workforce, safety, financial risk protection, and patient and community perceptions, as well as social and cultural factors.
- The "Three Delays" Framework can be useful to categorize barriers as those that delay the (1) *seeking* of care, such as knowing that a cleft palate is present and that it can be surgically treated, (2) *reaching* of care, including the costs of transportation and arranging childcare for other children at home, and (3) *receiving* care, which can be impeded by availability of ORs, anesthesiologists, or medications at the local hospital.
- Affordability is better seen not as the absolute cost of care, but as the cost of surgical care relative to the patient or family's ability to pay for it.
- As patients live farther from hospitals offering cleft care, are less educated, and have fewer resources, misconceptions about the availability, benefits, and cost of surgery are easily propagated.

C. A. Yao (✉) · D. T. Jumbam
Program in Global Surgery and Social Change, Harvard Medical School, Boston, MA, USA

Department of Plastic and Oral Surgery, Boston Children's Hospital, Boston, MA, USA

D. S. Corlew
Program in Global Surgery and Social Change, Harvard Medical School, Boston, MA, USA
e-mail: daniel_corlew@hms.harvard.edu

## Introduction

Many children born in lower and middle-income countries (LMICs) with facial clefts lack access to the surgical and other care necessary to correct these deformities. Even for children who can receive care, this leads to delays such that children are often older than is optimal when they do undergo surgical correction. This chapter addresses the barriers that prevent children in low-resource settings from accessing and receiving the care needed at critical ages for optimal lifelong results.

Unlike in high-income countries where cleft lips are generally repaired by 3–4 months of age and palates by 12 months, in low-resource settings care is often delayed significantly, to the detriment of the patient. In one study, the median age at initial presentation ranged between 17–35 months among 8 LMICs studied and between 14–66 months in 3 low-income countries. For every US$1000 decrease in Gross Domestic Product (GDP) per capita, there was a 70% increase in the probability of palatal surgery being delayed beyond 24 months [1]. A study in Vietnam showed that only 48% of patients presenting for cleft care were less than 18 months old [2].

Understanding the barriers patients face to access and receive care is the first step toward strengthening surgical healthcare systems to ensure that patients receive care that is timely and appropriate. The "three delays" framework was originally developed in the obstetric literature [3]. It also applies well to cleft care: the first delay being delay in seeking care, the second in getting to care, and the third in the provision of that care. Figure 3.1 summarizes the relationship between supply and demand of surgical care.

In the cleft setting, the first delay is often most significant. A patient may not get the surgical care they need for three major reasons: availability, affordability, and acceptability [4, 5]. Surgical care is not *available* when a country's healthcare system lacks the necessary infrastructure, workforce, supplies, and systems (Table 3.1) needed for service delivery.

© Springer Nature Switzerland AG 2021

J. W. Swanson, D. W. Low (eds.), *Global Cleft Care in Low-Resource Settings*, https://doi.org/10.1007/978-3-030-59105-2_3

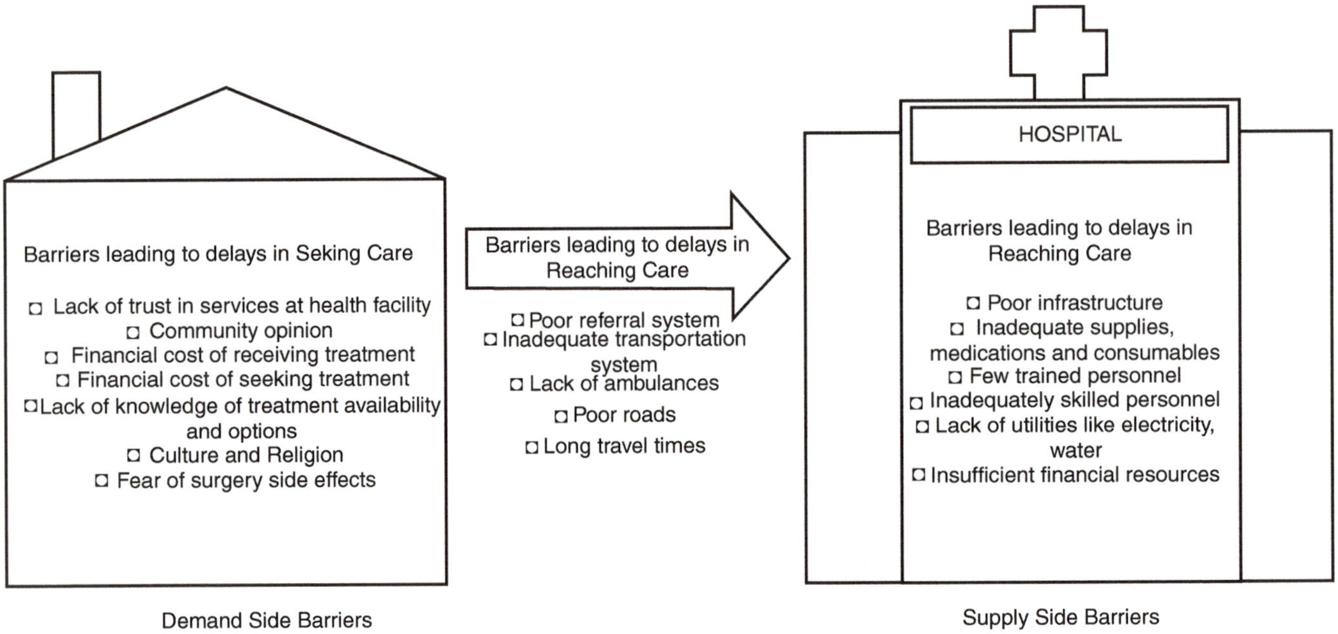


**Fig. 3.1** The "three delays" framework applied to surgical care

**Table 3.1** Types of Cultural, Financial, and Structural Barriers Experienced by Patients with Clefts [4]

| Barrier |
|---|
| Cultural (acceptability) |
| Fear of surgery/anesthetic and complications/rumors of bad outcomes |
| Lack of family/social support |
| Lack of time |
| No one to accompany |
| Role of decision maters |
| Social role (e.g., as beggars) |
| Too old for surgery |
| Acceptance of potentially correctable condition/no perceived need |
| Lack of understanding of severity of condition/un aware of danger signs |
| Cultural beliefs surrounding specific surgical conditions/use of traditional healers |
| Lack of information/understanding of disease process, surgical procedures, and aftercare |
| Financial (affordability) |
| Direct cost: surgical and inpatient fees, transport, food, clothes, accommodation for caregiver, emergency care, informal payments |
| Indirect costs: loss of earnings during surgery and recovery |
| Structural (accessibility) |
| Delayed diagnosis/decision to transfer |
| Distance to nearest treatment facility/service not available locally/poor quality of service |
| Lack of infrastructure: theaters, equipment, drugs, blood, laboratory equipment, radiography equipment |
| Lack of staff or knowledge/training of staff |
| Lack of appropriate transport to health facility and between health facilities |
| Poor roads |
| Poor communication between local and referral hospitals/difficulty navigating health care system to receive appropriate treatment |

Surgical care is not *affordable* if paying to access and receive surgery pushes patients and families deeper into poverty or financial ruin. *Acceptability* represents the patient demand for surgery. People may not seek appropriate surgical care because of lack of awareness, or incorrect information, or lack of community or cultural acceptance of surgical treatment. Lack of trust in the quality or dependability of surgical services at a health facility could also lead to low acceptability among the community.

The overarching picture of global surgical care is described by the Lancet Commission on Global Surgery, and is very applicable to cleft care. Five billion people worldwide were found to lack access to safe, timely, and affordable surgical care; 94% of people in LMICs were in this group. The lack of financial risk protection plays a major role in this access problem: the Lancet Commission found that 33 million people per year face financial catastrophe because of medical costs (defined as using more than 10% of their yearly spending money on surgical care), and 48 million people have catastrophic expenditures from paying for non-medical costs of surgery (e.g., transportation to the hospital, food needed while getting surgery, and wages lost from time away from work). None of these numbers included people who did not access their needed surgical care. The Lancet Commission found that roughly half of the global population is at risk of catastrophic expenditure if they needed surgery. Over 30 million people become impoverished (pushed into poverty or further into poverty) when paying for surgical care. Table 3.2 summarizes the goals for increasing delivery of surgical care in LMICs as set forth in the Lancet Commission [6].

**Table 3.2** Core indicators for monitoring of universal access to safe, affordable surgical and anaesthesia care when needed [6]

| | Definition | Target |
|---|---|---|
| Access to timely essential surgery | Proportion of the population that can access, within 2 h, a facility that can do caesarean delivery, laparotomy, and treatment of open fracture (the Bellwether Procedures) | A minimum of 80% coverage of essential surgical and anaesthesia services per country by 2030 |
| Specialist surgical workforce density | Number of specialist surgical, anaesthetic, and obstetric physicians who are working, per 100 000 population | 100% of countries with at least 20 surgical, anaesthetic, and obstetric physicians per 100 000 population by 2030 |
| Surgical volume | Procedures done in an operating theatre, per 100 000 population per year | 80% of countries by 2020 and 100% of countries by 2030 tracking surgical volume; a minimum of 5000 procedures per 100 000 population by 2030 |
| Perioperative mortality | All-cause death rate before discharge in patients who have undergone a procedure in an operating theatre, divided by the total number of procedures, presented as a percentage | 80% of countries by 2020 and 100% of countries by 2030 tracking perioperative mortality; in 2020, assess global data and set national targets for 2030 |
| Protection against impoverishing expenditure | Proportion of households protected against impoverishment 100% protection against impoverishment from direct out-of-pocket payments for surgical and anaesthesia care | 100% protection against catastrophic expenditure from out-of-pocket payments for surgical and anaesthesia care by 2030 |
| Protection against catastrophic expenditure | Proportion of households protected against catastrophic expenditure from direct out-of-pocket payments for surgical and anaesthesia care. | 100% protection against catastrophic from out-of-pocket payments for surgical and anaesthesia care by 2030 |

These indicators provide the most information when used and interpreted together; no single indicator provides an adequate representation of surgical and anaesthesia care when analysed independently

The World Health Organization (WHO), World Bank, and national governments have taken notice that people in LMICs tend to have the most trouble accessing surgical care. A number of countries, thus far including Tanzania, Ethiopia, Zambia, Pakistan, and Rwanda, have taken major steps to address barriers to surgical care as recommended by the WHO by introducing National Surgical Obstetric, and Anesthesia Plans (NSOAPs) as part of their overall National Health Plans. These plans outline a strategy to develop the six major areas needed for surgical capacity building: infrastructure and supplies, workforce, service delivery, information management, governance, and financing [6].

NSOAPs, while aimed at the greater picture of all surgical care, are particularly applicable to the barriers faced by people needing cleft care. *System* barriers, defined as a lack of expertise (i.e., workforce), infrastructure, facilities, and equipment are the most significant cause of low availability of cleft surgery [4]. The WHO created a standard survey to help assess a healthcare facility's capabilities. The survey can be repeated at different time intervals to assess a system's progress and challenges [7].

## Availability of Care (Supply)

### Workforce

The supply of surgeons qualified to perform surgery in LMICs is limited. WHO data indicate that the African, Eastern Mediterranean, and Southeast Asian regions account for 47% of the global population but only 17% of the licensed surgeons. More disturbing is that there is only one licensed anesthesiologist per 1 million people in Southeast Asia and Africa [8].

Internationally, cleft lip surgery is performed by plastic surgeons, oral surgeons, ear/nose/throat surgeons, and general surgeons who require specialized training beyond typical surgical training programs. A survey in Vietnam showed that 66% of patients did not receive cleft surgery because they perceived a lack of trained surgeons [9]. Many children with cleft lips and palates continue to receive surgical care from NGOs that bring temporary increases in workforce and resource availability. A comprehensive review reported that NGOs delivering care through supporting permanent surgical hospitals are the most cost-effective, safe, and sustainable vehicles for care delivery. They suggest that temporary, short-term platforms are efficient when no other surgical delivery platform is available [10].

The surgical and anesthesia workforce are not the only barriers to care. Even when surgeons are available, they may be hindered from providing quality cleft surgery by lack of other necessary personnel, lack of supplies, or financial realities of their practices. For example, it has been shown that the availability of cleft surgery decreases when surgeons capable of performing cleft surgery (typically plastic surgeons) earn more money to perform other types of surgery (e.g., cosmetic surgery), or have patients with more life-threatening surgical needs. Inequitable distribution of surgeons and other practitioners also constitutes a barrier for many people; most are based in urban areas where there are more opportunities for practice and for families. Few surgeons choose to work in rural areas where the need is greatest [11].

Safe anesthesia is an additional limiting factor for cleft and other surgeries in LMICs. The limited supply of trained anesthesiologists decreases the availability of surgery, especially for infants and small children for whom more specialized anesthesiology training is helpful or sometimes imperative. Consequently, anesthesia care in developing countries is often provided by non-physician providers with widely varied training and experience and associated safety concerns [12].

The underlying etiology of the barrier to care of the lack of a trained workforce is a reflection of a lack of training capacity of the country. Training of specialized practitioners such as surgeons requires a strong educational network, including a university or medical school, expert surgeons to serve as instructors and a hospital system that integrates surgeons in training. Specialized surgeons, who can perform cleft lip and palate surgery, require the above resources and have the added challenges of fewer expert instructors available and the relative rarity of patients born with a cleft lip and/or palate.

It is also important to acknowledge the network of support staff other than the surgeons and anesthesiologists that are required for safe surgical care provision. These include nurses, biomedical engineers, sterilization staff, speech therapists, and administrative staff. Limited numbers of these providers further limit care provision in LMICs.

### Infrastructure

Even when expertise to provide cleft surgery is available, inadequate infrastructure may be a barrier. Not only hospitals, but also basic public needs such as reliable roads, bridges, and public transport are major factors that decrease the availability of surgery [4]. Hospital buildings must have appropriately outfitted operating rooms, anesthesia capacity, hospital beds, laboratory facilities, and supply chains. Transportation infrastructure affects whether or not patients and families can safely and consistently travel to a hospital, and also whether or not supplies can be reliably delivered to hospitals.

Once patients arrive at a hospital facility, the facility must be functional, meaning it has space, durable equipment (medical machines) that is appropriate, available and functional, appropriate diagnostics (labs and imaging), and consumables (e.g., medicine, bandages, and other supplies). Inadequacies in any of these present further barriers to care and can lead to delays in care and adverse outcomes. Availability of basic utilities like water and electricity can determine the availability and even the quality of surgery provided. From cleaning and sterilizing surgical equipment to powering equipment such as anesthesia machines, water and electricity are essential for the provision of surgical care.

Most healthcare systems are designed such that basic and emergency curative and preventive services provided are lower tier primary health facilities while more complex care is provided at higher tier, secondary and tertiary hospitals. An effective referral system that allows patients in need of complex care to be effectively referred up the system is key. Referral systems rely on other medical practitioners to be aware of how to treat cleft deformities in order to refer appropriately and in a timely fashion. These practitioners also must know which hospitals or clinics are capable of providing cleft surgery and associated care. Referral systems must be effective, because poor communication between facilities, poor referral guidelines, and inadequate capacity at health facilities can be barriers to care. Without a functioning referral system, CLP patients may not receive the care they need.

While a majority of the deformities associated with cleft lip and cleft palate can be treated with a single operation, many cases need staged care, revision procedures, orthodontics, otologic care, and speech therapy. Without reliable transportation infrastructure, families taking care of a child with a cleft struggle to get to and from treatment facilities and the uncertainty of the time and cost of travel are compounded.

## Affordability and Acceptability of Surgical Care (Demand)

### Affordability

Once patients and families have decided to pursue surgical care for a cleft, affordability is often still a barrier [4, 9, 13, 14]. Affordability of surgical care includes not just the direct costs (cost of surgery, anesthesia, medications, supplies, laboratory tests, and overnight stays in the hospital) but also the indirect costs (transport to the surgery, transport of needed family members/caretakers, food and drink and the opportunity costs of missed work) (Table 3.3).

Affordability is better seen not as the absolute cost of care, but as the cost of surgical care relative to the patient or family's ability to pay for it [5]. The Lancet 2030 Commission defined two scenarios when this match is a problem: (1) When paying for surgery pushes a family into poverty, or

**Table 3.3** Direct and indirect costs of surgery [6]

| Direct | Indirect |
|---|---|
| Surgery<br>Anesthesia<br>Medications<br>Supplies<br>Laboratory, imaging, and other diagnostic tests<br>Hospital stay | Transport of patient and family to the facility<br>Food during treatment and travel<br>Opportunity costs of missing work |

further into poverty; or (2) When paying for surgery creates a catastrophic expense for the patient and family [6].

Often, affordability of surgical care is seen by patients and their families as the greatest barrier to surgical care. For example, 76.5% of patients observed in Cameroon reported cost of care as the most important reason for declining surgical care [15]. Similarly, Operation Smile and Smile Train surveys of surgeons, healthcare providers, and patients showed that patient travel costs were the most common barrier to accessing cleft surgical care [9, 14]. Research has shown that high travel costs are associated with low healthcare utilization. For those living in remote areas in LMICs, travel costs can be higher than the cost of surgery. Even in the United States, families report that traveling long distances to get cleft surgery is a burden [14].

**Barriers to Surgical Care from the Perspective of a Bangladeshi Family**

A boy in rural Bangladesh is born with a cleft lip and palate, and a small growth under his arm. He is one of four children. His family succeeded in seeking repair of his cleft lip when he was a young child. At age five, the axillary tumor has grown so large that his parents take him to the hospital many miles from their home. Surgery had to be delayed because the family was unable to pay for and arrange a blood transfusion. They return home to their jobs as garment workers. Five months later the tumor becomes infected and he is taken back to the hospital. He has an additional hospital stay and is treated for infections. One older sibling is sent out to work as a domestic help and the mother loses her job because she has missed too much work. Another child is injured. The father incurs substantial debt and eventually loses his job because of the frequent hospital visits by the time the treatment is finished (Fig. 3.2).

To finance the direct and indirect costs of surgery, patients are often forced to sell property or livestock or borrow from family and community members. 26% of households in LMICs must borrow money or sell belongings to pay for healthcare; the risk for needing to borrow or sell is higher as insurance coverage decreases and poverty increases [16]. It is therefore important to consider the cost to patients when developing programs to provide cleft surgery and associated care to the poorest and most disadvantaged populations.

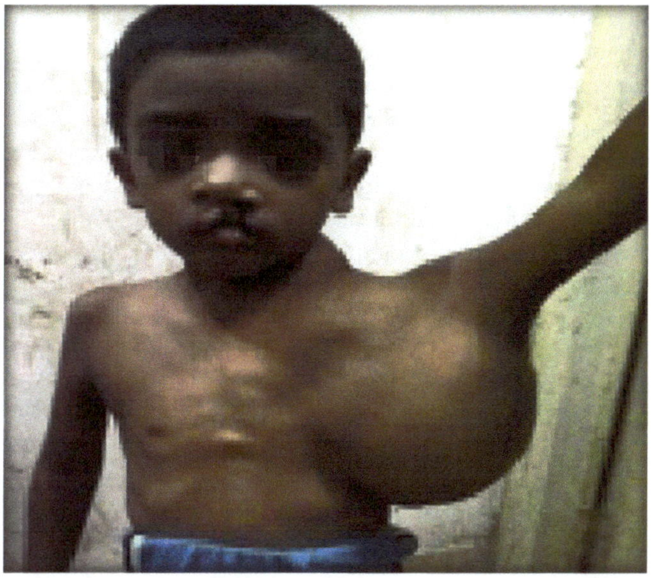

Fig. 3.2 Boy from Bangladesh. (Reprinted with permission of Dr. Banu. Professor Dr. Tahmina Banu, Pediatric Surgeon, Chittagong, Bangladesh)

## Acceptability

While cleft lip and palate is the most common craniofacial birth defect (affecting 1–2 per 1000 live births) [9], its relative rarity and the shortage of accessible surgical providers decreases community awareness toward the disease in LMICs. As patients live farther from hospitals offering cleft care, are less educated, and have fewer resources, misconceptions about the availability, benefits, and cost of surgery are easily propagated. Awareness of the ability for surgery to treat the disease may decline. Patients living in rural locations and far from cleft care centers are less likely to seek cleft care, and most (69%) of people in less developed countries live in rural areas [13]. Awareness that cleft lip and palate can be treated with surgery and speech therapy has been cited as a barrier to care by surgeons in LMICs around the world [14].

In many countries, especially where government corruption is significant, lack of trust in the healthcare system can present yet another barrier [4]. Surveys have found that patients seeking cleft care at an NGO-sponsored mission trip often did so because there was lack of trust in the country's medical system and providers, and that available treatment was perceived as poor [9]. Mistrust is propagated if patients cannot get care after arriving at local hospitals due to misinformation and bureaucracy.

Cultural norms may also prevent surgical care seeking. In many countries, female children are less likely to receive surgery than male children [17]. In some cultures the belief that deformities such as clefts are God's will or a punishment for sins can prevent care seeking [18]. In conjunction with these beliefs, some families may believe that they are meant to suffer through the deformity and to avoid surgical care. Acceptance of a potentially correctable condition leads to a lack of perceived need for surgical repair [4, 18].

It is important to recognize that patients and families view treatment options for a cleft through their own perceptions, which is like a lens that colors their every point of view. This perception is shaped by their education, community, family, culture, and religion. The ability to have accurate information affects patient and family perceptions. If a patient has inaccurate information about the costs, benefits, and risks of the surgery, they are not empowered to make the best decisions possible. "Fear" (of a procedure itself, complications, anesthesia, etc.) is a commonly cited reason that patients in LMICs do not pursue surgical care [4]. Improved education and outreach may bring patient perceptions closer to situational realities. Family and community perceptions regarding surgical care may evolve as each individual expands their knowledge.

## Conclusion

There are many barriers to obtaining cleft care in the developing world, including those related to infrastructure, workforce, safety, financial risk protection, and perceptions of all of these factors, as well as social and cultural factors. Cleft surgical care must be available, affordable, and acceptable in order for patients to receive it.

## References


1. Carlson LC, Hatcher KW, Tomberg L, Kabetu C, Ayala R, Vander Burg R. Inequitable access to timely cleft palate surgery in low- and middle-income countries. World J Surg. 2016;40(5):1047–52.
2. Swanson JW, Yao CA, Auslander A, Wipfli H, Nguyen TH, Hatcher K, et al. Patient barriers to accessing surgical cleft care in Vietnam: a multi-site, cross-sectional outcomes study. World J Surg. 2017;41(6):1435–46.
3. Thaddeus S, Maine D. Too far to walk: maternal mortality in context. Soc Sci Med. 1994;38(8):1091–110.
4. Grimes CE, Bowman KG, Dodgion CM, Lavy CB. Systematic review of barriers to surgical care in low-income and middle-income countries. World J Surg. 2011;35(5):941–50.
5. Weiser TGA. Excess surgical mortality: strategies for improving quality of care. In: Debas HT, Gawande A, Jamison DT, Kruk ME, Mock CN, editors. Disease control priorities. 1: essential surgery. Washington, D.C.: World Bank; 2015.
6. Meara JG, Leather AJM, Hagander L, Alkire BC, Alonso N, Ameh EA, et al. Global surgery 2030: evidence and solutions for achieving health, welfare, and economic development. Lancet. 2015;386(9993):569–624.
7. WHO-PGSSC Surgical Assessment Tool (SAT) Hospital Walkthrough Harvard Medical School Program in Global Surgery and Social Change. Available from: http://media.wix.com/ugd/346076_b9d8e8796eb945fe9bac7e7e35c512b1.pdf.
8. Global Health Observatory (GHO) data: World Health Organization. Available from: https://www.who.int/gho/health_workforce/surgical/en/.
9. Yao CA, Swanson J, Chanson D, Taro TB, Gura B, Figueiredo JC, et al. Barriers to reconstructive surgery in low- and middle-income countries: a cross-sectional study of 453 cleft lip and cleft palate patients in Vietnam. Plast Reconstr Surg. 2016;138(5):887e–95e.
10. Shrime MG, Sleemi A, Ravilla TD. Charitable platforms in global surgery: a systematic review of their effectiveness, cost-effectiveness, sustainability, and role training. World J Surg. 2015;39(1):10–20.
11. Bolkan HA, Hagander L, von Schreeb J, Bash-Taqi D, Kamara TB, Salvesen Ø, et al. Who is performing surgery in low-income settings: a countrywide inventory of the surgical workforce distribution and scope of practice in Sierra Leone. Lancet. 2015;385:S44.
12. Zoumenou E, Chobli M, le Polain de Waroux B, Baele PL. Twenty years of collaboration between Belgium and Benin in training anesthesiologists for Africa. Anesth Analg. 2018;126(4):1321–8.
13. Jenny HE, Massenburg BB, Saluja S, Meara JG, Shrime MG, Alonso N. Efficacy of facilitated capacity building in providing cleft lip and palate care in low- and middle-income countries. J Craniofac Surg. 2017;28(7):1737–41.
14. Massenburg BB, Jenny HE, Saluja S, Meara JG, Shrime MG, Alonso N. Barriers to cleft lip and palate repair around the world. J Craniofac Surg. 2016;27(7):1741–5.
15. Lerman BJ, Alsan M, Chia NJ, Brown JA, Wren SM. Beyond infrastructure: understanding why patients decline surgery in the developing world: an observational study in Cameroon. Ann Surg. 2017;266(6):975–80.
16. Kruk ME, Goldmann E, Galea S. Borrowing and selling to pay for health care in low- and middle-income countries. Health Aff (Millwood). 2009;28(4):1056–66.
17. Conway JC, Taub PJ, Kling R, Oberoi K, Doucette J, Jabs EW. Ten-year experience of more than 35,000 orofacial clefts in Africa. BMC Pediatr. 2015;15:8.
18. Ross E. A tale of two systems: beliefs and practices of South African Muslim and Hindu traditional healers regarding cleft lip and palate. Cleft Palate Craniofac J. 2007;44(6):642–8.

# 4 Innovations in Reaching Patients

Jordana Baron and Anjaramamy Ramamonjisoa

**Key Points**

- Design thinking is a structured problem-solving approach that can help guide the development of cleft outreach programs in a patient-focused way.
- A Cleft Patient Advocate program in Honduras follows Partner's in Health "accompaniment model" by training families of existing cleft patients to serve as ambassadors to identify and support families with new cleft diagnoses.
- A program in Madagascar reinforces deep community bonds by facilitating "patient villages" among families with cleft through specialized support groups and activities.
- Collaborative models in Alaska, Liberia, and Sudan explore the potential of partnering with community health workers to bring comprehensive care to rural patients.
- Several key themes of successful cleft outreach programs include defining the problem prior to developing a solution, focusing on the patient experience, partnering with community health workers and patient advocates, and using technology to support a strategy as opposed to being the strategy.

## Introduction

The purpose of this chapter is to introduce design thinking methodology as a tool for developing patient-centered, context-appropriate solutions for patient management, and to provide examples of innovative patient management

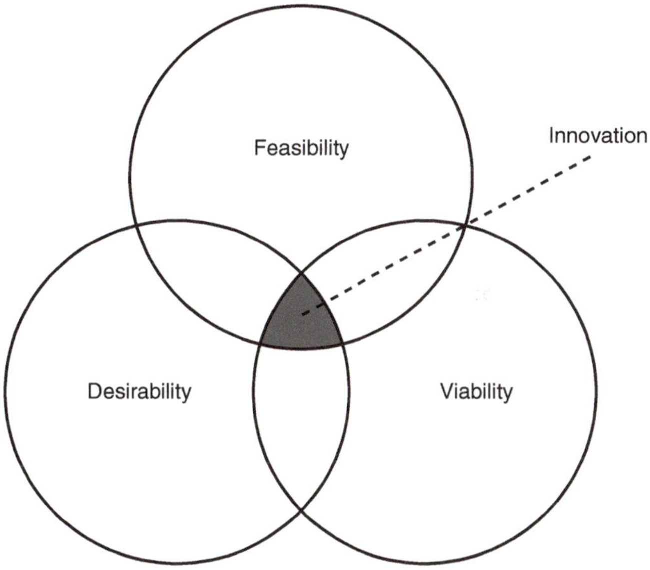


**Fig. 4.1** Standard design thinking conceptual model for innovative solutions

strategies and tactics that have been successful in low-resource settings. Borrowing from the design thinking field, we employ the term "innovation" as a solution that is simultaneously "feasible, desirable, and viable" (Fig. 4.1) [1]. The "patient experience" concept broadly represents a patient and their family's overall experience with healthcare during the course of care for a particular health condition or set of conditions. This experience is an integral part of how patients interact with an organization or system that delivers healthcare.

We segment patient management into three components: initial identification, sequencing into care, and ongoing case management (Fig. 4.2). We present and explore a number of practical examples from low-resource settings, each of which addresses multiple of these components. Though the examples were not explicitly developed using design thinking methodology, they embody patient-centricity, empathy, and

J. Baron (✉)
Johns Hopkins University Bloomberg School of Public Health (at time of writing), Washington, DC, USA

A. Ramamonjisoa
Operation Smile Madagascar, Washington, DC, USA

© Springer Nature Switzerland AG 2021

J. W. Swanson, D. W. Low (eds.), *Global Cleft Care in Low-Resource Settings*, https://doi.org/10.1007/978-3-030-59105-2_4

**Patient management**

Patient experience

1. Initial identification (outreach, building awareness)
2. Sequencing into care (primary surgery)
3. Ongoing case management (continuity of care / comprehensive care)

**Fig. 4.2** Patient management and patient experience framework

context appropriateness. With steadily increasing global access to platforms such as SMS and other media mechanisms, methods of communication and mass outreach are more widely available. They draw from a range of specialties including cleft lip and cleft palate, primary care, and infectious disease. And they tend to be purposefully "low-tech" so that they may be implemented anywhere and without expensive, often time-confusing investments in technology that can distract from patient-centered innovation.

## Design Thinking

Design thinking is a creative, empathy-driven, multi-disciplinary approach to problem solving that involves rapid prototyping and testing to develop "optimal solutions"—innovations that are simultaneously feasible, desirable, and viable (Fig. 4.1). It is "a multi-stage problem-solving process that optimizes solutions based on users' needs, behaviors, constraints, and operating contexts. Solutions are repeatedly tested and refined throughout the design and development process before implementation" [2]. Derived from product design, the design thinking process elicits creativity while keeping the end-user at the center of the process—a key reason why it is being used to address some of the most pressing challenges, like healthcare.

A systematic review of design thinking in healthcare revealed two important findings [3]. First, when compared to traditional interventions, those developed using design thinking experienced better health outcomes and higher usability and satisfaction (explored later in the chapter, and in Fig. 4.5). Second, design thinking may be particularly useful for underserved populations because it requires users to question assumptions and empathize with key stakeholders. This creates space for innovations to emerge, as is the case in global health.

In rural Tanzania, patients with HIV still have divergent health outcomes despite the existence of robust diagnosis and treatment dispensing systems [4]. To address this, an HIV program team turned to interdisciplinary tools, including design thinking, to gather insights on the patient experience. For instance, many patients concealed their HIV diagnosis from friends and family, and thus avoided nearby clinics and desperately sought confidentiality. The program team leveraged these insights and involved patients in developing and testing prototypes. What emerged were in-home and in-clinic solutions linked by a social message incorporating a Baobab tree image—an image that represented health and community: to improve patient–provider interactions and encourage patients not to skip or delay visits, clinics introduced "moments of praise and delight" in private and public settings. Patients were also given mobile phone-sized pillboxes to disguise their medication, or a calendar with images of "normal life" they could aspire to return to once achieving better health. The result is increased treatment retention and patient satisfaction. Though this is one small example, it demonstrates the potential of empathy-based insights to improve patient experiences and health outcomes.

## Examples from the Field

### Cleft Lip and Palate

#### Patient Accompaniment: Partners in Health and Operation Smile Honduras

**Problem Statement**
How to reach patients who may be unlikely or unable to seek or continue care for chronic conditions?

**Program Overview**
Beginning in Haiti, Partners In Health (PIH) pioneered the successful treatment of HIV and tuberculosis in low-resource settings by using community health workers (CHWs) to support patients on their path to health. The CHWs were individuals chosen by their communities to provide basic health services. Now known as "patient accompaniment", this concept is both a philosophy and program design that emphasizes meeting patients where they are, and walking—literally and figuratively—with them in solidarity throughout their healthcare journey. Inspired by the liberation theology of Peruvian priest Gustavo Gutierrez, accompaniment promotes a "preferential option for the poor" by providing social, psychological, and economic support to patients beyond medical care until patients decide otherwise [5]. The goal is to achieve "absolute equity of health outcomes for anyone, anywhere" [6].

With this in mind, Operation Smile, an international cleft lip and cleft palate organization, adapted PIH's publicly available *Accompagnateur Training Manual* to the cleft context and created a Patient Advocate (PA) program in Honduras. An *accompagnateur* is a person, usually a community health worker, who acts in the accompaniment role for patients as described above. With the goals of increasing equity of access to cleft care, and of regaining contact with patients who were lost to follow-up, the program equips parents whose children have received cleft treatment with Operation Smile to serve as links between

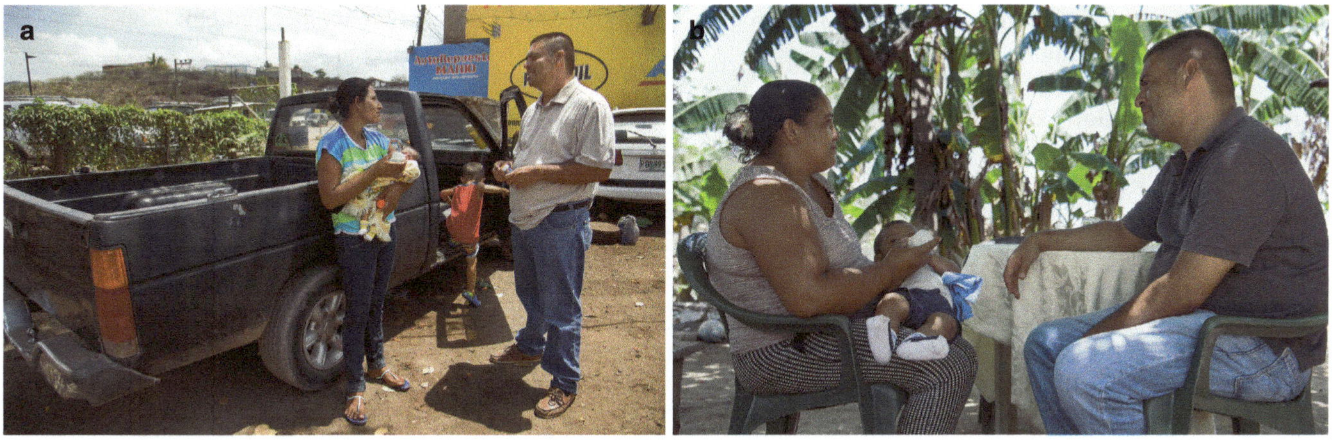

Fig. 4.3 Patient Advocate Alex Guerrero is a parent of a child with a cleft, and helps to teach parents of children with clefts to feed their children effectively (**a**) and access cleft care (**b**). (Photos courtesy of Operation Smile)

Table 4.1 Operation smile patient advocate materials

| |
|---|
| Polo shirts with program name and organization logo |
| Identification cards/nametags with program name and organization logo |
| Referral slips with Patient Advocate names |
| Hat and backpack with program name and organization logo |
| Cell phone with unlimited minutes and texting[a] |
| Notebook to track patient interactions and expenditures |
| Patient Advocate training manual |
| Flier with contact information of Patient Coordinator |
| Certificate of training completion |
| PowerPoint presentation/printouts of before and after photos |
| Annual report of the organization |

[a]Patient Advocates and program staff consider this to be the most important tool to facilitate the program

Table 4.2 Operation smile patient advocate toolkit

| |
|---|
| Role description for Patient Advocates |
| Job descriptions for Patient Coordinator and Program Manager |
| Framework for Patient Advocate meetings |
| Program budget |
| Guidelines for stipend disbursements |
| Confidentiality agreement |
| General release of liability |
| Brand resources |
| List of materials |

their communities and the organization. Patient Advocates (PAs) are selected based on demonstrated commitment to their own child's rehabilitation, a desire to support others on their journey with cleft care, and geographic diversity in order to connect with remote communities. A PA might help a young mother of a cleft patient to recognize that she will need to arrange care for her other children, or help arrange transportation, in anticipation of her child's upcoming surgery (Fig. 4.3a, b). This ability to anticipate problems, and help find practical solutions, helps overcome the myriad barriers that often prevent or delay cleft care from being sought and accessed. PAs are provided with essential materials (Table 4.1) and undergo an initial three-day training in conjunction with an Operation Smile surgical mission. Literacy is considered, but non-essential. Upon returning to their communities, PAs build awareness about cleft and opportunities for treatment, often through presentations at regular meetings of local organizations including health facilities, schools, and churches.

Human resources during the 1-year pilot phase consisted of seven PAs, one project manager, and one patient coordinator. The patient coordinator and PAs communicated regularly to schedule clinical appointments, coordinate logistics, troubleshoot challenges, and ensure continuity of care for patients. The project manager managed the budget, volunteer agreements with PAs, cell-phone contracts, supplies, and coordination of the PAs during medical missions and program meetings. The number of PAs has since expanded, and the program continues today. See Table 4.2 for a list of program tools.

### Why It Works

Solidarity and empathy are core tenets of Liberation Theology and PIH's accompaniment model. Through these efforts, PAs are innately capable of accompanying cleft patients through care precisely because they have done so with their own children. Their personal testimonies lend credibility to their efforts and those of Operation Smile. Frequency of communication and availability of support are also essential; PAs regularly contact each other, patients, and program staff to troubleshoot problems, schedule appointments, and provide logistical and emotional support. Additionally, building a referral network helps ensure long-term sustainability of access to cleft care among remote communities. Lastly, the program facilitates continuity of care, increasing the likelihood of optimal outcomes and full reintegration into society. Though Operation Smile's program is a vertical, condition-specific CHW program, it could feasibly be integrated into a country's existing CHW program for a broader set of conditions.

## Enhancing the Patient Experience: Operation Smile, Madagascar

### Problem Statement

How to integrate cleft care into communities to overcome barriers to care?

### Program Overview

#### Vision

A large island off the southeastern coast of Africa, Madagascar is a place where barriers to healthcare are extreme: only 20% of roads are paved, and the surgical specialist workforce density is only 0.78 per 100,000 (the World Health Organization recommends a minimum density of 20 per 100,000) [7]. Surgery is not only rare, it is largely unknown. For a mother of a newborn child with a cleft who has never left her village before, traveling to surgery can be extremely strenuous both logistically and emotionally. Operation Smile's team in Madagascar envisions a future where every cleft patient not only receives the right care at the right time, but has an experience worthy of sharing with their community. To that end, the strategic program components—a national awareness and registration campaign, a patient advocacy program, support groups, patient villages, feeding programs, and workshops—are grounded in the patient and community perspective. More than registering patients, organizing logistics, and determining surgical eligibility, enhancing the patient experience is about discovering who the patients are, where they come from, and enriching their lives beyond medical treatment. By designing programs from the patient perspective, patients become ambassadors for cleft care in their own communities—a solution that is simultaneously feasible, desirable, and viable.

#### National Registry

To build a national registry, Operation Smile works with regional and local branches of the Ministry of Public Health, as well as local non-governmental organizations/associations, churches, and schools, to register patients as early as birth. Early identification is critical both for patients' health as well as caregivers' well-being. A toll-free, 24-hour information/registration hotline is advertised through ongoing mass media campaigns. Registered patients are monitored, and those with low weight are enrolled in a feeding "bootcamp"; there, professionals provide advice, training, and demonstrations on how to prepare affordable, locally available foods that nourish the mother and child. Food supplements are provided if needed.

#### Support Groups

Support groups are another key program component to enhancing the patient experience. One type is a discussion group for parents of newborn babies with cleft, and parents of malnourished children. "Compassion booths" at medical missions serve a similar function. Run by parents of former patients, volunteers, or religious leaders, compassion booths are places where patients and families can process news about whether or not they will receive surgery, ask questions, get information about future programs, and be referred to alternative therapies such as feeding bootcamps, speech therapy sessions, and obturator fittings, among others.

#### Patient Villages

"Patient villages" are critical in creating a sense of solidarity and providing psychosocial support. In addition to providing free transportation, food, and lodging for the duration of a medical mission, Operation Smile partners with various organizations to organize daily workshops and activities aimed at improving health and well-being (Fig. 4.4). Offerings include oral hygiene, communicable disease education and prevention, yoga and dance classes, gardening, and crafting items to sell in marketplaces (Fig. 4.5). After spending time in the patient villages together, "cleft communities" begin to form, and families begin to naturally support each other. Upon returning to their home communities, they raise awareness and help identify other patients needing cleft care. They accompany each other when traveling to receive care to reduce anxiety of those who have never left their village, sharing best practices along the way.

### Why It Works

The concept of family, beyond blood relationships, plays a strong role in Malagasy communities. Incorporating this into patient management has resulted in patients taking an active, informed role in their journey—actions which empower them to help others navigate their journeys. Support groups and patient villages are essential to achieve this; they provide space for patients to empathize with each other, share meals together, embark on an unknown journey together, look after one another, and cheer and celebrate together. They help convert doubt and fear into excitement and mutual caretaking. Meaningful, high-quality patient experiences rooted in family and community transform patients and families into the ultimate ambassadors for cleft care.

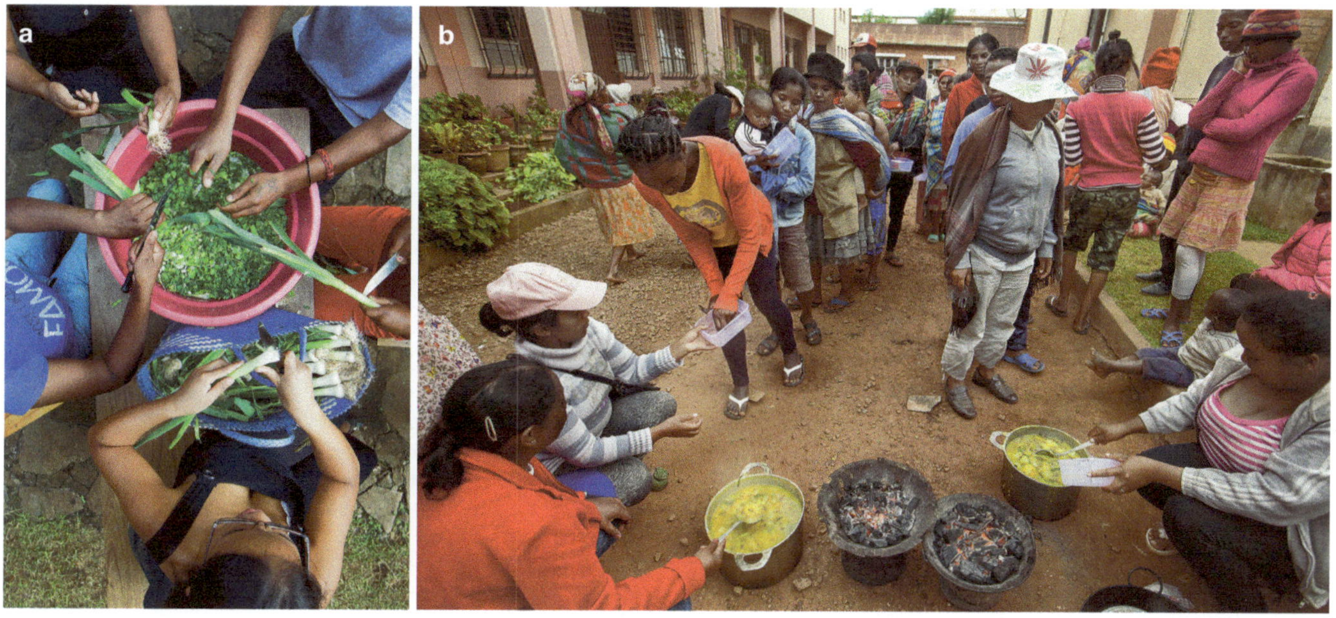

Fig. 4.4 A "patient village" of families coming together to prepare vegetables (**a**) then cook and eat (**b**) together in Antsirabe, Madagascar. (Photos courtesy of Operation Smile)

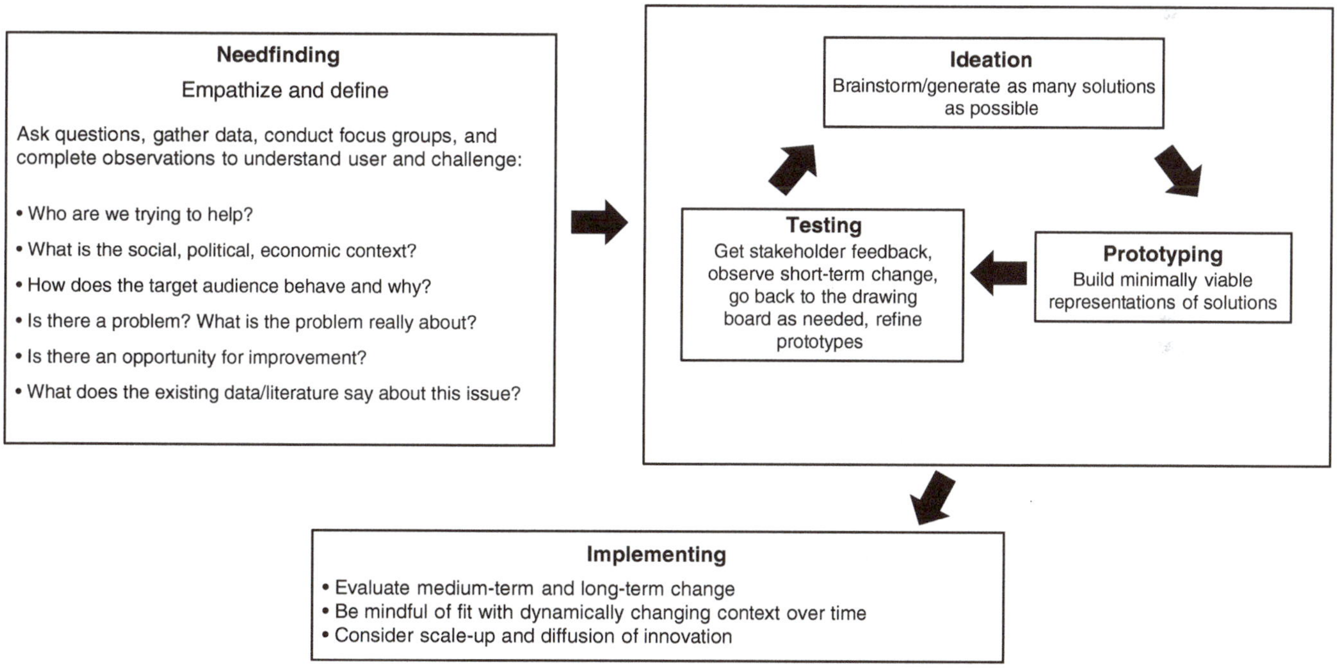


Fig. 4.5 "Design thinking process, stages of design thinking and examples of exercises used and questions asked in each stage, systematic review on Design Thinking in healthcare, search results through March 31, 2017" [3]

## Primary Care

### Nuka System of Care: Southcentral Foundation, Alaska, United States

#### Problem Statement

How to improve health outcomes among a historically marginalized native population?

#### Program Overview

The Nuka System of Care is a tribally managed healthcare system serving 60,000+ Alaska Natives from over 200 tribes. Spanning a geographic area roughly the size of Iran, the Nuka System represents a paradigm shift away from Alaska Natives being treated as beneficiaries/patients for/to whom things were being done, to a system where they are "customer-owners" who control the design and delivery of their own healthcare [8]. In 1999, the System was completely redesigned by Alaska Natives and the Southcentral Foundation (SCF) to work *for* Alaska Natives, and is jointly run by SCF and the Alaska Native Tribal Health Consortium.

Information for the System redesign came directly from Alaska Natives through extensive surveys, interviews, and focus groups with community members and tribal leaders [9]. The key result is an emphasis on Native beliefs that spiritual, social, and cultural connectedness is fundamental to physical health. From there emerged an integrated health system with coordinated care teams, a focus on primary care and prevention, redesigned facilities, and healthcare services and communications that blend Western medicine with "Native wisdom". For example, services for substance abuse, domestic violence, and other problems now target families and communities rather than individuals; native diets, food preparation, and spiritual and social elements are now incorporated into cancer treatment.

Health services are delivered through a variety of mechanisms, including in-office and at-home visits, telemedicine, email, and educational classes, among others. For villages not accessible by road, SCF partners with village health clinics and regularly deploys medical teams to provide health services. Through this model, SCF has achieved the seemingly impossible: significantly better health outcomes, reduced disparities, and reduced costs. The Nuka System is a clear example of an innovative solution that is truly patient-centered.

### Why It Works

Alaska Natives' participation as customer-owners in the design and delivery of their healthcare transformed not only their health system, but their health outcomes. The System now focuses on holistic care and multigenerational/multidimensional wellness, all made possible by strong relationships between customer-owners, healthcare providers, communities, and administrators [8]. Relationships are so important that the word "relationships" is also an acronym for Nuka System's operating principles (see Table 4.3). Further, the System's activities are guided by a shared vision, mission, and key points that emphasize shared responsibility, commitment to quality, and family wellness (see Table 4.4). SCF has also mastered the incorporation of customer-owner feedback through a variety of mechanisms, including in-person feedback, comment cards, surveys, 24-hour hotline and online forum, focus groups, advisory committees, and special events. Shared ownership and responsibility enable this system to flourish.

**Table 4.3** Southcentral Foundation's Nuka System of care operational principles

| |
|---|
| **R**elationships between the customer-owner, the family, and provider must be fostered and supported |
| **E**mphasis on wellness of the whole person, family, and community including physical, mental, emotional, and spiritual wellness |
| **L**ocations that are convenient for the customer-owner and create minimal stops for the customer-owner |
| **A**ccess is optimized and waiting times are limited |
| **T**ogether with the customer-owner as an active partner |
| **I**ntentional whole system design to maximize coordination and minimize duplication |
| **O**utcome and process measures to continuously evaluate and improve |
| **N**ot complicated but simple and easy to use |
| **S**ervices are financially sustainable and viable |
| **H**ub of the system is the family |
| **I**nterests of the customer-owner drive the system to determine what we do and how we do it |
| **P**opulation-based systems and services |
| **S**ervices and systems build on the strengths of Alaska Native cultures |

Gottlieb [8]

**Table 4.4** Nuka System of Care Framework

| |
|---|
| *Vision Statement*: A Native Community that enjoys physical, mental, emotional, and spiritual wellness. |
| *Mission Statement*: Working together with the Native Community to achieve wellness through health and related services. |
| **Key Points** |
| *Shared Responsibility* |
| We value working together with the individual, the family, and the community. We strive to honor the dignity of every individual. We see the journey to wellness being traveled in shared responsibility and partnership with those for whom we provide services. |
| *Commitment to Quality* |
| We strive to provide the best services for the Native Community. We employ fully qualified staff in all positions and we commit ourselves to recruiting and training Native staff to meet this need. We structure our organization to optimize the skills and contributions of our staff. |
| *Family Wellness* |
| We value the family as the heart of the Native Community. We work to promote wellness that goes beyond absence of illness and prevention of disease. We encourage physical, mental, social, spiritual, and economic wellness in the individual, the family, the community, and the world in which we live. |

Gottlieb [8]

## Community Health Workers: Last Mile Health, Liberia

### Problem Statement

How to deliver primary care to the most remote communities?

#### Program Overview

**Professionalization**

Last Mile Health (LMH) is an organization focused on delivering high-quality healthcare to remote communities in Liberia. Liberia is a West African country of approximately 4 million people, whose already weak health system left many without access to healthcare after the 2014–2015 Ebola epidemic [10]. LMH's program strategy is to professionalize—to recruit, train, equip, manage, and employ—community health workers (CHWs). LMH works with the Ministry of Health (MOH) to build and scale the National Community Health Workforce Program, which aims to have professional (CHWs) and clinical supervisors delivering healthcare to the most remote communities. Last Mile Health's Community Health Academy is an educational initiative to train hundreds of thousands of community health workers and health system leaders around the world to deliver healthcare to those without access.

**Community-Nominated Participants**

To become a CHW candidates must be nominated by their community, complete a literacy test, an in-person interview, and a training and skills assessment for which they are scored [11]. Candidates with the highest scores become CHWs. CHWs provide services both through active case-finding and patient self-presentation and are paid a monthly cash incentive of $70 USD for approximately 20 hours of work per week. Peer-supervisors visit CHWs weekly, while clinical nurse supervisors visit monthly. Both levels of supervisors visit CHWs in their home communities.

Although CHWs have historically focused on nutrition, vaccination, and hygiene, there is increasing evidence that they can play a critical role in surgical care delivery, including for cleft care [12].

#### Why it Works

The professionalization of CHWs differentiates LMH's model from other CHW programs. By focusing on performance management, supply chain strengthening, effective use of telecommunications, and patient transportation, LMH directly addresses the barriers that traditional CHW programs struggle to overcome [13]. Medical and digital technology also contributes to success; CHWs use inexpensive, rapid diagnostic tests for HIV and malaria, and an open source mobile data collection platform called Open Data Kit. Partnerships with the MOH and other organizations such as Partners In Health are also key. LMH supports the MOH in scaling the National Community Health Workforce Program; in doing so, efforts to deliver healthcare to remote communities are streamlined and strengthened rather than duplicated and diluted. Together, a decentralized healthcare system was designed with justice and equity at the center, utilizing nurses and CHWs to address specific health needs of remote communities [14].

## Infectious Disease

### Community-Based Surveillance System: CORE Group Polio Project, South Sudan

#### Problem Statement

How to monitor and control the risk of disease outbreaks in remote communities?

#### Program Overview

Community-based surveillance (CBS) systems are designed to detect specific health events in places with weak health systems and/or where populations have limited access to health facilities. The CORE Group Polio Project's CBS system for acute flaccid paralysis (AFP) was designed to identify AFP as a proxy for the poliomyelitis (polio) virus—a highly infectious disease that primarily affects young children and can cause permanent paralysis [15].

**Structure**

A common human resources structure for a CBS system consists of three levels: County Supervisors at the top, Sub-county Assistants in the middle, and Community Key Informants (CKIs) at the ground level. CKIs are responsible for detecting and reporting any suspected AFP cases within their village. They are selected among people who are known and respected within their communities, such as local leaders, healers, teachers, birth attendants, etc. Literacy is not required. Because AFP is rare, CKIs are not expected to conduct active surveillance, nor are they compensated. However, they are expected to report suspected cases to their Sub-county Assistant. The Sub-county Assistants supervise a minimum of 15 CKIs and are expected to visit each CKI within their jurisdiction once a week, verify suspected cases, and report them to a County Supervisor within 48 hours of verification of AFP. The County Supervisor visits each Sub-County Assistant within their jurisdiction each month and liaises with the World Health Organization (WHO) field representatives for polio global monitoring and management.

#### Why It Works

The CBS system is effective for many reasons. First, its simple three-tiered structure, clear reporting requirements, and effective training, coordination, and engagement with local communities allow for timely AFP detection and reporting; each village has a CKI in weekly contact with their Sub-county Assistant. Second, word of mouth is powerful in small, remote communities; rare health events like AFP typically catalyze health-seeking behavior, and news of such an event will likely reach a community leader and ultimately the CKI. Third, a confirmed case of AFP warrants a visit to the village from a County Supervisor and WHO field representative; this kind of visibility helps build trust because it conveys that people care about the health of these communities. Fourth, CBS systems are sustainable because they are designed to function in weak health systems; they do not rely on patients presenting at health facilities or on active surveillance mechanisms. Lastly, community-based surveillance for other serious health conditions could easily be incorporated into this same system, making it a valuable structure in which to invest. In the absence of a nearly collapsed health system, CBS systems are feasible, desirable, and viable.

## Conclusion & Key Takeaways

Improving access to cleft care is best approached through a patient-centric perspective. The examples described span cleft-specific programming to broader health system approaches for community engagement. Because a new cleft diagnosis is a fairly uncommon event at the community level, but patients with a cleft benefit from comprehensive and prompt care, success for many communities will likely involve a hybrid of these models. Furthermore, this poses an opportunity to strengthen an overall health system's outreach efforts, even as an organization or provider may be specifically focused on patients with clefts. A few key takeaways from the case studies are worth highlighting:

- *Define the problem prior to developing a solution.* Too often in global health, solutions are developed for the wrong problem. Spend time with stakeholders to truly understand the root of the challenge. Utilize methodologies such as design thinking to keep the primary stakeholder/s at the center of solution development, and continuously revisit commonly held assumptions.
- *Focus on the patient experience and CHWs/PAs.* Patient and CHW/PA involvement in solution development is critical to creating, implementing, and sustaining patient management strategies that work for the hardest to reach patients, as well as those attempting to reach them.
- *Technology is not the same thing as innovation.* Mobile applications are not silver bullets, but rather tools to support a strategy. Simple, low-tech solutions are often the most feasible, desirable, and viable. Building a robust word of mouth referral network can be more powerful than the shiniest gadget.

**Box: Additional Resources for Patient Engagement**

*Design Thinking*

- Design for Health www.designforhealth.org
- Ideo www.ideo.org, www.ideou.com
- Design Kit http://www.designkit.org
- USAID Center for Innovation and Impact https://www.usaid.gov/cii
- Dalberg Design https://dalberg.com/our-ideas/meeting-people-where-they-are-expecting-mothers
- The British Design Council https://www.design-council.org.uk/
- M4ID http://m4id.fi/
- D-Rev http://d-rev.org/

*Manuals and guidelines*

- Community-based surveillance https://www.afro.who.int/sites/default/files/2017-06/community-based-surveillance_idsr_training-manual.pdf
- Partners In Health Accompagnatuer Training Guide https://www.pih.org/practitioner-resource/accompagnateur-training-guide
- Last Mile Health Community Health Academy https://lastmilehealth.org/chacademy/

*Healthcare Delivery Organizations*

- Partners In Health www.pih.org
- Village Reach www.villagereach.org
- Last Mile Health www.lastmilehealth.org
- Nuka System of Care https://scfnuka.com/

*Other*

- www.empathyandinnovation.com
- Open Data Kit https://opendatakit.org/
- Journal of Patient Experience

**Acknowledgments** The authors would like to thank Operation Smile, Inc. for granting permission to include program information from Honduras and Madagascar. Thanks to Jeanie Barjum, Allison Bradshaw, Kristin Hatcher, and Erin McCrane, for facilitating a review of the Operation Smile sections. Thanks to Dr. Henry Perry at the Johns Hopkins Bloomberg School of Public Health for guidance. A special thank you to patients in Honduras, Madagascar, and around the world for inspiring this work. All materials referencing Operation Smile in the Cleft Lip and Cleft Palate section are the intellectual property of Operation Smile, Inc. Operation Smile, Inc. has granted permission for these materials to be used in this publication.

## References


1. IdeoU. Why design thinking? 2019. Image retrieved from https://www.ideou.com/pages/design-thinking.
2. Lee P. Before the backlash, let's redefine user-centered design. Stanf Soc Innov Rev. 2015:2–5. Retrieved from https://ssir.org/articles/entry/before_the_backlash_lets_redefine_user_centered_design#.
3. Altman M, Huang TT, Breland JY. Design thinking in healthcare. Prev Chronic Dis. 2018;15(180128):1–13. https://doi.org/10.5888/pcd15.180128.
4. Rao A, McCoy S. Optimizing on the edges. Stanf Soc Innov Rev. 2017:1–5. Retrieved from https://ssir.org/articles/entry/optimizing_on_the_edges.
5. Farmer P. Reimagining accompaniment: a doctor's tribute to father Gustavo Gutierrez. 2013. Partners In Health website. Retrieved from https://www.pih.org/article/in-the-company-of-the-poor.
6. Palazuelos D, Farmer PE, Mukherjee J. Community health and equity of outcomes: the partners in health experience. Lancet Glob Health. 2018;6(5):491–3. https://doi.org/10.1016/S2214-109X(18)30073-1.
7. Daniels K, Riesel J, Meara J. The scale-up of the surgical workforce. Lancet. 2015;385:S41. https://doi.org/10.1016/S0140-6736(15)60836-4.
8. Gottlieb K. The Nuka system of care: improving health through ownership and relationships. Int J Circumpolar Health. 2013;72. https://doi.org/10.3402/ijch.v72i0.21118.
9. Huhndorf S. Native wisdom is revolutionizing health care. Stanf Soc Innov Rev. 2017;15(3):18–23. Retrieved from http://search.ebscohost.com.proxy1.library.jhu.edu/login.aspx?direct=true&db=bsu&AN=123189939&site=ehost-live&scope=site.
10. Last Mile Health. General information. 2019. Retrieved from www.lastmilehealth.org.
11. White EE, Downey J, Sathananthan V, Kanjee Z, Kenny A, Waters A, Rabinowich J, Raghavan M, Dorr L, Halder A, Nyumah J, Duokie D, Boima T, Panjabi R, Siedner MJ, Kraemer JD. A community health worker intervention to increase childhood disease treatment coverage in rural Liberia: A controlled before-and-after evaluation. Am J Pub Health. 2018;108(9):1252. https://doi.org/10.2105/AJPH.2018.304555.
12. Last Mile Health. Strategic plan. 2019. Retrieved from https://lastmilehealth.org/our-strategy/.
13. Gualy S, Herrera C, Warden C, Valle T, Barnum J, Colman B, Siu A, Swanson JW. Enabling community health worker recognition and referral of surgical diseases: pilot study results of a pictorial guide. World J Surg. 2019;43(12):2949–58.
14. Panjabi R. A healthcare model for the world's most remote and impoverished: Dr. Paul Sax interviews Dr. Rajesh Panjabi. (P. Sax, Interviewer). Open Forum Infectious Dis. 2017;4(4):ofx221. https://doi.org/10.1093/ofid/ofx221.
15. Kisanga A, Abiuda B, Walyaula P, Losey L, Samson O. Evaluation of the functionality and effectiveness of the CORE Group Polio Project's community-based acute flaccid paralysis surveillance system in South Sudan. Am J Trop Med Hyg. 2019;101(4_Suppl):91–9.

# Part II

# Patient and Cleft Assessment

# Patterns, Anatomy, and Classification of Clefts

5

Renato da Silva Freitas, Isis Juliane Guarezi Nasser, Carrie Zimmerman, and Fabiola Grigoletto Lupion

**Key Points**

- The average worldwide incidence of cleft lip and palate is about 1/700 live births, with the highest incidence among Asian and Amerindian populations and lower rates among African populations.
- A thorough understanding of the embryology and anatomy of orofacial clefts is essential in approaching the surgical reconstruction and rehabilitation of such deformities.
- Orofacial clefts are caused by embryologic fusion defects and are affected by a complex interplay of genes and the environment.
- There is no international consensus regarding the best cleft lip or palate classification system.
- Cleft lip and palate (CL/P) presents on a spectrum from microform cleft lip to complete cleft lip and palate with nasal involvement. The severity of clefting correlates with functional outcomes and the complexity of surgical correction.

## Introduction

Cleft lip and/or palate (CL/P) is the most common congenital craniofacial malformation in the world with a worldwide incidence of about 1 in 700 births. Cleft patterns vary by ethnicity, and there is a sevenfold variation in CL/P prevalence between countries with the highest and those with the lowest rates. Multiple risk factors have been identified including family history, environmental exposures, and maternal nutrition – an interaction between genes and environmental factors that affect the fusion of midline facial tissue at 6–8 weeks of gestation. Careful physical exam of the entire face, nose, lips, alveolus, and palate characterizes the extent and severity of deformity. Involvement of each anatomic piece implicates functional consequences and need for surgical treatment: palate (feeding, speech, maxillary growth), lip (speech, appearance), nose (breathing, appearance), and alveolus (teeth). Rehabilitative treatment to optimize structure and function, and minimize stigmatization, demands a sound understanding of both embryology and anatomy of the deformity.

## Epidemiology

### Patterns of Cleft Lip and Palate

CL/P is the most common congenital anomaly of the face worldwide and constitutes about 13% of all reported congenital anomalies [3]. The most common orofacial cleft diagnosis is CL/P (46%), followed by isolated cleft palate (iCP) (33%) and isolated cleft lip (iCL) (21%). About 35% of orofacial clefts are associated with other congenital malformations, and this is more common for CP (about half of patients) than CL. Unilateral cleft is nine times more common than the bilateral. CL has a male predominance (OR 1.5:1 unilateral and 2:1 bilateral), but iCP is more common in females (2:1).

R. da Silva Freitas (✉)
Plastic Surgery Unit, Federal University of Parana, Curitiba, Brazil

Assistance Center for Cleft Lip and Palate (CAIF), Hospital do Trabalhador, Curitiba, Paraná, Brazil

I. J. G. Nasser
Assistance Center for Cleft Lip and Palate (CAIF), Hospital do Trabalhador, Curitiba, Paraná, Brazil

C. Zimmerman
Children's Hospital of Philadelphia, Philadelphia, PA, USA
e-mail: Zimmermac2@email.chop.edu

F. G. Lupion
Hospital de Clínicas, Federal University of Paraná, Curitiba, Brazil

© Springer Nature Switzerland AG 2021

J. W. Swanson, D. W. Low (eds.), *Global Cleft Care in Low-Resource Settings*, https://doi.org/10.1007/978-3-030-59105-2_5

Common abbreviations in cleft lip/palate care

| |
|---|
| CL – cleft lip |
| CP – cleft palate |
| CLP – cleft lip and palate |
| CL/P –cleft lip and/or palate |
| CL ± P – cleft lip with or without palate |
| u – unilateral |
| b – bilateral |
| i – isolated |

Genetically, CL ± P and iCP may be distinct entities: a family history of one may not increase risk of the other. If an affected child is born to a parent with a cleft lip and/or palate, the risk of recurrence in future pregnancies is 3% compared to 0.14% in the general population.

## Syndromic Clefts

CL/P can be further subdivided into syndromic and non-syndromic categories. The majority of cases (70% CL/P, 50% CP) are non-syndromic, meaning they are not part of an identified genetic syndrome. These tend to present sporadically but may have increased risk due to environmental exposure or genetic disposition [4]. Syndromic CL/P is most commonly caused by chromosomal abnormalities or single-gene mutations [4]. More than 275 identified syndromes are associated with CL/P [9].

Early examination by a physician experienced in rare genetic syndromes, and if appropriate genetic testing, can help identify other potential anomalies and appropriate specialist referrals, potentially reducing morbidity and mortality. The most common CL/P syndromes are outlined in Table 5.1. Associated symptoms often involve altered airway, cardiopulmonary, and renal systems that confer specific risks for cleft surgery if not identified and addressed prior.

**Table 5.1** Common cleft lip and palate syndromes [4]

| Syndrome/sequence | Characteristics | Other affected organ systems |
|---|---|---|
| Van der Woude | Most frequent CL/P syndrome<br>CL/P or CP, lower lip pits, hypodontia | None – only orofacial |
| Velocardiofacial syndrome (VCFS) or 22q11.2 | Wide variability in disease severity | Cardiac anomalies<br>Velopharyngeal insufficiency<br>Facial dysmorphia<br>Thymic hypoplasia<br>Learning disabilities |
| Stickler syndrome | May see with Robin sequence: micro-/retrognathia, glossoptosis, and airway obstruction | High-degree myopia<br>Hearing loss<br>Arthritis |
| Hemifacial microsomia | Unilateral underdeveloped face | Mandible hypoplasia<br>Facial palsy<br>Ear malformations<br>Hypoplastic cheek tissue |

## Racial and Ethnic Epidemiologic Variations

Data from EUROCAT [17], a large international database, between the years 1995 and 2007 show higher rates of CL/P in Latin America, China, and Japan and lower rates in South Africa, Southern Europe, and Israel. Canada and parts of Northern Europe displayed higher rates of CP with lower rates in Latin America and South Africa. There is a paucity of data from African countries, but the information that is available shows higher proportions of iCL and lower prevalence of CL/P and CP. More data collection is similarly needed from parts of India and the Middle East [12].

In developed nations, death from CL/P is very rare. However, in developing nations with limited access to surgical intervention, the mortality is higher. Incorrect parental perceptions of CL/P as an irreparable malformation and lack of education about cleft feeding techniques and oral hygiene lead to many infant deaths from neglect and malnutrition. The mortality rate of patients with clefts in one province with limited access to cleft care was estimated at over 90% [10].

A 2015 study stated there are between 400,000 and 2 million cleft patients awaiting the availability of cleft surgery globally. In sub-Saharan Africa, the average age of cleft repair is 10 years, compared to standards under 12 months of age in higher-resource settings. A recent study from the United States found that older age at time of surgical repair correlates with increased complications [18].

# Embryology

## The Gene-Environment Interplay

The embryological development of the face, and more specifically the oral region, relies on the interplay of different cell types (ectoderm and endoderm) and a vast range of cellular factors that impact cell differentiation, growth, apoptosis, adhesion, and signaling. A mutation in the genes controlling any one of these factors can lead to clefting.

Although there is a recognized genetic component of non-syndromic CL/P, its etiology appears to be multifactorial, and a variety of environmental factors have also been impli-

**Table 5.2** Facial prominences and derivatives

| Facial prominences | Derivatives |
|---|---|
| Frontonasal (1) | Forehead, nose apex<br>Medial nasal prominence: central nose, septum, philtrum, medial lip, primary palate<br>Lateral nasal prominence: nasal alae |
| Paired maxillary (2) | Secondary palate, lateral lip, lateral maxilla |
| Paired mandibular (2) | Mandible, lower lip |

cated in its cause. The most commonly cited exposures include teratogens, such as anticonvulsant drugs (phenytoin), maternal smoking, alcohol, and retinoids, and environmental pollutants, like ionizing radiation, ozone, pesticides, and secondhand smoke [11, 21].

## Facial Development

The development of the human face occurs between the 4th and 12th week of gestation (Table 5.2).

**Week 4** Starting in the fourth week of gestation, the ectoderm of the neural plate folds to form the neural tube. Neural crest ectodermal cells then differentiate into special ectomesenchymal cells which migrate around from the dorsal face and neck regions to form the developing face. The ectomesenchymal cells form five facial prominences which surround the developing mouth (stomodeum) [15]. Nasal placodes then form from the frontonasal prominence. Each nasal placode splits into a nasal pit and a medial and lateral nasal prominence (Fig. 5.1).

**Weeks 5–6** Each medial nasal prominence fuses with its contralateral counterpart to create the intermaxillary segment (primary palate). The intermaxillary segment also contributes to the labial component of the philtrum, the medial upper lip, and the upper four incisors. The fusion between primary palate and maxillary prominence initiates at the incisive foramen and proceeds anteriorly. The lateral nasal prominence forms into the nasal ala and alar base [14].

**Weeks 8–12** The maxillary prominences expand medially to give rise to the palatal shelves. The shelves move from a vertical to horizontal alignment as they grow and fuse in the midline to create the secondary palate around the eighth week, and closure proceeds from anterior to posterior, which helps to understand the spectrum of clefts of the secondary palate. The soft palate muscles are almost all derived from the fourth branchial arch and are innervated by X cranial nerve (vagus). The sole exception to this is the tensor veli palatini muscle, which arises from the first branchial arch and is innervated by V cranial nerve (trigeminal). The mandibular prominences form the mandible and lower lip [14, 15].

## Clefts as Failure of Fusion Events

Orofacial clefts form due to a failure of fusion of various embryologic prominences. The degree of cleft severity is dependent on the extent to which fusion is disrupted.

The structural interference of orofacial tissue can impair fusion leading to CL/P. For example, if a structure (tongue or tumor) sits between the two palatal shelves and obstructs their fusion, a cleft in the developing palate forms. The specific failed fusion events resulting in orofacial clefts are outlined in Table 5.3 [5].

## Cleft-Related Anatomy

### Nose: Tip, Alae, Columella, Nasal Sill, Paranasal Muscles

**Lip** There are many important landmarks in the upper lip that are measured and marked preoperatively to assure symmetry in cleft lip repair. The principal muscle of the lips is the orbicularis oris, a concentric "band-like" muscle that functions as a sphincter for the oral aperture (Fig. 5.2).

1. Philtral columns – Paired vertical, linear lip protuberances formed by contralateral fibers of orbicularis oris muscle as it crosses midline to insert into overlying dermis *(purple)*.
2. Philtrum, philtral dimple, or philtral groove – Central depression seen between philtral columns. This depression is created by less muscle fibers in this area *(light blue)*.
3. White roll – Inferior cutaneous skin border at the junction of vermilion, with anterior projection from the pars marginalis of the underlying orbicular oris *(white)*.
4. Vermilion – Keratinized mucous membrane of the outer lip composed of hairless, highly vascularized, stratified squamous epithelium. Also known as "dry vermilion."
5. Red line – Margin between vermilion and mucosa *(red)*.
6. Mucosa – Nonkeratinized mucous membrane of stratified squamous epithelium. When displaced out of the mouth, it becomes chapped. Also known as "wet vermilion."
7. Cupid's bow – Two peaks created by central white roll at inferior margin of philtral columns. Note the trough (nadir) of Cupid's bow *(yellow)* and the two peaks of the bow *(green)*.
8. Median tubercle – Central plumping of dry vermillion.

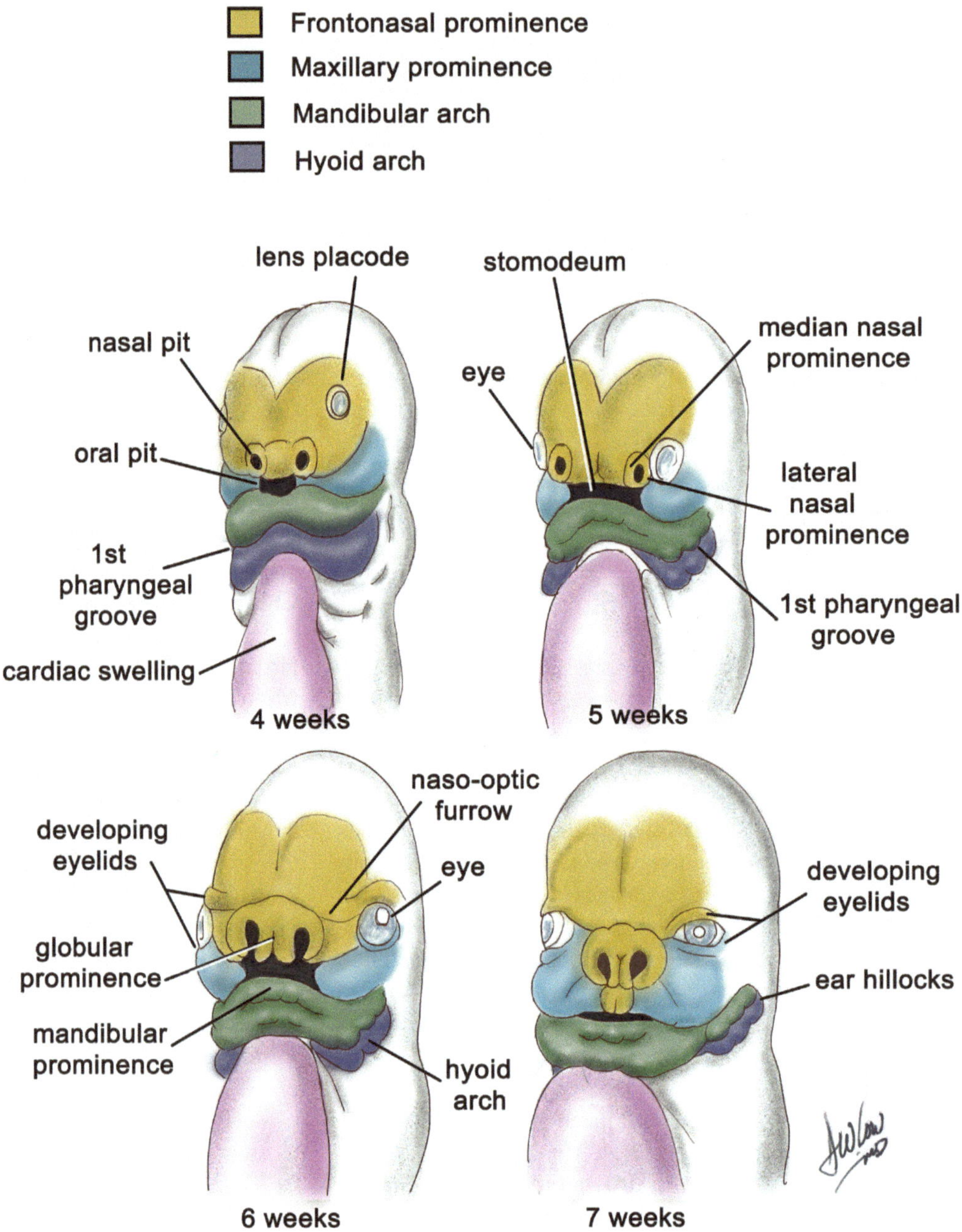


**Fig. 5.1** Embryologic facial formation

**Table 5.3** Orofacial clefts as failure of fusion

| Cleft | Failed fusion event |
|---|---|
| Unilateral cleft lip | Medial nasal prominence with maxillary prominence on one side |
| Bilateral cleft lip | Medial nasal prominence with maxillary prominence on both sides |
| Microform cleft lip | Failure of localized medial nasal process growth |
| Primary cleft palate | Medial nasal prominences |
| Secondary palate cleft | Closure of palatal shelves |

**Alveolus** The alveolar process is the thickened ridge of the bone from the maxilla from which teeth grow. Patients with alveolar clefts have a high prevalence of dental anomalies. The most common anomalies are an absence of the lateral incisors, displaced canine teeth, and supernumerary teeth.

## Palate

The palate forms the floor of the nasal cavity and roof of the oral cavity, in this way fulfilling its main function of separating the nasal and oral cavities from each other. This separation is essential for feeding, swallowing, and speech. The palate is made up of the anteriorly located hard palate and more posteriorly located soft palate (velum) [5].

**Hard Palate** The bony or hard palate (palatum osseum) is formed by the maxillary and palatine bones. The hard palate is subdivided into the primary and secondary palate with the incisive foramen between them.

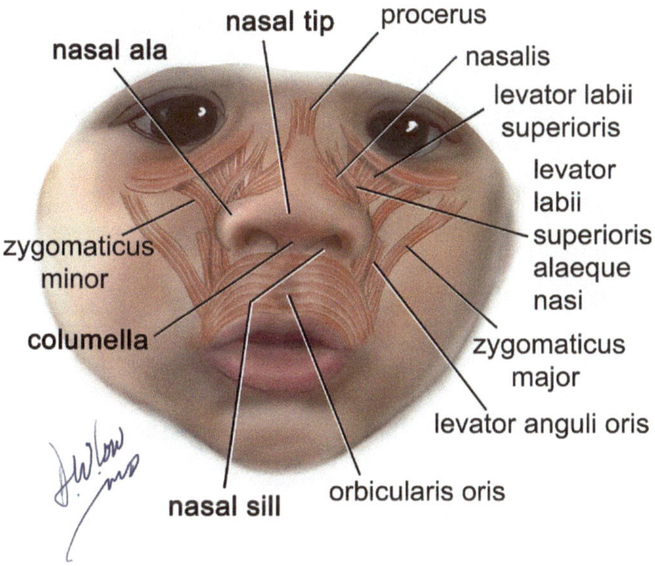


Fig. 5.2 Lip anatomy

Table 5.4 Soft palate musculature and function

| Muscle | Origin | Insertion | Function |
|---|---|---|---|
| Levator veli palatini | Petrous temporal bone Eustachian tube | Palatine aponeurosis | Elevation of the soft palate |
| Tensor veli palatini | Medial pterygoid plate of sphenoid Lateral cartilage of eustachian tube | Palatine aponeurosis | Tenses the soft palate Contracts to open the eustachian tube |
| Palatoglossus | Palatine aponeurosis | Lateral tongue | Pulls the soft palate toward the tongue |
| Palatopharyngeus | Palatine aponeurosis Hard palate | Upper border of thyroid cartilage | Tenses soft palate Draws pharynx anteriorly during swallowing |
| Musculus uvulae | Posterior nasal spine Palatine aponeurosis | Mucous membrane of uvula | Shortens the uvula |

**Soft Palate (Velum)** The soft palate is a collection of five muscles that work together to complete a variety of speech- and swallow-related functions and form part of the velopharyngeal sphincter. Four of the muscles are oriented bilaterally with the musculus uvulae muscle running longitudinally and midline between them. The functions of each individual muscle are outlined in Table 5.4.

## Classification

Although cleft lip and palate is a common abnormality, a universally accepted classification is still pending [1]. Historically there were many classifications proposed. The first classifications were in 1922 by Davis and Richie and in 1923 by Brophy, and they were based on anatomic and morphologic perspectives. In 1931, Veau proposed a simpler classification but left aside clefts of primary palate and did not differentiate incomplete from complete clefts (Fig. 5.3).

Fogh-Andersen [7] and Kernahan [8] based their classifications on embryologic perspectives, considering the incisive foramen to be a better dividing line to classify the clefts [1]. The Kernahan "striped Y" diagram, similar to the "LAHSHAL" classification, is used to visually denote the sidedness of a cleft (Fig. 5.4).

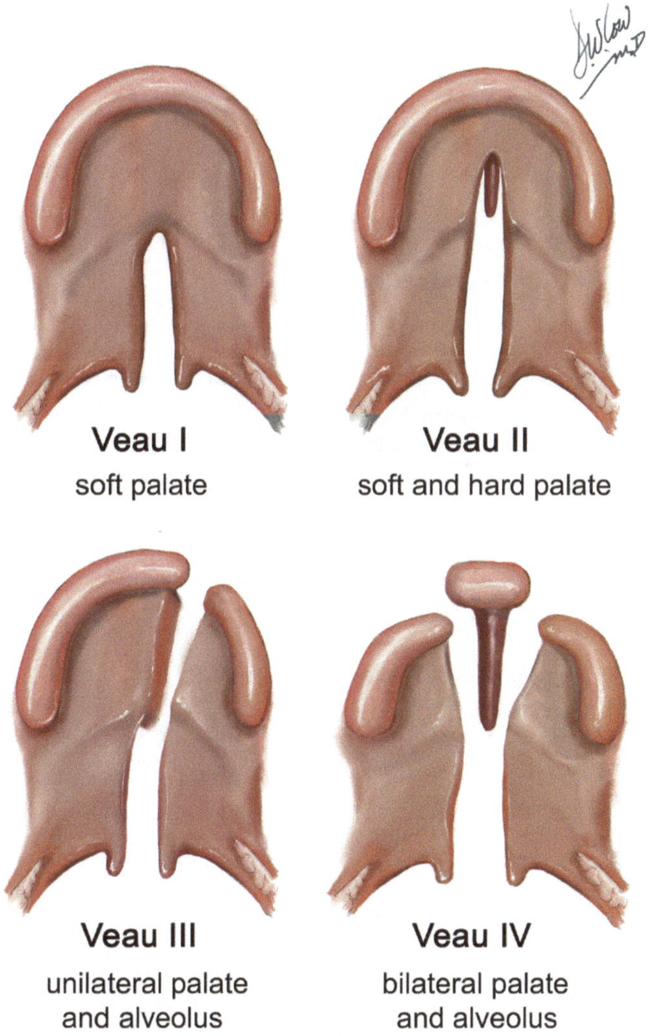


Fig. 5.3 Veau classification

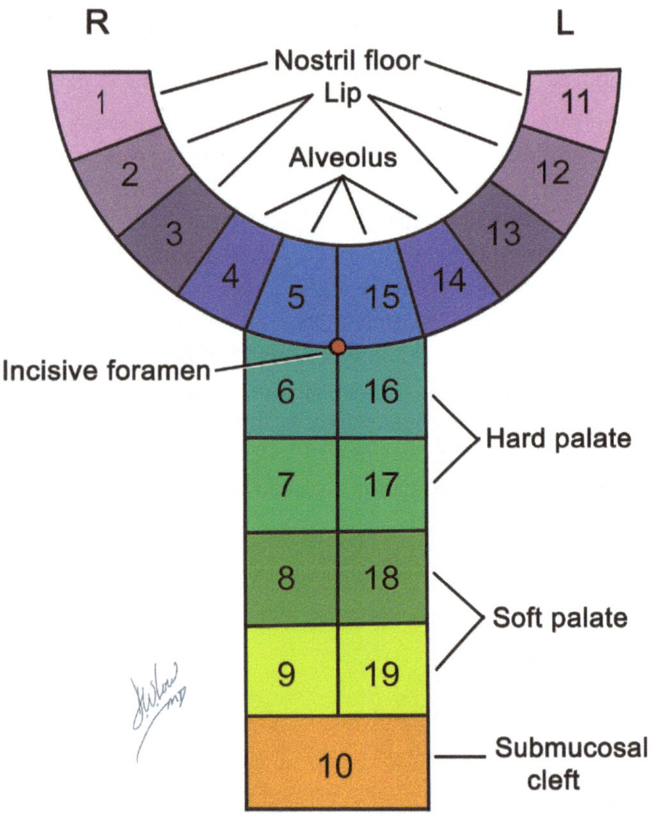


**Fig. 5.4** Kernahan classification

The most commonly used classification system in Brazil was created by Spina in 1973 [16] based on embryologic origins and categorizes presentation relative to the anterior incisive foramen as an anatomic reference to divide the facial malformations into four groups:

- Preforaminal (complete or incomplete) – cleft lip
  - Unilateral
  - Bilateral
- Transforaminal – cleft lip and palate
  - Unilateral
  - Bilateral
- Post-foraminal (complete or incomplete) – cleft palate
- Rare clefts – not associated with the incisive foramen

## Severity Classification

Recent work has sought to stratify severity of unilateral cleft lip deformities. Campbell et al. grade lips from 1 (incomplete, less than 50% of lip height) to 4 (complete, with nostril width ratio of cleft to noncleft side >2) (Fig. 5.5).

Among a study of 1800 patients from throughout the world, they found that 56% were incomplete (grades 1 and 2) and 44% were complete (Grades 3 and 4). Among both incomplete and complete types, the more severe type (Grades 2 and 4) were more common (Fig. 5.6).

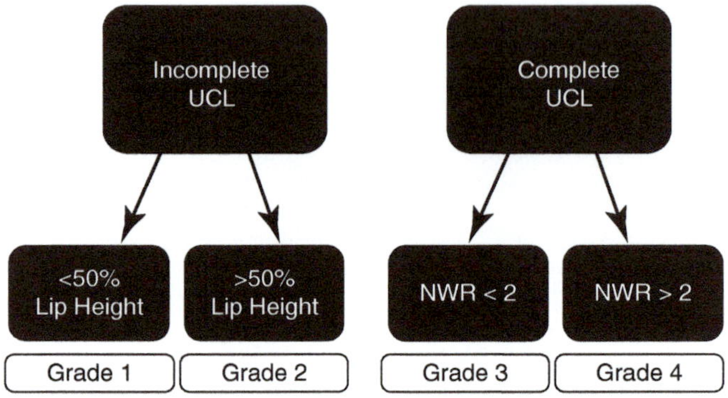


**Fig. 5.5** Classification of unilateral cleft lips from grades 1 to 4 based on severity. Unilateral cleft lip, UCL. Nostril width ratio (NWR) is the ratio of the width of the cleft to noncleft side

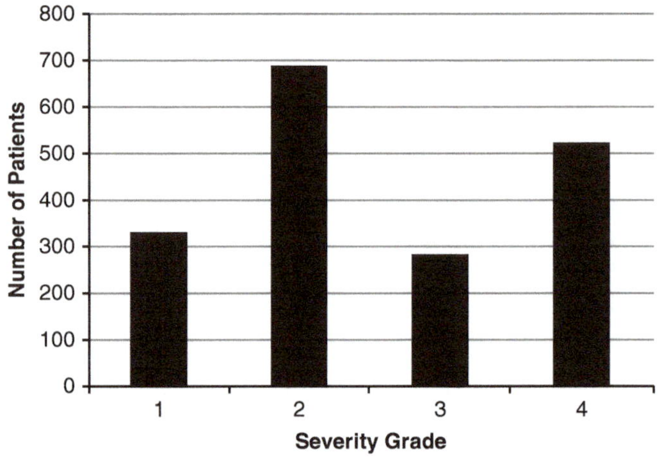


**Fig. 5.6** Distribution of UCL patients according to cleft severity

When cleft lip repair outcomes were assessed by a standardized photographic outcome tool in masked fashion, the aesthetic outcome was seen to be on an average higher when the severity grade was lower (Fig. 5.7).

Similarly, Yao et al. recently found that cleft width ratio (the ratio of the cleft width compared to commissure width), nostril width ratio, and philtral height ratio were most predictive of perceived cleft lip severity. A wide cleft width ratio (>0.5) is predictive of higher rates of unacceptable surgical results.

Finally, Rossell-Perry has proposed a "palatal index," in which the palatal cleft width at the hard-soft palate junction (x) is compared to the width of the palatal shelves [13]. In an assessment of 152 consecutive patients, he found palatal index to correlate significantly with frequency of postoperative fistula, although not with rates of velopharyngeal insufficiency (VPI) or poor speech.

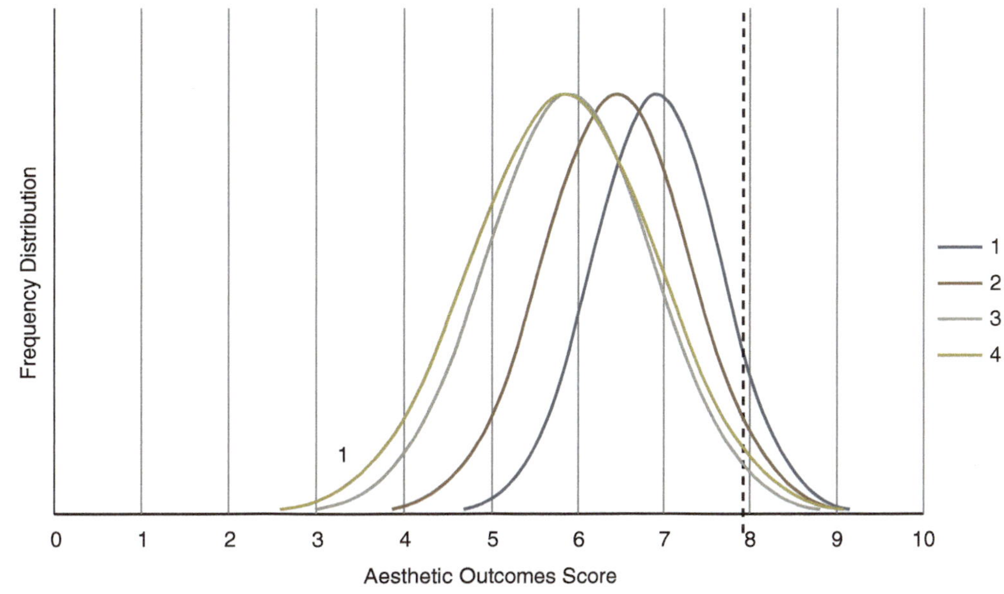


Fig. 5.7 Visual representation of the distribution of aesthetic outcome scores for each severity grade of unilateral cleft lip (dotted line represents highest possible score)

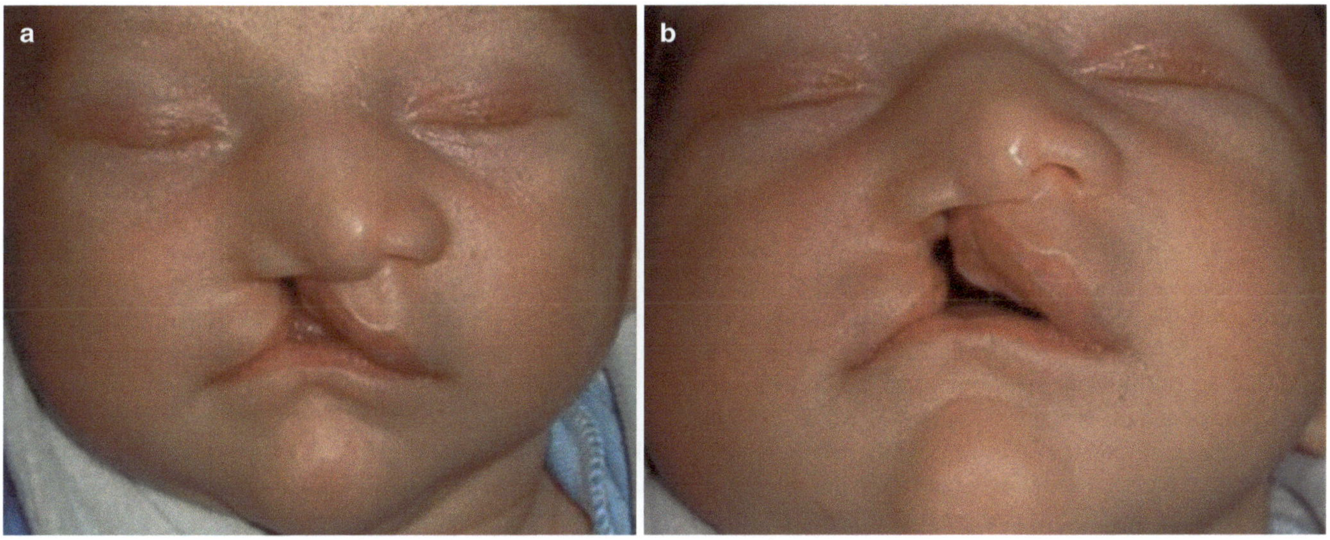


Fig. 5.8 Unilateral cleft lip. Notice alveolar splay, nasal deviation, and short ipsilateral upper lip

These indices of severity may help classify severity to modify clinical treatment/technique algorithms and draw increased attention to those patients at greater risk of poorer outcomes.

## Patterns

### Unilateral Cleft Lip and Palate (UCLPA): Main Features

In UCLPA, the vertical height of the lip is decreased on the cleft side. On the noncleft side, the philtral column, philtral dimple, and two-thirds of Cupid's bow are preserved. The orbicularis muscle is abnormally inserted with the superficial portion running parallel to the cleft margin and alar base on the cleft side and the base of the columella in the noncleft side. The deep portion of the orbicularis is interrupted but does not abnormally insert. This orbicularis muscle disruption is characteristic and persists even in microform clefts. The alveolar bridge may similarly be clefted and show lateral collapse. One may see projection and outward rotation of the maxilla (Fig. 5.8).

Regarding the nose in a UCLPA patient, the nasal tip deviates to the cleft side, and the side dome is depressed [19]. The alar cartilage is displaced caudally, creating an obtuse angle between medial and lateral crura and widening the nostril floor. The columella and anterior caudal septal border are deviated to the noncleft side. The posterior septum is convex on the noncleft side causing varying degrees of airflow obstruction.

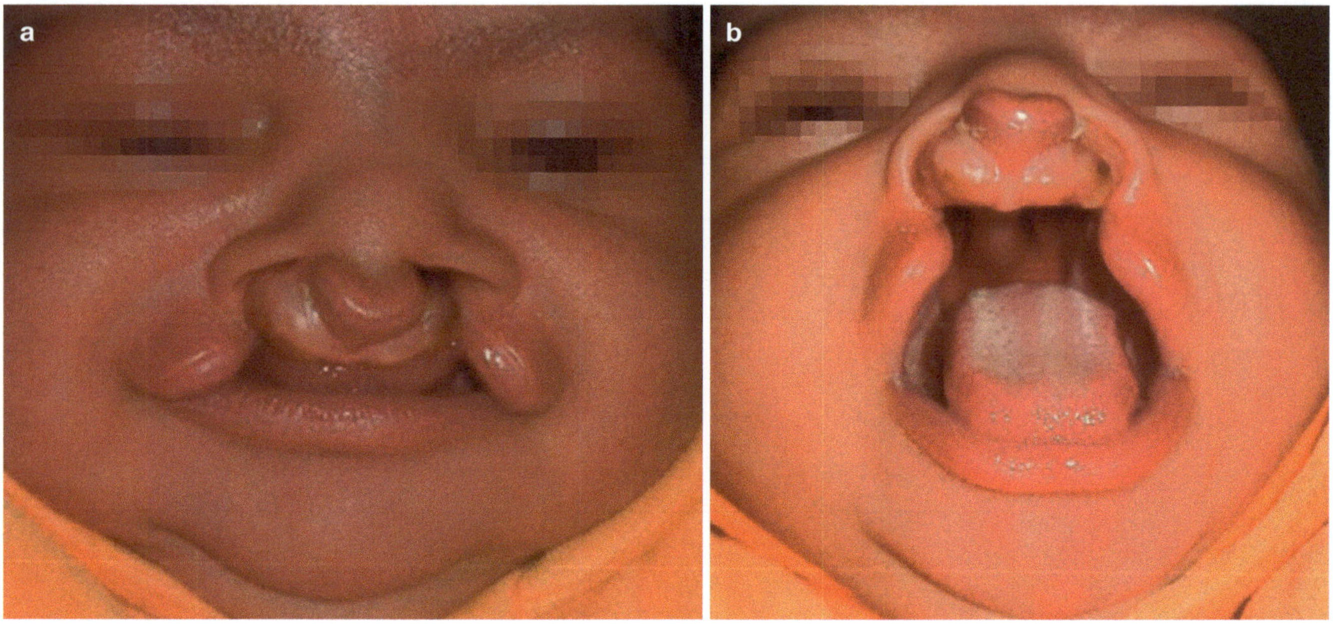


**Fig. 5.9** Bilateral cleft lip. Premaxilla and prolabium are two important anatomical structures that warrant consideration during BCLPA treatment

## Bilateral Cleft Lip and Palate (BCLPA): Main Features

The principal characteristic of bilateral cases is the presence of the prolabium and premaxilla; they are the end point of the frontonasal component. In complete cases, these structures are completely separated from the maxillary process in each side. Consequently, all the elements that come from the maxillary process are not present in the prolabium, for example, the orbicularis muscle. It also lacks Cupid's bow and philtral columns bilaterally. The vascularization and innervation are also altered, and instead of coming from the lateral elements, they come from the cephalic regions.

Each side of a bilateral cleft can display distinctive anatomical features. In the lateral segments, the orbicularis muscle behaves just as it does in a UCL. However, the premaxilla might display a wide scope of three-dimensional deformity as well as dental anomalies and a poorly formed or absent anterior nasal spine. Patients with BCLPA often have widened nostrils, a greatly shortened columella, and a broad and flat nasal tip (Fig. 5.9).

## Cleft Palate: Main Features

The severity of the cleft palate deformity is related to the cleft length and width. The CP abnormality is characterized by discontinuous midline palatal muscles [20]. These abnormally inserted muscles impair the velopharyngeal sphincter function, disrupting feeding, speech, and hearing (due to eustachian tube dysfunction) (Fig. 5.10).

**Hard Palate** Clefts of the hard palate might be preforaminal (primary palate), post-foraminal (secondary palate), or transforaminal (both).

**Soft Palate** Clefts of the soft palate can be submucous, incomplete, or complete.

**Submucous Cleft Palate** Submucosal cleft palates may not be obvious on oral inspection. Some cases display Calnan's classic triad: midline clear zone (zona pellucida), bifid uvula, and palpable notch in the posterior hard palate. Additionally, the levator veli muscles may be seen to insert on the hard palate with animation (Fig. 5.11).

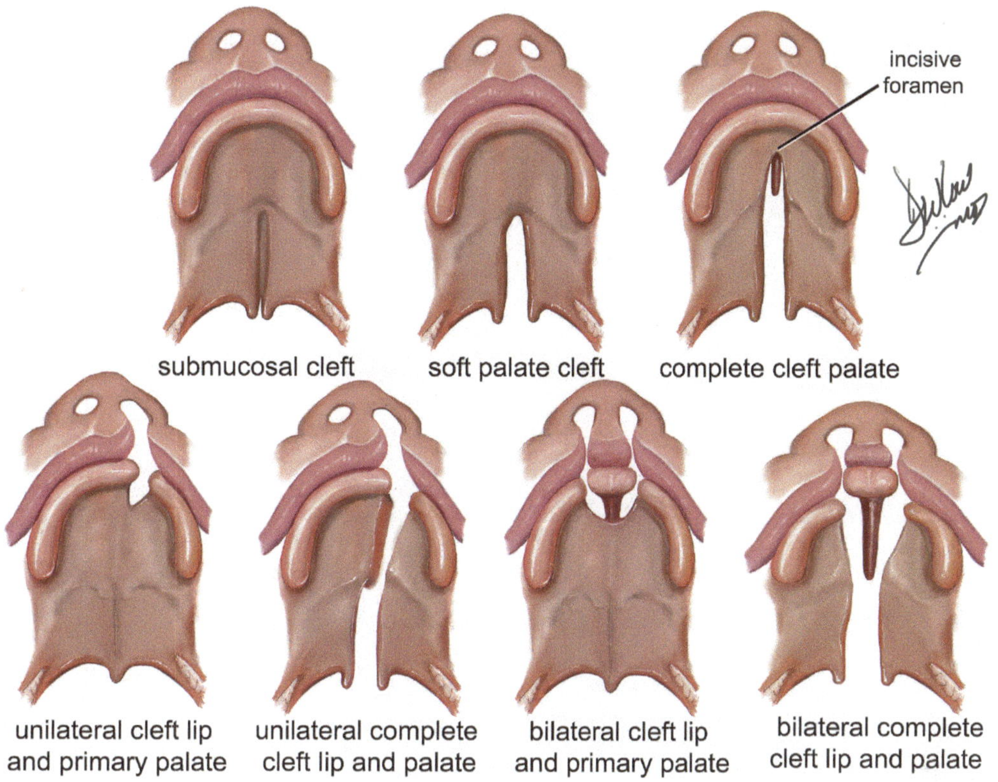


**Fig. 5.10** Patterns in cleft palate

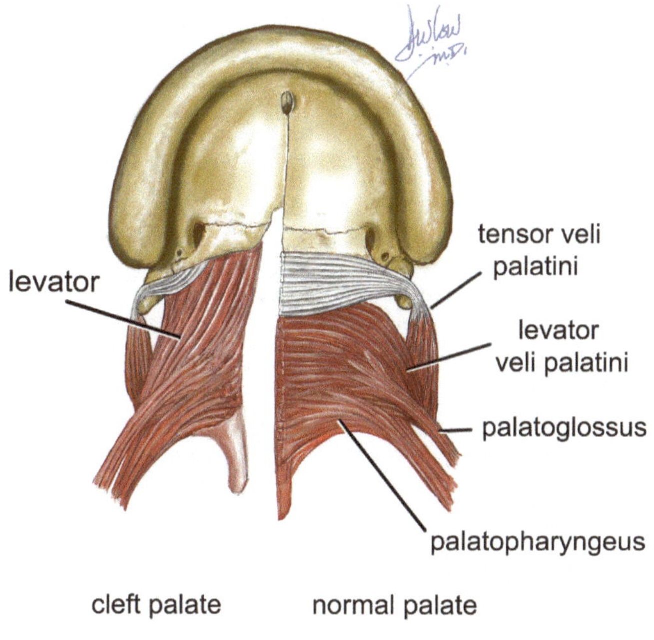


**Fig. 5.11** Palatal anatomy. Right side, cleft palate; left side, normal palate

**Pearls**

Incomplete UCL may display excess of upper lip volume. So, repair of incomplete unilateral cleft lip must take into consideration the related long lip. Due to less tension from the excess volume, patients with incomplete UCL often experience less scarring (Fig. 5.12).

Surgical correction of complete UCL, on the other hand, may lead to the development of a short upper lip. These surgical repairs, placed under high tension, often produce less aesthetically pleasing scars [2]. In addition, postoperatively, insufficient alar rotation may be seen [6]. One must take care to reduce risk of these poor outcomes during repair (Fig. 5.13).

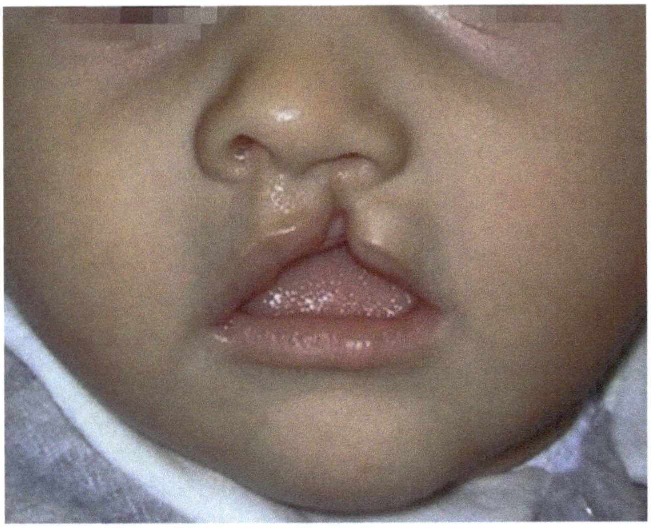

Fig. 5.12 Incomplete unilateral cleft lip

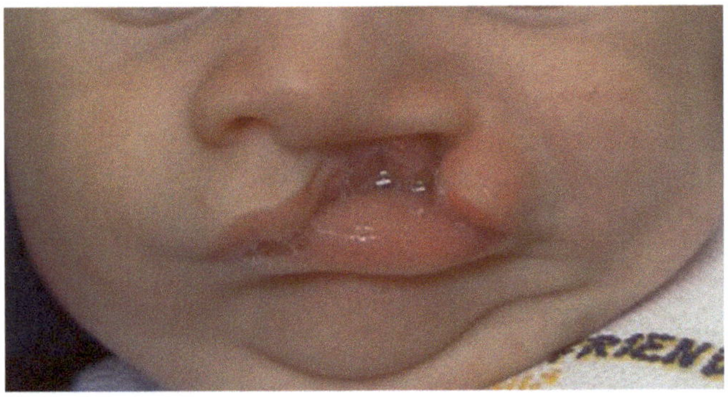

Fig. 5.13 Complete unilateral cleft lip

## References


1. Allori AC, Mulliken JB, Meara JG, Shusterman S, Marcus JR. Classification of cleft lip/palate: then and now. Cleft Palate Craniofac J. 2017;54(2):175–88. https://doi.org/10.1597/14-080.
2. Alonso N, Amaral CER d. Cleft lip and palate treatment: a comprehensive guide. Cham: Springer; 2018.
3. Batra P, Duggal R, Parkash H. Genetics of cleft lip and palate revisited. J Clin Pediatr Dent. 2003;27(4):311–20.
4. Brito LA, Meira JGC, Kobayashi GS, Passos-Bueno MR. Genetics and management of the patient with orofacial cleft. Plast Surg Int. 2012;2012:782821. https://doi.org/10.1155/2012/782821.
5. Campbell A, Restrepo C, eds. Essentials of Cleft Surgery. Cartagena: Global Surgical Arts; 2017.
6. Campbell A, Restrepo C, Park E, et al. Influence of severity on aesthetic outcomes of unilateral cleft lip repair in 1,823 patients. Plast Recon Surg Global Open. 2019;7:e2083.
7. Fogh-Andersen, P. Epidemiology and etiology of clefts. Birth Defects Orig Artic Ser. 1971;7(7):50–53.
8. Kernahan DA. The striped Y—a symbolic classification for cleft lip and palate. Plast Reconstr Surg. 1971;47:469–470.
9. Leslie EJ, Marazita ML. Genetics of cleft lip and cleft palate. Am J Med Genet C Semin Med Genet. 2013;163c(4):246–58. https://doi.org/10.1002/ajmg.c.31381.
10. Mossey P, Little J. Addressing the challenges of cleft lip and palate research in India. Indian J Plast Surg. 2009;42 Suppl:S9–s18. https://doi.org/10.4103/0970-0358.57182.
11. Mossey PA, Little J, Munger RG, Dixon MJ, Shaw WC. Cleft lip and palate. Lancet. 2009;374(9703):1773–85. https://doi.org/10.1016/s0140-6736(09)60695-4.
12. Mossey PA, Modell B. Epidemiology of oral clefts 2012: an international perspective. Front Oral Biol. 2012;16:1–18. https://doi.org/10.1159/000337464.
13. Rossell-Perry P, Nano EC, Gavino-Gutierrez AM. Association between palatal index and cleft palate repair outcomes in patients with complete unilateral cleft lip and palate. JAMA Facial Plast Surg. 2014;16(3):206–10.
14. Smarius B, Loozen C, Manten W, Bekker M, Pistorius L, Breugem C. Accurate diagnosis of prenatal cleft lip/palate by understanding the embryology. World J Methodol. 2017;7(3):93–100.
15. Sperber GH. In: Sperber SM, Guttmann GD, Sperber GH, editors. Craniofacial embryogenetics and development. 2nd ed. Shelton: People's Medical Pub. House USA; 2010.
16. Spina V. A proposed modification for the classification of cleft lip and cleft palate. Cleft Palate J. 1973;10:251–2.
17. World health Organization (WHO), I. C. o. B. D., European Surveillance of Congenital Anomalies (EUROCAT). World atlas of birth defects. 2nd ed. Geneva: World Health Organization; 2003.
18. Wu RT, Peck CJ, Shultz BN, Travieso R, Steinbacher DM. Racial disparities in cleft palate repair. Plast Reconstr Surg. 2019;143(6):1738–45. https://doi.org/10.1097/prs.0000000000005650.
19. Yao CA, Imahiyerobo T, Swanson J, Auslander A, De Cardenas D, Figueiredo JC, McCullough M, Costa M, Vanderburg R, Magee WP. The smile index: part 1. A large-scale study of phenotypic norms for preoperative and postoperative unilateral cleft lip. Plast Reconstr Surg. 2018;141(1):137–46.
20. Zhang Z, Stein M, Mercer N, Malic C. Post-operative outcomes after cleft palate repair in syndromic and non-syndromic children: a systematic review protocol. Syst Rev. 2017;6:1–7.
21. Zhao J, Zhang B, Yang S, Mei H, Qian Z, Liang S, . . . Du Y. Maternal exposure to ambient air pollutant and risk of oral clefts in Wuhan, China. Environ Pollut. 2018;238:624–630. https://doi.org/10.1016/j.envpol.2018.03.053.

# 6 Early Nutrition, Feeding and Management of Infants with an Oral Cleft

Patricia Bannister and Noreen Clarke

**Key Points/Pearls**

- Feeding and nutrition of infants born with cleft lip (CL) and/or palate (CLP/CP) is often challenging for parents and health professionals. Parents are central to infant health and need to be included in nutritional management and assessment.
- Suboptimal specialist training, variable healthcare infrastructure, and limited access to feeding equipment presents particular challenges in low-resource settings. Education, training, and support for all health workers regarding nutrition are important.
- Suboptimal feeding may lead to malnourishment, failure to thrive, postponement of primary surgery, and increased postoperative complication rates. Creative and innovative ways to deliver support are important. Early identification, communication, and intervention of feeding difficulties and malnourishment are essential for adequate development and delivery of timely and safe surgical care. Early registration plays a crucial role in the provision of responsive early care and prevents poor feeding habits from becoming established.
- For patients with malnutrition, collaboration and communication between hospital and community settings are essential for patient well-being.

P. Bannister (✉)
Retired Consultant Nurse, Pullum House, Beggars Ash, Ledbury, UK

University of Manchester, Manchester, UK

N. Clarke
Children's Hospital Los Angeles, Los Angeles, CA, USA

Keck Scholl of Medicine of USC, Los Angeles, CA, USA
e-mail: nclarke@chla.usc.edu

## Introduction

Infants born with a CL, CLP, or CP present with a variety of feeding challenges. Access to specialist knowledge, alternative feeding equipment, and a continuing supportive environment to help parents adapt to their new infant is not always available in many low-resource settings. This often results in a higher incidence of faltering growth. Careful attention to feeding assessment and management in infancy is essential particularly for infants with a cleft involving the palate. Regular monitoring growth is important to assure adequate nutrition. Primary surgery is usually undertaken within the first postnatal year, and poor nutritional status might may delay surgical reconstruction and increase complication rates.

## Feeding Guidance for Patients with Cleft Lip/Palate

### Normal Feeding

Infants are born with the natural ability to feed safely, utilizing an inborn set of reflexes which are organized in a sequential and timely manner [1] and are supported by functional respiratory, cardiac, and neurological systems. In bottle feeding, intraoral pressure is necessary to remove milk from the bottle, whereas in breastfeeding, intraoral pressure is required to position and stabilize the nipple in the infants' mouth allowing the tongue to rhythmically strip the elongated nipple [15]. An intact hard and soft palate is required for this increase in pressure to occur. Many health professionals lack sufficient knowledge about the mechanisms of normal feeding, so, consequently, they are unable to identify specific problems when feeding is interrupted by either mechanical or neurological problems. Breastfeeding is the recommended feeding method for all babies, particularly in LMIC where access to clean water can be problematic [17].

© Springer Nature Switzerland AG 2021

J. W. Swanson, D. W. Low (eds.), *Global Cleft Care in Low-Resource Settings*, https://doi.org/10.1007/978-3-030-59105-2_6

### Feeding Duration and Amounts

Infants usually complete a feed within 30–45 minutes. After that time, they often become tired and uncoordinated and may be expending more energy feeding than taken in for growth.

In the first 2 days, 70–90 ml/kg/day is generally advised and increased to 120–150 ml/kg/day within 3–4 days after birth [13].

### Initial Feeding Assessment

The use of a feeding assessment record is recommended to approach babies with potential feeding difficulties. Several assessment records have been developed taking into account feeding skills, systemic support (respiratory, cardiac, neurological), and maternal health. An example of this can be seen at http://www.eu-patient.eu/Members/The-EPF-Members/Associate-Member/European-Cleft-Association%2D%2D-ECO/. Used correctly, assessment guides the choice of feeding equipment, infant position for sleep and feeding, and frequency and volume of oral feeds. Specialist training, ongoing assessment, and parental teaching are essential for effective use [7].

## Specific Feeding Problems of Infants with CL+/− P

Although infants with a cleft may present with early difficulties, most full-term babies with a CL+/−P, and no additional morbidity, can learn to feed orally. To achieve this, they will require appropriate modifications to the chosen feeding method, whether breast or bottle feeding [2]. Accordingly, these infants can be nursed safely at home by their family and usually grow well.

The most frequently encountered problem is an inability to create sufficient intraoral pressure to effectively feed safely in an acceptable time frame. A baby with a cleft will typically initiate sucking but quickly move into non-nutritive sucking where little or no milk is delivered into the infant's mouth.

Infants born with an isolated CP may present with more complex difficulties and may require admission to hospital for further assessment. Upper airway obstruction, as found in Pierre Robin sequence, cardiac anomalies, and neurological issues may need to be addressed as the primary problem before oral feeding can be commenced as these issues often impact an infant's ability to feed safely and effectively. Feeding directly from the breast is difficult for infants where a cleft palate is involved, as the infant is unable to increase the intraoral pressure making elongation and stabilization of the nipple in the mouth particularly difficult.

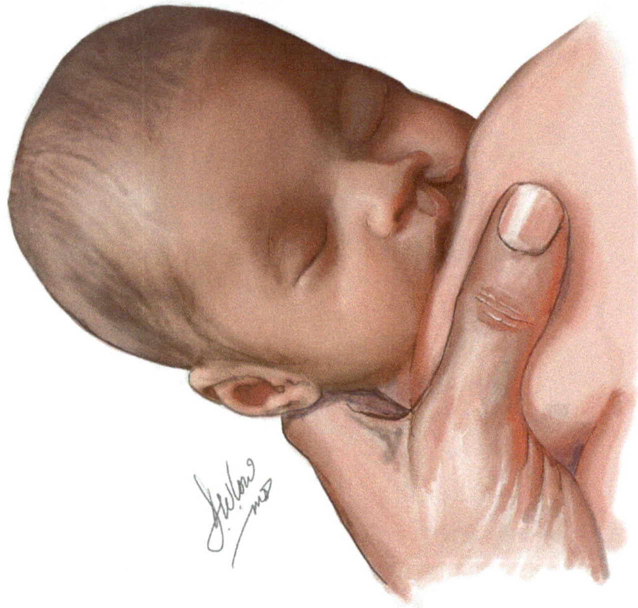

**Fig. 6.1** Latch-on and breast compression

### Cleft Lip

Babies born with isolated CL can usually feed directly from the breast and should be encouraged to do so. Mothers will usually need guidance to achieve a successful "latch-on" and maintenance of an adequate milk supply. Good latch-on is achieved by positioning the infant so that the cleft is under the breast tissue (Fig. 6.1). It is often useful to cradle the baby around the mother's body freeing the hand to support the adjacent breast in the baby's mouth throughout the feed. Breast compression during suckling increases milk flow [10]. Breastfeeding guidance for infants without a cleft is available [18], and with a number of additional elements, this remains relevant for babies with CL:

1. Massage the breast before a feed, with a little manual expression of milk.
2. Position the infant so that cleft is underneath the breast tissue.
3. Support the breast tissue in the mouth throughout the feed.
4. Using the thumb, gently compress the breast just above the areola to assist milk flow as the infant suckles.
5. Reposition the breast if attachment begins to falter.

### Cleft Palate with or Without Cleft Lip

Breastfeeding an infant with a CP is often a challenge as the lack of intraoral suction is more pronounced. In some instances, the mother may be able to manually express milk from the breast straight into her baby's mouth, but this is not always possible. Alternative feeding strategies are discussed below.

## Assisted Breast/Bottle Feeding and Devices

### Breastfeeding

When feeding directly from the breast is either not possible or only partially possible, expressed breast milk fed via a cup or teat and bottle is an option. Decisions to include additional feeding equipment are generally made over a period of several days when a baby fails to feed or gain adequate weight despite alterations in feeding technique. Several shaped cups are available for use with expressed breast milk (Figs. 6.2 and 6.3), and this is the advised method to support breastfeeding [19].

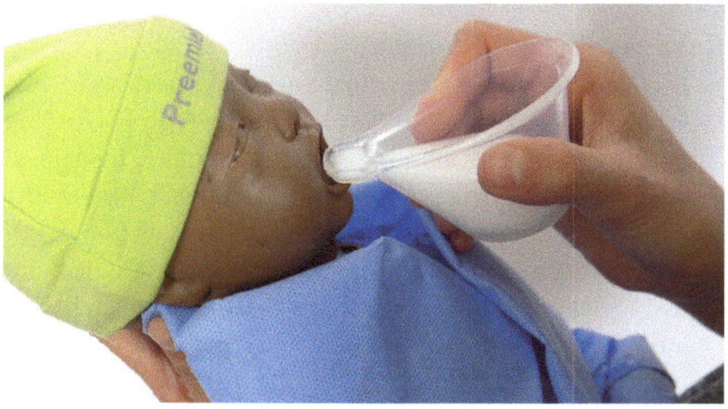


**Fig. 6.2** Nifty cup

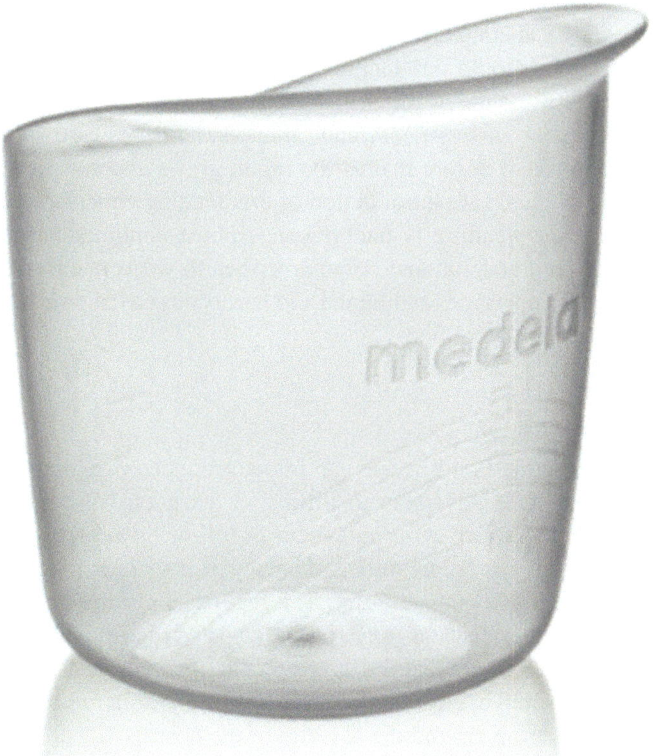


**Fig. 6.3** Medela cup

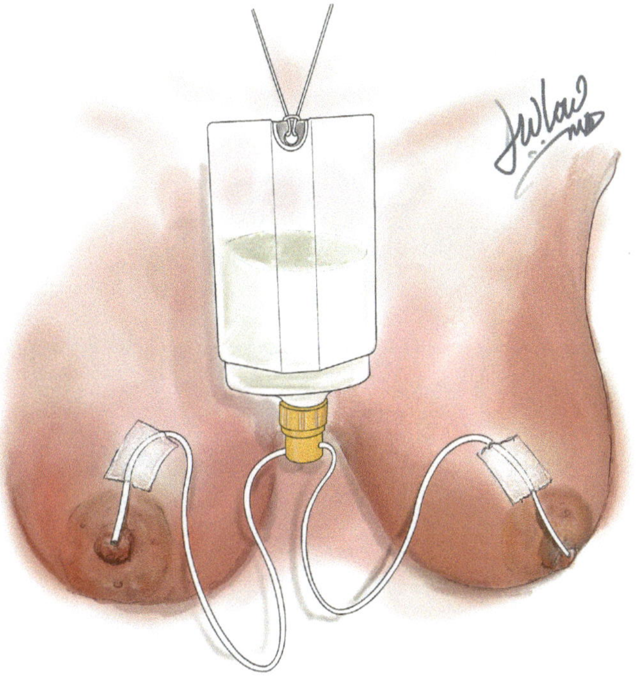

**Fig. 6.4** Medela Supplemental Feeding System. (https://www.medela.co.uk/breastfeeding)

- *Nifty Cup*. A small silicone cup in which the mother can express milk. The tapered end acts as a small reservoir and, when placed onto the infant's tongue, allows the infant to lap up the milk and control the pace of feeding (Fig. 6.2). It is manufactured by Laerdal and available in low-resource countries for approximately USD 0.50 each (https://laerdalglobalhealth.com/products/nifty-feeding-cup/).
- *Medela System*. The Medela Supplemental Feeding System (Fig. 6.4) has been developed to assist breastfeeding. A small tube is attached to the mother's nipple and to a bottle of breast milk seen here around the mother's neck. Milk from the bottle is delivered into the baby's mouth as the baby attempts to feed.

### Modified Bottles

There are no standard bottle/teats for infants with oral clefts, and a variety of bottles are used worldwide.

- Assisted feeding with soft flexible bottles (MAM and Mead Johnson) used with orthodontic teats (NUK/MAM) is widely used in HRS (Fig. 6.5). The caregiver is able to assist the delivery of milk by squeezing the sides of the bottle in either a continuous or pulse squeeze action [14], enabling the infant to gain adequate nutrition, within an acceptable time frame. The need for this help will vary within one feed, from one feed to the next, and from one infant to another. The frequency will depend on many factors such as the type of cleft, the presence of other anomalies, and the age of the infant.

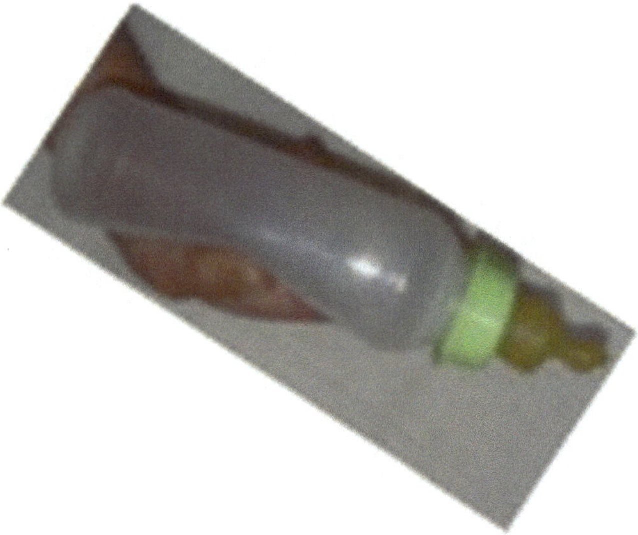

**Fig. 6.5** MAM bottle and NUK teat

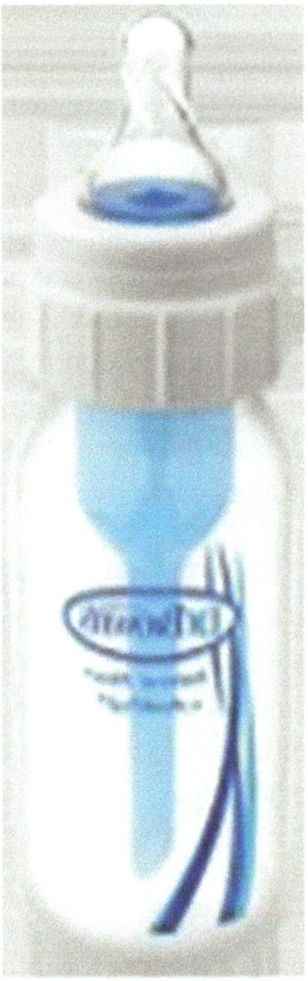

**Fig. 6.6** Dr. Brown bottle

- Dr. Brown bottle and teat (Fig. 6.6), with a one-way flow valve, has been used with some success. This system allows the infant to control the flow of milk and does not require caregiver to squeeze the bottle. The correct flow of milk results in a relaxed baby with no nasal regurgitation of milk while suckling. The introduction of either method of feeding follows a feeding assessment and is not advisable in the first 24–48 hours following birth. Assisted feeding is appropriate for the majority of newborn babies who have clefts but is not initially suitable where there is accompanied dysphagia or breathing problems.

## Oral Plates/Obturators

- These have been described by a number of teams as useful devises to assist with feeding. These plates occlude only the hard palate and not the posterior soft palate. They are an additional expense and require frequent remodeling as the infant grows adding to the burden of care for families, and they can cause mucosal ulceration on the sensitive nasal septum. Although some teams believe they are a helpful component in reshaping the cleft, for feeding purposes, there is no evidence that they are helpful.

## Nasogastric (NG) Feeding

- Some babies with CLP will be unable to safely and effectively feed and might require support with NG feeding during the first few months. Prematurity and/or associated developmental/anatomical conditions might cause failure to thrive, in spite of the use of noninvasive nutritional support measures. In such cases, hospital admission for assessment and management is indicated. Neonatal/pediatric specialist assessment should rule out additional comorbidities to provide specific management. To achieve adequate nutritional intake, the NGT would generally be used as a temporary feeding aid within a hospital admission. Only in settings with a safe water supply and the availability of adequate refrigeration and where parents can be adequately trained and supported with the NGT feeding should this method of feeding be considered for use outside the hospital.
- Frequent assessment and interdisciplinary care are required to ensure that as the infant grows and develops, the gradual safe introduction of oral feeding either before or after weaning is undertaken. Robust communication between hospital and community health workers ensures agreed plans are maintained and hazardous environmental issues are identified.

## Oral Hygiene

- During the first 8 weeks, an infant produces very limited saliva. It is advisable to offer 2–3 teaspoons of cooled boiled water after formula feeds or following nasal regurgitation. For breast milk-fed babies or if there is no cleft palate, this is unnecessary. The regular application of an edible lubricant on the exposed areas of the lip and premaxilla will prevent the development of soreness. A clean damp cloth using clean water may be helpful in removing debris from around the alar rim of the nostril.

## Positioning and Winding/Burping

- It is the easiest and most comfortable way for the baby to take in the milk and coordinate suckling and swallowing if they are in a forward facing semi-upright position. It is thought that this position lets gravity help with swallowing, limits nasal regurgitation, and helps prevent milk from entering into the Eustachian tubes connecting the mouth with the middle ear.
- If the flow of milk is correct, infants will have little problem with increased ingestion of wind; however, this may be a problem. If this happens, infants usually indicate their discomfort and may display frequent regurgitation. In the first few weeks, it may be necessary to wind the baby after every 1 oz of milk taken. It is recommended to stop two or three times during the feed to burp the baby.

## Sources of Milk and Milk Alternatives

There are several sources of human milk and milk alternatives to consider when planning the feeding care of the child with CLP where a mother's breast milk is insufficient or unavailable.

- *Mother's Milk.* It is crucial to educate the families and the community on the benefits of breastfeeding and mother's milk. These are the first choice for all infants.
- *Other Human Milk.* If the mother's milk is no longer available, human milk from a healthy wet nurse or a human milk bank is an alternative option. Milk from a wet nurse should be carefully considered within a given context, e.g., the risk of HIV or other diseases that may adversely affect the health of the infant. Human milk banking is currently rare in many LMICs. Acceptability of other human milk may vary from setting to setting, but if safely processed, this is a nutritional sound option.
- *Animal Milk.* Cow, goat, and other types of milk are reported sources of milk for children with oral clefts unable to effectively breastfeed. These milks are generally not suitable for infants and should only be used as a last resort. If the only viable source of milk is animal milk, caregivers should be instructed on boiling/sterilizing and storing milk to minimize infection risks. Every effort should be made to help to source a more complete source of nutrition, but if this is not possible, advice on additional supplements should be provided.
- *Formula and Powdered Milks.* Infant formula is often expensive and not widely available. In an effort to extend use, families may dilute the ratio of water to formula resulting in inadequate calories for growth. Guidance on the correct preparation and use of infant formula is available [16]. Other powdered milk can be used, though these might not be nutritional complete for infants and should not be advised. Additional boiled water given between feeds is advised where constipation becomes a problem.

## Weaning

From the age of 4–6 months, infants are able to supplement nutrition and are physiologically ready to accept the introduction of weaning foods. A balanced diet including adequate intake of carbohydrates, fats, protein, vitamins, and minerals is required to ensure sufficient nutrition for growth. In many parts of the world, roots and grains form the basis of nutrition [5]. Country- and locally specific weaning guidelines, for infants and young child, reflecting available foods, may be available. As a general guideline, the caregiver should be advised on including the following groups of foods within the infants' daily diet:

- Dairy – milk, yogurt, cheese
- Fruit and vegetables
- Meat, fish, or combined pulses/legumes (beans and peas)
- Cereal – wheat/oat/barley and rice products
- Fats – oil, butter, milk

Important aspects for children with unoperated cleft palate are developmentally appropriate textures (ranging from yogurt to mashed foods) and the amount of food presented to the child for each mouthful. These will help to prevent nasal regurgitation and choking and allow a child to learn to manage and enjoy foods.

## Nutrition and Growth Assessment

Families should be advised to hold their child's own record of growth and carry with them to the clinic or other health settings. Weight, height, and head circumference are recorded at birth and thereafter with each visit to identify if appropriate weight gain and growth have been established. Healthcare workers will be able to identify faltering growth and refer to a local pediatrician, a nurse, or, if available, a dietician for additional assessment and management.

### Growth Measurement

Adequate growth of infants and young children is an indication of appropriate nutrition. Monitoring and recording should adapt to WHO standards [17, 21]. Measurements of height, weight, upper mid-arm circumference (UMAC), and head circumference are recommended initially on a weekly basis and taken and recorded by a trained health worker [8]. Regular monitoring identifies infants who need extra support to grow. Growth is described in terms of Z-score (standard) deviations away from the median expected rather than as a percentage (e.g., 70%). Ideally two health workers are required, but this is not always possible, and parental help may be an alternative. Measurements are recorded in kilograms and centimeters using reliable equipment. Posters teaching health workers techniques to measure young children have been developed by Kat Hartman for UNICEF and available at https://www.kathartman.com/instructional#/instructional/unicef-anthropometric-nutrition-posters/.

## Weight Measure

A variety of scales are used to measure weight. Digital scales are more commonly used in high-resource settings, but these are not always available. In these settings, a Salter hanging scale (Fig. 6.7) can be used for children under 9 years/25 kg [12].

1. Weigh child without clothes or diaper.
2. Use the same scale at each measure.
3. When the baby is settled and weight value is stable, record to the nearest 100 g.
4. Assure that no one is touching the baby during weighing.
5. A caregiver may hold a baby on the scales. Subtract the weight of care from combined weight.
6. If the child is able to stand, a digital scale may be used.
7. Scales require frequent calibration (tested) using a 10 kg fixed weight and recalibration when the weights do not match.

## Length Measure

Children younger than 24 months are measured lying down. A measuring board/mat is used when available (Figs. 6.8 and 6.9), but when unavailable, a non-stretchable tape measure and a flat surface may be used.

1. Infants unable to stand are placed on their back on a measure board or flat surface.
2. Remove head and foot coverings.
3. First measurer places hands either side of the infants head and ensures the head remains touching either the measure board or wall/firm surface throughout the procedure.
4. Second measurer gently straightens the infants body and legs placing the soles of the feet on the footboard (Fig. 6.10) or against an upright book
5. Note the value on the board or make a mark where the heals meet the book.
6. When not using a measure board, lift the infant away and using a non stretchable tape measure, measure the length from the wall to the mark taken where the heal met the book.
7. Record the measurement in centimetres.

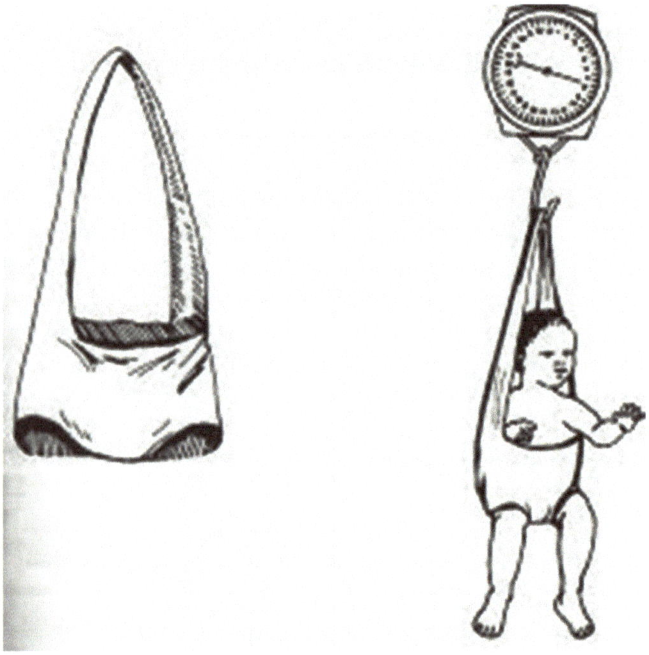

**Fig. 6.7** Salter hanging scale. (Motherchildnutrition.org)

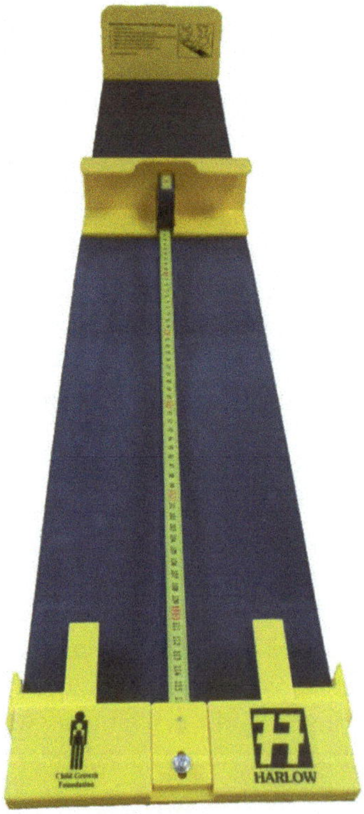


**Fig. 6.8** Neonatometre. (www.healthforallchildren.com)

## Head Circumference Measure

Head circumference is used to measure the volume of the growing underlying brain [4] (Fig. 6.11).

1. Wrap the tape around the widest circumference of the head above the eyebrow on the forehead and then across the most prominent part of the back of the head.
2. Reposition the tape and repeat the measurement three times.
3. Record the largest measurement to the nearest 0.1 cm.

## Mid-Upper Arm Circumference (MUAC) Measure

Mid-upper arm circumference (MUAC) measurement is a useful tool to detect if a child is malnourished (Fig. 6.12).

1. Identify the midpoint between the tip of the shoulder and the tip of the elbow of the left arm.
2. Place the tape measure around the arm at the midpoint.
3. Relax the arm.
4. Assure the tape measure is not too tight or too loose.
5. Record the value to the nearest 0.1 cm or 1 mm.

## Malnourishment: Diagnosis and Management

Malnutrition is a leading cause of mortality and morbidity worldwide. Severe malnutrition is primarily seen in countries with limited resources. Two forms of acute malnutrition are kwashiorkor (edematous malnutrition) and marasmus (wasting). Affected children may also have micronutrient deficiencies. Table 6.1 lists thresholds of malnourishment, and the WHO outlines Z-scores for height and weight based on sex and age (Figs. 6.13, 6.14, 6.15, and 6.16.)

WHO [17, 21] has developed criteria for the classification of moderate or severe malnutrition in children. These gauges are based upon the degree of wasting, stunting, and the presence of edema, which may occur separately or together. The goals of the clinical assessment are to distinguish between the types and severity of malnutrition and to identify compli-

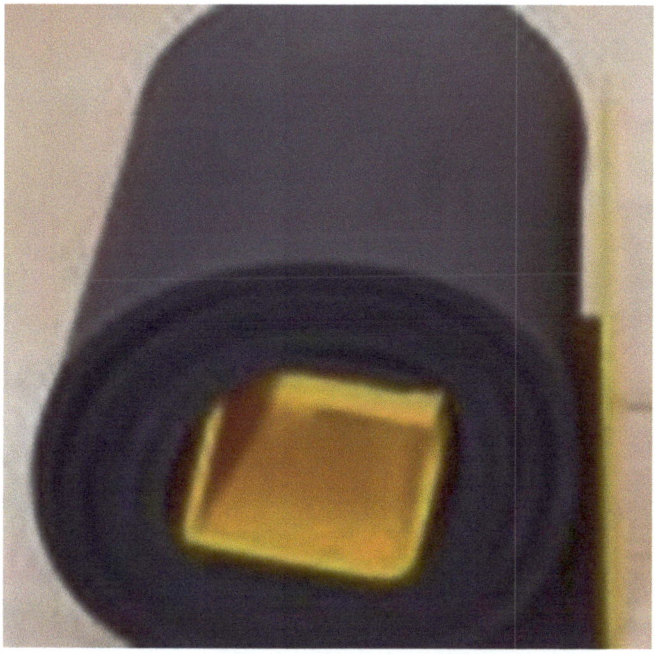

Fig. 6.9 Dunmow mat. (www.healthforallchildren.com)

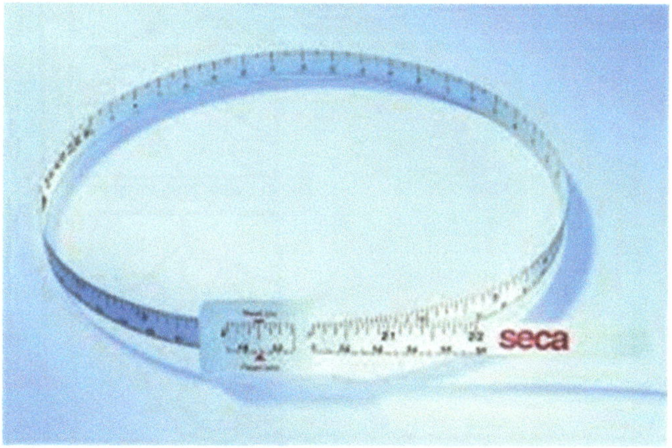


Fig. 6.11 Head circumference measure. (www.SECA.com)

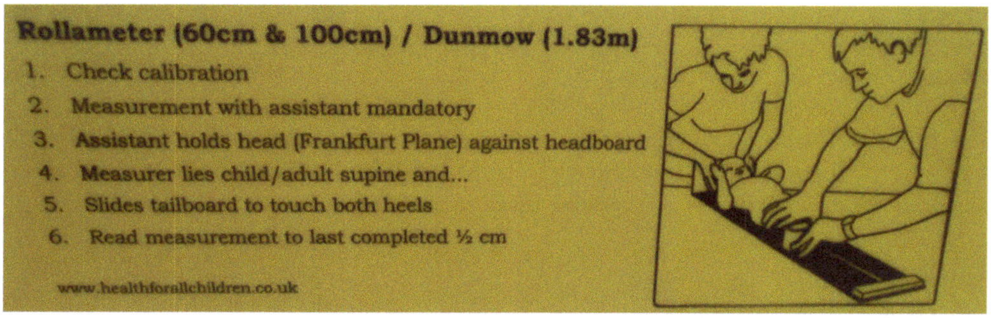


Fig. 6.10 Measuring length. (www.healthforallchildren.com)

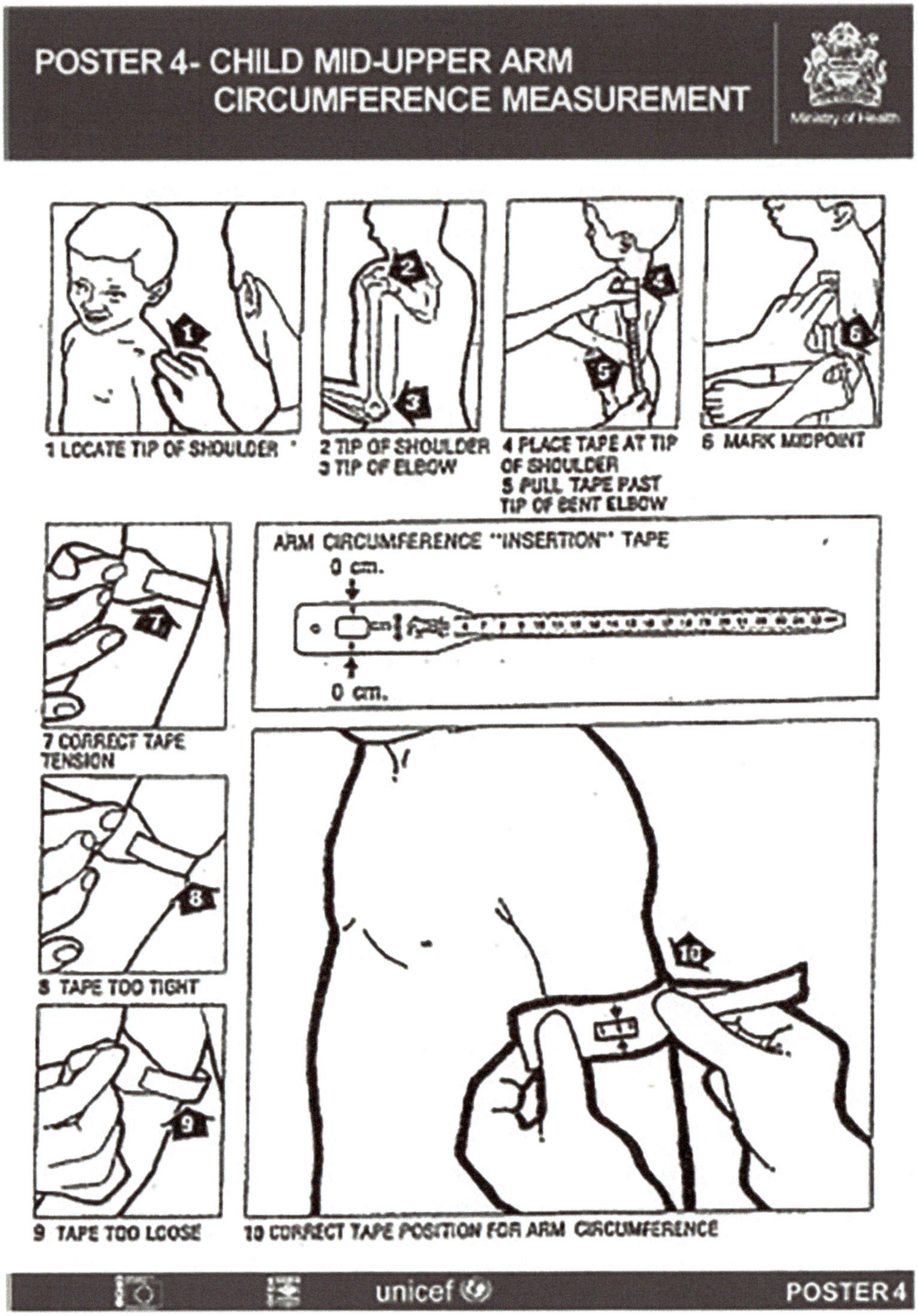


**Fig. 6.12** Mid-upper arm circumference. (motherchildnutrition.org)

cations that might be life-threatening (sepsis and acute dehydration).

First-line treatment of malnourishment is focused on adjusting feeding techniques and addition of supplementary calories. It is important not to introduce weaning foods too early as these are not easily digested in children under 4–6 months of age. For severely malnourished infants, it is important to establish a baseline of the amount taken in the prior 24 hours and then gradually increase the volume of feed until optimal amount for weight is reached. This allows the stomach to increase in size and avoid problems with vomiting.

**Table 6.1** World Health Organization classification of acute malnutrition

| Ages: 6–60 months[a] | | | |
|---|---|---|---|
| Clinical term | Measure | Moderate malnutrition (MAM) | Severe malnutrition (SAM) |
| Wasting | Mid-upper arm circumference (MUAC) | 11.5–12.4 cm[b] | <11.5 cm[b] |
| Wasting | Weight for height Z-score | −2 to −3[a] | <−3[a] |
| Kwashiorkor | Symmetrical pitting edema | Absent[a] | Present[a] |

[a]www.who.int/childgrowth/standards
[b]www.who.int/childgrowth/standards/ac_for_age/en/

## Perioperative Feeding Considerations

### Preoperative Nutritional Assessment

- Regular weight monitoring will identify persistent faltering growth. Additional calorie supplements need to be considered when preparing an infant for surgery.
- Parent-held records of growth measurements are easily transferred to hospital or other health settings.
- Iron deficiency anemia is common in LMICs. Hemoglobin of above 10 g/dl is advisable before surgery is considered. It may be necessary to consider the prescription of a liquid iron supplementation a few weeks before surgery, for all

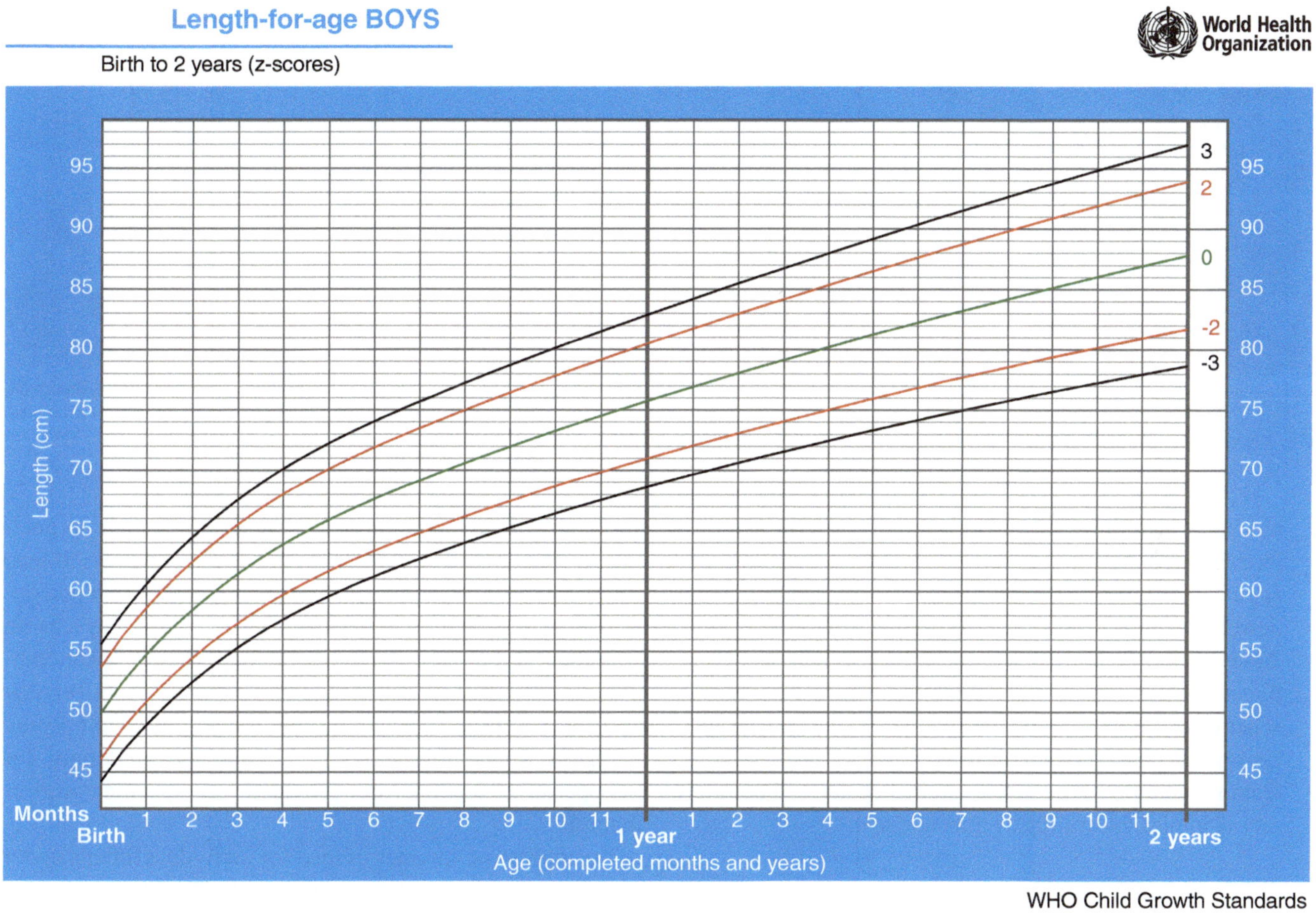


**Fig. 6.13** Length from Birth to 2 years (Boys)

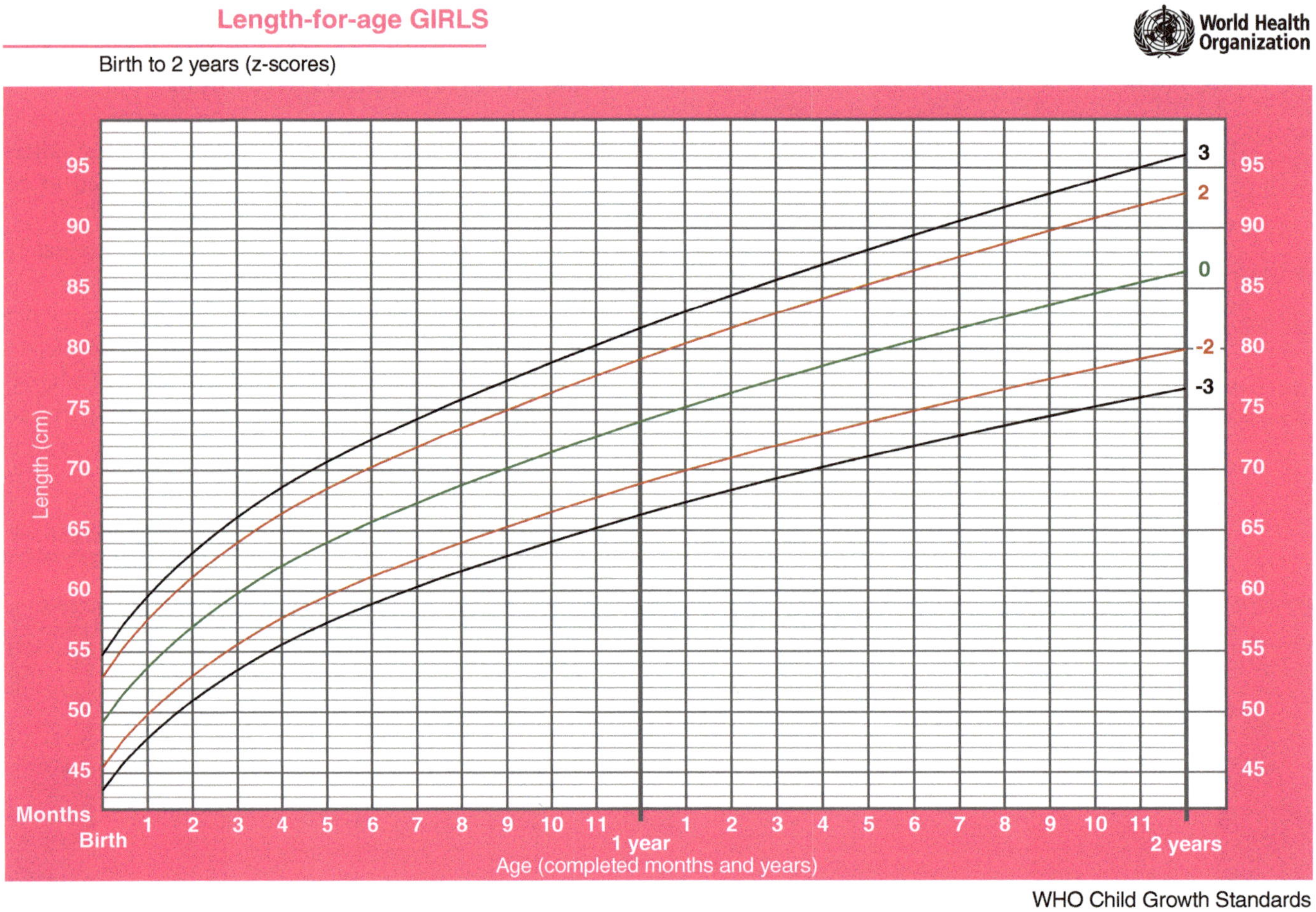


**Fig. 6.14** Length from Birth to 2 years (Girls)

newborns with low weight (including both term and preterm infants). For infants between 6 and 12 months, management may include weaning foods rich in iron [9] and deworming in addition to an iron supplementation [11].

- Assessment of additional comorbidities, which may complicate surgery, needs to be undertaken before surgery is scheduled. These may include a history of upper airway obstruction and cardiac concerns.
- Communication between the surgical center and community is important to support management.

## Postoperative Feeding

In both HRS and LMRS, infants are commonly discharged home within 24 hours after surgery, so establishing oral feeding quickly becomes important. Pain and a change in anatomy are factors that influence an infant's willingness to feed after surgery. Adequate scheduled intraoperative and postoperative pain relief, for a period of at least 5–7 days, is an important part of care. A recovering infant may appear comfortable until they are asked to feed. Feeding discomfort may result in a refusal to feed. Assuring feeding prior to hospital discharge after surgery is critical. Specific guidelines for postoperative feeding are provided on specific surgical chapters.

Postoperative volumes of feed for individual infants under weaning age need to reflect preoperative volumes as these may vary. For older infants who have already been weaned, soft mashed foods are frequently advised for the first 3 weeks following surgery. Discharge home is advisable only when feeding and pain relief are managed.

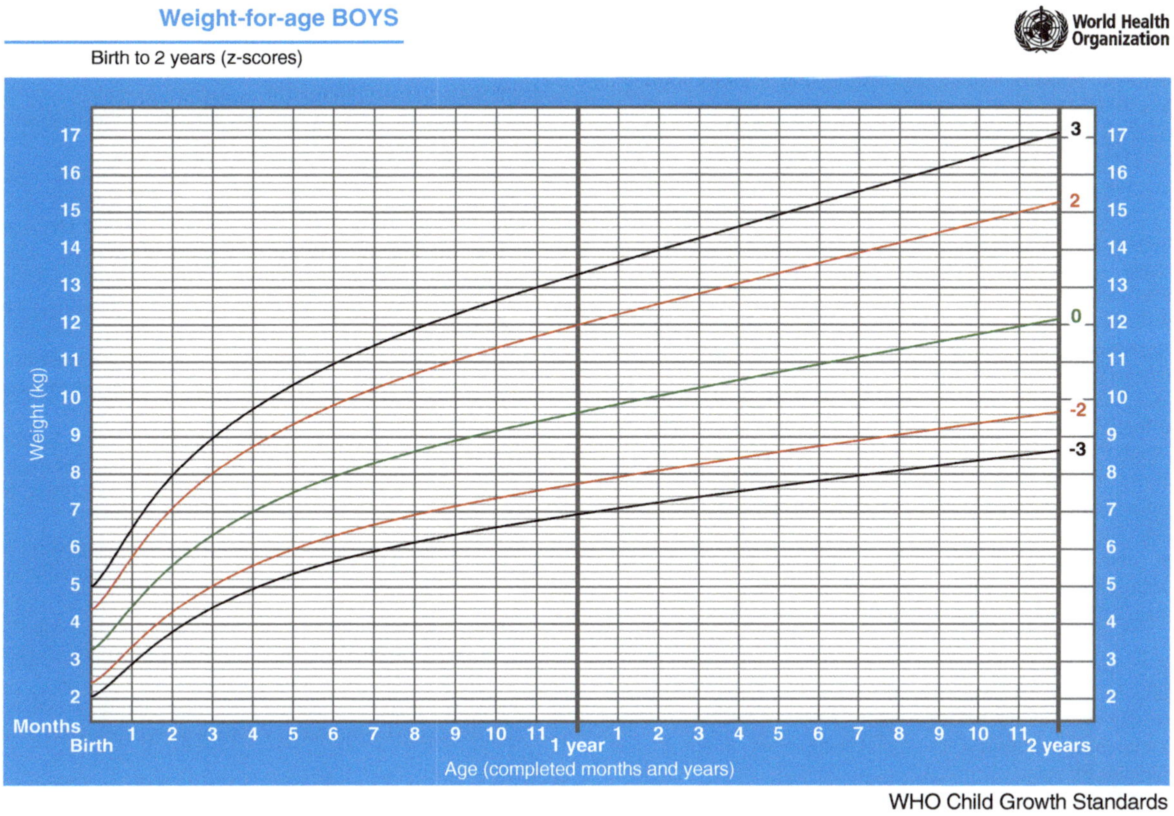


**Fig. 6.15** Weight from Birth to 2 years (Boys)

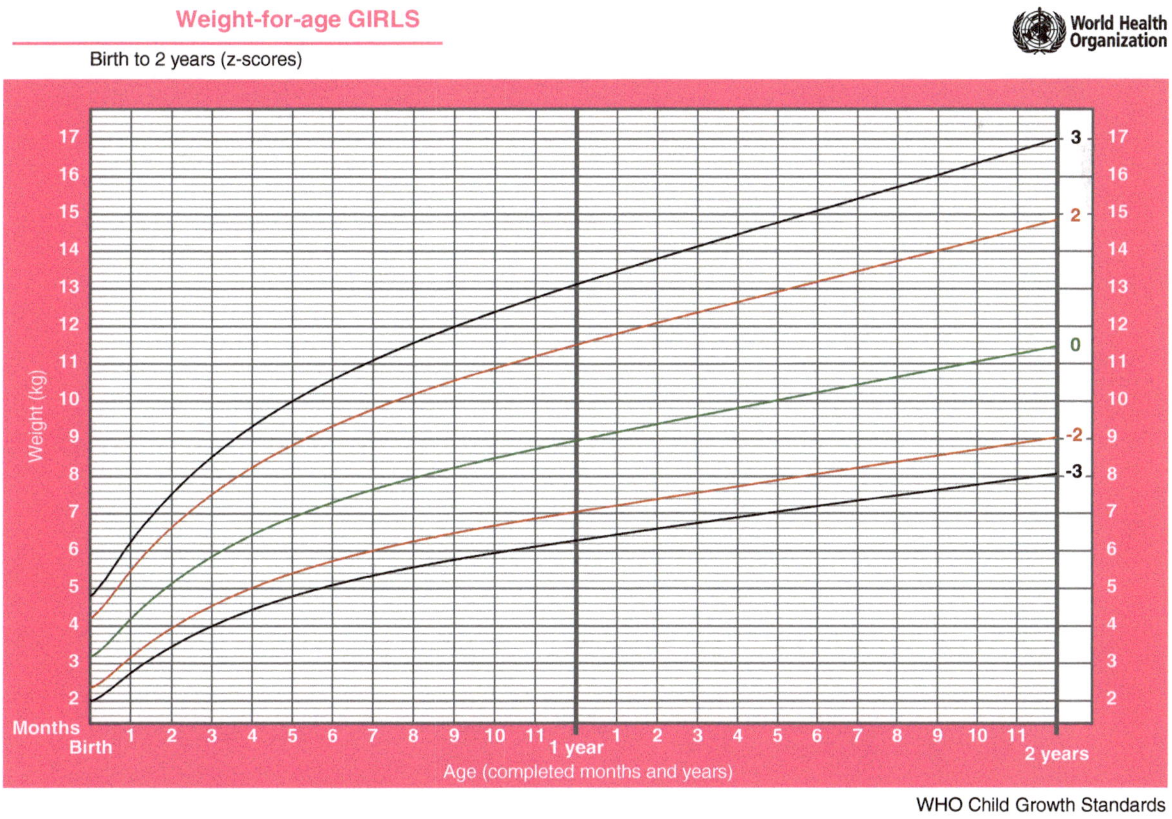


**Fig. 6.16** Weight from Birth to 2 years (Girls)

## References


1. Ardveson JC. Pediatric Feedingand Swallowing. Whurr Publishers. London. 1993.
2. Bannister T. Management of infants born with cleft. Infant. 2008;4(1) pp. 234–36.
3. Centers for Disease Control and Prevention (CDC). Measuring head circumference. 2016. Retrieved from https://www.cdc.gov/pregnancy/zika/testing-follow-up/documents/Microcephaly_measuring.pdf.
4. Centers for Disease Control and Prevention (CDC). Measuring infant head circumference: an instructional video for health-care providers. 2016. Retrieved from https://www.youtube.com/watch?v=HWV1JdAhsSo.
5. Cousens S, Nacro B, Curtiss V, Kanki B, Tall F, Traote E. Prolonged breast feeding: no association with increased risk of malnutrition. Publ Med. 1993;71:713–22.
6. Dunmow; Health for all Children. Retrieved from www.Healthforallchildren.com.
7. Feeding Assessment. European Committee for Standardisation (CEN) and written in conjunction with the European Cleft Organization. CEN/TR 16824. March 2015.
8. Hartman K. UNICEF: anthropometric nutrition posters. Retrieved from https://www.kathartman.com/instructional#/instructional/unicef-anthropometric-nutrition-posters/.
9. Lazzerin M, Rubert L, Pani P. 2013. Specially formulated foods for treating with moderate acute malnutrition in low and middle income countries. A review. The Cochrane Library. 6. http://www.cochranelibrary.com.
10. Lindberg N, Berglund AL. Mothers' experiences of feeding babies born with cleft lip and palate. Scand J Caring Sci. 2014;28(1):66–73.
11. Lutter CK. Iron deficiency in young children in low-income countries and new approaches for its prevention. J Nutr. 2008;138:2523–8.
12. Mother and Child Health and Education Trust. About essential nutrition actions at critical stages in the life cycle of women and children infants from birth to the first six months. 2017. Retrieved from http://motherchildnutrition.org/healthy-nutrition/about-essential-nutrition-actions/infants-from-birth-to-the-first-six-months.html.
13. Shelov SP, Remer AT. Caring for your baby and young child. American Academy of Pediatrics. New York: Bantam Books; 2014.
14. Shaw WC, Bannister RP, Roberts CJ. Assisted feeding is more reliable for infants with clefts—a randomized trial. Cleft Palate Craniofac J. 1999;36:262–8.
15. Woolridge MW. The anatomy of infant feeding. Midwifery. 1986;2(4):164–77.
16. World health Organization.How to prepare infant formula. 2007. https://www.who.int/foodsafety/document_centre/PIF_Care_en.pdf.
17. World Health Organization. Infant and young child feeding: model chapter for textbooks for medical students and allied health professionals. 2009. Library Cataloguing-in-Publication Data. ISBN 978 92 4 159749 4.
18. UNICEF, WHO. Capture the moment - early initiation of breastfeeding: the best start for every newborn. New York: UNICEF; 2018.
19. WHO guideline: protecting, promoting and supporting breastfeeding in facilities providing maternity and newborn services. 2017. ISBN 978-92-4-155008-6.
20. World Health Organization. The WHO child growth standards. 2006. Retrieved from https://www.who.int/childgrowth/standards/en/.
21. World Health Organization, United Nations Children's Fund. WHO child growth standards and the identification of severe acute malnutrition in infants and children, a joint statement. 2009. Retrieved from https://www.who.int/nutrition/publications/severemalnutrition/9789241598163_eng.pdf.

# Surgical Evaluation, Diagnosis, and Treatment Planning

7

Nicolas E. Sierra, Diana Bohórquez, Diógenes L. Rocha, and Marco A. Lopes-Gamborgi

**Key Points**

1. Evaluation and treatment planning for patients with cleft lip/palate (CLP) in low-resource settings, including the mission/outreach setting (MOS), must prioritize safety by anticipating specific logistical, clinical, and surgical challenges.
2. Surgical evaluation begins with a comprehensive diagnosis of each patient's cleft deformity and other medical problems, particularly for new patients.
3. An overall treatment plan through childhood should be created or updated and discussed with the patient's family.
4. Plans for specific procedures to be undertaken should match the patients' overall treatment strategy, their current state of health, and the provider team capabilities.
5. Prioritization is often necessary given the limited surgical capacity and can be aided by classification schemes, incorporating aspects of patient disease, patient geography, and team resources.
6. Surgical evaluation and treatment planning by a team or organization should be guided by a broader set of care standards, in order to ensure the best and safest possible surgical outcomes.
7. The protocols and techniques used in the MOS must adapt to the limitations of local infrastructure, the geographical and socioeconomic status of the population, and the barriers for accessing short- and long-term follow-up.

N. E. Sierra
Mobile Surgery International, Oaxaca, Mexico

Oral and Maxillofacial Surgery Department, Vall d'Hebron University Hospital, Barcelona, Spain

D. Bohórquez
Oral and Maxillofacial Surgery Department, Vall d'Hebron University Hospital, Barcelona, Spain

D. L. Rocha
Plastic and Reconstructive Department, Hospital das Clinicas, Universidade de Sao Paulo, Sao Paulo, Brazil

M. A. Lopes-Gamborgi (✉)
Centro de Atendimento Integral aof Fissurado Labiopalatal, Curitiba, Brazil

Núcleo de Pesquisa e Reabilitação de Lesões Lábio Palatais Prefeito Luiz Gomes, Joinville, Brazil

## Introduction

Treatment of patients with clefts in the mission/outreach setting (MOS) poses specific clinical, surgical, and logistical challenges. The team must first define the scope of a patient's surgical complexity and feasibility of safely meeting those needs. Patients with a wide scope of deformities, stages of development, and potentially previous treatment will be encountered during the screening process. In order to fully identify a patient's needs and risk profile, evaluation should be thorough and multidisciplinary. If surgical treatment is indicated, a patient's overall health and readiness must be assured, as well as the team capability and expertise, health system infrastructure, and postoperative follow-up to assure safe delivery. The chosen surgical approach ideally provides the best anticipated outcomes with the least possible burden of care and number of procedures.

In many situations, even after screening inappropriate surgical candidates, the number of patients needing and desiring care exceeds the surgical team capacity. Medications and medical supplies are limited, hospital bed capacity is limited, and even a hardworking surgical team must limit the number of cases performed in a day to ensure they do so safely. There is no single system for prioritizing patients, and several factors ought to be considered. Classification schemes

© Springer Nature Switzerland AG 2021

J. W. Swanson, D. W. Low (eds.), *Global Cleft Care in Low-Resource Settings*, https://doi.org/10.1007/978-3-030-59105-2_7

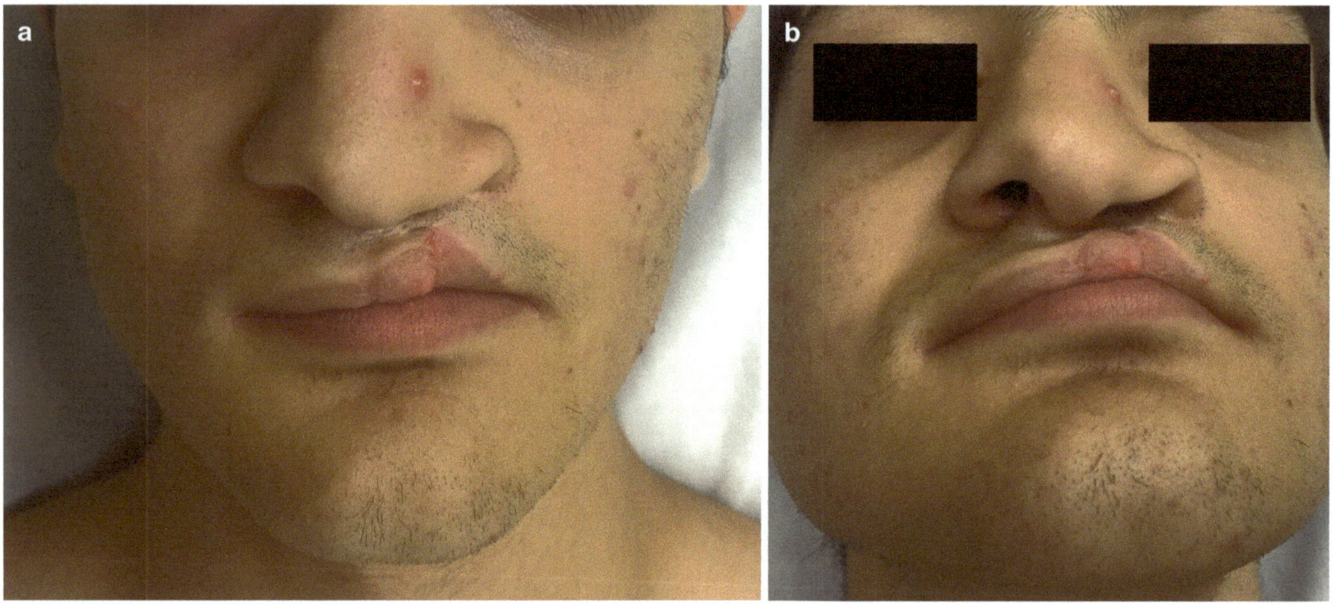


**Fig. 7.1** UCLP patient displaying anatomical features of a suboptimal primary repair: severe lip and nose asymmetry. (**a**) Front view. (**b**) Worm's eye view

may be useful to distinguish levels of surgical priorities and help focus care on the most needy patients [1].

Above all, protocols and techniques should adapt to the local health infrastructure and be part of a team or organization's broader set of care standards, in order to ensure the best and safest possible surgical outcomes.

## Surgical Diagnosis and Cleft Care Plan

Because cleft lip/palate (CLP) is a congenital condition and diagnosed primarily visually and physically, much of a patient's treatment needs can be anticipated and forecast into adulthood. A patient with an isolated soft palatal cleft is likely to need a palatal repair, ideally by 12–18 months of age, with a small chance of needing secondary revision or speech surgery. Conversely, an infant with a complete unilateral cleft lip and palate is likely to need at least four to six surgeries to correct their cleft lip, alveolar, palatal, nasal, and maxillary deformities through adolescence. The goal of this first stage of assessment is to fully characterize a patient's cleft deformity, anticipate their lifetime treatment needs, and communicate this information to the patient and parents while recording it accurately in the medical record.

### Cleft Diagnosis

Cleft deformity classification is described in detail in Chap. 6. A focused history from patient or family, other providers, or medical records can be useful but is often absent. The following are key features that should be assessed and tips for evaluation:

- Lip: Severity (complete, incomplete, minor form) and laterality. Check carefully for an asymmetric minor-form bilateral cleft lip even in the presence of a complete unilateral deformity. If previously repaired, assess for integrity of orbicularis oris muscle, alignment of white roll, tubercle fullness, and scar appearance (Fig. 7.1).
- Nose: Septal deviation, tip widening or lack of projection, alar rim slump, alar base malposition, internal valve collapse. If previously repaired, location of incisions.
- Alveolus: Notching or clefting, dental arch appearance, and continuity of teeth. If previously repaired lip, assess for presence of a nasolabial/ nasoalveolar fistula and associated symptoms (regurgitation, hypernasality) (Fig. 7.2).
- Palate: Overt clefting of the hard/soft palate and laterality. Bifid uvula, zona pellucida (pallor of soft palate), notched hard palate suggestive of submucous cleft palate. Assess motion. The palate is best examined in infants with the surgeon sitting opposite of the parent and infant's head on the surgeon's lap and body on parent's lap, with tongue depressor and light source, and viewed from over the infant's head (Fig. 7.3).
- Craniofacial: Other facial clefts (rare craniofacial clefts, hypertelorism, lateral facial cleft), micrognathia (small jaw suggests Robin sequence), other facies suggestive of craniofacial syndromes.

### Surgical Treatment Pathway

The standards of care for assessing overall surgical treatment needs of a patient with CLP in the MOS are not different from those established at comprehensive centers. Protocols vary by

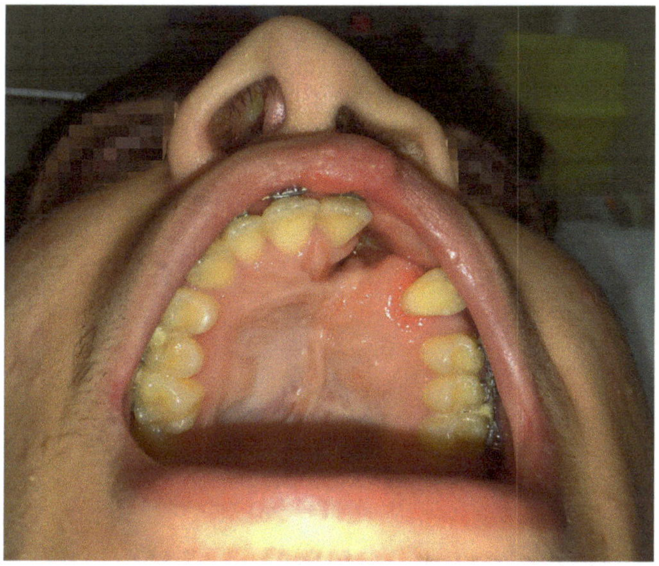

**Fig. 7.2** UCLP patient with nasoalveolar fistula after suboptimal primary lip repair

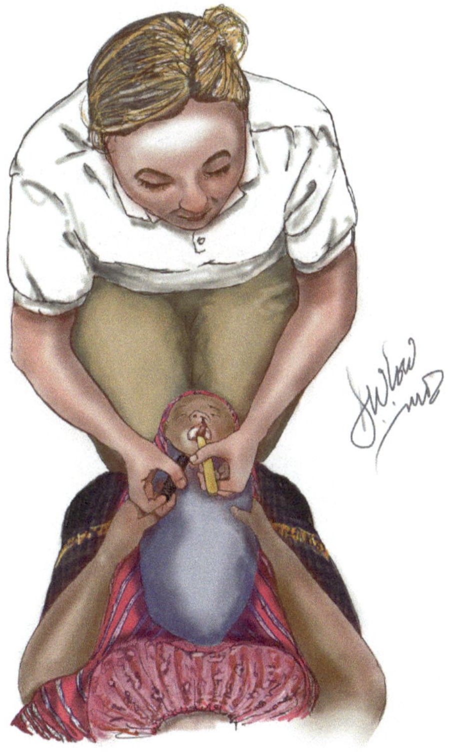

**Fig. 7.3** The palate is best examined in infants with the surgeon sitting opposite the parent and infant's head on the surgeon's lap and body on parent's lap, with tongue depressor and light source, and viewed from over the infant's head

**Table 7.1** Procedures included in most CLP treatment protocols

| Age | Procedure | Age | Procedure |
|---|---|---|---|
| 0–12 months | Preoperative orthopedics and NAM[a] | 4–7 years | Secondary CP/VPD surgery[b] |
| 3 months | Lip adhesion | >4 years | Other secondary CL procedures |
| 3–6 months | Primary CL repair | 6–12 years | (Secondary) Alveolar bone graft |
| 9–18 months | Primary CP repair | >16/18 years | Orthognathic surgery |
| 18–24 months | Delayed hard palate repair | >16/18 years | Rhinoplasty |

[a]*NAM* Nasoalveolar molding
[b]*VPD* Velopharyngeal dysfunction

team, but common approaches and technique follow (Table 7.1). Any selected protocol should pursue the best surgical outcomes with the smallest burden of care and number of procedures. Utilizing all opportunities to counsel patients and families on treatment progress and plans, coupled with quality surgical outcomes, is likely to improve compliance with subsequent procedures [8]. Listed technical difficulty is meant to be a general indicator and relative guide – all cleft cases are potentially technically challenging, and the quality of outcome likely depends in part on the quality of technique.

- *Preoperative Orthopedics and NAM (PO/NAM)*

  *PO/NAM is a non-surgical molding of the alveolar segments and/or nose, performed by a dentist/orthodontist for several months with biweekly visits to modify the intraoral splint – moderate technical complexity, moderate material resource need, and high need for patient follow-up.*

  Recent evidence suggests that PO/NAM might improve surgical outcomes in severe CLP deformities. The use of PO/NAM demands structured and stable local staff and infrastructure. Some organizations provide continuous non-surgical care (dentistry, speech therapy, psychology) through comprehensive outreach. Such settings are suitable for developing PO/NAM programs [9, 10].

- *Lip Adhesion (LAd)*

  *LAd is typically a short (1-hour) surgical procedure with low expected blood loss, low airway risk, and lower to moderate technical complexity.*

  LAd may be beneficial for BCLP patients with severe premaxillary protrusion and/or prolabium deficiency, particularly when access to PO/NAM programs is not available. LAd can transform a severe/wide cleft into a mild/narrow deformity facilitating the primary reconstruction [9]. In the MOS, LAd might replace PO/NAM techniques with a reduced burden of care, lesser cost, and fewer number of hospital visits. In severe BCL deformities, the use of LAd might reduce the risk of postoperative lip dehiscence and also premaxillary fracture, necrosis, and atrophy [9]. In the long term, the LAd might reduce the severity of secondary dentofacial deformities (Fig. 7.4)

- *Primary CL Repair*

  *Unilateral CL repair is typically a short to medium (1–2-hour) surgical procedure with low expected blood*

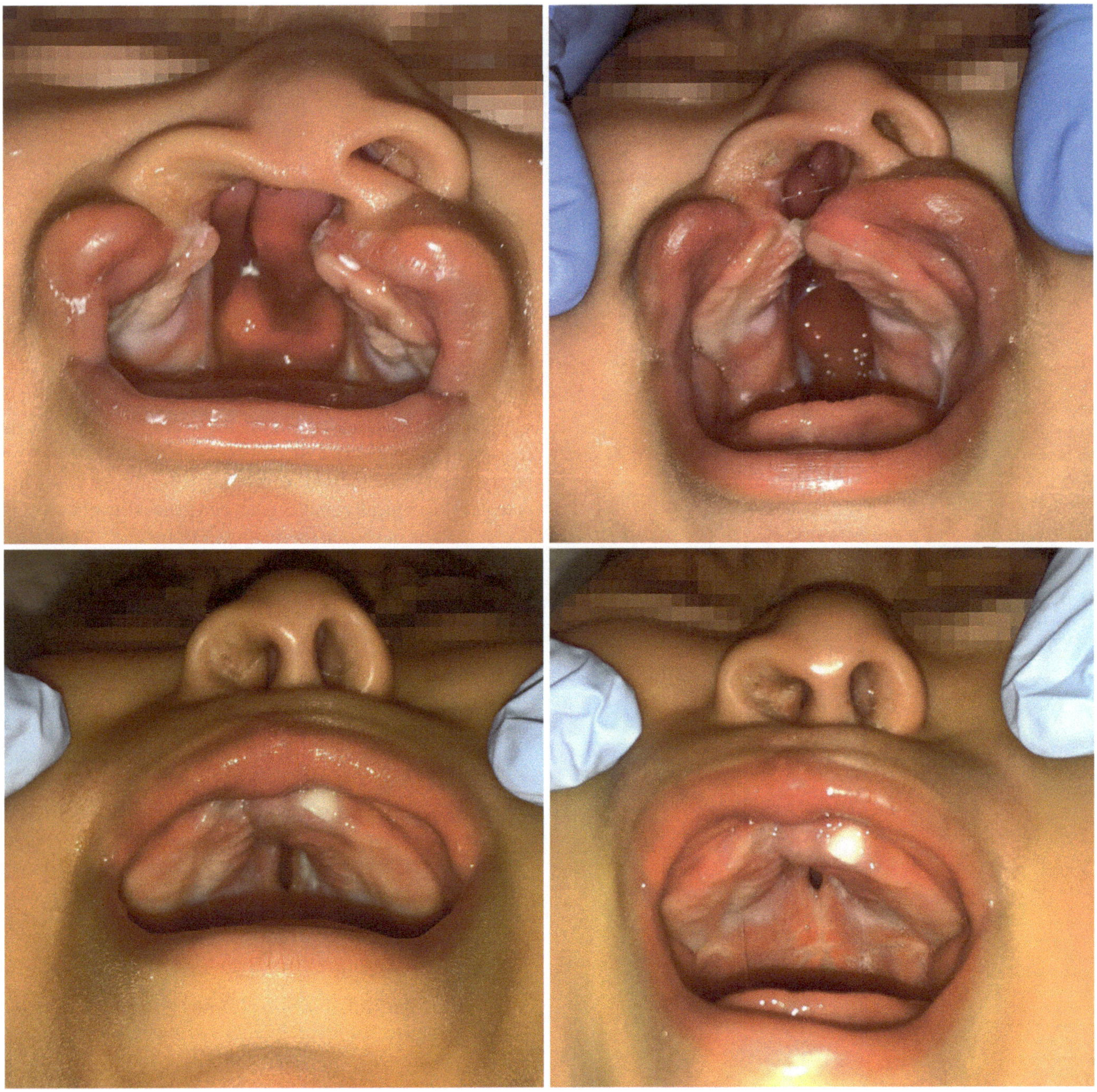

Fig. 7.4 UCLP patient. Above left: severe deformity with a wide cleft and a severe primary nasal asymmetry. Above right: post-treatment outcome after PMO/NAM. Below left/right: postoperative outcome after lip-nose-soft palate repair. The hard palate has been left unrepaired to promote maxillary growth

*loss, low airway risk, and moderate to high technical complexity. Bilateral CL repair is typically a medium (2+ hour) surgical procedure with low expected blood loss, low airway risk, and moderate to high technical complexity.*

Any chosen technique must pursue the best possible functional and cosmetic outcomes, ideally in a single procedure. In choosing a technique, the surgical team might consider anatomical incision when possible to improve cosmetic outcomes, primary rhinoplasty to improve aesthetics through childhood (including caudal septum repositioning to improve nasal symmetry and maxillary leveling and alignment through growth) based on surgeon experience [12], and anterior nasal floor closure with anterior vomer/primary hard palate flaps to prevent pre-/post-alveolar fistulas. Postoperative complications (lip dehiscence, prolabial necrosis, premaxillary ischemia, etc.) might not be suitable for timely revision [10] in the MOS.

- *Primary CP Repair*

  *CP repair is typically a medium-length (2–3 hour) surgical procedure with moderate expected blood loss, moderate airway risk, and moderate to high technical complexity.*

  Primary CP repair should provide a reliable palate closure with functional levator veli muscle repositioning while promoting mid-facial growth [12], regardless of technique. The surgical team should consider the use of adequate intravelar veloplasty and adequate tissue dissection and release to enable tension-free closure and recognize that some maneuvers such as double-opposing Z-plasty are difficult without loupe magnification, that wide palatal clefts increase the risk of dehiscence and fistula, and that pushback techniques may increase the risk of anterior fistulas and restricted mid-facial growth due to single-layer closure and wide residual raw surfaces. Minimally invasive techniques (that avoid lateral releasing incisions and may improve mid-facial growth or reduce bleeding) are best done by experienced hands, because inadequate dissection and residual tension risk dehiscence and/or fistula. Postoperative complications (flap necrosis and palate dehiscence) might be more suitably addressed in a delayed fashion [3].

- *Delayed Hard Palate Repair*

  The use of staged palatal repairs to favor maxillary growth remains controversial. In the MOS, access to surgery, speech therapy (ST), and prosthodontics is limited. Accordingly, protocols including a delayed hard palate repair should only be implemented when local teams can offer close and long-term follow-up [13, 14] (Fig. 7.5).

- *Secondary CP Repair/VPD Surgery*

  *Secondary CP repair/VPD surgery can range from short to long duration (1–3 hour), with variable expected blood loss, up to high potential airway risk, and up to high technical complexity.*

  A wide variety of morpho-functional scenarios can be found in CP patients with velopharyngeal dysfunction (VPD). The diagnostic approach of VPD is best performed jointly by experienced speech pathologists (SPs) and cleft surgeons [15], as outlined in Chaps. 21 and 29. VP incompetence is managed with speech therapy rather than surgery [16]. VP insufficiency is treated surgically, based on the etiology, which may include palatal fistula, inadequate muscular reconstruction (intravelar veloplasty), or short or scarred palate. Pharyngoplasty or pharyngeal flap creates particular potential risks of bleeding and airway occlusion peri- and postoperatively, as well as obstructive sleep apnea in the long term.

- *Secondary CL Surgery*

  *Secondary CL repair is typically a short to medium (1–2 hour) surgical procedure with low expected blood loss, low airway risk, and low to moderate technical complexity.*

  Patients with inadequate oral competence and function (orbicularis discontinuity), symptomatic nasolabial fistula, or poor aesthetic outcomes after primary CL repair are candidates for secondary procedures. At the time of screening, the main aesthetic concerns should be clearly disclosed with both the patient and the family [13]. Selection and treatment of these patients is further discussed in Chap. 16. Procedures in adult patients can be efficiently scheduled under locoregional anesthesia +/− sedation. Minor revisions are best avoided for severe secondary deformities; instead, consider total lip re-do procedures with simultaneous correction of anterior oronasal fistula if present (Fig. 7.1).

- *Alveolar Bone Graft*

  *ABG is typically a medium (2-hour) surgical procedure typically requiring preoperative patient preparation, two surgical fields, low expected blood loss, low airway risk, and moderate to high technical complexity.*

  ABG procedures demand multidisciplinary preparation, often involving transverse palatal expansion, and close follow-up by qualified local staff within a comprehensive care team. While demanding of surgeon technical experience, orthodontic collaboration and appropriate patient selection, the intra-operative risk profile typically minimal and instrumentation requirements straightforward. A hip nerve block and postoperative antibiotics should be considered.

- *Orthognathic Surgery*

  *Orthognathic procedures are long (4–8 hours) and require extensive multidisciplinary patient preparation, with high expected blood loss, high airway risk, high technical complexity, and extensive instrumentation needs.*

  Mid-facial retrusion and malpositioned maxillary segments are common in CLP patients due to their underlying deformity and surgical treatment [16]. Orthognathic surgery (OS) repositions the facial skeleton to correct both occlusal function and aesthetics. The LeFort I maxillary advancement with 3D reposition is the procedure of choice in most patients, sometimes in combination with mandibular repositioning and/or rotation of the occlusal plane [16]. OS planning, preparation, execution, and follow-up require the coordinated approach between experienced (orthodontics, speech pathology, cleft/craniofacial surgery) specialists within a comprehensive team. The stability of surgical out-

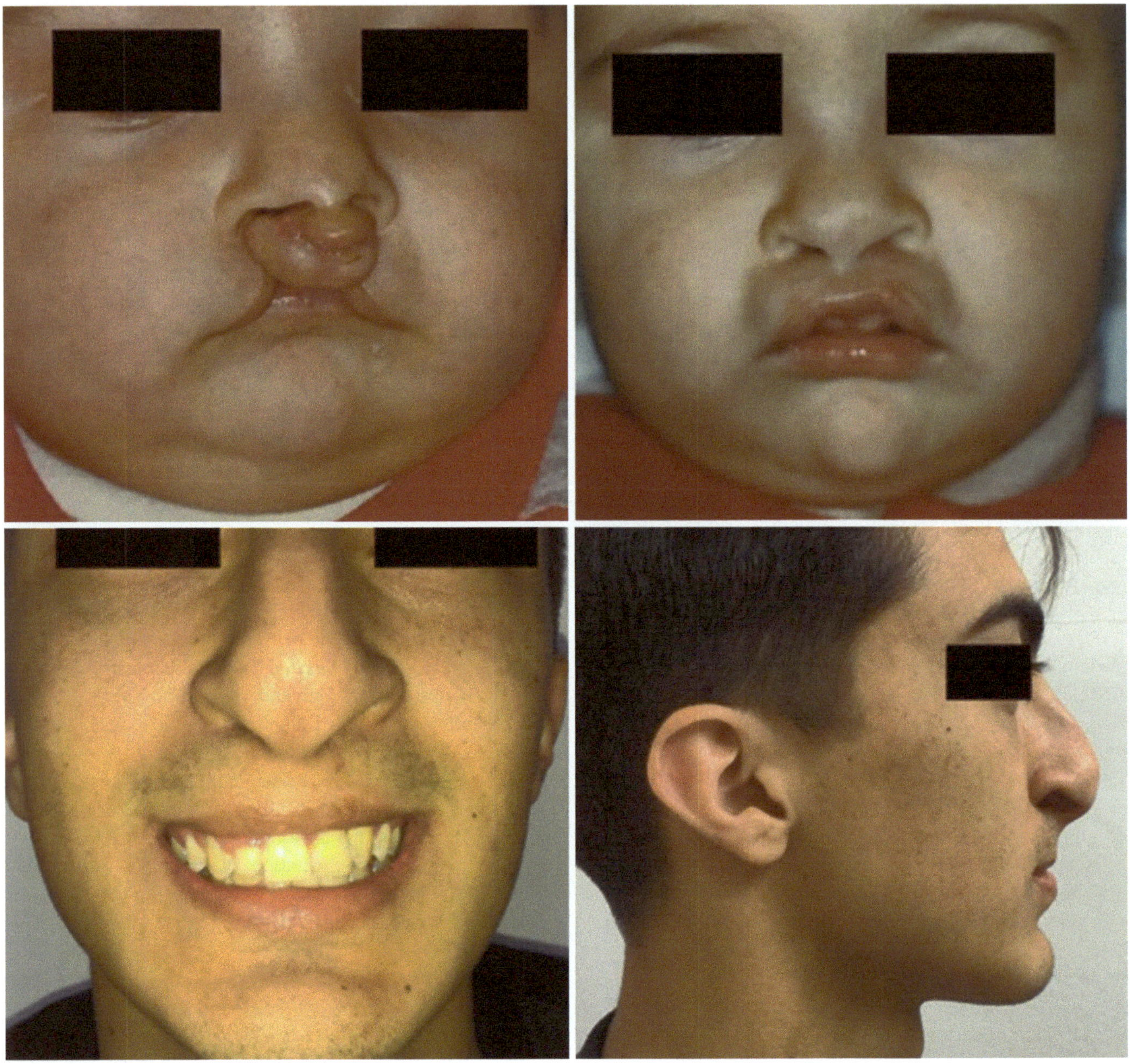

**Fig. 7.5** BCLP patient. Above left: severe deformity with premaxillary protrusion and prolabium deficiency. Above right: postoperative outcome after lip adhesion. Below left: front view of long-term treatment outcome, after definitive lip repair. Below right: lateral view of long-term treatment outcome, after definitive lip repair

comes highly depends on a close orthodontic postoperative follow-up.

- *Rhinoplasty*

  *Rhinoplasty is typically moderate length (2–3 hours), with low airway risk, low expected blood loss, and high technical complexity.*

  Simultaneous primary cleft lip and nasal reconstruction improves nasal aesthetics and function through growth. However, the cleft nasal deformity typically causes restricted nasal airflow and difficulty breathing, as well as appearance-related concerns, and residual nasal deformities are common among CLP patients. Secondary nasal procedures are generally performed either at elementary age, to improve psychosocial development in severe cases, or at skeletal maturity (14–18 years) [12, 13]. Surgical maneuvers typically address septal deviations and malpositioned upper/lower lateral cartilage causing obstruction, as well as asymmetry and lacking nasal projection. Some minor procedures (alar reposition, alar stenosis correction, etc.) can provide important improvements and be performed under local anesthesia.

## Surgical Patient Screening and Specific Treatment Plan

Moving beyond the overall cleft care plan, the patient's fitness to undergo surgical treatment must be carefully evaluated in conjunction with anesthesia and pediatric colleagues. Patients and their families arriving to mission sites and hospitals in LICs present with a wide scope of surgical complexities and potentially high rates of undiagnosed underlying conditions. CLP reconstructive procedures are elective procedures and should expose patients to only minimum perioperative risks. A sound preoperative surgical (and interdisciplinary) assessment will help to identify baseline abnormalities with increased risks that may prompt delay, further workup, or transfer to a more tertiary facility if available [2]. Several types of factors should be considered (Table 7.2).

Among presenting issues, some are likely to be transient and resolve with time. Others will pose ongoing risks; in settings of limited diagnostic or therapeutic capabilities, with no realistic option for external transfer, the risks and benefits of surgical treatment must be carefully assessed and balanced. For every selected case, the surgical team should be experienced and equipped sufficiently to provide predictable and quality surgical outcomes in both [4].

Although in many teams it is the pediatrician or anesthesiologist who diagnoses a concerning condition and suggests deferring surgery, it is important for the surgeon to understand specific risks to surgical outcomes. For instance, one recent study suggested that a medial upper arm circumference <12.5 cm or a leukocyte count of >11.5 k was each associated with increased rates of postoperative lip or palatal dehiscence, respectively, even though these cutoffs did not necessarily meet the criteria for severe malnutrition or leukocytosis [20]. Therefore, it is incumbent to surgical outcomes.

## Prioritizing Patients

Even after screening out unsuitable surgical candidates, in LICs, there is frequently a mismatch between demand for cleft surgery and capacity to provide it. Several factors are sometimes taken into account when considering the priority of surgical patients for care, when there are limited spaces:

1. Urgency of patient disease (e.g., delaying primary palate repair beyond 18 months of age carries greater functional risk to speech development than delaying a cleft lip revision)
2. Addressing complications (such as a palatal fistula, particularly when the primary surgery was performed by the same surgical team)
3. Continuity of comprehensive cleft care (for instance, performing an alveolar bone graft in a patient who has just undergone orthodontic preparation for the procedure)
4. Geography/distance (a patient who has traveled a long distance may have fewer other opportunities for care)

**Table 7.2** Conditions and comorbidities with increased surgical risk that may prompt delay, further workup, or transfer to a more tertiary facility

| Type of factor | Examples | Management |
|---|---|---|
| 1. Acute illness | Upper respiratory infection | Patients with signs of infection, especially affecting the respiratory tract, should not be scheduled for surgery [3]<br>Acute treatment as necessary, delay surgery (>4–6 weeks generally) |
| 2. Inappropriate age | Inadequate size/age for cleft lip repair (generally 3–6 months) or palate repair (>9 months)<br>Immature for alveolar bone graft (>7 years), definitive rhinoplasty (>14 years)<br>Benefit of certain procedures in older patients (palate repair >10 years of age, bone graft >14 years of age) controversial | Delay until older age<br>"Age deviation" can be considered in borderline cases with multidisciplinary input<br>Benefits and risks of certain procedures in older patients warrant discussion with patient/family and multidisciplinary team as necessary |
| 3. Nutrition/delay | Malnourishment<br>Anemia (can be sign of the above) | Malnourished patients should not be scheduled for surgery. In the MOS, it is common to screen patients with adequate weight and selective protein malnourishment (Kwashiorkor) [2]<br>These patients should be addressed to specific nutritional support/counseling programs in preparation for future surgery |
| 4. Conditions requiring further workup | Anemia<br>Coagulation disorders<br>Heart murmur | Surgery should not be performed until further workup<br>Referral should be made to tertiary hospital/pediatrician |
| 5. Dysmorphic features/comorbidities | Severe developmental delay<br>Associated syndromes (e.g., 22q11 deletion, craniofacial microsomia) | Should be referred to a pediatrician/hospital for workup and to rule out associated anomalies/syndromes<br>Can potentially be "cleared" if risks deemed low<br>Can potentially receive cleft care at a tertiary facility able to mitigate increased surgical and anesthetic risk<br>May ultimately not be surgical candidates |

**Table 7.3** Surgical priority classification scheme

| Priority | Diagnosis | Comments |
|---|---|---|
| 0 | Complication/sequelae of previous surgery | Surgical treatment of major complications (e.g., palatal fistulae) is often considered utmost priority, particularly when previous treatment has been by the same surgical team/organization |
| 1 | Primary cleft lip | CL repair is often considered highest surgical priority, reasoning that the social repercussion of an unoperated CL may be higher than CP. In addition, for complete cases, the orthopedic action of the CL repair and nasal floor closure improves maxillary arch anatomy facilitating CP repair. However, this may increase risk that patients not receive CP repair in timely fashion<br>Some rare (Tessier) facial clefts can be classified into Priority 1 category<br>CL repair in younger patients (aged 3–6 months) may increase risks and depends on the mission/center infrastructure, the experience level of the anesthesia staff, and team capability for postoperative monitoring of patients |
| 2 | Primary cleft palate | Some teams/organizations classify the primary CP repair into Priority 1 to increase compliance for the subsequent (CL) surgery<br>The best functional (speech) outcomes seem to be achieved when primary CP repair is performed before 18 months; younger in this window (9–12 months) may favor speech outcomes and later in this window (12–18 months) may favor mid-facial growth<br>CP repair in younger patients (aged 6–12 months) may increase risks and depends on the mission/center infrastructure, the experience level of the anesthesia staff, and team capability for postoperative monitoring of patients |
| 3 | Late primary cleft palate (Over 10 years of age) | CP repair in older patients is relatively deprioritized by some teams, because although high patient satisfaction, improved resonance, and reduced nasal regurgitation are often seen, speech problems such as misarticular often persists [21] and surgery may have higher blood loss |
| 4 | Secondary CL/CP repair All ages | Some organizations emphasize that *secondary CL/CP repairs/revisions* should be performed *by experienced cleft surgeons* because the procedure *must* offer a clear improvement of the patient aesthetics and/or function<br>Candidates for *secondary CP repair* should be preoperatively analyzed by both surgery and speech pathology. The use of fibronasoendoscopy highly improves the accuracy of assessment and surgical indications |
| 5 | Other CLP procedures: *Alveolar bone graft, speech surgery, rhinoplasty, orthognathic surgery* | Those locations with sustained cleft care programs will accumulate patients with surgical needs different than CL/CP repair: alveolar bone graft, secondary speech surgery, orthognathic surgery, and rhinoplasty<br>With increased recognition of the importance of these procedures to completion of cleft care and obtaining optimal patient outcomes, many teams are integrating them into higher priority positions<br>These procedures depend on specific surgeon expertise, equipment, patient continuity, and other considerations; specific outreach efforts dedicated exclusively for these procedures sometimes best address the needs of these patients |

5. Team-specific capabilities (for instance, a team may be particularly trained/equipped to perform speech surgery, whereas this is usually not available)

Classification schemes can be useful when screening a large volume of patients, in order to denote surgical priorities (Table 7.3). Typically in practice, schemes such as this are only one of several factors used in prioritizing patients. One limitation of the classification shown in Table 7.3 is that it may prioritize lip and palatal revisions over procedures such as speech surgery, ABG, and rhinoplasty that are less familiar to some teams in LICs but important to completing cleft treatment.

Regardless of how patients are prioritized and screened, a family or patient learning that they will not receive surgery can be devastating. There is understandable disappointment for those who have spent time and resources seeking care to not receive care. However, particularly in cases of screening, it is often out of concern for the patient's well-being that surgery is being deferred. Yet frequently this is not effectively communicated to the patient or family, causing misunderstanding and exacerbating resentment. "Tips and Tricks: When Surgery Isn't Possible" proposes some useful ways to handle these situations.

In some settings with high numbers of primary CL/CP patients, there can be fewer slots for patients who need revision or later-stage surgery. These later-stage procedures are often associated with higher (surgical/anesthetic/infrastructural) complexity and longer surgical times; often, these patients undergo repeated rejection from missions and progressively accumulate with few chances to be scheduled. Teams might consider developing specific programs for these patients in hospitals with adequate facilities and with participation of highly experienced volunteers [5].

**Tips and Tricks: When Surgery Isn't Possible**

When patients or families learn they are not able to receive surgical treatment, they are often upset, and misunderstanding is common. The following may help improve communication:

- Patients who have been assessed or screened and who are not scheduled for surgery should sit down with a physician, ideally a surgeon, to learn why.
- For patients who had a concern raised at screening, this needs to be communicated to the family with a follow-up plan:
  - For an acute illness, the findings need to be shared, treatment (e.g., antibiotics, rehydration solution) offered if appropriate, and timing for surgical eligibility reviewed.
  - For inappropriate age, risks of proceeding should be discussed and optimal timing for surgery reviewed to assure appropriate follow-up.
  - For malnutrition, a feeding plan needs to be created as well as identifying mechanisms for obtaining appropriate foods and following progress.
  - For conditions requiring further workup, a clear explanation and referral paperwork need to be given to the family, ideally with a point of contact at the tertiary hospital.
- A patient coordinator or social worker can be helpful to addressing family barriers to care and follow-up.
- A medical record system that tracks who did not receive surgery can be important to give priority at future occasions.
- In a mission setting, "announcing" who has made it into the operating schedule makes those who have not feel excluded and should be avoided.

Finally, efforts can potentially be made to reduce the need for prioritization, particularly in a mission setting. For instance, better identifying and anticipating need at a certain time and place can allow better planning for staffing, equipment, and schedule availability. Further, improved planning and patient communication with a cleft team may enable virtual screening, routing appropriate patients to year-round cleft centers, or other interventions.

## Structuring Safe Surgery in the Mission/Outreach Setting

### Surgical Schedule

Every available moment of the OR should be maximally and efficiently used. A coordinated approach of the schedule by the nursing, surgical, and anesthesia specialist should account for:

- The youngest infants have poorer tolerance to fasting. Accordingly, the daily surgical schedule should start with the youngest patients.
- Complex/prolonged procedures (primary CL/CP cases with severe deformities, secondary CP repairs, orthognathic surgery, etc.), procedures with high risk of postoperative bleeding, and procedures requiring prolonged postoperative observation/recovery should be scheduled early in a multi-day mission and, also, early on the daily schedule.
- Patients with surgical or medical conditions requiring prolonged/close early postoperative follow-up (rare facial clefts, flaps, grafts, orthognathic surgery, etc.) should be scheduled at the beginning of the mission.
- The geographical origin of the patient/family should be considered on the mission schedule. Some patients arriving from distant locations deserve special consideration if safety and time permit.
- Some organizations avoid scheduling operations the day before team departure out from the country. Alternatively, only minor procedures under local anesthesia might be scheduled. It is highly recommended to avoid any palatal surgery during the last day of the mission program.

The surgical schedule should equally focus on efficiency, safety, and quality [6]. Every available moment of OR time should be maximally and efficiently used to perform clinical care, with teaching opportunities as able and without any rush to emphasize speed over quality. Accordingly, the number of cases per table/day should allow enough time for the anesthesia and surgery specialists to perform the best possible technique/procedure [11]. Efficiency is highly improved by good communication and speedy coordination of the OR in-and-out process [7].

Performing combination procedures (i.e., primary cleft lip and palate repair at the same time) under a single anesthetic increases the operating time and perioperative risk;

Table 7.4 Example of a weekly surgical schedule for an operating table

| Day 1 | Day 2 | Day 3 | Day 4 | Day 5 | Day 6 |
|---|---|---|---|---|---|
| 1ry BCL | 1ry BCL | 1ry BCL | 1ry UCL | 1ry UCL | 2ry CL re-do |
| 1ry CP | 1ry CP | 1ry UCL | 1ry UCL | 1ry UCL | Lip scar revision |
| 1ry CP | 2ry CP | 1ry UCL adult | 1ry CP | 1ry UCL | ----0---- |
| 1ry CP adult | 1ry CP adult | 2ry CP | Septo-rhino | 1ry UCL adult | ----0---- |
| Lip scar rev. | Lip scar rev. | 2ry CL re-do | Lip scar rev. | 2ry CL re-do | |

however, it might be beneficial in sites/settings with either high treatment dropout rate or with limited opportunities to access a forthcoming mission program. Simultaneous procedures are feasible in experienced hands, but the risks must be acknowledged. While either a lip or palate repair may have inconsequential blood loss, the combined blood loss may induce a consequential anemia; the combined anesthetic duration could trigger a postoperative pneumonia. Thus the decision must reflect mission/center infrastructure, experience level of the surgical and anesthesia staff, and team capability for postoperative monitoring of patients [17].

CL procedures in select adult patients can be performed under local anesthesia (LA), regional blocks, and sedation. If the number of such procedures is high, the team can schedule one operating table for procedures under LA. However, it should be noted that safe and efficient sedation techniques demand highly skilled anesthesia specialists [2] (Table 7.4).

## Avoiding Complications

A thoughtful program on a surgical mission is essential to enabling safe and high-quality surgical care. Any issues or doubts with respect to the safety of any intervention/procedure should be discussed at any time [18].

The multidisciplinary screening process should optimally select patients for providing safe surgical care. The surgical team should discuss and agree on the surgical standards of reconstructive techniques for primary CL and CP repair. Complex cases should be discussed to establish agreement on the surgical approach to provide the best outcomes. Surgical team members should openly expose their skill limitations, and complex cases should be directed to more experienced members [6, 19]. In this way, the mission becomes a good setting for teaching and learning new techniques.

Surgeons should be encouraged to avoid operating out of their comfort zone. Throughout the surgical program, surgeons should review the charts of assigned patients to identify potential issues deserving further discussion [6]. Surgeons should physically reexamine the patient and review the treatment plan on the day of surgery, including communicating with the patient and family, particularly in cases when a surgeon colleague examined the patient previously. Cases of divergent plans should be discussed before inducing anesthesia.

On the day of surgery, the patient's health status should be reassessed to exclude the onset of concurrent illness. The surgical team members must systematically use the surgical safety checklist. The checklist is highly beneficial for unfamiliar settings such as in MOCs by improving communication and relationships among team members, overcoming language barriers, and completing the health assessment of the screening [19].

## Postoperative Care Planning

The postoperative team and plans put into place for each patient should reflect the nature of the surgical care provided. Before starting the surgical program, the team members (cleft surgeon, pediatric anesthetist, pediatrician, pediatric intensivist, PACU nurse, and post-op nurse) must agree on the postoperative management (feeding, wound care, medication, etc.) for each type of procedure, and handoffs occur for each patient appropriately [6].

The hospitalization time should adapt to the complexity and risk of the procedure, the geographical and social background of the patient, and the early postoperative findings (Table 7.5).

Even in the MOS, at all times, an on-call team should be designated, including one cleft surgeon, one surgical assistant, one OR nurse, one pediatric anesthetist, one anesthesia assistant, and one PACU nurse [6].

Postoperative rounds should include at least one member from the surgical, pediatric, and post-op nursing teams. Two postoperative rounds are recommended every day: one before starting the surgical program and another at the end of the surgical program before team departure from hospital

Table 7.5 Average hospitalization time for CLP surgical procedures

| Time for discharge | Procedures |
|---|---|
| Ambulatory | Minor surgery (CL scar revision) under local anesthesia |
| Post-op Day 1 | Lip adhesion, CL repair, some CP repair, rhinoplasty, some alveolar bone grafting |
| Post-op Day 2 | Some CP repair, some alveolar bone grafting, VPD surgery, orthognathic surgery |
| Longer hospitalization | Syndromic patients<br>Perioperative airway/hemodynamic events<br>Early postoperative bleeding<br>Postoperative fever<br>Wound care concerns<br>Nutritional concerns |

facilities. Thorough examinations might prevent and detect potential OR returns.

Upon discharge, the caregiver (and the patient) should receive clear and detailed instructions to warrant adequate postoperative wound care and medication compliance. The use of forms with clear but simple instructions coupled with depictions/illustrations highly improves compliance [6].

The team/organization should arrange for aftercare and follow-up. In addition, the caregiver and/or the patient should be instructed on detection and immediate basic management of postoperative complications: fever, bleeding, hematoma, seroma, wound infection, dehiscence, necrosis, etc. In addition, the team/organization should provide a 24-h telephone number to contact local staff and report any potential complication after discharge. In most locations, emailing or SMSing a postoperative photo might be possible and will be very helpful to initially assess the event. The local staff must instruct the caregiver on remote/immediate management of such events and should coordinate patient assessment and management by the local staff members or by the appropriate reference hospital [6].

## References


1. Berger JH, Jian Z, O'Reilly EB, Christman MS. First do no harm: predicting surgical morbidity during humanitarian medical missions. World J Surg. https://doi.org/10.1007/s00268-018-4720-9.
2. Melookaran AM, Rao SA, Antony SB, Herrera A. Anesthesia for children with craniofacial abnormalities in the developing countries: challenges and future directions. J Craniofac Surg. 2015;26:1069–72.
3. Calis M, Aral AM, Sencan A, Kanbak M, Vargel I, Ozgur F, Iscen D. Humanitarian activities of Interplast Turkiye: 6 years of experience in Uzbekistan for surgical treatment of cleft patients and related secondary deformities. Ann Plast Surg. 2016;77:494–8.
4. Moses JJ, Rochelle WJ. Cleft and craniofacial mission care management of facial clefts: international missions. Oral Maxillofac Surg Clin North Am. 2016;28:203–20.
5. Operation smile. Resource manual. Global standards of care.
6. Braun TL, Louis MR, Dickey RM, Buchanan EP. A sustainable and scalable approach to the provision of cleft care: a focus on safety and quality. Plast Reconstr Surg. 2018. https://doi.org/10.1097/PRS.0000000000004580.
7. Chao TE, Riesel JN, Anderson G, Mullen JT, et al. Building a global surgery initiative through evaluation, collaboration, and training: the Massachusetts General Hospital experience. J Surg Ed. 2015. https://doi.org/10.1016/j.jsurg.2014.12.018.
8. Carlson LC, Stewart BT, Hatcher KW, Kabetu C, VanderBurg R, Magee WPA. Model of the unmet need for cleft lip and palate surgery in low- and middle-income countries. World J Surg. 2016;40:2857–67.
9. Zaidi SH, Rehman JU, Rahman HU, Ahmed N. Lip adhesion– a viable alternative to pre-surgical orthodontics for the management of wide cleft lips in third world countries. J Ayub Med Coll Abbottabad. 2018;30(2):171–4.
10. Grayson BH. Discussion: limited evidence for the effect of presurgical nasoalveolar molding in unilateral cleft on nasal symmetry: a call for unified research. Plast Reconstr Surg. 2013;131:75e–6e.
11. Rosell-Perry P, Segura E, Salas- Butinza L, Cotrina-Rabanal O. Comparison of two models of surgical care for patients with cleft lip and palate in resource-challenged settings. World J Surg. 2013. https://doi.org/10.1007/s00268-013-2395-9.
12. Monson LA, Kirschner RE, Losee JE. Primary repair of cleft lip and nasal deformity. Plast Reconstr Surg. 2013;132:1040e.
13. Marcus JR, Allori AC, Santiago PE. Principles of cleft lip repair: conventions, commonalities, and controversies. Plast Reconstr Surg. 2017;139:764e.
14. Agrawal K, Panda KA. Modified surgical schedule for primary management of cleft lip and palate in developing countries. Cleft Palate Craniofac J. 2001;48:1.
15. Hughes C, Campbell J, Mukhopadhyay S, McComrmack S, Silverman R, Lalikos J, Babigian A, Castiglione C. Remote digital preoperative assessments for cleft lip and palate may improve clinical and economic impact in global plastic surgery. Cleft Palate–Craniofac J. 2017;54:535–9.
16. Roy AA, Rtshiladze MA, Stevens K, Phillips J. Orthognathic surgery for patients with cleft lip and palate. Clin Plast Surg. 2019;46(2):157–71.
17. Laub DR. Globalization of craniofacial plastic surgery: foreign Mission programs for cleft lip and palate. J Craniofac Surg. 2015;26:1015–31.
18. Hughes CD, Babigian A, Alkire BC, Wong A, Papp SA, Vincent JR, Meara JG, Castiglione C, Silverman R. The clinical and economic impact of a sustained program in global plastic surgery: valuing cleft care in resource-poor settings. Plast Reconstr Surg. 2012;130:87e.
19. Best DL, Gauger TL, Dolan LA, Donnelly A, Ranganathan K, Ulloa-Marin C, Sung-Hsieh HH. Orofacial cleft management by short-term surgical missions in South America: literature review. 2018. Int J Oral Maxillofac Surg. https://doi.org/10.1016/j.ijom.2018.05.025.
20. Swanson MA, Auslander A, Morales T, et al. Predicators of complication following cleft lip and palate surgery in a low-resource settings: a prospective outcomes study in Nicaragua. Presentation at the European Cleft Palate Association. Utrecht; June 2019.
21. Murthy J, Sendhilnathan S, Hussain SA. Speech outcome following late primary palate repair. Cleft Palate Craniofac J. 2010;47(2):156–61.

# Pediatric and Anesthesiologic Evaluation

8

Anna Kolentz, Anne Hing, and Plinio Sierra

**Key Points**

1. Team care begins at the time of diagnosis of a cleft lip/palate with a comprehensive assessment for early detection and management of CLP-related syndromes and comorbidities.
2. A thorough assessment of feeding and breathing functions, particularly in the neonatal period, should rule out malnutrition and obstructive breathing disorders and enable adequate and timely counseling and assistance.
3. Pediatrician assessment is focused on identifying signs/symptoms of comorbid disease or related syndromes and directing additional diagnostic testing or specialist workup as needed.
4. Anesthesia evaluation is directed at systemic readiness to undergo surgery, taking into account a child's personal and family anesthetic history, and anticipating potential challenges of the airway and respiratory system or ability to withstand general anesthesia and prevent potential perioperative events.
5. Surgical candidates within the low-resource/outreach setting are CLP patients who:
   (a) Are healthy, well nourished, and with adequate weight gain at the time of presentation for surgery
   (b) Are free of concurrent infections
   (c) Do not show evidence of airway obstruction
   (d) Have normal screening lab results
   (e) Fall within what the local team/infrastructure capabilities can safely manage through the perioperative process if they display minor comorbidities

## Introduction

Initiation of team care for a patient with cleft lip/palate (CL/P) should occur at the time of diagnosis. Parental counseling should ideally be started at the time of prenatal detection. However, in the low-resource/outreach (LRO) setting, where prenatal diagnosis is seldom available, public hospitals or humanitarian organizations might mobilize local teams to provide counseling and treatment coordination shortly after birth. Parental counseling empowers the caregivers by explaining the cleft and its anticipated treatment. By outlining the importance of their child's general health and nutritional status at the time of each surgery, treatment outcomes can be improved.

The initial visit focuses on providing an overall treatment strategy adapted to the children's deformity, the associated comorbidities, and the provider team capabilities. An overview of the indicated surgical interventions and their timing should be discussed. If locally available, non-surgical assessments (audiometry, dental, and speech) should be indicated. The clinical and nutritional/feeding assessment will guide the follow-up schedule to assure that the child is thriving. The frequency of monitoring should be determined by current health status and the provider's concern for associated health concerns.

If associated anomalies are suspected, appropriate imaging, laboratory, and clinical referrals should be indicated and reviewed with the parents and the interdisciplinary team. For

A. Kolentz
Hospital Casa de Saúde Bon Jesus, Caruaru, Pernambuco, Brazil

A. Hing (✉)
Seattle Children's Hospital, Seattle, WA, USA
e-mail: anne.hing@seattlechildrens.org

P. Sierra
Department of Pediatric Anesthesia, King Abdullah Specialized Children's Hospital, Riyadh, Saudi Arabia

© Springer Nature Switzerland AG 2021

J. W. Swanson, D. W. Low (eds.), *Global Cleft Care in Low-Resource Settings*, https://doi.org/10.1007/978-3-030-59105-2_8

infants with confirmed comorbidities and/or syndrome diagnoses, surgical reconstruction may be referred to a more tertiary facility if available or should be delayed until the child is determined to be ready for surgery. For older patients, a thorough assessment of deformities, associated health concerns, and comorbidity diagnosis is similarly important.

## Overall Health and Nutrition

Infants and children with CL and/or CP are at an increased risk for weight faltering, malnutrition, upper airway obstruction, obstructive sleep apnea, and dysphagia with secondary impact on lower airway due to chronic aspiration. Feeding and nutritional assessment are discussed in further detail in Chap. 7.

Orofacial clefting can be grouped into three general categories: (1) isolated CL/P, (2) isolated CP, and (3) CLP. Infants born with isolated CL may be able to adequately seal (at breast) to create sufficient negative intraoral pressure during feeding. However, the infant's mother may need assistance with infant positioning and latch for effective breastfeeding. On the other hand, patients with CP *will not be able to generate negative intraoral pressure to transfer milk from the breast effectively.* These infants often require special feeding support, sometimes including the use of devices such as a specialized infant cleft feeder or cup. As is recommended that infants receive expressed breastmilk, mothers will need assistance with breast pumping.

The assessment of the infant's feeding at the clinic setting is important to assure effective and safe feeding (Table 8.1). Attention to the infant's suck, swallow, and breathe cycle is important when using cleft feeders and infant cups. Coughing, choking, or color change could be indicator of dysphagia and risk for aspiration.

Malnourishment is frequently found among CLP patients in the LRO setting and is associated with increased risks for postoperative complications (site infection, wound dehiscence, etc.) and mortality.

Malnutrition might be related to a combination of factors:

- Feeding difficulties caused by the deformity
- Lack of knowledge/training of the caregivers on feeding positioning, techniques, and aids
- Lack of financial and/or feeding resources

Anthropometric measurements: Height, length, MUAC, etc., are useful parameters to identify and monitor patients with malnourishment and are discussed in Chap. 7. This information can help make formal diagnosis of malnutrition (Table 8.2). Patients with confirmed malnutrition should not be scheduled for surgery. Instead, the family should be provided with counseling and educational programs, nutritional resources if available, and a follow-up calendar by the local team. Surgery can be scheduled upon correction of the nutritional status of the patient. Occasionally, pediatric and

**Table 8.1** General feeding goals for an infant (birth–2 months)

| *General feeding goals for an infant (birth–2 months)* |
|---|
| 7–8 feedings/24 hours |
| Each feeding <30 minutes |
| Total intake/day: 150 ml/kg |
| Example: A 4 kg infant should take 600 ml/24 h (75 ml/feeding × 8 feedings) |

**Table 8.2** Types of pediatric malnutrition

| Pediatric malnutrition type | Definition | Example | Management |
|---|---|---|---|
| Marasmus | Global nutritional deficiency | Infants <24 months<br>No weight gain/weight loss<br>Weight-for-length < 2 SD<br>MUAC <2 SD | Delay surgery<br>Nutritional assessment<br>Nutritional program/follow-up<br>Counseling/education<br>Feeding technique training<br>Resource support |
| | | Children >24 months<br>Weight loss<br>BMI < 2 SD<br>MUAC <2 SD | |
| Protein deficiency Kwashiorkor | Severe protein deficiency with normal caloric intake | Short height<br>Normal weight<br>Hair/nail/skin changes | |
| Obesity | Overweight | Children and adolescents with age- and sex-specific BMI > 85th and < 95th percentiles | Nutritional assessment<br>Nutritional program/follow-up<br>Counseling/education<br>Surgery could be scheduled according to local team capabilities |
| | Severe | Children and adolescents with age- and sex-specific BMI > 95th percentile | Nutritional assessment<br>Nutritional program/follow-up<br>Counseling/education<br>Delay surgery |

adult CLP patients with obesity may attend a center/program.

Within the malnutrition spectrum, obese patients deserve special considerations. Obese infants and toddlers should raise attention for congenital endocrinological conditions that may need specific medical and perioperative management. On the other hand, obese adult patients may associate a combination of chronic conditions within the metabolic syndrome spectrum (hypertension, heart disease, diabetes, etc.) that demand specific medical and anesthetic perioperative management. Finally, the concurrence of obesity, adenotonsillar hypertrophy, and postoperative swelling highly increases the risk for perioperative obstructive airway emergencies. The readiness of potential emergency airway adjuncts, avoiding the use of narcotics, and utilizing nasopharyngeal tubes during the early postoperative period are specific recommendation for such patients.

## Ruling Out Syndromic Conditions and/or Associated Congenital Anomalies

25–30% of CL/P patients are found to have associated anomalies, chromosome imbalance, or an underlying syndromic diagnosis, and up to 50% for patients with CP and Robin sequence. Such patients face an increased risk for perioperative morbidity including but not limited to cardiovascular dysfunction, pituitary insufficiency, and/or cervical spine instability. Ruling out comorbidities is important for the overall health approach but especially for ensuring safety of the CL/P patient undergoing surgical reconstruction. There are >200 genetic syndromes associated with CL/P deformities. Resources to assist identification of a specific syndrome diagnosis in lieu of formal clinical genetic consultation include access to textbooks and use of online facial recognition/clinical feature programs (Table 8.3).

A set of screening questions can help identify potential risk factors as part of the history and review of systems (Table 8.4.) If a syndromic diagnosis is reported or suspected, focus should be on the identification of potential associated risk factors (hypopituitarism, cervical spine instability, cardiac and/or renal anomalies) that would impact the child's safety for surgery (Table 8.5). For instance, a child with CLP and additional features of cutis aplasia, hypotelorism, murmur, and postaxial polydactyly should be suspected to have trisomy 13, or Patau syndrome. Such patients have frequent and severe cardiac anomalies, low muscle tone, and central apnea; they are at very high operative risk and often do not survive beyond 12 months of age. In another example, a patient with CL/P, wide spaced eyes, and hypospadias would raise concern for Opitz oculo-genital-laryngeal syndrome. Such patients often have laryngeal clefts and often suffer chronic aspiration and pose increased anesthetic risk.

**Table 8.3** Online resources to assist in genetic syndrome diagnosis

| Genetic references |
|---|
| NORD: https://rarediseases.org/ |
| OMIM: https://www.omim.org/ |
| Gene Tests: https://www.genetests.org/ |
| Genetic Alliance: http://www.geneticalliance.org/ |
| Disease Information Search: http://www.diseaseinfosearch.org/ |
| Face2Gene: http://www.fdna.com/face2gene-for-geneticist-healthcare-providers/ |
| Oxford Desk Reference Clinical Genetics (Oxford Desk Reference Series) 1st Edition; Jane A. Hurst and Helen V. Firth |

**Table 8.4** Screening questions to identify potential risks in patients with cleft lip/palate

| |
|---|
| Has your child had difficulties breathing, cough, or fever in the past month? |
| Has your child had a diarrheal or vomiting illness in the past 2 weeks? |
| Has your child been growing OK? Do you have a record of any prior measurements? |
| Does your child fall asleep during feeding? Is he/she sleepy most of the day? |
| Does your child cough and/or turn blue with feedings? |
| Does your child nurse and use a bottle (if so what type) or cup? |
| Does your child struggle to breathe when awake or upset? |
| Does your child struggle to breathe while sleeping? |
| Do you observe snoring or pauses in breathing? |
| Does your child have a murmur? |
| Has your child ever had a convulsion? |
| Are you worried about your child's developmental progress? Vision? Hearing? Activity level? |
| Have you been told, or are you concerned, that your child has health problems in addition to their cleft lip/palate? |
| Is there a family history of life-threatening events with anesthesia? |
| Is your child specially prompt to develop bruises with minor trauma or prolonged bleeding with skin lacerations/cuts? |
| Has your child undergone surgery in the past (and were there any complications with bleeding, anesthesia, or infection)? |
| Has your child been hospitalized previously? |
| Has your child been prescribed with medications or is under any current conventional or traditional treatment? |
| For children with breastfeeding, it is important to rule out current or recent maternal intake of medications or traditional/indigenous medicine/herbs |
| Has your child been identified as allergic for any food/medication, or has had skin/airway reactions upon ingestion/injection of specific foods/medications? |

## Cleft Palate and Pierre Robin Sequence

Pierre Robin sequence (PRSq) is the triad of (1) a small jaw (micrognathia), (2) a tongue with low tone (glossoptosis), and (3) airway obstruction (Fig. 8.1). A cleft palate is not a component of PRSq, although approximately 40% of patients with PRSq have a cleft palate and 25% of patients with an isolated cleft palate have PRSq. Infants with PRSq have an increased risk for upper airway obstruction, hypoxia, aspiration, feeding difficulties, inadequate intake, and nutritional

**Table 8.5** Factors to consider in safe surgical management of patients with cleft lip/palate based on history and physical exam features

| System evaluation | Finding | Health/syndrome concern | Potential implications for surgical readiness |
|---|---|---|---|
| Constitutional | Short stature | Condition with thyroid/GH deficiency | Abnormal metabolism, hypothermia, hypoglycemia |
| | Large | Hydrocephalus | Increased intracranial pressure |
| Head size | Small | Brain malformation, holoprosencephaly | Seizures, developmental delay, hypopituitarism (adrenal crisis, hypernatremia, hypoglycemia) |
| Eyes | Sparse lashes/ eyebrows | Ectodermal dysplasia | Inability to sweat – hyperthermia, if associated with ectrodactyly – at risk for renal anomalies |
| | Eyelid defect | Craniofacial microsomia (upper lid)<br>Treacher Collins syndrome (lower eyelid)<br>Kabuki syndrome (long fissures with lateral lid eversion)<br>Burn-McKeown syndrome | Craniofacial microsomia (mandibular hypoplasia and difficult airway, at risk for cervical spine anomalies/instability/cardiac and renal anomalies); Kabuki syndrome (multiple anomalies including cardiac, renal, immunodeficiency); Burn-McKeown (choanal atresia/cardiac anomalies) |
| | Coloboma (iris or retina) | Chromosome 22q duplication; CHARGE syndrome | Chromosome 22q dup (cardiac defect); CHARGE syndrome (dysphagia and aspiration, upper airway obstruction at choanae, cardiac and renal anomalies, immunodeficiency) |
| | Cataract | Smith-Lemli-Opitz syndrome (microcephaly, micrognathia, cleft palate, 2–3 toe syndactyly, postaxial polydactyly) | Upper airway obstruction, adrenal insufficiency due to low cholesterol |
| | Microphthalmia | Holoprosencephaly (HPE); CHARGE syndrome | HPE: hypopituitarism (adrenal crisis, hypernatremia, hypoglycemia)<br>CHARGE syndrome (dysphagia and aspiration, upper airway obstruction at choanae, cardiac and renal anomalies, immunodeficiency) |
| | Hypotelorism | Holoprosencephaly (HPE) | Hypopituitarism (adrenal crisis, hypernatremia, hypoglycemia) |
| | Hypertelorism | Opitz syndrome<br>Aarskog syndrome<br>Frontonasal dysplasia | Opitz syndrome (laryngeal cleft with aspiration of oral feedings, cardiac anomaly)<br>Aarskog syndrome (cervical spine anomaly)<br>Frontonasal dysplasia (many forms – cardiac anomalies, brain malformation) |
| Nose | Nasal mass | Encephalocele, teratoma | Airway obstruction |
| | Narrow | Holoprosencephaly (HPE) | Hypopituitarism (adrenal crisis, hypernatremia, hypoglycemia) |
| | Bifid nose | Frontonasal dysplasia | Cardiac anomalies, brain malformation |
| Ears | Microtia | Craniofacial microsomia (CFM)<br>Treacher Collins syndrome (TCS)<br>Branchio-oto-renal (BOR) syndrome | CFM (mandibular hypoplasia and difficult airway, cervical spine anomalies/instability/cardiac and renal anomalies); TCS (mandibular hypoplasia and difficult airway)<br>BOR (renal insufficiency/malformation) |
| | Asymmetric | CHARGE syndrome<br>Craniofacial microsomia | CHARGE syndrome (dysphagia and aspiration, upper airway obstruction at choanae, cardiac and renal anomalies, immunodeficiency)<br>CFM – mandibular hypoplasia and difficult airway (at risk for cervical spine anomalies/instability/cardiac and renal anomalies) |
| | Preauricular tags/pits | Craniofacial microsomia (CFM)<br>Branchio-oto-renal (BOR) syndrome | CFM (mandibular hypoplasia and difficult airway, cervical spine anomalies/instability/cardiac and renal anomalies)<br>BOR (renal insufficiency/malformation) |
| Lips | Midline cleft | Frontonasal dysplasia<br>Holoprosencephaly<br>Oral-facial-digital syndrome | Frontonasal dysplasia (cardiac anomalies, brain malformation)<br>Holoprosencephaly (hypopituitarism with adrenal crisis, hypernatremia, hypoglycemia)<br>Oral-facial-digital syndrome (renal insufficiency, brain malformations) |
| | Lower lip pits | Van der Woude syndrome; Kabuki syndrome | Van der Woude syndrome (no increase in risk); Kabuki syndrome (multiple anomalies including cardiac, renal, immunodeficiency) |

**Table 8.5** (continued)

| System evaluation | Finding | Health/syndrome concern | Potential implications for surgical readiness |
|---|---|---|---|
| | Macroglossia | Congenital hypothyroidism<br>Beckwith-Wiedemann syndrome | Hypothyroidism (slowed metabolism)<br>Beckwith-Wiedemann syndrome (macroglossia/cleft palate, hypoglycemia, airway obstruction, increase in risk for childhood malignancy) |
| Mouth and tongue | Microglossia | Hypoglossia-hypodactyly syndrome | Airway obstruction; dysphagia with aspiration pneumonia |
| | Accessory buccal frenula | Smith-Lemli-Opitz syndrome (microcephaly, micrognathia, cleft palate, 2–3 toe syndactyly, postaxial polydactyly)<br>Oral-facial-digital syndrome | Smith-Lemli-Opitz syndrome (upper airway obstruction, adrenal insufficiency due to low cholesterol)<br>Oral-facial-digital syndrome (renal insufficiency, brain malformations) |
| Mandible | Small | Robin sequence (many syndromes/ chromosome imbalance) | Tongue-based airway obstruction/difficult intubation |
| | Asymmetric | Craniofacial microsomia | Mandibular hypoplasia and difficult airway, cervical spine anomalies/instability/cardiac and renal anomalies |
| Faces | Asymmetric | Craniofacial microsomia | CFM (mandibular hypoplasia and difficult airway, cervical spine anomalies/instability/cardiac and renal anomalies) |
| Neck | Webbed and/or short | Cervical spine fusion anomalies | Unstable cervical spine, difficult intubation |
| | Torticollis | Cervical spine segmentation anomalies | Unstable cervical spine, difficult intubation |
| Cardiovascular | Murmur | Congenital heart defect – syndrome or chromosome imbalance | At risk for overcirculation, heart failure, and cyanosis, preload dependent |
| Respiratory | Chest wall size/ asymmetry | Skeletal dysplasia<br>Poland anomaly (absent pectoralis muscle) | Skeletal dysplasia (at risk for restrictive lung disease, cervical spine instability)<br>Poland anomaly (can be associated with Moebius – VI and VII cranial nerve palsies with possible dysphagia/aspiration risk) |
| Abdomen | Umbilical hernia | Beckwith-Wiedemann syndrome | Macroglossia/cleft palate, hypoglycemia, airway obstruction, increase in risk for childhood malignancy |
| Genitourinary | Ambiguous genitalia | Chromosome imbalance<br>Smith-Lemli-Opitz syndrome (microcephaly, micrognathia, cleft palate, 2–3 toe syndactyly, postaxial polydactyly) | Upper airway obstruction, adrenal insufficiency due to low cholesterol |
| | Hypospadias | Smith-Lemli-Opitz syndrome (microcephaly, micrognathia, cleft palate, 2–3 toe syndactyly, postaxial polydactyly)<br>Opitz syndrome (hypertelorism/ widow's peak) | Smith-Lemli-Opitz syndrome (upper airway obstruction, adrenal insufficiency due to low cholesterol); Opitz syndrome (laryngeal cleft with aspiration of oral feedings, cardiac anomaly) |
| | Shawl scrotum | Aarskog syndrome | Cervical spine anomaly |
| | Bifid scrotum | Opitz syndrome | Laryngeal cleft with aspiration of oral feedings, cardiac anomaly |
| Musculoskeletal | Scoliosis | Syndrome or skeletal dysplasia | Skeletal dysplasia (at risk for restrictive lung disease, cervical spine instability) |
| | Polydactyly | Skeletal dysplasia<br>Smith-Lemli-Opitz syndrome (microcephaly, micrognathia, cleft palate, 2–3 toe syndactyly, postaxial polydactyly)<br>Chromosomal (trisomy 13) | Skeletal dysplasia (at risk for restrictive lung disease, cervical spine instability)<br>Smith-Lemli-Opitz syndrome (upper airway obstruction, adrenal insufficiency due to low cholesterol)<br>Chromosomal (multiple anomalies including cardiac) |
| | Syndactyly | Ectodermal dysplasia | Inability to sweat – hyperthermia, if associated with ectrodactyly – at risk for renal anomalies |
| | Ectrodactyly | Ectodermal dysplasia | Inability to sweat – hyperthermia, if associated with ectrodactyly – at risk for renal anomalies |
| | Terminal transverse deficiency | Moebius sequence | Moebius sequence (dysphagia with increase aspiration risk) |
| | Congenital limb contractures | Arthrogryposis | Malignant hyperthermia |

(continued)

**Table 8.5** (continued)

| System evaluation | Finding | Health/syndrome concern | Potential implications for surgical readiness |
|---|---|---|---|
| | Disproportionate limbs/trunk | Skeletal dysplasia | Skeletal dysplasia (at risk for restrictive lung disease, cervical spine instability) |
| Neurologic | Hypotonia | Metabolic condition, multiple syndromes, chromosome imbalance | If severe hypotonia, concern for an increased risk for airway obstructive symptoms, dysphagia |
| | Tetany | Chromosome 22q11 deletion | Hypocalcemia, immunodeficiency, cardiac and renal anomalies, cervical spine instability |
| | Facial palsy | CHARGE syndrome<br>Craniofacial microsomia<br>Moebius sequence (if abducens palsy) | CHARGE syndrome (dysphagia and aspiration, upper airway obstruction at choanae, cardiac and renal anomalies, immunodeficiency)<br>CFM (mandibular hypoplasia and difficult airway, cervical spine anomalies/instability/cardiac and renal anomalies)<br>Moebius sequence (dysphagia with increased aspiration risk) |
| | w = weakness | Myopathy | Malignant hyperthermia |
| Infectious | Frequent infections | Chromosome 22q11 deletion<br>CHARGE syndrome<br>Kabuki syndrome | Chromosome 22q11 deletion (hypocalcemia, immunodeficiency, cardiac and renal anomalies, cervical spine instability)<br>CHARGE syndrome (dysphagia and aspiration, upper airway obstruction at choanae, cardiac and renal anomalies, immunodeficiency)<br>Kabuki syndrome (multiple anomalies including cardiac, renal, immunodeficiency) |
| Endocrine | Short stature/slowed rate of growth with normal weight | Growth hormone deficiency | Abnormal metabolism, hypoglycemia |
| | Polyuria | Diabetes insipidus, renal insufficiency | Diabetes insipidus (hypernatremia; additional pituitary hormone deficiency); renal failure |
| Skin | Cutis aplasia | Trisomy 13 | Cardiac anomaly, dysphagia, apnea |

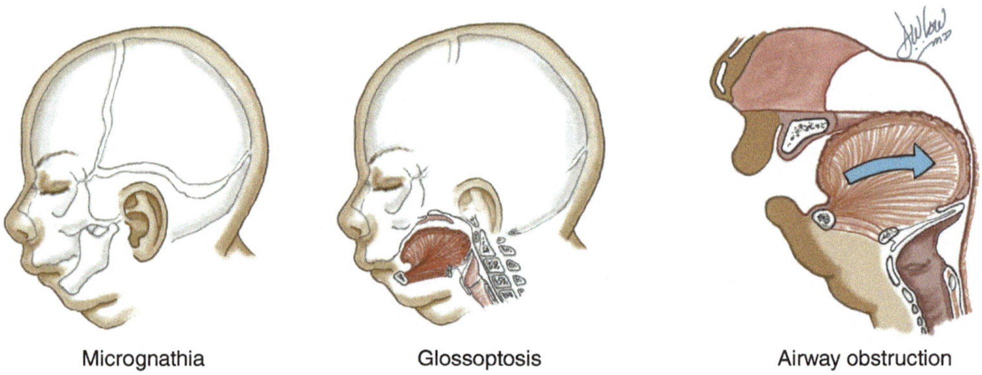


**Fig. 8.1** Triad of Pierre Robin sequence: micrognathia, glossoptosis, and airway obstruction

compromise with weight faltering. A lateral skull X-ray typically shows collapse of the airway stripe (Fig. 8.2). The degree of mandibular hypoplasia variably affects breathing and feeding functions, which are the two main clinical concerns of PRSq patients.

The clinical and surgical management will depend on the severity of airway obstruction, the feeding functional impairment, and their clinical repercussion (hypoxia-hypercapnia/failure to thrive) (Table 8.6), and this is further discussed in Chap. 25.

**Box: Solutions from the Field**

In remote settings where a symptomatic child is encountered and an expedient referral is not possible, a nasopharyngeal airway can be placed. This will at least stent open the airway past the tongue-based airway obstruction. If a nasopharyngeal airway is not available, one can be improvised from an infant endotracheal tube or an adult-sized nasogastric tube (Fig. 8.3a, b).

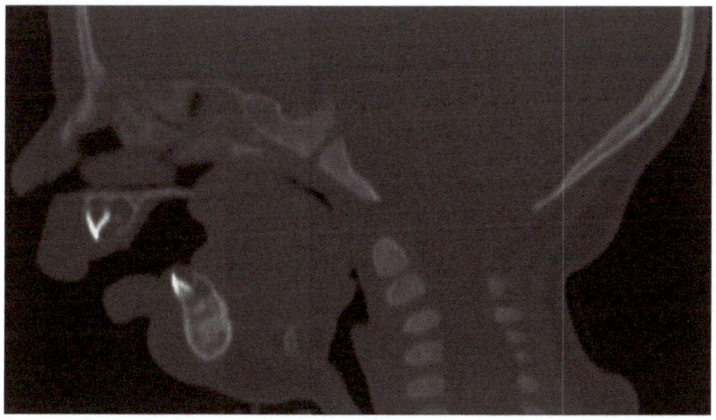

**Fig. 8.2** Cross-sectional view of the nasopharynx showing prolapse of the tongue base and collapse of airway stripe

**Table 8.6** Pierre Robin sequence management according to clinical severity

| Clinical severity | Management |
|---|---|
| Mild | Regular CP management<br>Thorough assessment of feeding and breathing<br>Close clinical follow-up |
| Mild-Moderate | Positional therapy: prone position prevents the tongue from obstructing the airway<br>Specific feeding/nutritional support |
| Moderate-severe | Invasive management to secure airway/feeding<br>Airway<br>Nasopharyngeal airway (can fashion from NP tubing) (Fig. 8.3)<br>Mandibular distraction<br>Tongue-lip adhesion<br>Tracheostomy<br>Feeding<br>Nasogastric tubing<br>Gastrostomy |

## Preoperative Assessment of the CLP Patient

The assessment of the overall health status, the specific health concerns related to the deformity, and the detection of potential comorbidities should be adapted to the patient's age and the geographic setting. Children living in regions where specific conditions or infections such as thalassemia or malaria are prevalent should have appropriate laboratory studies.

### Review of Systems: Medical History

Specific screening surveys (Table 8.4) might be helpful for systematizing the clinical assessment in the preoperative screening setting. Positive responses to the proposed questions may lead to additional laboratory and/or imaging studies. Systematized surveys, when coupled with standardized medical records/forms, ease the information exchange between team members and increase patient safety.

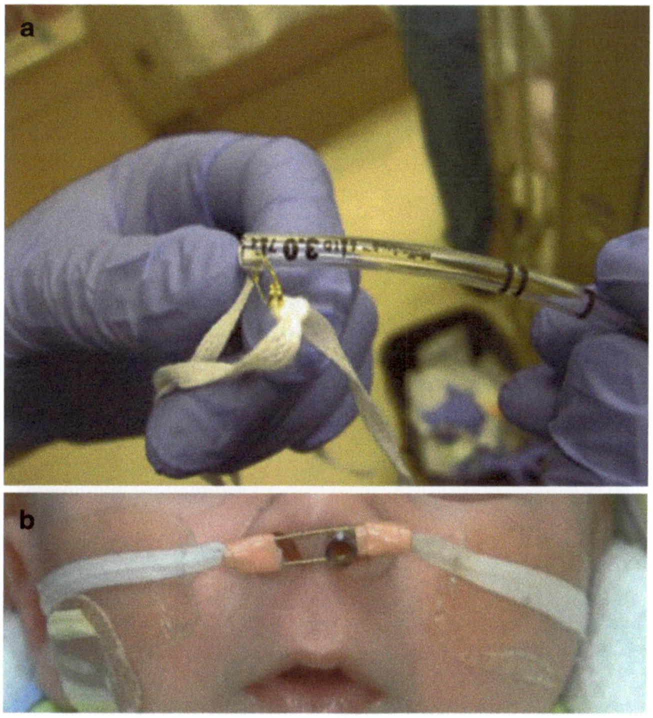


**Fig. 8.3** (**a**, **b**) A nasopharyngeal (NP) airway, can be fashioned from a pediatric endotracheal tube or larger nasogastric tube. A nasoendoscope can verify that the distal tip is below the tongue base but above the glottis. It is secured externally, and patency can be maintained using normal saline and suctioning every 4 hours. The diameter/length of the NPA is adjusted periodically, according to the recurrence of clinical findings of airway obstruction. Caregivers are instructed on NPA maintenance and detection of obstruction symptoms and signs

### Review of Systems: Physical Examination

It is important to observe the child's level of alertness, overall activity level, and breathing while awake and asleep and during feeding (if possible). If the child is awake, observe for age-appropriate activity. A sleepy/lethargic infant may reveal significant malnutrition, illness, or neurologic impairment. During child's sleep, check for loud snoring or torturous breathing – carefully remove the blanket/clothes to observe the child's work of breathing (look for tracheal tug, head bobbing, subcostal retractions, and skin color). If the child is feeding, check for signs of aspiration: cough, sputter, color change, or tachypnea. The physical examination should be tailored to specific risks of patients with cleft lip/palate (Table 8.7). Vital signs including temperature, heart rate, and respiratory rate should be recorded and compared to age-specific normal values (Table 8.8).

Measurement of oxygen saturation is increasingly seen as standard in low-resource settings. It is highly sensitive to detect cardiopulmonary disease that is clinically significant in patients with cleft lip/palate, and small pulse oximeters can be obtained for under $50.

**Table 8.7** A systematic physical examination scheme for patients with cleft lip/palate

| | |
|---|---|
| Anthropometric measurements | Weight, length, MUAC |
| Vital signs | Temperature, heart rate, respiratory rate, Sat-$O_2$ |
| Skin and annexes | Asses for cyanosis, pallor, jaundice, mottling, edema, turgor, dryness, and amount of subcutaneous fat |
| Head and neck | Assess the fontanelle and overall head size. A bulging fontanelle with macrocephaly suggests hydrocephalus, whereas a bulging fontanelle with lethargy is concerning for meningitis Ophthalmologic and/or external ear anomalies (microphthalmia/microtia and/or preauricular pits/tags) should raise concerns for syndromic diagnosis |
| Cleft deformity | Type and severity. Midline clefts should raise concerns for associated neurological midline deformities, and further assessment of neurologic status (brain imaging) and pituitary function is recommended |
| Upper airway | Nasal patency and overall assessment for obstruction; nasal congestion, stertor, stridor, etc. |
| Cardiovascular and respiratory | Respiratory dynamics, breathing retractions, auscultation for air movement, wheezing, and rales, cardiac (murmurs, capillary refill) |
| Abdomen | Scars of previous surgeries; assess for organomegaly |
| Genitourinary | Rule out ambiguity of genitalia, cryptorchidism, or hypospadias as it might associate hormone imbalance, adrenal insufficiency, or syndrome diagnosis |
| Neuromuscular | Overall muscle tone/strength and cranial nerve function. Infants with myopathy (muscle weakness) associate an increased risk for malignant hyperthermia. Infants with hypotonia may struggle with apnea and/or airway obstruction following anesthesia |
| Spinal | Rule out scoliosis and torticollis. Fixed head tilt with short neck is concerning for cervical spine segmentation anomalies, placing the child at risk for cervical spine injury and difficult intubation |
| Limbs | Distal limb anomalies such as polydactyly/ syndactyly are suggestive of syndrome diagnosis |

Nutritional and feeding assessment is further discussed in Chap. 7. The child's weight, length, and head circumference should be measured and compared to age-specific values to determine if the development is appropriate and if weight-for-length ratio is normal. If the growth rate is slow with weight-for-length ratio <10%, then the MUAC (mid-upper arm circumference) should be obtained.

## Further Workup: Laboratory and Imaging Studies

Most children with isolated CLP deformities do not require laboratory studies or imaging studies other than basic blood test (Hb/Hct, WBC, platelets) and coagulation parameters (PTT, PT, INR).

Specific blood tests should be indicated by specific risk factors based on local epidemiology/endemics (malaria/thalassemia/Mediterranean fever), personal history, family history, and/or examination findings.

Further laboratory studies to assess metabolic and endocrinological functions (electrolytes, glucose, cortisol, thyroid levels) should be requested upon suspected associated comorbidities and/or syndromes.

Imaging studies are not necessary for healthy CLP patients undergoing surgery. Chest/abdominal X-rays, head/neck CT scans, echocardiography, etc. should also be requested upon suspected associated comorbidities and/or syndromes.

Congenital cardiac anomalies are reported in up to 3–16% of CLP children. Accordingly, in those patients showing abnormal cardiac examination, in the LRO setting, where echocardiogram is not readily available, a pulse oximetry detecting hypoxemia could be highly suggestive of a cardiac anomaly that is clinically significant.

**Table 8.8** Reference vital signs by age

| General vital signs and guidelines | | | |
|---|---|---|---|
| Age | Heart rate (beats/mins) | Blood pressure (mmHg) | Respiratory rate (breaths/min) |
| Premature | 110–170 | SBP 55–75, DBP 35–45 | 40–70 |
| 0–3 months | 110–160 | SBP 65–85, DBP 45–55 | 35–55 |
| 3–6 months | 110–160 | SBP 70–90, DBP 50–65 | 30–45 |
| 6–12 months | 90–160 | SBP 80–100, DBP 55–65 | 22–38 |
| 1–3 years | 80–150 | SBP 90–105, DBP 55–70 | 22–30 |
| 3–6 years | 70–120 | SBP 95–110, DBP 60–75 | 20–24 |
| 6–12 years | 60–110 | SBP 100–120, DBP 60–75 | 16–22 |
| >12 years | 60–100 | SBP 110–135, DBP 65–85 | 12–20 |

*SBP* Systolic blood pressure, *DBP* Diastolic blood pressure

## CLP Surgery, Anesthesia, and Comorbidities

Confirmation of comorbidities should guide the team to schedule for surgery with adequate facilities, infrastructure, and perioperative monitoring or, alternatively, to refer the patient into special programs or subspecialized reference centers.

### Ruling Out Concurrent Infections

General anesthesia and surgical trauma cause stress and, secondarily, endocrinological, metabolic, and immunological changes in patients [1, 2]. Accordingly, surgical site infection and/or worsening of concurrent infections could occur throughout the perioperative period. Any evidence of active local infection on oral and/or facial soft tissues (perioral impetigo, active herpes infection at any stage of evolution, acute adenotonsillitis, etc.) forces the cancellation of the scheduled surgery, until the infected areas are fully recovered.

#### Otitis Media

Otitis media with effusion (OME) and acute otitis media (AOM) must be differentiated. OME occurs when non-infected fluid on the middle ear is accumulated as a result of an upper respiratory tract infection. OME is a common finding in the general population, and up to 60% of non-cleft children might display episodes of OME during the first 2 years of life. On the other hand, CP patients feature Eustachian tube dysfunction, which further alters the adequate ventilation and clearance of fluid from the middle ear. Consequently, up to 97% of CP patients develop episodes of OME during the first 2 years of life [3]. Accordingly, the clinical finding of an OME in a patient during the preoperative assessment should not be a cause for delay or cancelation of a surgical procedure. Conversely, in the setting of AOM, adequate treatment should be initiated, and delay of surgery should be considered until the acute infection improves. In both cases, OME and AOM, caregivers should be instructed on adequate prevention and management of further episodes and also on early detection of AOM. Ideally, the local team should provide otologic clinical follow-up because optimal speech outcomes depend on an adequate hearing function.

#### Respiratory Tract Infections (RTIs)

*Acute upper respiratory tract infections (URTIs)* are the most frequent human illness and the most common infection in childhood, associating an increased risk of perioperative respiratory adverse events (PRAEs). Thus, a rigorous respiratory clinical assessment can prevent devastating perioperative complications. The acute viral URTI or "common cold" clinical picture groups a constellation of signs and symptoms including variable degrees of sneezing, nasal congestion and discharge (rhinorrhea), sore throat, cough, low-grade fever, headache, and/or malaise.

Airway manipulation under general anesthesia causes local trauma, and the patient with concurrent or recent URTI that is taken to surgery under general anesthesia might develop PRAEs during induction and extubation and even during the early postoperative period. The hyperreactive airway can develop obstruction at different levels causing PRAEs including laryngospasm, bronchospasm, atelectasis, and ventilation insufficiency, which might lead to apnea and cardiorespiratory arrest. In fact, according to data from the Pediatric Perioperative Cardiac Arrest Registry, PRAEs were the second most common cause of perioperative cardiac arrests in children, with laryngospasm being the most likely cause for respiratory-induced cardiac arrests. In addition, the surgical patient with acute URTIs associates an increased risk of postoperative PRAEs including pneumonia.

The differential diagnosis of URTIs includes other infectious and non-infectious pathologies with similar clinical manifestations:

- Infectious: streptococcal pharyngoamigdalitis, croup, epiglottitis, herpangina, bronchiolitis, pneumonia
- Non-infectious: allergic/vasomotor rhinitis, asthma, gastroesophageal reflux, foreign body aspiration

*Viral bronchiolitis (VB)* is an RTI with a spectrum of clinical manifestations ranging from minimal symptoms to respiratory insufficiency requiring mechanical ventilation. *VB is the most common cause of hospitalization in children under 2 years of age with respiratory infection. In* 80% of cases, the etiological agent is respiratory syncytial virus (RSV). After the infection, most of these patients remain with degrees of airway hyperreactivity, increased secretions, wet cough, rhonchus, wheezing, and respiratory muscle retractions for a prolonged period of time, usually 3–6 weeks. Such patients are on major risk of severe PRAEs, and accordingly, *CLP* patients under 2 years, who are candidates for surgery, presenting with signs or symptoms of bronchial obstruction, should be carefully evaluated to rule out a recent acute bronchiolitis.

#### RTIs and the CLP Surgical Patient

In the context of surgical programs carried out by Humanitarian Organizations in the mission/outreach setting, it is mandatory to count with highly experienced pediatric assessment.

The perioperative risk for PRAEs increases exponentially in a patient undergoing general anesthesia with a recent or concurrent respiratory tract infection; the team should provide a patient-specific management plan for such patients presenting for surgical reconstruction. Even in patients that have recently recovered, assessment and management by experienced pediatric anesthesia and pediatric specialists, with the skills to identify clinical manifestations of recent RTIs, is critical to best prevent, identify early, and efficiently handle potential PRAEs (Table 8.9).

### Other Respiratory Comorbidities

#### Asthma

Allergic asthma is a leading cause of morbidity, and the most common cause for hospital admission, in the pediatric population. The condition is a chronic inflammatory disease of the

**Table 8.9** Management of cleft lip/palate patients with recent infection

| |
|---|
| *Proceeding with the surgical plan* in patients with recent infection should be determined by factors such as the patient's age, the overall health status, the type and intensity of the infection, the time of evolution, the skills and knowledge of the anesthesia provider, and the availability of adequate infrastructure and equipment for perioperative monitoring and support. The anesthetic protocol should be adjusted and modified to further prevent PRAEs in such patients |
| *Postpone and reschedule the procedure* for patients with symptomatic RTI<br>2–4 weeks: Common cold, flu and flu-like viral infections (rhinovirus, parainfluenza, influenza, H1N1, COVID-19)<br>6–8 weeks: In the case of RSV infection and bronchiolitis, surgery should be postponed between 6 and 8 weeks<br>For both types of infection, the period is generally estimated from the time the patient is fully recovered and is asymptomatic |
| *Cancel and refer to a local hospital* those patients with comorbidities or when the infrastructure or the human resources are insufficient to provide adequate perioperative monitoring and support |

**Table 8.10** Management of patients with asthma

| | |
|---|---|
| *Symptomatic patients* (wheezing, prolonged exhalation, etc.)<br>Postpone and reschedule the procedure until the symptoms are controlled and the patient is fully asymptomatic<br>Counseling for identification and prevention of potential triggers<br>Adjust prescription: Long-term controllers and/or crisis/rescue medication<br>*Asymptomatic patients*<br>Proceed with the surgical plan if experienced anesthesia providers and adequate infrastructure and equipment for perioperative monitoring and support are available<br>Continue with the current prescription throughout the perioperative process<br>Specific anesthetic management according to the severity of the condition | |
| Crisis: occasional<br>Symptoms: mild<br>Therapy: on demand | Crisis: frequent<br>Symptoms: severe<br>Therapy: daily/long term |
| Inhaled BD during induction and prior extubation | Preparation with systemic corticosteroid therapy for 48 h<br>Dexamethasone PO: Once daily, 0,6 mg/kg, max 16 mg/dose<br>Stress doses of corticosteroids during induction<br>Dexamethasone IV: 0,5 mg/Kg, max 12 mg/dose<br>OR<br>Hydrocortisone IV: 2 mg/kg. Adjusted to weight<br>Inhaled BD during induction and prior extubation |

airways characterized by three main partially reversible features: airway obstruction, airway inflammation, and airway hyper-responsiveness. Asthma is characterized by recurrent episodes of cough, wheezing, dyspnea, and chest tightness.

Asthma can be challenging to diagnose. The frequency and severity of clinical manifestations are highly variable among patients displaying only one or a combination of symptoms. Most patients are >4 years old at the time of onset…, are regularly exposed to smoke (tobacco, wood fire cooking, etc.), and/or have history of allergic rhinitis and/or atopic dermatitis. The condition is rare in patients under 2 years of age, and accordingly, patients displaying wheezing within this age range should raise the suspicion of a recent infection of RSV. In fact, an association between RSV bronchiolitis and subsequent wheezing and asthma has been documented.

During the preoperative assessment of a patient with asthma, the triggers and the severity of the condition, the frequency of events, and the type and intensity of symptoms should be investigated. Also, the specialist should inquire on the latest crisis and the preventive and treatment strategies, specifically about adherence and effectiveness. The planning and management for surgical CLP patients with asthma is summarized in Table 8.10.

### Obstructive Sleep Disorders (OSDs)

Children are at risk for obstructive sleep apnea caused by rapid growth of adenotonsillar tissue in early childhood. In fact, the prevalence of OSD in the pediatric population ranges from 1.2% to 5.8%. Typically, pharyngeal lymphoid tissue shrinks after 8 years of age; however, in a subset of children, adenotonsillar hypertrophy and hyperplasia might persist. CLP patients display additional primary and secondary anatomical alterations (nasal deformity, maxillary retrognathia, palate lengthening, pharyngeal flaps) that increase the risk of chronic airway obstruction. *Thus, relative to the non-cleft population, children with CL/P are seven times more likely to develop OSDs* [4].

**Table 8.11** Signs and symptoms of obstructive sleep apnea in children

| |
|---|
| Signs and symptoms of OSA in children include |
| Snoring |
| Labored breathing during sleep |
| Mouth breathing |
| Apnea |
| Gasping or snorting during sleep |
| Restless sleep with movements |
| Frequent awakening during sleep |
| Enuresis |
| Morning headache |
| Daytime sleepiness |
| Learning difficulties |

Airway obstruction coupled with untreated OSD morbidity (failure to thrive, developmental neurocognitive disorders, cardiovascular dysfunction, pulmonary hypertension, blood hypercoagulability, etc.) significantly increases the perioperative morbimortality risk of affected patients. Targeted history questioning, coupled with a thorough physical examination, will aid the clinicians to suspect and rule out OSDs and indicate further work-up consultations and tests (Table 8.11). In the LRO setting, with limited access to sophisticated tests such as polysomnography, the pediatric Sleep-Related Breathing Disorder (SRBD) questionnaire can be a useful screening tool and is available for free online [5].

Patients with OSD have much higher perioperative morbimortality risks. When under general anesthesia, patients with OSD have major risk for developing PREs, especially when opioids are administered, including laryngospasm, bronchospasm, excessive sedation responses, and postoperative apnea. In addition, the anatomical modifications of CLP reconstructive surgery, and the secondary soft tissue edema, dramatically modify the airflow dynamics within the upper airway. Hence, the general anesthesia protocol in CLP patients with OSDs should exclude the use of opioids. Instead, the use of locoregional nerve blocks (infraorbital and/or suprazygomatic), with short- and long-acting local anesthetics (Lidocaine/Bupivacaine), offers effective analgesia during and after surgery, reducing the needs for general anesthetics (propofol/sevoflurane). Furthermore, close postoperative monitoring for 24 hours with oxygen saturation monitoring and potentially intensive care unit admission should be provided for these patients.

## Surgical Timing and Surgical Readiness

Surgical protocols for reconstruction of CLP deformities include timely interventions to achieve the best possible surgical outcomes (Table 8.1). As time-sensitive but non-urgent procedures, CLP reconstructive surgeries should expose patients to only minimum perioperative risks. Early CL repair (<6 months) should be avoided in the LRO setting given the increased perioperative and anesthetic risks. However, borderline patients (4–6 months) could be scheduled according to the local team and infrastructure capabilities, after an interdisciplinary discussion and agreement.

On the other hand, patients presenting at later stages of development for reconstruction of primary and/or secondary CLP deformities are common in the LRO setting. It is often more challenging to obtain satisfactory functional (i.e., speech/dental) and aesthetic (i.e., nasal shape) outcomes when surgical reconstruction is initiated at an older age; however, in many cases, major improvements can be offered to confirm the surgical indication.

Readiness for surgery is determined by completion of the assessments that have been discussed throughout this chapter, addressing development, cleft-related risk factors, and laboratory markers (Table 8.12).

**Table 8.12** Assessment for surgical readiness

| |
|---|
| Assessment of an infant or child with cleft lip and/or palate for surgery readiness includes: |
| 1. Assessments of developmental status |
| Gestational vs postnatal age and developmental status at the time of surgery |
| 2. Assessment of cleft-related risk factors: |
| (a) Breathing function and airway obstruction |
| (b) Feeding function, nutritional status, and development |
| (c) Rule out associated anomalies |
| 3. Clinical assessment and physical examination by systems |
| 4. Blood (and additional patient-specific) test results |

*Different tools have been developed to predict the perioperative morbimortality risk of children undergoing surgery. Classically, surgeons applied the* Musgrave's rule of 10s to determine a child's readiness for cleft lip repair. This rule of 10s was proposed according to the results of a 1960 study that found a fivefold increase in perioperative complications in CL infants undergoing CL repair and did not meet three criteria: (1) weight > 10 lbs, (2) Hb >10 grams, and (3) WBC count <10 k [6]. In 1976, Millard modified the rule of 10's changing the third criteria for age > 10 weeks. More recently, a study from 50 major US institutions found that only a weight < 10 lbs was an independent risk factor for postoperative complications and prolonged postoperative stay [7]. While the rule of 10s may be less relevant now in US hospitals, it may still serve as a reasonable rule of thumb in lower-resource settings where other risks may be higher.

While the American Society of Anesthesiologists' Physical Status (ASA PS) classification is extensively used to characterize the preoperative status of surgical patients, the tool was not designed to predict perioperative risks of morbidity or mortality or adverse events. Furthermore, the ASA PS classification may be less applicable to children than adults. The Pediatric Respiratory Assessment Measure (PRAM) is one tool that is currently being explored, but is not yet validated. In the absence of validated classifications, predicting the pediatric perioperative risks and defining readiness for surgery demand the integrated findings by a pediatrician and a pediatric anesthesiologist with sound experience providing care for patients with facial deformities in the LRO setting.

## References

1. Nasr VG, DiNardo JA, Faraoni D. Development of a pediatric risk assessment score to predict perioperative mortality in children undergoing noncardiac surgery. Anesth Analg. 2017;124(5):1514–9.
2. Yuki K, Matsunami E, Tazawa K, Wang W, DiNardo JA, Koutsogiannaki S. Pediatric perioperative stress responses and anesthesia. Transl Perioper Pain Med. 2017;2(1):1–12.

3. Kuo C-L, Lien C-F, Chu C-H, Shiao A-S. Otitis media with effusion in children with cleft lip and palate: a narrative review. Int J Pediatr Otorhinolaryngol. 2013;77(9):1403–9.
4. Silvestre J, Tahiri Y, Paliga JT, Taylor JA. Screening for obstructive sleep apnea in children with syndromic cleft lip and/or palate. J Plast Reconstr Aesthet Surg. 2014;67(11):1475–80.
5. Chervin RD, Hedger K, Dillon JE, Pituch KJ. Pediatric sleep questionnaire (PSQ): validity and reliability of scales for sleep-disordered breathing, snoring, sleepiness, and behavioral problems. Sleep Med. 2000;1(1):21–32.
6. Wilhelmsen HR, Musgrave RH. Complications of cleft lip surgery. Cleft Palate J. 1966;3:223–31.
7. Chow I, Purnell CA, Hanwright PJ, Gosain AK. Evaluating the rule of 10s in cleft lip repair: do data support dogma? Plast Reconstr Surg. 2016;138(3):670–9.

# Part III

# Complete Surgical Treatment

# 9 Anesthesia for Patients with Cleft Lip and Palate

Gaston Echaniz, Plinio Sierra, and Adrian Bosenberg

## Introduction

Lack of facilities and technical resources together with untrained anesthesia providers mitigates against safe surgery. Anesthesia for cleft patients is associated with several potential complications which may be life-threatening if not recognized and managed properly.

## Anesthesia Challenges

### Epidemiological Public Health Issues

The general guidelines for the perioperative care of CLP patients should be in strict accordance with the current recommendations listed in the International Standards for a Safe Practice of Anesthesia. The contribution of anesthesia to the burden of surgical disease is difficult to evaluate, but it is integral to surgery and may contribute to disability and death. Within this framework outlined by WHO, Safe Surgery Saves Lives project, and national governments, it is unacceptable to provide anesthesia that does not guarantee safe surgery. Medical missions to countries where there is a lack of human resources, equipment, medications and supplies need to bring their own supplies to provide anesthesia to acceptably safe standards. The supply of anesthesia medications must be cost-effective and requires an efficient supply chain. In LMICs, it is common to find adults who have not had reconstructive surgery.

G. Echaniz (✉)
Department of Pediatric Anesthesia, Sant Joan de Déu Barcelona Children's Hospital, Barcelona, Spain

P. Sierra
Department of Pediatric Anesthesia, King Abdullah, Specialized Children's Hospital, Riyadh, Saudi Arabia

A. Bosenberg
Department Anesthesiology and Pain Management, Seattle Children's Hospital, University Washington, Seattle, WA, USA

## Timing of Surgery and Anesthesia Implications

Despite the global health priorities by the United Nations Millennium Development Goals in 2008 and the World Health Organization Global Initiative for Emergency and Essential Surgical Care in 2005, timely access to corrective surgery remains unequal, sometimes absent, and almost always late. In LMICs, the surgical treatment for cleft lip and/or palate is delayed beyond the international standards adopted and accepted by international academic organizations. The airway and cardiovascular management are the main anesthetic challenges. These are different for the same patient at different age; the younger the patient is, the higher will be the risk for airway and cardiovascular morbidity. The main development of the respiratory system is between the week 35 of intrauterine life until 2 or 3 years of age. The anatomical and physiological development of the thoracic cage, lung tissue, and air conduction systems from the mouth to the alveoli are deeply involved in the response to anesthesia medications. All available anesthesia medications have a profound effect on cardiovascular and respiratory performance in infants and children. Additionally, all these medications have a very important interaction and potentialization of their pharmacological effects. Inhalation of anesthetic gases with an inspired fraction of oxygen 21% and less than or equal to 100% produces atelectasis and risk for hypoxemia. The children's thoracic cage has a much greater compliance than the adults' ones. This further facilitates the development of atelectasis increasing the ventilation pressure, which may affect the cardiac output by decreasing venous return. To this is added a relative or absolute state of hypovolemia derived from fasting, sometimes very long during medical missions in LMICs.

© Springer Nature Switzerland AG 2021

J. W. Swanson, D. W. Low (eds.), *Global Cleft Care in Low-Resource Settings*, https://doi.org/10.1007/978-3-030-59105-2_9

## Preoperative Assessment

A preoperative evaluation offers the opportunity to evaluate potential risks and institute management to reduce these risks as well as a complete medical history and physical examination. Particular attention should be paid to associate abnormalities. Infants and craniofacial abnormalities increase the risk of a difficult airway. Retrognathia is a common feature that should be evaluated in each child. It is also important to rule out obstructive sleep apnea (OSA) and to differentiate between rhinorrhea frequently seen in cleft patients and an acute upper respiratory tract infection (URI). At the end of the preoperative evaluation, the following questions should be answered (Fig. 9.1).

### Upper Respiratory Tract Infection (URI)

Upper respiratory infections are common in children. Chronic rhinorrhea is common in children with CLP due to food reflux into the nasal passages. The information provided by parents and caregivers must differentiate a child with hyperactive airway and a child with URI (Table 9.1). Surgical repair reduces rhinorrhea and URI. The risk of postoperative respiratory complications (PRC) increases with the severity of the defect. If surgery is postponed due to URI, the patient should be rescheduled in at least 4 weeks, prior reevaluation.

### Nutrition and Hydration

Children with poor nutrition are at risk of poor surgical outcomes. Severe acute malnourished (SAM) patients have 5–20-fold increased risk of mortality. A clinical assessment and the anthropometric measurements are mandated to evaluate the nutritional status. Another aim of the preoperative assessment is to identify malnourished patients and monitor and provide treatment and education with the goal of improving the nutritional status to an acceptable level to reduce the risk of perioperative complications.

**Key Tips**
- Although surgery can improve breastfeeding, severe malnutrition is not a surgically-treated disease.
- Improving the nutritional status prior to the surgical repair may significantly reduce the perioperative morbidity and improve outcomes.

### Associated Conditions and Anesthesia Implications

CLP is listed as a feature of more than 200 specific genetic syndromes (Table 9.2). 10–60% CLP is associated with other anomalies or medical conditions. The time between birth and the initial repair allows for a thorough workup of other comorbidities and evaluation of any underlying syndromes. Cardiac and airway abnormalities are the major concerns for the anesthesiologist.

Children with CP are prone to middle ear effusions and recurrent otitis media, as well as gastroesophageal reflux and pulmonary aspiration. Obstructive sleep apnea is a common problem, and supraglottic airway obstruction can occur on induction or emergence from anesthesia.

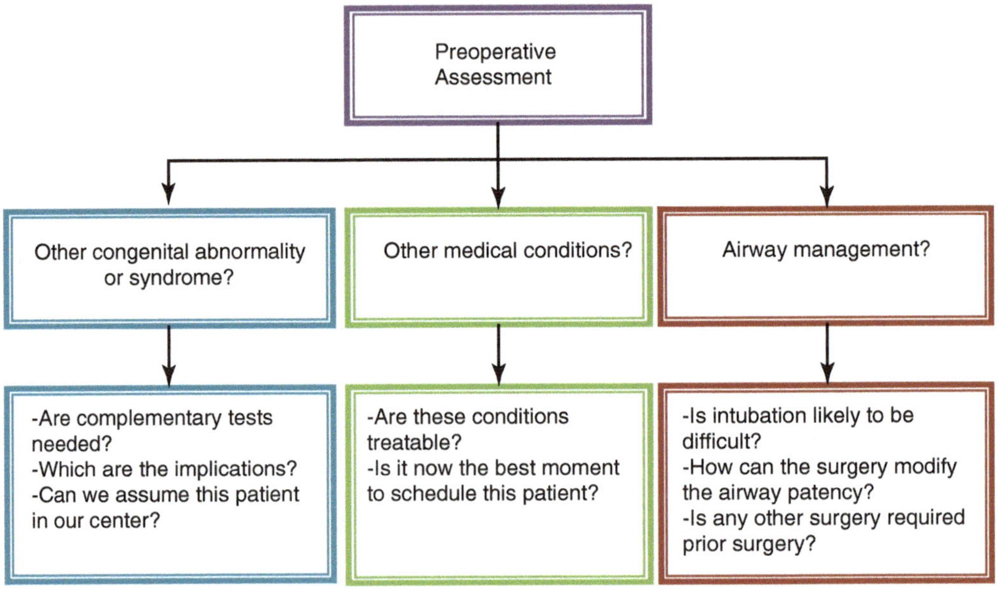


**Fig. 9.1** Schematic representation of the main concerns to be answered during preoperative evaluation

**Table 9.1** Differential diagnosis of allergic rhinitis and respiratory tract infection

| | Mild URI | Severe URI | Lower RI | Allergic rhinitis |
|---|---|---|---|---|
| History | No fever<br>Minimal cough<br>Clear runny nose<br>Sneezing | Malaise<br>Fever<br>Purulent coryza<br>Sneezing<br>Cough | Severe cough<br>Sputum production<br>Wheezing<br>+/− Fever | Atopy<br>Seasonal history<br>Sneezing |
| General exam | Non-toxic appearance<br>Clear runny nose | Toxic appearance<br>Malaise<br>Fever | Rales<br>+/− Toxic appearance<br>+/− Irritability | No fever<br>Allergic shiners |
| Pulmonary exam | Clear lungs<br>+/− Upper airway congestion | Clear lungs<br>Upper airway congestion | Rales<br>Rhonchi | Clear lungs |

**Table 9.2** Syndromes related with CLP and their main anesthesia implications

| Syndrome | Clinical findings | Considerations |
|---|---|---|
| Treacher Collins | Bilateral symmetrical abnormality of the 1st and 2nd branchial arch<br>*Ear*: anomalies of the external, middle, and inner ear. Hearing loss<br>*Eye*: ptosis of upper eyelid, coloboma of lower eyelid, down-slanting palpebral fissures<br>*Facial bones*: hypoplastic maxilla, zygoma, and mandible<br>Tongue retro-positioned<br>Pharyngeal hypoplasia | Airway obstruction<br>Difficult intubation. It may become less difficult with increasing age<br>Postoperative intensive care |
| Pierre Robin sequence | Micrognathia<br>Glossoptosis<br>Isolated cleft palate<br>Group of conditions:<br>*34%* Stickler syndrome<br>Pierre Robin sequence plus (retinal detachments, myopia, glaucoma, stiff or hypermobile joints. early osteoarthritis, scoliosis, mitral valve prolapse)<br>*17%* non-syndromic<br>*11%* velocardiofacial syndrome<br>*10%* fetal alcohol syndrome | Severe airway obstruction<br>Feeding difficulties<br>Jaw shows catch-up in growth Intubation may become easier with age |
| Goldenhar (oculo-auriculo-vertebral spectrum) | Unilateral defect of the 1st and 2nd branchial arches. Mostly sporadic<br>Facial asymmetry with maxillary and/or mandibular hypoplasia<br>Unilateral deformity of external ear<br>Coloboma of upper eyelid<br>Vertebral anomalies | Difficult airway (ventilation and/or intubation). Intubation may become more difficult with increasing age |

Children with craniosynostosis (Apert, Crouzon, and Pfeiffer syndromes) have abnormalities that limit neck motion and require a smaller endotracheal tube.

**Key Tips**

- Most syndromes may cause a difficult airway; attention should be focused on airway stability during perioperative period.
- Accidental extubation, bleeding, or swelling of the airway may be especially catastrophic in this group of patients.
- Intensive care unit should be available.

## Airway Management: Relevant Facts for Surgeons

A perioperative airway management plan is essential, following a valid pediatric difficult airway management algorithm in both predictable and unpredictable situations. Appropriate airway devices, face masks, and endotracheal tube (ETT) should be available, and a real-time monitoring is mandatory (SpO2 and EtCO2) (Fig. 9.2).

Difficult cases should be performed by the most experienced anesthesiologist. Since the airway is shared by anesthesiologist and surgeon during the surgical procedure, a good team communication is the cornerstone to avoiding preventable complications.

CLP may be related with difficult face mask ventilation (abnormal facial configuration, midface hypoplasia, severe OSA) and difficult intubation (mandibular hypoplasia, poor mouth opening, cleft defect, prominent premaxilla, and facial asymmetry). Older patients have a wider and deeper cleft defect with a large alveolar defect. When CLP is left sided, laryngoscope blade may fall into the defect making laryngoscopy challenging. In patients with a bilateral CLP,

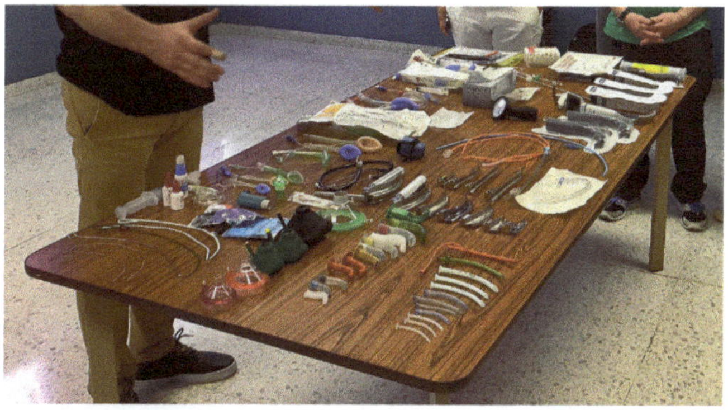

**Fig. 9.2** Helpful airway adjuncts for cleft patients, including stylets (left), laryngeal mask airways (LMAs, top), videolaryngoscopes (right), and nasopharyngeal and oral airways (bottom)

premaxilla is prominent making laryngoscopy and visualization of the vocal cords truly difficult.

A piece of gauze can be placed into the cleft defect to avoid the laryngoscope blade falling into the cleft (Fig. 9.3). Having a ETT stylet or a bougie may also help. Finally, videolaryngoscopes are extremely useful, although most of the time they are not available in LMICs.

Airway reactivity during head or ETT manipulation may be reduced by intravenous or topical lidocaine and/or systemic narcotics.

Due to the risk of aspiration, a throat pack (TP) should be used and correctly identified with a radiopaque or silk suture; insertion time and withdrawal time must be documented in anesthesia record (Fig. 9.4).

Airway and ETT positioning must be reassessed (bilateral breath sound, respiratory system compliance, capnography, SpO2) after each airway manipulation such as insertion and removal of the Dingman gag (DG) and throat pack (TP). Endobronchial intubation, accidental extubation, and ETT kinking may occur (Fig. 9.5). A needle cap may be placed beside the ETT to prevent its compression during DG placement (Fig. 9.6).

Minimizing airway manipulation may reduce postoperative airway edema and obstruction: choose the appropriate ETT size (avoid high cuff pressure on tracheal mucosa and unnecessary ETT exchanges); carefully introduce and remove DG and TP; and avoid unnecessary head and neck movements during surgery (Fig. 9.7). Perioperative dexamethasone use has been shown to reduce pain, edema, and PONV (postoperative nausea and vomiting) after oral surgery.

Direct visual inspection should be done prior to extubation to verify hemostasis and the absence of secretions. If aspiration is required, this should be done under direct laryngoscopy to avoid trauma to the surgical field.

Although surgery may be performed under general anesthesia in spontaneous breathing, manual assisted or control ventilation is recommended in infants and small children to reduce the work of breathing.

Closure of the palate defect may result in upper airway obstruction. Syndromic patients and those with preoperative OSA are at higher risk of airway obstruction. Extubation should be done when the infant is fully awake and airway reflexes have returned. Moreover, airway obstruction after

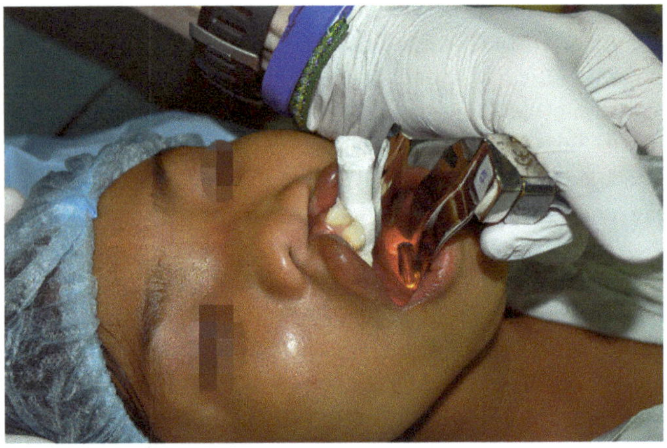

**Fig. 9.3** A gauze piece is placed into the cleft defect to improve laryngoscopy

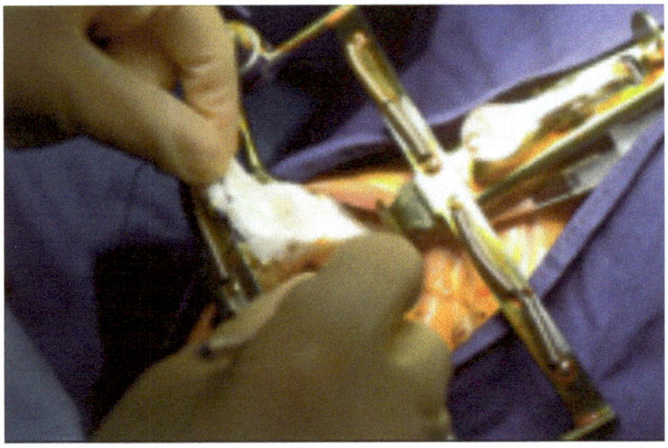

**Fig. 9.4** Throat pack insertion

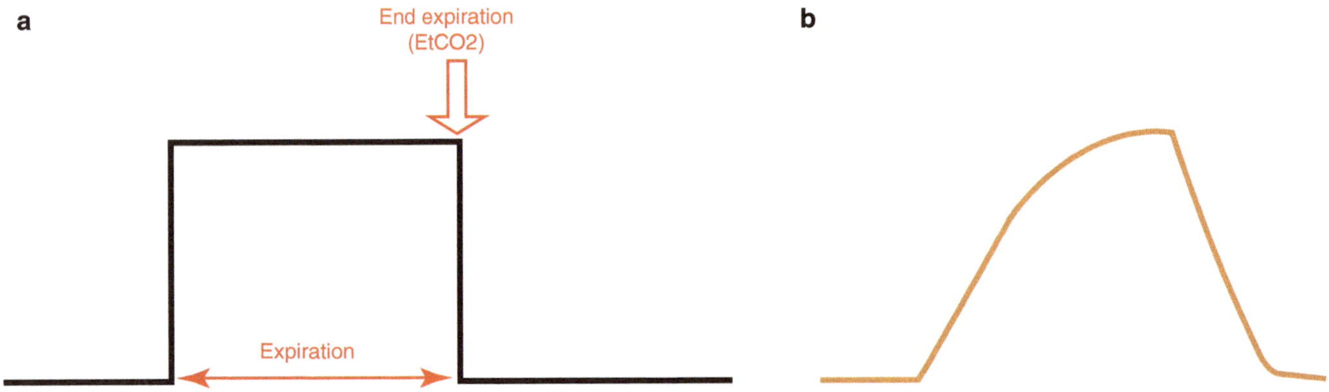


**Fig. 9.5** Normal capnography pattern (**a**) and obstructive pattern (**b**) after DG placement

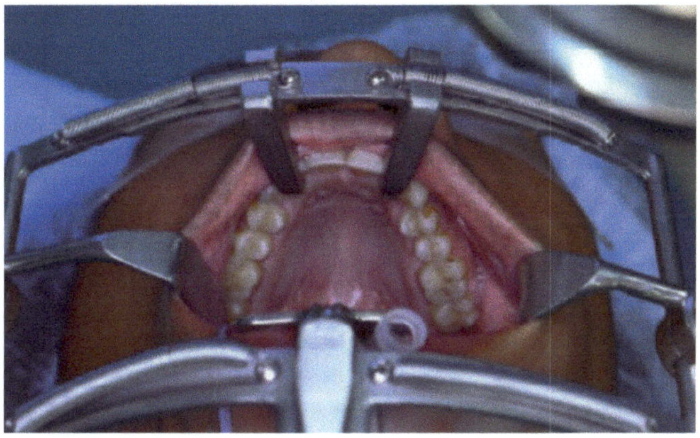

**Fig. 9.6** A needle cap is placed between the Dingman blade and the lower teeth to avoid ETT compression

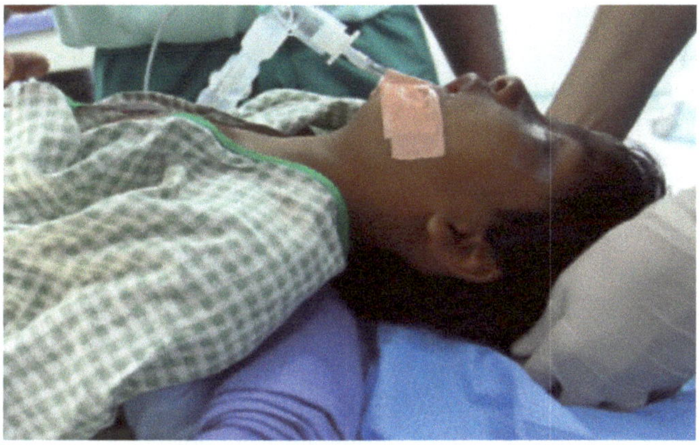

**Fig. 9.7** Shoulder roll placement during cervical extension

extubation may be due different factors (swelling, inadequate mouth breathing, laryngospasm, retained throat pack, blood clot, etc.). A short period of continuous positive airway pressure (CPAP) may be sufficient as may be turning the child lateral or prone. Nasopharyngeal airway (NPA) can provide a cleared airway and a route to perform suction. This device is well tolerated, and it should be placed in the nostril contralateral to the cleft defect. In patients at high risk of postoperative airway obstruction, the NPA may be inserted prior to extubation and removed the following day once swelling has subsided and the child has mastered mouth breathing. Oropharyngeal airways are not well tolerated and can cause damage of the surgical field. In our practice, a tongue stitch is placed at the end of all cleft palate repairs and kept overnight until there is little risk of airway obstruction (Fig. 9.8). Although reintubation is usually not necessary, all drugs and devices must be prepared to face this potential complication. All CLP patients should be observed closely during the early postoperative period. Ideally a specialized postoperative care unit with experienced medical and nursing staff is required.

As a last resort in the event of loss of airway, with inability to ventilate or reintubate, needle cricothyrotomy can be a lifesaving option to enable ventilation. The needle is inserted

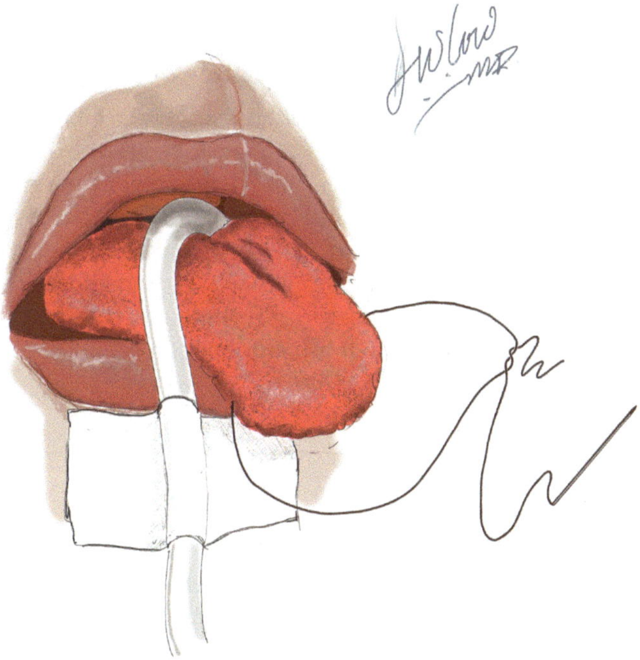

**Fig. 9.8** Use of tongue stitch in a case of postoperative airway obstruction after CP surgery

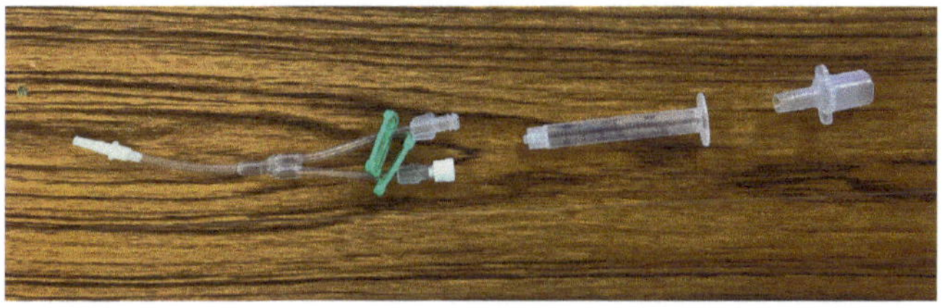

**Fig. 9.9** Needle cricothyrotomy device can be improvised using a 14 gauge angiocatheter or hypodermic needle, attached to a peripheral IV Y-connector, to a 3 mL syringe with plunger removed, and to a size 7 endotracheal tube connector. (Courtesy of Marcelo Texiera, MD.)

through the skin and cricothyroid membrane in the midline of the neck, just below the thyroid cartilage ("Adam's apple"). Figure 9.9 shows a technique using supplies typically available in a low-resource setting.

**Key Tip: Upper Airway Obstruction After Extubation May Occur Due to Different Causes**

1. Critical reduction in size of a previously tenuous airway
2. Presence of the throat pack or a piece of gauze
3. Excessive sedation
4. Laryngeal edema due to a large ETT size or ETT movement
5. Tongue swelling secondary to vascular compression by the retractor
6. Laryngospasm

## Antibiotic Prophylaxis

Delayed healing and palate fistula formation are more common in wide cleft defects, poor surgical technique, and surgical site infection (SSI). CLP surgery can be classified as a clean contaminated case. It is known that antibiotic prophylaxis significantly reduces the risk of surgical site infection (SSI). Although antibiotic prophylaxis is generally recommended as a single preoperative dose, Aznar and colleagues showed that the use of postoperative antibiotic prophylaxis can reduce the incidence of fistulae after primary CP repair in a developing area.

## Anesthesia Technique

A craniofacial center with an interdisciplinary team would be ideal to manage CLP patients. This is not always available in many countries, so practice should be modified by experience and available facilities. Surgical repair under general anesthesia with endotracheal intubation is recommended, although cleft lip may be repaired under local anesthesia in older and cooperative patients.

In case of general anesthesia, either an intravenous or inhalation induction may be undertaken, depending on the age, intravenous access, and risk of difficult airway. Inhalation induction with a volatile agent (e.g., sevoflurane, halothane) in oxygen is a common practice; ketamine given intramuscularly or intravenously (1–2 mg/kg) is an alternative. Intravenous access should be obtained as soon as the child is asleep and face mask ventilation confirmed. A standard intravenous induction may be appropriate for older children or adults without anticipated difficult airway (e.g., propofol 2–3 mg/kg, thiopentone 3–5 mg/kg). When intubation is expected to be difficult, maintaining spontaneous ventilation is essential and is the safest approach.

Spontaneous ventilation alternated with intermittent manually assisted ventilation intervals is safer in the event of a disconnection or inadvertent extubation. Maintenance with inhalational anesthesia is more common. Intravenous ketamine boluses may also be given for maintenance (0.25 mg/kg/dose). Ketamine produces dissociative anesthesia and has the advantage of maintaining respiration and cough reflex. Disadvantages of ketamine include sialorrhea and emergence phenomena.

Existing fluid deficits and intraoperative losses are replaced with crystalloids. CP repairs have the potential risk for significant blood loss. Facilities for cross-matching and blood transfusion must be available.

Infiltration with a local anesthetic solution containing epinephrine 1:200.000 by the surgeon is a common practice at our institution in order to reduce blood loss.

Careful monitoring after surgery allows early detection of any airway obstruction or postoperative bleeding. Patients at particular risk should be cared for in an intensive care unit. Children may be reluctant to feed after surgery, and intravenous fluids should be continued until adequate oral intake is established.

## Intraoperative and Postoperative Pain Management

### General Consideration

Cleft surgery, especially CP repair, may cause significant pain up to 24–48 h postoperatively. Emergence agitation is also common after CLP surgery. A multimodal approach, using multiple analgesics with additive or synergistic effects as well as local and regional analgesia, is frequently used to maximize pain control while minimizing side effects of individual drugs or techniques. The emotional component of pain must also be addressed using instinctive comforting measures, distraction techniques, and non-pharmacological treatments to complement safe and effective use of analgesic drugs. A loading dose of rectal paracetamol (30–40 mg/kg) is recommended in infants and should be administered as early as possible after anesthesia induction. Intravenous paracetamol (15 mg/kg) is a good alternative when available. Metamizole or dipyrone has analgesic, spasmolytic, and antipyretic effects. The recommended IV dose is 20–40 mg/kg every 8 h. Due to the risk of agranulocytosis after long-term use, it is recommended for short-term use and in a hospital setting only. Ibuprofen is another alternative for perioperative pain management. It may be administered orally or IV at 10 mg/kg every 8 h.

Perioperative opioid analgesics have the advantage of promoting a smoother emergence with less crying, which may reduce swelling and bleeding from the surgical site. However, CP surgery is associated with a high risk of postoperative airway obstruction, which may be increased with administration of opioids. There is a justifiable concern about using opioids in infants with respect to postoperative sedation, respiratory depression, and consequent airway compromise.

### Regional Anesthesia in Cleft Surgery

#### Infraorbital Nerve Block

The infraorbital nerve is the terminal branch of the maxillary nerve and exits the skull through the infraorbital foramen. The foramen is located approximately 8 mm below the inferior orbital rim on a vertical line that passes through the mid-

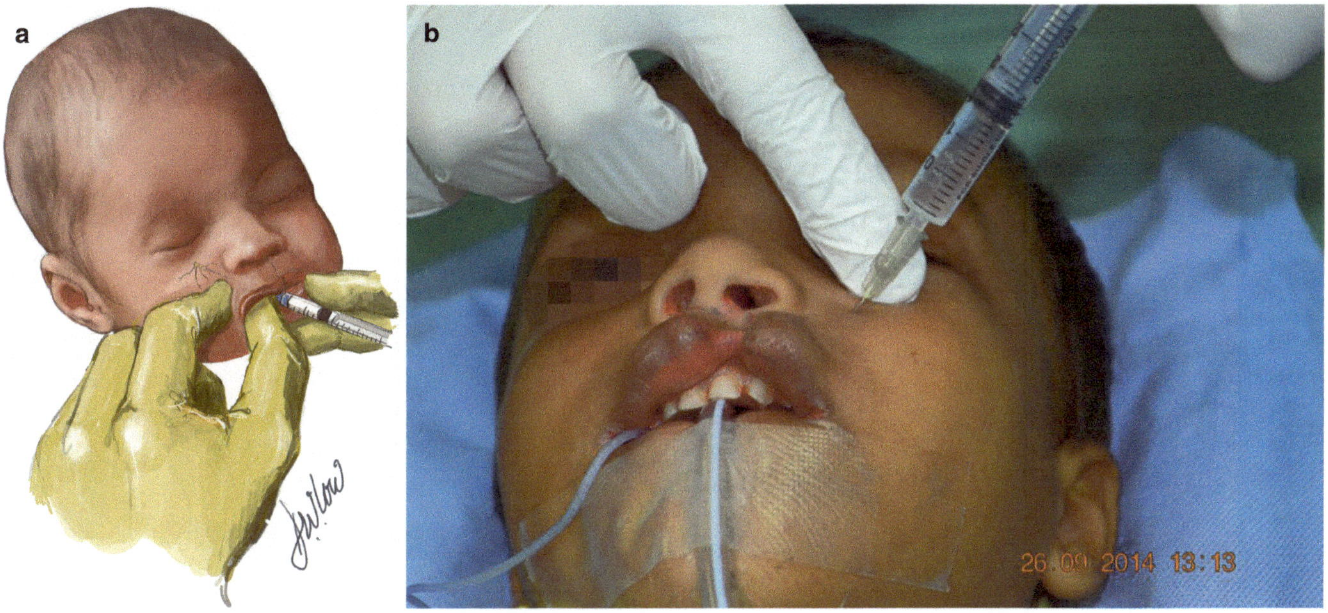


**Fig. 9.10** Infraorbital nerve block. Intraoral (left) and extraoral (right) approaches

point of pupil in adults (2–3 mm below the rim in infants). Two different approaches (intraoral and extraoral) have been described (Fig. 9.10). For the extraoral approach, the puncture site in infants is located at the midpoint of a line drawn between the mid-palpebral fissure and ipsilateral lip commissure, about 7.5 mm lateral to the ala of the nose. In adult patients, the puncture site is located at 7 mm lateral and 15 mm above the ala of the nose. It is our practice to orientate the needle at 45° angle in an inferior and medial direction to avoid entering the infraorbital foramen and to allow the local anesthetics to spread in the direction of the branches of the infraorbital nerve. Once bony contact with the maxilla is made and after negative aspiration, the local anesthetic is injected. Manual pressure may be applied to favor the caudal distribution of the local anesthetics. Digital pressure at the puncture site is maintained for about 2 min to minimize hematoma formation. For the intraoral approach, puncture point is in the sub-sulcal groove at the level of the canine or first premolar. Needle is oriented toward the infraorbital foramen, and, once the maxilla is contacted and after negative aspiration, the local anesthetic is injected. Manual pressure is also applied at the infraorbital foramen to favor the caudal distribution of the local anesthetic and to protect the orbital contents. For both techniques, a 27 G needle can be used, and 0.5–3 ml of local anesthetics is injected per side.

### Palatal Nerve Blocks

Sensory innervation of the posterior two-thirds of the palate is provided by the greater palatine nerves (GPN) and lesser palatal nerves (LPN), while nasopalatine nerve (NPN) supplies the anterior one-third. Palatal nerve block can be performed after patient positioning and once the Dingman retractor is in place. The GPN is blocked on the hard palate in the region of the greater palatine foramen (about 1 cm medial to the third upper molar) using a standard dental cross mouth injection technique. When dentition is not present, the injection is performed 0.5 cm anterior to the rear edge of the hard palate and 1 cm medial to the palatal aspect of the alveolar process. The needle should not be inserted into the greater palatine canal to avoid vascular pedicle injury. The LPN is blocked immediately posterior and lateral to the greater palatine foramen, generally at the midpoint between the rear edge of the hard palate and the pterygoid hamulus. The NPN is blocked by a single injection of local anesthetic in the incisive papilla at the level of the incisive foramen. In cases of complete CL and CP in which a nasopalatine foramen does not exist, local anesthetic solution is injected into the incisor on both sides of the slit pulp (Fig. 9.11).

### Bilateral Maxillary Nerve Block by Suprazygomatic Approach

The maxillary nerve leaves the skull through the foramen rotundum and passes through the pterygopalatine fossa (PPF) before entering the inferior orbital fissure, which the nerve traverses anteriorly, to finally reach the midface by the infraorbital foramen. Maxillary nerve is responsible for the sensory innervation of the midface, including the hard and soft palate, upper jaw, upper dental arch, and upper lip. The suprazygomatic maxillary nerve block approach may be performed with a 27 gauge 38 mm needle or a 22 G 50 mm needle in older children. Following aseptic preparation of the skin, the puncture site is at the frontozygomatic angle formed by the zygomatic arch and posterior orbital rim. After inserting the needle perpendicular to the skin and contacting the

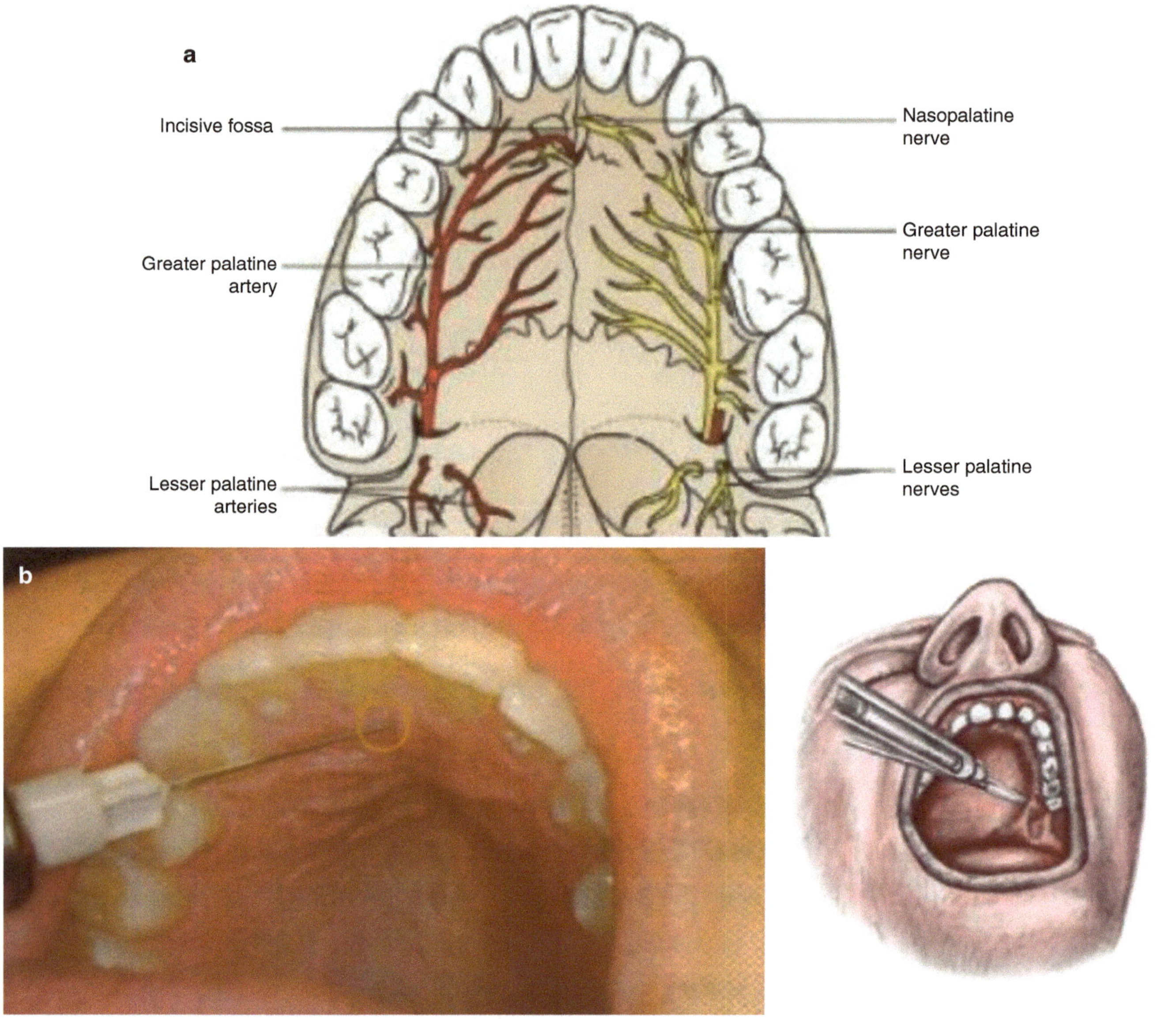


**Fig. 9.11** (**a**) Anatomy of palate innervation and vessels. (**b**) NPN block (left) and GPN and LPN blocks (right)

greater wing of the sphenoid (approximately 15–20 mm deep), the needle is partially withdrawn, reoriented toward "Cupid's bow" approximately 20° anterior and 10° inferior, and advanced to 35–38 mm depth to direct the needle into the pterygopalatine fossa (Fig. 9.12). Following a negative aspiration test, 0.15 ml/kg of local anesthetic is injected (maximum of 5 ml per side).

## Particular Considerations

### CL Repair

Ideally, CL repair should be done before 6 months of age. Presurgical infraorbital nerve block reduces or eliminates the need for narcotics. Postoperative pain control can be supplemented with acetaminophen.

### Primary CP repair

Ideally, CP should be repaired by about 12 months of age for speech reasons. Palatorrhaphy may require more than one surgery. Older patients might have wider defects with marked mucoperiosteal fibrosis increasing the risk of bleeding. CP repair is a painful procedure, and these patients may need high doses of opioids perioperatively. The ideal anesthetic plan should guarantee an emergence from anesthesia with the patient calm, without pain or PONV, and with complete recovery of the airway reflexes. Multimodal analgesic approach including narcotics and non-narcotic drugs as well as regional anesthesia can help ensure optimal pain control. Opioids can be used intraoperatively to smooth the hemodynamic response to endotracheal intubation and surgical pain. Fentanyl 1–2 mcg/kg, nalbuphine 100–200 mcg/kg, or morphine 50–100 mcg/kg has been used. Remifentanil (0.05–0.2 mcg/kg/min)

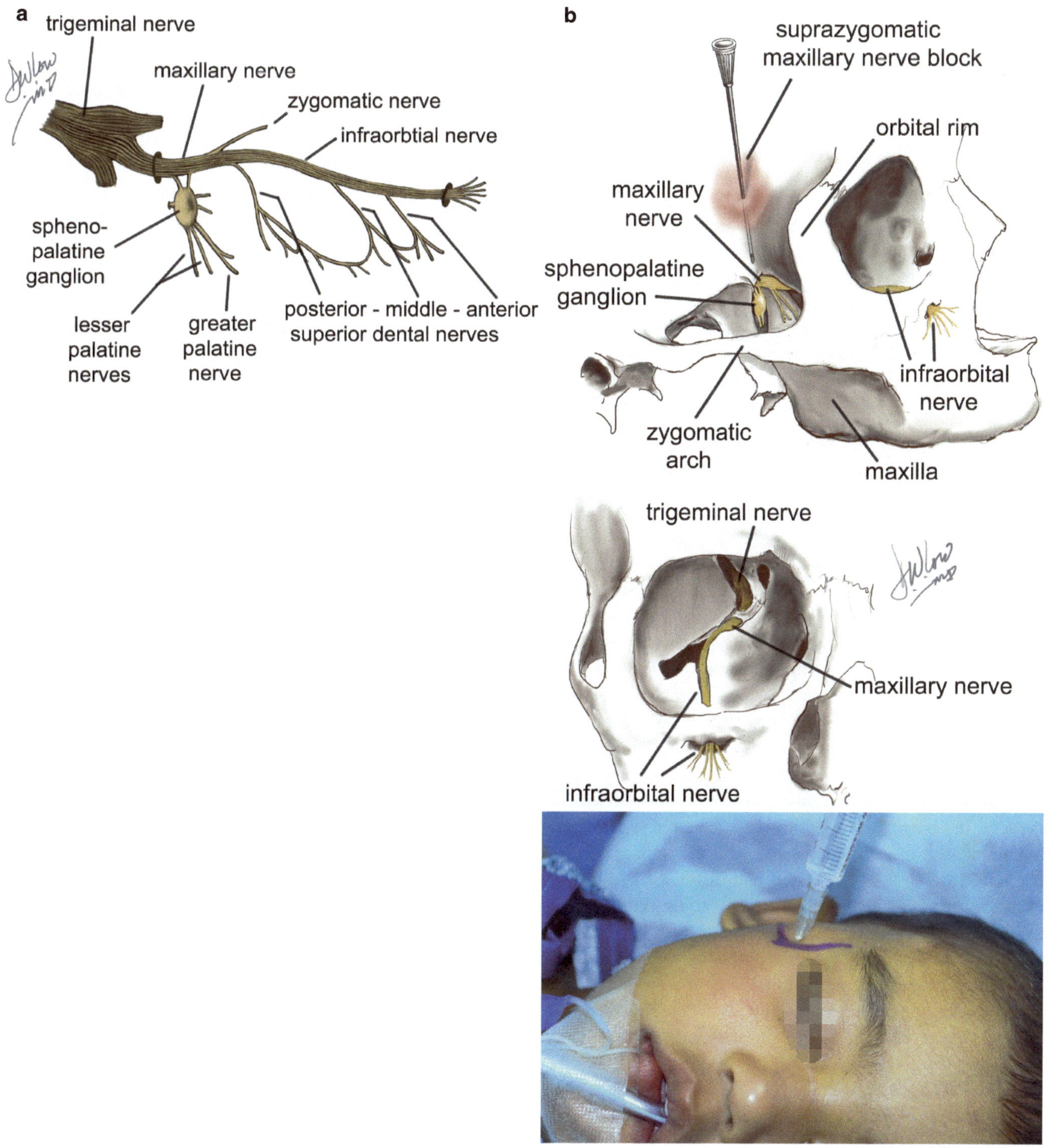


**Fig. 9.12** (**a**) Anatomy of maxillary nerve and its branches. (**b**) Maxillary nerve block by suprazygomatic approach

as continuous infusion has also been used for intraoperative pain management. Regional anesthesia options include different techniques such as local infiltration, palatal nerve block, or maxillary nerve block by suprazygomatic approach.

Use of intravenous clonidine (2–3 mcg/kg) or dexmedetomidine (0.5–1 mcg/kg) as adjuvant in perioperative anesthesia reduces opioid consumption and hypnotic medication. Alpha-2 agonists have analgesic, sedative, anti-shivering, and anti-emetic effects and have shown to reduce the incidence of emergence agitation. Moreover, they prolong the duration of the regional nerve blocks when administered as adjuvant of local anesthetics.

Postoperative nausea and vomiting prophylaxis is also recommended.

High dose of dexamethasone 0.2–0.4 mg/ kg at the time of induction is useful as an analgesic adjuvant and to reduce swelling and PONV.

Tranexamic acid (10–15 mg/kg) has been used to reduce or treat perioperative bleeding.

### Secondary CP Repair

CP revision and closure of oronasal fistulae (ONF): ONF may remain after primary palatoplasty. One approach to repair the ONF is to reopen the palate around the fistulous path, debride the tissues, and make a new closure by planes. Anesthesia considerations are similar to the primary CP repair with an increased risk of bleeding. Antifibrinolytics may be useful, considering the risk of bleeding when dissecting fibrous tissues with high fibrinolytic activity.

Another surgical option for ONF is to perform a tongue flap division, in which a flap is taken from the dorsum of the tongue and sutured to the CP fistulae. Postoperative airway obstruction may be expected since the flap will limit the mouth opening and an oropharyngeal airway cannot be used. Careful extubation with scrupulous hemostasis is mandatory, and extubation should be performed with utmost care and with the presence of the surgeon in the OR, in case of airway obstruction that cannot be solved by face mask ventilation. In this scenario, advanced airway management is impossible by conventional laryngoscopy or even videolaryngoscopy. The immediate technical resources would be a Bonfils retromolar laryngoscope or a flexible fibrobronchoscopy intubation. In both cases, it is required to be very skilled with the devices. In case of failure of this plan, the rapid separation of the tongue flap must be considered. This is a quick procedure but with high risk of aspiration and difficult laryngoscopy due to bleeding. Emergency tracheotomy kit must be available.

A second surgery is required to perform the division of the flap from the tongue. Evaluation of the airway may be difficult. The anesthetic considerations are similar to the previously described, but in this case, it will be an elective situation.

Velopharyngeal insufficiency (VPI) is a common complication after primary palatoplasty. Surgical options to solve the VPI include one of the following procedures, based on a multimodal evaluation: Furlow palatoplasty (double-opposing Z-plasty), overlapping intravelar veloplasty with oral Z-plasty, pharyngeal flap, and sphincter pharyngoplasty. Anesthesia considerations are similar to those for primary CP repair. However, these procedures involve an important modification of the airway anatomy, especially on the soft palate and nasopharynx. Postoperative airway obstruction must be expected, and a special management should be planned in case the patient with a pharyngeal flap requires a nasotracheal intubation for future procedures. Therefore, there should be a complete medical history, with detailed surgical description and report of clinical findings including preoperative nasal endoscopy. A detailed discussion with the surgeon is necessary for the best airway approach (nasal intubation, submentonian intubation, etc.).

### Alveolar Bone Graft Surgery

This surgery adds bone to the alveolar gum ridge and is usually performed at the age of 7–9 years. Bone is typically harvested from the anterior part of the iliac crest. Acute pain following iliac crest bone graft is common and multifactorial, and a multimodal analgesic approach is recommended. Ipsilateral ultrasound-guided transversus abdominis plane (TAP) block +/− subcutaneous field infiltration provides good pain control.

### Secondary Correction of Nasal Deformities in CLP Patients: Open Rhinoplasty

This surgery is usually performed around the age of 18 years old. It is a painful procedure, and a multimodal analgesic approach is necessary. Local anesthetic infiltration by the surgeon, infraorbital nerve block, or maxillary nerve block by suprazygomatic approach can be used. Intraoperative permissive and induced hypotension anesthesia approach may be required to reduce bleeding. High dose of dexamethasone 0.2–0.4 mg/ kg at the time of induction is usually given to reduce pain, inflammation, swelling, and PONV. Postoperative nausea and vomiting prophylaxis (dexamethasone, ondansetron). Tranexamic acid (10–15 mg/kg) has been used to reduce or treat perioperative bleeding.

### Orthognathic Surgery

This procedure is usually performed around the age of 18 years old. Specialized maxillofacial surgeons and technical resources are needed. The type of endotracheal intubation must be discussed with the surgeon (nasotracheal, orotracheal, and submentonian intubation). Securing the ETT and connections is critical. A rescue protocol of the airway should be previously discussed in case of damage or rupture of the endotracheal tube during surgery. Special attention should be paid to the medical history to rule out the presence of velopharyngeal flap (anesthesia consideration previously discussed). These are usually long procedures (careful patient positioning, securing IV access, prevention and correction of hypothermia).

Postoperative pain may be an important concern and a multimodal pain management is required. Local anesthetic infiltration with epinephrine by surgeons is usually performed. Regional anesthesia techniques such as maxillary nerve block for Lefort 1 osteotomy or a combination of maxillary nerve block and mandibular nerve block can be used. These surgeries have a *high risk of bleeding*. Different anesthesia techniques that guarantee a fast and safe control of the patient's cardiovascular conditions have been used (TIVA,

**Table 9.3** General recommendations for local anesthetic doses

| Drug | Onset of effect (min) | Duration without epinephrine (min) | Duration with epinephrine (min) | Maxim dose without epinephrine | Maxim dose with epinephrine |
|---|---|---|---|---|---|
| Lidocaine | 10–20 | 30–120 | 60–400 | 5 mg/kg | 7 mg/kg |
| Bupivacaine | 15–30 | 120–240 | 240–480 | 2.5 mg/kg | 3.2 mg/kg |
| Mepivacaine | 10–20 | 30–120 | 30–120 | 4.5 mg/kg | 7 mg/kg |
| Ropivacaine | 15–30 | 180–720 | 240–720 | 2–3 mg/kg | 3–4 mg/kg |

TIVA-TCI, alpha-two agonists, short-lived narcotics, etc.). Carefully manage fluids and electrolyte balance. *Intraoperative permissive or induced hypotension anesthesia approach as well as prophylaxis of hyperfibrinolysis has been used. Tranexamic acid 10–20 mg/kg is used as the loading dose after induction of anesthesia followed by 10 mg/kg/h as continuous infusion. Blood products must be available.*

*Posterior pharyngeal swelling may occur and prolonged intubation may be necessary.* High dose of dexamethasone 0.5–1 mg/ kg after anesthesia induction. Postoperative nausea and vomiting prophylaxis.

Postoperative care protocols must be strict in the management of pain, PONV, bleeding, airway compromise, infection control, etc. Conventionally various types of tooth-mounted devices like arch bars, dental and interdental wiring, and metallic and nonmetallic splints are used to achieve intermaxillary fixation. The current tendency is to use nonmetallic material for fixation. In any case, the patient must keep at the head the necessary instruments to immediately remove the intermaxillary fixation in case of an emergency (Table 9.3).

## Conclusion

- Preoperative evaluation is particularly important to rule out associated medical conditions or syndromes related with cleft defects. Airway and cardiac assessment are some of the most relevant considerations.
- Life-threatening complications may occur during the perioperative period.
- Good team communication is essential throughout the entire perioperative period in order to avoid complications and to improve outcomes.

## Bibliography


1. Kempthorne P. The WFSA global anesthesia workforce survey. Anesth Analg. 2017;125:981–90.
2. Weiser TG, et al. An estimation of the global volume of surgery: a modeling strategy based on available data. The Lancet. 2008;372(9633):139–44.
3. Funk LM, et al. Global operating theatre distribution and pulse oximetry supply: an estimation from reported data. Lancet. 2010;376:1055–61.
4. Hadler RA, et al. Anesthesia care capacity at health facilities in 22 low- and middle-income countries. World J Surg. 2016;40(5):1025–33.
5. Higashi H, Barendregt JJ, Kassebaum NJ, Weiser TG, Bickler SW, Vos T. The burden of selected congenital anomalies amenable to surgery in low and middle-income regions: cleft lip and palate, congenital heart anomalies and neural tube defects. Arch Dis Child. 2015;100(3):233–8. https://doi.org/10.1136/archdischild-2014-306175. Epub 2014 Sep 26. PMID: 25260520.
6. Carlson L. A model of the unmet need for cleft lip and palate surgery in low- and middle-income countries. World J Surg. 2016;40:2857–67.
7. Mukhopadhyay S, Ojomo K, Nyberger K, G. Meara J. Lancet Commission on Global Surgery, Iran J Pediatr. 2017;27(4):e11273. https://doi.org/10.5812/ijp.11273.
8. Meara JG, et al. Global surgery 2030: evidence and solutions for achieving health, welfare, and economic development. Lancet. 2015;386(9993):569–624.
9. Adrian WG, et al. World Health Organization-World Federation of Societies of Anaesthesiologists (WHO-WFSA) international standards for a safe practice of anesthesia. Anesth Analg. 2018;126(6):2047.
10. Kempthorne P, et al. The WFSA global anesthesia workforce survey. Anesth Analg. 2017;125(3):981–90.
11. Nickerson J, et al. Access to controlled medicines for anesthesia and surgical care in low-income countries: a narrative review of international drug control systems and policies. Can J Anesth. 2017;64:296–307.
12. Mukhopadhyay S, et al. Lancet commission on global surgery. Iran J Pediatr. 2017;27(4):e11273.
13. de Beer DAH. The Universal Anaesthesia Machine (UAM): assessment of a new anesthesia workstation built with global health in mind. Anesthesia. 2016;72(4):444–51.
14. Spritz RA. The genetics and epigenetics of orofacial clefts. Curr Opin Pediatr. 2001;13(6):556–60.
15. Milerad J, Larson O, Hagberg C, Ideberg M. Associated malformations in infants with cleft lip and palate: a prospective, population-based study. Pediatrics. 1997;100(2Pt1):180–6.
16. Gunawardana RH. Difficult laryngoscopy in cleft lip and palate surgery. Br J Anaesth. 1996;76(6):757–9.
17. Dubreuil M, Ecoffey C. Laryngeal mask guided tracheal intubation in paediatric anaesthesia. Paediatr Anaesth. 1992;2:344.
18. Bosenberg AT, Kimble FW. Infraorbital nerve block in neonates for cleft lip repair: anatomical study and clinical application. Br J Anaesth. 1995;74(5):506–8.
19. Mesnil M, Dadure C, Captier G, Raux O, Rochette A, Canaud N, et al. A new approach for perioperative analgesia of cleft palate repair in infants: the bilateral suprazygomatic maxillary nerve block. Paediatr Anaesth. 2010;20:343–9.
20. Captier G, Dadure C, Leboucq N, Sagintaah M, Canaud N. Anatomic study using three-dimensional computed tomographic scan measurement for truncal maxillary nerve blocks via the suprazygomatic route in infants. J Craniofac Surg. 2009;20:224–8.
21. Chiono J, Raux O, Bringuier S, Sola C, Bigorre M, Capdevila X, et al. Bilateral suprazygomatic maxillary nerve block for cleft palate repair in children: a prospective, randomized, double-blind study versus placebo. Anesthesiology. 2014;120:1362–9.
22. Anderson B. Acetaminophen analgesia in infants. Anesth Analg. 2001;93(6):1626–7.
23. Roulleau P, Gall O, Desjeux L, Dagher C, Murat I. Remifentanil infusion for cleft palate surgery in young infants. Paediatr Anaesth. 2003;13(8):701–7.
24. Antony AK, Sloan GM. Airway obstruction following palatoplasty: analysis of 247 consecutive operations. Cleft Palate Craniofac J. 2002;39(2):145–8.
25. Bell CN, Macintyre DR, Ross JW, Pigott RW, Weller RM. Pharyngoplasty: a hazard for nasotracheal intubation. Br J Oral Maxillofac Surg. 1986;24(3):212–6.

26. Liao YF, Noordhoff MS, Huang CS. Comparison of obstructive sleep apnea syndrome in children with cleft palate following Furlow palatoplasty or pharyngeal flap for velopharyngeal insufficiency. Cleft Palate Craniofac J. 2004;41(2):152–6.
27. Habel A, Sell D, Mars M. Management of cleft lip and palate. Arch Dis Child. 1996;74(4):360–6.
28. Sommerlad BC. Management of cleft lip and palate. Curr Paediatr. 2002;12:43–50.
29. Frawley G, Espenell A, Howe P, et al. Anesthetic implications of infants with mandibular hypoplasia treated with mandibular distraction osteogenesis. Paediatr Anaesth. 2013;23(4):342–8.
30. Hosking J, Zoanetti D, Carlyle A, et al. Anesthesia for Treacher Collins syndrome: a review of airway management in 240 pediatric cases. Paediatr Anaesth. 2012;22(8):752–8.
31. Augsornwan D, Pattangtanang P, Pikhunthod K, et al. Postoperative pain in patients with cleft lip and palate in Srinagarind Hospital. Med Assoc Thai. 2011;94 Suppl 6:S118–23.
32. Aznar ML, Schönmeyr B, Echaniz G, et al. Role of postoperative antimicrobials in cleft palate surgery: prospective, double-blind, randomized, placebo-controlled clinical study in India. Plast Reconstr Surg. 2015;136(1):59e–66e.

# Principles of Cleft Lip Repair

# 10

Sashank K. Reddy, Nima Khavanian,
Kusezweni Kevin Nduku, and Richard J. Redett III

**Key Points**

- With the use of contemporary techniques in cleft lip repair, careful planning and skillful execution can yield excellent results, even in the most challenging of cases.
- The unilateral and bilateral cleft lip and nasal deformities result in a predictable series of anatomic differences involving the skin, muscle, mucosa, and bony/cartilaginous framework that must be addressed at the time of repair.
- Presurgical orthopedics or lip adhesions can be used to reduce a wide cleft and better align the bony/cartilaginous framework prior to repair.
- Timing of cleft lip repair varies by center from as early as several days after birth to 3 or 4 months of age. The "rule of 10s" serves as a reasonable guideline for when a child can safely undergo surgery.
- Excellent results can be achieved with all commonly used methods of cleft lip repair, including rotation advancement and anatomic subunit approaches.
- Surgeons vary with regard to the extent to which they address the cleft nasal deformity at the time of lip repair. Commonly addressed issues include nostril size and alar shape and positioning.
- Anticipating secondary deformities may enable the cleft surgeon to minimize the need for secondary revision. Nonetheless, patients will occasionally require revisions, and the decision to undergo secondary surgery and its timing are often based on patient, family, and surgeon preferences.

## Introduction

Care of the patient with cleft lip is among the most challenging and rewarding problems in plastic surgery. Achieving a functional, aesthetically pleasing primary repair profoundly benefits child and family. By contrast, errors introduced early are hard to overcome, as scar burden and decreased developmental plasticity mitigate against ideal results. With contemporary repair techniques and presurgical orthopedics, even patients with severe deformities can obtain near-anatomic restoration. Excellent results can be achieved with a variety of methods, but certain elements of diagnosis, planning, and skillful execution are invariant. It is these principles that we highlight in this chapter – aesthetic considerations in diagnosis and surgical planning, presurgical care and timing of repair, and marrying appropriate technique to anatomical substrate. Our hope is that attention to these principles can yield more effective and lasting outcomes for surgeons and our smallest patients.

## Aesthetics and Functional Considerations

Cleft lip and nasal deformities disrupt facial harmony because they fall in the most visually central and projecting portion of the patient's face. Even subtle distortions in these features are readily noticed. Below we describe features of the aesthetically pleasing nose and lips and how these are altered by facial clefting. We further describe methods to analyze cleft lip nasal deformities so that an adequate framework is established to formulate repair.

Aesthetics of the nose and lip should be considered together when planning repairs. Except in the most subtle microform cleft lips, a noticeable component of nasal deformity is present in patients with cleft. The aesthetically pleasing infant nose is centrally placed in the face within the second horizontal third and third vertical fifth (Fig. 10.1). The pleasing nose is symmetric, with soft contours between

S. K. Reddy · N. Khavanian · R. J. Redett III (✉)
Department of Plastic and Reconstructive Surgery, Johns Hopkins School of Medicine, Baltimore, MD, USA
e-mail: rjr@jhmi.edu

K. K. Nduku
Department of Plastic and Reconstructive Surgery, University of Zimbabwe, Harare, Zimbabwe

© Springer Nature Switzerland AG 2021

J. W. Swanson, D. W. Low (eds.), *Global Cleft Care in Low-Resource Settings*, https://doi.org/10.1007/978-3-030-59105-2_10

its constituent subunits and preservation of symmetry. On anteroposterior view, the tip is not excessively wide. On lateral view, the infant nose will have a gradual and soft slope toward the tip without a prominent supratip break. Worm's eye view reveals a nearly equilateral triangle formed by the nasal base and ala. The alae themselves are oval and can be more horizontally oriented than they are in adults. The columella and septum are straight with adequate length to ensure good tip projection.

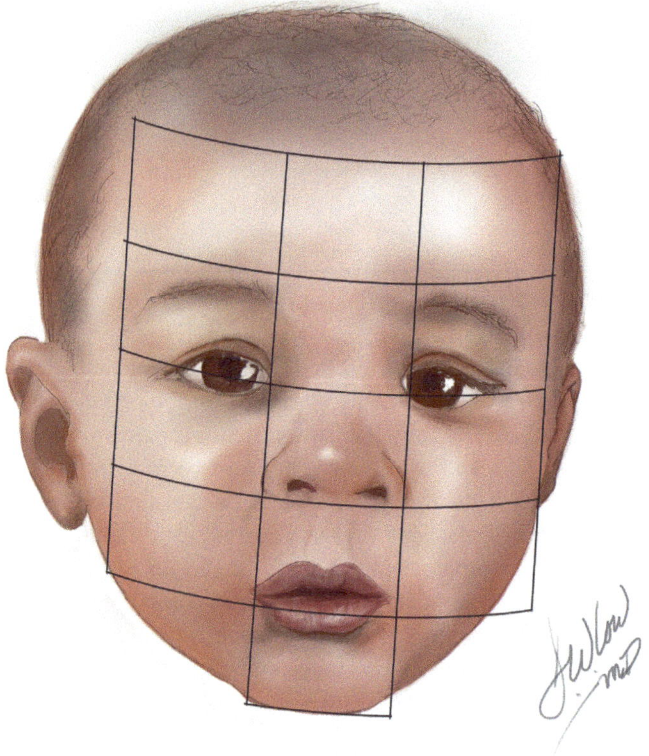

**Fig. 10.1** Normal face

In patients with unilateral or bilateral cleft nasal deformity, a number of departures from this aesthetic ideal are present. Unilateral patients display asymmetries with the bridge of the nose deviated to the cleft side and the tip deviated to the non-cleft side (Fig. 10.2). The septum may also be deviated to the cleft side. Abnormal widening of cleft-side ala is observed, and the affected side is deprojected as it falls onto the deficient pyriform of the cleft maxilla. Bilateral nasal deformities retain symmetry but present a number of further challenges due to the abnormally projecting premaxilla (Fig. 10.3). These patients have a short, wide columella. Both alae are excessively wide as is the poorly projecting tip. Careful noting of the types and degrees of nasal deformity present is critical to plan for nasal repair at the time of the initial operation and throughout the arc of the patient's care.

Aesthetically pleasing upper lips result from symmetry and proportionality of disparate anatomic elements. The most prominent portions of the cutaneous lip are the philtral columns. These ridges arise from the inner ala and diverge gently as they extend down in equal length to terminate in the peaks of Cupid's bow. Between the philtral columns, the philtral dimple is not excessively wide. The white roll of non-hair-bearing skin marks the boundary between the cutaneous and vermillion lip. It proceeds in a smooth line paralleling the vermillion with no step-offs or discontinuities. The

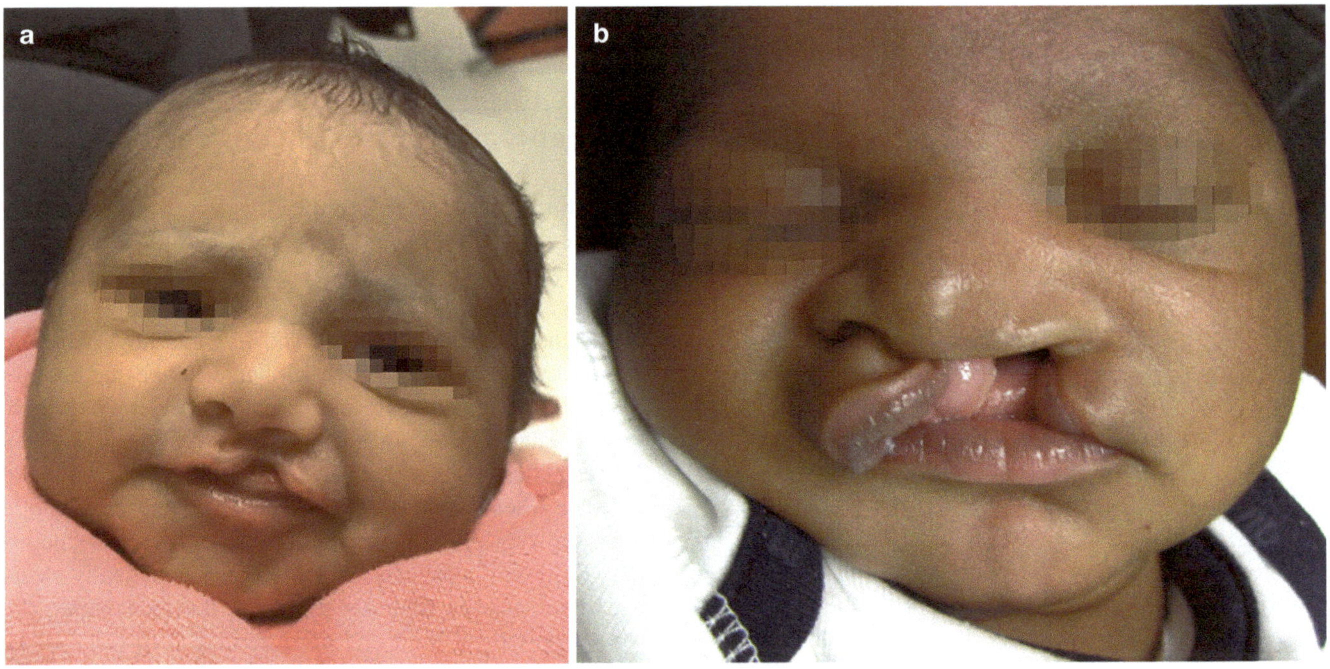


**Fig. 10.2** Child with a unilateral cleft lip: (**a**) incomplete and (**b**) complete

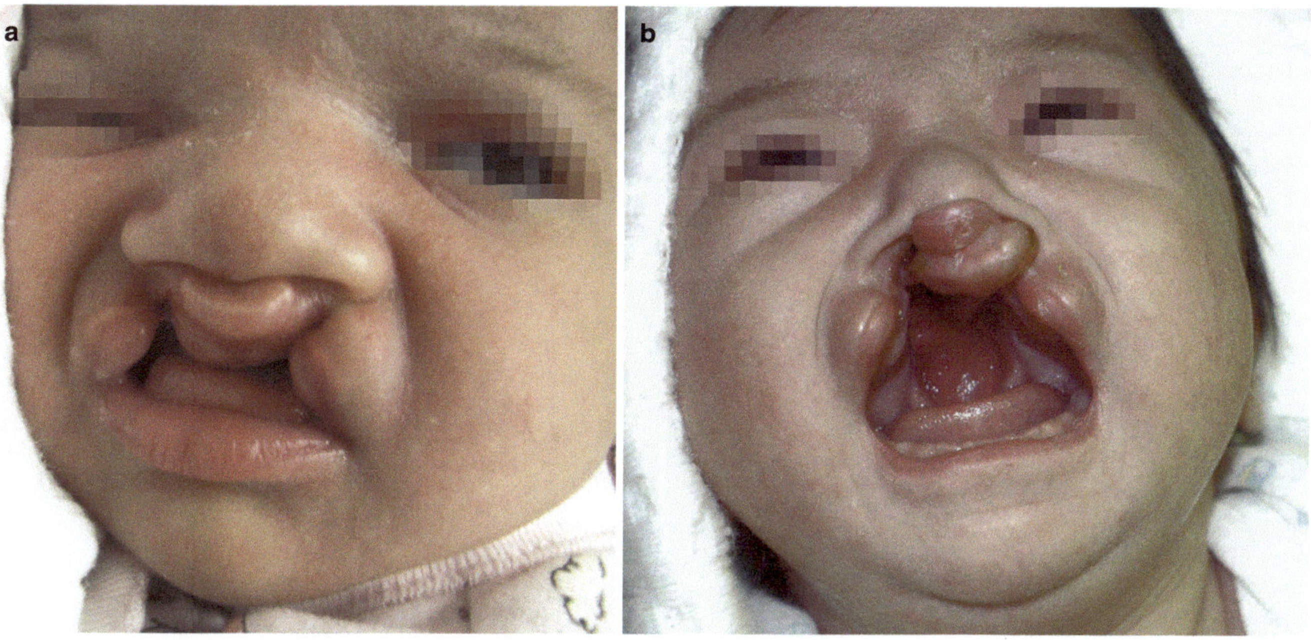

Fig. 10.3 Child with a bilateral cleft lip: (a) incomplete and (b) complete

vermillion lip is marked by wet and dry components with the wet, mucosal portion extending into the oral cavity.

Cleft lips suffer varying degrees of distortion in these elements. In unilateral cleft lips (uCL), they range from microform variants demarcated by a mere notch in the vermillion cutaneous junction to wide complete cleft lips with major nasal deformities and large alveolar clefts. All but microform variants have a marked discontinuity in Cupid's bow. The cleft-side philtral column is shorter. Both the medial and lateral lip elements are canted upward as one looks medially from the commissures. In very wide unilateral cleft lips, the lateral lip element can be short (Fig. 10.2). Bilateral cleft lips (bCL) are characterized by an often short prolabium with no true philtral columns. In severe cases, the premaxillary element protrudes at a nearly right angle to the vertical plane of the face with wide nasoalveolar gaps on either side (Fig. 10.4).

In addition to analyzing the aesthetic subunits of the lip and nose, careful attention has to be paid to constituent tissue types. The situation is analogous to nasal reconstruction in which one plans to restore lining, support, and cover. Similarly, in lip repair, one must pay attention to mucosa, orbicularis oris muscle, and cutaneous/vermillion cover. These components can be variously missing or malpositioned during cleft development. Failure to properly release and restore these components can have functional consequences later in life. In unilateral cleft lips, the orbicularis oris muscle originating on the non-cleft side does not typically terminate below Cupid's bow peak as one might expect. Rather it extends and attaches to the base of the nose. Similarly, the lateral orbicularis elements are tethered to the alar base obliterating the physiologic "empty triangle" between the alar base and orbicularis on animation. Release of these developmentally abnormal attachments is necessary to get rotation and lengthening of both the cleft and non-cleft sides and to allow tension-free repair of the orbicularis muscle. Additionally, sutures placed to affect this repair must span the orbicularis only and not extend to the overlying skin to avoid dimpling when the patient subsequently smiles. Crusting and chapping of the lip can result from extending the wet mucosa into the normal domain of the dry vermillion.

## Timing of Repair, Nasoalveolar Molding, and Lip Adhesion

Determining the timing of definitive lip repair begins with a consideration of procedures to optimize cleft geometry. Presurgical orthopedics with nasoalveolar molding (NAM) or cleft lip adhesion serve to decrease cleft width and to place the lip and nose onto a better aligned bony framework. There is a paucity of literature directly comparing long-term results with these two modalities; however, both techniques may be cost-effective and offer distinct advantages [1, 2]. Improvements have been noted with both techniques in intersegment distance; nasoalveolar molding more effectively addresses nasal height and columella height at the cost of a higher burden of care on families and providers [3–5]. Outcome studies have demonstrated improvement in aesthetic and functional outcomes, with possible improvements in speech and feeding as well [6–10]. Dec et al. have demonstrated lower oronasal fis-

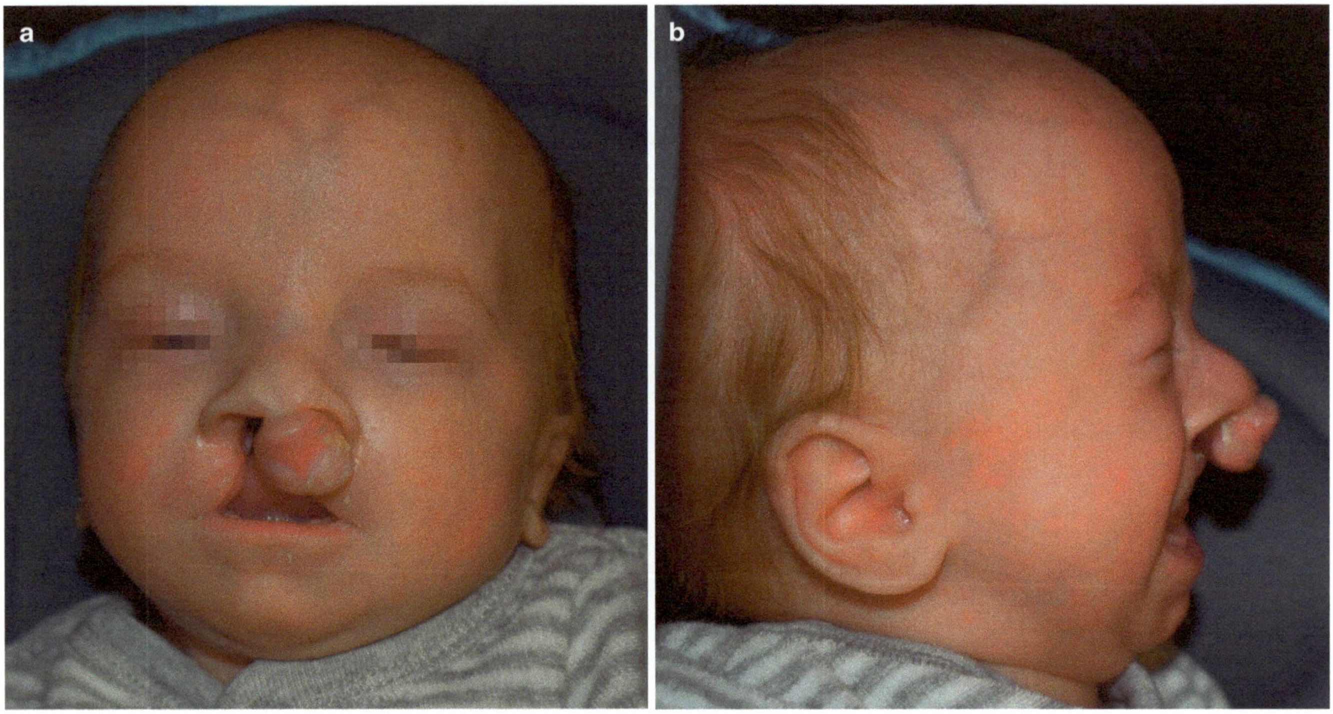


Fig. 10.4 Severely protruding premaxilla in patient with a bilateral cleft lip

tula rates in cleft lip and palate patients treated with preoperative nasoalveolar molding [11]. Although the best results are obtained in children who undergo molding before 1 month of age, improvements may be obtainable up to an age of 1 year or more [5]. In settings where NAM is available, we recommend considering this modality for children with complete cleft lip. If nasoalveolar molding is not available, a cleft lip adhesion can be performed.

## Cleft Lip Adhesion

Cleft lip adhesion essentially converts a wide complete cleft lip to an incomplete cleft lip, thereby narrowing the alveolar cleft and reducing the tension of the final repair. In many centers, lip adhesion is employed for two patient groups: (1) patients with wide cleft lips with splayed alveolar segments (uCL) or premaxilla (bCL) in which high tension is expected after primary repair and (2) patients with medical comorbidities with expected wound healing difficulty.

Cleft lip adhesion is performed under general anesthesia and typically at 3–6 months of age. It is undertaken early in this window when there is concern for increasing splay and widening of alveolar segments and occasionally later if need be delayed for medical comorbidities (e.g., cardiac anomalies that prevent earlier surgery) or delayed patient presentation. Key principles of cleft lip adhesion are described in Table 10.1 and shown in Fig. 10.5.

Table 10.1 Key principles of cleft lip adhesion

| |
|---|
| Incisions are made through the skin, muscle, and mucosal layers to enable their apposition |
| Incisions are optimally made in tissue that will be subsequently discarded in the definitive lip repair, to minimize additional scarring. This generally means along the cleft margins |
| Undermining is kept to a minimum to reduce scarring and impaired tissue perfusion |
| The orbicularis oris muscle layer provides the greatest tissue strength, and approximating this layer generally gives the most durable repair in a wide cleft |
| Many surgeons attempt to independently repair all three tissue layers: skin, muscle, and mucosa |
| Longer-lasting suture material (e.g., polydioxanone (PDS)) can be utilized, as the incisional scar is typically excised at definitive lip repair |

## Timing of Definitive Repair

Definitive cleft lip repair can be accomplished at any point when the child is old enough to tolerate anesthesia. Historically, surgeons have been guided by the "rule of 10s" for patients with clefts to undergo surgery: 10 pounds of weight, 10 weeks of age, and 10 g/dL hemoglobin. A recent study based on US patients has questioned whether this traditional mantra is still followed or necessary [12]. Nonetheless, given the more limited anesthesia and resuscitative infrastructure in low-resource settings, the "rule of 10s" still provides a reasonable guide.

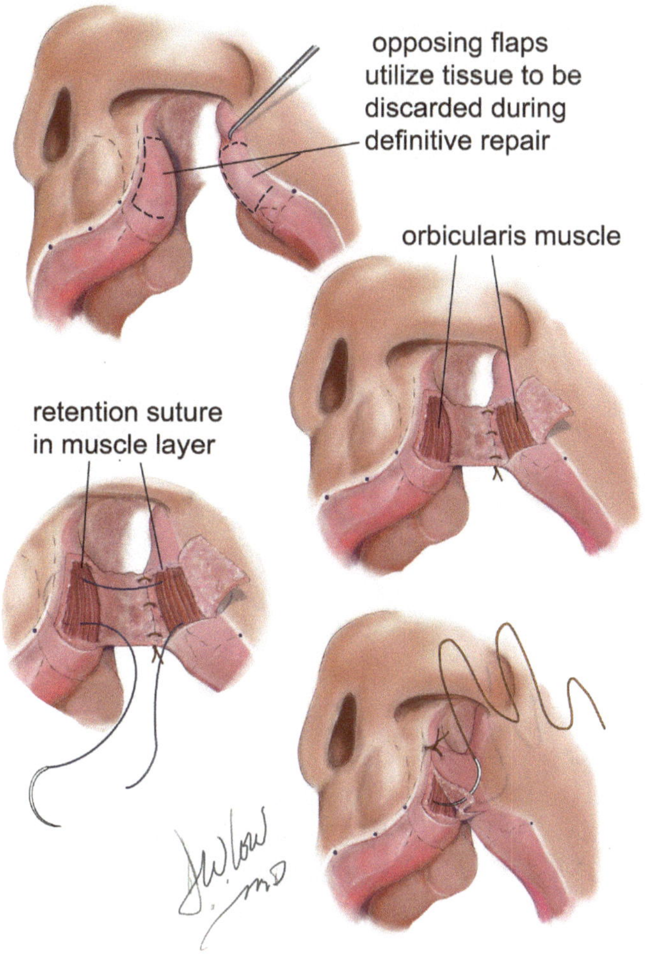


**Fig. 10.5** Cleft lip adhesion technique: incisions and tissue approximation

Generally, we perform repair around 3–4 months of age when tissues have adequate integrity to tolerate manipulation and suture placement but are still disposed to favorable scarring. Advocates of earlier repair at several days to 1 month of age point to potential improvements in scar appearance, ease of manipulating nasal tissues due to more malleable cartilage, and family satisfaction [13]. However, lip and nasal structures in very young infants are considerably smaller, placing greater demands on technical execution, and anesthesia and bleeding risks greater; thus this should be considered with caution in low-resource settings. We feel equivalent results can be obtained with skillful repair in the 3–6-month window commonly employed. A further benefit of waiting is the ability to incorporate presurgical remodeling with nasoalveolar molding or lip adhesion. These procedures may have a more marked impact on final outcomes than a 2-month head start, particularly for wider clefts. In patients with cleft lip and palate, accomplishing lip repair at 3–6 months also allows sufficient time for lip healing prior to palate surgery.

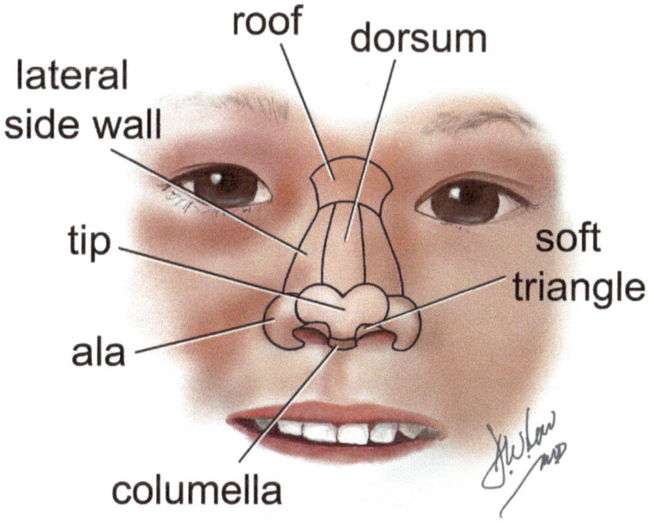


**Fig. 10.6** Anatomic subunits of the nose and lip

Finally, in settings where cleft surgery is only performed periodically, timing of needed future surgical procedures should be taken into account with surgical services offered. For a healthy 3-month-old girl with a cleft lip and palate, whose only access to care is during annual outreach missions, every effort should be made to repair her cleft lip so that she can undergo palate repair 1 year later at 15 months of age, which is when the ideal window for palatoplasty begins to close in order to obtain optimal speech outcomes. In all cases, suitability for surgery should be assessed in conjunction with anesthesiology and pediatric specialists.

## Technical Considerations

Excellent results can be achieved with all commonly used methods of cleft lip repair provided the surgeon employs meticulous technique and respects certain principles. General technical points are presented here with details of individual techniques reserved for subsequent chapters.

## Anatomic Subunits of the Nose and Lip

In planning repair of cleft lip nasal deformities, it is helpful to use the concept of anatomic subunits. First introduced by Burget and Menick in nasal reconstruction [14], the method entails division of facial features into their constituent subunits defined by natural points of contour transition (Fig. 10.6). In the nose, these subunits are the midline dorsum, tip, and columella as well as the sidewalls, ala, and soft triangles. Reconstructions are planned so that subunit boundaries are respected and when necessary recreated. Scars within subunits are avoided when possible. Reconstructions performed this way are more aesthetically pleasing because scars are placed at points where the beholder is expecting them and where natural shadows provide masking.

Subunits of the lip include the philtral columns, the cutaneous-vermillion junction or white roll, and the junction between the wet and dry vermillion [15]. Meticulous, contiguous, and symmetric restoration of these subunits is paramount. Step-offs or length discrepancies are readily perceived. As with nasal reconstruction, scar placement in lip repair should be along anatomic subunits when possible and avoid crossing them except where necessary such as in the vermilion. Modern methods of lip repair including modified Millard, Mohler, and Fisher techniques all place cutaneous scars along the perceived cleft-side philtral column. Of these approaches, the Fisher repair is perhaps the most exact in respecting the philtral column across its entire length. Although the Millard and Mohler repairs carry the cranial most portion of the cutaneous scar between the philtral columns to varying degrees, this also allows recruitment of more cutaneous tissue for rotation.

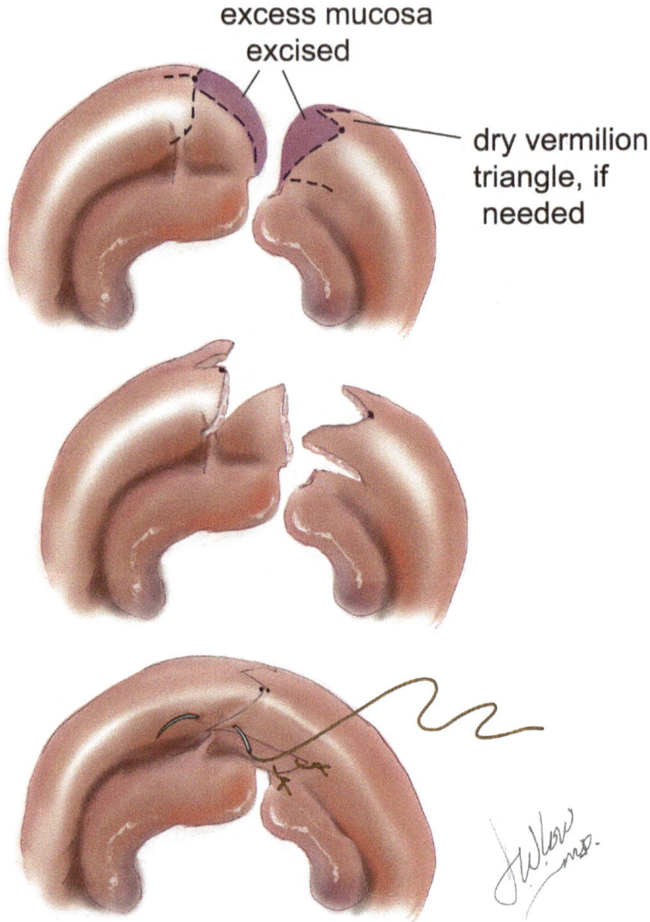


Fig. 10.7 Technique for mucosal-side closure in the rotation-advancement technique, to prevent excess mucosal bunching

## Cleft Severity and Tension of Repair

A further principle is to minimize tension across the repair. This can prove challenging in wide clefts and is greatly aided by presurgical orthopedics or lip adhesion. Increased tissue tension may play a role in the finding it is more difficult to obtain an optimal lip repair in lips that have a more severe cleft deformity [16]. In a borderline case, one school of thought is to use a lip adhesion, and another is to anticipate an early lip revision to address a widened scar or thinned muscle layer. In cases where this is not possible and the cleft remains wide, use of a technique such as the modified Millard or Mohler techniques provides greater reach by virtue of the backcut. To accomplish this using the Fisher anatomic subunit repair, one can move the position of the mark corresponding to Noordhoff's point to obtain greater length. Regardless of technique, more extensive dissection and mobilization is required in more severe clefts in order to adequately release and reposition tissue. Another technical refinement relates to closing of the mucosa. Rather than performing a straight-line closure to a point within the upper lip sulcus which can lead to bunching of the wet mucosa at the lip edge, we are careful to precisely measure and mark the mucosal distance, eliminating this excess tissue primarily (Fig. 10.7).

## Nasal Floor Repair

One aspect of cleft repair that deserves special consideration is the repair of the anterior nasal floor. The prevention of fistulas in the nasal floor or anterior palate following cleft repair is not a subject that is often discussed in the literature, although they are identified in up to 30–75% of cases. Some surgeons address this area at the time of cleft repair, whereas others delay it until the time of cleft palate repair or even at the time of alveolar bone grafting [17]. Those that defer correction argue that the use of local flaps at the time of lip repair may distort the tissues in the region and complicate subsequent operations. This delay however comes at the cost of more difficult visualization at the time of palate repair and the patient having to live with a symptomatic fistula, particularly if repair coincides with alveolar bone grafting.

Several techniques have been described in closing the anterior nasal floor with the details often varying between surgeons; in general flaps are elevated from either the medial and lateral lip elements, nasal lining, or mucoperiosteum. Two recent studies [17, 18] independently found relatively low fistula rates (3–8%) with the use of nasal lining flaps at the time of lip repair, with one group identifying a tenfold reduction in nasolabial fibulas. On the medial cleft side, nasal mucosa as a septal or vomer mucoperichondrial flap can be elevated off of the cartilaginous septum. On the lateral cleft side, nasal mucosa anterior and inferior to the inferior

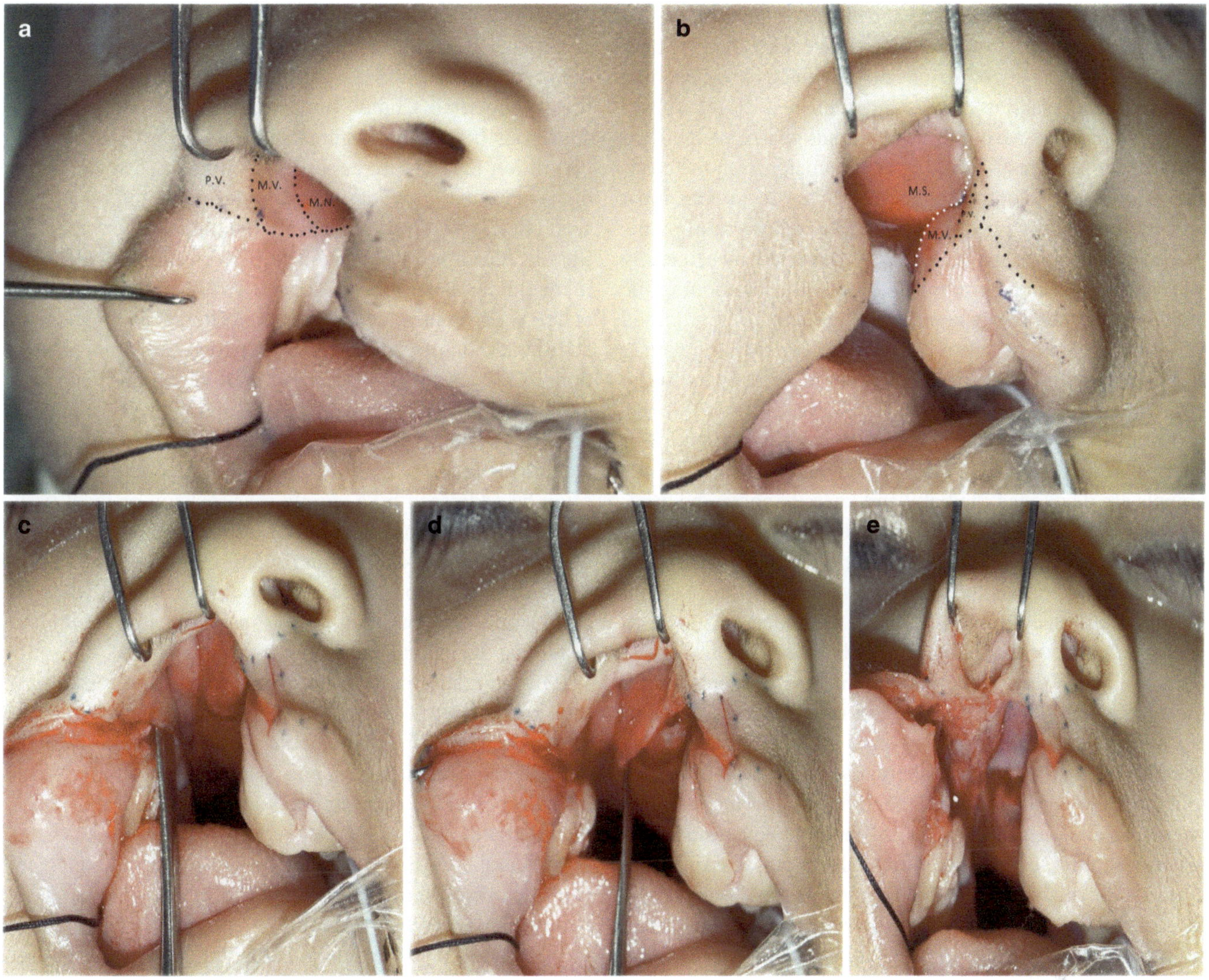


**Fig. 10.8** Lateral (**a**) and medial (**b**) nasal wall views show the vestibular mucosa (M.V.) and nasal mucosa (M.N.) which are each incorporated into the nasal flaps with undermining; the nasal skin (P.V.) is not. After mobilization of the lateral (**c**) and medial (**d**) flaps, they are approximated in the mid-nostril (**e**). (Photos and technique description courtesy of Edwar Alvarez, MD, and Moises Fernández, MD)

turbinate can be raised off of the piriformis as a mucoperiosteal flap (Fig. 10.8). These flaps are thick and well vascularized and can be approximated in the mid-nostril to recreate nasal floor. The flaps are generally dissected down to the junction of the nasal and oral mucosa. In bilateral clefts, an inferior strip of mucosa should be left on the vomer to prevent devascularizing the premaxilla. Nasal floor repair can be performed with any type of lip markings and can therefore be used with any skin repair technique.

## Rhinoplasty at Primary Lip Repair

Surgeons vary widely in the extent to which they perform nasal correction (rhinoplasty) at the time of primary lip repair [19–21]. Proponents of extensive primary intervention argue that the more malleable nasal cartilages allow for ready reshaping that is harder to achieve later. Furthermore, they rightly point to the psychosocial burden attending unaddressed nasal deformity as the child enters school. Factors favoring delay include the considerable growth and changes to nasal shape that occur from infancy to adulthood [22, 23]. Arguments that major manipulation disrupts nasal growth centers do not appear to be borne out by long-term data [20, 24–26]. However, it is difficult to adequately predict and account for this evolution in infancy. Extensive early repair carries more significant scar burden which can render subsequent modifications more challenging.

We favor a balanced approach with precise adjustments to nostril size and shape and position of the base of the ala at the time of primary repair, open-tip rhinoplasty at approximately age 6, and definitive septorhinoplasty in the teenage years. Achieving pleasing size and shape of the cleft nostril can be challenging. At primary repair, we focus on reducing size discrepancy, recognizing that adjunctive procedures such as Weir resection can be accomplished during subsequent rhinoplasty. We use urethral sounds to size each nostril and resect the corresponding excess diameter from the cleft-side nostril base prior to closure. At primary repair, one must also ensure that both nostrils are on a level horizontal plane. A cant at this stage cannot be easily corrected subsequently without redoing the entire repair. To aid in repositioning the cleft-side ala, the lower lateral cartilage should be released by inserting a small scissors into the lip incision and spread along the pyriform. To preserve these modifications to the nose, we suture elastomer splints into the nostrils for 4 weeks.

Primary cleft rhinoplasty begins by mobilizing the lower lateral cartilage off its overlying skin envelope. Subcutaneous tunnels are developed medially and laterally above the cartilage and connected to one another, allowing for its independent repositioning in a more symmetric fashion. One must take care to not violate the overlying vestibular skin envelope during this dissection so as to avoid complications such as nostril stenosis or the creation of adhesions. The lower lateral cartilage is then reshaped using mattress sutures and/or transcutaneous plication/suspension sutures aimed at creating a lifted and more projected nasal dome [27, 28]. Tajima and Maruyama describe an alternative inverted-U approach to the cleft lower lateral cartilage, proposing an incision that begins medially at the junction of the columella and membranous septum, extending onto the dorsal nasal skin before crossing the alar rim again and terminating on the inner surface of the lateral ala. The skin is widely undermined, and several sutures are placed to reposition and secure the cleft lower lateral cartilage to the contralateral lower lateral cartilage and bilateral upper lateral cartilages [29].

## Revisions

Despite the best planning and execution, suboptimal outcomes are occasionally encountered. Anticipating common secondary deformities may enable the cleft surgeon to perform the primary repair in a way to minimize the chance of need for secondary revision. The incidence of secondary lip surgery is varied with reports ranging from 16 to over 50% of all patients [30]. The decision to undergo secondary surgery is often subjective and based on patient, family, and surgeon preferences without any clear indications for the type or timing of revision required.

Outcomes that may require revision can be divided into superficial deformities or deeper, muscle-related deformities. This simple diagnostic criterion helps to not only frame the approach to secondary revision but can also guide the timing of surgical intervention in order to optimize patient outcomes [30]. Superficial deformities include poor scarring as well as step-offs or irregularities along the various aesthetic subunits such as a wide or asymmetric philtrum, short lip, asymmetry in Cupid's bow, irregularity in the vermillion-cutaneous border, mucosal excess, or bulging of the lateral vermillion [31–33]. Excessively prominent scarring can be managed initially by massage. If inadequate improvement is seen after 3–6 months, topical steroid cream can be initiated. Steroid injections are difficult to perform on this age group in the office. In our practice, operative revision is delayed for at least 12 months when possible. Others have described additional non-operative techniques such as the use of fractional $CO_2$ lasers in resurfacing cleft scars, particularly in adolescent and adult patients [34]. Although an exciting avenue for future research, we do not currently employ these techniques in our practice. Other superficial deformities can often be addressed by a simple scar revision or local tissue rearrangement consisting of z-plasties and V-Y advancements. Given the relative minor nature of these procedures, some authors advocate for these to be performed while the child is growing, particularly if it may help with social integration at the patient and/or family's request [30].

Muscle-related deformities often require a more extensive revision or complete redo of the primary repair. Timing of these procedures should again be a group decision involving the surgeon, patient, and family. However, in some cases, it may be beneficial to postpone such cases until the end of facial growth [30].

Bilateral cleft lip repairs are particularly challenging and can often result in inadequate long-term results, even in the most experienced hands. A full revision at the end of facial growth can be a powerful procedure that improves the surgical scar, lengthens the upper lip, corrects any whistle deformity, improves symmetry at the nasal sill, and adds volumes to a deficient upper vermillion [30, 35]. Other techniques such as modification of the Abbe flap or pedicled prolabial island flaps have also been described and can similarly add volume to the vermillion and reconstruct Cupids' bow while also adding horizontal length to the upper lip [32, 33]. Autologous fat grafting and hyaluronic acid fillers can also improve lip volume and symmetry and represent appealing alternatives when major revision is not desired or warranted. Secondary lip repair is discussed in detail in Chap. 16.

## Conclusions

As much as any operation in plastic surgery, repair of cleft lip and nose rewards careful analysis and skillful execution. In many cases, presurgical orthopedics or lip adhesion should be considered. For definitive repair, surgeons should adopt a repair technique that is most comfortable for them while remaining adaptable to requirements of individual patient anatomy. Plans are made to restore aesthetic subunits of the lip and nose in harmonious fashion. Scars are placed at natural boundaries whenever possible. Abnormal attachments of cleft tissues are released. Tissue constituents – mucosa, muscle, and skin – are individually addressed. Care is taken to minimize tension. Nasal repair takes a balanced approach addressing critical elements at primary repair that set the stage for subsequent rhinoplasty. Parents are instructed in scar management, and any revisions are delayed until tissue healing has fully evolved. Respecting these principles can lead to better outcomes for this most challenging and rewarding operation.

## References


1. Shay PL, Goldstein JA, Paliga JT, et al. A comparative cost analysis of cleft lip adhesion and nasoalveolar molding before formal cleft lip repair. Plast Reconstr Surg. 2015;136(6):1264–71.
2. Zide BM, Jelks GW. Surgical anatomy of the orbit. 1st ed. Philadelphia: Lippincott Williams & Wilkins; 1985.
3. Vander Woude DL, Mulliken JB. Effect of lip adhesion on labial height in two-stage repair of unilateral complete cleft lip. Plast Reconstr Surg. 1997;100(3):567–72; discussion 573–564.
4. Liou EJ, Subramanian M, Chen PK. Progressive changes of columella length and nasal growth after nasoalveolar molding in bilateral cleft patients: a 3-year follow-up study. Plast Reconstr Surg. 2007;119(2):642–8.
5. Shetty V, Thakral A, Sreekumar C. Comparison of early onset nasoalveolar molding with patients who presented for molding up to 1 year of age. J Oral Maxillofac. 2016;74(4):811–27.
6. Prahl C, Kuijpers-Jagtman AM, van't Hof MA, Prahl-Andersen B. A randomised prospective clinical trial into the effect of infant orthopaedics on maxillary arch dimensions in unilateral cleft lip and palate (Dutchcleft). Eur J Oral Sci. 2001;109(5):297–305.
7. Ross RB, MacNamera MC. Effect of presurgical infant orthopedics on facial esthetics in complete bilateral cleft lip and palate. Cleft Palate Craniofac J. 1994;31(1):68–73.
8. Konst EM, Prahl C, Weersink-Braks H, et al. Cost-effectiveness of infant orthopedic treatment regarding speech in patients with complete unilateral cleft lip and palate: a randomized three-center trial in the Netherlands (Dutchcleft). Cleft Palate Craniofac J. 2004;41(1):71–7.
9. Uzel A, Alparslan ZN. Long-term effects of presurgical infant orthopedics in patients with cleft lip and palate: a systematic review. Cleft Palate Craniofac J. 2011;48(5):587–95.
10. Maillard S, Retrouvey JM, Ahmed MK, Taub PJ. Correlation between nasoalveolar molding and surgical, aesthetic, functional and socioeconomic outcomes following primary repair surgery: a systematic review. J Oral Maxillofac Res. 2017;8(3):e2.
11. Dec W, Shetye PR, Grayson BH, Brecht LE, Cutting CB, Warren SM. Incidence of oronasal fistula formation after nasoalveolar molding and primary cleft repair. J Craniofac Surg. 2013;24(1):57–61.
12. Chow I, Purnell CA, Hanwright PJ, Gosain AK. Evaluating the rule of 10s in cleft lip repair: do data support dogma? Plast Reconstr Surg. 2016;138(3):670–9. https://doi.org/10.1097/PRS.0000000000002476.
13. Hammoudeh JA, Imahiyerobo TA, Liang F, et al. Early cleft lip repair revisited: a safe and effective approach utilizing a multidisciplinary protocol. Plast Reconstr Surg Glob Open. 2017;5(6):e1340.
14. Burget GC, Menick FJ. The subunit principle in nasal reconstruction. Plast Reconstr Surg. 1985;76(2):239–47.
15. Fisher DM. Unilateral cleft lip repair: an anatomical subunit approximation technique. Plast Reconstr Surg. 2005;116(1):61–71.
16. Campbell A, Restrepo C, Park E, Navas G, Deshpande G, Swanson J, Schonmeyr B, Wendby L, Ayala R. Influence of severity on aesthetic outcomes of unilateral cleft lip repair in 1,823 patients. Plast Reconstr Surg Glob Open. 2019;7(1):e2083. https://doi.org/10.1097/GOX.0000000000002083.
17. Mittermiller PA, Sethi H, Morbia RP, et al. Anatomical nasal lining flaps for closure of the nasal floor in unilateral and bilateral cleft lip repairs reduce fistulas at the alveolus. Plast Reconstr Surg. 2018;142(6):1549–56.
18. Mendoza M, Perez A. Anatomical closure technique of the nasal floor for patients with complete unilateral cleft lip and palate. J Plast Surg Hand Surg. 2013;47(3):196–9.
19. Tan SP, Greene AK, Mulliken JB. Current surgical management of bilateral cleft lip in North America. Plast Reconstr Surg. 2012;129(6):1347–55.
20. Lonic D, Morris DE, Lo LJ. Primary overcorrection of the unilateral cleft nasal deformity: quantifying the results. Ann Plast Surg. 2016;77(Suppl 1):S25–9.
21. Mulliken JB. Correction of the bilateral cleft lip nasal deformity: evolution of a surgical concept. Cleft Palate Craniofac J. 1992;29(6):540–5.
22. Broadbent TR, Woolf RM. Cleft lip nasal deformity. Ann Plast Surg. 1984;12(3):216–34.
23. Allori AC, Mulliken JB. Evidence-based medicine: secondary correction of cleft lip nasal deformity. Plast Reconstr Surg. 2017;140(1):166e–76e.
24. Salyer KE, Genecov ER, Genecov DG. Unilateral cleft lip-nose repair: a 33-year experience. J Craniofac Surg. 2003;14(4):549–58.
25. Anderl H, Hussl H, Ninkovic M. Primary simultaneous lip and nose repair in the unilateral cleft lip and palate. Plast Reconstr Surg. 2008;121(3):959–70.
26. Haddock NT, McRae MH, Cutting CB. Long-term effect of primary cleft rhinoplasty on secondary cleft rhinoplasty in patients with unilateral cleft lip-cleft palate. Plast Reconstr Surg. 2012;129(3):740–8.
27. McComb H. Primary correction of unilateral cleft lip nasal deformity: a 10-year review. Plast Reconstr Surg. 1985;75(6):791–9.
28. Sykes JM, Tasman AJ, Suarez GA. Cleft lip nose. Clin Plast Surg. 2016;43(1):223–35.
29. Tajima S, Maruyama M. Reverse-U incision for secondary repair of cleft lip nose. Plast Reconstr Surg. 1977;60(2):256–61.
30. Garland K, Matic D. Current approaches to cleft lip revision. Curr Opin Otolaryngol Head Neck Surg. 2019;27(4):287–93.
31. Yotsuyanagi T, Yamashita K, Yamauchi M, et al. New technical method to correct secondary vermilion deformities with cleft lip. J Plast Reconstr Aesthet Surg. 2018;71(12):1810–5.
32. Lee JW, Lee SJ, Suh IS, Lee CK. Modified Abbe flap for reconstruction of Cupid's bow and vermilion tubercle in secondary cleft lip deformity. Arch Craniofac Surg. 2018;19(1):13–9.
33. Mokal NJ, Desai MF. A novel technique using a subcutaneously pedicled islanded prolabial flap for the secondary correction of bilateral cleft lip and nasal deformity. Indian J Plast Surg. 2017;50(3):251–9.
34. Mossaad A, Kotb A, Abdelrahaman M, Ahmady HA. Post-surgical repair of cleft scar using fractional CO2 laser. Open Access Maced J Med Sci. 2018;6(7):1231–4.
35. Rossell-Perry P, Gavino-Gutierrez AM. Surgical technique for whistler deformity repair in bilateral cleft lip patients: an anthropometric study. Ann Plast Surg. 2016;77(2):183–9.

# Unilateral Cleft Lip repair: Rotation-Advancement Technique

# 11

Philip Kuo-Ting Chen and Vikram Pandit

**Key Points**
Five reasons for performing lip repair:

1. To restore normal lip appearance
2. To restore normal lip function
3. To restore normal nasal appearance
4. To restore normal nasal function
5. To reduce psychological impact

**Key Points**
- Careful markings for the anatomical landmarks
- Design of incisions to restore the anatomical subunits
- Mucosal flaps for nasal floor reconstruction
- Adequate release of muscles for alar base mobilization and repositioning
- Philtral reconstruction by overlapping muscle sutures
- Restore the white skin roll by white skin roll flap
- Correct vermilion deficiency by vermilion flap
- Primary nasal reconstruction by semi-open rhinoplasty, septal release, cartilage repositioning, and primary septal cartilage graft

## Introduction

Primary cleft lip and nasal reconstruction is the most important procedure during the long journey of total cleft care. Even in the presence of low-resource settings, cleft surgeons should still try their best to achieve an optimal result to reduce the number and difficulty of secondary revisions and reduce the psychological problems in these patients.

## Patient Selection and Clinical Planning

### Timing of Surgery

The authors obey the concept of "rule of tens." The timing for lip repair is around 3 months of age with body weight around 10 pounds (roughly 5 kg), with hemoglobin more than 10 g% and white blood cell count less than 10,000/mcL.

### Operative Planning

In low-resource setting areas, it will be relatively difficult to have presurgical nasoalveolar molding [1] to improve the presurgical condition. However, the wide alveolar cleft can still be narrowed down with prone sleep position and lip taping [2].

Surgery and anesthesia should have no difference compared to "high-resource setting areas."

The nasal deformity can be corrected with a delicate surgery. Low resources should not be the excuse of leaving nasal deformity till adolescence or adulthood.

Most of the postoperative care should be the same in both low-resource and high-resource settings.

P. K.-T. Chen (✉)
Craniofacial Center, Taipei Medical University Hospital, Taipei, Taiwan

Department of Surgery, Taipei Medical University, Taipei, Taiwan

V. Pandit
Pandit Clinic, Pune, India

© Springer Nature Switzerland AG 2021

J. W. Swanson, D. W. Low (eds.), *Global Cleft Care in Low-Resource Settings*, https://doi.org/10.1007/978-3-030-59105-2_11

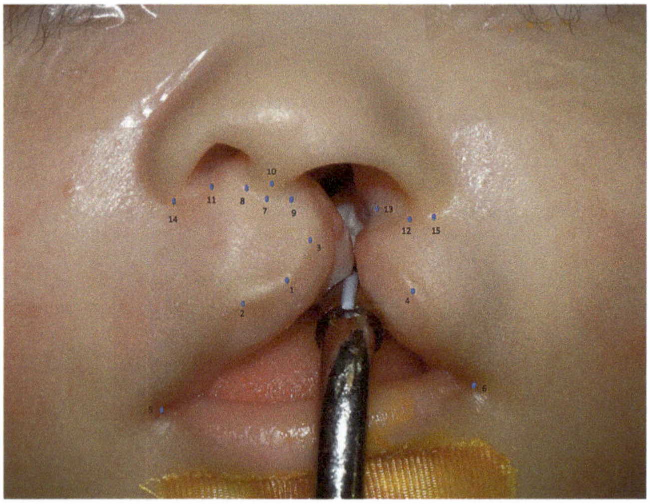

**Fig. 11.1** Anatomical markings

## Relevant Surface Anatomy

There are several surface anatomical points that should be marked for surgical planning (Fig. 11.1).

For unification, the "left" means the cleft side and "right" means the non-cleft side [3–5]:

1. LS: labiale superius, midpoint of Cupid's bow
2. CPHIR: crista philtri inferior, right side, peak of Cupid's bow on non-cleft side
3. CPHIL: crista philtri inferior, left side, peak of Cupid's bow on cleft margin of the non-cleft side
4. CPHIL′: crista philtri inferior, left, peak of Cupid's bow on cleft-side lateral lip
5. CHR: cheilion, right side, commissure on non-cleft side
6. CHL: cheilion, left side, commissure on cleft side
7. SN: subnasale, midpoint of columella
8. CPHSR: crista philtri superior, right side, upper point of philtral column on non-cleft side
9. CPHSL: crista philtri superior, left side, upper point of philtral column on cleft side
10. CPHSL′: the new crista philtri superior, left side, after rotation incision
11. MNSR: medial nasal sill point on non-cleft side
12. MNSL: medial nasal sill point on cleft side
13. SNLG: the split point of nasolabial groove – the point in nasal vestibulum where the skin-mucosa junction changes its direction
14. SBALR: subalare, the most inferior point of each alar base on the non-cleft side
15. SBALL: subalare, the most inferior point of each alar base on the cleft side

## Key Equipment

The instruments used for cleft lip repair are fairly simple. The author's preferred instruments include big single hooks, small double hooks, and small single hooks, fine-tipped Adson forceps, Adson forceps, caliper, and ruler. Also suture scissors, blunt-tip tenotomy scissors, scalpel handles, handle for #67 blade, fine-tipped needle holders, and fine-tipped clamps are used. A Dingman mouth gag is needed if an anterior palate repair is combined with lip repair. Sutures used are 5-0 polyglactin, 5-0 polydioxanone, and 7-0 polyglactin.

## Anesthesia

Even in low-resource area, primary lip repair in early childhood should be performed under general anesthesia with endotracheal intubation with RAE tube and anesthetic machine suitable for infants. Local anesthesia with or without heavy sedation is not encouraged for safety concern even in older children.

After inducing general anesthesia, bilateral infraorbital nerve blocks can be given with 5% bupivacaine for intra-/postoperative pain management. After skin markings, 1% lidocaine with 1:200,000 epinephrine can be injected for better hemostasis during the surgical procedure.

## Procedural Technique

### Incisions on the Non-cleft Side

The authors use two kinds of incision on the non-cleft side: (1) Mohler's incision if the discrepancy between CPHIR and CPHIL is more than 2 mm [6] and (2) simple rotation incision if the discrepancy between the two points is less than 2 mm.

**Mohler's Incision** (Fig. 11.2)
The incision is marked as a curvilinear line from CPHIL extending upward into the base of columella and then makes a 90-degree back-cut to the point of CPHSR. The turning point of the back-cut is the new upper point of the philtral ridge on the cleft margin, i.e., CPHSL′. The incision across the free border of the lip at CPHIL, is made at right angle to the white skin roll axis so as to include more tissue at the free border. This incision can be applied to most patients except the median facial dysplasia patients with very narrow columella.

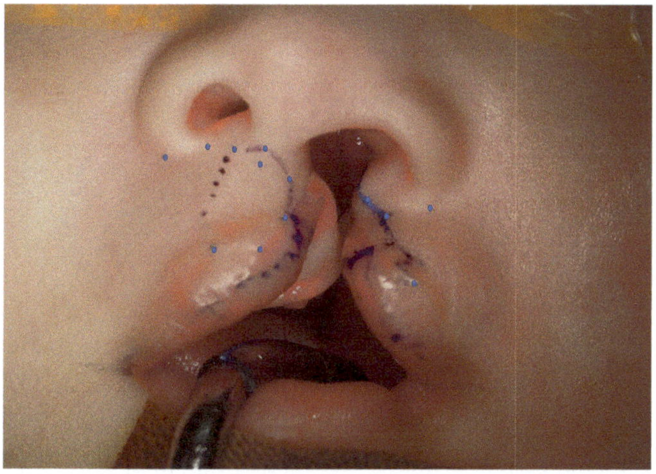

**Fig. 11.2** Skin markings for Mohler's incision

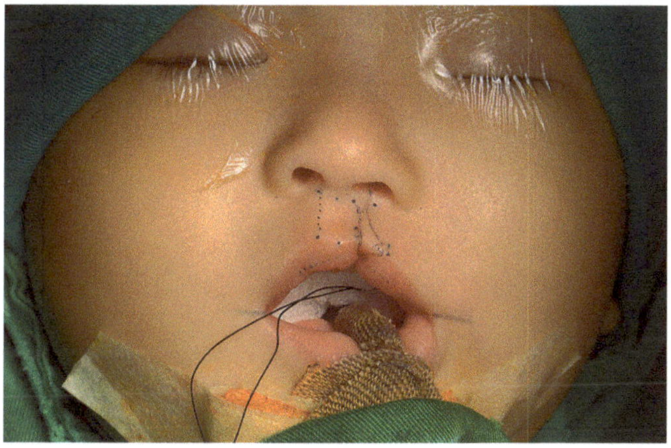

**Fig. 11.3** Skin markings for simple rotation incision

## Simple Rotation Incision (Fig. 11.3)

This is a shorter curvilinear incision from CPHIL to CPHSL. This will avoid the scar across the nasolabial junction which is usually more obvious than the vertical scar on the lip. If the amount of rotation is inadequate, the incision line can be easily converted into a Mohler's incision with extension into the columellar base.

The lip is stabilized with hooks and finger, while incision is made with #67 blade. The incision across the free border of the lip at CPHIL should be right angle to the axis of the white skin roll to include more tissue in free border.

## Adequate Rotation

The abnormal muscle insertion to the columellar base is released with a pair of tenotomy scissors (Fig. 11.4).

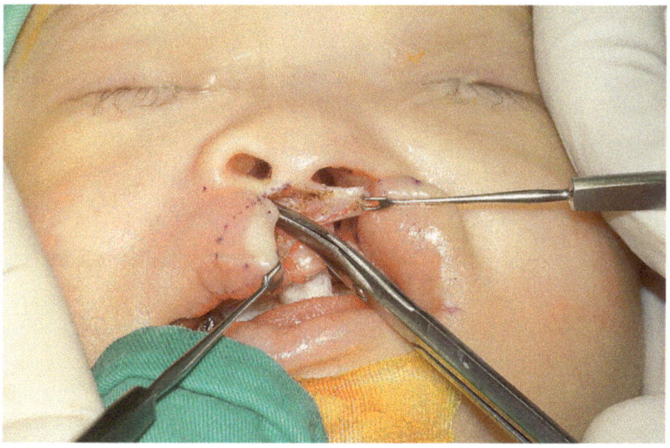

**Fig. 11.4** Release of muscle insertion under columellar base

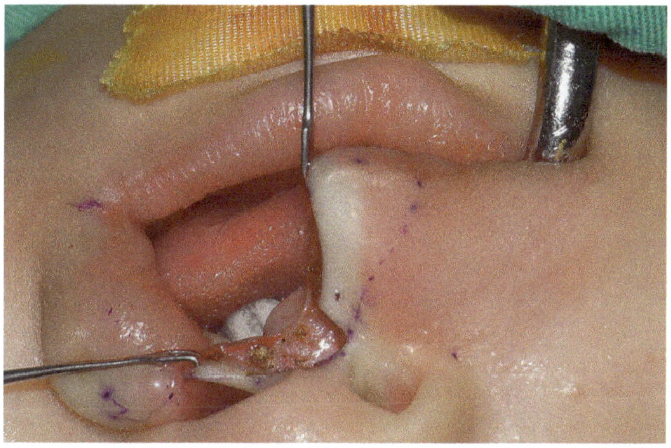

**Fig. 11.5** Check the adequacy of rotation

Downward traction of the lip with a small double hook will determine if the points CPHIR and CPHIL are at the same level (Fig. 11.5). The back-cut advocated by Millard is not suggested even if the rotation is not adequate as this will leave a wider and lower defect at the apex of the rotation as compared to Mohler's incision. Closure of this wider defect is always more difficult than a Mohler's incision, and the resultant scar is always more conspicuous.

The authors routinely insert a white skin roll (WSR) flap for lip subunit repair. An additional 1–2 mm Cupid's bow (CPHIL) lowering can be achieved with this 2 mm WSR flap, thus decreasing the necessity of a back-cut.

## Muscle Dissection on the Rotation Flap

The muscle layer is dissected along the skin edge initially with blade (Fig. 11.6) and then continued with a pair of tenot-

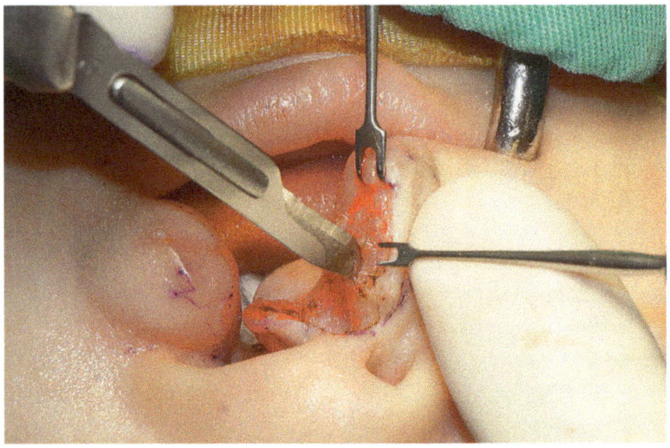

Fig. 11.6 Muscle dissection on the rotation flap

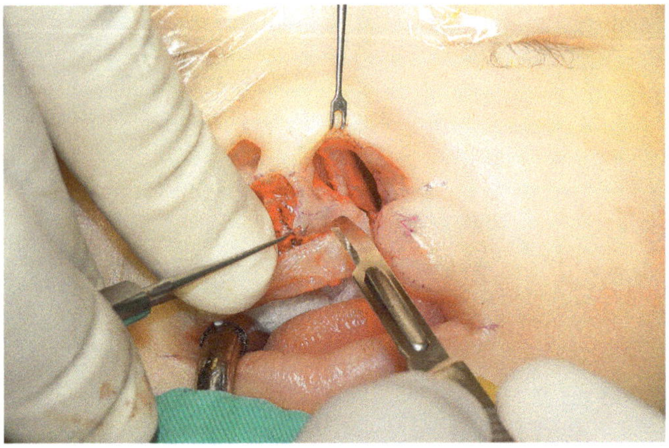

Fig. 11.7 Incision for C-flap

omy scissors. The muscle attachment to the skin is released in the subdermal plane till the midline of the philtrum. The dissection plane is deeper initially leaving a cuff of muscle on the incision edge for better philtral ridge morphology.

## C-Flap and Footplate of Medial Crura

The C-flap incisions are made in the line extending from point CPHIL along the skin and mucosa junction to the deepest point of the skin on the premaxilla (Fig. 11.7). Then the incision turns superiorly for 5 mm or even longer along the columellar skin and septum-mucosa junction. The intercrural space beneath the columella is separated by tenotomy scissors (Fig. 11.8). This allows mobilization of the C-flap and repositioning the downward displaced medial crural footplate on the cleft-side lower lateral cartilage (LLC).

The medial tip of the C-flap (at point CPHIL) will be used to fill in the defect at the columellar base created by Mohler's incision. On the other hand, it will be trimmed accordingly in patients with simple rotation incision.

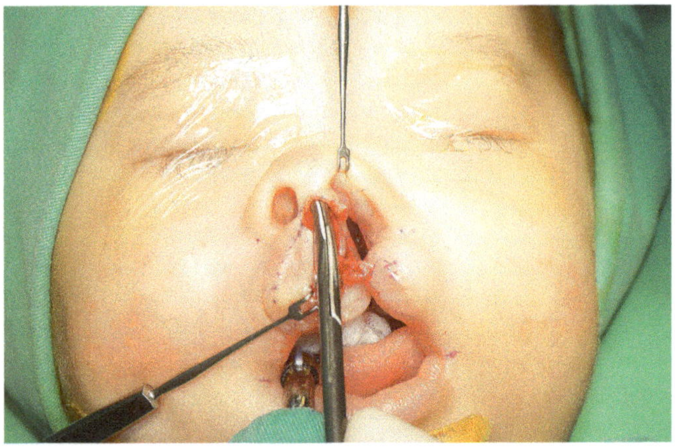

Fig. 11.8 Separation of space between right and left medial crura by tenotomy scissors

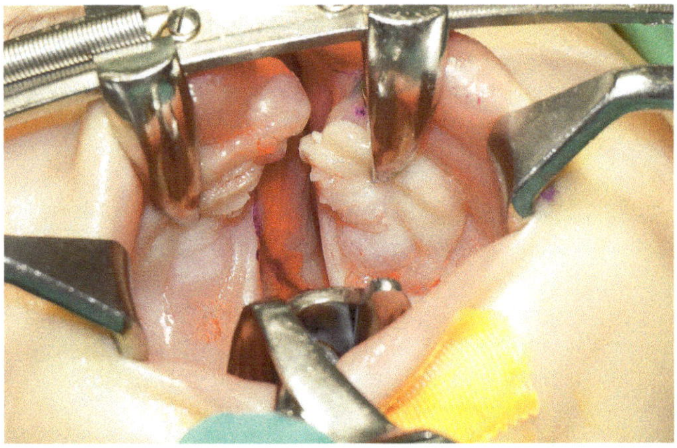

Fig. 11.9 Markings for vomer-septal flap

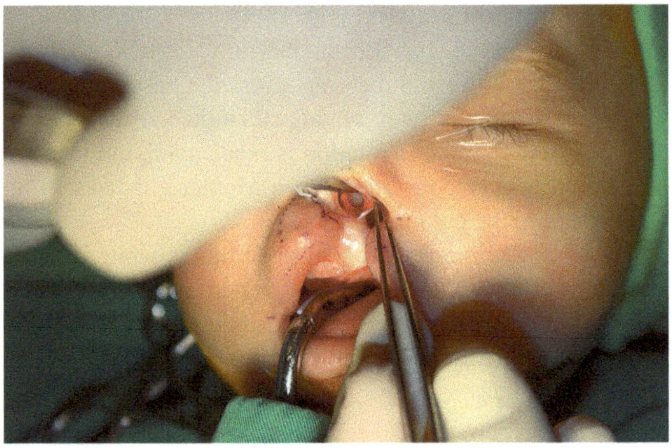

Fig. 11.10 Raising of septal mucoperichondrial flap

## Nasal Septal Dissection

The authors favor anterior palate repair during primary lip repair. The septal incision behind the C-flap is further extended downward behind the premaxilla (Fig. 11.9). A septal mucoperichondrial flap is raised in continuity with the vomer flap used for the anterior palate repair (Fig. 11.10).

The dislocated caudal part of the septum can be easily mobilized from the vomer bone and repositioned through this septal dissection.

## Incisions on the Cleft Side

A triangular WSR flap is designed at the point CPHIL′, in accordance to the width of the WSR at point CPHIR (Fig. 11.11). Usually the width and length are around 2 mm in a 3–6-month-old baby. Then a curvilinear incision is designed connecting the upper point of the WSR flap and the point MNSL. The incision is extending inward to the point SNLG and then turns its direction along the piriform junction of nasal vestibular skin and nasal mucosa (Fig. 11.12) to the base of inferior turbinate, turning inward to include an inferior turbinate (T) flap.

The incision line at the point CPHIL′ is right angle to the WSR moving downward for 1 mm, then moving medially to include the 3–4 mm of vermilion, and then moving at a right angle further downward to the mucosa.

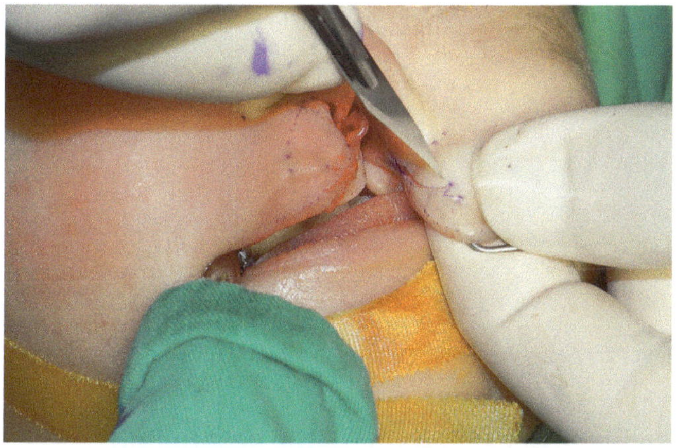

Fig. 11.11 Incision for white skin roll (WSR) flap

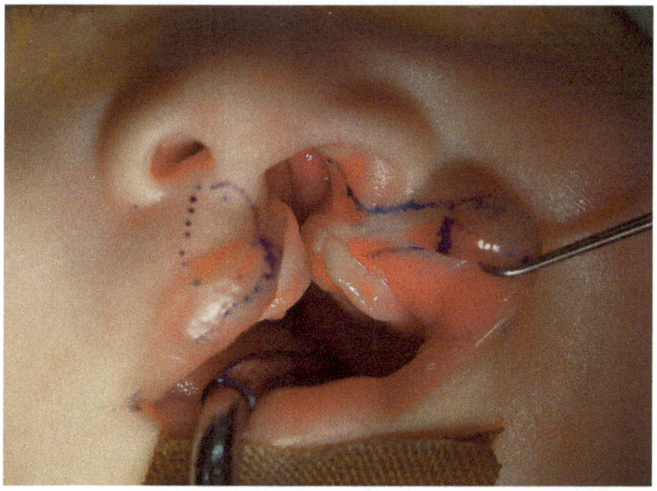

Fig. 11.12 Incision markings along the pyriform rim on cleft side

## L-Mucosal Flap

An L-flap is marked based on the alveolar margin, with its upper margin being the incision line of the advancement flap and its lower margin on the mucosa. The width of the L-flap is around 5 mm. The length of this flap varies depending on the length required for the reconstruction on the medial lip vermilion.

## Inferior Turbinate Flap

The incision line on the inferior turbinate extends from the piriform rim inward on the lower and upper edges of the inferior turbinate for a distance of 1.5 cm. The base of this flap is on the vestibular skin. This flap is helpful to fill the mucosa defect after releasing the alar base from the retropositioned lesser segment.

## Incision and Dissection

The lateral lip is stabilized with a big single hook and fingers. The WSR flap is made with #11 blade followed by #67 blade for the rest part (Fig. 11.11). The L-flap is raised by tenotomy scissors leaving a layer of muscle to ensure adequate blood supply (Fig. 11.13). The T-flap is elevated in a retrograde fashion with small double hooks and tenotomy scissors.

The alar base and the lateral lip are well mobilized from the maxilla above the periosteum plane using tenotomy

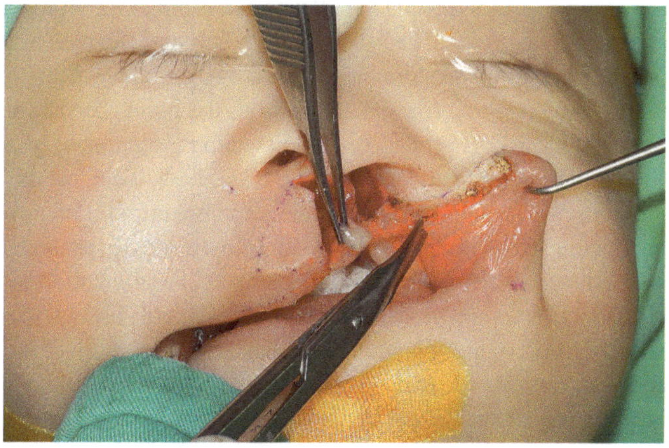

Fig. 11.13 Raising of L-flap

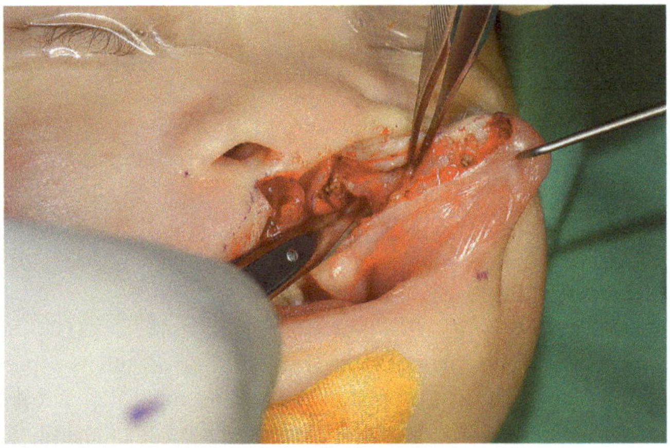

Fig. 11.14 Dissection of the muscle on maxilla on lateral (cleft) segment

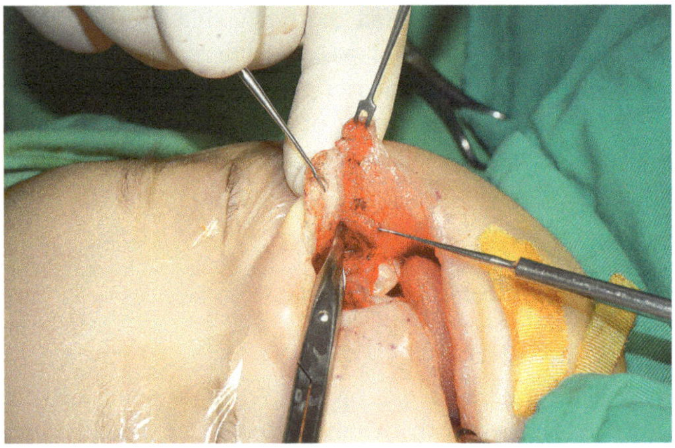

Fig. 11.16 Extent of muscle dissection: till angular artery on the cleft side

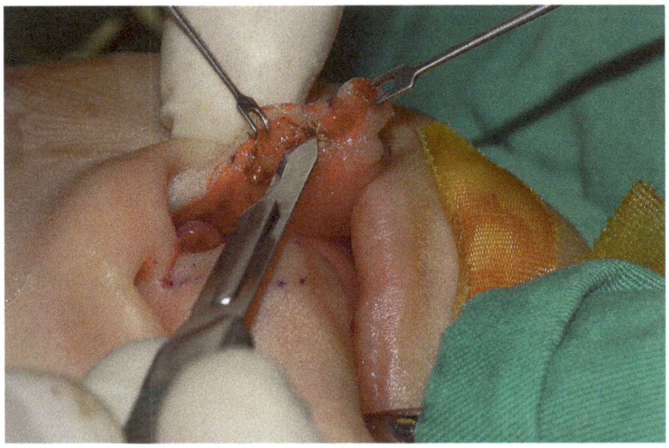

Fig. 11.15 Dissection of the muscle on skin side

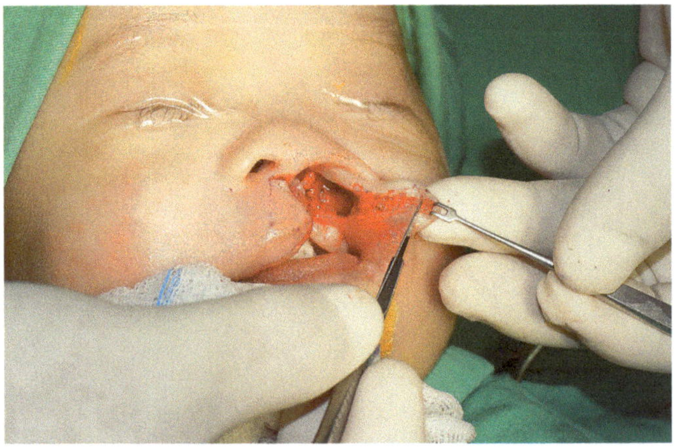

Fig. 11.17 Raising of orbicularis marginalis flap

scissors (Fig. 11.14). The extent of the maxillary dissection is usually close to the infraorbital foramen. Even in wide clefts, mobilization of the lip and alar base can be accomplished with a more extensive dissection over the maxilla.

The lateral lip mucosa is dissected 2 mm from the edge. Excessive mucosal dissection will result in submucosal fibrosis and should be avoided. Using a tenotomy scissors, the bunched orbicularis peripheralis muscle is dissected from the skin along the wound edge to a line extending from the point SBALL to the point CPHIL′ (Fig. 11.15). The dissection is continued on a subdermal plane superiorly around the alar base. This releases the abnormal muscle insertions of the paranasal muscles including the transverse portion of the nasalis muscle, depressor septi, and levator muscles of the upper lip and ala. The extent of muscle dissection should be lateral to the angular artery (Fig. 11.16), ensuring most of the abnormal muscle insertions to the alar base are completely released. Adequate muscle release allows lengthening of the lateral lip in both vertical and horizontal dimensions. Similar to the non-cleft side, a cuff of muscle is left on the wound edge for better philtral ridge morphology.

## Removal of Fat Pad Under the Vestibulum

After mobilizing the alar base from the maxilla, the vestibular webbing will be aggravated. This vestibular webbing is a common deformity seen after primary lip repair.

Usually upon adequate muscle dissection beneath the alar base, a cuff of fat pad will bulge out from the nasal vestibule. Removal of this fat pad will decrease the tissue thickness at nasal vestibule, thus improving the vestibular webbing.

## Elevation of Orbicularis Marginalis Flap

The orbicularis marginalis (OM) flap is incised (Fig. 11.17) along the free border of the lip to include the orbicularis marginalis muscle, the vermillion medial to point CPHIL′, and the corresponding mucosa posteriorly. The incision line of the OM flap is perpendicular to the skin, and the muscle volume at CPHIL′ is preserved similar to the volume at the point

CPHIR on the non-cleft side. Gentle downward traction of the OM flap can determine the tissue adequacy along the free margin, and the lip contour should be in a smooth line (Fig. 11.18). It is important to preserve all vermilion tissue medial to CPHIL′ at the beginning for more flexibility in designing the vermilion flap later on.

## Nasal Floor Reconstruction and Alar Base Repositioning

### Lip Repair with Anterior Palate Repair

When an anterior palate repair is performed simultaneously with primary lip repair, a vomer flap is raised and imbricated beneath the mucoperiosteal edge of the lesser segment (Fig. 11.19) [7]. The vomer flap is extending forward as a septal flap. The nasal floor is reconstructed by the septal and L-flap to achieve a complete mucosal closure from nasal floor to the junction of hard and soft palate. The septal flap is sutured to the lower margin of the L-flap (Fig. 11.20), while the upper margin of the L-flap is sutured to the lower margin of the piriform incision. The alar base is advanced medially and superiorly. The upper margin of the piriform incision is sutured to the septal/L-flaps (Fig. 11.21). The vertical position of the alar base should be at the same level of the non-cleft side. Final positioning of the alar base can be adjusted after nasal reconstruction.

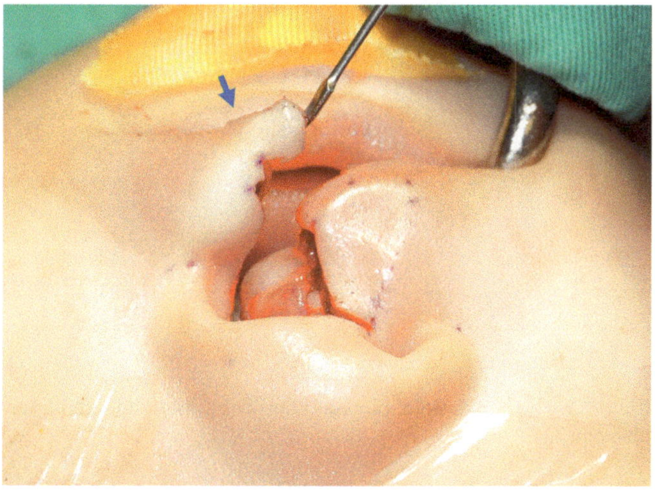

**Fig. 11.18** Check the adequate thickness of the free border flap

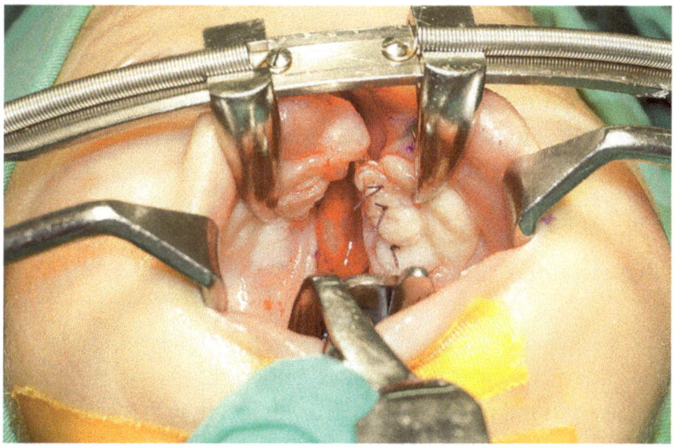

**Fig. 11.19** Imbricating of vomer flap under mucoperiosteal layer of lesser segment for anterior palate repair

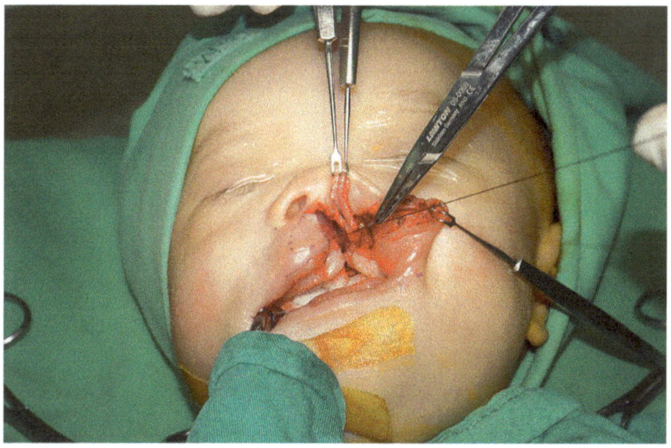

**Fig. 11.20** Closure of nasal floor with septal flap and L-flap

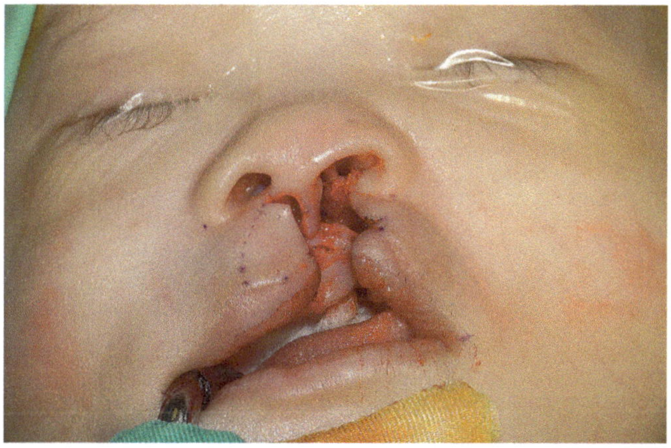

**Fig. 11.21** Closure of vestibular skin to the L-flap and septal flap

### Lip Repair Without Anterior Palate Repair

The T-flap based on vestibular skin is rotated 90° caudally to fill in the defect on piriform rim. Its superior edge is sutured to the inferior edge of the piriform incision. T-flap corrects the mucosal deficiency and allows repositioning of the LLC and alar base without restriction. The L-flap is brought medially behind the columella and sutured to the mucoperichondrial flap of the posterior septal incision. The inferior edge of the T-flap is sutured to the superior edge of the L-flap. The mucosal side of the inferior turbinate flap and L-flap is facing superiorly to create the mucosal side of the nasal floor

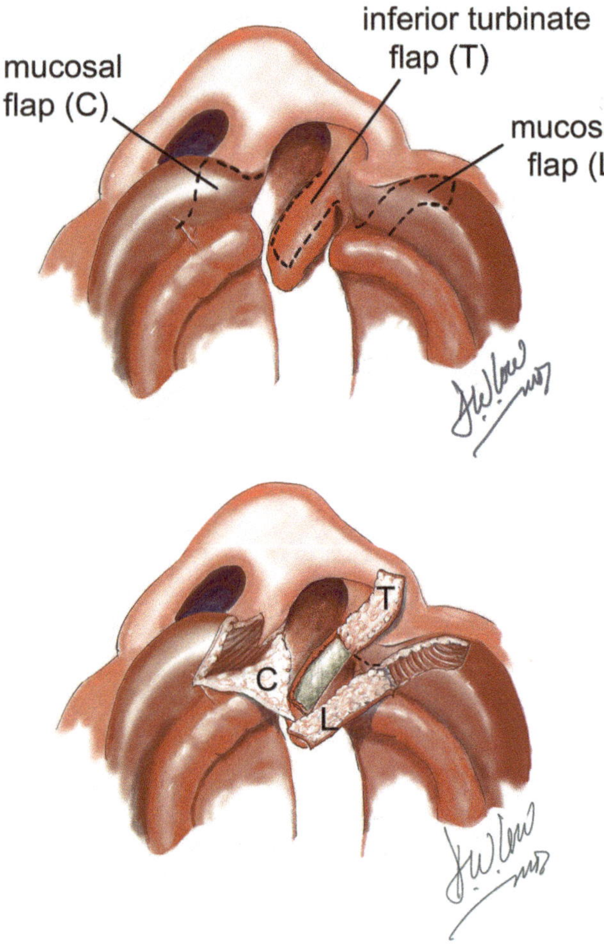


Fig. 11.22 Incision lines for L-flap and inferior turbinate flap

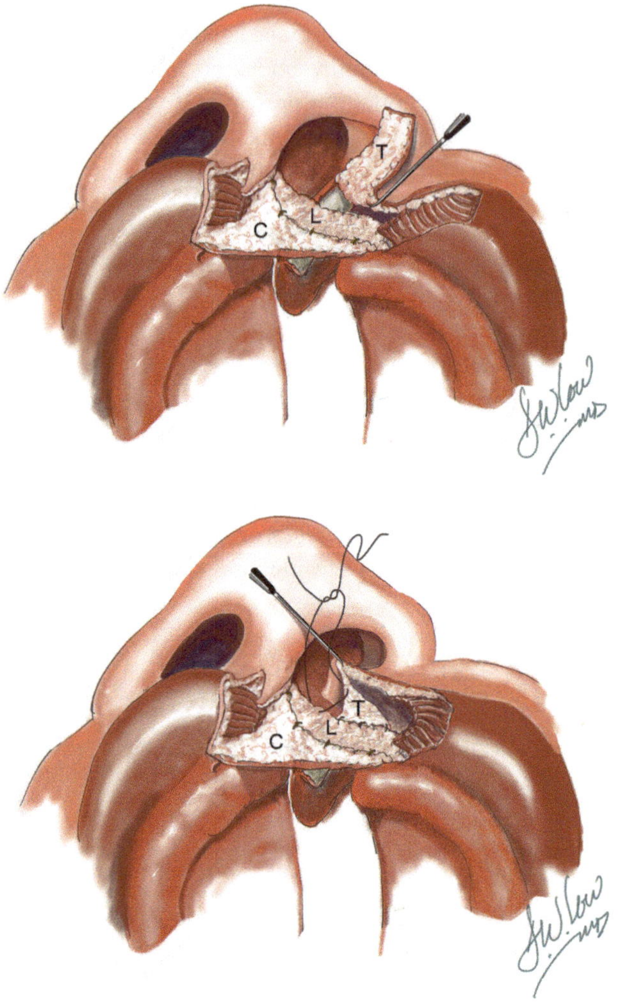


Fig. 11.23 Reconstruction of nasal floor with L-flap and inferior turbinate flap

The C-flap mucosa is turned laterally and placed below the L-flap. Its tip is sutured to the base of L-flap, and its upper margin is sutured to the inferior edge of the L-flap. This gives good mucosal closure of the nasal floor and lateral nasal wall without leaving any raw surface. The vestibular skin with attached ala is advanced as described previously (Figs. 11.22 and 11.23).

## Sequence of Operation When an Anterior Palate Repair Is Combined with Lip Repair

Vomer flap is used for all patients with combined anterior palate repair and a lip repair. The sequence of the operation is to do septal incision first to raise a septal flap. The dissection is carried backward to the junction of the premaxilla and septum that is curved inward. Then attention is drawn to the oral cavity where a vomer flap is raised from its most posterior part carried forward until the two incisions are met. The edge of the mucoperiosteum on lesser segment is raised to its alveolar margin. The vomer is imbricated underneath the lesser segment to the alveolus to finish the anterior palate repair. Then the attention is drawn back to lip incision.

## Closure of the Base of Columella

The medial tip of the C-flap is brought medially to fill the defect on columella base after a Mohler's incision, or it is trimmed in a simple rotation incision.

## Muscle Reconstruction

The muscle layer is approximated with 5-0 polydioxanone. A key suture is placed in the muscle apposing points CPHIL to CPHIL′. With downward traction, Cupid's bow is leveled. This can assure the correct placement of subsequent muscle suture. The tip of the muscle in the advancement flap is anchored to the caudal edge of nasal septum (Fig. 11.24) [8]. This anchoring

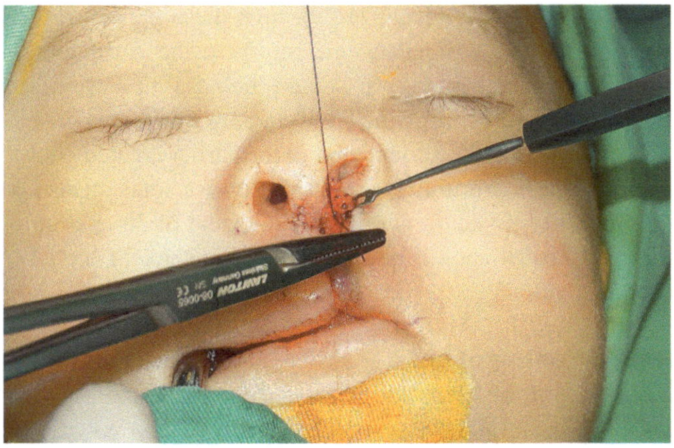

Fig. 11.24 Septal anchoring suture

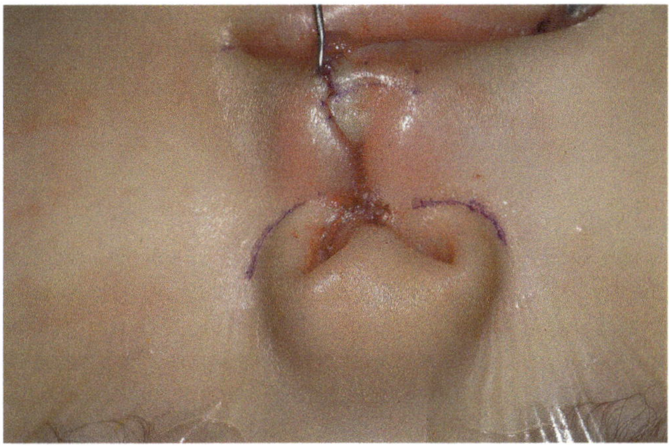

Fig. 11.25 Insertion of WSR flap and vermilion flap

suture helps to pull the lateral lip medially to centralize Cupid's bow. The muscle sutures are placed with lateral muscle above the medial muscle to simulate a philtral column. Catching hold of the subdermal layer at the midline of philtrum during muscle approximation helps to restore the philtral dimple. The orbicularis marginalis muscle is carefully sutured to avoid any depression in the free border after surgery.

## Insertion of the WSR Flap

Points CPHIL and CPHIL′ are approximated with 5-0 polydioxanone subcuticular suture followed by 7-0 polyglactin suture for the skin. The width of the WSR is measured and marked at the point CPHIL following the WSR contour. An incision line according to the length of WSR flap is carefully designed to place the WSR flap tip at the horizontal groove of the lip contour line (Fig. 11.25) as advocated by Onizuka [9]. The natural contour line is right on the upper margin of the WSR. This helps to restore the continuity and fullness of the white skin roll. The author uses WSR flap in every case. If the rotation is not enough, it can lengthen the lip by inserting this WSR flap. If the rotation is adequate, a WSR flap is still used (with trimming of the tissue on medial lip for "lip contour line").

## Incisions for Triangular Vermillion Flap

The vermillion flap is marked and incised on the OM flap under tension with a #11 blade [10]. It is inserted into an incision made along or above the red line beneath the point CPHIL. The main purpose of this vermilion flap is to correct the vermilion deficiency beneath Cupid's bow instead of increasing the tissue bulk on the central free border (Fig. 11.25). The tip of the vermillion flap should not cross the natural lip tubercle that is always present in a unilateral cleft. This vermilion flap is needed in most of the cleft patients with vermilion deficiency below the point CPHIL.

## Closure of the Free Border of the Lip

The excess mucosa below the vermilion flap and on the lateral lip is trimmed accordingly to approximate the free border of the lip. Incisions on the vermillion are closed with continuous 7-0 polyglactin suture. The mucosa is closed with interrupted 5-0 polyglactin sutures. The upper edge of the buccal mucosa is sutured to the lower edge of C-flap mucosa that bridges the alveolar gap. This gives a complete mucosal closure without tension.

## Closure of the Nasal Floor and the Lip Skin

A single hook is used for traction at the upper margin of the WSR flap to level Cupid's bow. Then the points MNSL and CPHSL′ are approximated with 5-0 polydioxanone subcuticular suture followed by 7-0 polyglactin suture for the skin. This creates a suture line that mimics the philtral ridge.

The lateral tip of the C-flap is brought laterally inside the nasal sill to preserve the natural nasal sill. The excessive tissue inside the nasal sill is carefully trimmed to preserve the natural "pedestal" appearance of the columella. The nasal floor is closed with 5-0 polyglactin sutures.

The final skin closure is achieved by 5-0 polydioxanone subcuticular suture followed by 7-0 polyglactin suture for the skin.

## Semi-open Rhinoplasty

During the past 30 years, several techniques have been used for nasal reconstruction in unilateral clefts by the senior author [11–13]. In the authors' experience, semi-open rhinoplasty can achieve a clean and less traumatic dissection over the cartilaginous framework besides better visualization and repositioning of the displaced cartilages. It can elongate the columella through a reverse U incision on the alar rim of the cleft-side nostril.

### Incision

A rim incision is marked on the non-cleft nostril, while a reverse U incision is marked on the cleft nostril. The reverse U incision is made 2 mm higher than the alar rim on the non-cleft side to achieve an over-correction on the cleft nostril (Fig. 11.26a). The lateral part of this incision is always across the alar rim into the nasal vestibulum to avoid alar rim kicking after approximation of the lower lateral cartilages.

### Release of Fibrofatty Tissue from LLCs

Incisions are made with #67 blade while stabilizing the alar rim with two small double hooks. Dissection of the lower lateral cartilages (LLCs) is performed between the skin and cartilage using tenotomy scissors. The caudal edges of both LLCs can be easily visualized through these incisions, thus avoiding any risk of iatrogenic injury to the cartilaginous framework. The fibrofatty tissue on the nasal tip is released from both LLCs through incisions on both sides. This dissection pocket should be connected to the earlier created pocket through the intercrural space dissection for total release of the fibrofatty tissue on nasal tip. The extent of dissection on the cleft nostril should be lateral to the groove of the LLC caudal edge.

### Repositioning of LLCs

The LLC on the cleft side is rotated medially and approximated to the LLC on the non-cleft side with 5-0 polydioxanone mattress sutures. The stitches are placed 5 mm more laterally on the cleft-side cartilage for over-correction (Fig. 11.26b). A second through-and-through suture is placed on the medial crus lower than the first stitch for further crural support (Fig. 11.26c). A firm "cartilage-to-cartilage" adhesion can only be achieved after total releasing of the fibrofatty tissue from both LLCs through incisions on both nostrils.

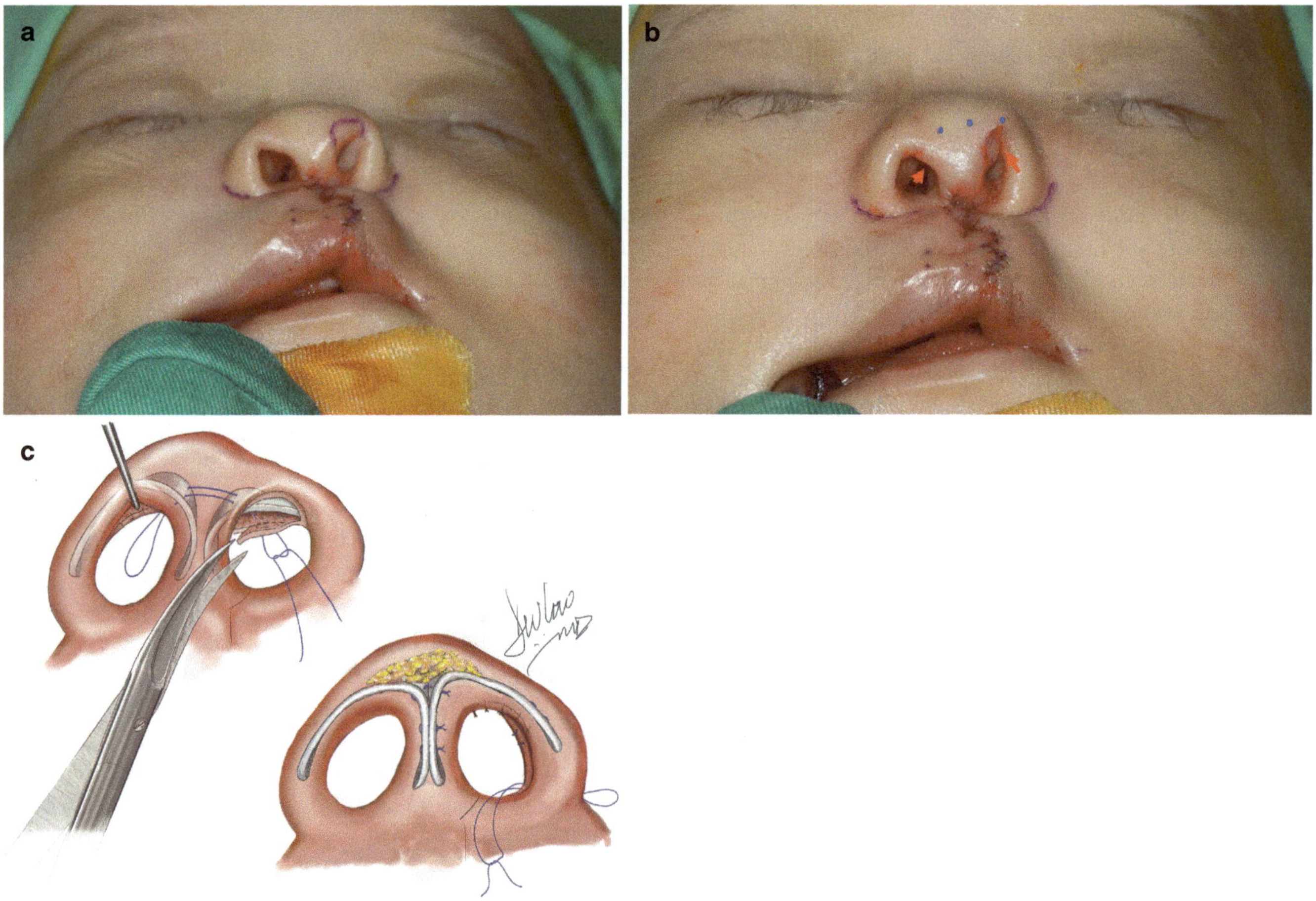

**Fig. 11.26** (**a**) Reverse U incision on cleft side and alar rim incision on non-cleft side. (**b**) A pair of dots are marked at both alar domes, roughly at the distance according to the columellar width. Another dot is marked about 5 mm lateral to the dome of the cleft side. The suture for approximation of the lower lateral cartilages is placed at the dome of the non-cleft side and lateral point of the cleft side. Thus the lower lateral cartilage is advanced more medially on the cleft side. (**c**) After approximating the LLCs, the skin under the reverse U incision will be moved medially to form the upper columella on the cleft side. Some excessive skin can be trimmed accordingly. Two sutures are placed on medial crura and another two sutures (the alar transfixion sutures) are placed on the alar-facial groove on the cleft side

### Trimming the Excessive Skin

After repositioning of the LLCs, the columella on the cleft side will be lengthened by the tissue along the medial limb of the reverse U incision. There is always excess skin under the reverse U incision. This excessive skin is trimmed with a sharp scissors, and the wound is closed with 5-0 polyglactin sutures.

### Primary Septal Cartilage Graft

A piece of septal cartilage graft can be obtained from the caudal edge of the deviated septum after raising the septal/vomer flap for anterior palatal closure and septal repositioning. The size of the graft is around 3 × 15 mm (Fig. 11.27). This cartilage is scored and placed on the alar rim of the cleft side as an internal splint [14].

### Alar Base Position

The cleft-side alar base should be at the same level with its counterpart after surgery. The most important factor in achieving alar base symmetry is adequate release of the abnormally attached paranasal muscles and good approximation of the lip musculature.

### Creation of the Alar-Facial Groove

Dissection between the skin and LLC releases the fibrous attachments and leaves behind a significant dead space. Furthermore, mobilization of the cleft-side alar base will accentuate the vestibular webbing within the nostril. Removal of the fat pad and two alar transfixion sutures help in solving these problems while defining the alar-facial groove. The lower suture obliterates the dead space and tacks down the vestibular webbing. The upper suture catches the leading edge of the LLC and provides support to the LLC. Skin dimpling from these sutures usually disappears 2 weeks after surgery (Fig. 11.26c).

**Tips and Tricks**

- Use Mohler's/simple rotation incision for symmetric philtral morphology.
- Use mucosal flaps for nasal floor closure.
- Adequate release of the abnormal muscle insertion.
- Alar base repositioning.
- Muscle reconstruction to form the philtral ridge.
- White skin roll flap for lip contour line.
- Vermilion flap for vermilion deficiency.
- Semi-open rhinoplasty to facilitate cartilage repositioning.
- Primary septal cartilage graft as internal splinting.

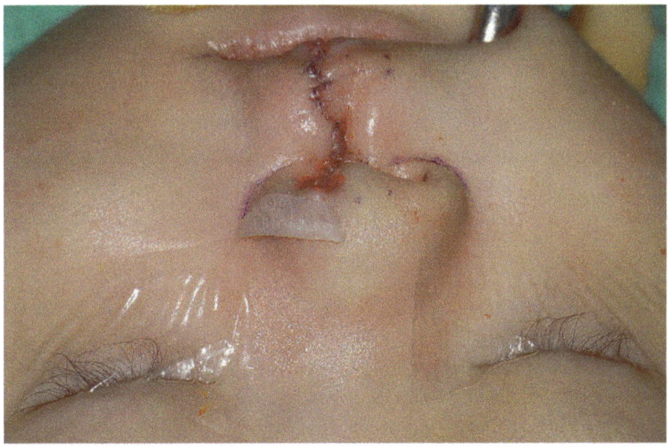

**Fig. 11.27** Size and position for placement of primary septal cartilage graft

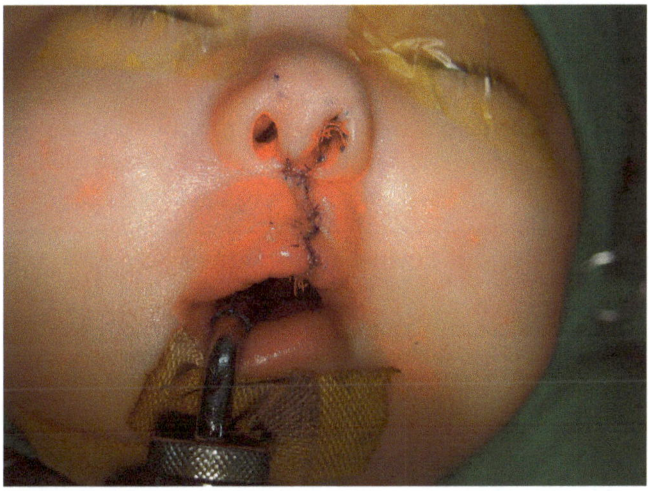

**Fig. 11.28** Complete skin closure

The final appearance of the lip and nose after surgery is shown in Fig. 11.28.

## Postoperative Care

### Wound Care

The lip and nasal wounds should be cleansed with normal saline cotton buds every 3–4 hours, and then apply antibiotic ointment over the wound. The author prefers changing the normal saline wet dressing every 3–4 hours for better wound care if there is plenty of discharge. The normal saline wet dressings should be continued until the wounds are clean.

## Stitch Removal

The sutures are removed after 5–7 days. The procedure was done in outpatient clinic under sedation with chloral hydrate. The patients should be kept for monitoring for a period of time until their vital signs are stable.

## Aftercare

The lip scar is stabilized with micropore tape for about 6 months. Silicone sheet or silicone gel is suggested for better scar care if available [15].

The authors prefer using a silicone nasal conformer to maintain the shape of the nose for at least 6 months [16]. These conformers can be put at the appointment for suture removal at 7th postoperative day. Although these conformers are not popular in most part of the world, they are recommended if available. However, it should be mentioned that these conformers are not mandatory as the aforementioned surgical techniques were used in other parts of the world and could get similar results without using the conformers.

## Follow-Up and Complication Management

The complications of primary lip and nasal repair include the following:

1. Wound infection: This complication can be avoided by careful wound care and oral antibiotics.
2. Stitch abscess: This complication is caused by the long-lasting absorbable sutures in subcutaneous layer. It can be handled with conservative wound care if it happens.
3. Wound dehiscence: This complication can be avoided by good surgical technique, adequate release of muscles and careful approximation of muscle layer to reduce the tension across the suture lines, and good wound care. Normal saline wet dressing is used for minor wound separation. For major wound separation, wound re-approximation usually will result in re-dehiscence; thus it is not recommended. It should be managed with wound care. Re-operation can only be done after the wound heals.
4. Hypertrophic scar: This complication is not uncommon in Orientals and Africans. It is managed with taping, local pressure, and moisturization with silicone sheet or silicone gel. Dye laser or local steroid injection can be considered if the previous managements are ineffective.
5. Nasal infection: This complication is caused by nasal conformer and the long-lasting absorbable sutures inside the nose. It can be avoided by adequate nasal hygiene.
6. Nasal stenosis: The basic thing to prevent nasal stenosis is not to make the nostril too small. The mucosal flaps for nasal floor reconstruction can provide ample tissue to prevent subsequent scar contracture and stenosis. Stenting with urinary catheter is a good way to correct nostril stenosis even in low-resource setting areas if a silicone nasal conformer is not available.

Even in low-resource setting areas, these patients should be followed on a regular basis until their facial growth is complete. Only by regular follow-up, surgeons can know their results and make necessary modifications for their techniques or protocols.

The examples of the result of this technique are shown in Figs. 11.29, 11.30, 11.31, 11.32, 11.33, 11.34, 11.35, and 11.36.

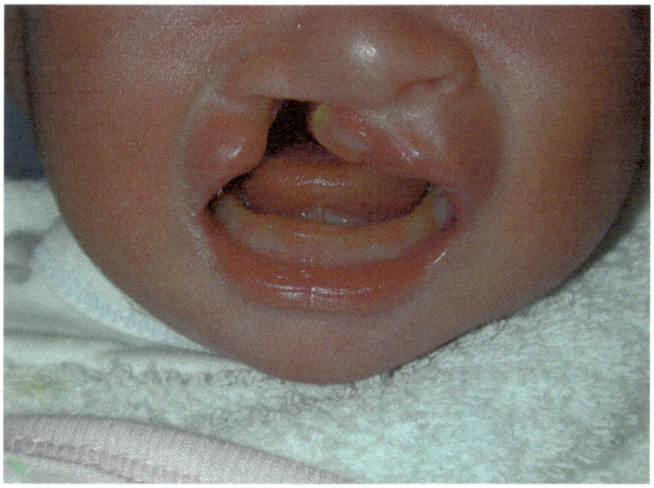

**Fig. 11.29** Patient A: Right complete cleft lip and palate, front view

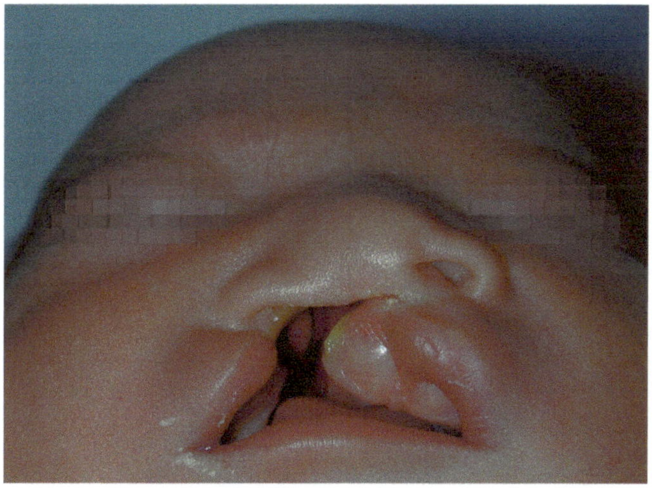

**Fig. 11.30** Patient A: Right complete cleft lip and palate, submental view

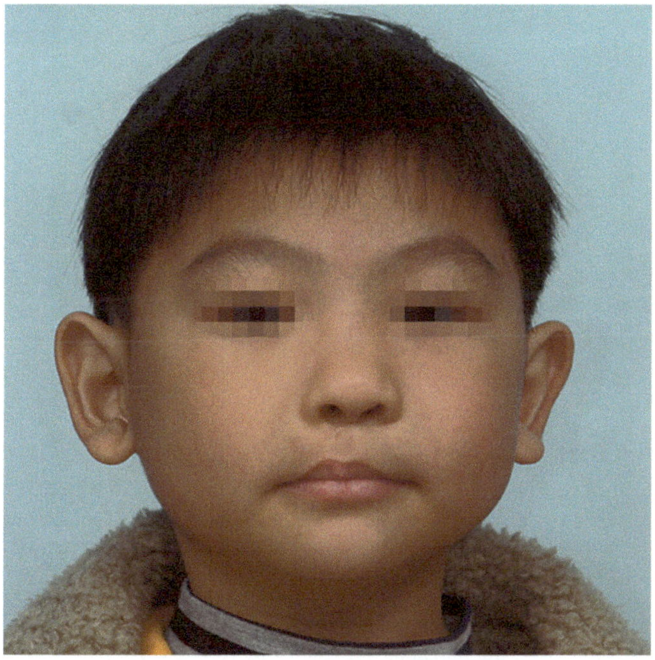

**Fig. 11.31** Patient A: 6 years after lip repair, front view

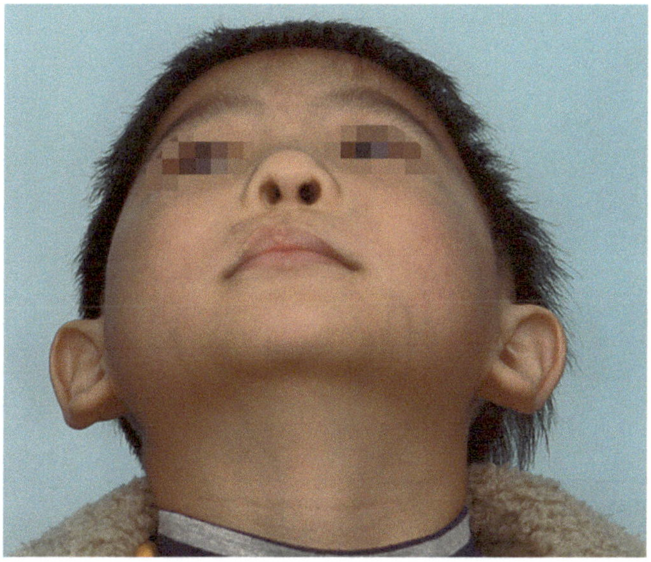

**Fig. 11.32** Patient A: 6 years after lip repair, submental view

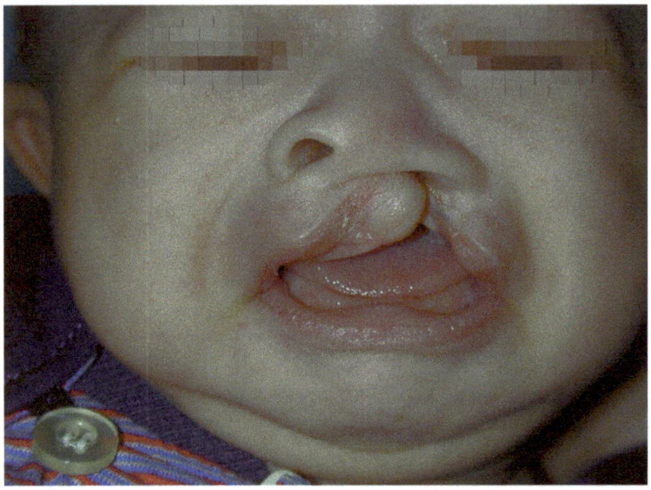

**Fig. 11.33** Patient B: Left complete cleft lip and alveolus, front view

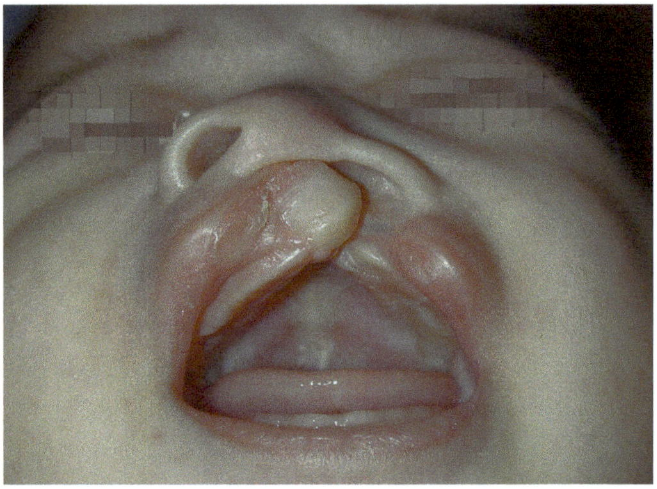

**Fig. 11.34** Patient B: Left complete cleft lip and alveolus, submental view

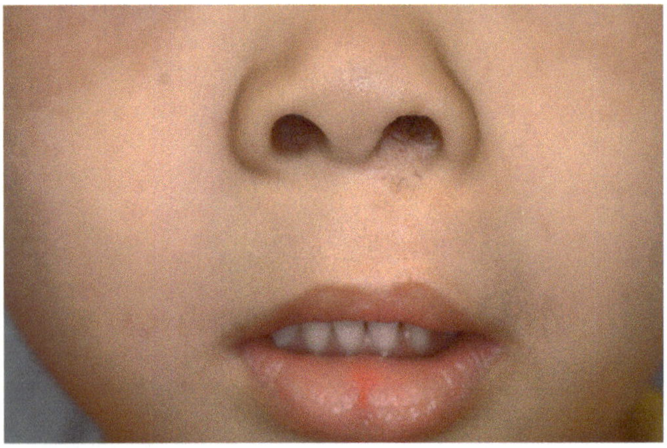

**Fig. 11.35** Patient B: 6 years after lip repair, front view

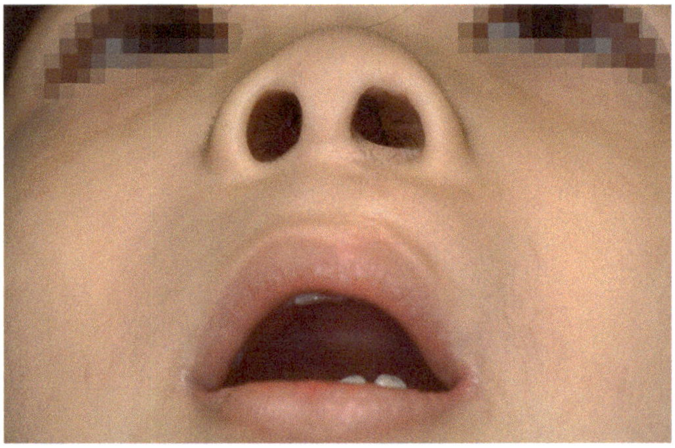

**Fig. 11.36** Patient B:-6 years after lip repair, submental view

## References


1. Grayson BH, Santiago PE, Brecht LE, et al. Presurgical nasoalveolar molding in infants with cleft lip and palate. Cleft Palate Craniofac J. 1999;36(6):486–98.
2. Pool R, Farnworth TK. Preoperative lip taping in the cleft lip. Ann Plast Surg. 1994;32(3):234–49.
3. Noordhoff MS, Chen YR, Chen KT, Hung KF, Lo LJ. The surgical technique for the complete unilateral cleft lip-nasal deformity. Oper Techn Plast Reconstr Surg. 1995;2(3):167.
4. Chen PK, Noordhoff MS, Kane A. Chap 23. repair of unilateral cleft lip. In: Neligan P, editor. Plastic surgery, vol. 3. 3rd ed. London: Elsevier-Saunders; 2012.
5. Chen PK, See JUC, Noordhoff MS. Chap 21.2. Rotation advancement cheiloplasty. In: Neligan P, editor. Plastic surgery, vol. 3. 4th ed. London: Elsevier;2018.
6. Mohler L. Unilateral cleft lip repair. Plast Reconstr Surg. 1987;80(4):511–6.
7. Liao YF, Lee YH, Wang R, Huang CS, Chen PK, Lo LJ, Chen YR. Vomer flap for hard palate repair is related to favorable maxillary growth in unilateral cleft lip and palate. Clin Oral Investig. 2014;18(4):1269–76.
8. Lu TC, Filson S, Yao CF, Chen PK. Septal anchoring suture: a key suture to improve the nasolabial symmetry in unilateral cheiloplasty. Int J Oral Maxillofac Surg. 2018;47:1106–13.
9. Onizuka T, Ichinose M, Hosaka Y, Usui Y, Jinnai T. The contour lines of the upper lip and a revised method of cleft lip repair. Ann Plast Surg. 1991;27(3):238–52.
10. Noordhoff MS, Millard DR. Reconstruction of vermillion in unilateral and bilateral cleft lips. Plast Reconstr Surg. 1984;73(1):52–61.
11. Liou EJW, Subramanian M, Chen PK, Huang CS. The progressive change of nasal symmetry and growth after nasoalveolar molding: a three-years follow-up study. Plast Reconstr Surg. 2004;114:858–64.
12. Chang CS, Por YC, Liou EJW, Chang CJ, Chen PK, Noordhoff MS. Long term comparison of four techniques for obtaining nasal symmetry in unilateral complete cleft lip patients: a single surgeon's experience. Plast Reconstr Surg. 2010;126:1276–84.
13. Lu TC, Lam WL, Chang CS, Chen PK. Primary correction of nasal deformity in unilateral incomplete cleft lip: a comparative study between three techniques. J Plast Reconstr Aesthet Surg. 2012;65:456–63.
14. Lu TC, Yao CF, Lin S, Chang CS, Chen PK. Primary septal cartilage graft for the unilateral cleft rhinoplasty. Plast Reconstr Surg. 2017;139(5):1177.
15. Chang CS, Wallace CG, Hsiao YC, Huang JJ, Chen ZC, Chang CJ, Lo LJ, Chen PK, Chen JP, Chen YR. Clinical evaluation of scar gel in the treatment of cleft lip scars. Sci Rep. 2018;8:7422.
16. Yeow VKL, Chen PK, Chen YR, Noordhoff MS. The use of nasal splints in the primary management of unilateral cleft nasal deformity. Plast Reconstr Surg. 1999;103(5):1347–54.

# Unilateral Cleft Lip Repair: Modified Mohler Technique

12

Chen Shen and Roberto L. Flores

**Key Points**

- The apex of the Cutting-Mohler back-cut should be placed on the columella at least 1.5–2 mm superior to the base of the nose, as novice surgeons often underestimate the vertical height of this critical mark, leading to some of the shortcomings of this repair.
- The L-flap should be based on the lateral nasal wall and not the alveolus, as originally described by Millard, for an alveolar-based L-flap will create a nasolabial fistula.
- The addition of a Noordhoff triangular flap of vermillion will help to prevent notching and to restore fullness to the medial lip vermillion.
- The best time to close the floor of the nose is during cleft lip repair; therefore, this should be attempted in every case.
- Primary cleft lip and nasal reconstruction has been made more predictable through presurgical manipulation of the nose and alveolus with NAM.
- Achieve a tension-free reconstruction in the critical aesthetic areas of the nose and upper lip skin, as even mild amounts of tension will result in relapse of the cleft deformity.
- Primary cleft rhinoplasty is critical to aesthetic and functional results; however, excessive dissection should be prevented, as it may result in excessive scar of the nasal tip that may be prohibitive to predictable rhinoplasty in the future.

## Introduction

The principles of Millard rotation-advancement were founded on the realization that the Cupid's bow is preserved in patients with unilateral cleft lip deformities. A back-cut was placed on the superior aspect of the upper lip which allowed for inferior rotation of the philtrum and Cupid's bow. The defect created by the back-cut was filled by an advancement flap from the lateral element. Although the Millard repair effectively positioned Cupid's bow, the resulting scar wound veers across the philtrum border at the superior aspect and risks creating a micronostril in cases of a wide unilateral cleft. In 1987, Lester Mohler improved on Millard's technique by relocating the back-cut from the upper lip to the columella [1], creating a scar which adhered to the subunit principles of the upper lip. In addition, the Mohler's repair utilizes the C-flap, rather than the lateral lip element, to fill the defect created by the downward rotation of the Cupid's bow, decreasing the need for medial advancement of the lateral lip element and thus decreasing the risk of creating a micronostril.

In Mohler's original design, the back-cut extended to the middle of the columellar base, limiting the downward rotation of Cupid's bow (Fig. 12.1). Millard accurately criticized Mohler's original description of his columellar back-cut as being inadequate for use in complete clefts and likely useful only in incomplete clefts [2]. In Cutting's variation, the apex of the Mohler incision was extended to just beyond the midline of the columella. The back-cut was then brought down to the opposite philtral column but no further (Fig. 12.2). This modification allows for full downward rotation of the Cupid's bow in any unilateral cleft lip patient, regardless of severity. Cutting's popularization and modification of the Mohler repair justify the appropriate description of the technique as the Cutting-Mohler repair.

C. Shen (✉) · R. L. Flores
Hansjörg Wyss Department of Plastic Surgery, NYU Langone Health, New York, NY, USA
e-mail: Chen.Shen@nyulangone.org; Roberto.Flores@nyulangone.org

© Springer Nature Switzerland AG 2021

J. W. Swanson, D. W. Low (eds.), *Global Cleft Care in Low-Resource Settings*, https://doi.org/10.1007/978-3-030-59105-2_12

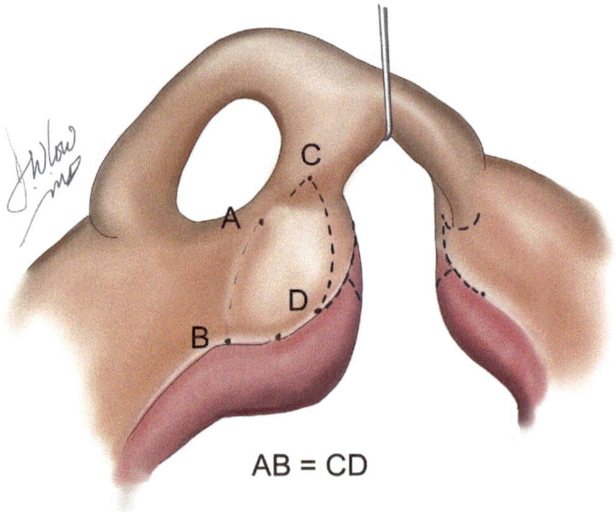


Fig. 12.1 Original markings for Mohler unilateral cleft lip repair

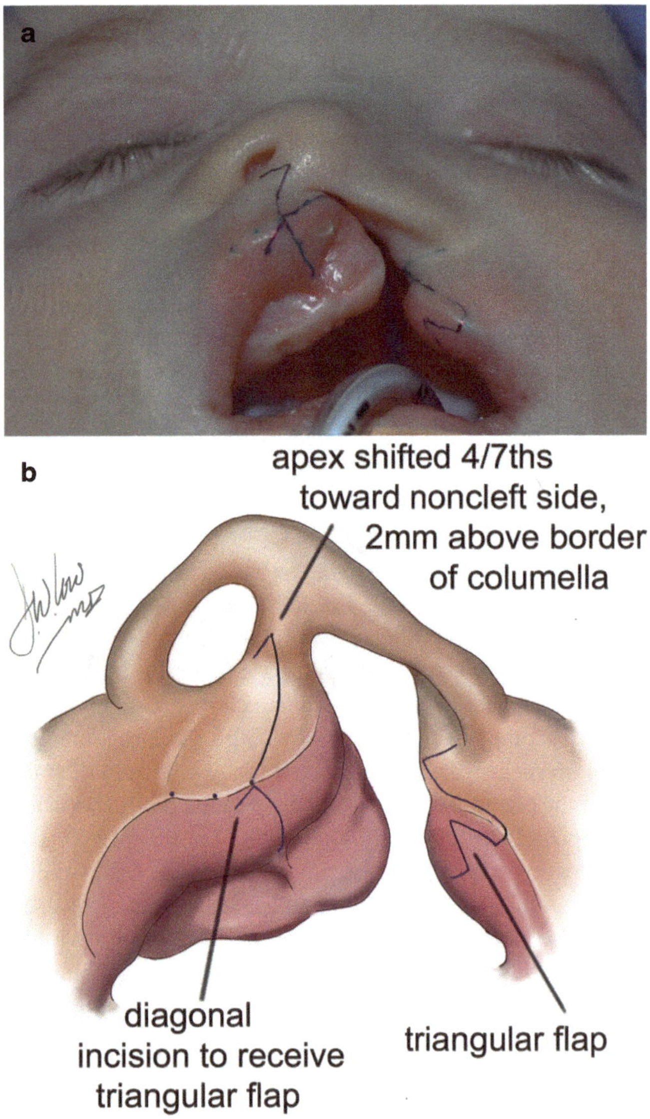


Fig. 12.2 Final markings for the Cutting-Mohler unilateral cleft lip repair on table (**a**) and schematically (**b**)

## Anatomy

The orbicularis oris sphincter is maintained in resting position through multiple attachments with the muscles of facial animation of the lower face. Interruption of the orbicularis oris sphincter by a cleft deformity results in distortion of the upper lip and nose by the unopposed action of the zygomaticus major and minor, the risorius, and the orbicularis oris itself.

In the medial lip element, disruption of the orbicularis oris results in vertical shortening of the medial upper lip, superior rotation of the Cupid's bow, and vertical shortening of the vermillion. The columella and philtral column are shortened on the cleft side.

In the lateral lip element, the height and transverse length are shortened. Disruption of the pars superficialis on the lateral lip alters the direction of this muscle to run almost vertically in the area below the ala, leading to aberrant attachments to the nostril and periosteum of the piriform aperture. This leads to a vertically foreshortened lateral lip, sometimes producing a bulge in this area.

Separation of the orbicularis oris results in unopposed action of the ipsilateral zygomaticus major. This results in lateralization of the alar base, depression of the nostril rim, and canting of the columella toward the cleft side. Unilateral attachment of the orbicularis oris to the medial crura footplates, anterior nasal spine, and caudal septum on the noncleft side exacerbates the columellar tilt and contributes to deviation of the caudal septum toward the noncleft side. The cumulative effects on the underlying cartilaginous structures include shorted medial crus of the lower lateral cartilage, elongated and inferiorly displaced lateral crus, and dislocated septum out of the vomer that bows toward the cleft side.

The alveolus of the upper jaw is normally intact, and a standard U shape is appreciated when looking at this structure from below. In the affected patient, the greater segment of the alveolus is rotated anteriorly and laterally due to fetal protrusion of the tongue. The lesser segment of the alveolus rotates posteriorly. The medial buttress of the maxilla can be hypoplastic and posteriorly displaced. As the maxilla is the foundation of the nose, these bony aberrations have a cumulative effect on the cleft nasal deformity.

## Preoperative Planning

Preoperative assessment of a patient with unilateral cleft lip includes complete physical examination with assessment for other comorbidities. Facial exam includes laterality (left, right, or midline), severity of cleft lip (microform, minor form, incomplete, or complete), and extent of nasal deformity.

Presurgical orthopedics such as nasoalveolar molding (NAM) can make primary cleft lip repair and primary rhinoplasty more predictable, especially in patients with complete cleft or significant nasal deformity [3–5]. NAM can help correct the outwardly rotated greater segment and posterolaterally displaced lesser segment, realigning the skeletal platform into a more anatomic position. In addition, if the alveolar segments are aligned within 1 mm, a gingivoperiosteoplasty (GPP) can be performed, which can avoid a secondary bone grafting procedure in 60–73% of patients [6–8]. NAM typically commences 2 weeks after birth and is completed after 10 weeks of therapy in patients with unilateral cleft. Although a potentially useful presurgical intervention, it is not a requirement for primary cleft lip repair.

**Field Solutions**

Although the Cutting-Mohler repair can be applied to any complete unilateral cleft lip deformity, regardless of severity, NAM increases nasal symmetry [9–11], decreases need for nasal and facial dissection during primary cleft rhinoplasty, facilitates gingivoperiosteoplasty [12], and decreases requirement of secondary "touch-up" surgery. Alternatively, lip taping, Latham device, other forms of presurgical orthopedics, or lip adhesion may be pursued.

Multidisciplinary care is essential for optimal outcomes. Members of the team include plastic surgeons, pediatricians, orthodontists, pediatric dentists, oral-maxillofacial surgeons, speech pathologists, otolaryngologists, audiologists, child psychologists, pediatric geneticists, nurse team coordinators, and social workers.

## Surgical Management

Quality of the primary repair establishes initial function and appearance for the patients and has great bearing on their future quality of life. Initial lip and nose repairs are performed at approximately 3 months of age.

**Tips and Tricks**

The goal of primary cleft lip and nasal repair is to obtain the most lasting result with the least amount of surgery possible. The ideal goal is one surgery at the time of infancy and a final touch-up surgery on the lip or nose (if needed) at the time of facial maturity.

When considering the delicate reconstruction of the three-dimensional form of the lip and nose, even mild amounts of tension will result in relapse of the cleft deformity, can cause widened scars, and predispose the patient to further surgery that may result in additional scars in the area. Therefore, tissues should be adequately freed until tension is completely eliminated in the critical aesthetic areas of the nose and upper lip skin to achieve a tension-free reconstruction. In cases when presurgical orthopedics is not used, extensive dissection may be required.

**Tips and Tricks**

Even a small amount of tension on soft tissue closure will result in relapse. It is important to surgically release soft tissue attachments to prevent tension on closure. These points of attachment include the orbicularis oris attachment to the anterior nasal spine on the noncleft side, the orbicularis oris attachment to the pyriform aperture on the cleft side, the release of the alar base and possibly the nasal lining from the pyriform rim on the cleft side, and, when appropriate, composite release of the lateral lip element from the face of the maxilla. This is even more critical when no presurgical orthopedics is performed.

Previous studies have demonstrated the aesthetic benefit of primary cleft rhinoplasty [13, 14] as well as the safety of infant rhinoplasty to subsequent nasal growth, but primary cleft rhinoplasty should be directed and limited in dissection to prevent excessive scar in the nasal tip and result in a challenging nasal repair in the future. Therefore, the goal is to anatomically reposition the displaced lower lateral cartilages with the least amount of surgery. Ideally, patients would receive effective primary cleft rhinoplasty at the time of cleft repair followed by a secondary rhinoplasty at the time of facial maturity. Proper planning, surgical technique, and appreciation of the larger picture can avoid repeated nasal revisions and potentially insurmountable hurdles of an aggressively dissected or over-operated scarred nose.

## Surgical Approach

### Positioning

The patient should be placed in a supine position with gentle neck extension from a shoulder roll.

## Markings

Surgical markings for the Cutting-Mohler unilateral cleft lip repair initially follow the traditional white roll markings as described by Millard. In the medial lip element, the height and depth of the Cupid's bow are marked on the unaffected side (Fig. 12.1). These two points are used to mark the height of the Cupid's bow on the cleft side, where the white roll usually disappears. If Cupid's bow is wide or indistinct, the marks can be placed more narrowly so that less downward rotation is required.

In the lateral lip element, the white roll mark can be determined by three methods. The distance between the height of the Cupid's bow and the lateral commissure may be measured and used to locate the corresponding white roll point, as advocated by Millard [15], but this can prioritize lip width over vertical height of the lip. Even small discrepancies in vertical lip height are visible at conversation distance, while discrepancies in horizontal width are less easily noticed and correct over time [16, 17]. Noordhoff describes using the widest point of the vermillion (Noordhoff point) [18], but use in patients with a wide cleft may result in a vertically foreshortened lip. Therefore, the third method, which uses the height of the cutaneous upper lip on the noncleft side (typically 10 mm), should be employed. This distance is measured on the lateral lip from the medial aspect of the alar base to determine the mark made on the white roll.

The apex of the back-cut is then marked on the columella approximately 2 mm superior to the border of the columella in the upper lip and 4/7th across the columella toward the noncleft side. Care is taken not to extend the marked back-cut below the columella onto the upper lip, as this would elongate the upper lip during repair and extend the C-flap to the upper lip, disrupting the subunit borders. The apex of the back-cut is directed by the height of the Cupid's bow on the cleft side while bowing this line out to the same degree as the philtral column of the unaffected side to recreate the subtle curve (Fig. 12.2). The back-cut is marked as a straight line to the height of the philtrum on the noncleft side and no further. The angle formed by these two lines will affect the degree of downward rotation of the Cupid's bow. Subtle modifications in the location of these two points can have profound effects on the extent of downward rotation of Cupid's bow, the width of the philtrum, and the resulting shape of the columella.

**Tips and Tricks**
Small changes in the location of the base and apex of the Cutting-Mohler back-cut can have large effects on the extent of downward rotation of Cupid's bow possible, the width of the columella, and the shape of the philtrum. Regarding placement of the apex of the back-cut, placing the point too inferior will limit the degree of downward rotation of Cupid's bow; too far to the cleft side will result in a wide superior philtrum and an exceedingly narrow columella; and too far to the noncleft side will result in a narrow philtrum with a poor blood supply. Regarding placement of the base of the back-cut, placing the point too inferior (on the lip) will lengthen the upper lip; too superior will limit the extent of the downward rotation of Cupid's bow; and too far to the cleft side will limit the extent of the downward rotation of Cupid's bow and comprise the width of the superior philtrum. Failure to work through the learning curve of proper point placement leads to some of the reported shortcomings of the repair.

The C-flap and M-flap are marked in the usual fashion (Fig. 12.2). Care is taken to incorporate as much white lip into the C-flap as possible while avoiding the mucosa. The vermillion of the medial lip element can include a receiving incision for a Noordhoff triangular vermillion flap which is drawn as a diagonal line on the dry lip 1 mm inferior to the white roll, toward the red line.

**Tips and Tricks**
A Noordhoff triangular vermillion flap is included to restore fullness to the vermillion at the area of the tubercle, prevent a whistling deformity, and anatomically reconstruct the red line of the upper lip [18].

A small incision is marked along the alar crease on the cleft side with care not to extend this incision around the alar base. The border of the L-flap is then marked by first marking an incision 1 mm inferior to the white roll mark on the lateral lip element. This mark then transects the white roll perpendicularly and then curves swiftly to meet the medial edge of the previously made mark on the alar crease. The remainder of the L-flap can then be made with or without the addition of a Noordhoff triangular flap. Care should be taken to extend inferior border of the L-flap just superior to the alveolus, as this will base the L-flap off of the lateral nasal wall and not the alveolus, as originally described by Millard (Fig. 12.2).

All premarked incisions are made full thickness through the skin and mucosa.

## Surgical Technique

The M-flap is elevated in a submucosal plane, and the C-flap is elevated in the subcutaneous plane with care to preserve

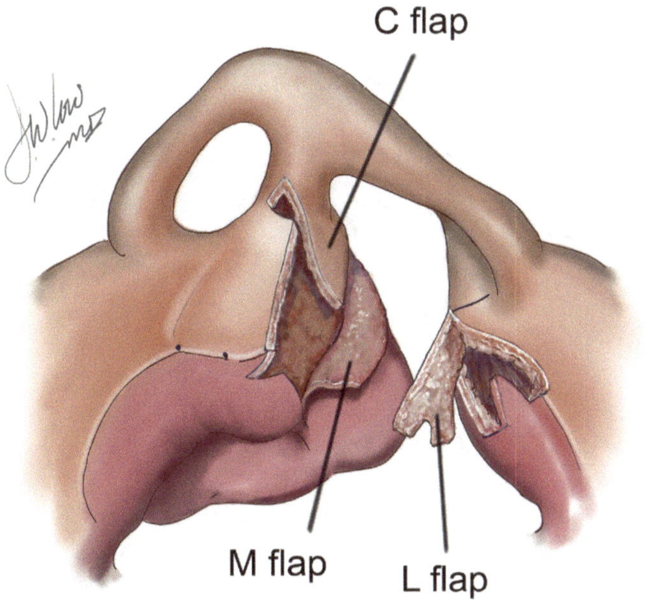


Fig. 12.3 C-, M-, and L-flap dissection

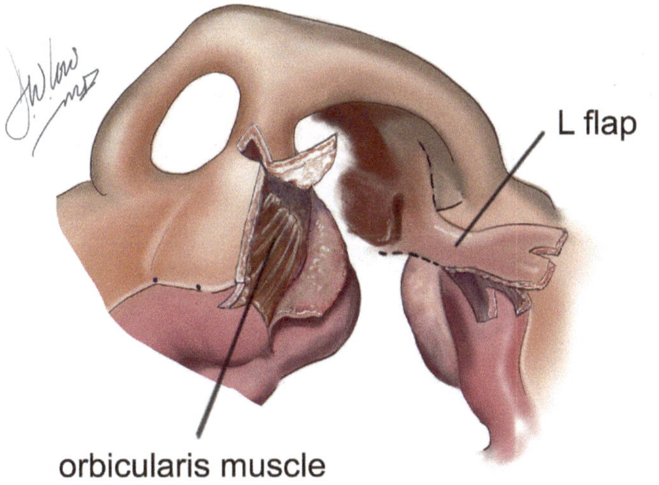


Fig. 12.4 Sharp dissection of the L-flap from the orbicularis oris and extension to the lateral nasal wall

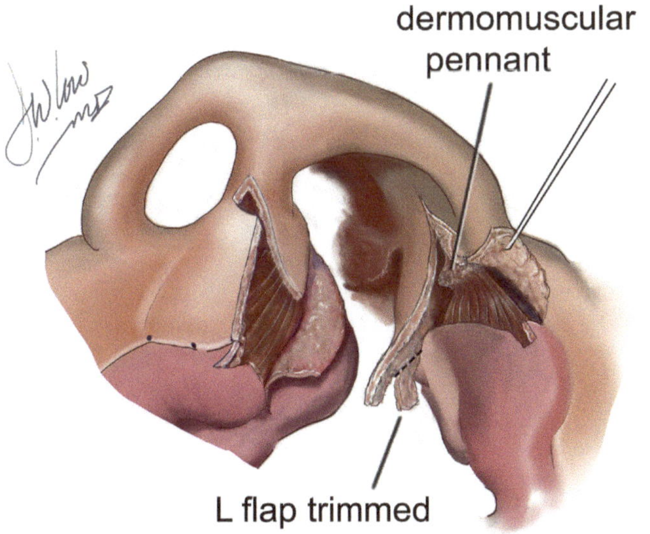


Fig. 12.5 L-flap trimming and creation of the dermomuscular pennant

the underlying orbicularis oris. The dissection is continued into the apex of the Cutting-Mohler incision within the columella (Fig. 12.3). Complete full-thickness horizontal transection of the orbicularis oris is then made at the junction between the upper lip and columella and not the apex, or else the medial crura will be transected (Fig. 12.4). The oral mucosa should be preserved underneath the upper lip muscle. Tension-free, full downward rotation of the Cupid's bow should be appreciable at this time. If additional rotation is still required, the labial frenulum can be horizontally transected in a hockey-stick fashion (long limb of the incision parallels the frenulum, while the short limb transects it), and the defect may be filled by base of the M-flap. The medial lip element is prepared by mobilizing the philtral skin from the muscle in a subcutaneous plane up to but no further than the philtral dimple. This will aid in aesthetic reconstruction of the philtrum and precise placement of the Cupid's bow.

The L-flap is sharply dissected from the orbicularis oris in the subcutaneous and submucosal plane and should be based on the lateral nasal wall and not the alveolus, as previously described by Millard, to prevent creation of a nasolabial fistula (Fig. 12.4). As one approaches the area of the piriform aperture, the dissection plane changes from submucosal to subperiosteal. A Woodson elevator is then used to create a subperiosteal pocket in the area of the piriform aperture. A vertical intranasal incision is made at the border of the nasal mucosa and squamous skin to meet the superior border of the L-flap (Figs. 12.4 and 12.5). The depth of this piriform aperture incision should extend to the bone. Subperiosteal dissection will complete the elevation of the L-flap posteriorly until it is based off the lateral nasal wall. A horizontal incision is made at the exact border of the lateral nasal wall with the nasal floor. An incision is made at the base of the vomer to elevate a vomer flap using the periosteal elevator. The lateral nasal wall and vomer flaps will be used later to close the anterior nasal floor. A gingivobuccal sulcus incision is made in continuity with the piriform aperture incision, with care to preserve the L-flap (Fig. 12.5). A supraperiosteal dissection is made across the maxilla to fully mobilize the alar base and lateral lip element. In patients with incomplete clefts or those who underwent NAM, there will be a limited need for this incision and dissection; otherwise the dissection across the face of the maxilla may be extensive. Tension-free translation of the alar base flap to the anterior nasal spine will demonstrate adequate dissection, as even a small amount of tension at the

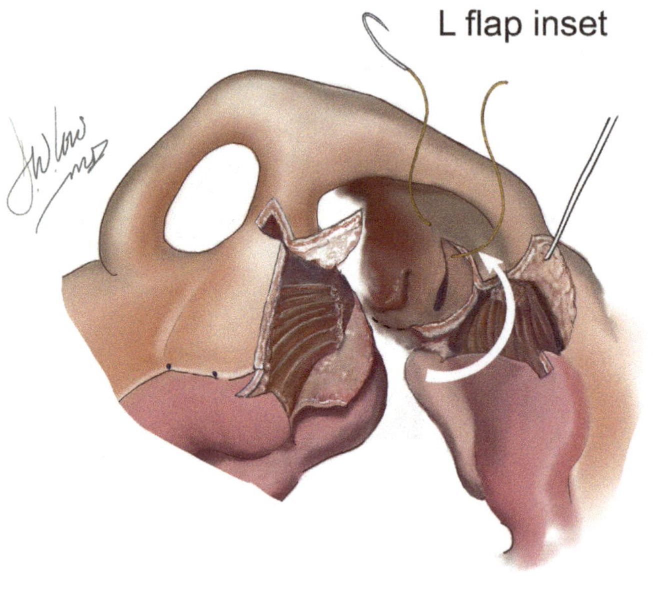


**Fig. 12.6** L-flap sutured under tension to the base of the piriform aperture incision

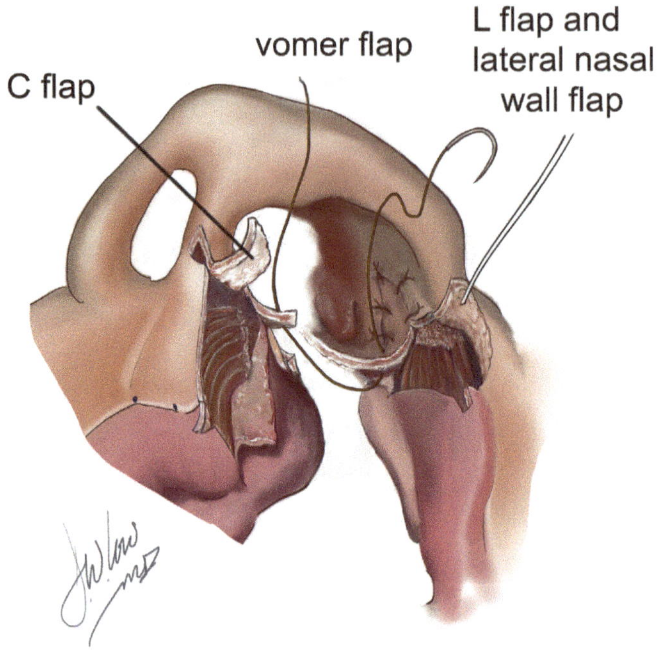


**Fig. 12.7** Nasal floor closure

time of closure will result in relapse of the deformity. The alar base skin should be elevated in a thick split-thickness skin graft plane, so a layer of the dermis is present on the underlying muscular flap. This dermomuscular pennant will be used to relocate the alar base. The lateral lip skin is mobilized from the orbicularis oris as far lateral as the alar base incision.

The L-flap is sutured under tension to the base of the piriform aperture incision (Fig. 12.6). Excess L-flap is trimmed, and the remainder is sutured into the defect created by the piriform aperture incision. A gingivoperiosteoplasty is performed at this time if desired. The lateral nasal wall flap/L-flap is sutured to the vomer flap using several absorbable sutures to close the anterior nasal floor and facilitate successful gingivoperiosteoplasty and/or alveolar bone grafting (Fig. 12.7). Sutures should first be placed in a simple fashion and then in a horizontal mattress to create a watertight closure of the nasal floor. The gingivobuccal sulcus incision is closed using several oblique sutures to relieve tension from the midline of the mucosal reconstruction, preventing dehiscence. The mucosa of the upper lip is then closed with simple sutures, with care not to incorporate muscle.

The rhinoplasty portion of the procedure will elongate the columella and elevate the depressed lower lateral cartilage. A hemimembranous septum incision is first made on the cleft side (Fig. 12.8). Through the apex of the Cutting-Mohler back-cut, blunt dissection is performed to create a dissection pocket between the medial crura with care not to damage the lower lateral cartilages. Converse scissors are then inserted underneath the nasal tip skin and over the upper and lower lateral cartilages on the cleft and noncleft sides. Careful blunt dissection will create a subcutaneous pocket over the

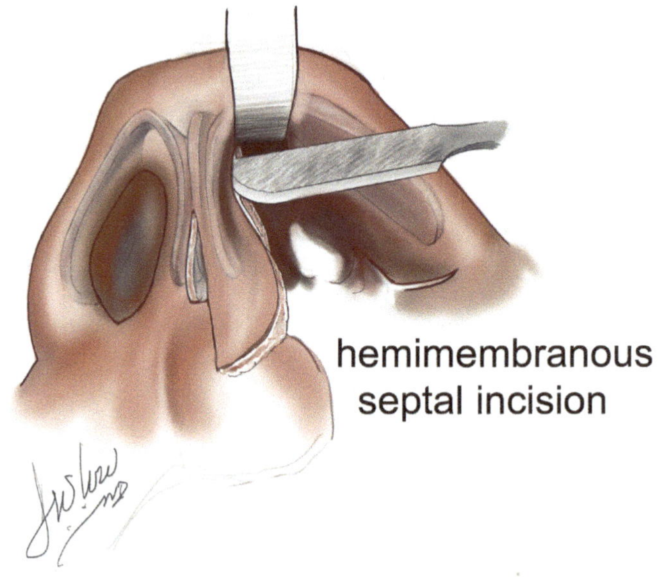


**Fig. 12.8** Hemimembranous septum incision first made on the cleft side

upper and lower lateral cartilages in preparation for rhinoplasty (Fig. 12.9). Care is taken not to close the dissection scissors in the pocket, as it can lead to damage to the lower lateral cartilages. If no NAM was performed, an additional nostril rim incision and a dissection pocket are made to connect the rim incision to the subcutaneous pocket underneath the nasal tip. A Ragnell retractor is used to elevate the depressed lower lateral cartilage in a super-corrected position. Several horizontal mattress sutures are then placed

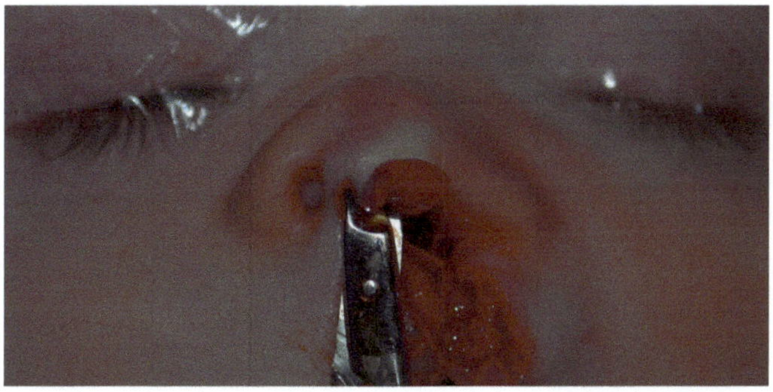

Fig. 12.9 Blunt dissection with Converse scissors creates a subcutaneous pocket over the upper and lower lateral cartilages in preparation for rhinoplasty

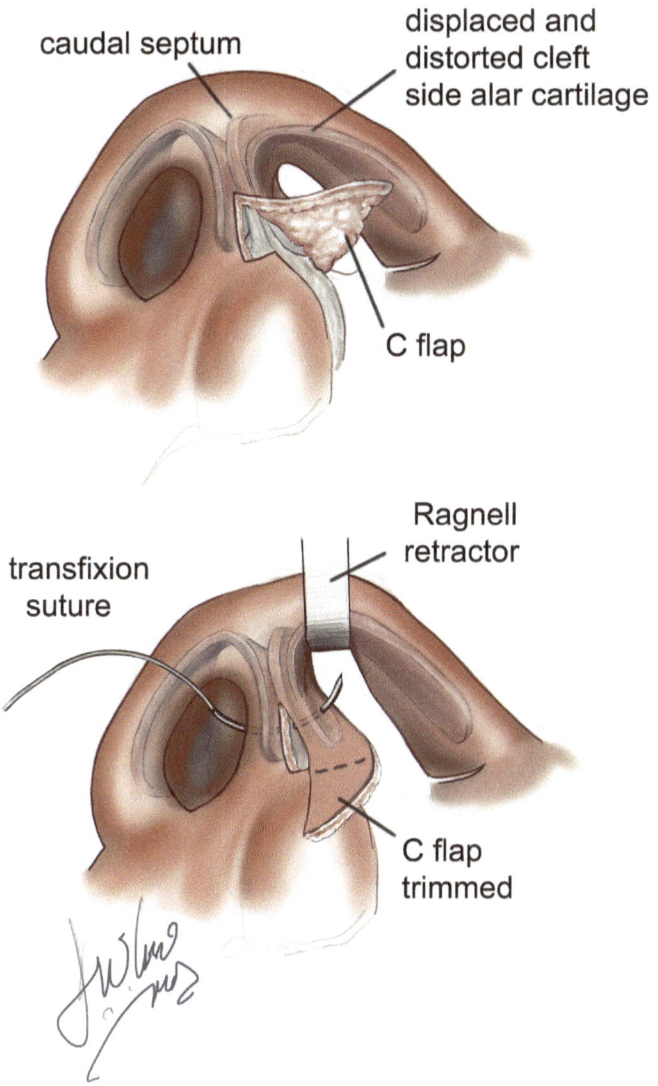


Fig. 12.10 Tip rhinoplasty. Trimming and inset of the C-flap

using long-lasting absorbable transfixion sutures to affix the medial crura to the cartilaginous septum (Fig. 12.10). These sutures also shape the columella, so precise placement is essential. The columellar length on the cleft side should equal that of the noncleft side. If a nostril rim incision is used, a suture is placed from the cleft-side lower lateral cartilage to the upper cartilage to further reinforce the former's elevated position. Overcorrection of the vertical position of the lower lateral cartilage is critical to a long-lasting aesthetic result.

> **Tips and Tricks**
> Primary cleft rhinoplasty should be performed in all patients regardless of the use or non-use of presurgical orthopedics. There should be an overcorrection of the vertical height of the lower lateral cartilage on the cleft side whenever possible. The height of the lower lateral cartilage typically falls over time.

The alar base is first repositioned using long-lasting absorbable suture placed through the dermomuscular pennant underneath the alar base and then the caudal septum and medial crus on the noncleft side (Fig. 12.11). This suture and a second reinforcing suture will set the alar base in an anatomic position, medialize the columella, and straighten the anterior septum. The orbicularis oris is carefully trimmed so that the skin edges perfectly oppose at the completion of the muscular reconstruction to eliminate all tension from the upper lip skin repair (Fig. 12.12). The lip is closed through superior to inferior reconstruction of the orbicularis oris and reconstruction of the white roll and then vermillion. The Noordhoff triangular flap, if used, is trimmed and inset at this time. The C-flap is trimmed and inset to fill the defect by downward rotation of the Cupid's bow with closure (Fig. 12.10). Excess alar skin is trimmed, and the nostril floor is closed in a stair-step fashion to avoid confluence of four corners of the C-flap and alar base flaps with the medial and lateral elements of the upper lip skin flaps.

If NAM was implemented, the nostril apex overhang is addressed using a long-lasting absorbable suture placed obliquely (laterally and posteriorly) just behind the nostril rim, through the lower lateral cartilage, underneath the skin of the nasal tip, and out of the nostril on the opposite side (Fig. 12.13). The suture is then returned 2 mm behind the exit suture hole on the noncleft side, parallel to the first suture, and returning to the cleft nostril, thus elevating and medializing the depressed lateral crura as well as adding tip definition. If no NAM was used, the lower lateral cartilage is elevated by the previously placed suture from the lower lateral to upper lateral cartilage. A small rim of overhanging skin at the nostril apex is trimmed, and the rim incision is closed. Regardless of technique, the depressed lower lat-

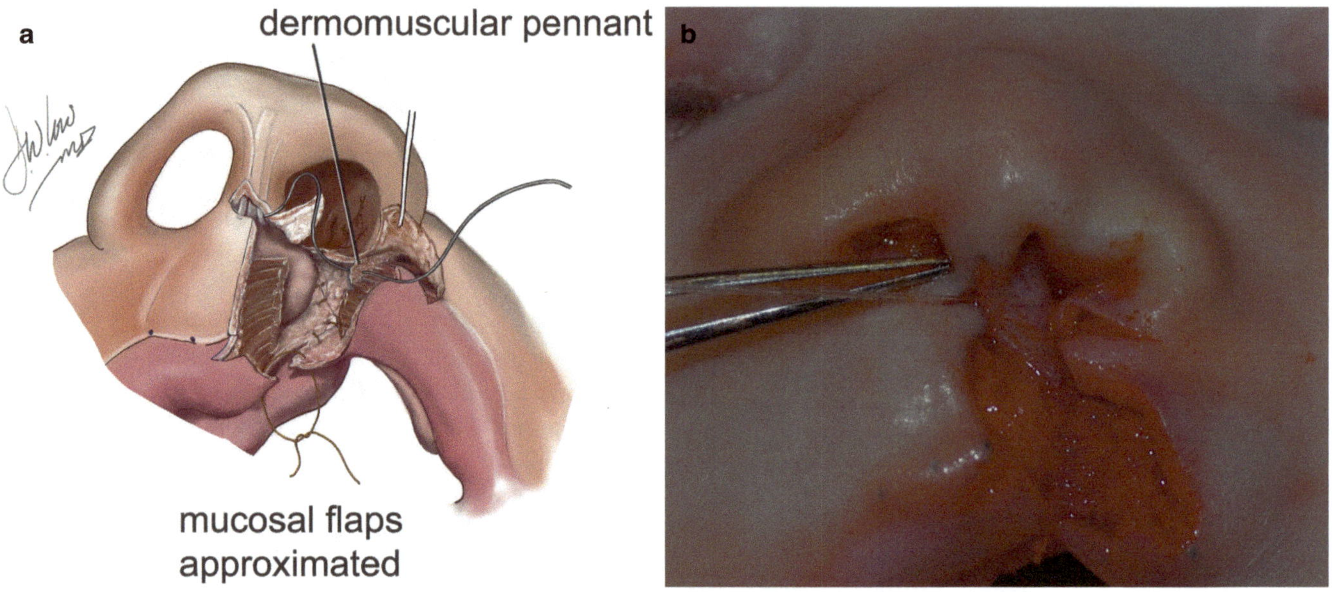


**Fig. 12.11** Repositioning of the alar base by approximating to the caudal septum and medial crus on the noncleft side (**a**). Manual repositioning of the caudal septum helps medialize the columella (**b**)

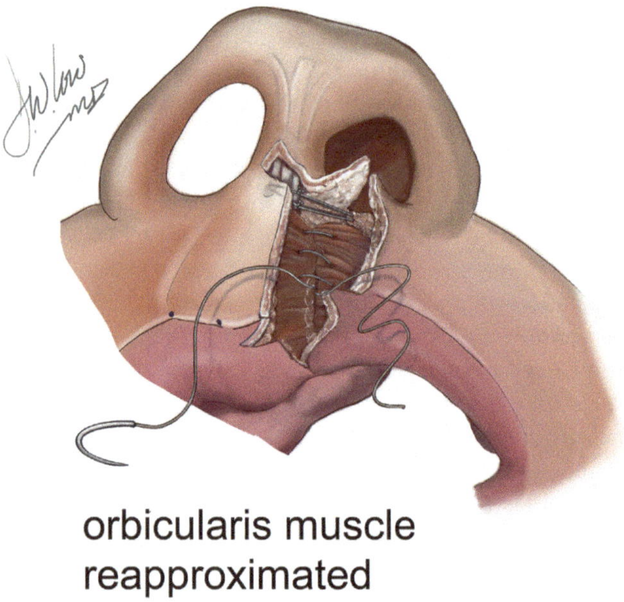


**Fig. 12.12** Trimming and reconstruction of the orbicularis oris muscle

eral cartilage should be overcorrected such that the cleft side is higher than the noncleft side. The vestibular web obliteration is performed using internal retention sutures placed behind the web out of the nasal facial groove (Fig. 12.13). The suture can then be returned through the same cutaneous hole and back into the nostril anterior to the vestibular web, thus obliterating the web and accentuating the nasal facial groove. Multiple suture may be required, especially in cases of complete and wide unilateral cleft nasal deformity.

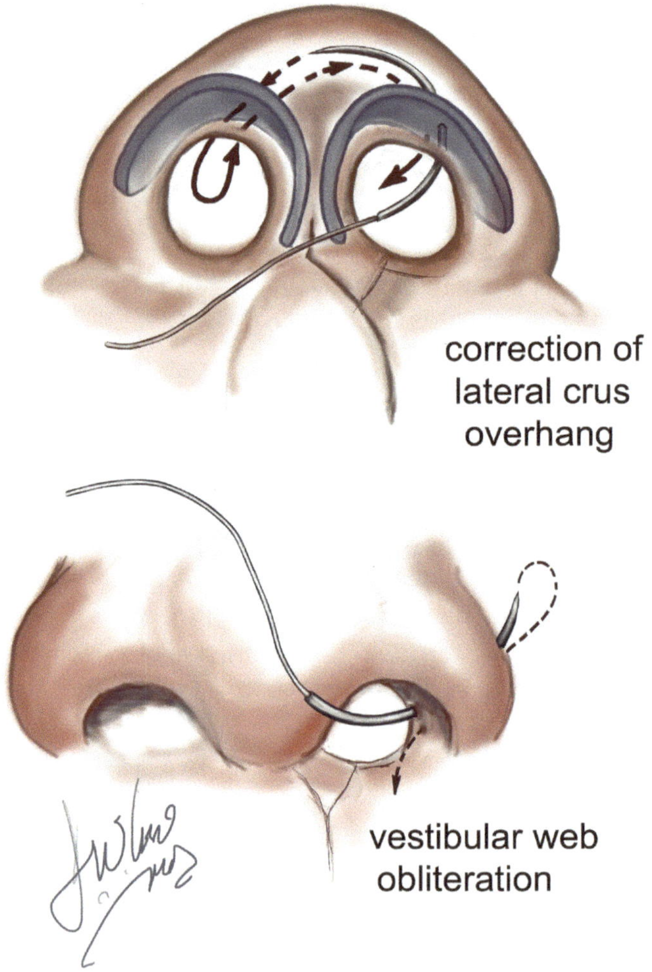


**Fig. 12.13** Correction of the nostril apex overhang and vestibular web obliteration

## Postoperative Care

Unilateral cleft lip repair is commonly performed as outpatient surgery. Parents are instructed to clean the upper lip twice daily with soap and water as well as dilute hydrogen peroxide. Children are placed in hand mittens for 5–7 days to protect the reconstructed site. No pacifier is used for a 1-week period, and bottle feeding as well as breastfeeding can continue normally. All permanent sutures are removed 5–7 days postoperatively, and the lip is taped in compression for 5 weeks to prevent microshearing at the incision line.

## Outcomes

In experienced hands, patients undergoing the Cutting-Mohler repair can obtain lasting symmetry to the lip and nose with scars strategically placed within the subunit borders of the face (Fig. 12.14a–f). Long-term clinical outcomes demonstrate restoration of the upper lip height on the affected side [16]. Surgeons and parents should appreciate initial shortening of the upper lip height on the affected side, peaking at 6–8 weeks postoperatively and eventually elongating over the course of 1 year as the scar softens and remodels.

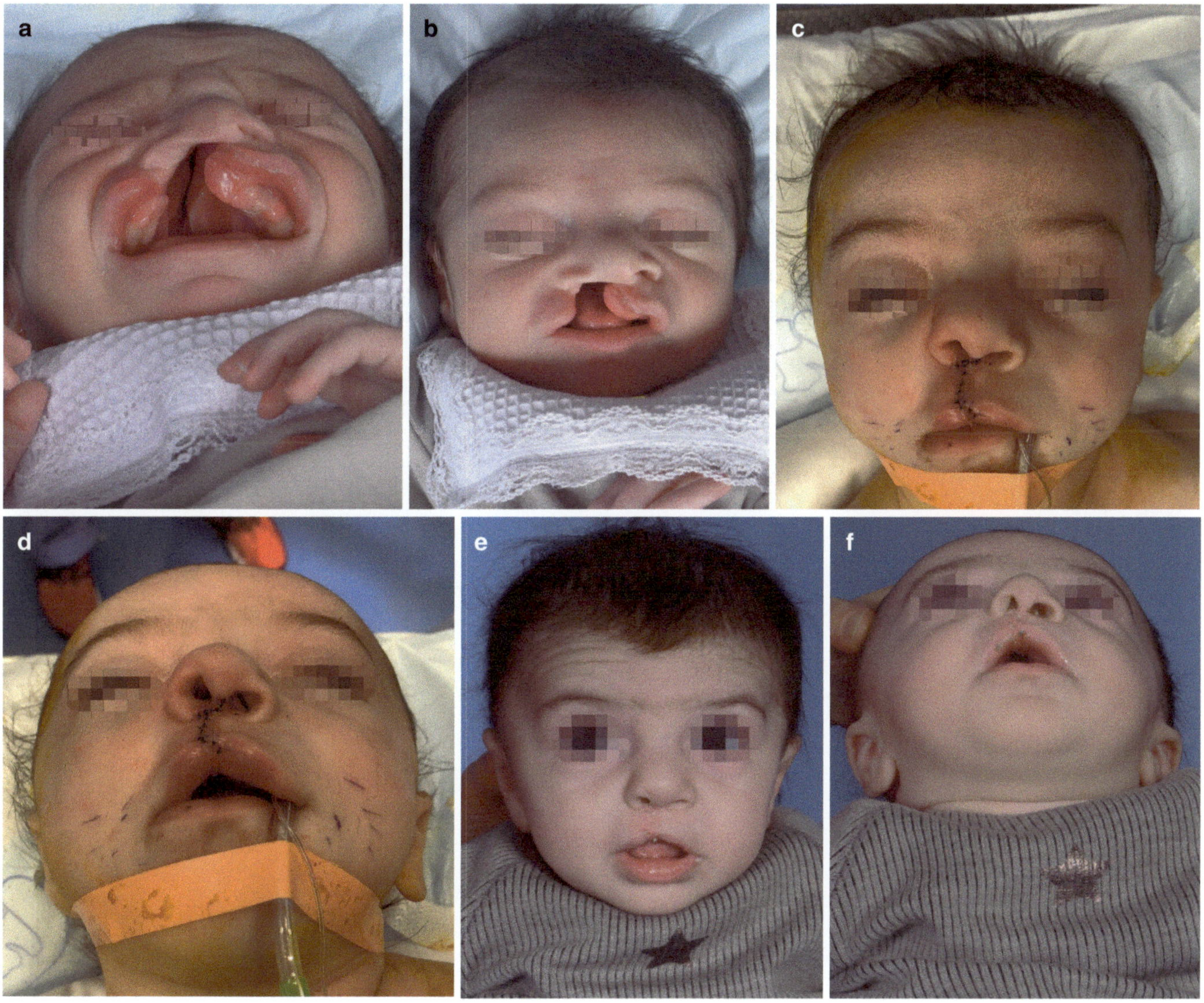


Fig. 12.14 Right unilateral complete cleft lip repair using this technique is shown (preoperative, **a** and **b**; immediately postoperative, **c** and **d**; and a 3-week early postoperative result, **e** and **f**)

## Complications

Complications include relapse of the nasal deformity, scar contracture/widening, inadequate multidisciplinary care and follow-up during growth, and maxillary growth inhibition.

## References

1. Mohler LR. Unilateral cleft lip repair. Plast Reconstr Surg. 1987;80(4):511–6.
2. Millard DR Jr. Discussion: unilateral cleft lip repair. Plast Reconstr Surg. 1987;80(4):517.
3. Grayson BH, Santiago PE, Brecht LE, Cutting CB. Presurgical nasoalveolar molding in infants with cleft lip and palate. Cleft Palate Craniofac J. 1999;36(6):486–98.
4. Grayson BH, Garfinkle JS. Early cleft management: the case for nasoalveolar molding. Am J Orthod Dentofacial Orthop. 2014;145(2):134–42.
5. Grayson BH, Cutting C, Wood R. Preoperative columella lengthening in bilateral cleft lip and palate. Plast Reconstr Surg. 1993;92(7):1422–3.
6. Santiago PE, Grayson BH, Cutting CB, Gianoutsos MP, Brecht LE, Kwon SM. Reduced need for alveolar bone grafting by presurgical orthopedics and primary gingivoperiosteoplasty. Cleft Palate Craniofac J. 1998;35(1):77–80.
7. Pfeifer TM, Grayson BH, Cutting CB. Nasoalveolar molding and gingivoperiosteoplasty versus alveolar bone graft: an outcome analysis of costs in the treatment of unilateral cleft alveolus. Cleft Palate Craniofac J. 2002;39(1):26–9.
8. Wang YC, Liao YF, Chen PK. Outcome of gingivoperiosteoplasty for the treatment of alveolar clefts in patients with unilateral cleft lip and palate. Br J Oral Maxillofac Surg. 2013;51(7):650–5.
9. Barillas I, Dec W, Warren SM, Cutting CB, Grayson BH. Nasoalveolar molding improves long-term nasal symmetry in complete unilateral cleft lip-cleft palate patients. Plast Reconstr Surg. 2009;123(3):1002–6.
10. Gomez DF, Donohue ST, Figueroa AA, Polley JW. Nasal changes after presurgical nasoalveolar molding (PNAM) in the unilateral cleft lip nose. Cleft Palate Craniofac J. 2012;49(6):689–700.
11. Chang CS, Por YC, Liou EJ, Chang CJ, Chen PK, Noordhoff MS. Long-term comparison of four techniques for obtaining nasal symmetry in unilateral complete cleft lip patients: a single surgeon's experience. Plast Reconstr Surg. 2010;126(4):1276–84.
12. Sato Y, Grayson BH, Garfinkle JS, Barillas I, Maki K, Cutting CB. Success rate of gingivoperiosteoplasty with and without secondary bone grafts compared with secondary alveolar bone grafts alone. Plast Reconstr Surg. 2008;121(4):1356–67; discussion 1368–9.
13. McComb H. Primary correction of unilateral cleft lip nasal deformity: a 10-year review. Plast Reconstr Surg. 1985;75(6):791–9.
14. Salyer KE. Primary correction of the unilateral cleft lip nose: a 15-year experience. Plast Reconstr Surg. 1986;77(4):558–68.
15. Millard DR Jr. Cleft craft: the evolution of its surgery. Volume 1 - The unilateral deformity, vol. 1. Boston: Little, Brown, and Company; 1976.
16. Cutting CB, Dayan JH. Lip height and lip width after extended Mohler unilateral cleft lip repair. Plast Reconstr Surg. 2003;111(1):17–23; discussion 24–6.
17. Mulliken JB, LaBrie RA. Fourth-dimensional changes in nasolabial dimensions following rotation-advancement repair of unilateral cleft lip. Plast Reconstr Surg. 2012;129(2):491–8.
18. Noordhoff MS. The surgical technique for the unilateral cleft lip-nasal deformity. Taipei: Noordhoff Craniofacial Foundation; 1997.

# Unilateral Cleft Lip Repair: Anatomic Subunit Approximation Technique

# 13

Raymond W. Tse and David M. Fisher

## Introduction

The *anatomic subunit approximation approach* to unilateral cleft lip repair [1, 2] involves a measured, landmark-based plan that provides multiple opportunities to verify the design prior to each successive step. Given that it is based upon landmarks, it can be applied to clefts along the full spectrum of presentation. Although the many landmarks may initially seem cumbersome, the carefully measured design allows for efficient surgical execution and avoids the need to revise incisions. Each point in the repair is a standard anthropometric landmark that new surgeons should learn and that experienced surgeons should already recognize [2]. For the less experienced surgeon, the well-thought-out plan helps with confidence. For the more experienced surgeon, the overt identification of nasolabial features can help to fine-tune the surgical repair.

The original design is a hybrid that includes key elements of several surgical techniques and incorporates them into a clever design. It was influenced by Dr. Samuel Noordhoff who used a modification [3] of Millard's rotation-advancement repair [4, 5] and by Dr. Hugh Thomson who performed a modification [6] of the Randall-Tennison inferior triangle repair [7, 8]. It follows the concept that facial structures are composed of recognizable anatomic subunits and that placement of the closure along the borders of subunits makes the eventual scars less visible.

This chapter will review principles, design details, and modifications [2, 9] that can help to produce reliable outcomes.

## Principles

1. Common to all approaches to cleft lip repair is the need to lengthen the vertically short medial lip. The anatomic subunit approximation achieves this via the Rose-Thompson effect [10, 11] whereby the straight-line closure of a diamond-shaped excision results in elongation. If further lengthening is needed, a laterally-based triangular flap is placed above the white roll, where the lip transitions from a vertical to horizontal surface, When a lower triangle flap is used, the Rose-Thompson effect allows for a small triangle to be used.
2. At first glance, it may appear that the approach involves excision of excessive tissue. However, the repair produces a scar that lies intermediate in position to that produced by the *rotation-advancement repair* and the *inferior triangle repair* (Fig. 13.1). The scar of the *inferior triangle repair* is more lateral in the upper part of the lip indicating that more lateral lip skin is discarded with this repair. On the other hand, the *rotation-advancement repair* discards more medial lip in the form of the *c-flap*, which is truly discarded in many incomplete cleft cases and is displaced from the lip into the sill in complete cases. Further discard of valuable red lip occurs in the case of a vertically short lateral lip when transverse length is sacrificed to achieve vertical height. The *anatomic subunit approximation approach* more equally distributes discard of cleft marginal tissues from the medial and lateral lip. Given that anatomic landmarks, including Noordhoff point, are never compromised, transverse lateral lip element length is never sacrificed to achieve vertical height. Preservation of lateral lip tissues is

R. W. Tse (✉)
Division of Plastic Surgery, Department of Surgery, University of Washington, Seattle, WA, USA

Division of Craniofacial and Plastic Surgery, Department of Surgery, Seattle Children's Hospital, Seattle, WA, USA
e-mail: raymond.tse@seattlechildrens.org

D. M. Fisher
Division of Plastic & Reconstructive Surgery, University of Toronto, Toronto, ON, Canada

The Cleft Lip and Palate Program, Division of Plastic & Reconstructive Surgery, The Hospital for Sick Children, Toronto, ON, Canada

© Springer Nature Switzerland AG 2021

J. W. Swanson, D. W. Low (eds.), *Global Cleft Care in Low-Resource Settings*, https://doi.org/10.1007/978-3-030-59105-2_13

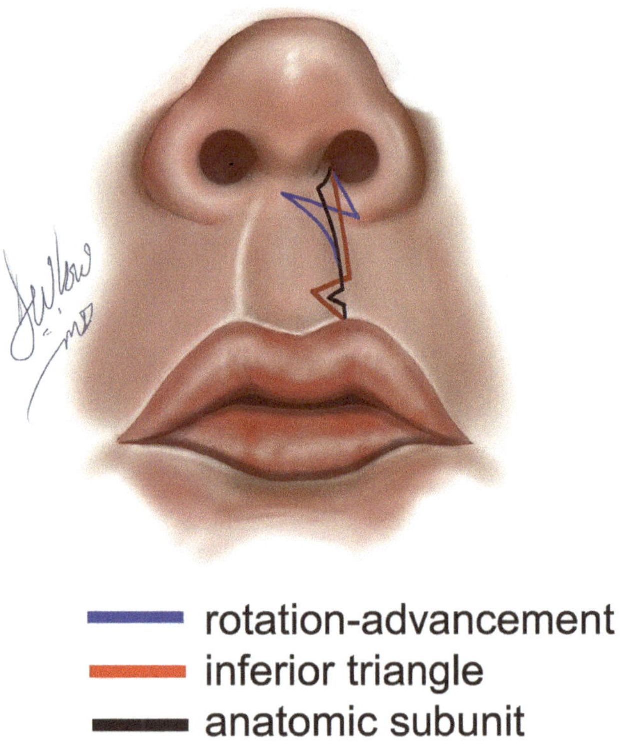


**Fig. 13.1** The anatomic subunit approximation produces a scar in the upper half of the lip that lies intermediate in position to those produced by rotation-advancement repair and the inferior triangle repair

important given that vertical deficiencies are often accompanied by existing horizontal deficiency [12].

3. Repair follows an orderly progression to allow surgeons to "measure twice and cut once." Landmarks and measurements guide the plan for incisions and help to determine if the triangular flap is unnecessary (i.e., some incomplete clefts) or if nasal sill excision isn't needed (i.e., some microform cleft). Checkpoints allow the surgeon to verify the subsequent steps through progressive stages of surgical release.
4. Rather than producing specific tissue movements, the goals of surgery should be to *centralize* midline structures and to *balance* nasolabial form. While the non-cleft side may appear more natural, recent study has confirmed that neither side of the cleft is normal [13]: Uncoupled growth of the premaxilla results in lateral deviation of anterior nasal spine, a squished non-cleft nostril sill, and an upward and outward displacement of the non-cleft alar base. The philtrum follows the premaxilla and rotates away from the cleft. Meanwhile, the cleft alar base has been left behind (normal in vertical and horizontal position but retruded). The combination of incision design, adequate release, muscle repair, and component reconstruction can produce the appropriate tissue tensions to balance form, placing key structures in symmetric position and rotation.

## Technique

### Plan

Landmarks are described using terminology from the original description [1] as well as standard anthropometric names [2] (Fig. 13.2).

Marks are placed starting at midline, identifying the non-cleft side, and then reflecting the known landmarks, to define the less distinct cleft-side landmarks.

#### Lip Points

The center of the columella (*subnasale*, sn) and the height of the non-cleft philtral column (*crista philtri superioris*, cphs) are identified along the nasolabial crease. The proposed height of philtral column incision (cphs′) is identified using the corresponding non-cleft-side landmark such that it is equidistant to *subnasale*.

Cupid's bow is identified along the vermilion border and is defined by the two peaks (*crista philtri inferioris*, cphi, and cphi′) and its low or midpoint (*labiale superioris*, ls). Given that transitions in contours and concavities hide scars better, the philtral column points, cphi and cphs, are identified along the medial border of the philtral ridge, where the convexity of the column transitions to the concavity of the philtral dimple (Fig. 13.2a). Note that the non-cleft point, cphi, is not the highest point of the curve of the lip but is rather where the straight portion of the bow meets the curve/convexity of the lateral lip element (Fig. 13.2a). On the other side of the bow, adjacent to the cleft, there is no such convexity, and thus cphi′ is marked equidistant to the center of the bow (ls).

The lateral point of lip closure, cphi″, is identified based upon tissue adequacy according to *Noordhoff* and is defined as the point along the vermilion border at which the vermilion border and vermilion-mucosal junction (red line) begin to converge medially (Fig. 13.2a). At this point, there will be adequate vermilion height, and the remaining lateral cutaneous white roll will be of optimal quality. Moving this point medially will result in central vermilion deficiency and will leave a cutaneous roll of poor quality. If this point is moved laterally, lateral lip transverse length, which is most often deficient, will be further compromised. Furthermore, there is a natural anterosuperior convexity of the white roll that can be preserved if cphi″ is placed according to Noordhoff's recommendations, thereby providing tissue for a more natural-appearing lip.

Once all of the landmarks along the vermilion have been identified, corresponding points (Fig. 13.2d) above the white roll (black dots with white outline) and along the mucosa-vermilion border (red dots with black outline) can be identified (perpendicular to the lip).

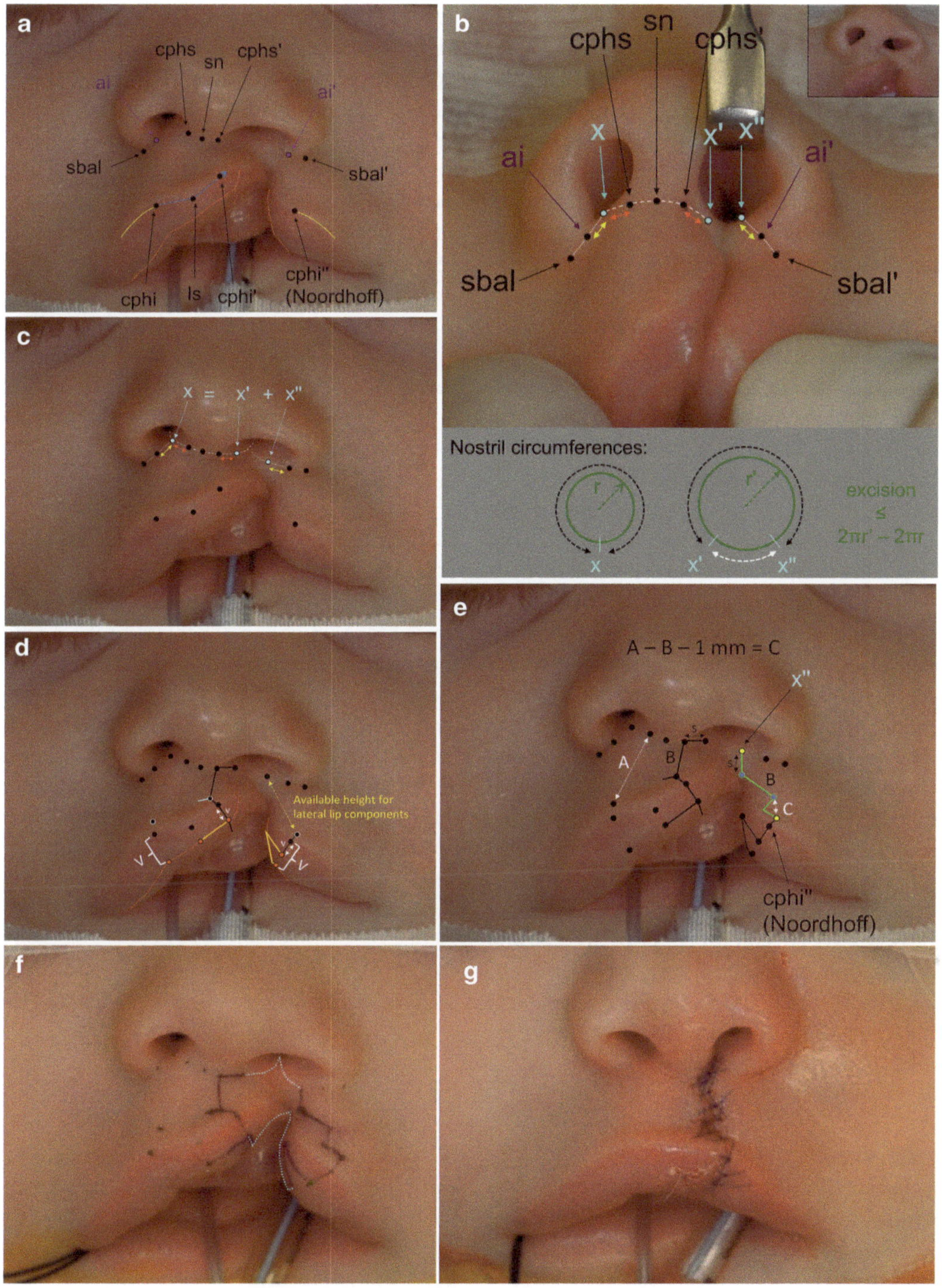


**Fig. 13.2** Design on child with complete cleft with Simonart band. (**a**) Points are standard anthropometric landmarks (subnasale, sn; christa philtri superioris, cphs; subalare, sbal; labialis superioris, ls; christa philtri inferioris, cphi). Cupid's bow peak is defined at the medial junction of the straight (blue) and convex curved (yellow) regions of the vermilion border. Noordhoff point is defined at the level of convergence of red line with vermilion. Alar insertion (ai) point is defined by following the nostril rim to its intersection with the nasal sill. (**b**) Manual correction of the lip and nose result in a symmetric configuration of landmarks. Nostril diameter can be measured using "urethral sounds" so that nostril circumferences can be calculated. Nostril sill excision should not exceed the measured difference in nostril circumference to avoid creating a micronostril. (**c**) x is the intersection of the alar-sill crease and the columellar-labial crease on the non-cleft side. Corresponding landmarks are identified along corresponding creases on the cleft side to define x' and x", the points of nasal sill closure. (**d**) Corresponding landmarks are placed along the vermilion-mucosal junction (red dots with black outline) and above the white roll (black dots with white outline). Landmarks on the medial lip are connected to define the medial incisions. A lateral lip vermilion flap is designed to augment the deficient vermilion on the medial side (orange). The lateral design needs to match the medial lip incisions. The available lateral lip height (yellow arrow) is defined by the lateral point of nasal closure (x") and the point above the white roll at Noordhoff point (cphi"). (**e**) Lateral lip markings are designed to match medial lip incisions and augment height. (**f**) Actual markings with nasal floor and lip mucosa incision (dotted white lines). (**g**) immediate result after closure. (**g**) Appearance immediately following repair. Modified with permission from Tse R, Lien S. Unilateral Cleft Lip Repair Using the Anatomical Subunit Approximation: Modifications and Analysis of Early Results in 100 Consecutive Cases. *Plast Reconstr Surg.* 136, 119–30 (2015)

### Nose Points

Points of nostril sill closure on either side of the cleft are defined (Fig. 13.2b, c) so that when they are approximated, two goals are accomplished: (1) the nares are of equal circumference and (2) alar bases are symmetric from the anterior view. Several landmarks are used to identify these points. *Subalare* (sbal), the lowest point along the ala, is found along the ala-sill crease. The *alar insertion point* (ai), which was not part of the initial description, is found at the intersection of the alar rim with the nasal sill, along the nose-lip crease [2]. The landmarks are identified on the non-cleft side and used as reference when identifying the same landmarks on the cleft side. When identifying cleft-side landmarks, the nasal deformity should be manually corrected by bringing nasal base elements together and gently supporting the dome with a retractor (Fig. 13.2b). The orientation of sbal-ai on both sides should be similar when the nose has been corrected (Fig. 13.2b). That orientation will become asymmetric as the surgeon allows the nose and lip slump back down to the uncorrected position (Fig. 13.2b, c).

On the non-cleft side, columella-sill and ala-sill creases are followed to their intersection to define the "arbitrary" point, x. On the cleft side, corresponding points (x′ and x″) need to be defined so that when they are manually approximated (i.e., to mimic x), the nasal deformity should be corrected (Fig. 13.2b). Those points are found along the corresponding columella-sill and ala-sill creases such that the distances from sn-cphs′ and sbal′-ai′ mirror those on the non-cleft side (Fig. 13.2b, c).

In the case of an incomplete cleft or cleft with Simonart band, the nasal floor will be intact but excessively wide. Appropriate excision can be confirmed prior to incision (Fig. 13.2b). Urethral sounds are used to measure diameter (circumference = diameter × π). The distance between x′ and x″ should not exceed the difference in circumferences (approximately the difference in diameters multiplied by 3) as over-resection can produce a micronostril.

### Medial Markings: Connect the Dots

The medial lip markings (Fig. 13.2d) simply connect the landmarks along the *nasal sill* (x′-cphs′), along the *philtral column* (cphs′-cphi′), and across the *white roll*, *vermilion border*, and *vermilion-cutaneous junction* (red line) at cphi′. This last line is made perpendicular to the lip so that its incidence with the proposed philtral column incision (cphs′-cphi′) forms an angle that will open once incised (Rose-Thompson effect). A small back-cut is designed above the white roll (blue line, Fig. 13.2d) and is oriented to provide maximal vertical release (usually perpendicular to the proposed philtral column incision). The length of the back-cut is based upon the size of the calculated equilateral triangle from the lateral lip that will be needed to augment medial lip height. Another incision is designed along the red line (orange line, Fig. 13.2d) so that the deficient vermilion height may be augmented with a lateral lip vermilion flap.

### Lateral Lip Vermilion Flap

Vermilion is almost universally deficient below the cleft-side half of Cupid's bow [14]. An opening incision has already been marked along the vermillion-mucosa junction below the cleft-side half of Cupid's bow (orange line, Fig. 13.2d). This incision will receive a laterally based *vermilion triangular flap* (orange triangle, Fig. 13.2d) from the lateral lip element. A line equal in length to the height of vermillion below the *cleft-side bow peak* is drawn below *Noordhoff point* (v, Fig. 13.2d). These lines will approximate upon closure. Because the vermilion heights (V, Fig. 13.2d) below the *non-cleft-side bow peak* (cphi) and below *Noordhoff point* (cphi″) are usually similar (within 0.5 mm in most cases), the remaining height of vermilion is all that is required to augment the vermilion deficiency of the medial lip element.

### Determining Base Width of Lateral Lip Inferior Triangle Flap

Measurements are taken from the heights of the philtral columns at the lip-columella crease to the points marked above the peaks of Cupid's bow above the white roll (Fig. 13.2e); the height along cphi-cphs is the *total lip height, A*; the height along cphi′-cphs′ is the *greater lip height, B*. The *total lip height* is measured with the lip at rest. The *greater lip height* is measured with gentle downward traction on the lip to unfurl the medial lip and predict the tension on the lip after repair. The *lesser lip height, C* (base width of the *small inferior triangle*), is equal to the *total lip height* minus the *greater lip height* and less 1 mm:

$$\begin{aligned}&\textit{Lesser lip height}\\&= \textit{total lip height} - \textit{greater lip height} - 1\text{ mm}\\&= \textit{base width of the small inferior triangle}\end{aligned}$$

The 1 mm accounts for the approximate length achieved by the Rose-Thompson effect. The *lesser lip height* is usually between 1 and 1.5 mm and 2.5 mm at the greatest. For minor clefts, an *inferior triangle* may not be necessary.

### Fitting the Lateral Lip Markings to the Available Lateral Lip Height

All of the points thus far have been anatomic landmarks and do not vary. Between the *lateral point of closure in the nostril sill* (x″) and the white roll at Noordhoff point (cphi″), three limbs need to be positioned (the *nasal sill*, the *greater lip height*, and the *inferior triangle*). The spatial configuration of the three limbs will vary based upon the vertical height of the lateral lip (yellow dashed arrow, Fig. 13.2d). The components can articulate open or close in order to fit the available height (Fig. 13.3).

In the case of a vertically short lateral lip (Fig. 13.3a), as is often the case in complete clefts, the *greater lip height* incision will be more horizontal, and its lateral extreme

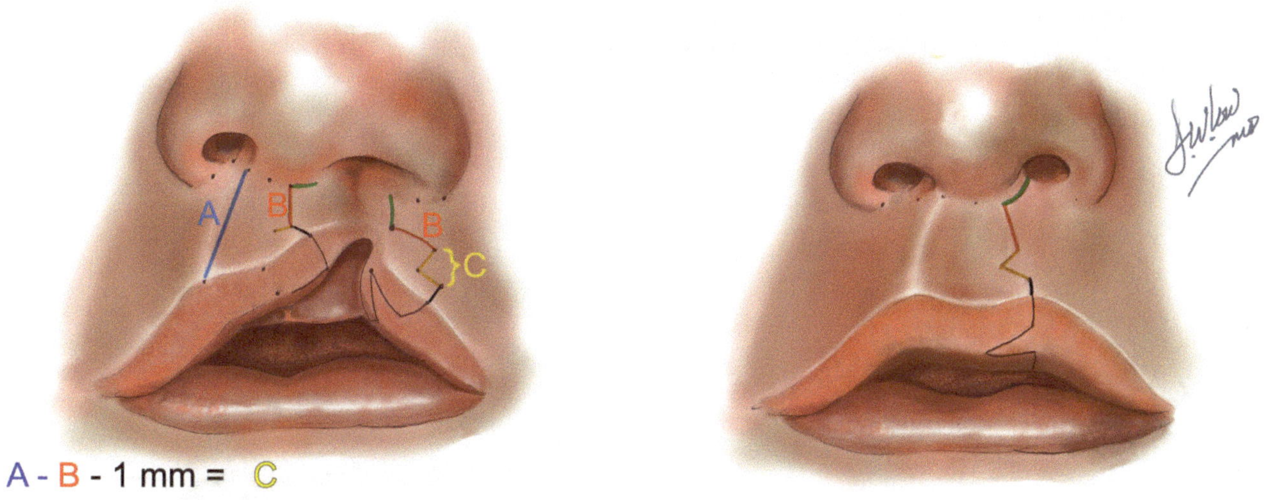


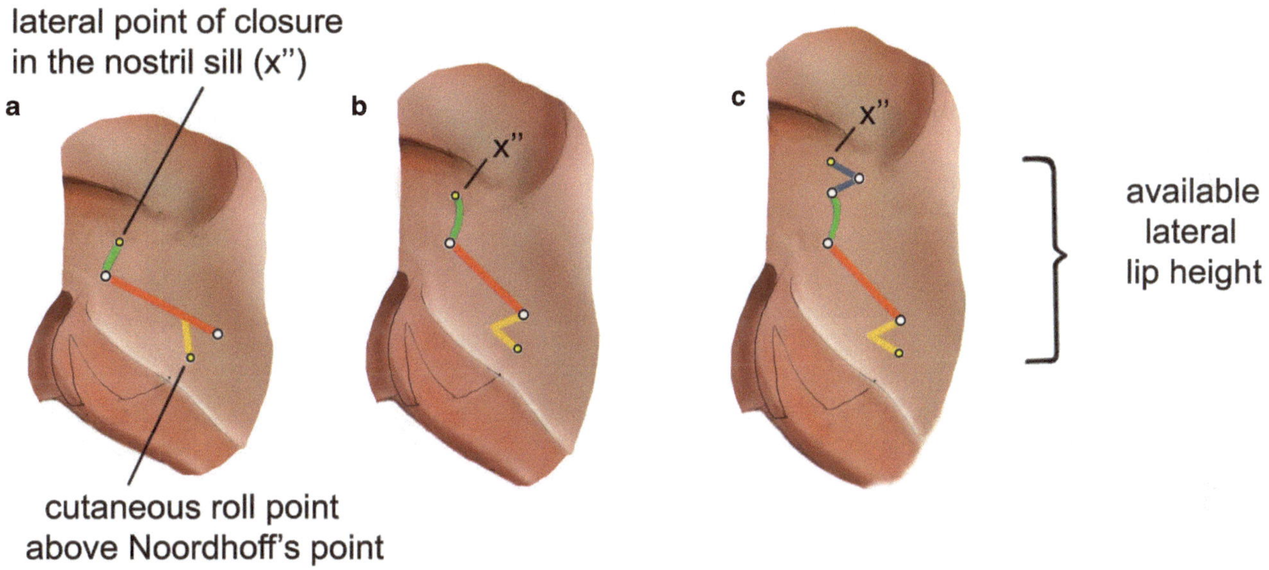


**Fig. 13.3** Variations in lateral lip height and alterations in design. Between the lateral point of closure (x″) and the white roll at Noordhoff point (cphi″), three components need to be included. A triangle with base width C (yellow), the greater lip height B (red), and the nasal sill closure (green). (**a**) Short lateral lip height. The "B" or greater lip height limb is coincident with one surface of the triangle. (**b**) Moderate lateral lip height. The angle between limbs match those of the medial lip design. (**c**) Excessive lateral lip height. Excess lateral lip height is removed as a wedge excision (blue) so that the angle between limbs match those of the medial lip design

may need to be coincident with the upper incision of the *inferior triangle,* which will require an upward pointing orientation.

In the case of a vertically moderate lateral lip (Fig. 13.3b), as is often the case in complete clefts with Simonart band and some incomplete clefts, the *greater lip height* incision will be more vertical, and the *inferior triangle* will have a more horizontal pointing orientation. The angle between the *nasal sill* and *greater lip height* limbs should be made to match the angle between these two limbs on the medial lip.

In the case of excessive lateral lip height (Fig. 13.3c), as is often the case in incomplete or minor-form clefts, opening the angle between the nasal sill and greater lip height incision can produce an overly obtuse configuration that does not match the medial lip incision. In these cases, a wedge of the upper lip can be excised just below the *lateral point of closure in the nostril sill* (x″). The excision is placed so that the scar will lie along the alar crease with the lateral apex of this wedge excision extending no further than subalare. Although many surgeons may be reluctant to commit to excision, there are several ways to confirm that the lateral lip height is indeed excessive. First, the vertical position of Noordhoff point (cphi″) may be lower than the non-cleft Cupid's bow peak (cphi). Second, the cleft lateral lip height (cphi″-sbal′) is equal or greater than the non-cleft lateral lip height (cphi-sbal). Third, and most important, the angle

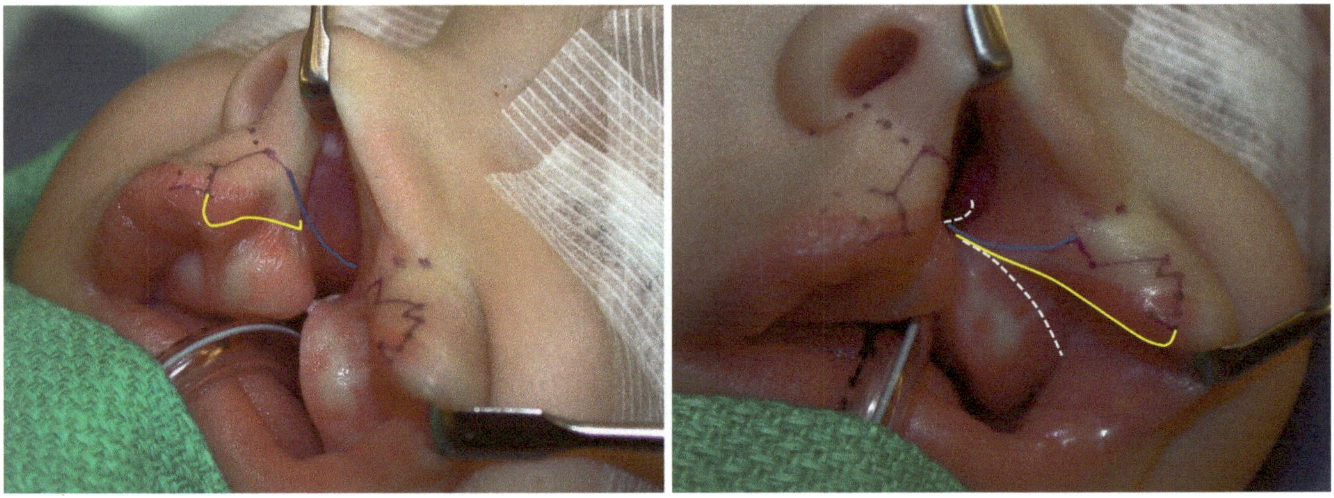

Fig. 13.4 Nasal floor and lip mucosa incisions for complete cleft. Corresponding yellow and blue incision lines will be approximated. Upper buccal sulcus and nasal sidewall incisions (white dotted lines) used to mobilize lip and alar base, respectively

between the nasal sill and the greater lip height limbs doesn't match that of the medial lip markings.

## Connecting the Two Sides

For complete clefts (Fig. 13.4), incisions from the points of nostril closure (x′ and x″) extend intranasally along the cleft margins for closure of the nasal floor. Mucosal incisions extend cranially to the points of attachment of each lip element to the alveolus. Extending laterally from the attachment point of the lateral lip element, an upper sulcus incision is made, usually with the addition of a back-cut.

For incomplete clefts, a wedge excision of nostril sill above the *medial* and *lateral points of nostril closure* (x′ and x″) is performed (Fig. 13.2f). Mucosa of the cleft margins is removed by wedge excision, with the peak above the level of the cleft. Occasionally, a short lateral upper buccal sulcus advancement incision is helpful.

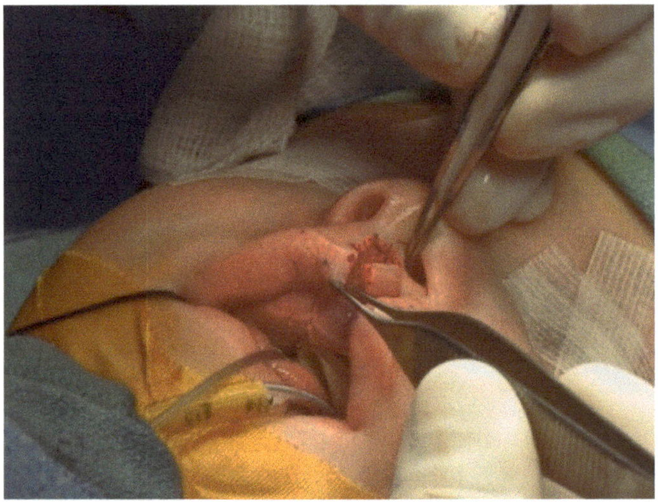

Fig. 13.5 Checkpoints. Following excision of medial lip marginal tissues and muscle dissection, correct the nose and level Cupid's bow to confirm that back-cut is needed. After making the back-cut, level the bow and re-measure the size of triangle needed. Adjust the lateral lip markings if needed

## Surgical Release and Re-measure

It is critical that dissection begins with the medial lip. Incisions are made with scalpel and completed with scissors. The opening incision above the cutaneous roll is not made at this point. Dissection frees the muscle from the overlying skin and vermilion and from the underlying mucosa. Dissection between the skin and muscle is limited to 1 mm from the cut edge to preserve the philtral dimple. The orbicularis is freed from its upturned insertion in the region of the columellar base and upper alveolar cleft margin. CHECKPOINT #1: The columellar base is positioned to mimic its final position, and gentle downward rotation of the cleft-side peak of Cupid's bow is performed in an attempt to level Cupid's bow by the Rose-Thompson effect alone. The requirement of an opening incision to level Cupid's bow is confirmed (Fig. 13.5). If required, the opening incision is made through the skin and subcutaneous tissue but not through the muscle. CHECKPOINT #2: Again the columellar base is positioned to mimic its final position, and gentle downward rotation of the cleft-side peak of Cupid's bow is performed in an attempt to level Cupid's bow. If insufficient, the opening incision can be extended as needed. With the

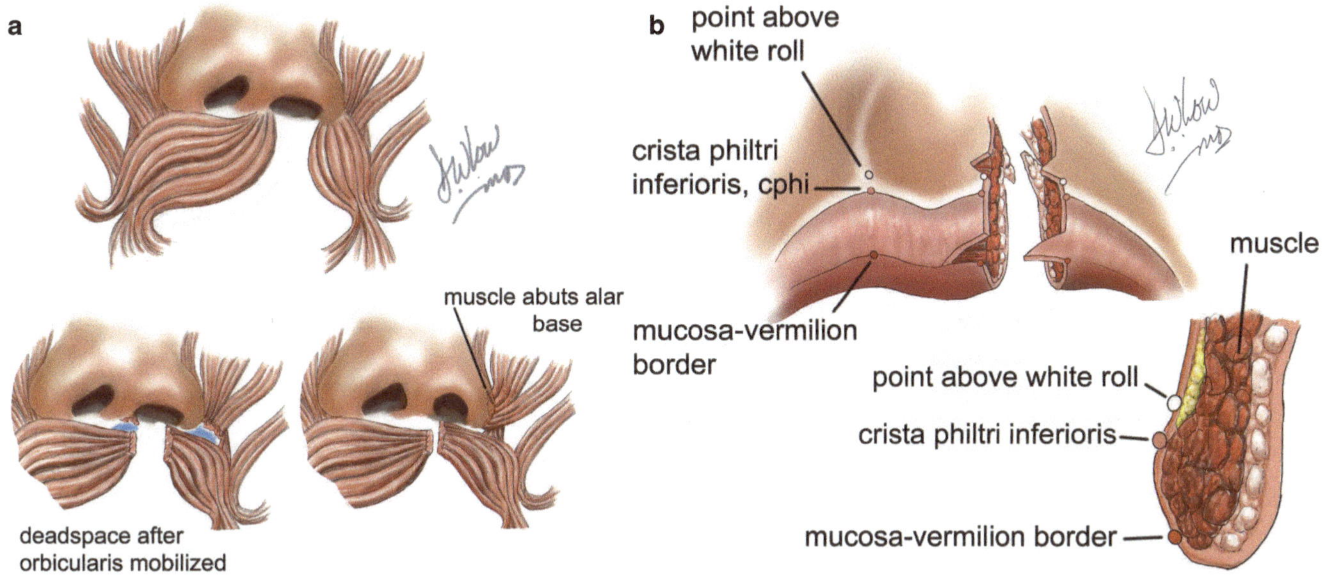


**Fig. 13.6** Muscle. Release of muscle at the base of columella and nasal ala produces areas devoid of muscle on either side. Muscle on the medial side rotates downward, while muscle on the lateral side advances to fill the dead pace under the columella. Note the "J" shape of the pars marginalis along the lower part of the lip. Careful approximation on either side of the cleft preserves the pout of the lip

bow now level, the size of the triangular defect created by the opening incision is measured and compared to the size of the inferior triangle drawn on the lateral lip element. If there is any discrepancy, the size of the inferior triangle can be redrawn such that it exactly matches the size of the opening defect required to level the bow.

Dissection continues with the lateral lip. For complete clefts, it is helpful to start with the mucosal incisions. The upper sulcus incision and the piriform marginal incision are made, and the lateral lip and alar base are mobilized in an supra-periosteal plane. CHECKPOINT #3: Before lateral lip skin incisions are made, the medial and lateral lip elements, now fully mobilized, are manipulated, and the *medial point of closure in the nostril sill* (x′) and the *lateral point of closure in the nostril sill* (x″) are approximated. Symmetry of the nostril margin circumference and of alar base positioning is checked. If need be, the *lateral point of closure in the nostril sill* (x″) can be repositioned before the skin incisions of the lateral lip are made. Cleft marginal tissue is discarded. Dissection frees the muscle from the overlying skin and vermilion and from the underlying mucosa (Fig. 13.6). On the lateral lip element, dissection between the skin and muscle is more extensive, extending laterally as far as the alar base to relieve the orbicularis muscle bulge. Orbicularis is freed from its upturned insertion in the region of the alar base and upper alveolar cleft margin. Dissection deep to the muscle and in an supra-periosteal plane frees the alar base from the underlying maxilla. Wide dissection minimizes tension at repair. The vestibular web, formed by the caudal margin of the lower lateral cartilage's lateral crus, the accessory cartilages, and investing perichondrium, is released from its posterolateral attachment to the piriform rim (Fig. 13.7). When this release from the piriform rim is sufficient, the alar base can now be correctly positioned without accentuating the buckling of the alar rim and of the lateral alar flare.

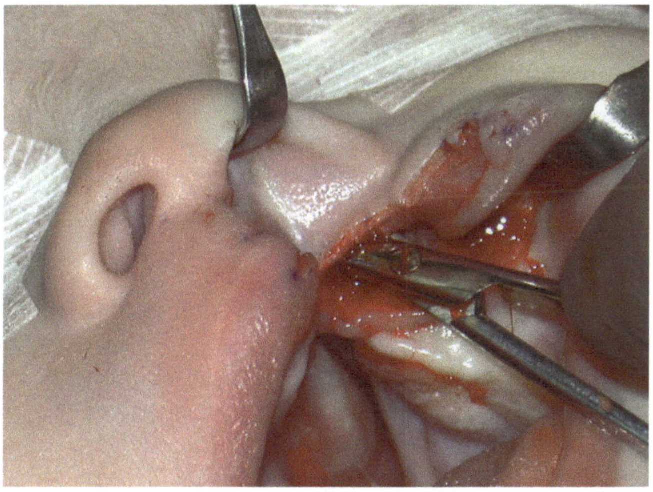

**Fig. 13.7** Release along piriform aperture

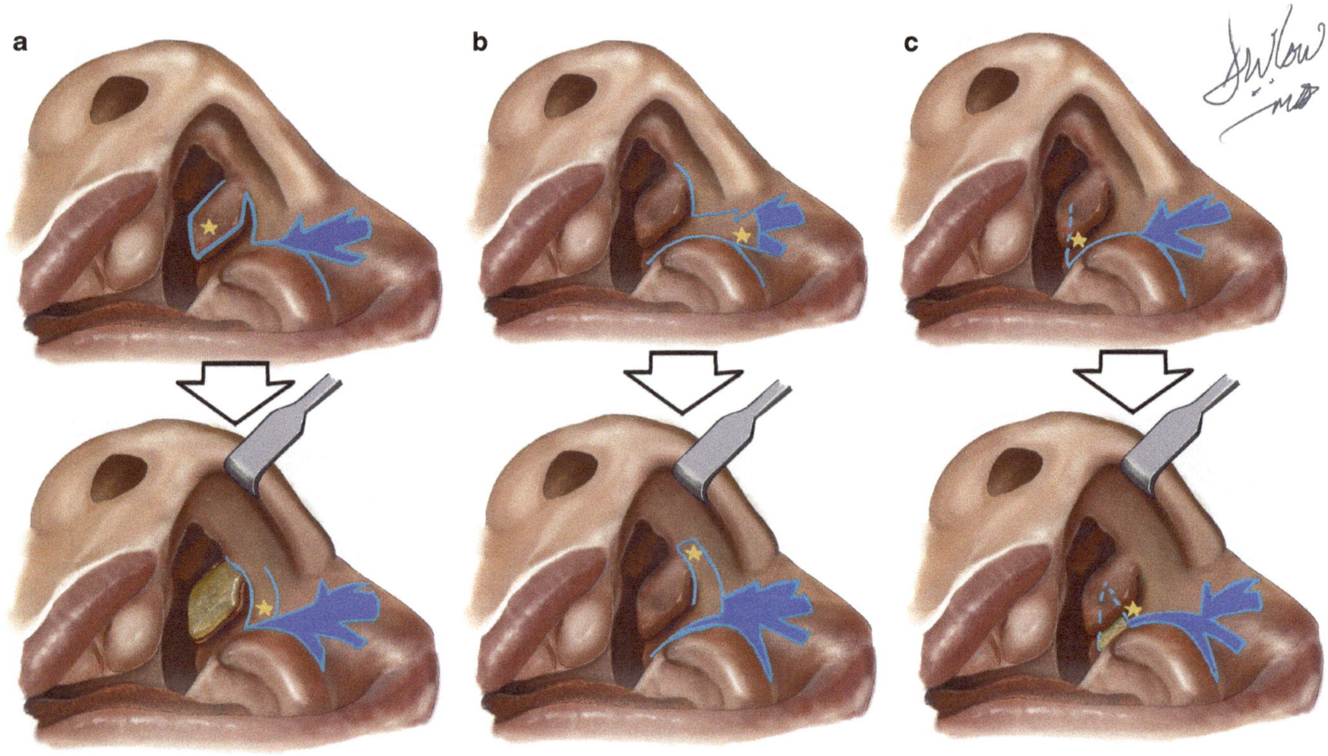


**Fig. 13.8** Reconstruction of lateral nasal sidewall and closure of the floor with any of the three options: (**a**) turbinate flap; the anteriorly based flap is transposed into the defect produced by the releasing incision along the piriform aperture, (**b**) L-flap; tissue along the lateral cleft margin that would otherwise be excised is left in continuity with mucoperiosteum along the lateral nasal wall so that it can be transposed into the defect produced by the releasing incision along the piriform aperture, and (**c**) lateral nasal sidewall advancement; mucoperiosteum along the lateral nasal wall is elevated with an incision along the cleft margin and backcut far posterior so that the lining can be advanced en-block with the alar base

## Component Reconstruction

Release and component reconstruction are equally as important as the design and incisions.

Primary septoplasty can be performed during primary repair via the medial lip incision [14]. Having freed the lip and columellar base from the premaxilla in an supra-periosteal plane, the anterior nasal spine is identified. The septospinal attachments are divided transversely, and the septum is freed from caudal attachments with an elevator. Direct release involves submucoperichondrial dissection on the non-cleft side of the caudal septum to allow repositioning of the caudal septum to the sagittal plane. By maintaining the cleft-side mucoperichondrium attachment of the caudal septum, the extended nostril sill closure will keep the caudal septum in its straightened position. An indirect release involves subperiosteal dissection along nasal floors and release of the periosteum on the non-cleft side to allow centralization of the septum.

If there is a significant anteroposterior distance between the greater and lesser maxillary segments, anterior advancement of the alar base will leave a dead space between the piriform margin and the new position of the alar base. Reconstruction of the sidewall can prevent subsidence and may involve a turbinate flap, L-flap, or lateral nasal wall flap (Fig. 13.8) [15, 16]. The flap is used to close nasal floor as far back as the mid-palatal shelf. Although all of these flaps are effective, we have started to favor the lateral nasal wall flap as it provides a continuous layer of nasal closure across the alveolar defect that may facilitate alveolar bone grafting [15, 16]. The closure progresses anteriorly to the nasal sill and the two points of closure (x′ and x″).

Placement of intranasal sutures is easier prior to full closure of the nasal floor. From within the nasal vestibule, forceps are used to reposition the cleft-side dome anteromedially and to grasp the caudal margin of the upper lateral cartilage (Fig. 13.9). Although no incision or dissection is performed, the tissues advance easily. One or two internal nasal valve plication sutures are placed to maintain the anteromedial advancement of the lateral crus and to create the normal overlap of the lower lateral cartilage and the upper lateral cartilage. Alar transfixion sutures are placed to obliterate any dead space created by the release of the vestibular web from the piriform rim and to maintain anteromedial advancement of the lateral crus (Fig. 13.10).

If an upper buccal sulcus mucosal incision has been made, the lateral lip mucosa is advanced to the premaxillary mucosa and closed progressing from the sulcus, to the free margin, and up to the mucosa-vermillion junction.

Muscle approximation can have profound effect on lip form (Fig. 13.6). The orbicularis muscle that was previously

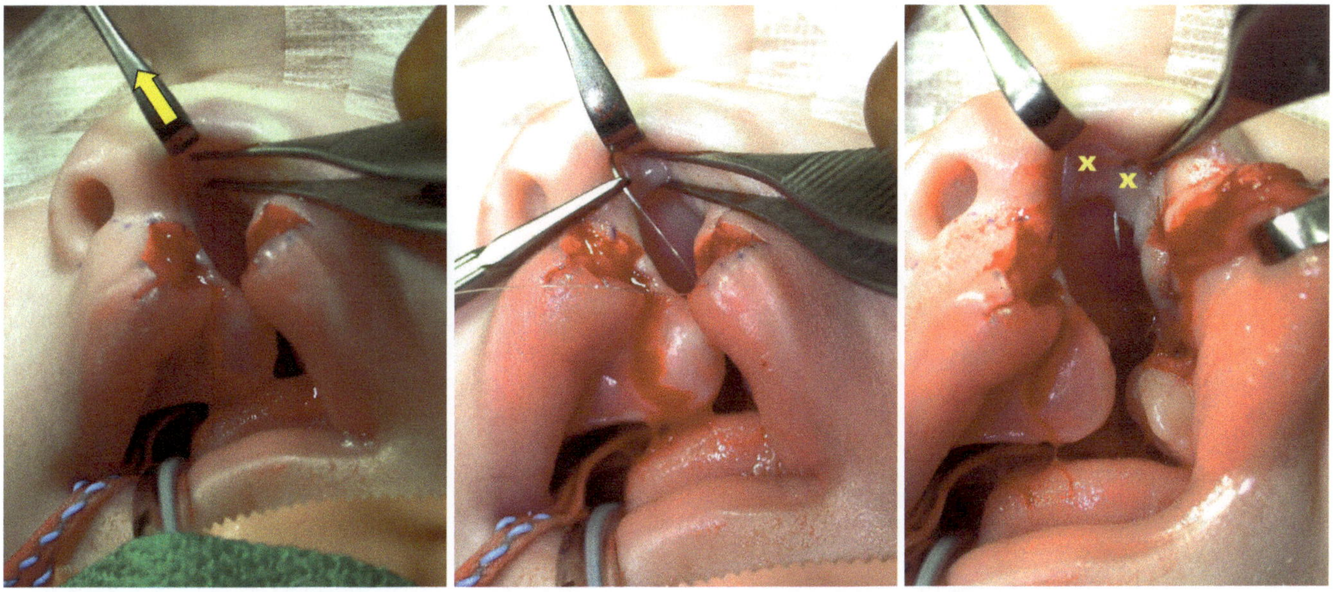

Fig. 13.9 Horizontal mattress to secure lower lateral cartilage overtop of upper lateral cartilage, thereby establishing the scroll region. Modified with permission from Tse RW, Mercan E, Hopper RA, Birgfeld CB, Fisher DM. Reply: Unilateral Cleft Lip Nasal Deformity: Foundation-Based Approach to Primary Rhinoplasty. Plast Reconstr Surg. 2020 Sep;146(3):373e–5e

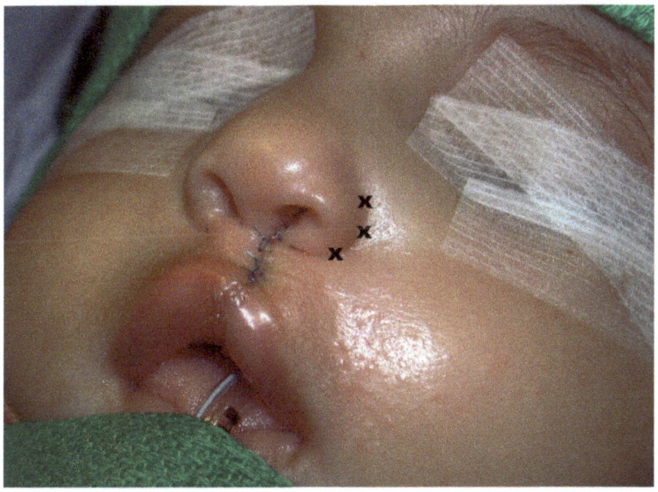

Fig. 13.10 Alar transfixion sutures to lateralize the internal nasal lining, stabilize the alar advancement, and accentuate the alar crease

inserted into alar base is brought across the nasal floor/sill and inset into the base of the columella. This acts as alar cinch stitch. Careful placement of this suture will allow the alar bases and columellar base to be positioned in the appropriate horizontal plane. The rest of the muscle is approximated from cranial to caudal with special care to preserve the "J" shape of the pars marginalis as it contributes to the pout of the lip. Given that the orbicularis has a deep and superficial layer with distinct functions, we use simple sutures in hopes of opposing each layer.

The lateral vermilion flap is debulked of underlying muscle, trimmed to size, and inset into the opening incision along the red line of the medial lip.

## Final Closure

The skin is approximated with deep dermal and then simple interrupted sutures. A 5-0 or 6-0 absorbable suture (polyglactin or poliglecaprone) is used for the muscle, mucosa, and dermis. A slowly absorbing suture (polydioxanone) is used for the septum and alar cinch. A non-absorbable 7-0 polypropylene suture is used for surface skin when there is an option for suture removal under sedation. An alternative is to use a 6-0 polypropylene running intracuticular along the vertical limb of the philtral column (that can be easily removed without sedation) and 8-0 polyglactin in a simple interrupted manner for everything else.

## Case Examples

Figure 13.2 illustrates the lip design in a case of complete cleft with Simonart band. Figure 13.11 illustrates the planning for a wide complete cleft. Figure 13.12 illustrates the planning for an incomplete cleft. Figure 13.13 illustrates planning for a microform cleft; the upper components of repair were not needed given the existing nasal base symmetry (as confirmed by landmarks).

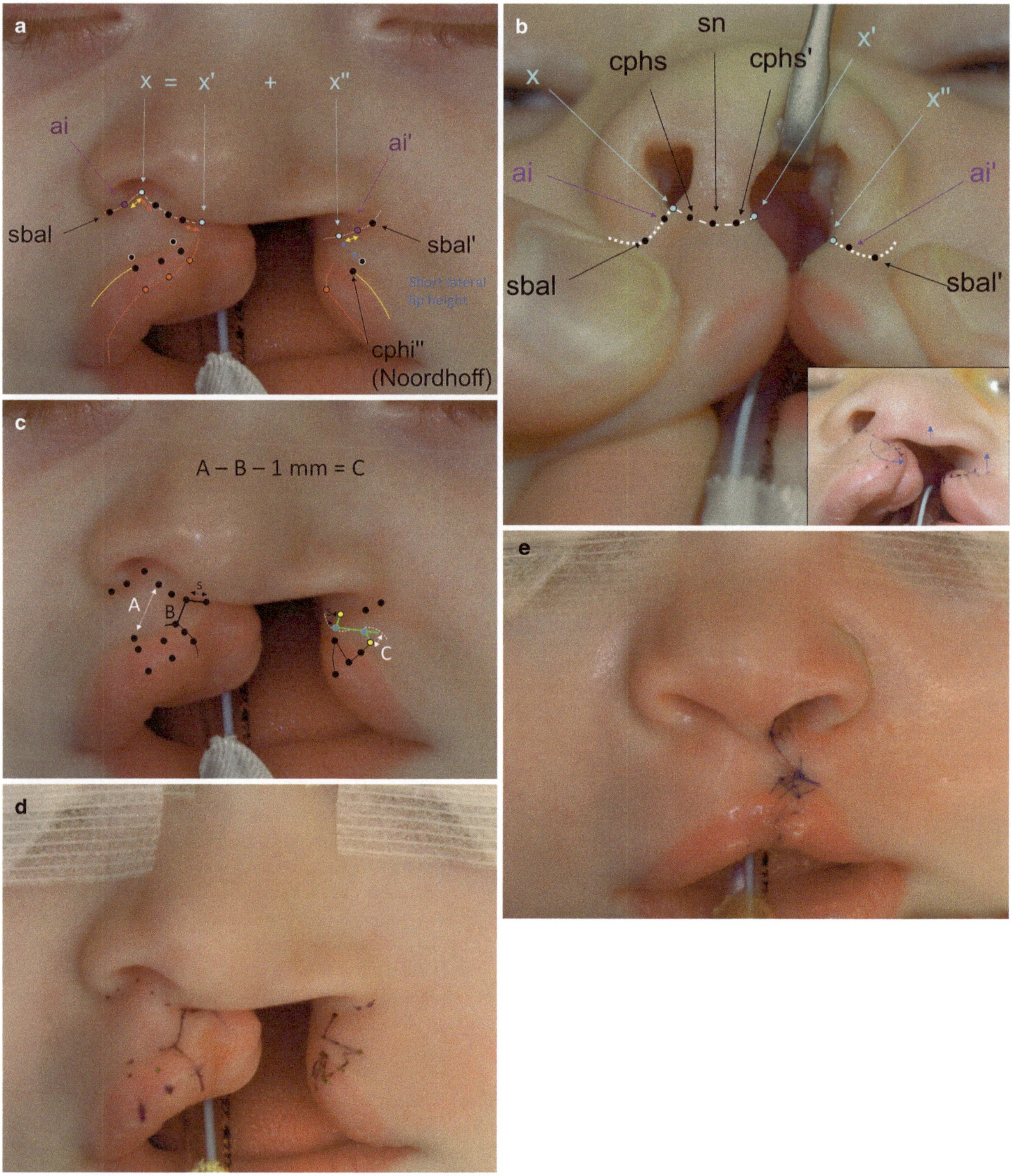


**Fig. 13.11** Design and repair for child with a wide complete cleft: (**a**) Points of nasal floor closure (x' and x'') are defined along nose-lip creases using the intersection of those corresponding creases on the non-cleft side (x). Cupid's bow and Noordhoff point, and their corresponding landmarks above the white roll (black dots with white outline) and along the red line (red dots with black outline) provide the rest of the landmarks. The vertical height between the white roll landmark above Noordhoff point and the lateral point of nasal closure (x'') defines the available lateral lip height for the lateral lip elements. This height is short in patients with complete clefts. (**b**) When the points of nasal closure (x' and x'') are approximated, the desired nasal change should be produced and the landmark configuration should appear symmetric. The laterally deviated columella needs to be centralized and the cleft alar base needs to be advanced anteriorly (**c**) Medial lip incisions are derived by connecting the dots. Given the limited lateral lip height, lateral lip elements are collapsed together so that the edge of the triangle flap is coincident with the philtral limb (i.e. B). (**d**) Actual markings. (**e**) Appearance immediately following closure

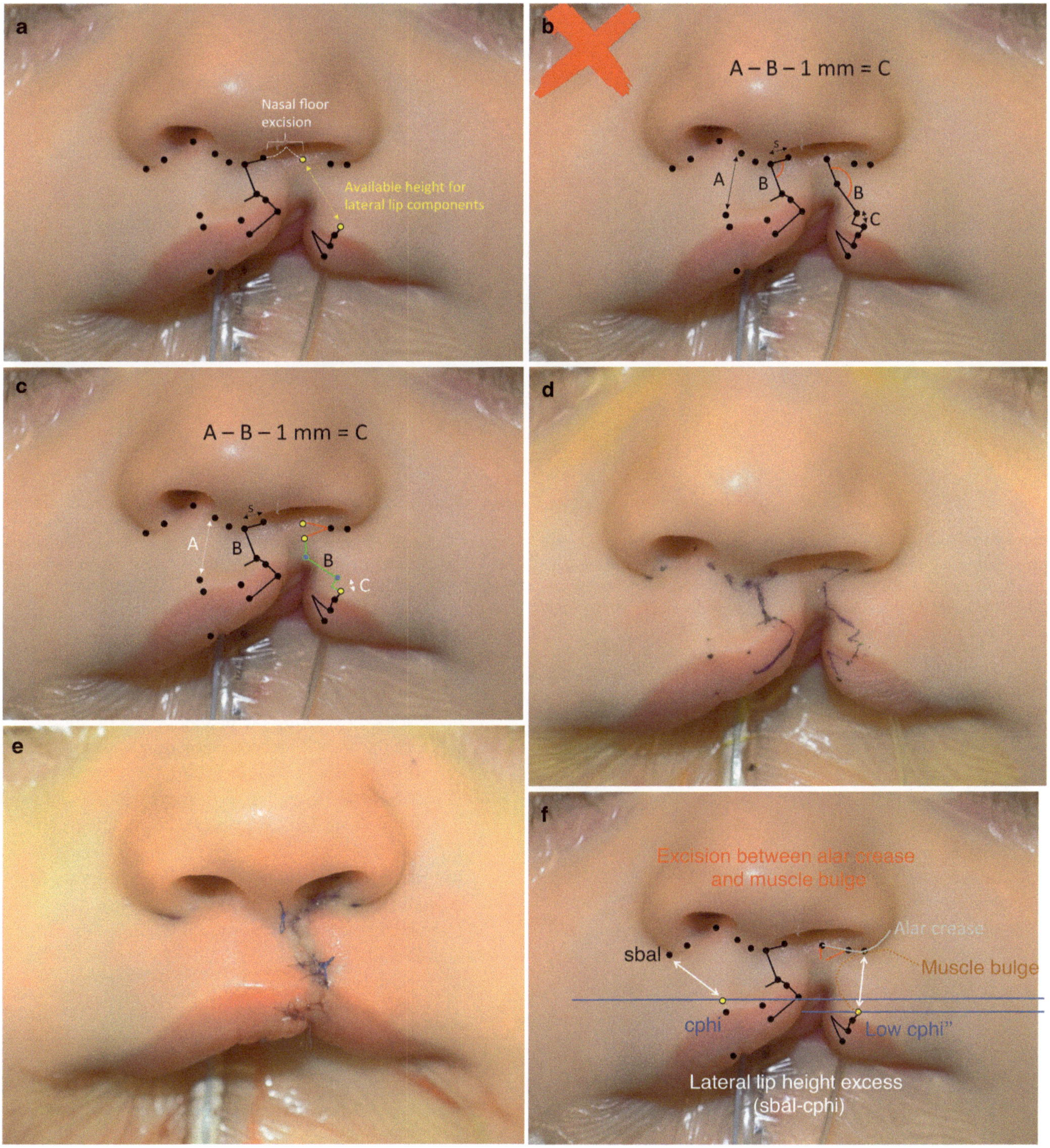


**Fig. 13.12** Design and repair for child with an incomplete cleft and lateral lip height excess; (**a**) Excess lateral lip height. (**b**) If lateral lip elements simply span the available lateral lip height, the angle between limbs on the lateral side will not match those on the medial side. (**c**) The philtral limb, B, is made more horizontal so the the angle it forms with the sill limb, s, matches that on the medial side. The excess height is excised as a wedge (red lines). (**d**) Actual markings. (**e**) Appearance immediately following closure. (**f**) The closure from wedge excision hides along the alar crease and involves skin that is beyond the muscle bulge of orbicularis. Indicators that a wedge needs to be excised includes the low position of cphi" relative to cphi; the tall lateral lip height (white arrows); and, most importantly, the an obtuse angle between limbs of the lateral lip markings relative to the medial lip markings

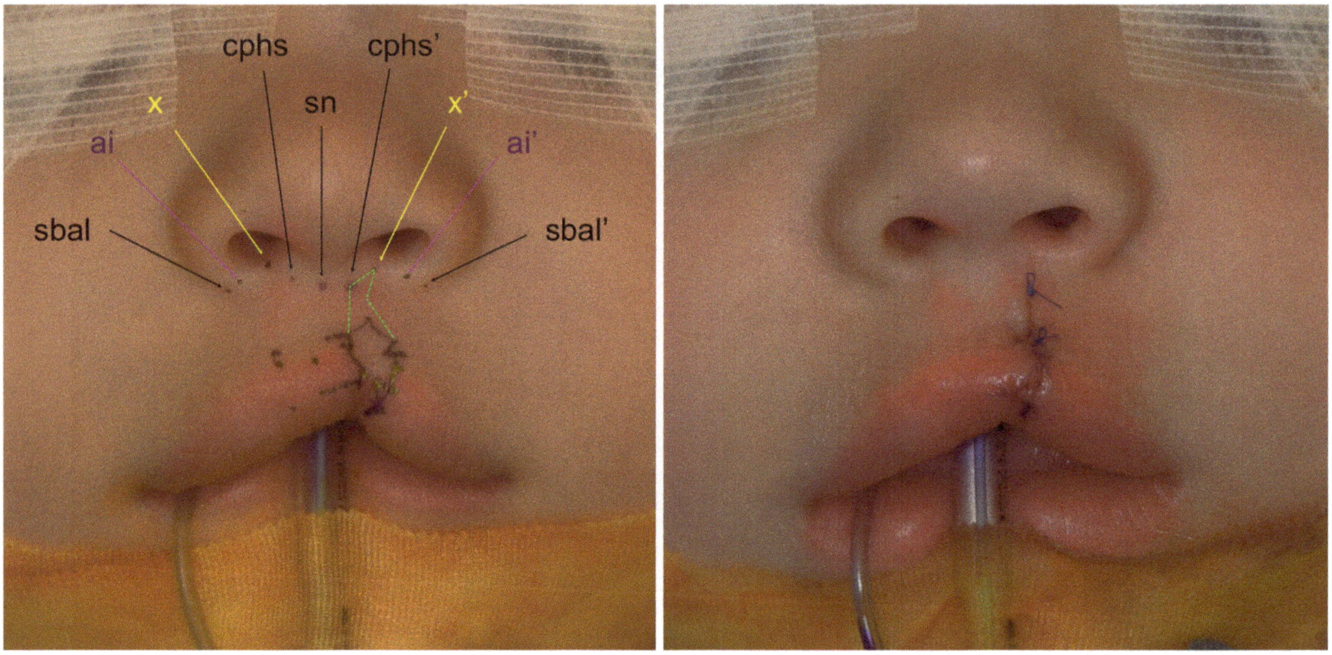


**Fig. 13.13** Design and repair for child with microform cleft. Landmark placement confirmed nasal base symmetry (i.e., x′ and x″ were the same point). Given that the upper lip incisions were not needed (green dotted lines), the lower lip incisions were tapered to an apex to limit the height of scar. Reproduced with permission from Tse R. Reply: Unilateral Cleft Lip Repair Using the Anatomical Subunit Approximation: Modifications and Analysis of Early Results in 100 Consecutive Cases. Plast Reconstr Surg. 2015 Dec;136(6):855e–7e

**Pearls and Pitfalls**

1. Neither side (cleft vs non-cleft) is normal. The cleft-side dome and nasal tip are collapsed because the non-cleft alar base and columella are displaced laterally, whereas the cleft alar base is retruded [9]. Correction involves movement of non-cleft alar base medial, centralization of the columella, and anterior repositioning of the cleft alar base. Those movements should be made when "correcting the nose" and identifying anatomic landmarks (Figs. 13.2b and 13.11b). The correction can be retained via muscle dissection and repair that "balances" the components of the lip and nose.
2. Do not compromise on landmarks to make up for lateral lip deficiencies. Moving the vertical level of the *lateral point of closure in the nostril sill* (x″) to elongate the lateral lip height should be avoided, as it will compromise the final vertical position of the alar insertion. Moving the *lateral point of lip closure* (cphi″) beyond *Noordhoff point* to increase the available lateral lip height should be avoided, as it results in excessive tissue discard, greater tension at closure, and reduction in lip fullness. Variations in lateral lip height can be addressed by altering the configuration of elements in the lateral lip design.
3. Do not make Cupid's bow too wide. Identify the peak of the bow along the medial border of philtral ridge at the transition from the straight to convex vermilion border.
4. Do not be afraid to excise vertical excess, especially if incomplete lip and sometimes with complete cleft lip with soft tissue band (Fig. 13.12c). Excessive lateral lip height results either in lip asymmetry or cephalic displacement of the cleft alar base.
5. Use checkpoints to verify successive steps.

## References


1. Fisher DM. Unilateral cleft lip repair: an anatomical subunit approximation technique. Plast Reconstr Surg. 2005;116:61–71.
2. Tse R, Lien S. Unilateral cleft lip repair using the anatomical subunit approximation: modifications and analysis of early results in 100 consecutive cases. Plast Reconstr Surg. 2015;136:119–30.
3. Noordhoff MS. The surgical technique for the unilateral cleft lip-nasal deformity. Taipei: Noordhoff Craniofacial Foundation; 1997.
4. Millard DR. Complete unilateral clefts of the lip. Plast Reconstr Surg. 1960;25:595.
5. Millard DR. Extensions of the rotation-advancement principle for wide unilateral cleft lips. Plast Reconstr Surg. 1968;42:535.
6. Thomson HG. Unilateral cleft lip repair. Oper Tech Plast Reconstr Surg. 1995;2:175.

7. Tennison CW. The repair of the unilateral cleft lip by the stencil method. Plast Reconstr Surg. 1952;9:115.
8. Randal P. A triangular flap operation for the primary repair of unilateral clefts of the lip. Plast Reconstr Surg. 1959;23:331.
9. Tse R. Reply: unilateral cleft lip repair using the anatomic subunit approximation: modifications and analysis of early results in 100 consecutive cases. Plast Reconstr Surg. 2015;136(6):855e–7e.
10. Rose W. On harelip and cleft palate. London: HK Lewis; 1891.
11. Thompson JE. An artistic and mathematically accurate method of repairing the defect in cases of harelip. Surg Gynaecol Obstet. 1912;14:498.
12. Boorer CJ, Cho DC, Vijayasekaran VS, Fisher DM. Presurgical unilateral cleft lip anthropometrics: implications for the choice of repair technique. Plast Reconstr Surg. 2011;127:774–80.
13. Tse RW, Knight R, Oestreich M, Rosser M, Mercan E. Unilateral Cleft Lip Nasal Deformity: Three-Dimensional Analysis of the Primary Deformity and Longitudinal Changes following Primary Correction of the Nasal Foundation. Plast Reconstr Surg. 2020;145(1):185–99.
14. Sitzman TJ, Fisher DM. Presurgical unilateral cleft lip anthropometrics: incidence of vermilion height asymmetry. Plast Reconstr Surg. 2013;131:935e–6e.
15. Tse RW, Mercan E, Fisher DM, Hopper RA, Birgfeld CB, Gruss JS. Unilateral Cleft Lip Nasal Deformity: Foundation-Based Approach to Primary Rhinoplasty. Plast Reconstr Surg. 2019;144(5):1138–49.
16. Tse R. Unilateral cleft lip - principles and practice of surgical management. Seminars Plast Surg. 2012;26:145–55.

# Bilateral Cleft Lip Repair

# 14

David K. Chong and Nicolas S. Dhooghe

## Introduction

Bilateral lip repair remains one of the great challenges of cleft surgery. Unlike the unilateral lip cleft, which is often more like a jigsaw puzzle, the bilateral lip deformity can present itself in many different forms and severity. The position of the premaxilla, the size of the prolabium, the extent of asymmetry, and the severity of the nasal deformity are highly variable. Some of the confronting anatomy that challenges even seasoned cleft surgeons includes the severely protruding premaxilla and the often associated shortened columella.

With regard to the approach to the lip, there are two main schools of thought. One is to bring the red lip together entirely from the lateral lip elements. The other is to incorporate some of the red lip repair from the prolabial element (Manchester) [1]. We choose to present the technique from the former as it is our belief that long-term results are better and avoid the "patch"-like appearance of the prolabial vermillion mismatch which often becomes more apparent as the patient ages.

The nose remains the main stigma for patients with complete bilateral lips. Surgeons differ about the amount of primary intervention at primary lip repair. Some will do almost no work on the nose at the time of lip repair, preferring to defer surgery to later in life when the cartilage is more developed. Others are more aggressive, attempting to delineate the lower lateral cartilages through various incisions and shape the diminutive cartilages with direct suture fixation techniques [2]. Some respected surgeons recommend excision of the soft triangle in attempt to minimize the stigma of the nasal deformity [3].

We use a largely closed approach to nasal shaping and feel that we are able to improve the shape of the nose enough without introducing scars or damage that will complicate later interventions. We agree that the cartilages are too delicate to attempt to do significant dissection and to influence the shape. When one looks at the maneuvers required in definitive rhinoplasty, it's hard to conceive the effect that one could have in a primary procedure at 6 months of age.

## Goals of Surgery

- To achieve symmetry. Any primary asymmetry should be addressed at the time of repair.
- Place scars along the seams of the anatomical nasolabial subunits.
- Creation of an upper labial sulcus by using the mucosa of the prolabium.
- Achieving continuity of the orbicularis oris muscle by connecting the muscle of the lateral lip elements across the midline.
- Creation of a philtrum of the right dimension, taking into account changes that occur with growth, as the philtrum is known to grow faster than the columellar length and nasal tip protrusion [3].
- Create continuity and symmetry of the lip vermillion arch, with creation of the Cupid's bow and a median tubercle of sufficient height and fullness. This is done by using tissue from the lateral lip elements.
- We consider correction of the nasal deformity just as important as the lip repair, and both deserve the same amount of time and attention. Surgery in bilateral cleft lip is a nasolabial repair, not a lip repair. However, this should be done without creating visible scars on the nose, which in our opinion potentially replaces one stigma with another and compromising the result of the later, often

D. K. Chong (✉)
Plastic and Maxillofacial Surgery Department, Royal Children's Hospital, Melbourne, VIC, Australia

N. S. Dhooghe
Plastic, Reconstuctive and Esthetic Surgery, Ghent University Hospital, Ghent, Oost-Vlaanderen, Belgium
e-mail: Nicolas.dhooghe@uzgent.be

© Springer Nature Switzerland AG 2021

J. W. Swanson, D. W. Low (eds.), *Global Cleft Care in Low-Resource Settings*, https://doi.org/10.1007/978-3-030-59105-2_14

needed, open rhinoplasty. In a low-resource setting, this secondary rhinoplasty is often not possible, making primary correction of the nose of even greater importance.

## Timing and Indications for Surgery

There is no medical urgency to repair a bilateral cleft lip. It is indicated at any age if the child is healthy. A good guideline for assessing if a child is considered healthy is the "rule of tens" in which the child is 10 weeks of age, weighs 10 pounds (4,53 kg), and has a hemoglobin level of 10 g/dl [4]. Few repairs are carried out before the age of 3 months, and we prefer performing the repair at the age of 6 months, as the landmarks are larger and easier to identify. If the child is near 1 year of age or older and has a cleft lip and palate, speech becomes the first priority and closure of the palate before or simultaneously with the lip repair is indicated [3]. If a child is older and learning how to walk or at a difficult age for cooperation with postoperative care, it might disrupt the repair and make postoperative scar management more challenging.

## Our Technique for Bilateral Complete Cleft Lip Repair

We use the technique for bilateral cleft repair as described by Fisher, however with some modifications [5].

The day of a bilateral cleft lip repair is one of the most important days in the patient's life. The surgeon must take as much time as necessary and avoid distractions [3]. The procedure requires a high level of attention and concentration. Making sure all the necessary instruments and sutures are present and the whole operating team is well prepared for the procedure is therefore essential. Loupe magnification is helpful for accurate identification of anatomical landmarks, for precise tissue dissection and for perfect approximation. Make sure you can move around the patient and observe the lip repair from different angles.

### Patient Preparation and Setup

The procedure is generally performed under general anesthesia. The patient is positioned supine with the neck neutral and head stabilized in a head ring. An oral tube is used and taped to the chin in the midline. A throat pack is inserted to further fixate the tube and prevent aspiration of fluids. The head is prepped and draped, and corneas are protected with transparent tape to still enable the plane of the eyes in the surgical field to be visualized as an aid to assessing labial and nasal symmetry. The transparent tape should still allow the cheek to move freely. The surgeon must have the ability to freely examine the face from all angles throughout the procedure to ensure that three-dimensional balance is achieved.

Presurgical photographs are taken, which usually consist of a front and lateral view of the face as well as a worms-eye view to evaluate the lip projection, vermillion arch, and symmetry and projection of the nose.

### Markings (Fig. 14.1)

The labial cleft closure is designed, measured, and determined prior to skin incision. The operation is the execution of a formulated plan. It is important that the surgeon spends enough attention on marking and measuring and is commit-

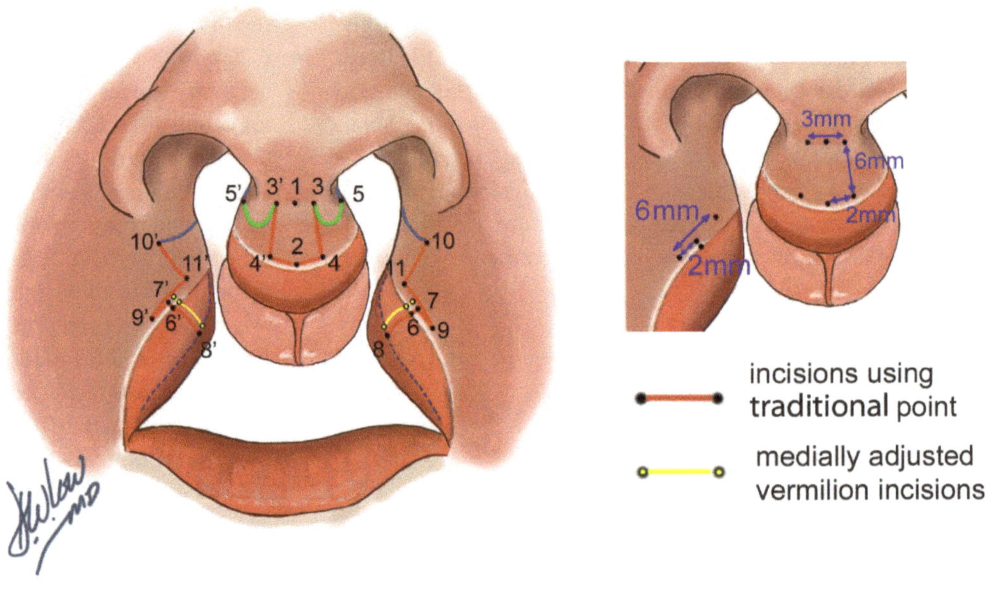


**Fig. 14.1** Markings for bilateral cleft lip repair

ted to his plan. This eliminates the potential of compromising landmarks and removes the fear of height or length discrepancies. Precise measurements and markings are a supplement to the surgeon's "artistic eye" and a great support throughout the surgical procedure.

Markings are performed with methylene blue dye after the patient is prepped and draped. Markings of landmarks and anatomic contours are made with dots at the landmarks listed below and along the lines of interest for measurement, incision, or alignment of elements. Tattoo all points to prevent loss of landmarks.

## We Start by Making the Markings on the Prolabium

- Mark the midline at the lip-columellar junction [1].
- Design the philtral tie. The measurements apply for patients around 6 months of age.
- The width of the philtral tie at the lip-columellar junction is 3 mm (point 3–3′).
- The length of the vertical legs is 6 mm (point 3–4 and point 3′–4′).
- Make the angle of the tip at point 2 as acute as possible. This will determine the shape of Cupid's bow. Point 2 can be on or above the white roll but not caudal to it. The white roll marks the junction between the red vermillion and the skin. All cuts must be made above the white roll of the prolabium, as the white roll after the repair is made from the lateral lip elements. The white roll of the prolabium will be discarded. The distance between point 2–4 and 4′ is 2 mm.
- Point 5 and 5′ are located on the junction between skin and mucosa, at the level of the lip-columellar crease. Mark two semi-circular C-flaps on each side of the philtral tie. These flaps will be rotated upward between 90 and 180 degrees into the nostril and are of great importance to create a nice angle between the lip and the columella. This may create excess skin in the nostril sill but can either be tucked into the nostril during the repair or trimmed if necessary.

## Markings on the Lateral Lip Elements

- Start by marking the wet dry junction of the vermillion with a dotted line. This is the line between the wet mucosa and the dry vermillion. In a cleft lip repair these lines must be made continuous and perfectly aligned.
- Mark the point of medial lip closure (point 6 and 6'). We feel that in a natural lip, the vermillion is thinner at the median tubercle compared to the vermillion at the points of Cupid's bow. We therefore place our points that will be joined at the midline (point 6 and 6′), to create the median tubercle, more medial than Noordhoff's point. Acknowledging the fact that Noordhoff's point marks the peak of the cupid's bow in a unilateral lip repair. Point 6 and 6' should still be at the thickest part of the red lip, even though the vermillion portion of the red lip has narrowed Point 7 and 7′ are placed at the same level as point 6 and 6′, just above the white roll.
- Draw a vertical line across the white roll (point 6 and 6′ to 7 and 7′) and then a line, slightly convex medially, across the vermillion (point 7 and 7′ to 8 and 8′).
- Mark a back cut (point 9), at the cranial edge of the white roll, parallel to it, with a length equal to lower leg of the philtral tie (point 2 to 4 and 4′, 2 mm).
- Mark point 11 and 11′, by drawing a line along the same axis, starting from point 9 and 9′, with the same length as the vertical height of the philtral tie (point 3 and 3′ to 4 and 4′, 6 mm).
- Marking point 10 and 10′ is difficult because it does not represent a specific anatomic point and requires decision-making by the surgeon marking 10 and 10' may be difficult for the novice surgeon but using the insertion of the alar base is a good guide (Fig. 14.2). Point 10 and 10′ will join point 5 and 5′ to create a symmetric position of the alar base at an appropriate level compared to the lip-columellar crease, and by doing so, nostrils are created with a symmetric width and

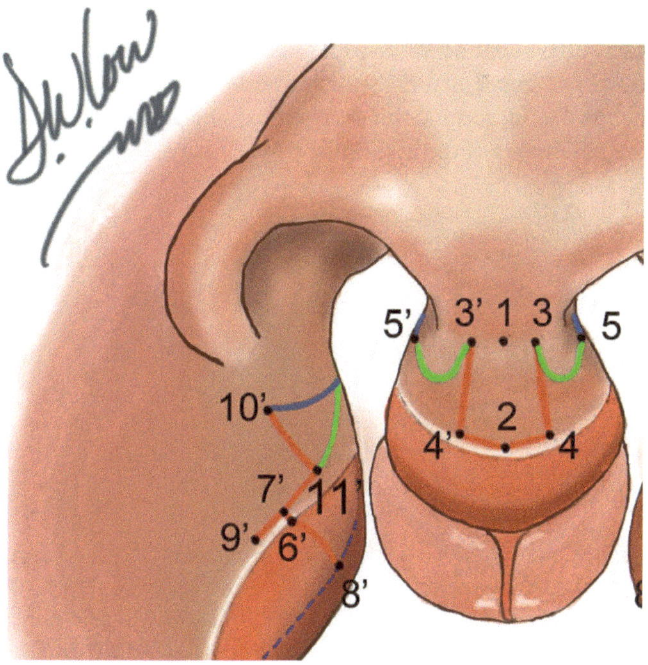


Fig. 14.2 Marking point 10 and preserving an excess skin triangle for more freedom in nostril shaping

circumference. Remember that creating a good shape of the nose is just as important as the repair of the lip and any discrepancy in the height of the alar base will be noticeable and very hard to correct later in life. Although visualizing and marking point 10 and 10′ is very important, we do not mark a cutting line from point 10 and 10′ to 11 and 11′. Instead, we draw a line from point 11 and 11′ along the skin mucosa junction into the nose. The skin above the line between 10 and 11 and 10′ and 11′ will be rotated upward into the nose during the lip repair and joined to the skin of the C-flaps. Any excess skin can be trimmed later in the repair and as a surgeon gains confidence in his repair he will begin to gain the courage to excise the skin triangle between the blue and red lines determined by point 10. This gives the surgeon more freedom in the creation of the right nostril width, which is of utmost importance in a bilateral cleft lip repair.

All markings have now been made. However, before proceeding, double check every marking and measurement. When you are ready to commit to your plan, tattoo the points with a needle and ink so you don't lose your precious landmarks. When cutting, avoid cutting away and losing your marks.

## Surgery: the Execution of Your Plan

Infiltrate the lateral lip elements, nose and prolabium with a local anesthetic solution with adrenalin. Performing a block of the infraorbital nerve with a local anesthetic can be useful. The infraorbital nerve provides sensation for the upper lip, nose, and cheek and exits the infraorbital foramen 4–7 mm below the infraorbital rim on a vertical line at the level of the medial limbus of the iris [6].

## Creation of the Philtral Tie and Posterior Wall of the Upper Buccal Sulcus

Incise the philtral tie and the C-flaps. Elevate them as a superiorly based thin skin flap onto the level of the nasal spine. It is important to adequately release the philtral tie and to release the angles between the C-flaps and the philtral tie.

Discard the vermillion and white roll of the prolabium.

Thin the prolabial mucosa using scissors, and fold it upward to create the posterior wall of the upper labial sulcus. Suture it at the level of the nasal spine with a resorbable suture (Fig. 14.3).

## Incision of the Lateral Lip Markings

By holding the lateral lip between your thumb and index, you can reduce bleeding by compressing the labial artery. When incising over the vermillion, remember to follow the medially convex curve. Once you are across the wet dry junction, it is important to preserve as much mucosa as possible to avoid a whistle notch deformity, caused by shortness of the lip at the level of the midline (Fig. 14.4).

## Release of the Lateral Lip Elements and Alar Bases

Release the gingivobuccal sulcus and lateral nose at the level of piriform aperture to facilitate the lip and nasal closure. Incise along the gingivobuccal sulcus and extend this incision medially toward the piriform aperture along the skin mucosa junction. Laterally a back cut can be made to improve mobilization. Dissect the lateral lip element and alar base off of the maxilla in a supra-periosteal plane. Ensure you place

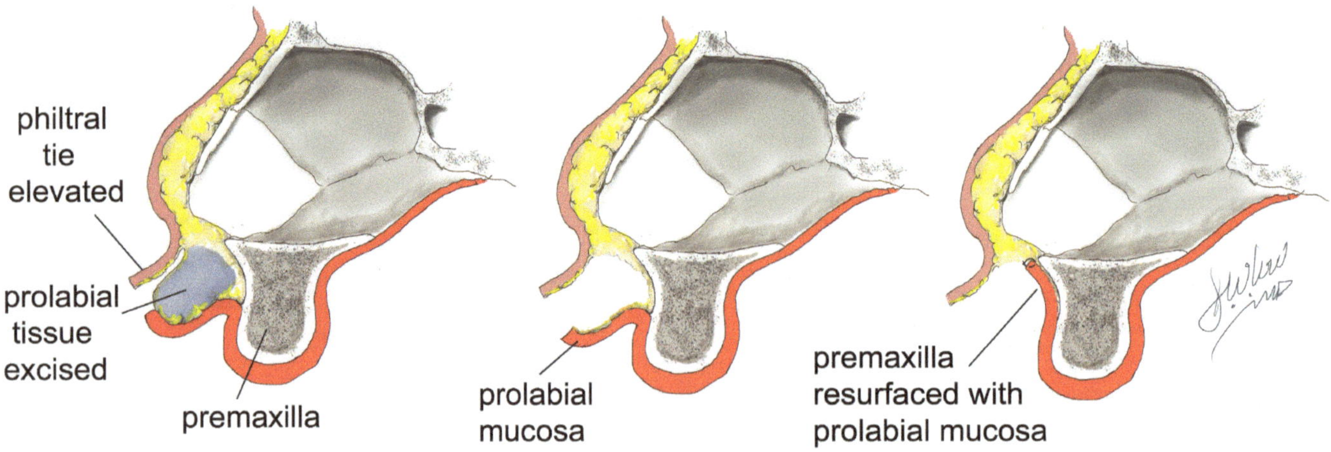


**Fig. 14.3** Elevation of the philtral tie and creation of the posterior wall of the upper buccal sulcus

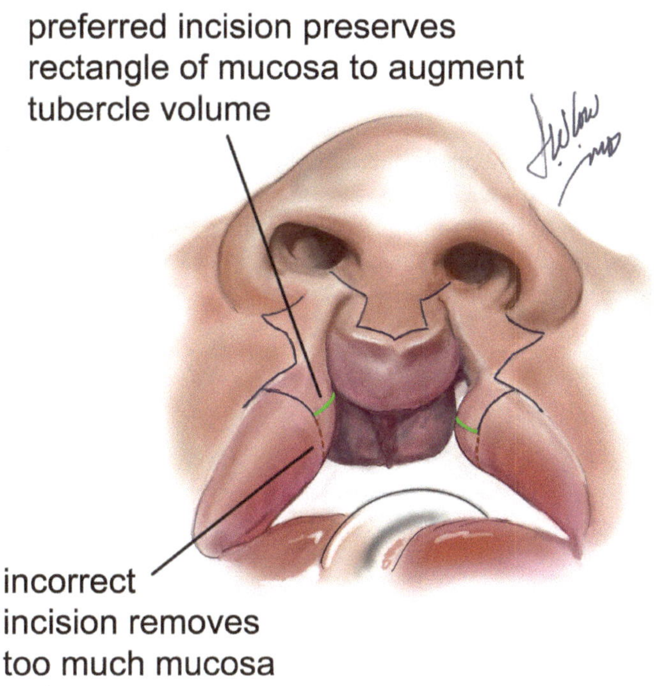


**Fig. 14.4** Correct design of the incision lines of the mucosa of the lateral lip elements. Green indicates the correct incision lines, whereas the red lines will result in deficiency of mucosa resulting in vertical shortness at the level of the midline

one digit along the inferior orbital rim to help control the extent of dissection needed while preventing inadvertent entry into the orbit, as the maxilla is vertically short in this age group. Blunt dissection with the scissors in a vertical orientation will prevent infraorbital nerve injury.

Ensure that you dissect all attachments off the lateral and inferior portions of the piriform aperture to ensure that the aberrant connection between the lower lateral cartilage and the maxilla is released. Release is complete once the lateral lip elements and alar bases are sufficiently mobile to allow for tension-free repositioning of the alar bases and closure of the lip. The amount of lower lateral cartilage dissection varies according to surgical preference. If nasal degloving is to be performed, place scissors carefully in the plane between the skin and medial crura. Gently dissect in this plane between the skin and the cartilage from the medial crura toward the lateral crura (performed by Dr. Chong based on the influence of Drs. McComb and Salyer) [7, 8]. Likewise, a dissection between the cartilage and skin can be performed from lateral to medial. Opponents of nasal cartilage degloving consider the risk of cartilage injury; subsequent scarring and impaired growth outweigh the benefit achieved with this degloving. In the primary nasal correction without cartilage degloving, the correction is achieved with release of abnormal ligamentous attachments at the piriform and suture techniques, avoiding the risks listed above.

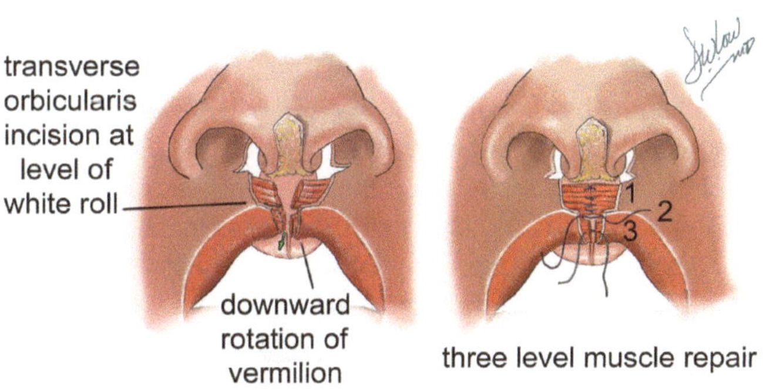


**Fig. 14.5** With a transverse incision of the orbicularis muscle and muscle repair in three levels, with different amounts of tension, a good three dimensional lip shape can be achieved

## Muscle Release

Release the orbicularis oris muscle in the lateral lip elements from the alar base. Release it from the skin to achieve sufficient advancement for a good approximation of the orbicularis muscle from both lateral lip elements at the midline, without creation of a muscle bulge. Perform only a limited release of the muscle from the mucosa.

Performing a small cut in the orbicularis muscle, at the level of the white roll and parallel to it, will allow better downward rotation of the vermillion and the lip vermillion to roll out more and create a bulge relative to the lip skin (Fig. 14.5).

## Evaluation of Alar Base Position with Muscle Closure

In our opinion, the position of the alar bases with approximation of the orbicularis muscle is a key point of any bilateral cleft lip repair. You can mimic the effect of this closure by approximating the muscle with two forceps. If the alar bases move too much upward and cause the typical pinched, cat- or bunny-like nose deformity, typical of previous bilateral cleft lip repair, this needs to be addressed before continuing with the lip repair. *We feel it is of utmost importance to achieve an optimal correction of the cleft nasal deformity, before starting with closure of the muscle.* One can either use a cinching stitch to each alar base or fixate the alar base in the right position by suturing it to the premaxilla depending on the vector required. We do this by suturing the soft tissue at the base of the lower laterals to each other or to the periosteum of the premaxilla with a slow resorbable suture (PDS 4.0).

Only when you are satisfied of the correct and symmetrical position of the alar bases should you start closing the lip elements. Often the tension of the nose is different in amount and direction as compared to the lip closure and hence may require separate attention than just that which is achieved by the orbicularis muscle repair.

## Closure of the Lip Mucosa

First the mucosa is joined and sutured at the midline with a resorbable suture (Chromic Gut 5.0). If desired, one or more stitches can be used to close the releasing incisions in the gingivobuccal sulcus, although this is not mandatory. The mucosa is then progressively closed doing ones best to use bites to attain symmetrical lengths of closure.

## Muscle Repair

The muscle release, repositioning, and approximation are the foundation of the lip repair. Repair the muscle beginning superiorly. The muscle repair is divided in three levels (Fig. 14.5). The upper level is sutured using a non-resorbable suture (Prolene 4.0) and extends from the upper edge of the orbicularis until the level of the transverse releasing incision. The initial stitch placed superiorly should set the lip to be repaired in a balanced fashion. Each successive muscle stitch is placed to ensure the lip points of closure at the level of the white roll are well matched. The alignment of the points of closure is checked after each successive muscle stitch.

The second level of the repair is done by approximating the muscle at each edge of the transverse "opening" incisions in the muscle which is approximately at the level of the white roll. This stitch is very important to define the shape of the lip in its three dimensions, as it can give the lip a pout and ensure that the arc of the repaired lip has is a harmonious continuous nice bow and not a tip. At this level we use slow resorbable stitch (PDS 4.0).

The third level of the muscle repair is done by suturing the orbicularis at the level of the lip vermillion less tightly with a resorbable suture (Monocryl 4.0).

## Anterior Closure of the Lip Skin and Vermillion

Suture the lip vermillion using a resorbable suture and ensure that the wet dry junction is correctly aligned.

The skin is stitched, matching the length of the skin of the philtral tie to the length of the lateral lip elements and suturing the tip of the philtral tie to the continuous white roll. Point 2 will be joined to point 7 and 7′, point 9 and 9′ to point 4 and 4′, and point 11 and 11′ to point 3 and 3′ (Fig. 14.1). Because of accurate and precise preoperative measurement, a seamless and perfect approximation of the labial elements is reached. The only "cut-as-you-go" occurs at the nasal sill where some adaptation is often required to ensure the right diameter and shape to the nostril opening as well as tailoring the scar to sit in the shadow of the nostril sill. If necessary, excess skin can be trimmed. It is very important to rotate the C-flaps in a cephalad direction bilaterally in order to create a well-defined angle between the columella and the lip (Fig. 14.6). Proportions of the tubercle should be symmetric at completion of repair (Fig. 14.7). Fast resorbable sutures can be used, avoiding the need to remove the sutures after 5–7 days under sedation, often difficult in a low-resource setting.

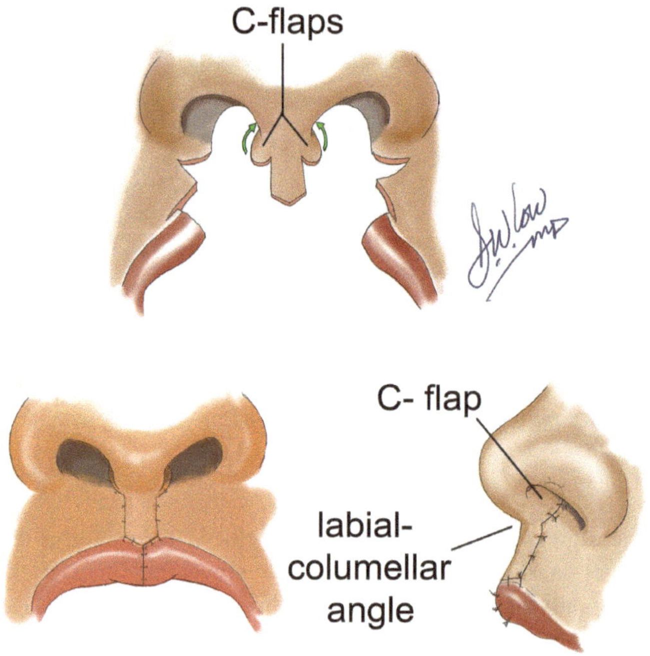


Fig. 14.6 Cephalad rotation of the C-flaps defines the lip-columellar angle

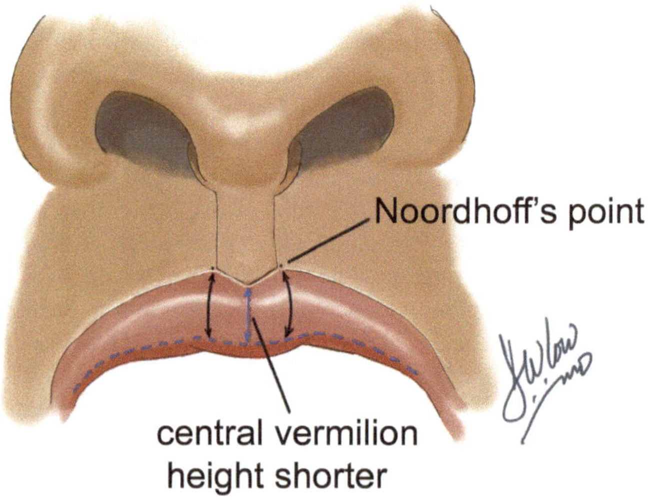


Fig. 14.7 Balanced proportions of the reconstructed tubercle

## Primary Nasal Correction

In a low-resource setting, a secondary rhinoplasty is often not possible, making a good primary nasal correction even more important. Although many techniques have been described for primary nasal correction, we wish to avoid creating an additional scar on the nose or creating a new stigma in an attempt to avoid another. Our primary nasal correction consists of release of the lower lateral nasal cartilage, as described above, and shaping of the nose with stitches. First we place two suspension stitches, suspending the lower laterals to the periosteum of the nasal bone and creating projection of the nasal tip. A 23 gauge needle is placed diagonally from the nasal dorsum through the lower lateral cartilage, at the level of the alar domes (Fig. 14.8). A Monocryl 4.0 suture is passed through the needle and retrieved at the other end. The needle is drawn back at a level just underneath the skin and then pushed back through the lower lateral cartilage, creating a mattress suture with a not inside the nose and no visible sutures on the nasal dorsum. This suture is placed on both sides to achieve symmetry. The same technique is used to define the alae by placing the sutures just above the lower lateral cartilage, to eliminate dead space and define the shape of the alae (Fig. 14.9).

If possible, nasal stents are placed in the nostrils and secured to prevent aspiration. These stents will keep the nostrils in the desired shape and counteract possible deformation of the nostrils due to scarring.

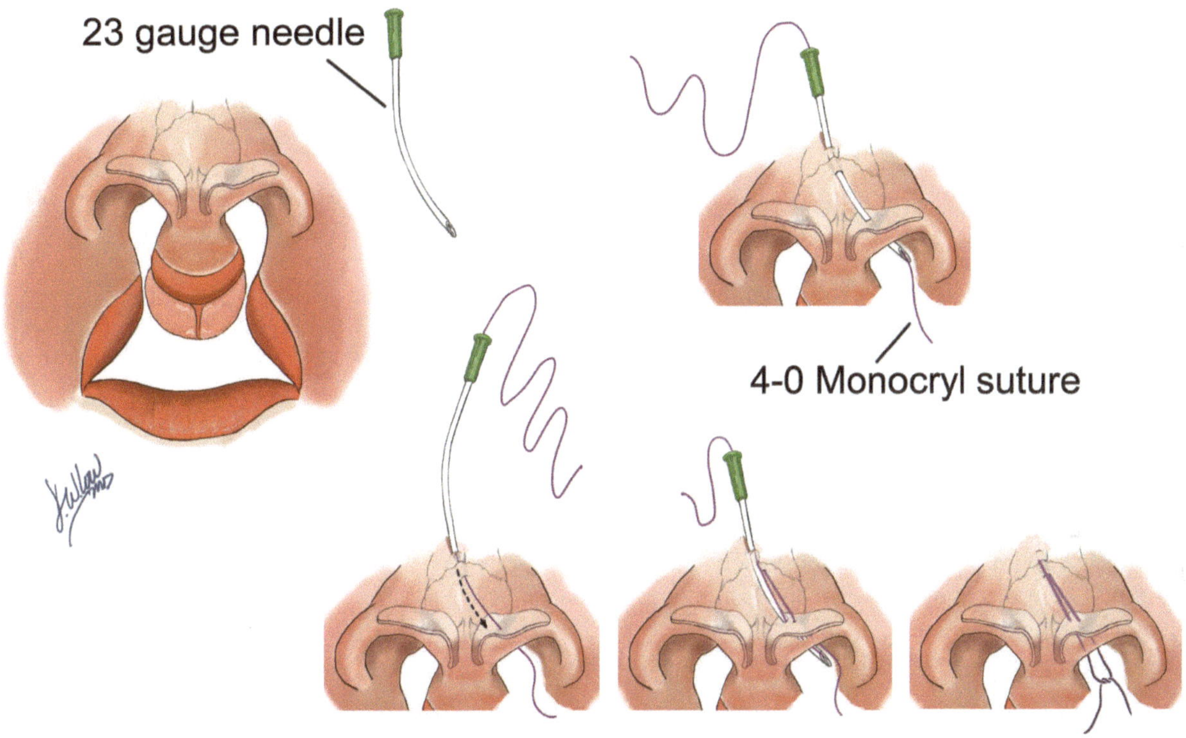


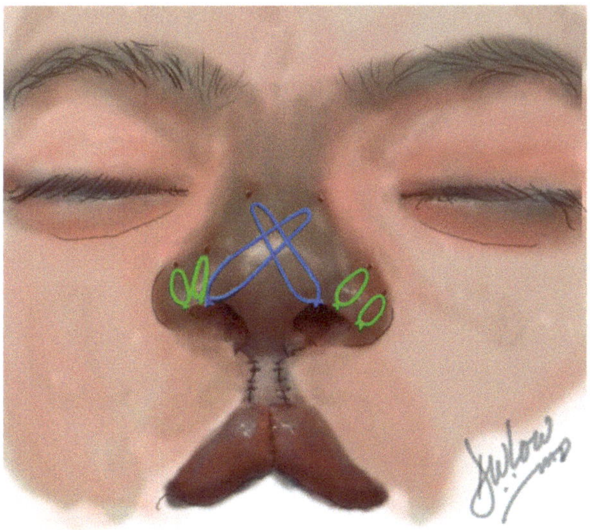

**Figs. 14.8 and 14.9** primary nasal correction by degloving of the lower lateral cartilages and placement of suspension stitches

## Postoperative Care

Ointment is regularly applied to the suture lines to prevent crusting and improve scarring.

If necessary, sutures are best removed after 5 days to prevent visible suture marks. If nasal stents are available, these should be used for a minimum of 6 weeks and up to 3 months.

One must warn the parents of the "look" of the patient postoperatively. Unlike unilateral cases, where the facial balance is immediate, the bilateral patient will look tight, overdone, and potentially the upper lip overly projected due to the position of the premaxilla. Parents should be prepared for this appearance and assured that there will be improvement in the tightness and protrusion with time. There is a much greater evolution of the facial appearance as compared to unilateral cleft lips.

**Tips and Tricks**

- Do not make your philtrum too large, as it is known to grow faster.
- Use two semi-circular skin flaps on each side of the philtrum, which are rotated in a cephalad direction into the nostril sill, to create a distinct angle between the lip and the columella.
- Assess the median tubercle of the parents. You must avoid a whistle notch deformity but also making it too full.
- To avoid central mucosal deficiency, preserve enough mucosa when incising the lateral lips.
- Aim for an optimal correction of the cleft nasal deformity, before starting with the lip closure and without creating a new scar.
- The muscle repair is the foundation of your lip repair.
- Warn the parents of the postoperative look.

## References


1. Zhang JX, Arneja JS. Evidence-based medicine: the bilateral cleft lip repair. Plast Reconstr Surg. 2017;140(1):152e–65e.
2. Henry C, Samson T, Mackay D. Evidence-based medicine: the cleft lip nasal deformity. Plast Reconstr Surg. 2014;133(5):1276–88.
3. Mulliken JB. Repair of bilateral cleft lip and its variants. Indian J Plast Surg. 2009;42 Suppl:S79–90.
4. Bentz ML, Bauer BS, Zuker RM. Principle and practice of pediatric plastic surgery. 2nd ed. Boca Raton: CRC Press, Taylor & Francis Group. 2016
5. Fisher DM, Sommerlad BC. Cleft lip, cleft palate, and velopharyngeal insufficiency. Plast Reconstr Surg. 2011;128(4):342–60.
6. Zide BM, Swift R. How to block and tackle the face. Plast Reconstr Surg. 1998;101(3):840–51.
7. Salyer KE. Primary correction of the unilateral cleft lip nose: a 15-year experience. Plast Reconstr Surg. 1986;77(4):558–68.
8. McComb H. Primary repair of the bilateral cleft lip nose: a 15-year review and a new treatment plan. Plast Reconstr Surg. 1990;86:882–9.

# Secondary Cleft Lip Repair

# 15

Alexis Rothermel and Donald R. Mackay

**Key Points**

- A thorough analysis of the secondary cleft deformity is essential in planning corrective surgery. The common deformities are asymmetries of:
  1. Misalignment of the vermillion-cutaneous junction (white roll)
  2. Misalignment of the vermillion-mucosal junction (red line)
  3. Misalignment of the orbicularis oris muscle which can result in abnormal muscle bulges
  4. Short lip at the repair (whistle deformity)
  5. Residual cleft nose deformities are common
- Secondary corrections should be tailored to the defect.
- Minor defects may require simple procedures such as a z-plasty or diamond-shaped scar excision.
- Fat grafting is a useful tool in treating volume deficits.
- Severe deformities are best addressed by completely redoing the lip repair.
- The residual lip and nose deformities are often best addressed by performing a lip revision and cleft nose rhinoplasty at the same time. (Cleft nasal deformities are dealt with in the Septorhinoplasty Chap. 22).

## Introduction

Although we strive to produce perfect lip repairs at the primary surgery, the truth is that most children with clefts of the lip have a secondary defect that can be improved with a secondary surgery [1].

A. Rothermel · D. R. Mackay (✉)
Division of Plastic Surgery, PennState Hershey College of Medicine, Hershey, PA, USA
e-mail: dmackay@pennstatehealth.psu.edu

**Table 15.1** Systematic outline of the underlying causes of secondary unilateral cleft lip deformities and solutions to the problems

| Unilateral cleft lip deformities | |
|---|---|
| Problem | Solution |
| *Asymmetry* | |
| *Scar* | |
| Wide, hypertrophic | Scar excision, postop massage |
| Position – in line of philtral column | Re-excise and suture |
| Philtral column flattened | "scar graft," fat graft |
| *Vermillion-cutaneous – "roll"* | |
| Mismatch (Figs. 15.1 and 15.2) | Diamond excision, suture, Z-plasty |
| *Vermillion-mucosal – "red line"* | |
| Mismatch (Figs. 15.1 and 15.2) | Excise and realign, Z-plasty |
| *Deficiency* | |
| *Vertical – short lip* | Redo the repair |
| "Whistle deformity" | Excise scar, "scar graft," fat graft |
| *Horizontal – tight lip* | Fat graft |
| *Combination – severe* | Abbe flap |
| *Excess* | |
| *Lateral vermillion* | Elliptical excision on red line |
| *Muscle derangement* | |
| *Lateral muscle bulges* | Excise scar, undermine, align muscle, resuture |

Most of these secondary operations can be performed as outpatient procedures.

Unilateral secondary cleft lip deformities all result in an asymmetry. It is helpful to define the cause of the asymmetry (Table 15.1), which helps in planning the surgical correction.

Bilateral cleft lip deformities may also include asymmetries, but either tissue excess or deficiency in the philtrum frequently defines the defect (Table 15.2).

Although not part of this chapter, it is important to consider the nose and lip as a unit both at the primary surgery and when secondary surgery is performed [2–4].

© Springer Nature Switzerland AG 2021

J. W. Swanson, D. W. Low (eds.), *Global Cleft Care in Low-Resource Settings*, https://doi.org/10.1007/978-3-030-59105-2_15

**Table 15.2** Systematic outline of the underlying causes of secondary bilateral cleft lip deformities and solutions to the problems

| Bilateral cleft lip deformities | |
|---|---|
| Problem | Solution |
| *Asymmetry* | |
| *Scar* | |
| Wide, hypertrophic | Scar excision, postop massage |
| Position – in line of philtral column | Re-excise and suture |
| Philtral column flattened | "scar graft," fat graft |
| *Vermillion-cutaneous – "roll"* | |
| Mismatch | Diamond excision |
| *Vermillion-mucosal – "red line"* | |
| Mismatch (Figs. 15.1 and 15.2) | Excise and realign, Z-plasty |
| *Deficiency* | |
| *Vertical – short lip* | Redo the repair |
| *Horizontal – tight lip* | Fat graft |
| *Combination – severe* | Abbe flap |
| *Excess* | |
| *Vertical – long upper lip* | Moustache shaped excision under nostril sill (Figs. 15.13 and 15.14) |
| *Muscle derangement* | |
| *Lateral muscle bulges* | Excise scar, undermine, align muscle, resuture |

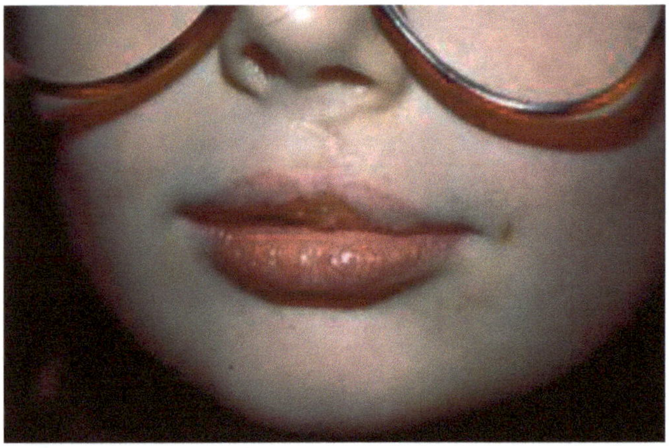

**Fig. 15.1** This is an example of a misalignment problem. Mucosa has been incorporated into the central part of the lip that would normally consist of vermillion. The exposed mucosa is red and crusted in obvious contrast to the paler vermillion. The scar of the lip repair crosses the line of the philtrum column

## Patient Selection and Clinical Planning

### Timing of Surgery

There are no hard and fast rules in the planning and timing of secondary lip surgery and considerable variation is the norm.

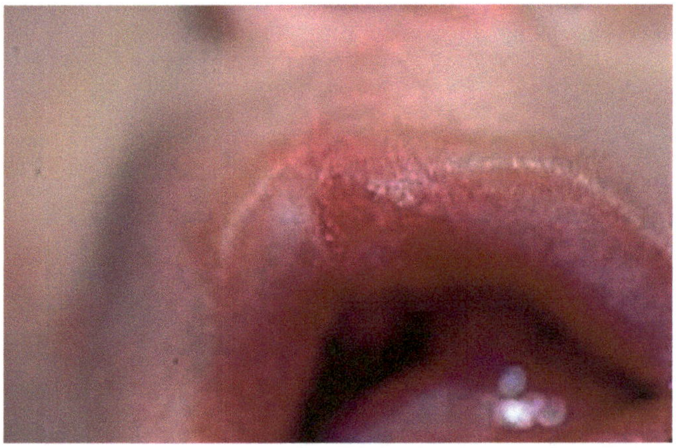

**Fig. 15.2** In this example there is misalignment of both the vermillion-cutaneous junction (white roll) and the vermillion-mucosal junction

In centers that have the luxury of reliable long-term follow-ups, secondary surgery can be part of a long-term treatment plan. The wishes of the family and the patient can be considered. There will be obvious cultural differences but our philosophy has been to perform these secondary procedures when the child expresses a desire to proceed.

In situations where follow-up is rare and resources are limited, the best possible secondary surgery should be performed when the patient presents for surgery, assuming they are medically fit.

Practical considerations such as getting as much secondary surgery as possible done for each anesthetic and each visit must be weighed against sacrificing quality and safety.

### Planning Surgery

Most of these secondary operations can be performed as outpatient procedures. Many of the procedures including fat grafting can be performed under local anesthetic.

Careful assessment of the secondary deformity allows the surgeon to plan the secondary surgery (Fig. 15.3a).

The surgeon should use a skin marker to draw the proposed incisions and mark the key anatomic points including the vermillion-cutaneous junction (the "white" roll) and the vermillion-mucosal junction (the "red" line or erroneously called the "wet dry" vermillion junction) [5] (Fig. 15.3b).

### Relevant Anatomy

Understanding the abnormal anatomy and especially the abnormal muscle attachments in both unilateral and bilateral

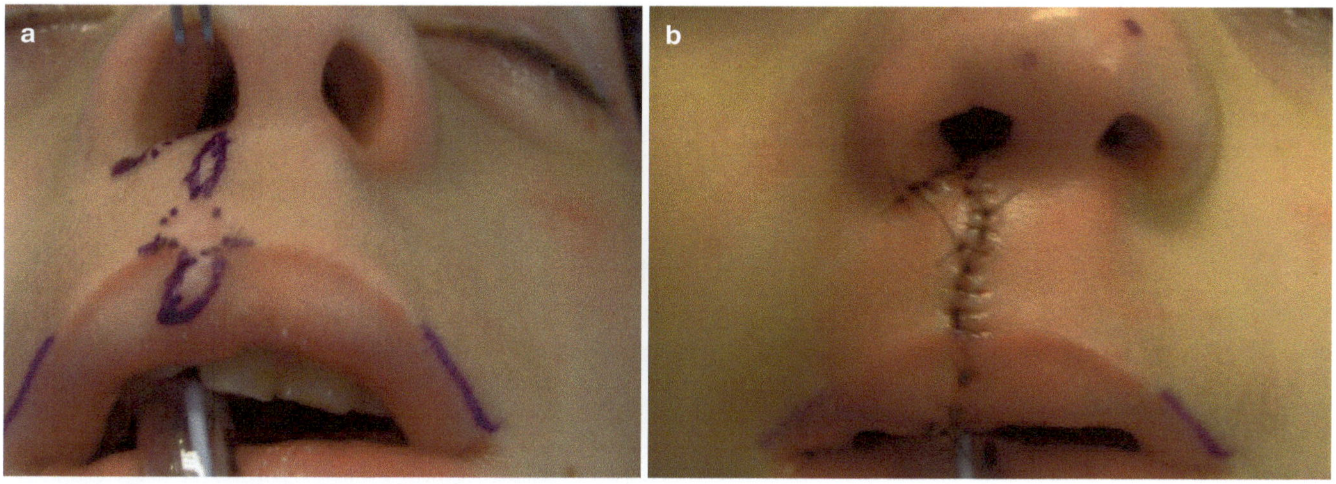


**Fig. 15.3** (**a**) Preoperative markings of the vermillion-cutaneous junction, and the widened scar on the lip and vermillion guide the surgery. (**b**) The immediate postoperative result. The vermillion-cutaneous junction is accurately aligned and the lip scar is placed in the line of the philtral column. The author seldom uses nylon sutures now. After accurate dermal apposition, either rapidly absorbing sutures or skin glue is preferred

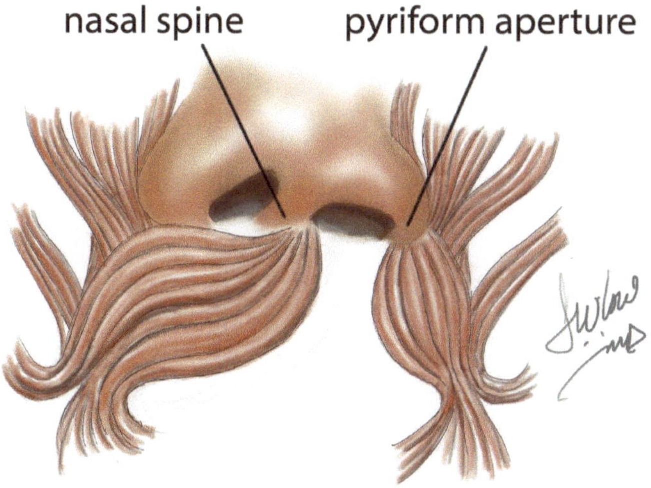


**Fig. 15.4** The orbicularis oris muscle attaches to the nasal spine and pyriform aperture in a unilateral cleft lip. Inadequate release and mobilization of the muscle will result in a short lip. This must be addressed when undertaking a secondary revision

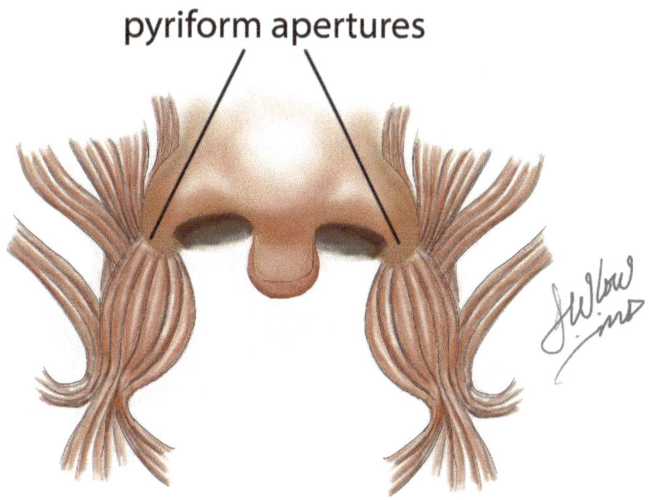


**Fig. 15.5** The orbicularis oris attaches to the both pyriform apertures in a bilateral cleft lip. There is no muscle in the prolabium. The muscle must be mobilized across the midline to establish continuity if this was not done at the primary repair

clefts helps the surgeon understand the secondary defect and guides the revision [6, 7] (Figs. 15.4 and 15.5). For example, inadequate release of the muscle from the nasal spine and the lateral pyriform aperture in a unilateral cleft results in a short lip and whistle deformity or a short upper lip with a muscle gap in a bilateral clefts. Inadequate mobilization and approximation of the muscle results in obvious muscle bulges on either side of the repair.

Appreciation of normal lip symmetry and the position of the skin-vermillion (roll) and vermillion-mucosal (redline) junctions are essential in guiding secondary surgery [7] (Fig. 15.6).

## Key Equipment

Lip revisions (Fig. 15.4)

- Scalpel
- Fine forceps
- Small dissecting scissors
- Skin hooks

Small-volume liposuction and fat grafting (Fig. 15.5)

- 10 cc syringe
- Fine liposuction cannulas
- Small bore, blunt fat injection needles

Standard tumescent fluid

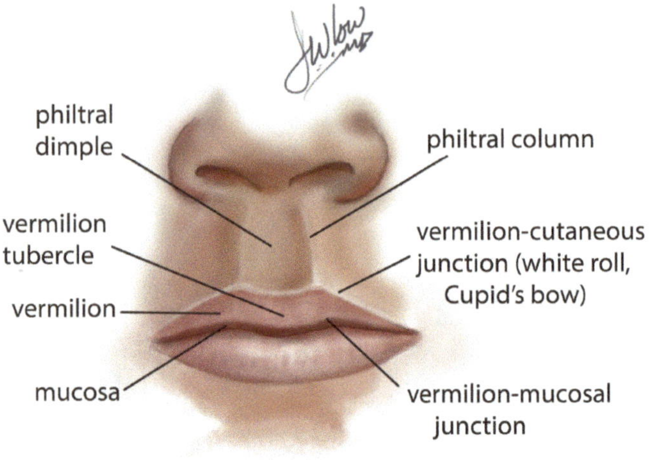


**Fig. 15.6** The goal for any revision is to reestablish the anatomic landmarks and critical junctions. Ideally the lip scar should lie along the philtral column. It is essential to accurately realign the vermillion-cutaneous and vermillion-mucosal junctions

## Anesthesia

Many of the revisions including small volume fat grafts can be performed under local anesthesia.

Young patients and patients undergoing more extensive revisions will have general endotracheal anesthesia.

## Procedural Technique

Where local anesthesia is appropriate, these procedures do not need full sterility in an operating room but can be performed using regional sterility in clean rooms.

The operating room setting should be reserved for the more extensive cases requiring general anesthesia.

There is nothing special about the surgical technique used for these operations. Meticulous planning, careful dissection and tissue handling, and precise approximation are hallmarks for successful outcomes. We now routinely use 4-0 or 5-0 absorbable sutures for muscle and mucosal approximation and fine (6-0 or 7-0) absorbable sutures or cyanoacrylate glue to approximate the skin.

There is no good evidence for the use of antibiotics in these cases. Minor revisions do not need any antibiotics. The current recommendation for more extensive and lengthy operations is to give a single dose of prophylactic antibiotic immediately preoperatively (Figs. 15.7 and 15.8).

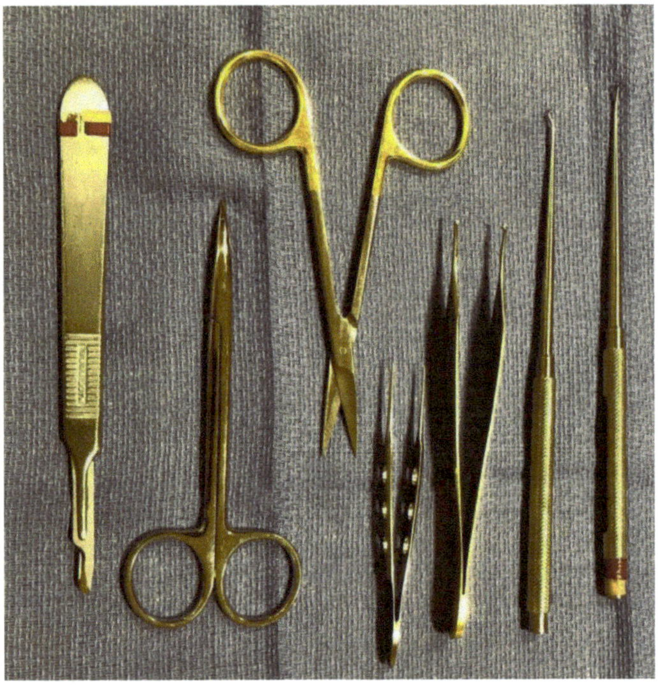

**Fig. 15.7** Basic instruments used to revise cleft lip defects include a scalpel, fine forceps, scissors, and skin hooks

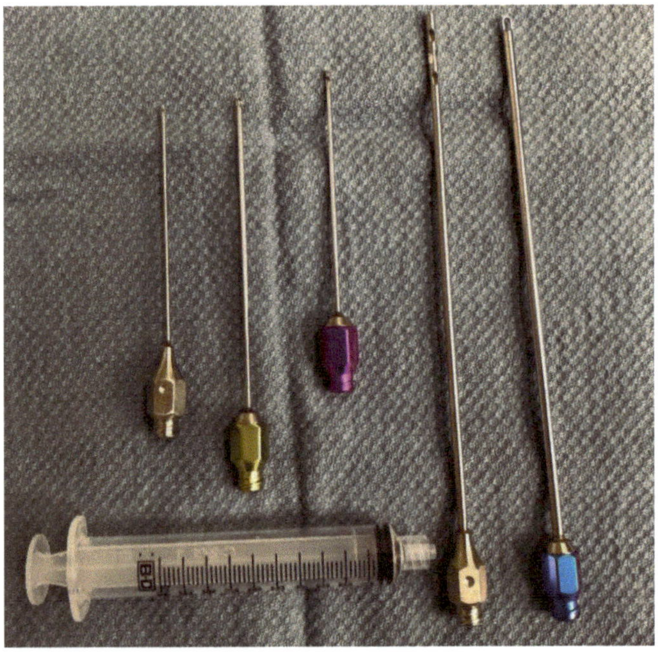

**Fig. 15.8** Liposuction instruments. A 10 cc syringe and small-bore liposuction cannula are all that is needed to suction a small volume of fat. Blunt narrow bore fat injection needles attached to the 10 cc syringe are used to deposit the fat in small aliquots to achieve the desired result

## Unilateral Cleft Lip Deformities

### Clinical Examples of Unilateral Cleft Lip Deformities

Small length discrepancies can be corrected by excising the scar in a diamond pattern (Fig. 15.9a, b).

Minor contour deficiencies can be corrected with small volume lipo-aspirated fat grafts (Fig. 15.10a, b).

Inferiorly pedicled "scar-grafts" provide a useful volume augmentation for whistle deformities (Fig. 15.11a, b). Fat grafts will provide additional volume augmentation when needed (Fig. 15.12a, b).

Severe deformities where the lip is short need a complete redo of the lip repair where all layers including the mucosa and muscle are carefully approximated (Fig. 15.13a, b).

Some patients with severe deformities will still be left with relative thin upper lips even after secondary surgery that has corrected other deformities. A vermillion-switch procedure is a useful technique that can correct the thin upper lip and provide a balanced appearance by reducing a full lower lip [8] (Fig. 15.14a, b).

## Bilateral Cleft Lip Deformities

### Clinical Examples of Bilateral Cleft Lip Deformities

Minor secondary bilateral cleft lip deformities can be corrected using the techniques described for unilateral deformities. Fat grafts are very useful for addressing volume deficiencies [2, 9].

Severe bilateral lip deformities will need a redo of the entire lip repair (Fig. 15.10). Careful alignment of the muscle, skin, vermillion, and mucosa is essential with attention to correctly aligning the cutaneous-vermillion and vermillion-mucosal junctions. The philtrum in bilateral clefts is often too wide and needs to be narrowed. These severe deformities often require staged and repeated revisions (Fig. 15.15a–c).

Two patterns of secondary bilateral cleft lip deformity that we encounter are lips that are either too long or conversely too short and tight.

Long lips are treated by excising the excess under the nostril sills (Fig. 15.16) or as part of revision that includes the philtral columns (Fig. 15.17).

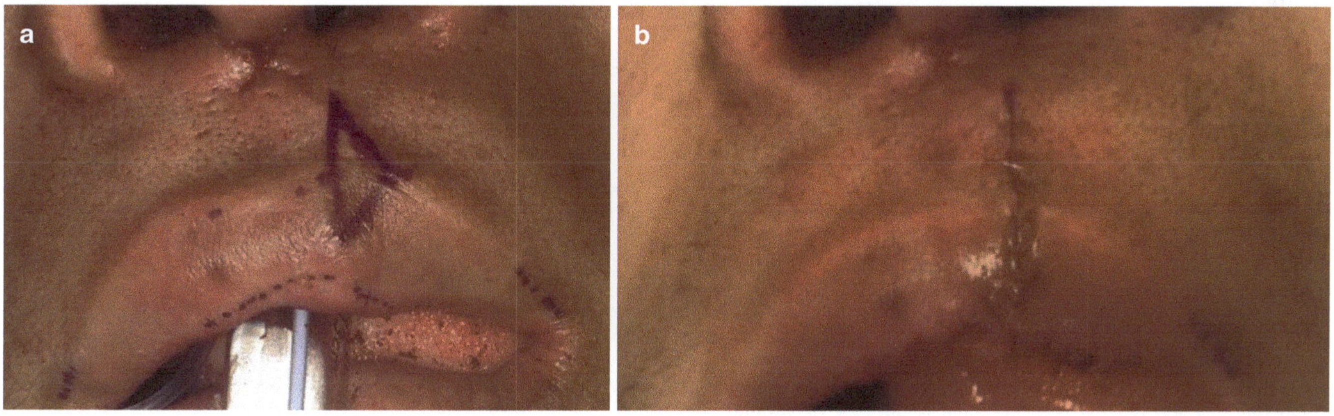


**Fig. 15.9** (**a**) Relatively minor misalignment of the vermillion-cutaneous junction. Planned correction with a diamond-shaped excision. (**b**) After resection, the vermillion cutaneous junction is now aligned

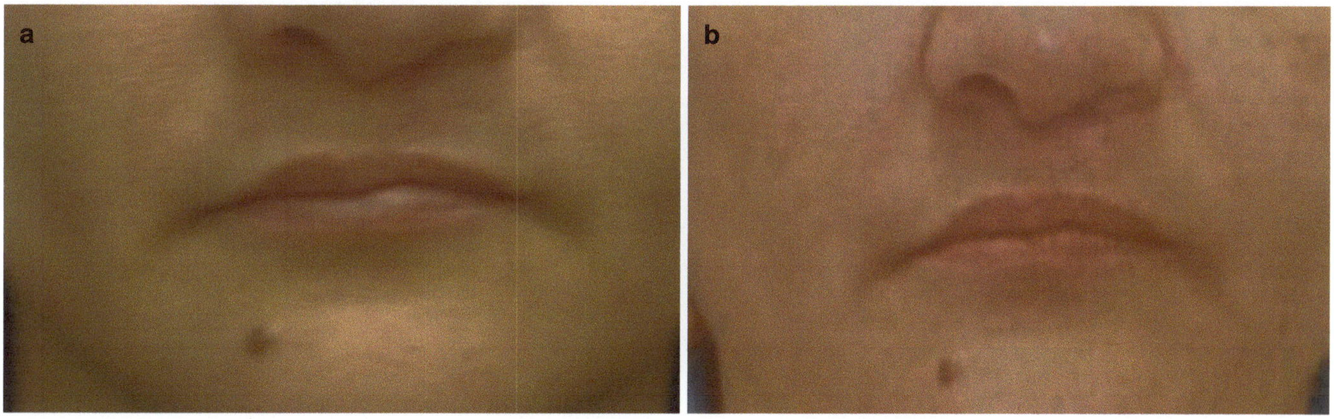


**Fig. 15.10** (**a**) Minor lip deformity with lack of volume on the left cleft side. (**b**) Deformity corrected with 2 cc of liposuctioned fat

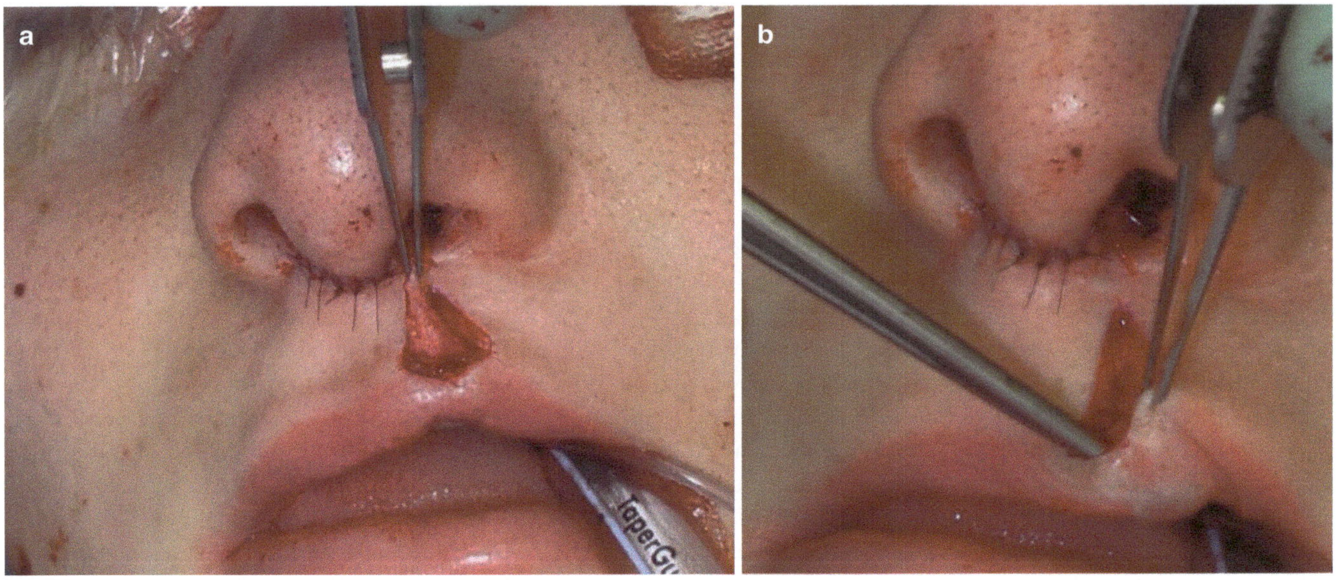


**Fig. 15.11** (**a**) Example of "scar graft." The incisions for the scar revision are made either side of the scar and down to the muscle layer. The scar is de-epithelialized and dissected down to the lip margin keeping an inferior pedicle. (**b**) A pocket is dissected at the site of the vermillion deficiency and the scar flap if tucked into the site before the wound is closed

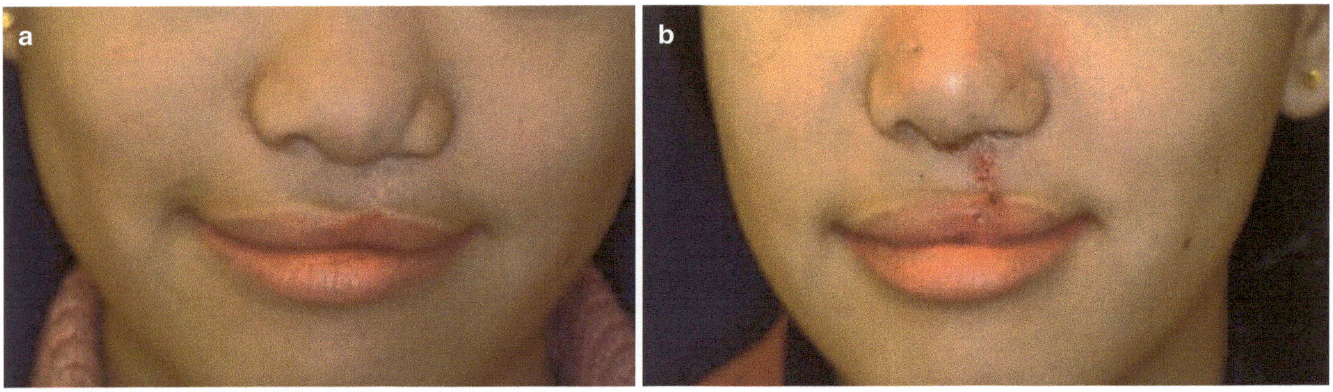


**Fig. 15.12** (**a**) This patient has a slight misalignment of the vermillion-cutaneous junction but the main problem is the lack of volume and height of the vermillion. (**b**) The early result after a rhinoplasty and lip revision. The vermillion was augmented with an inferiorly based "scar graft" and fat injections

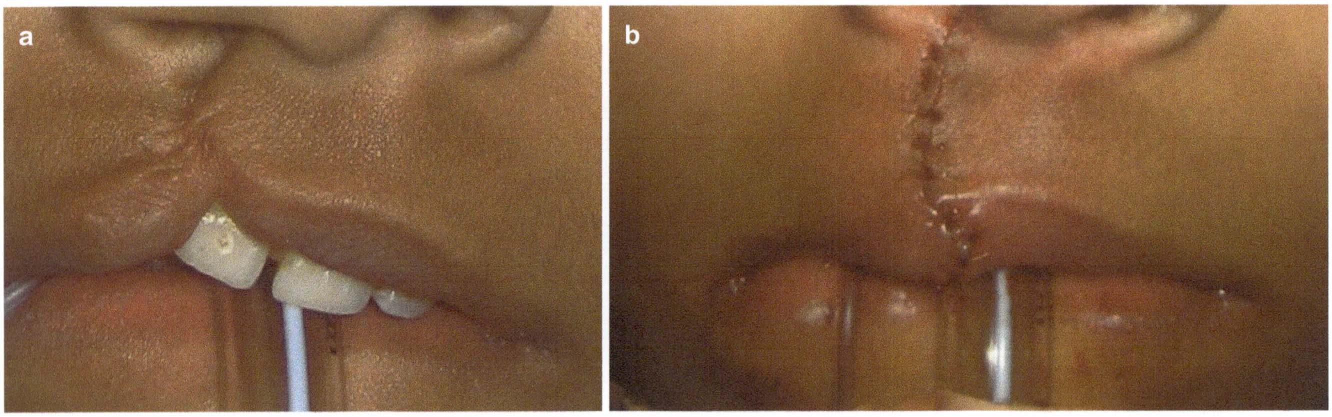


**Fig. 15.13** (**a**) Unilateral repair with short lip, muscle defect at the repair, no alignment of the vermillion-cutaneous junction or the vermillion-mucosal junction, and a prominent whistle deformity. (**b**) Improvement attained by completely redoing the lip. The muscle, vermillion-cutaneous junction, and vermillion-mucosal junction were all carefully approximated. The repair line is more in line with the philtral column

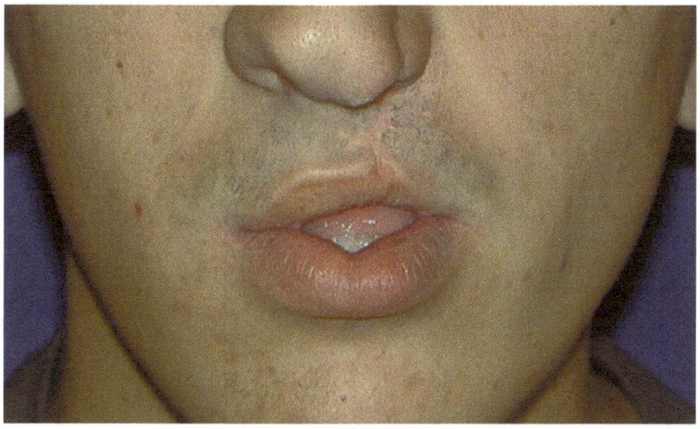

Fig. 15.14 Severe unilateral deformity. This patient underwent a rhinoplasty and lip revision. He still had a relative thin upper lip and full lower lip. This patient underwent a vermillion switch procedure as outlined below

An Abbe flap may be the ideal solution for bilateral lips that are too short and tight [10] (Fig. 15.18a–c).

## Follow-Up and Complication Management

Patients and families should be warned about possible infections and bleeding both of which are fortunately rare. It is important to manage the patients and family's expectations of the surgery. Many of these patients will need additional procedures to get the best result. The reconstructions are often staged.

In resource-poor settings, a multi-staged approach may be impractical and the approach will be adapted to get the maximum benefit from a single operation (Figs. 15.19, 15.20, and 15.21).

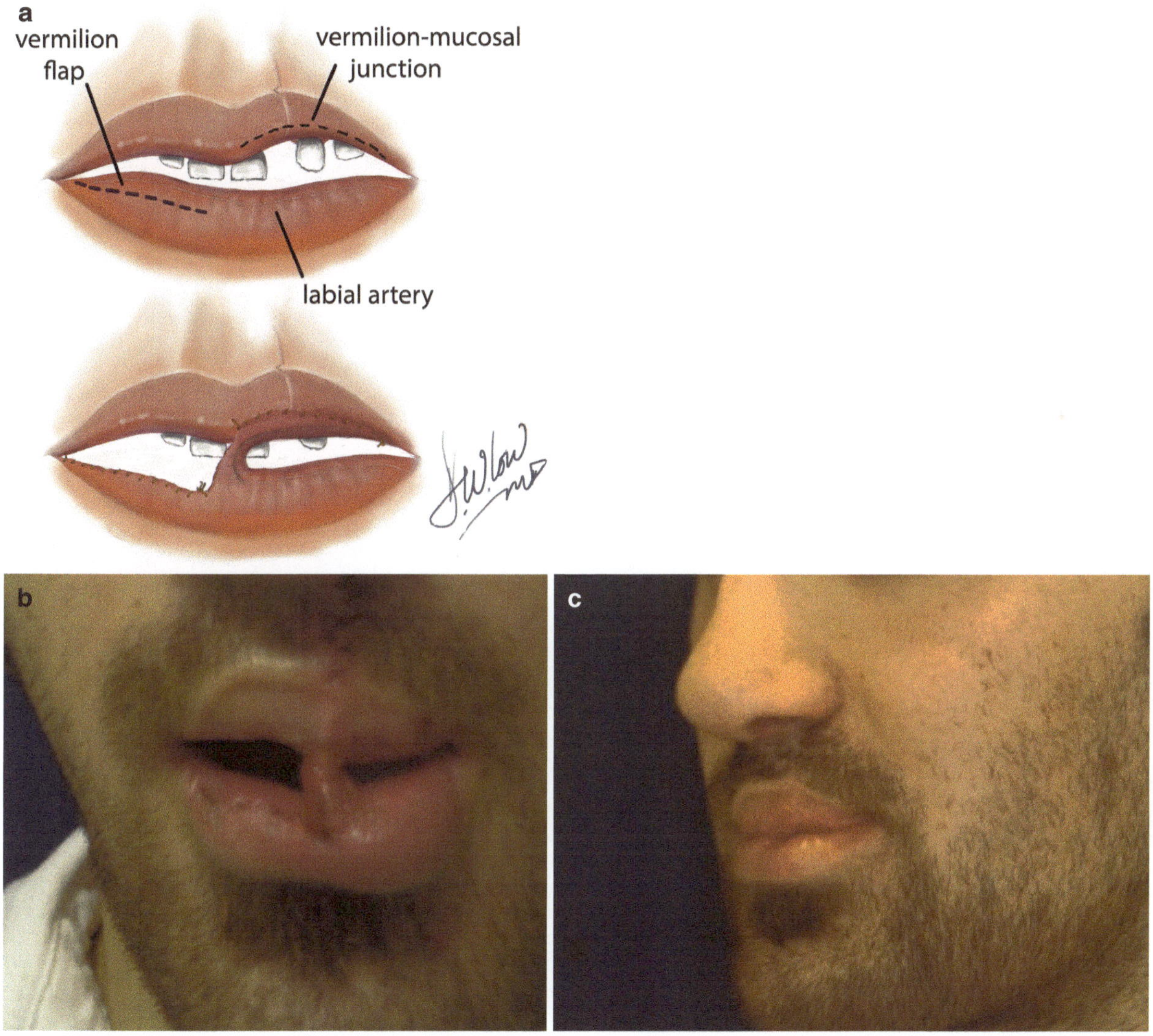


Fig. 15.15 (a) Vermillion switch operation. A flap of vermillion and mucosa based on the labial artery is elevated to the midline and inset into the opposite upper lip. The recipient site is made by incising along the vermillion mucosal junction. The remaining lower lip is elevated 2–3 weeks later and used to augment the oppposite side of the upper lip if needed. (b) Patient with vermilion switch flap in place before second stage. (c) Late result after final division and inset of vermillion switch

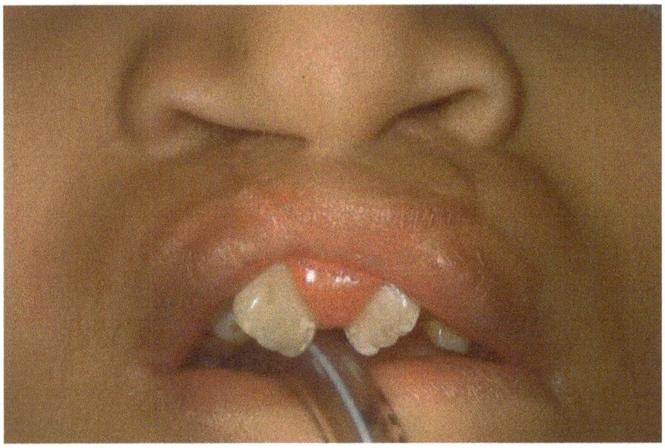

Fig. 15.16 Example of a severe bilateral lip deformity with malalignment of the vermillion-mucosal and vermillion-cutaneous junctions. The philtrum is too wide, the muscle has not been approximated as evidence by the bulges on either side of the philtrum

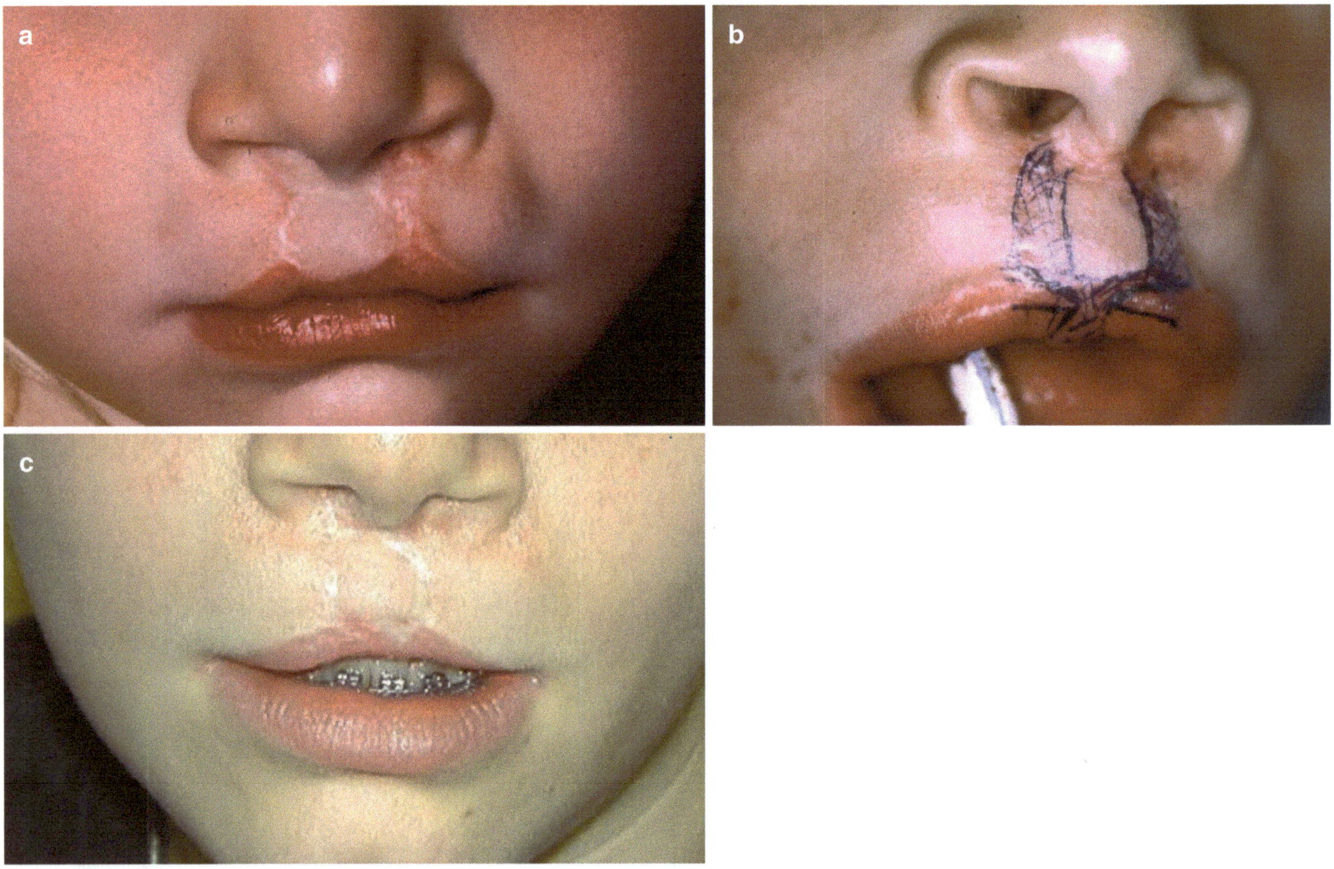


Fig. 15.17 (a) Bilateral lip with widened philtrum, irregular scars, and central vermillion deficiency. (b) Surgical plan includes excision of scars, narrowing the philtrum, and advancing vermillion flaps across the midline at the same time as a corrective rhinoplasty. (c) Result after surgery with improved symmetry but obvious central vermillion deficiency

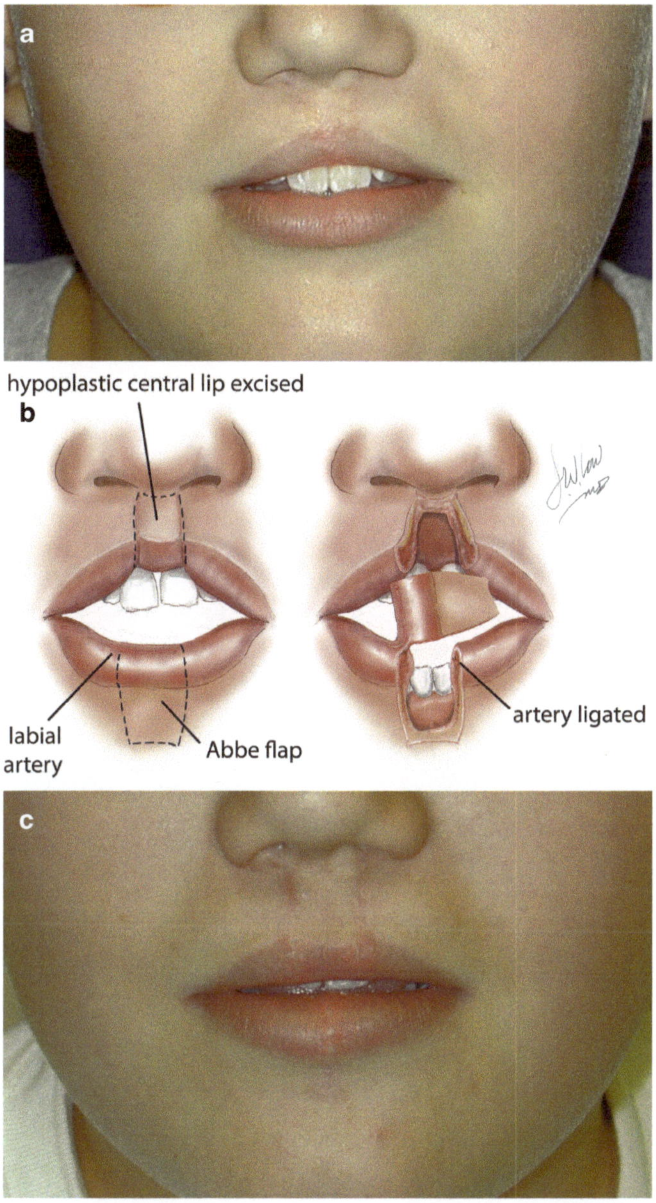


Fig. 15.18 (**a**) Example of bilateral cleft with residual short upper lip. An Abbe flap is a good solution for this problem. (**b**) Abbe flap design. (**c**) Final result after division and inset of Abbe flap

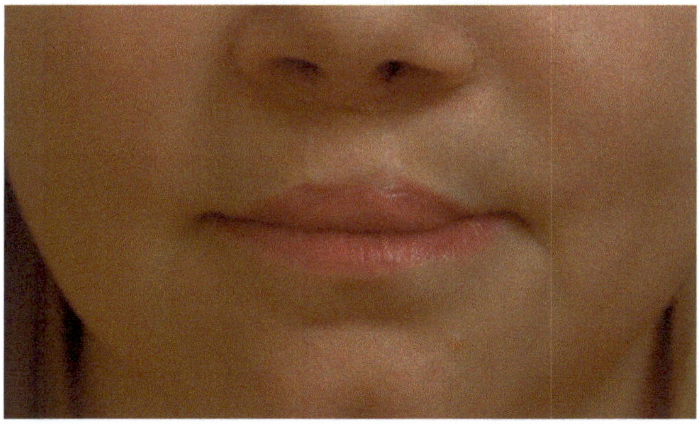

Fig. 15.19 Final result after vermillion switch and further scar revision

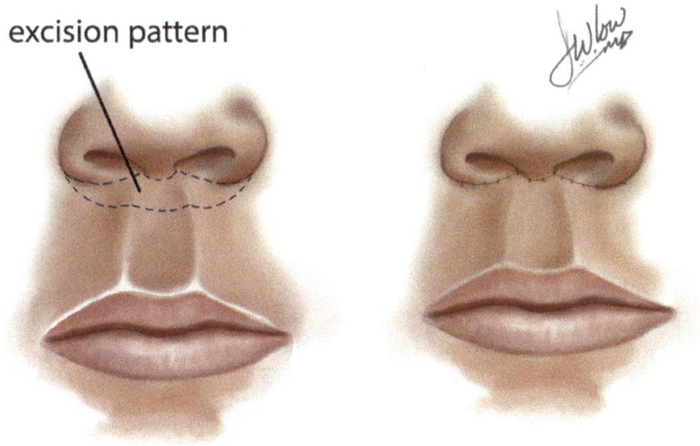


Fig. 15.20 Upper lip skin excision pattern to correct a long lip

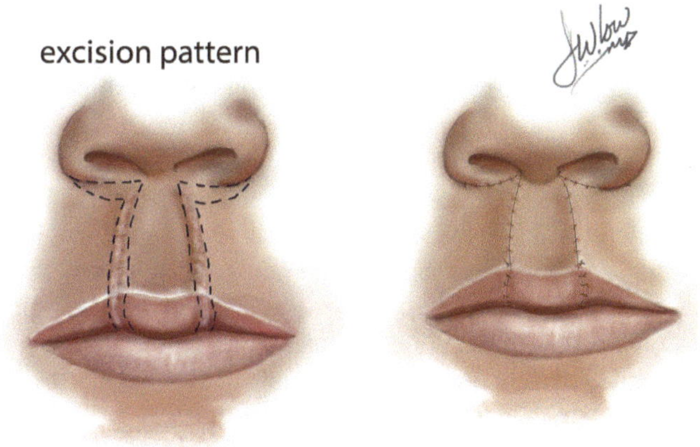


Fig. 15.21 Excision pattern to correct long lip as well as correction of widened scar and philtrum

## Cleft Lip Revision, Case 1

### Case Study: Whistle-Notch Cleft Lip Deformity with Unrepaired Nasal Deformity

Edwar Alvarez and David Alvarez

#### Case Analysis

This adult with bilateral cleft lip has undergone previous lip repair, and presents with a whistle-notch deformity of the lip, a shortened philtrum, a poorly defined cupid's bow, and a shortened columella with ptotic nasal tip.

Goals of care are to reconstruct his orbicularis oris muscle patency, lengthen and define his philtrum, and create columellar height with nasal tip projection.

#### Treatment Considerations

Planning cleft lip revision in conjunction with tip rhinoplasty enables columellar and philtral subunits to be improved without compromising the blood supply to the other.

In this case, elongation of the columella was performed with fork flaps, which also facilitated exposure for septorhinoplasty with use of septal cartilage for tip graft. The philtrum was left vascularized as an island on the orbicular oris muscle. After reconstructing the inferior orbicularis oris muscle continuity, correction of the whistle-notch deformity was performed utilizing the philtral island flap in Fleur-de-Lis fashion

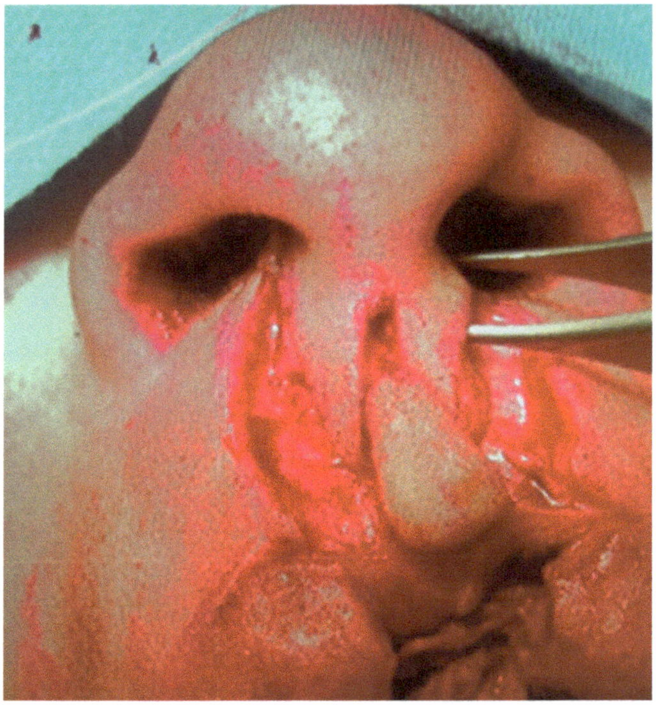

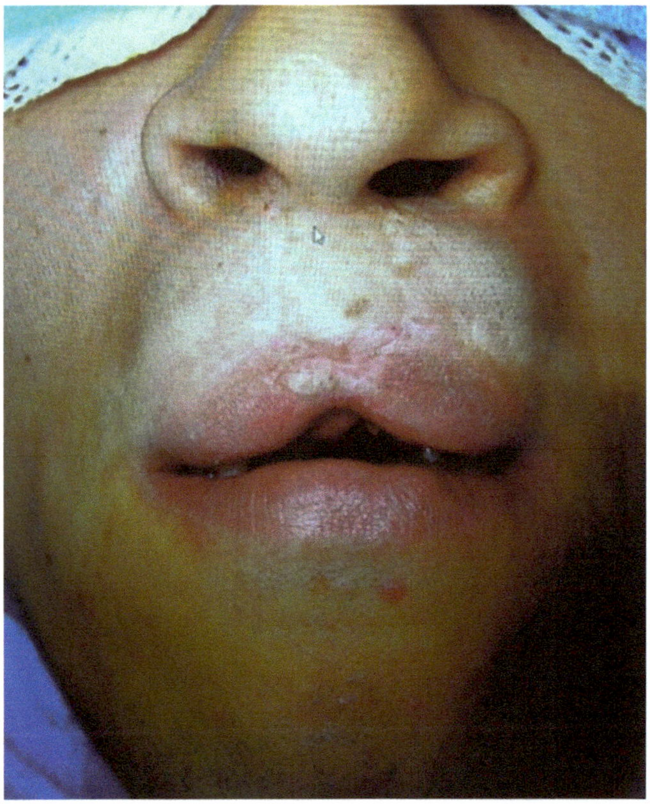

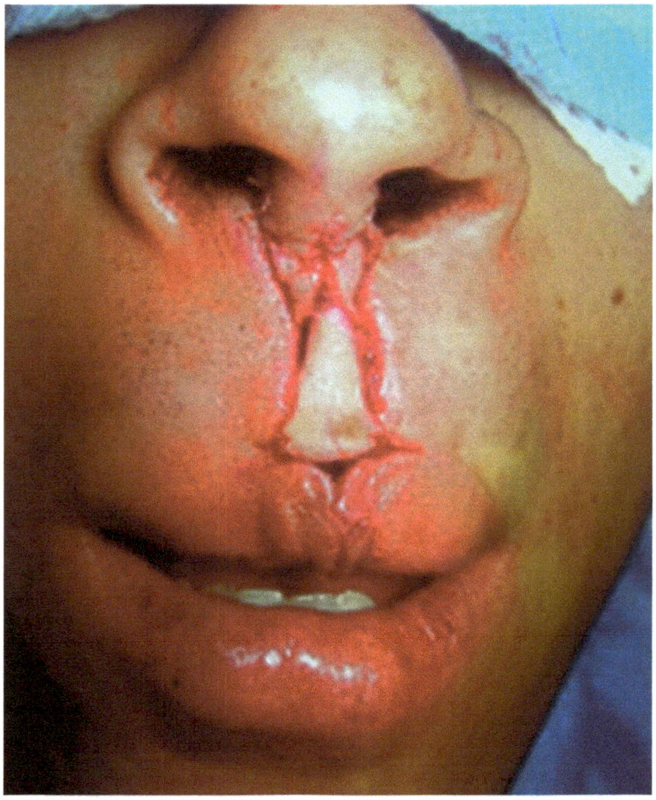

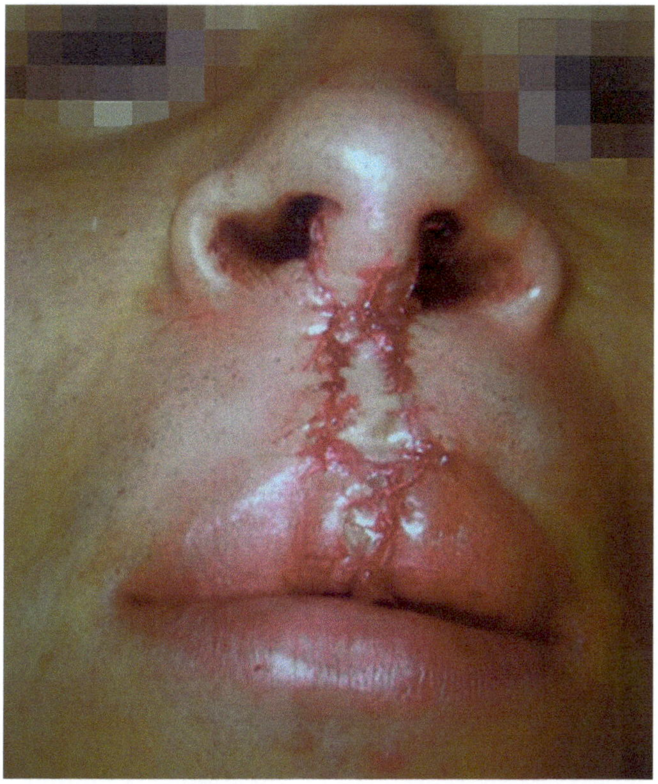

## Cleft Lip Revision, Case 2

### Case Study: Enlarged Philtrum

Edwar Alvarez and David Alvarez

#### Case Analysis

This 3-year-old boy with previously repaired bilateral cleft lip, likely of Manchester type technique, and presents with discontinuity of the orbicularis oris muscle, a widened and poorly-defined philtrum, and severe premaxillary exposure. Continued anterior projection of the premaxilla is frequently seen after primary repair when continuity of the orbicularis muscle is not established.

Goals of care are to reconstruct his orbicularis oris muscle patency, recreate the philtrum, and recreate the gingivobuccal sulcus.

#### Treatment Considerations

A straightforward lip revision can maintain a superiorly-based philtral flap, which is narrowed considerably. This provides anterior exposure to excise vestigial prolabial orbicularis oris muscle remnants and approximate viable orbicularis muscle from each side. The gingival mucosa can be divided in a "T" technique (see Case 22.2) to enable interposition of buccal mucosa, and recreation of a gingivomucal sulcus and frenum.

Premaxillary setback can also be considered, although this may have a negative impact on maxillary growth, particularly in a young child. If the orbicularis oris can be approximated primarily, this is likely to create a tether effect that drives the premaxilla into better apposition with the alveolar segments.

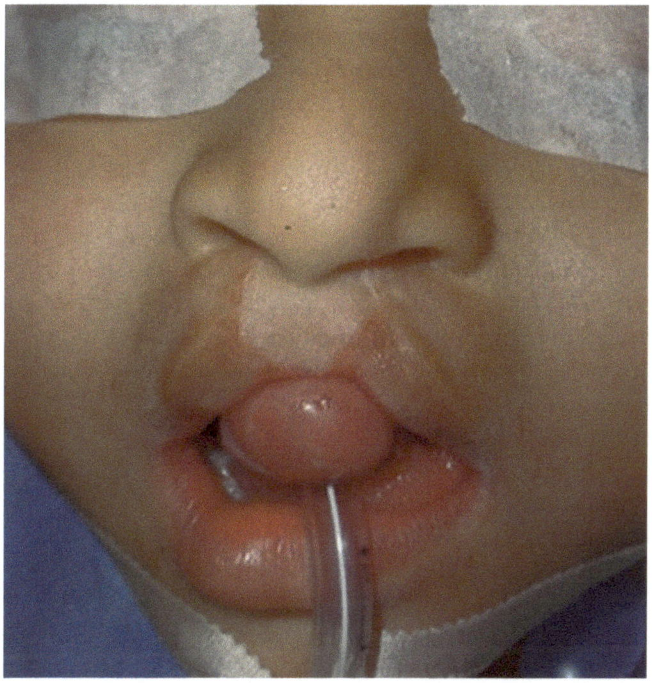

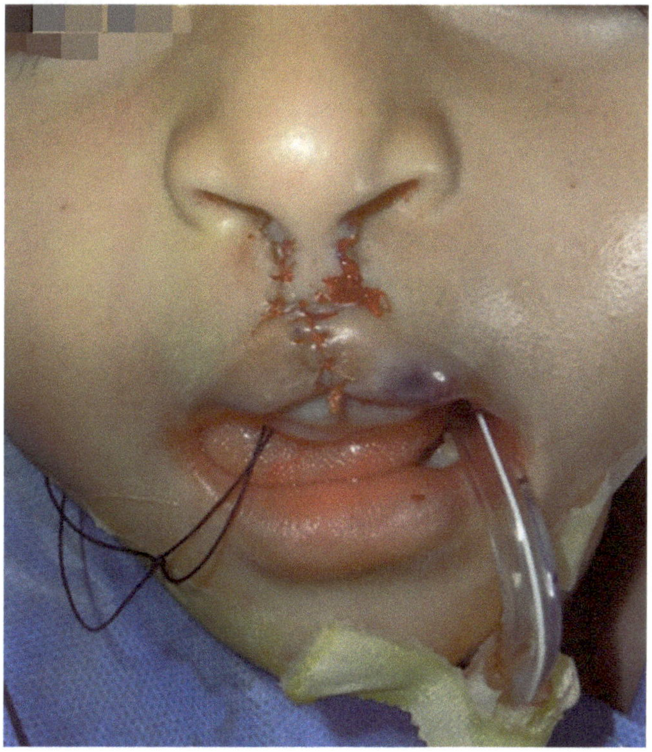

## Cleft Lip Revision, Case 3

### Case Study: Hypertrophic Cleft Lip Scar

Edwar Alvarez and David Alvarez

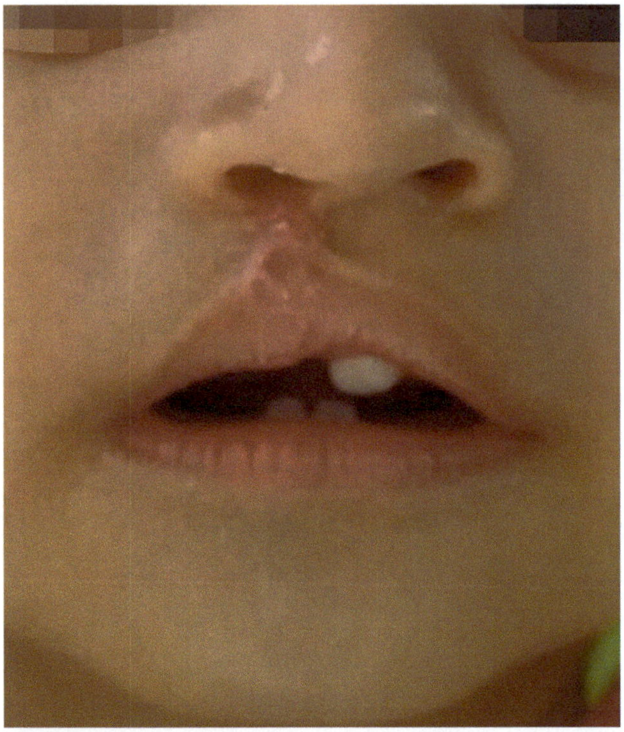

#### Case Analysis

This young boy with previously repaired right unilateral cleft lip presents with hypertrophic lip scar and severe lip retraction, with loss of anatomical lip elements.

Goals of care are to eliminate the scar hypertrophy, and restore balanced lip appearance.

Hypertrophic scarring is often graded by degree of thickness, pain, elevation of the skin surface, and darkened color. It can arise from excessive tension on the incision margins postoperatively, inflammation or infection, or genetic predisposition. Hypertrophic scar can be distinguished from keloid because the hypertrophy is contained within the margins of the incision or wound, rather than expanding beyond them. Hypertrophic scar can sometimes be prevented by scar massage following surgery.

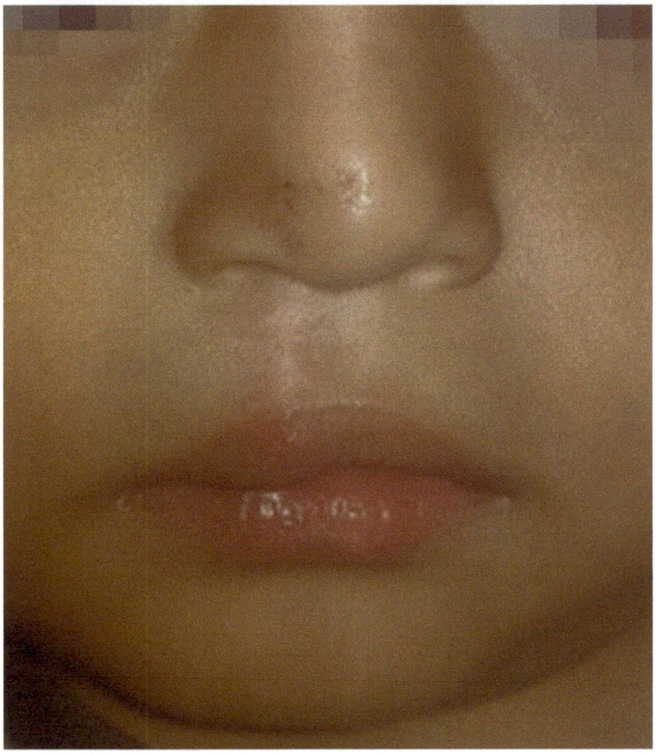

#### Treatment Considerations

Mild scar hypertrophy can often be treated by steroid injection. Kenalog 40 (40 mg per mL) is often diluted 50:50 with lidocaine, and administered intradermally using a 27 or 30 gauge needle. It stings for several moments, then subsides. It can be done in clinic, even with young children.

Given the severity of this hypertrophic scar, surgical resection of the hypertrophic scar tissue can be performed with reconstruction of Cupid's bow and neo-creation of adequate lip length using the Rose-Thompson technique.

## References


1. Stal S, Hollier L. Correction of secondary cleft lip deformities. Plast Reconstr Surg. 2002;109(5):1672–81; quiz 82.
2. Byrd HS. Correction of secondary unilateral cleft lip and nose deformity. In: Losee JE Kirschner, RE, editors. Comprehensive cleft care. 2. 2nd ed. Boca Raton: CRC Press; 2016. p. 1029–45.
3. Sadove AM, Eppley BL. Correction of secondary cleft lip and nasal deformities. Clin Plast Surg. 1993;20(4):793–801.
4. Salyer KE, Genecov ER, Genecov DG. Unilateral cleft lip-nose repair: a 33-year experience. J Craniofac Surg. 2003;14(4):549–58.
5. Noordhoff MS. Reconstruction of vermilion in unilateral and bilateral cleft lips. Plast Reconstr Surg. 1984;73(1):52–61.
6. Burt JD, Byrd HS. Cleft lip: unilateral primary deformities. Plast Reconstr Surg. 2000;105(3):1043–55; quiz 56–7.
7. Mulliken JB, Pensler JM, Kozakewich HP. The anatomy of Cupid's bow in normal and cleft lip. Plast Reconstr Surg. 1993;92(3):395–403; discussion 4.
8. Kawamoto HK Jr. Correction of major defects of the vermilion with a cross-lip vermilion flap. Plast Reconstr Surg. 1979;64(3):315–8.
9. Warner JP. Secondary deformities of the cleft lip and nose. In: Michael L, Bentz BSB, Zuker RM, editors. Principles and practice of pediatric plastic surgery. 1. 2nd ed. Boca Raton: CRC Press; 2017. p. 499–510.
10. Koshy JC, Ellsworth WA, Sharabi SE, Hatef DA, Hollier LH Jr, Stal S. Bilateral cleft lip revisions: the Abbe flap. Plast Reconstr Surg. 2010;126(1):221–7.

# Principles of Cleft Palate Repair

# 16

Percy Rossell-Perry

**Key Points**

- Cleft palate assessment characterizes the extent of deformity, which influences the strategy for repair, as well as cleft severity, which influences outcomes.
- There are several approaches to timing and staging of cleft palate repair: single-stage repair of the hard and soft palate, repair of the hard palate at time of lip repair followed by later soft palate repair, or repair of soft palate followed by delayed hard palate repair. The first is most common.
- Common options for hard palate repair include elevating two mucoperiosteal flaps, one mucoperiosteal flap, hybrid forms of palatoplasty, or single-layer closure with a vomer mucoperichondrial flap. The author describes his favored single-flap technique and rationale.
- Common options for soft palate repair include straight-line repair with intravelar veloplasty or double-opposing Z-plasty interposition technique.
- Unilateral uvuloplasty may also convey additional aesthetic and functional benefits based on the personal experience of the author.
- Palatal approach and technique should be oriented to maximizing key outcomes: good speech and auditory function, maxillary growth, and absence of fistula.

**Electronic Supplementary Material** The online version of this chapter (https://doi.org/10.1007/978-3-030-59105-2_16) contains supplementary material, which is available to authorized users.

P. Rossell-Perry (✉)
E. Rebagliati Martins Hospital ESSALUD Lima PERU, Lima, Peru

## Introduction

Cleft palate results from failure of mesenchymal penetration during embryologic development of the face and affects about one in every 700 children [1]. Multiple risk factors have been associated with this congenital disease and include genetic factors, maternal alcohol and tobacco abuse, certain medications, and infections during pregnancy. This palatal defect impairs speech, feeding, hearing, and oral hygiene, requiring early surgical correction. The cleft palate can involve only the secondary palate to varying degrees (described as incomplete cleft palate) or both the primary and secondary palates at one or both sides (described as unilateral or bilateral complete cleft palate). Although the focus of this review is on the specifics of surgical repair, the more individualized diagnosis and management of the cleft palate and prevention of complication are emphasized. A surgical protocol based on the proposed classification of severity and innovative surgical techniques is presented in this chapter, based on our 25-year experience in Peru caring for children with clefts in both an urban comprehensive cleft center and regular outreach programs.

## Anatomy

Congenital hypoplasia is defined as underdevelopment or incomplete development of a tissue or organ. This condition may affect the different components of the palate, mucosa, skeleton, muscles, and vessels, and has implications for the diagnosis, treatment, and prognosis of cleft palate. In complete unilateral cleft palate, the vomer is attached to the maxilla on the non-cleft side, stimulating the normal development of this segment. The cleft side (non-attached to the nasal septum) is hypoplasic in different degrees. Spriestersbach [2] proposed a theory (confirmed later by Maher) [3] about the association between aberrant craniofacial morphogenesis and commensurate aberrant blood supply. We agree that ele-

© Springer Nature Switzerland AG 2021

J. W. Swanson, D. W. Low (eds.), *Global Cleft Care in Low-Resource Settings*, https://doi.org/10.1007/978-3-030-59105-2_16

mental hypoplasia within the cleft palate may be associated with postoperative non-desirable outcomes such as velopharyngeal insufficiency, mucoperiosteal flap necrosis, and palatal fistulas.

Maher performed one of the few studies of vascular supply in a cleft palate [3]. He described variations in the palate arteries of cleft palate patients and observed arterial anastomoses between the greater palatine artery and the following arteries: infraorbital, superior alveolar, sphenopalatine branches from the maxillary artery, and superior labial branches from the facial artery in cleft and non-cleft palate fetuses (Figs. 16.1, 16.2, and 16.3) [3]. The main blood supply of the palate is provided by the greater palatine artery. This artery reaches the mucoperiosteum of the hard palate and runs anteriorly (continuing its pathway into an osseous groove until it reaches the retroincisive zone) in the lateral portion of the palate near its junction with the alveoli. Additional branches are provided by the descending palatine artery (lesser palatine arteries), ascending palatine (from the facial artery), tonsillar branch (branch of the ascending palatine artery), and ascending and recurrent pharyngeal arteries (both from the external carotid artery) [3]. There is a large network of anastomoses between the vessels that supply the hard palate and soft palate. One of the most important manifestations is the anastomoses between the ascending palatine branch and lesser palatine arteries (in variable number). We believe the key surgical implication of these vascular abnormalities is to minimize unnecessary incisions and dissection particularly around the more fragile hypoplasic elements of a cleft.

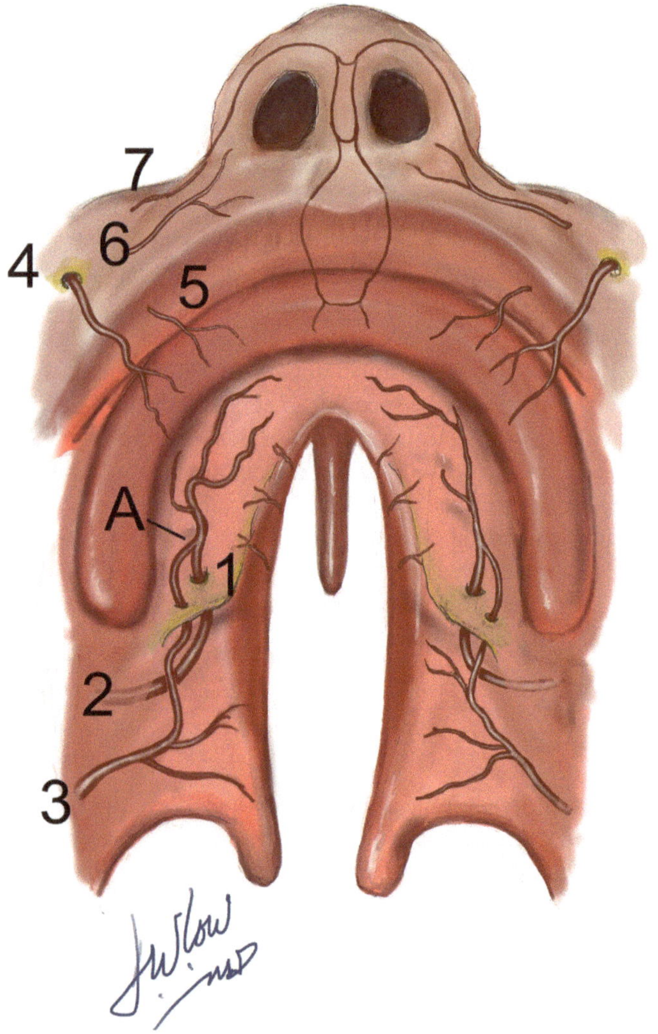


**Fig. 16.1** Incomplete cleft palate vascularization. 1. Greater palatine artery. 2. Descending palatine artery. 3. Ascending palatine artery. 4. Branches from infraorbital artery. 5. Superior alveolar artery. 6. Branches from superior labial artery. 7. Dorsal nasal artery. A. Vascular anastomosis between descending palatine artery and ascending palatine artery through lesser palatine vessels

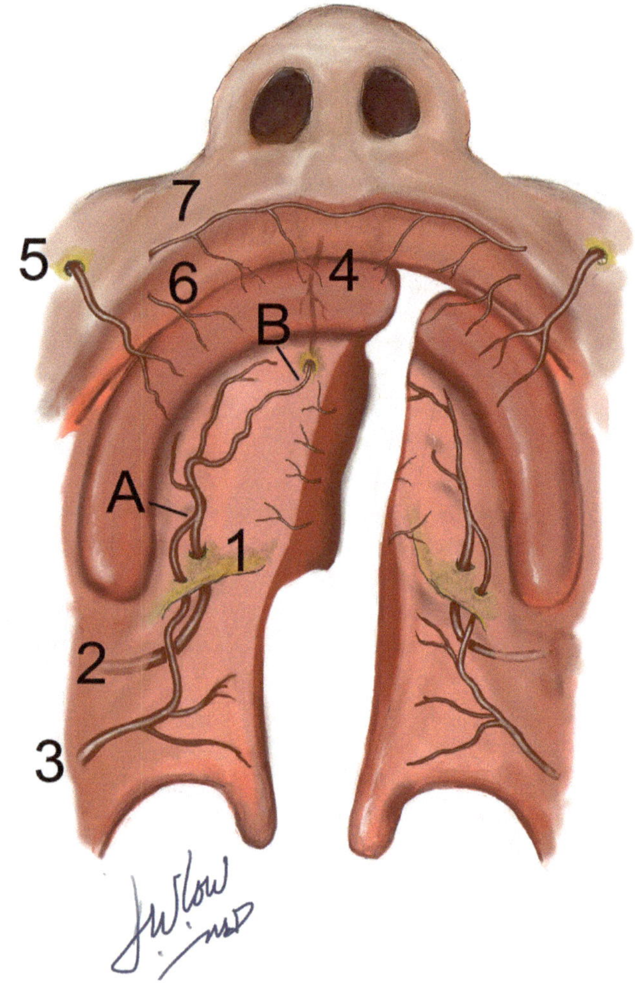


**Fig. 16.2** Unilateral cleft palate vascularization. 1. Greater palatine artery. 2. Descending palatine artery. 3. Ascending palatine artery. 4. Anterior palatine artery. 5. Branches from infraorbital artery. 6. Superior alveolar artery. 7. Branches from superior labial artery. A. Vascular anastomosis between descending palatine artery and ascending palatine artery through lesser palatine vessels. B. Vascular anastomoses between greater palatine artery and anterior palatine artery

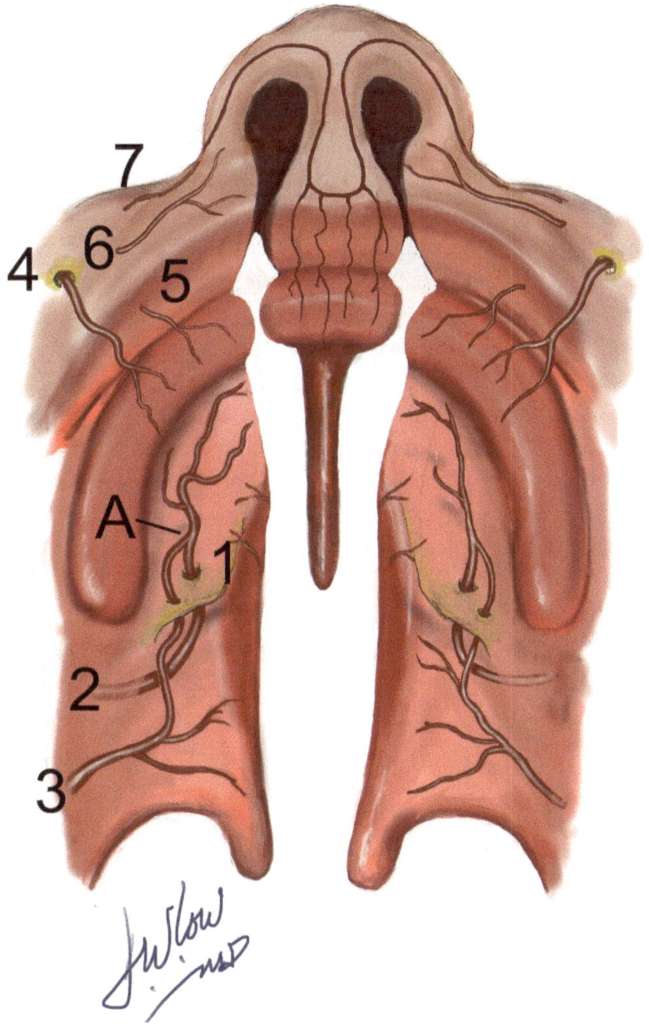


Fig. 16.3 Bilateral cleft palate vascularization. 1. Greater palatine artery. 2. Descending palatine artery. 3. Ascending palatine artery. 4. Branches from infraorbital artery. 5. Superior alveolar artery. 6. Branches from superior labial artery. 7. Dorsal nasal artery. A. Vascular anastomosis between descending palatine artery and ascending palatine artery through lesser palatine vessels

## Classification and Protocols

The Veau classification is commonly used to *categorize* palatal clefts into their four most common overt forms: (1) isolated soft palate only, (2) isolated hard and soft palate, (3) unilateral complete cleft lip and palate, and (4) bilateral complete cleft lip and palate – see Chap. 5.

The cleft palate index – a proportion between the cleft's width (tissue deficiency) and width of both palatal segments (amount of tissue available for cleft repair) – indicates the *severity* of the cleft. This distance is measured at the level of the junction of the hard and soft palates (Fig. 16.4) [4].

Based on these measurements, the index classifies three degrees of severity for the cleft palate:

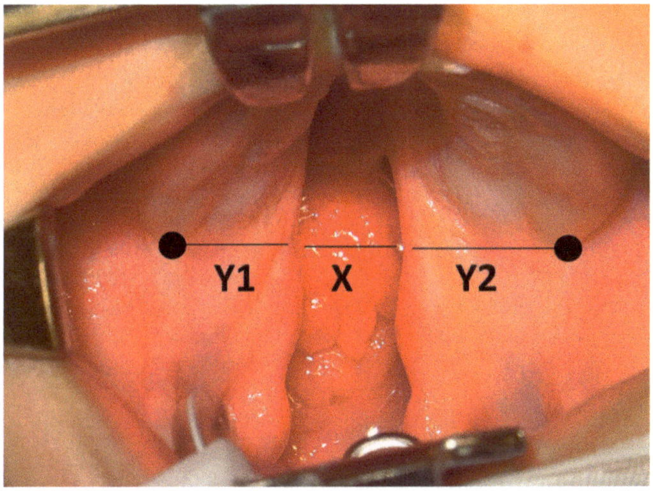


Fig. 16.4 The cleft palate index. This is estimated using the proportion between the cleft's width (X) and the sum of the width of the palatal segments (Y1 + Y2)

(a) Mild (cleft palate index less than 0.2)
(b) Moderate (cleft palate index of 0.2–0.4)
(c) Severe (cleft palate index more than 0.4)

Our surgical protocol (the Lima cleft palate repair protocol; see Reference 4) is based on this classification; each type has specific characteristics that should be considered for its surgical repair. Different studies have established the association between the severity of the cleft (based on cleft width and cleft palate index) and non-desirable outcomes after primary cleft palate repair [4]. The cleft palate surgical protocol proposed by the author is based on this protocol to prevent surgical complications as palatal fistulas and mucoperiosteal flap necrosis.

There are several approaches to timing and staging of cleft palate repair:

- Single-stage repair of the hard and soft palate. Typically performed at 9–12 months of age, with hard palate repair by mobilizing unilateral or bilateral mucoperiosteal flaps and soft palate repair by intravelar veloplasty (IVV) or double-opposing Z-plasty. Potential advantages of one-stage repair are the reduced rate of fistulas and better speech development.
- Repair of the hard palate at time of lip repair (typically 3–6 months) followed by later soft palate repair (9–12 months): "Oslo protocol" [5]. Potential advantages of early anterior palate repair narrowing the palatal cleft and reducing nasolabial fistulas.
- Repair of soft palate at time of lip repair (typically 3–6 months) followed by delayed hard palate repair (2–3 years): "Gothenburg protocol" [6]. Potential advantages of earlier palatal muscle reconstruction for speech and reduced dissection of hard palate until after more growth is attained.

**Table 16.1** Comparison of four surgical techniques used for primary unilateral cleft palate repair

| | Surgical techniques | | | |
|---|---|---|---|---|
| Parameters | Two flap | One flap | Delayed soft palate repair | Delayed hard palate repair |
| Subperiosteal dissection | Extended | Extended | Most extended[a] | Reduced[b] |
| Relaxing incisions | Bilateral | Unilateral | Required in severe forms | Not required[b] |
| Surgical stages | One | One | Two | Two |
| Rate of fistula | Low | Low | Increased | Increased |
| Velopharyngeal insufficiency | Similar | Similar | Increased[c] | Similar |
| Maxillary growth disturbance | Similar | Similar | Similar | Similar |

[a]Subperiosteal dissection is extended bilaterally during second stage and performed twice over the cleft side
[b]Outcome observed only when soft palate closure is performed before 6 months of age
[c]Some studies reported increased rate of velopharyngeal insufficiency using this protocol [27]

The delayed soft palate repair (Oslo protocol) and delayed hard palate repair (Malek) are used in different centers around the world [5, 6].

Table 16.1 describes the most common protocols and the accepted advantages and disadvantages of each. Different cleft teams continue to gather evidence and refine techniques on different protocols as we seek the best, most consistent outcomes.

## Preoperative Considerations

In our population, the preoperative analysis can be outlined in a "cleft palate's rule of ten" (10 kilos in height, 10 grams of hemoglobin per deciliter, and 10 months of life). This concept is supported practically and not by scientific evidence.

Presurgical evaluation is completed using the following tests:

- Pediatric evaluation (through preoperative history, physical examination, and health clearance) is necessary to determine the nutritional status and acute or chronic infections.
- Full blood count, PT (prothrombin time), and ASA grade estimation.
- Chest X-ray is indicated only if the patient's history or physical examination suggests pulmonary abnormalities.

All patients undergoing routine primary cleft palate repair should be of the American Society of Anesthesiologists (ASA) physical status class 1 or class 2. Syndromic patients (ASA 3 or 4) should receive individual management developed by the medical board with special considerations in psychosocial aspects and family interaction.

Nothing per oral (NPO) guidelines are very important to be fulfilled by the parents as follows: breast milk (4 hours) and solids (6 hours).

## Surgical Techniques for Hard Palate Repair

In complete clefts, surgeons can elect among a hard palatal technique and soft palatal technique; these techniques are unpaired.

Common hard palate repair techniques include:

- Bilateral monopedicled mucoperiosteal flaps – "Bardach repair." Has the advantage of being able to extensively mobilize tissue medially, such as for a wide cleft palates; disadvantage of extensive dissection, limited flap vascularization, and leaving raw surfaces to mucosalize (Chap. 17; Fig. 17.2).
- Unilateral monopedicled mucoperiosteal flap. Which is the author's preferred technique for unilateral cleft palate repair, described subsequently (Figs. 16.5, 16.6, and 16.7).

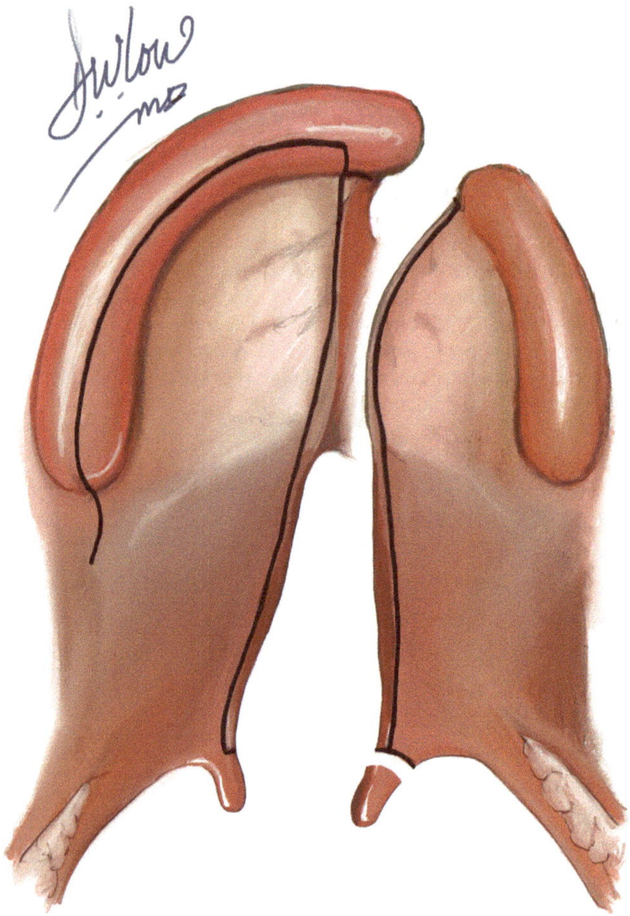

**Fig. 16.5** The one-flap technique for unilateral cleft palate repair. A. Surgical incisions

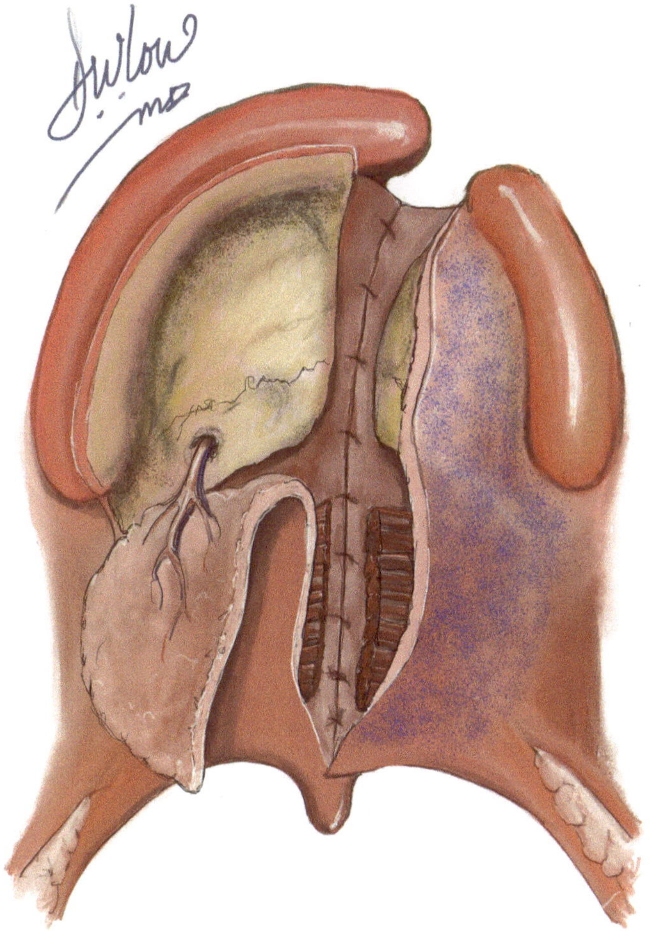


Fig. 16.6 The one-flap technique for unilateral cleft palate repair. B. One-flap elevation. Dotted area: Oral mucosa elevation at the cleft side

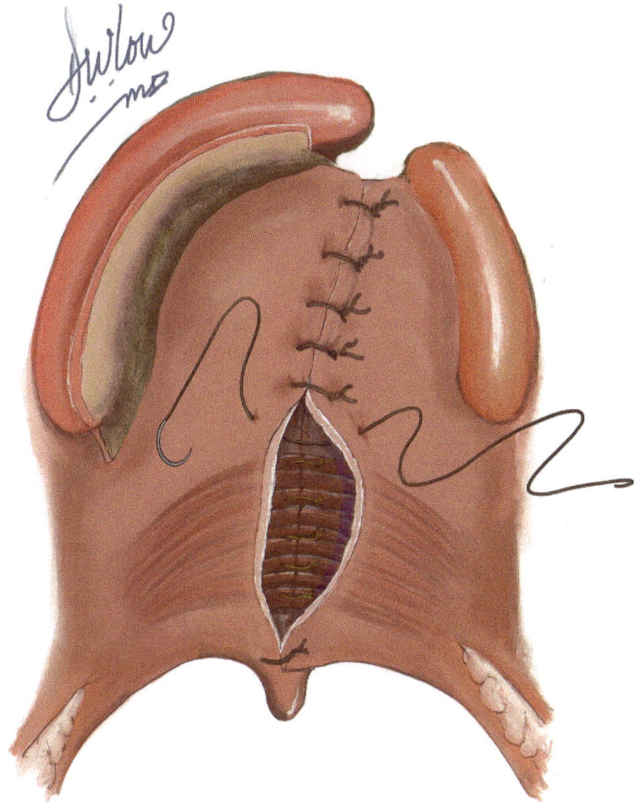


Fig. 16.7 The one-flap technique for unilateral cleft palate repair. C. Oral mucosa closure

- Bilateral RELAXING incisions – "Von Langenbeck repair." Advantage of maintaining perfusion to bipedicled mucoperiosteal flaps but limits degree of anterior medial transposition (Chap. 17; Fig. 17.3).
- Hybrid palatoplasties, as described by Gillet and Clarke combining extended and limited relaxing incisions [7].
- "Minimal incision" (no lateral relaxing incisions). Entire dissection done through incision at medial cleft margin. Avoids relaxing incisions but high risk of inadequate mobilization and fistula.
- Vomer flap. Closure of nasal mucosa with mucoperichondrial flap can be unilateral or bilateral. Can be done as a single-layer closure of hard palate at time of lip repair, oral surface allowed to mucosalize secondarily. It is described in detail in Chap. 17. Further study may be needed in low-resource settings, as variable results were noted in one center in India [8].
- The vomer flap can be done as the nasal layer closure at time of single stage palatoplasty, with use of one of the above techniques for oral mucosa.

## One-Flap Palatoplasty (Figs. 16.5, 16.6, and 16.7)

The method is indicated for unilateral cleft palates using healthy non-cleft tissues for cleft palate closure. This technique evolved from that described in 1996 by Gillett and Clarke [7], however with some major differences. Gillett uses the lesser segment for monopedicled flap, in order to minimize surface area dissection near the incisive foramen. Our technique places the monopedicled flap on the greater segment, in order to avoid devascularization of the hypoplasic lesser segment. Only a small relaxing incision rather than an extended release on the contralateral side is used for severe forms of unilateral cleft palate (cleft palate index more than 0.4). The quality of the greater palatine artery is more predictable to be safer in the greater segment of a unilateral cleft palate. A comparison study has been performed between one- and two-flap palatoplasty for unilateral cleft palate repair without surgical outcome differences [9].

### Surgical Technique

The Dingman mouth is applied with the patient in the supine position and neck extended. Local anesthesia plus a vasoconstrictor is infiltrated into the palatal tissues 5 minutes before

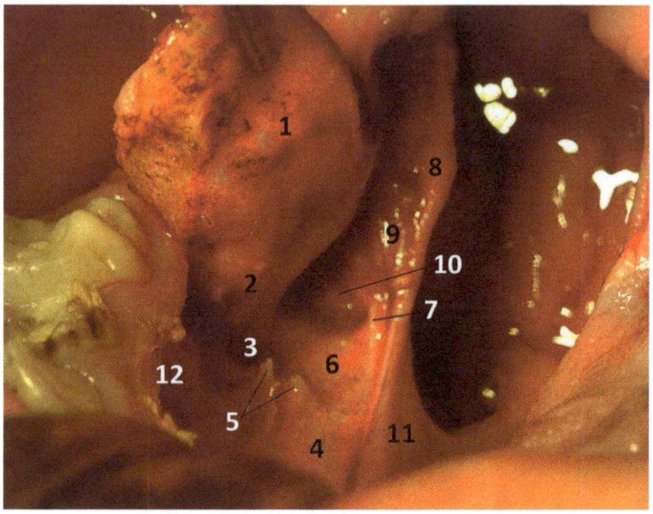


Fig. 16.8 Surgical anatomy of the greater palatine vessels. 1. Mucoperiosteal flap. 2. Greater palatine vessels. 3. Greater palatine foramen. 4. Palatine process of maxilla. 5. Palatal spines. 6. Horizontal plate of palatine bone. 7. Posterior nasal spine. 8. Nasal mucosa. 9. Palatoglossus muscle. 10. Palatine aponeurosis. 11. Vomer. 12. Relaxing incision

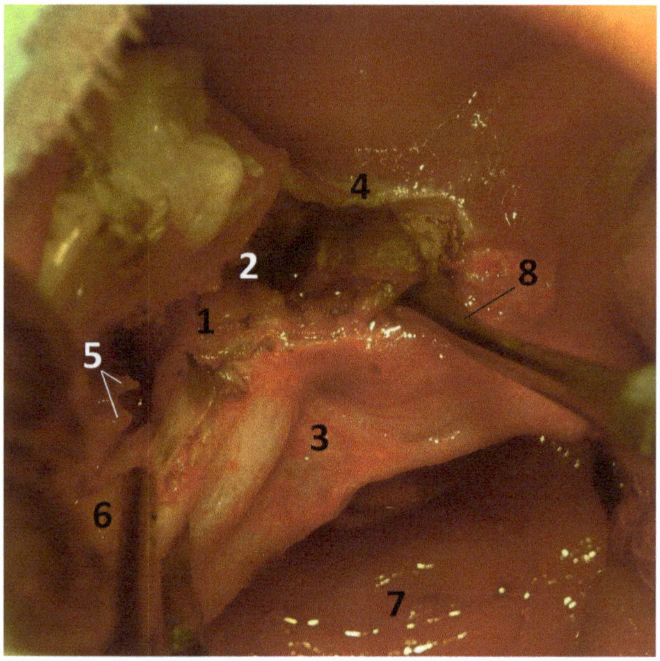


Fig. 16.9 Intraoperatory view of the greater palatine vessels before its surgical dissection at the non-cleft side. 1. Greater palatine vessels. 2. Greater palatine foramen. 3. Mucoperiosteal flap. 4. Relaxing incision. 5. Palatine spines. 6. Palatine process of maxilla. 7. Adenoids. 8. Surgical elevator

surgery. A lateral relaxing incision at the non-cleft side is performed using cautery.

This incision is placed along the edge of the palate just medial to the line of dental eruption and 1 centimeter extended over the soft palate to prevent any tension on midline closure at this level. Medial cleft incisions are performed using 15 blades from the alveolar cleft to the base of the uvula.

The greater segment mucoperiosteal flap is easily elevated and continued up to the greater palatine pedicle. Next, skeletonization of this vascular bundle is required using blunt dissection with firm but gentle traction to loosen it from the greater palatine foramen (Figs. 16.8, 16.9, 16.10 and Video 16.1). Surgery of the cleft palate is surgery of the greater palatine artery – this is a key point. Subperiosteal dissection without relaxing incisions is required of the lesser segment to facilitate midline closure (Fig. 16.11). A small relaxing incision is necessary on the side of the greater segment for severe unilateral cleft palates (cleft palate index more than 0.4). Closure of the cleft palate starts with the uvular repair and continues with nasal mucosa closure and muscle repair performed via non-radical intravelar veloplasty (Video 16.2).

At completion, the oral mucosa is carefully closed using an absorbable 5-0 suture for border-to-border edge approximation. This type of closure confirms to the surgeon that the tension of the closure is appropriate. Careful hemostasis should be performed, and Surgicel is placed over the lateral raw surface (Figs. 16.12, 16.13, and 16.14).

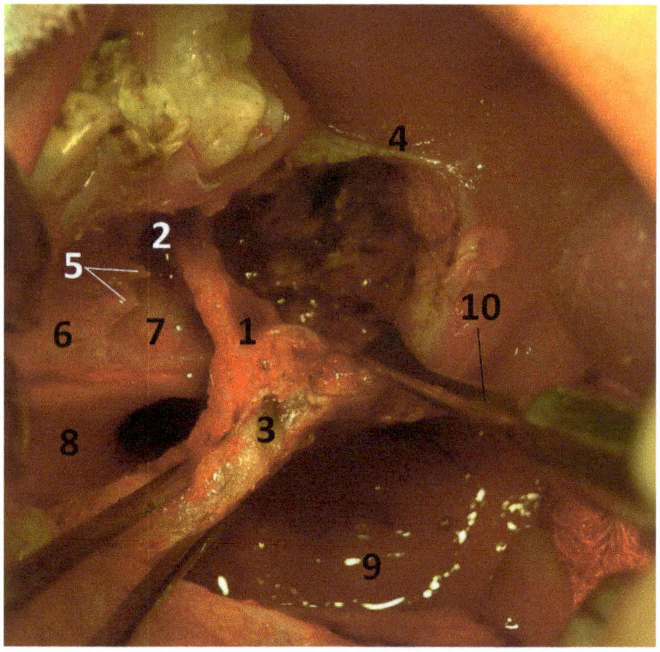


Fig. 16.10 Intraoperatory view of the greater palatine vessels after its surgical dissection at the non-cleft side. 1. Greater palatine vessels. 2. Greater palatine foramen. 3. Mucoperiosteal flap. 4. Relaxing incision. 5. Palatine spines. 6. Palatine process of maxilla. 7. Horizontal plate of palatine bone. 8. Vomer. 9. Adenoids. 10. Surgical elevator

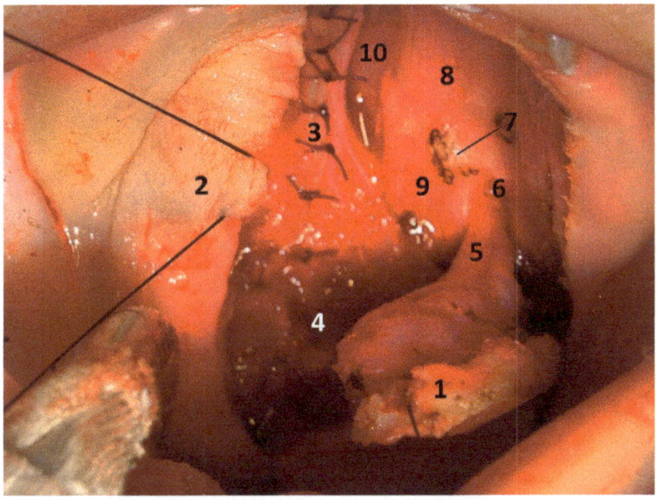


**Fig. 16.11** Subperiosteal dissection and mucoperiosteal flap elevation at the cleft (left in this photo) and non-cleft side (right in this photo). 1. Mucoperiosteal flap at the cleft side. 2. Mucoperiosteal flap at the non-cleft side. 3. Nasal mucosa repaired. 4. Muscular repair. 5. Greater palatine vessels. 6. Greater palatine foramen. 7. Palatine spines. 8. Palatine process of maxilla. 9. Horizontal plate of palatine bone. 10. Vomer

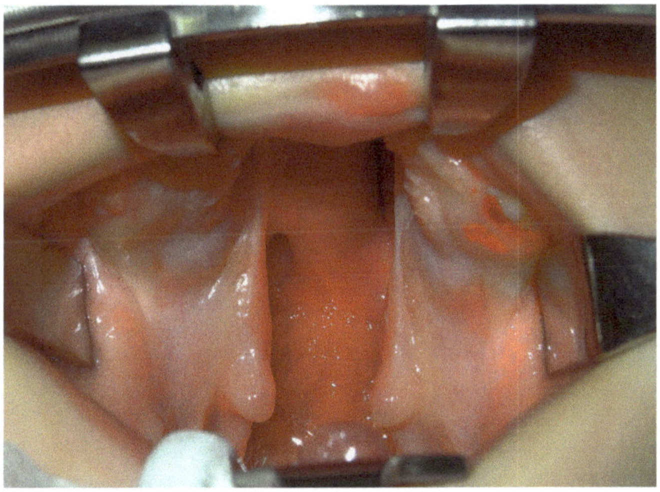

**Fig. 16.12** Preoperative view of severe unilateral cleft palate repair. (Cleft palate index: 0.45)

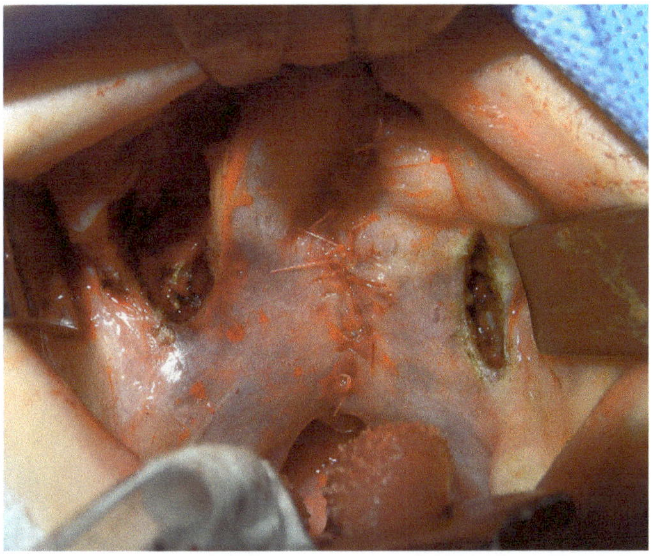

**Fig. 16.13** Immediate postoperative view of the repaired unilateral cleft palate using the one-flap plus relaxing incision (hybrid palatoplasty) technique

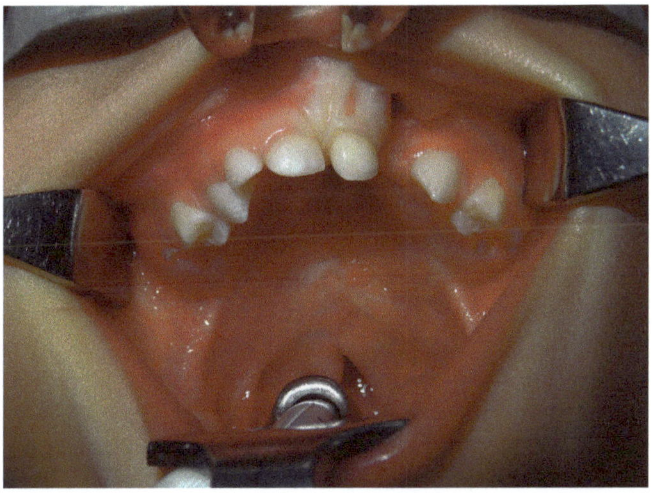

**Fig. 16.14** Postoperative view of the repaired unilateral cleft palate using the one-flap plus relaxing incision (hybrid palatoplasty) technique

Using a Foley catheter balloon is a simple method for hemostasis when bleeding cannot be completely controlled after surgery and is coming from the soft palate (Fig. 16.15) [10]. The device is gently advanced into the nostril until the catheter tip is visualized in the back of the throat. Next, the balloon is inflated with up to 10 milliliters of sterile water depending on the patient's age. This device is left in place for 12–24 hours and is then deflated; if the bleeding does not return, the catheter may be removed.

## Surgical Techniques for Soft Palate Repair

Muscle reconstruction of the levator sling is a key element of soft palate repair, and two predominant techniques are utilized:

- Radical intravelar veloplasty has been popularized by Brian Sommerlad and is used in many centers (described in Chap. 18).

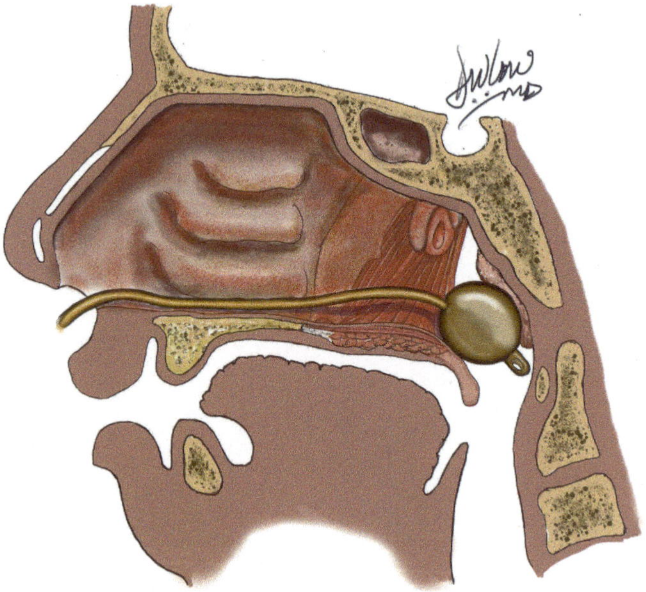

Fig. 16.15 Location of the balloon using the Foley method for the management of the bleeding during or after palatoplasty

- Double-opposing Z-plasty was first described by Leonard Furlow and is described in Chap. 19.

Several trials have sought to compare the two techniques, and each can demonstrate good outcomes. Concerns that the Furlow repair was associated with higher fistula rate may have been mitigated by Peter Randall, whose modified Furlow repair employs lateral releasing incisions.

The author employs a non-radical intravelar veloplasty in order to attain muscular reconstruction (Video 16.3).

Preservation of the tendon of the tensor veli palatini muscle may be associated with better middle ear function [11].

The submucous cleft palate is defined as an abnormal development of the palatal muscles with intact oral and nasal mucosa. The classic submucous cleft palate triad was described by Calnan in 1954. The diagnostic Calnan's triad of bifid uvula, translucent zone in soft palate, and bony notch in the posterior edge of the hard palate can be variable. Ultrasound imaging is indicated to identify occult forms of submucous cleft palate.

This condition may not be diagnosed until later age. Almost 50% of patients with this condition may remain asymptomatic into adulthood [12].

The surgical treatment is indicated only when velopharyngeal insufficiency, feeding problems, and unremitting ear disease have been demonstrated. Different studies have observed that Furlow palatoplasty can satisfactorily correct this type of cleft palate.

## Unilateral Uvuloplasty (Fig. 16.16 and Video 16.4)

Although little evidence exists to inform whether or how to best reconstruct the uvula, uvuloplasty has been suggested to both favorably decrease the velopharyngeal aperture and enlarge the posterior velum. Based on initial description of Carlos Navarro, the author developed a uvuloplasty technique that appears to show reduced nasality and improved palatal competency in a preliminary study [13]. The technique is based on the preservation of the larger hemi-uvula and excision of the other one. The uvular tissue excision should be extended laterally to the junction between the soft palate and top of the tonsillar pillars to prevent the lateralization of the repaired uvula (a common mistake observed using the original technique). The mobilization of the preserved uvula reduces the velopharyngeal space, improving its function. A mucosal incision at the preserved uvula side is made along the cleft margin and extended up to the base of this hemi-uvula. Next, the incision is turned 90 degrees for 1 centimeter and includes only oral mucosa, preserving the uvularis muscle. Nasal and oral mucosa are carefully repaired with absorbable 5-0 sutures, and unilimb Z-plasty is performed in which a triangle of mucosa from the excised side

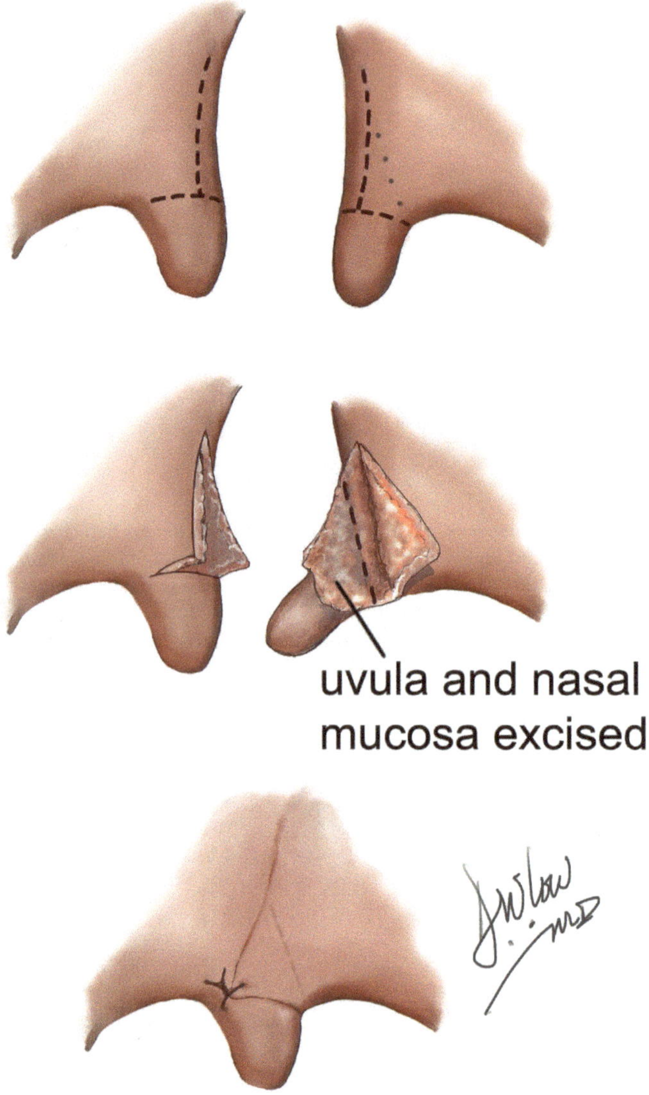


Fig. 16.16 Surgical technique for uvular repair in patients with cleft palate using the unilateral uvuloplasty. Preoperative view. Dotted line: Area of nasal mucosa excision

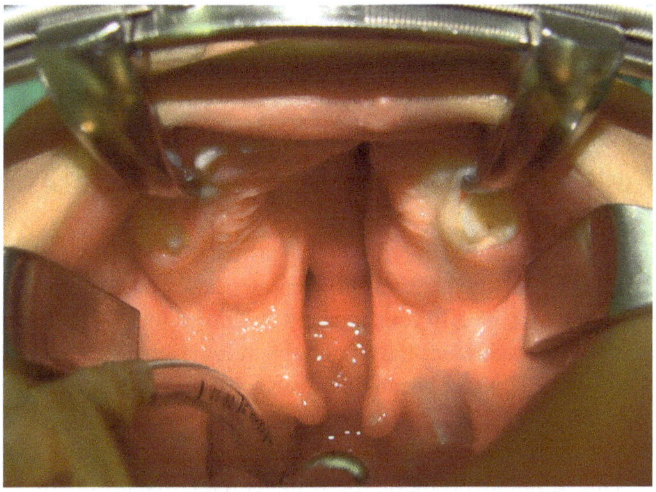

**Fig. 16.17** Preoperative view of unilateral cleft palate repair

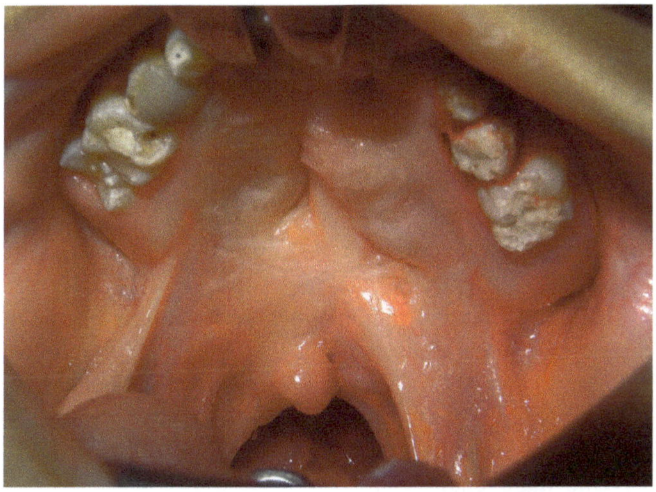

**Fig. 16.18** Postoperative view of the repaired uvula using the unilateral uvuloplasty after 4 years

is placed over the preserved uvula to provide additional length and prevent scar retraction of the repaired soft palate (Figs. 16.17 and 16.18). Velar function is thought to improve in this technique because of three mechanisms: (a) intravelar veloplasty muscle reposition, (b) velopharyngeal space reduction, and (c) lengthening of the soft palate using an unilimb Z-plasty.

## Postoperative Care

After surgery, the patient is observed at post-anesthetic care unit (PACU) until the patient is awake and oral feeding is assured. The start of liquid feeding is recommended 3 or 4 hours after anesthesia; the use of spoons during the first 24 hours is recommended, avoiding bottle feeding with nipples and syringes to prevent the risk of bleeding and aspiration.

Different preventive methods are usually recommended for postoperative care after cleft lip and palate repair. Some of these include tongue stitching, nasopharyngeal airway tube placement, and arm splint placement; we do not like to recommend these methods because of the absence of scientific support.

There is unclear scientific evidence concerning the use of antibiotic prophylaxis after cleft palate repair. Although their use is being reduced in high-resource settings, a recent randomized controlled trial from a low-resource setting in India suggested reduced fistula and complication rates with a 5-day postoperative prophylactic course of amoxicillin [14].

Fever is commonly observed during the first 24 hours after cleft palate repair; however, this procedure is rarely associated with infection, and fever typically resolves spontaneously.

The use of paracetamol in combination with a nerve block is usually sufficient to achieve adequate analgesia after surgery. The patient can be discharged the following day after demonstrating sufficient oral intake.

## Outcome Assessment

Available evidence suggests that palate repair outcomes are related to surgeon factors (quality of technique, volume of procedures regularly performed), patient factors (cleft severity, nutritional status), and surgery facility/environment. There is insufficient scientific data concerning the impact of a surgeon's skills on the cleft palate repair outcome. However, intuitively we consider this a most important factor. The main outcomes to be considered for assessment after cleft palate repair include palatal fistulas, speech, and maxillary growth.

### Palatal Fistulas

Recent meta-analysis have observed widely varying rates of palatal fistulas after primary cleft palate repair, from 2% up to 57% in surgical missions [15].

Reddy et al., in 2017 [16], concluded that due to the lack of high-quality studies, there is no conclusive evidence of a relationship between one- or two-stage palatoplasty and facial growth, speech, and fistula formation in patients with unilateral cleft lip and palate. However, a meta-analysis published by Stein et al. [17] observed less fistula development after primary cleft palate repair using the one-stage type of repair. An early single-stage, two-layer closure (oral and nasal mucosa) and the use of relaxing incisions may be associated with lower rates of postoperative fistulas [18].

## Speech

A well-repaired velopharyngeal mechanism is needed for proper speech development this being one of the primary goals of cleft palate repair. Surgical repositioning of the levator palatini muscle during palatoplasty creates a competent velopharyngeal sphincter [19, 20]. The surgical technique, type of cleft (Veau score), and age at the time of surgery seem to be the most important factors to consider in terms of adequate speech production.

Better functional outcomes have been reported using radical intravelar veloplasty and Furlow techniques.

Two randomized clinical trials compared the Furlow palatoplasty with the classical Von Langenbeck technique. Both of them observed significantly better velopharyngeal function for speech was obtained using Furlow technique [21, 22].

A meta-analysis observed less velopharyngeal insufficiency using one-stage repair than using two-stage repair [23].

Time of primary repair is considered as key point for proper speech development in these patients.

Sullivan et al. observed association between age at the time of surgery and the need for surgical management of velopharyngeal insufficiency [24].

This study concluded that early cleft palate repair reduces the development of compensatory misarticulations.

## Maxillary Growth

A systematic review published by Zhang et al. in 2017 [23] concluded that evidence regarding the optimal surgical technique and rate of maxillary hypoplasia is lacking with no gold-standard technique to date.

A similar study published by Reddy et al. in 2017 [16] observed no conclusive evidence of an association between the surgical protocol and facial growth.

A recent meta-analysis observed that one-stage repair is associated with less risk of fistula formation and velopharyngeal insufficiency than two-stage repair [17].

Another meta-analysis published by Bichara et al. [25] suggested that impaired maxillary sagittal growth appears to be consequence of lip repair rather than primary cleft palate surgical repair.

A multicenter clinical trial study (from Denmark, Finland, Norway, Sweden, and the United Kingdom) known as the SCANDCLEFT study included three clinical trials of primary surgery for unilateral cleft lip and palate that compared dental arch relationships at 8 years of age after using one and two stages [26]. The results did not provide any statistical evidence that one surgical technique for cleft palate repair was superior to the other.

The development of maxillary growth impairment seems to be multifactorial. Related factors include primary cheiloplasty, age, use of relaxing incisions, subperiosteal dissection of the palate, presence of raw bony surfaces, surgical technique, surgeon's performance, cleft type, and genetics.

## Author's Approach and Supporting Evidence

The proposed surgical protocol for primary cleft palate repair has been evaluated through different studies and published by the author in different indexed scientific journals. These are the observed outcomes: palatal fistulas (from 6.25% up to 8.6%) [4, 27], velopharyngeal insufficiency (from 3.10% up to 9.90%) [4, 27], and maxillary growth (2.8 using the Attack 5 year old's scale for dental arch relationship) [28].

Our surgical protocol for primary cleft palate repair is based on the proposed classification of severity. The main concepts are as follows:

(a) Non-use of presurgical orthopedics

The lack of scientific evidence and associated complications using presurgical orthopedics are the main reasons why these treatments were not typically used except for severe bilateral cleft lip and palate cases [29, 30].

(b) Early surgical correction (9–12 months old)

Different scientific publications have supported that the early correction of nonsyndromic cleft palate repair (around 9–12 months old) is associated with better functional outcomes, particularly speech [24, 31]:

(c) One-stage repair

One versus two stages for primary cleft palate repair is still under intense scientific debate. A recent systematic review and meta-analysis did not find differences between these two protocols in relation to facial growth. In addition, this study concluded that the one-stage protocol is associated with a lower risk of fistula formation and velopharyngeal insufficiency than the two-stage protocol [15]. Other systematic reviews and meta-analysis concluded that more well-designed studies are necessary to establish differences between the protocols [17, 23].

(d) More individualized selection of the surgical technique. Based on the used surgical protocol, a more individualized surgical treatment is proposed by the author, as follows:

*Incomplete cleft palate:* Furlow technique and Von Langenbeck technique for severe clefts. *Unilateral cleft palate:* One-flap palatoplasty. A small relaxing incision at the cleft side is necessary only for severe clefts. *Bilateral cleft palate:* Von Langenbeck technique. A hybrid palatoplasty would be used for severe clefts.

A similar individualized protocol has been proposed later by Tse et al. [32] with major differences for unilateral and bilateral cleft palate repair. Their protocol uses unipedicled flaps at the cleft side for unilateral and bilateral cleft palates without any consideration about the severity of the cleft.

(e) Preservation of the blood supply for the mucoperiosteal flaps of the cleft side. The cleft side tissues are congenital hypoplasic tissues and should receive a different treatment than the non-hypoplasic side. The blood supply may be better preserved with bipedicled rather than unipedicled flaps at the cleft side. Severe complications such as mucoperiosteal flap necrosis seem to be observed in more hypoplasic clefts (bilateral, incomplete) probably because of the use of unipedicled flaps [33–35].
(f) Unilateral uvuloplasty

For a long time, we have used the conventional technique for uvular repair without good aesthetic and functional outcomes. It is very difficult to repair the uvula using a straight-line closure because of the higher rate of retraction. The new technique we describe using one hemi-uvula for uvular repair allowed us to obtain better cosmetic and functional outcomes [13].

The proposed surgical protocol for primary cleft palate repair is presented in Table 16.2 [36].

The author does not consider significant differences about primary cleft palate repair outcomes between countries with low- and high-resource settings. Observed differences are not related with the country income, these are more associated with the used model of surgical care. Different studies are supporting this hypothesis. Increased rate of complications has been observed in association with surgical mission model [37, 38]. Primary cleft palate repair is not a "high tech" treatment, and quality of surgical outcomes is associated mostly to surgeon's performance and volume of procedures regularly performed over a period of time. Low- and middle-income country cleft palate treatment is characterized by a large number of patients operated by single surgeon, predominance of surgical missions as model of surgical care, and the lower number of follow-up patients.

**Table 16.2** The Lima Surgical Protocol for primary cleft palate repair

| |
|---|
| *Incomplete cleft palate* |
| *Veau I*: Furlow technique |
| *Veau II: Mild,* Furlow technique |
| *Moderate:* Hybrid technique |
| *Severe:* Von Langenbeck technique |
| *Unilateral cleft palate* |
| *Mild:* Hybrid technique |
| *Moderate:* One-flap technique |
| *Severe:* One-flap technique plus relaxing incision at the cleft side |
| *Bilateral cleft palate* |
| *Mild:* Hybrid technique |
| *Moderate:* Von Langenbeck technique |
| *Severe*[a]: *Before 6 months old:* Delayed hard palate closure (uranorraphy at 1 year). *After 6 months old:* Hybrid palatoplasty, one-flap technique combined with relaxing incision |

[a]The strategy in this type is to transform the severe form in a moderate or mild form. The soft palate closure may change the width of the cleft if this is repaired before 6 months. Then the hard palate can be closed using Von Langenbeck technique at 1-year-old. If the soft palate closure is done after 6 months, the width of the cleft is not changed, and a hybrid palatoplasty is required to close the cleft without palatal fistulas

## Conclusion

Cleft palate management involves multiple disciplines and a course that lasts from birth to adulthood. Careful and individualized analysis of each cleft palate type based on its severity allows the selection of appropriate treatment. The usefulness of the proposed classification and surgical protocol may require additional studies to better illustrate its impact on cleft palate management. Professional training and expertise and team management performed in a reference center model represent the key points to guarantee optimal surgical outcomes.

## References


1. Global registry and database on craniofacial anomalies: report of a WHO Registry Meeting on Craniofacial Anomalies: Baurú, Brazil, 4–6 December 2001/main editors, Mossey P, Castilla E.
2. Spriestersbach D, Dickson D, Fraser F, et al. Clinical research in cleft lip and cleft palate: the state of the art. Cleft Palate J. 1973;10:113–65.
3. Maher W. Distribution of palatal and other arteries in cleft and non-cleft human palates. Cleft Palate J. 1977;14(1):1–12.
4. Rossell-Perry P, Caceres Nano E, Gavino-Gutierrez A. Association between palatal index and cleft palate repair outcomes in patients with complete unilateral cleft lip and palate. JAMA Facial Plast Surg. 2014;16:206–10.
5. Abyholm F, Borchgrevin H, Eskeland G. Cleft lip and palate in Norway. III. Surgical treatment of CLP patients in Oslo 1954–75. Scand J Plast Reconstr Surg. 1981;15:15–28.
6. Malek R, Psaume J. New concept of the chronology and surgical technique on the treatment of cleft lip and palate. Results in 220 cases. Ann Chir Plast Esthet. 1983;28:237–47.
7. Gillett DA, Clarke HM. The hybrid palatoplasty: a preliminary report. Can J Plast Surg. 1996;4:157–60.
8. Deshpande G, Wendby L, Jagtap R, Schonmeyr B. The efficacy of vomer flap for closure of hard palate during primary lip repair. J Plast Reconstr Aesthet Surg. 2015;68(7):940–5.
9. Rossell-Perry P, Cotrina-Rabanal O, Caceres-Nano E. One flap palatoplasty: a cohort study to evaluate a technique for unilateral cleft palate repair. Plast Reconstr Surg Glob J. 2015;3(4):e373.
10. Rossell-Perry P, Schneider WJ, Gavino-Gutierrez AM. A comparative study to evaluate a simple method for the management

of postoperative bleeding following palatoplasty. Arch Plast Surg. 2013;40(3):263–6.
11. Flores R, Jones B, Bernstein J, Karnell M, et al. Tensor veli palatini preservation, transection and transection with tensor tenopexy during cleft palate repair and its effects on Eustachian tube function. Plast Reconstr Surg. 2010;125(1):282–9.
12. Mc Williams B. Submucous clefts of the palate: how likely are they to be symptomatic? Cleft Palate Craniofac J. 1991;28(3):247–51.
13. Rossell-Perry P, Navarro-Gasparetto C, Caceres-Nano E, et al. A prospective, randomized, double-blind clinical trial study to evaluate a method for uvular repair during primary palatoplasty. J Plast Surg Hand Surg. 2014;48:132–5.
14. Aznar M, Schnmeyr B, Echaniz G, Nebeker L, Wendby L, Campbell A. Role of postoperative antimicrobials in cleft palate surgery. Prospective double blind randomized placebo controlled clinical study in India. Plast Reconstr Surg. 2015;136(1):59e–66e.
15. Bykowski M, Naran S, Winger D, Losee J. The rate of oronasal fistula following primary cleft palate surgery: a meta-analysis. Cleft Palate Craniofac J. 2015;52(4):e81–7.
16. Reddy R, Gosla Reddy S, Vaidhyanathan A, Berge S, et al. Maxillofacial growth and speech outcome after one-stage or two-stage palatoplasty in unilateral cleft lip and palate. A systematic review. J Craniomaxillofac Surg. 2017;45(6):995–1003.
17. Stein M, Zhang Z, Fell M, Mercer N, Malic C. Determining postoperative outcomes after cleft palate repair: a systematic review and meta-analysis. J Plast Reconstr Surg. 2019;72(1):85–91.
18. Salyer K, Sng K, Sperry E. Two flap palatoplasty: 20 year experience and evolution of surgical technique. Plast Reconstr Surg J. 2006;118(1):193–204.
19. Sommerlad BC. A technique for cleft palate repair. Plast Reconstr Surg. 2003;112:1542–8.
20. Andrades P, Espinosa-de-los-Monteros A, Shell DH IV, et al. The importance of radical intravelar veloplasty during two-flap palatoplasty. Plast Reconstr Surg. 2008;122:1121–30.
21. Wiliams W, Seagle M, Pegoraro-Krook M, Souaza T, et al. Prospective clinical trial comparing outcome measures between Furlow and Von Langenbeck palatoplasties for UCLP. Ann Plast Surg. 2011;66(2):154–63.
22. Spauwen P, Goorhuis-Brouwer S, Schutte H. Cleft palate repair: furlow versus Von Langenbeck. J Craniomaxillofac Surg. 1992;20(1):18–20.
23. Zhang Z, Stein M, Mercer N, Malic C. Postoperative outcomes after cleft palate repair in syndromic and non-syndromic children: a systematic review protocol. Syst Rev. 2017;6(1):52.
24. Sullivan SR, Marrinan EM, LaBrie RA, Rogers GF, Mulliken JB. Palatoplasty outcomes in nonsyndromic patients with cleft palate: a 29-year assessment of one surgeon's experience. J Craniofac Surg. 2009;20(Suppl 1):612–6.
25. Bichara L, Araujo R, Flores-Mir C, Normando D. Impact of primary palatoplasty on the maxillomandibular sagittal relationship in patients with unilateral cleft lip and palate: a systematic review and meta-analysis. J Oral Maxillofac Surg. 2015;44(1):50–6.
26. Heliovaara A, Skaare P. Kuseler A. Shaw W. et al. Scandcleft randomized trials of primary surgery for unilateral cleft lip and palate. Dental arch relationships in 8 year-olds. Eur J Orthod. 2019. Epub ahead of print. https://doi.org/10.1093/ejo/cjz067.
27. Rossell-Perry P. Two methods of cleft palate repair in patients with complete unilateral cleft lip and palate. J Craniofac Surg. 2018;29(6):1473–9.
28. Rossell-Perry P, Cotrina-Rabanal O, Figallo-Hudtwalcker O, Gonzalez-Vereau A. Effect of relaxing incisions on the maxillary growth after primary unilateral cleft palate repair in mild to moderate cases: a randomized clinical trial. Plast Reconstr Surg Glob. 2017;5(1):e1201.
29. Hamid Reza H, Eleftherios K, Athanasios A. Treatment outcomes of presurgical infant orthopedics in patients with non-syndromic cleft lip and/or palate: a systematic review and meta-analysis of randomized controlled trials. PLoS One. 2017;12(7):e0181768.
30. Papadopoulos M, Koumpridou E, Vakalis M. Effectiveness of presurgical infant orthopedics treatment for cleft lip and palate patients: a systematic review and meta-analysis. Orthod Craniofac Res. 2012;15(4):207–36.
31. Rohrich R, Love E, Byrd H, Steve M. Optimal timing of cleft palate closure. Plas Recons Surg J. 2000;106(2):413–21.
32. Tse R, Siebold B. Cleft palate repair: description of an approach, its evolution and analysis of postoperative fistulas. Plast Reconstr Surg. 2018;141(5):1201–14.
33. Rossell-Perry P, Cotrina-Rabanal O, Barrenechea-Tarazona L, Vargas-Chanduvi R, Paredes-Aponte L, Romero-Narvaez C. Mucoperiosteal flap necrosis after primary palatoplasty in patients with cleft palate. Arch Plast Surg. 2017;44(3):217–22.
34. Rossell-Perry P, Figallo-Hudtwalcker O, Vargas-Chanduvi R, Calderon-Ayvar Y, Romero-Narvaez C. Risk factors leading to mucoperiosteal flap necrosis after primary palatoplasty in patients with cleft palate. J Plast Surg Hand Surg. 2017;51(5):348–51.
35. Rossell-Perry P. Flap necrosis after palatoplasty in patients with cleft palate. Biomed Res Int. 2015;2015:516375. https://doi.org/10.1155/2015/516375.
36. Rossell-Perry P, Luque-Tipula M. The Lima Surgical Protocol for Cleft Palate Repair. J Craniofac Surg. 2020;31(6):1533–8.
37. Maine R, Hoffman W, Palacios-Martinez J, Corlew D, Gregory G. Comparison of fistula rates after palatoplasty for international and local surgeons on surgical missions in Ecuador with rates at a craniofacial center in the United States. Plast Reconstr Surg. 2012;129(2):319e–26e.
38. Rossell-Perry P, Segura E, Salas-Bustinza L, Cotrina-Rabanal O. Comparison of two models of surgical care for patients with cleft lip and palate in resource-challenged settings. World J Surg. 2015;39(1):47–53.

# 17 Cleft Palate Repair: Early Anterior Palatal Closure and Intravelar Veloplasty Techniques

Brian C. Sommerlad

**Key Points**

- Primary palate repair is the most important event in the management of a child with a cleft of lip and palate or isolated cleft palate. A less than satisfactory primary lip repair can often be improved by revision. A poor palate repair sometimes cannot be.
- Management of the hard palate can be separated from the management of the soft palate but each is related and affects outcome. The technique used for management of the hard palate primarily affects maxillary growth and the management of the soft palate primarily affects speech. However, the technique used for hard palate closure will influence the soft palate repair.
- In clefts involving lip and palate, the author carries out a single-layered closure of the hard palate with vomerine flap at the same time as performing lip repair. This greatly facilitates the subsequent soft palate repair.
- All cleft palates have abnormal anterior insertion of muscles – the palatopharyngeus into the back of the hard palate and the levator to the cleft margins more anteriorly than the normal insertion. Repair involves separating muscles from oral and nasal mucosa, and retropositioning and reconstructing them more posteriorly in the soft palate.
- The technique of palate repair is important not only for speech but also for hearing and maxillary growth (and therefore appearance).

B. C. Sommerlad (✉)
Great Ormond Street Hospital for Children, London, UK
e-mail: BSommerlad@Sommerlad.co.uk

## Introduction

Cleft palate repair is the single most important event in the management of a patient with cleft lip and palate or isolated cleft palate. This is even more important in low-resource countries, where patients may never return after initial surgery. It is also technically demanding.

The technique used in low-resource countries needs to be safe and to have outcomes which are as reliable as possible.

In patients with unilateral clefts of lip and palate, single layer vomerine flap closure of the hard palate at the time of lip repair [1] makes the lip operation a little more time-consuming and demanding but greatly facilitates the palate repair. The advantages of the vomerine flap are:

- Less destructive subsequent repair of the soft palate, with reduced need for further surgery on the hard palate.
- Reduced incidence of postoperative hard palate fistulae.
- More effective closure of the alveolar cleft.

Disadvantages include:

- The possibility of postoperative bleeding (reduced by the use of intravenous tranexamic acid 10 mg per Kg at the time of the lip repair).
- Possible effect on maxillary growth. However, to date, follow-up of the author's patients up to the age of 15 has not shown a deleterious effect on growth.

Simultaneous bilateral vomerine flaps in bilateral clefts may compromise the blood supply to the premaxilla. For that reason, the author usually prefers a complete vomerine flap on one side (usually the wider) and an incomplete vomerine flap (posterior to the pre-vomerine suture) on the other side. An attempt is made to close the remaining defect at the time of palate repair but if this is not possible, at the time of alveolar bone grafting.

© Springer Nature Switzerland AG 2021

J. W. Swanson, D. W. Low (eds.), *Global Cleft Care in Low-Resource Settings*, https://doi.org/10.1007/978-3-030-59105-2_17

Fig. 17.1 The incisions for a 3-flap VWK pushback

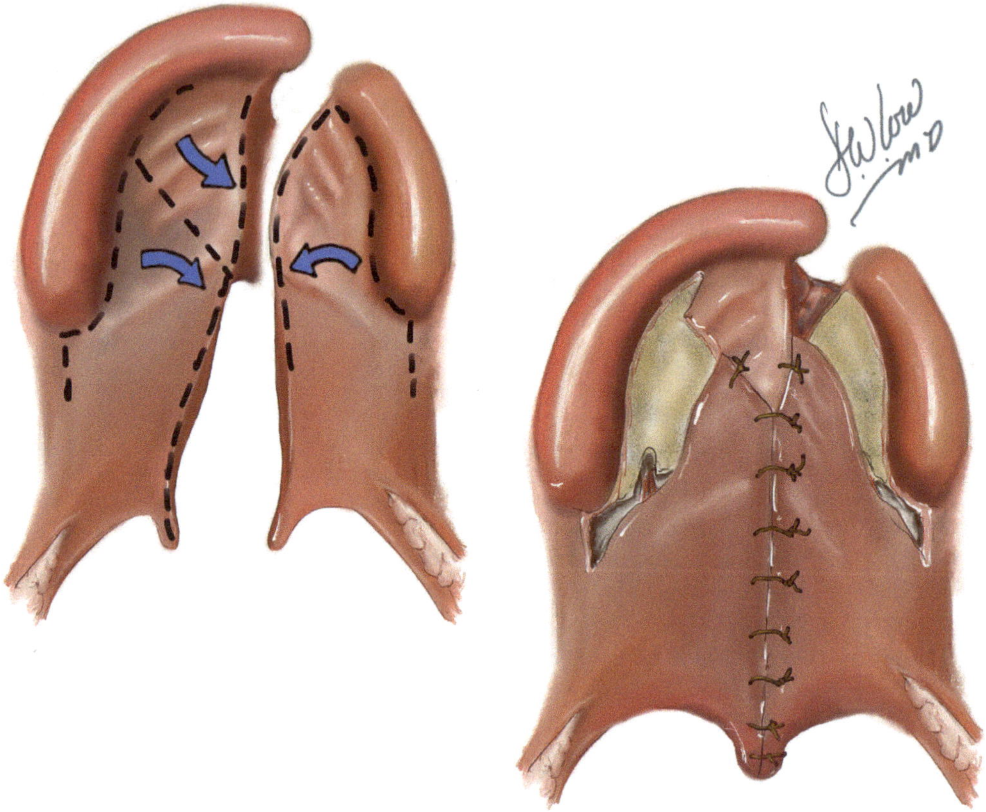

The 3- or 4-flap Veau-Wardill-Kilner (Fig. 17.1) pushback procedure [2–4]:

- Has not been shown to produce effective lengthening with improved speech.
- Produces maxillary arch collapse.
- Almost certainly impairs forward maxillary growth.
- Frequently results in fistulae at the junction of the flaps, which can be very difficult to repair.
- This technique has been used commonly in low-resource countries and has resulted in many disadvantaged patients.

The two-flap (Bardach) (Fig. 17.2) repair is less damaging but, in the author's view, the anterior incisions are unnecessary.

After single-layer vomerine flap closure at lip repair, many palates can be repaired without any hard palate mucoperiosteal incisions (approximately 90% in the author's experience) [5]. If necessary, lateral releasing incisions (von Langenbeck) [6, 7] (Fig. 17.3) can be used.

The author repairs the soft palate with radical retropositioning and reconstruction of the soft palate musculature. If at all possible, this is done with the operating microscope. In many low-resource countries, it is possible to have access to an operating microscope which is suitable for palate repair. There is the potential to do great harm in radical muscle dissection. There is a long learning curve and correct visualisation and equipment is essential. It is better to do no muscle repair than a repair which results in devascularisation and/or denervation of the palate muscles. At least this leaves the option for further surgery in the future. Radical muscle repair is not appropriate for occasional operators or those without appropriate training and skill.

## Timing

In patients with *unilateral clefts of lip and palate and bilateral clefts where the premaxilla is not prominent*, the author personally prefers to repair lip and anterior palate at 3 months and the remainder of the palate at 6 months. There is good evidence that repair of the soft palate before the age of 12 months optimises speech outcomes. A current trial (the TOPS trial) is looking at a comparison between repair at 6 and 12 months.

In patients with *bilateral clefts and a very prominent premaxilla*, the author carries out a two-stage lip repair but still aims to complete primary surgery in two operations.

- *First operation at the age of 3 months – extended lip adhesion*
- This involves radical lateral subperiosteal dissection for mobilisation, linking the muscle through the prolabium with long sutures but not carrying out muscle dissection,

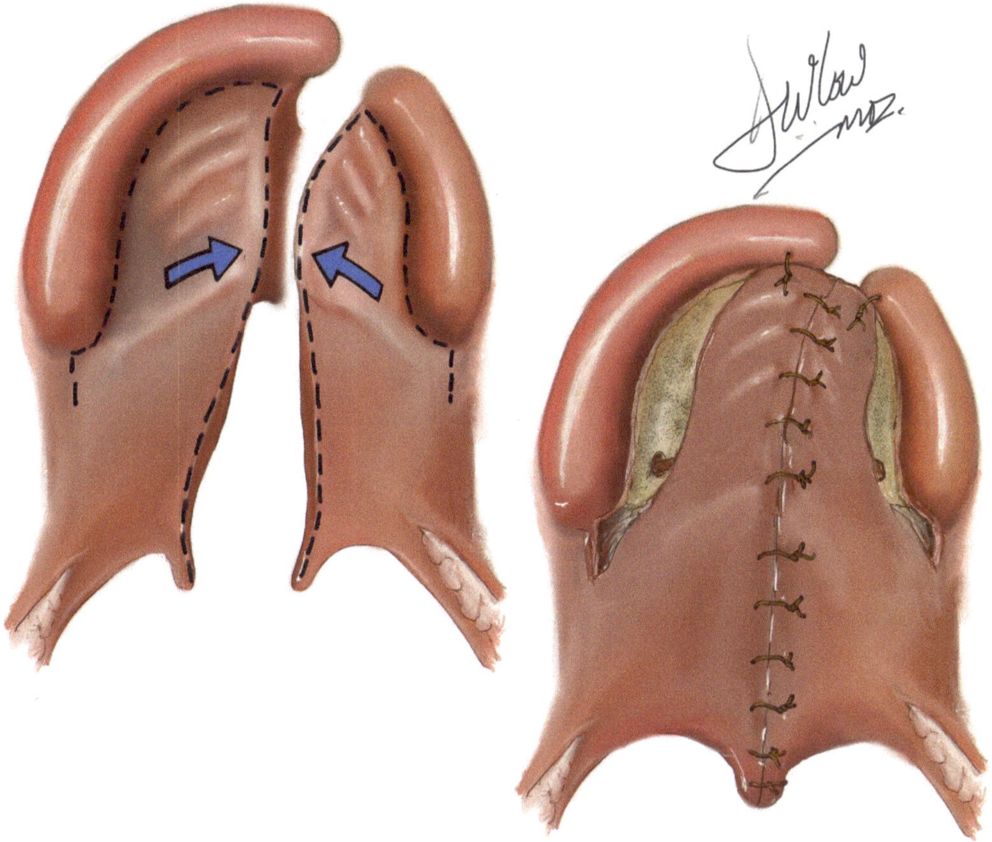

Fig. 17.2 The incisions for a 2-flap Bardach repair

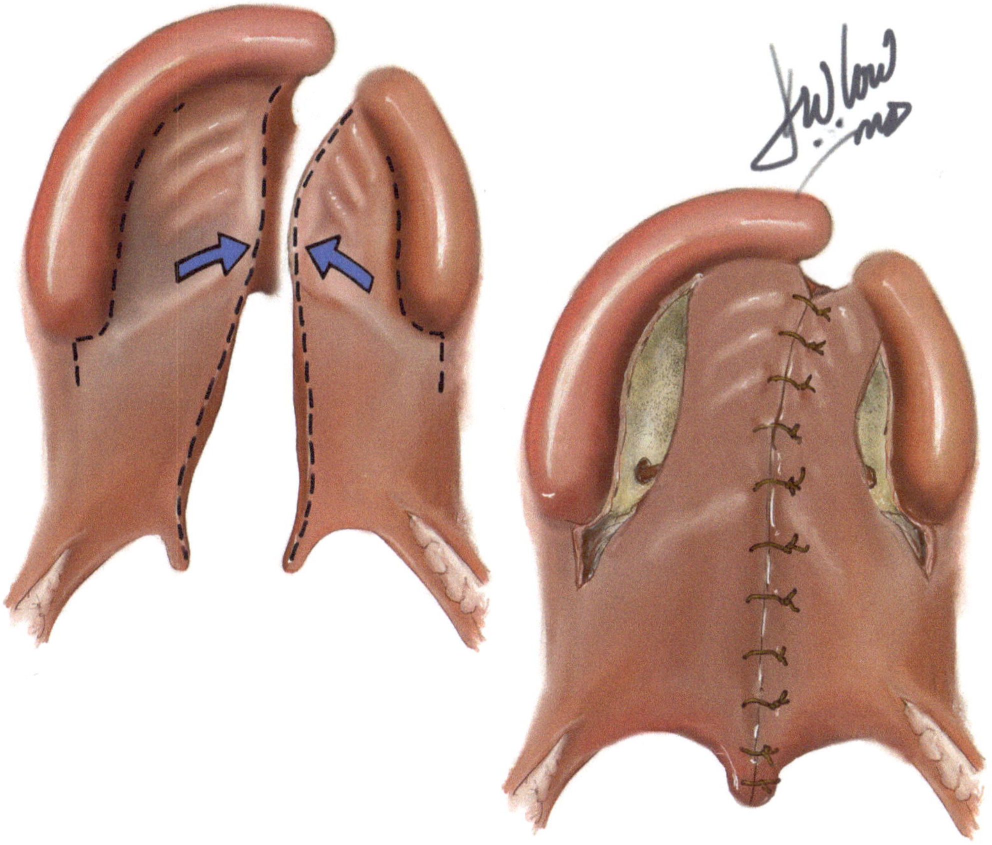

Fig. 17.3 The incisions for the traditional von Langenbeck repair. The extensions behind the alveolus are not necessary

not narrowing the prolabium or carrying out nasal dissection. Complete vomerine flap is performed on one side and an incomplete on the other.

- *Second operation at the age of 9 months – the remainder of the repair is carried out*
- Soft palate repair is performed. The lip is reopened, the vomerine flap on the incomplete side completed, the prolabium narrowed, the lip muscles dissected and united and closed nasal dissection performed. This is a particularly useful protocol in low-resource countries, where presurgical orthopaedics may not be available.
- This protocol therefore involves two stages – closure of lip and anterior palate, followed by closure of soft palate.

In patients with *isolated clefts of the palate,* the author usually carries out the repair at the age of 6 months but extends this until up to 12 months in Robin sequence babies with potential airway compromise.

Alternative protocols favoured by other surgeons for repair of *clefts of lip and palate* are:

- Closure of lip and soft palate followed by closure of hard palate (delayed hard palate closure). This is mainly done by surgeons who believe it improves maxillary growth. The evidence for this is not strong.
- Closure of palate, followed by closure of lip. This is carried out by some surgeons in low-resource countries, on the basis that if the lip is repaired patients may not come back for repair of the palate. This is a good argument.
- Closure of lip followed by closure of hard and soft palate. This is still probably the most common protocol throughout the world and was the author's until 1993 when he began using the vomerine flap at lip repair.

## Preparation

### Presurgical Orthopaedics/NAM

The author and colleagues have been involved in a randomised controlled trial of the use of an active form of presurgical orthopaedics versus none and at 10 years have shown no benefits of PSO in terms of appearance, maxillary growth or speech. It has now been abandoned by our team.

The jury is still out on the long-term benefits of nasoalveolar moulding (NAM). However, it is not available in most low-resource settings.

### Patient Selection

Many patients in low- and middle-income countries may be under-nourished, anaemic and suffering from conditions such as malaria. Patient assessment, in collaboration with a skilled paediatric anaesthetist, is therefore critical. The traditional "rule of tens" – 10 weeks, 10 lb (4.5 kg), haemoglobin 10 g/dl – is still a good guide but it may be necessary to operate on patients who are less than optimal.

It is important to recognise syndromic patients, particularly where the syndrome may be associated with cardiac, respiratory or endocrine conditions.

### Instruments and Equipment

All cleft surgery should ideally be carried out with appropriate magnification and illumination. As stated above, the author uses an operating microscope for palate repair whenever available [8] and encourages other surgeons to do so if at all possible. The requirements for a microscope are:

- Focal length variable or 250–300 mm
- Adjustable angle of binoculars
- Easy adjustment of position
- Sideways rotation
- Side arm for assistant
- Side arm for video (if for demonstration)

If an operating microscope is not available, the author uses 3.5 × 40 cm focal length loupes with headlight if necessary. Power failure is common in many less developed countries and a headlight can be invaluable.

Appropriate instruments, of which sharp scalpel blades are the most important, are essential (Fig. 17.4).

The essential instruments are:

- A mouth gag which facilitates exposure but minimises obstruction [9] (Fig. 17.5)
- An easily rotatable scalpel handle
- Ideally, a scalpel handle to which can be fitted angled blades

Sharp dissectors are important and knife rather than scissor dissection is to be encouraged.

Arguably more important than the surgical instruments are the anaesthetic and monitoring equipment – to be used by an experienced and skilled paediatric anaesthetist.

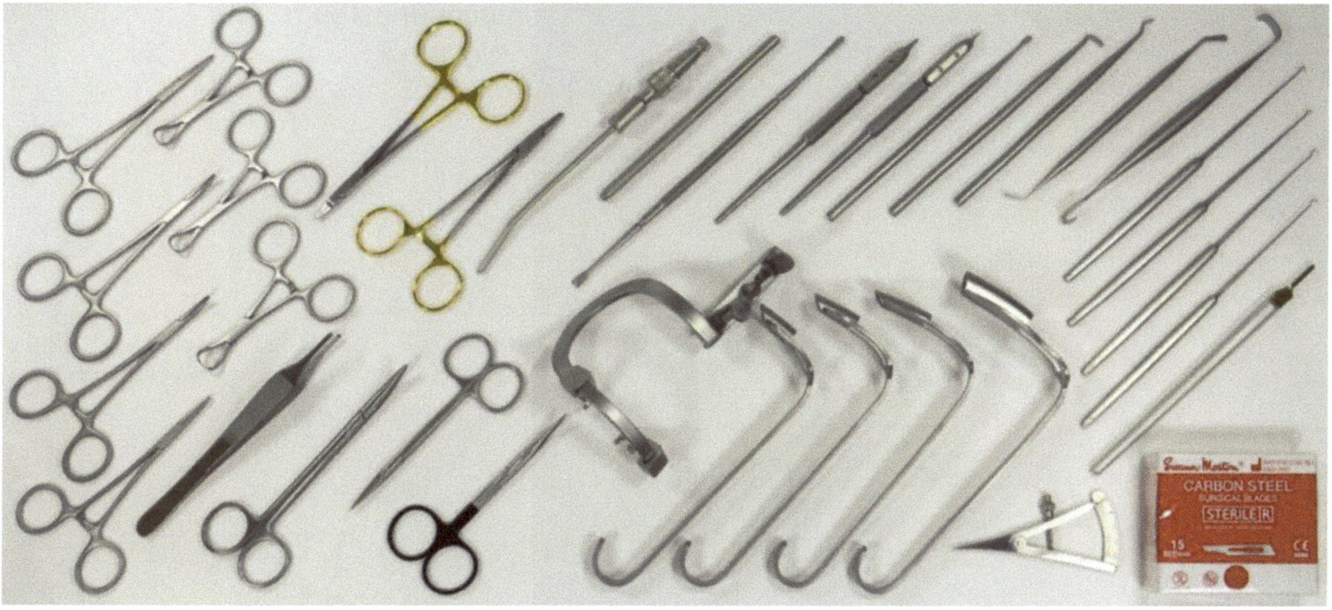


**Fig. 17.4** A cleft instrument set. (Courtesy of S. Murray and Co, Surgical Instrument Makers – www.smurray.co.uk)

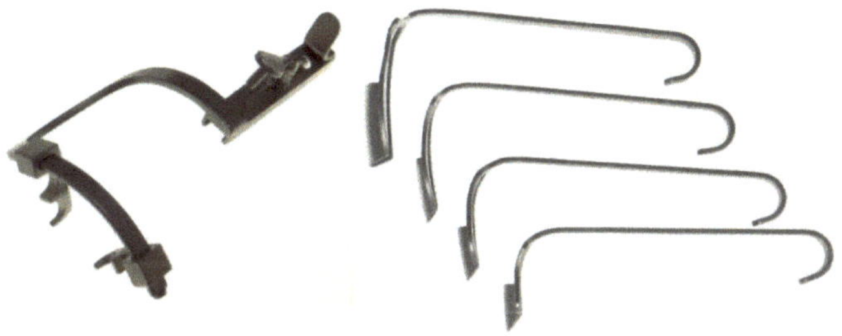

**Fig. 17.5** A modified mouth gag suitable for use with an operating microscope. (Courtesy of S. Murray and Co, Surgical Instrument Makers – www.smurray.co.uk)

## Surgical Techniques

### First Stage – Lip and Vomerine Closure of the Hard Palate

#### Unilateral Cleft Lip and Palate (UCLP)

Local anaesthetic with adrenalin is infiltrated into the vomerine mucosa (as well as the lip). Tranexamic acid, 10 mg/kg IV, is given routinely.

At the time of the lip repair, the medial incision in the lip extends back along the side of the premaxilla, caudal to the groove between vomer and premaxilla (Fig. 17.6) to reach the hard palate and is then extended at the junction of the palatal and vomerine mucosa to the point where the vomer is no longer connected to the palate (Fig. 17.7). The incision then continues at the inferior margin of this component of the vomer to the skull base and sometimes a releasing incision is made at the junction of vomer and adenoid tissue.

It is important that the incision on the side of the premaxilla is inferior to (oral to) the groove which exists between the premaxilla and the vomer (Fig. 17.6). Making the incision in this line is anatomically accurate but the dissection is more difficult. Prior infiltration and hydro-dissection of the vomerine mucoperiosteum, especially in the region of this groove, facilitates dissection. Elevation of the mucoperiosteum begins anteriorly over the premaxilla to reach the groove and then begins in the hard palate with the dissection reaching forward to the groove and, with care, the mucoperiosteum can be elevated out of the groove without perforation.

The vomerine flap usually hinges at the angle where the almost horizontal part of the vomer meets the vertical component.

An incision is then made at the edge of the palatal shelf laterally, extending forward to link with the dissection in the lateral segment of the lip. The use of an angled (69) Beaver blade is often very helpful. The oral mucoperiosteum is then elevated for about 5 mm.

The first step in lip closure is to interdigitate the vomerine mucosa beneath the oral mucoperiosteum with horizontal mattress sutures, to produce a two-layer repair (Fig. 17.8). This ensures a high success rate.

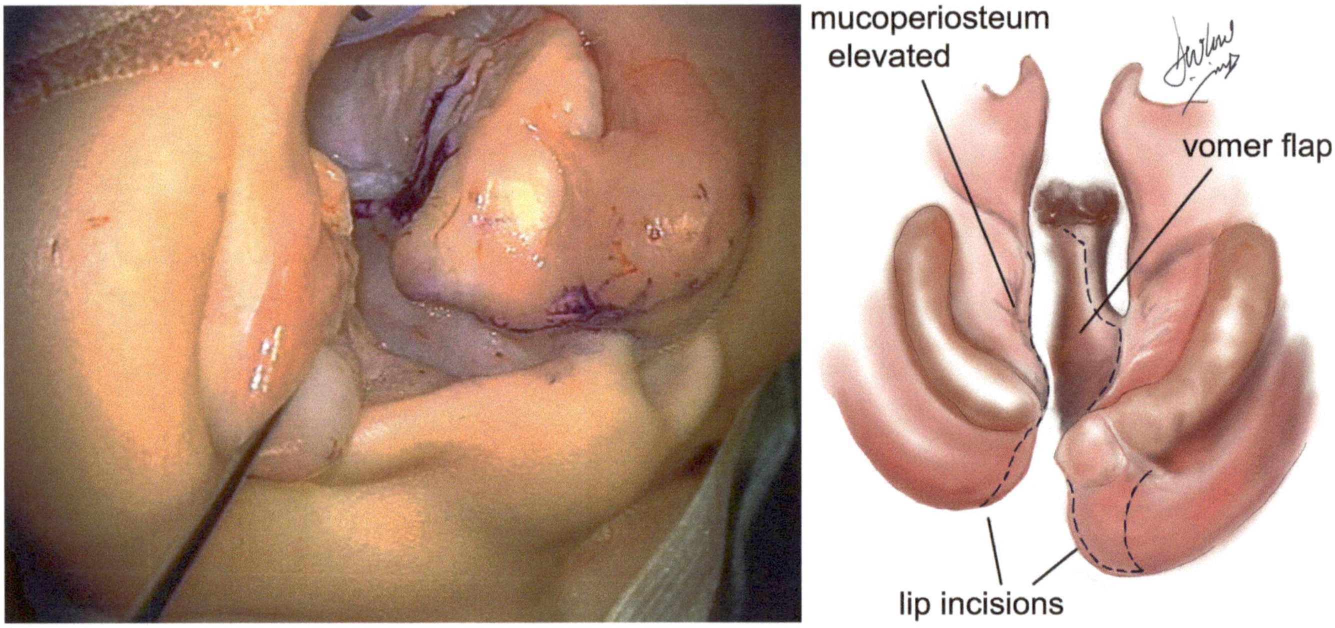


**Fig. 17.6** The vomer flap incision from the lip extending posteriorly in a left unilateral complete cleft – caudal to the groove between the vomer and the premaxilla

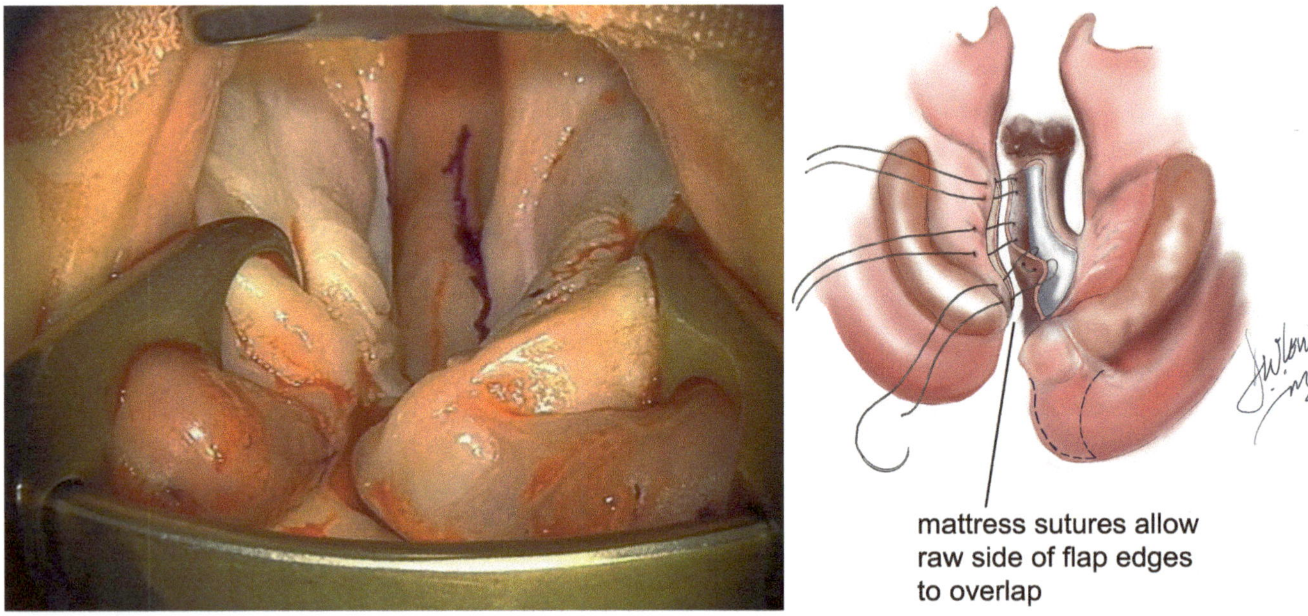


**Fig. 17.7** The incision at the junction of the vomer and hard palate mucosa

### Bilateral Cleft Lip and Palate (BCLP)

A similar technique is used on one side (usually the wider). However, there is less vomerine mucosa available in most bilateral clefts. On the other side, the author only dissects the vomerine mucosa posterior to the pre-vomerine suture to avoid damaging the blood supply of the premaxilla.

In bilateral clefts with a very prominent premaxilla, the two-stage protocol described above is very helpful and allows the uncompleted vomerine flap to be completed.

## Second Stage: Closure of the Remainder of the Palate with Muscle Dissection 3–6 Months Later

### Unilateral Cleft Lip and Palate (UCLP)

The raw surface of the vomerine flap should have epithelialised. This enables a flap of this new epithelium, based posteriorly, to be turned back to facilitate closure of the nasal layer of the soft palate.

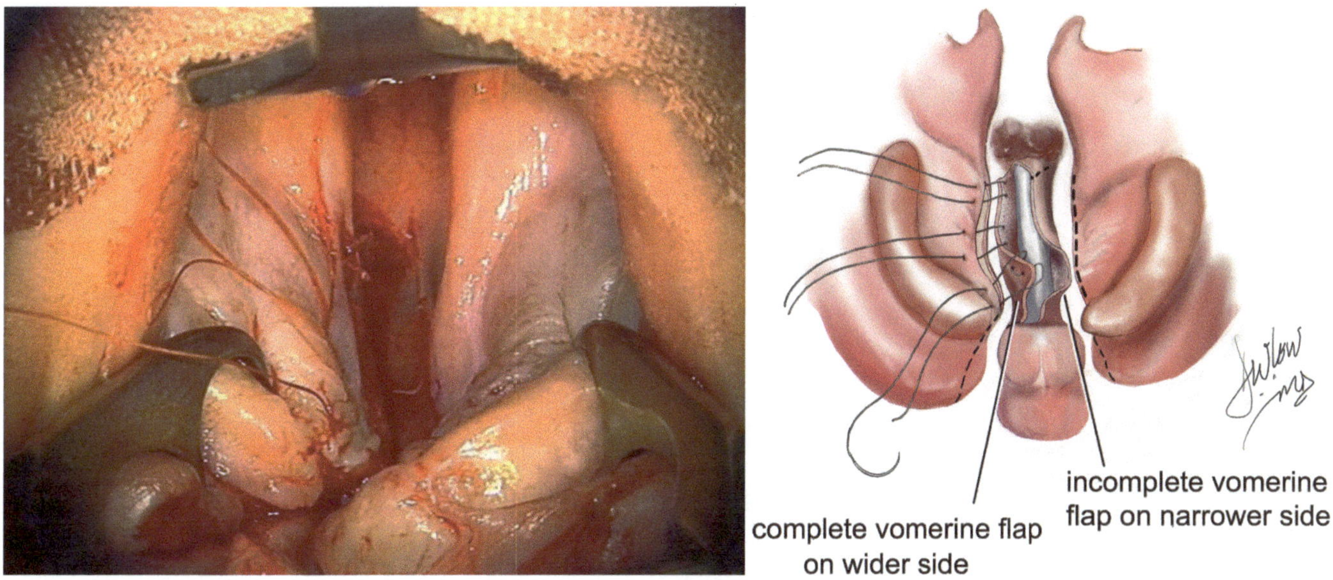


Fig. 17.8 The superiorly based vomerine flap is overlapped beneath the oral mucosa of the lesser palatal segment with horizontal mattress sutures

The technique of repair is then the same as repair of an isolated cleft palate which is described below.

### Bilateral Cleft Lip and Palate

The technique of soft palate dissection is similar. The differences are that:

- The cleft is likely to be wider
- Vomerine flap closure may have been less complete
- There is less neomucosa available for a posteriorly based flap
- Following the author's technique, there will be a residual defect on one side in front of the pre-vomerine suture where the vomerine flap was not raised. An attempt is made to raise it at this stage.

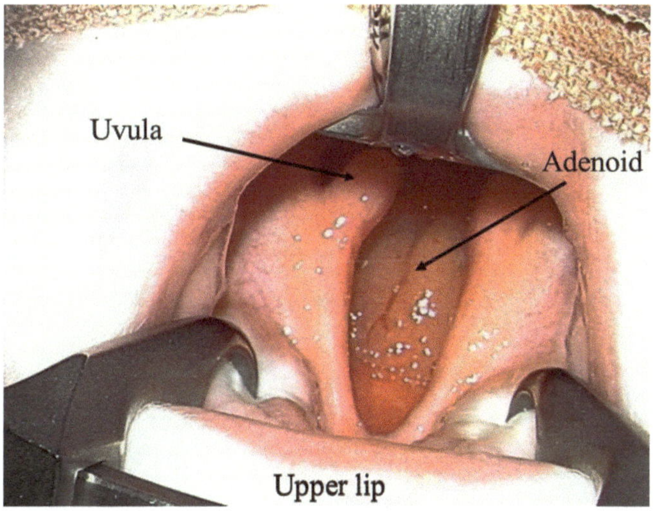


Fig. 17.9 A cleft involving the posterior third of the hard and the soft palate

## Isolated Cleft Palate (and Unilateral and Bilateral Clefts of Lip and Palate After Vomerine Flap Closure of the Hard Palate at Lip Repair)

Incisions are made at the junction of the oral and nasal mucosa of the soft palate. This can usually be identified by colour, the nasal mucosa usually being more pink (Fig. 17.9) and darker in darker skinned individuals. There may also be small polyps at the junction between oral and nasal mucosa. The incision extends in the midline onto the hard palate (Fig. 17.10) even in soft palate-only clefts. In more complete clefts bilateral vomerine flaps are raised with posterior releasing incisions at the junction of the vomerine mucosa and the adenoids if necessary.

The oral mucoperiosteum is then elevated on both sides. Medially, it is essential to enter the subperiosteal plane. Laterally, it is important to elevate the mucoperiosteum from the back of the hard palate. On both sides, the subperiosteal dissection then continues to the back of the hard palate and, very importantly, oral mucosal glands are identified at this point – adherent to the back of the hard palate and the tensor tendon/palatal aponeurosis of the anterior soft palate. Initially by knife dissection and then by sharp dissection, the oral mucoperiosteum with these glands is elevated (Figs. 17.11 and 17.12) to expose the white triangular tendinous insertion at the nasal component of the tensor tendon laterally and the palatopharyngeus insertions into the back of the hard palate medially. (Contrary to many reports, the levator does not insert into

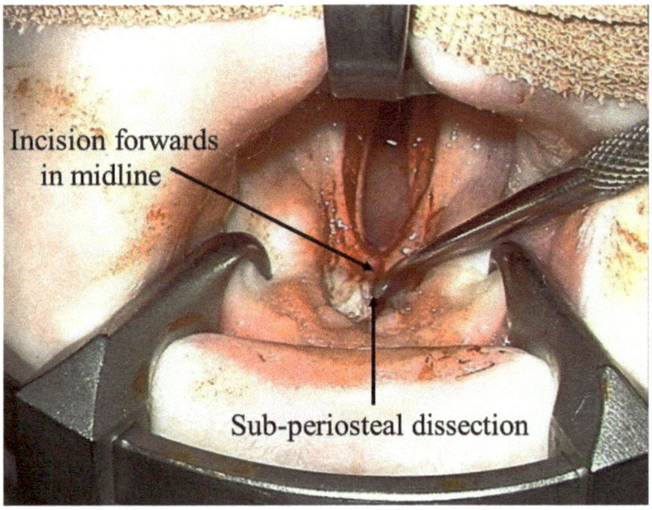


Fig. 17.10 The incision at the junction of oral and nasal mucosa extending onto the hard palate where subperiosteal dissection is performed

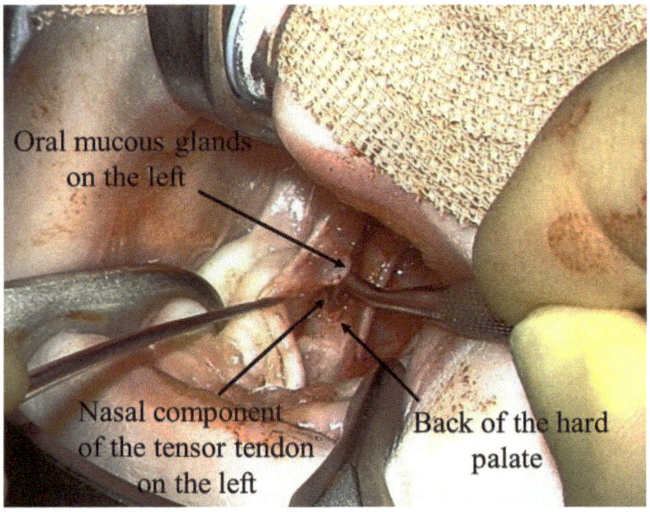


Fig. 17.11 Elevation of mucous glands from the back of the hard palate on the left to expose the nasal insertion of the tensor

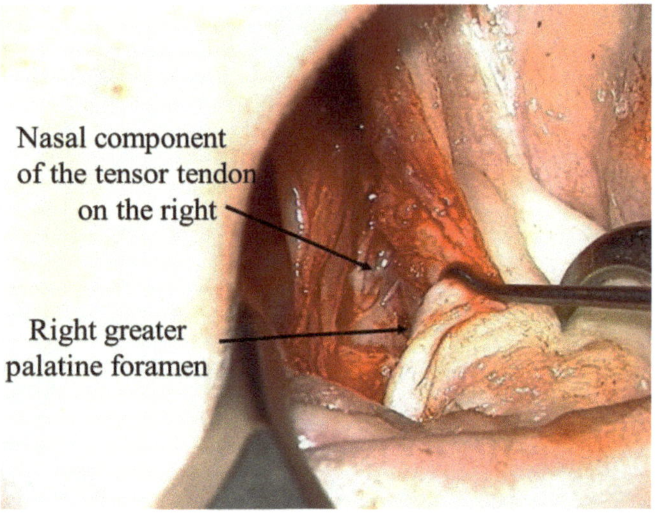


Fig. 17.12 Repeating the process on the right to expose the tensor insertion and the greater palatine neurovascular bundle

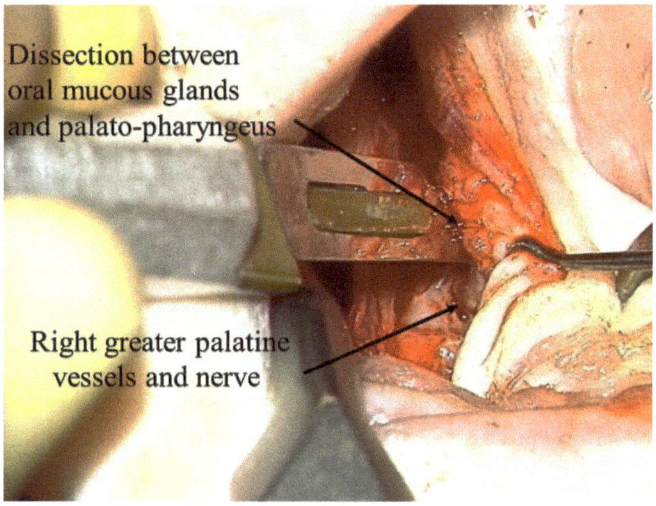


Fig. 17.13 Then continuing the dissection of oral mucosa from the muscle on the right

the back of the hard palate in a cleft palate but it does insert more anteriorly than normal into the margin of the cleft.)

The greater palatine neurovascular bundle can be visualised and freed (Fig. 17.12). There is often a tight structure just behind this pedicle which, if divided, frees the oral mucosa significantly.

The dissection then continues, dissecting in a plane between the oral mucosa and mucous glands and the underlying muscle (palatopharyngeus) (Fig. 17.13). The dissection extends laterally to the pterygoid hamulus.

The nasal myomucosal layer is then sutured (Fig. 17.14) (with the posteriorly based neomucosal flap from the vomer aiding closure anteriorly in clefts of lip and palate). Closure of the nasal myomucosal layer before muscle dissection makes the muscle dissection (largely by scalpel) easier by providing some tension. Anteriorly, the vomerine mucosa is sutured to the lateral nasal mucosa. Between the two, an attempt is made to place a suture through all four components of the nasal layer closure.

A paramedian incision is then made, usually about 4 mm lateral to the midline posteriorly (leaving mucous glands on the nasal layer) and becoming closer to the midline anteriorly but leaving the sutures used for nasal closure intact. This dissection continues vertically until the nasal mucosa layer is reached. It can be identified by bluish discolouration and by a plexus of small vessels well seen under the operating microscope. The aim is to leave this layer intact. The dissection then continues laterally between this nasal mucosa layer with its vascular plexus and the palatal musculature

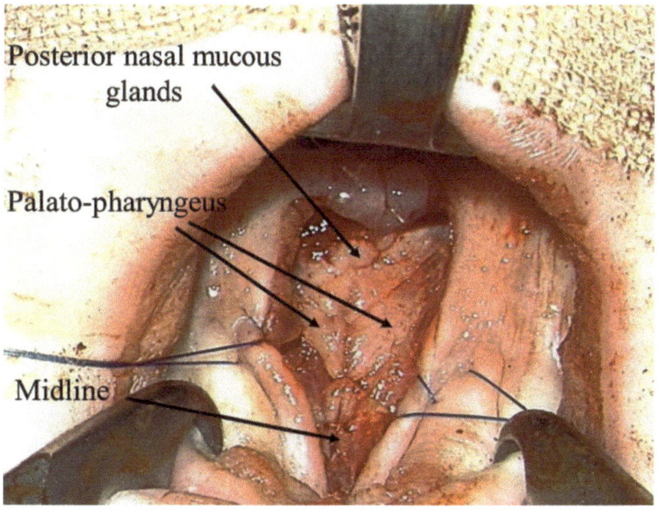


**Fig. 17.14** Closure of the nasal myomucosal layer

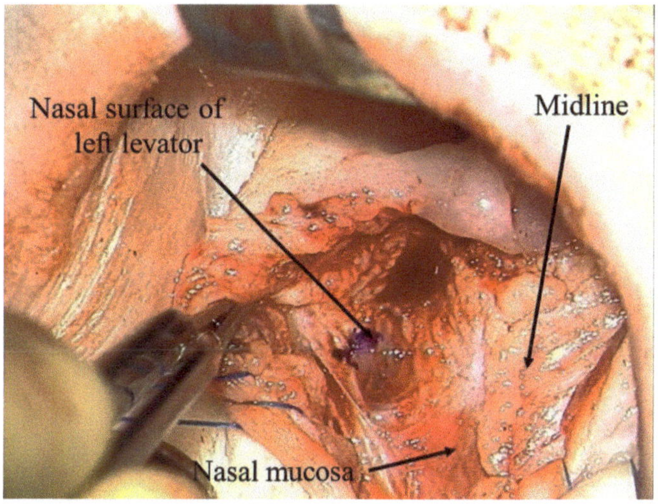


**Fig. 17.15** After paramedian incisions down to the bluish nasal mucosa, dissection continues in a plane between the muscle and the nasal mucosa to expose the nasal surface of the levator

(Fig. 17.15). The levatorpalati muscle, which is closely applied to the nasal layer, is then identified if possible. Dissection of this layer facilitates the subsequent retropositioning of the palatal musculature.

An incision is then made transversely, dividing the muscle (palatopharyngeus) from the back of the hard palate medially and then at least part of the tendinous nasal component of the tensor palati laterally from the back of the hard palate. The incision then passes posteriorly, medial to the pterygoid hamulus, to divide most of the tensor tendon. Part is left and the remainder of the tensor palati muscle does not retract. The tensor palati muscle itself is not seen in the palatal dissection and is not primarily a palatal muscle.

Following release of the tensor from the pterygoid hamulus, blunt dissection then continues to split the palatopharyngeus fibres (part of which remain oriented anteriorly and inserted in

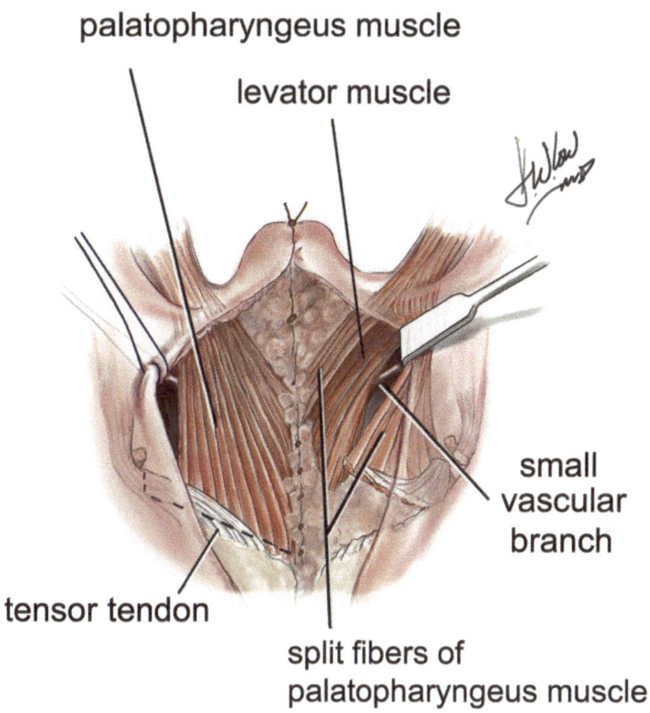


**Fig. 17.16** Splitting palatopharyngeus to expose the left levator

the region of the maxillary tuberosity). The splitting of these fibres should expose the anterior surface of the levatorpalati muscle (Fig. 17.16), which is then further freed from the nasal layer (Fig. 17.17) and retropositioned into at least the posterior half (and sometimes the posterior third) of the velum. A constant blood vessel anterior to the levator can be freed anteriorly (Fig. 17.18) and also retropositioned. If no accidental holes have been made in the nasal mucosa, cruciate incisions are made laterally in the nasal mucosa (Fig. 17.19) to allow escape of blood and minimise the risk of haematoma and subsequent infection.

Closure of the muscle (the levator with the postero-medial fibres of the palatopharyngeus) is then performed (Fig. 17.20). The author uses non-absorbable 4/0 nylon sutures. A posterior muscle orientating stitch is then inserted and then at least two sutures are passed clearly through the levator muscle on each side (with the knots nasal). The final muscle suture incorporates the retropositioned tensor tendinous component, which strengthens the repair.

A twisted loop mattress suture [10] (Figs. 17.21 and 17.22) is inserted, through the oral layer and picking up the tissue on the nasal layer near the midline, to close the oral to the nasal layer in front of the repaired muscle. This helps to avoid a dead space and to ensure that the muscle remains retrodisplaced.

Finally, the remainder of the oral layer is closed without lateral releasing incisions if there is no significant tension (Fig. 17.23) but with as limited lateral releasing incisions as possible if necessary.

A suction test performed at the end of the procedure will confirm whether or not the palate is sufficiently long to reach the posterior pharyngeal wall.

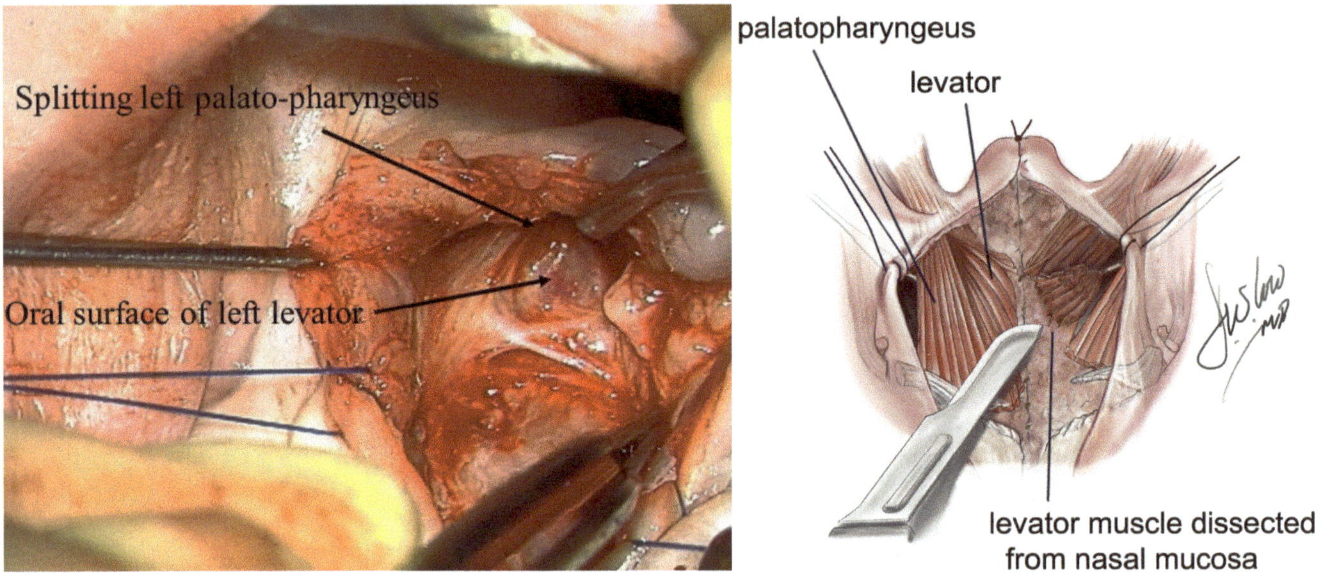


**Fig. 17.17** Dissection between the levator and the nasal mucosa shown on the right

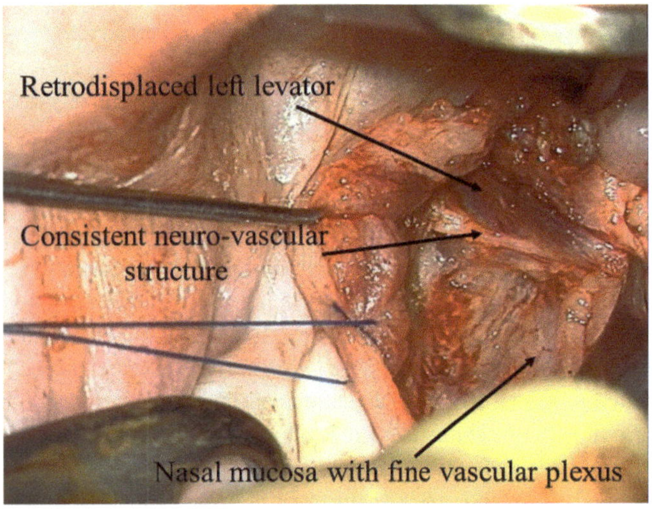


**Fig. 17.18** The left levator is further retrodisplaced by freeing a restraining neurovascular structure

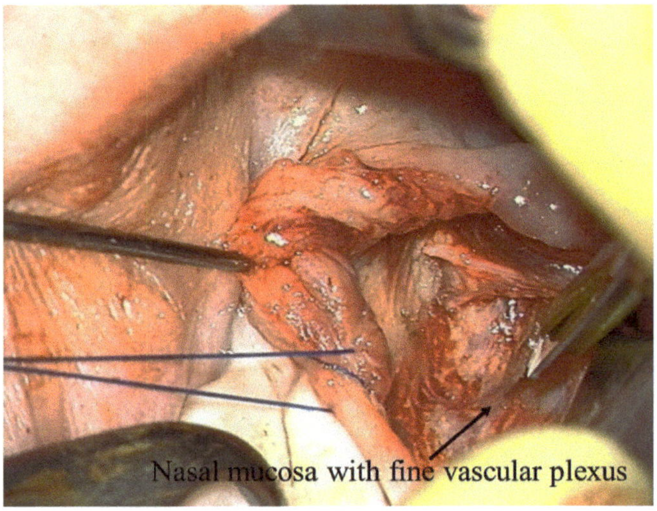


**Fig. 17.19** If a hole has not been accidentally made in the nasal mucosa, it is made laterally, avoiding the small vessels within the nasal layer

The oral mucosa is then closed. The first suture is a twisted loop mattress suture which closes the oral mucosa to the nasal mucosa in the midline in front of the muscle. This helps to reduce dead space and to maintain the position of the posteriorly displaced muscles. The remainder of the oral mucosa is closed but no attempt is made to close the oral mucoperiosteum very anteriorly, where the vomerine flap will already have achieved closure.

## Illustration

If necessary, limited lateral releasing incisions are performed. These are made at the junction of the palatal and the gingival mucosa, curving around the back of the alveolus but not extending back into the soft palate. In wide clefts where it is obvious that lateral releasing incisions will be necessary, it is better to perform them early so that bleeding from them should have stopped by the end of the operation.

## Submucous Cleft Palate

Again, the dissection is similar, except that the aim is to keep the nasal mucosa intact [11]. This can be very challenging in patients where the translucent zone is thin. Prior hydro-dissection and careful knife dissection should allow elevation of the oral mucosa without making a hole in the nasal mucosa.

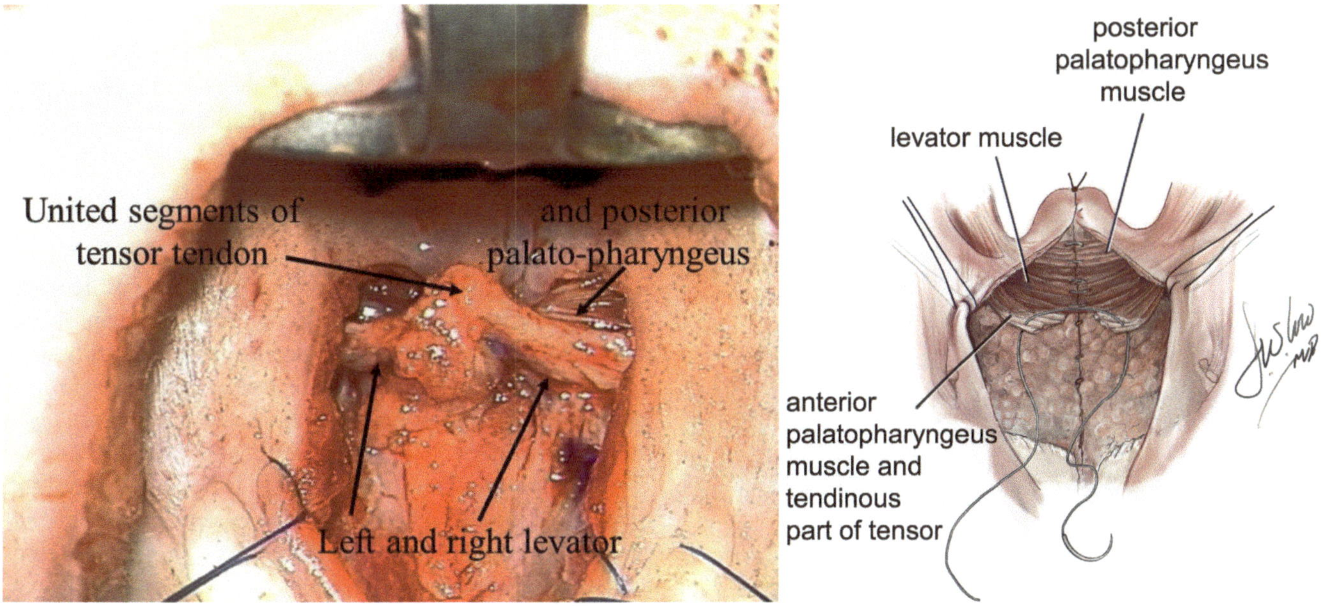


**Fig. 17.20** The retrodisplaced muscles (levator with some fibres of palatopharyngeus) are united in the posterior soft palate with non-absorbable sutures

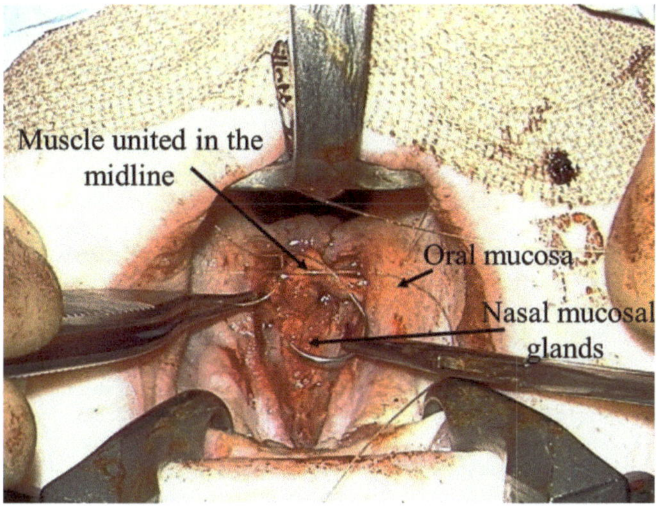


**Fig. 17.21** A twisted loop mattress suture is inserted, closing the oral to the nasal mucosa in front of the repaired muscle

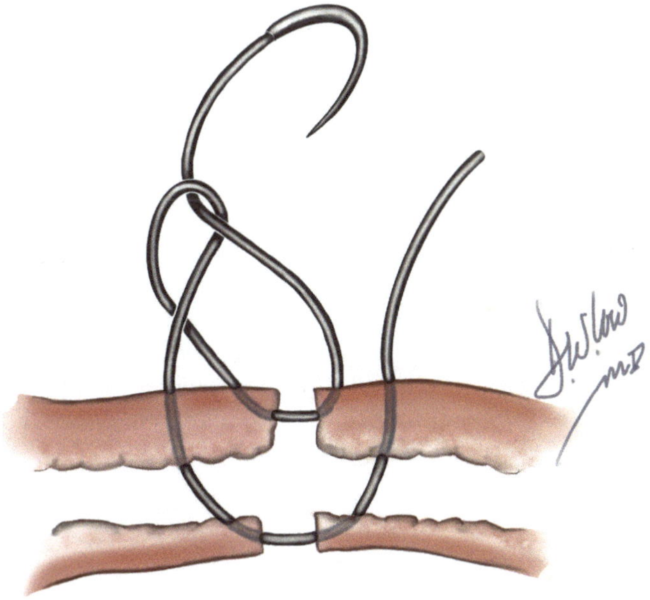

**Fig. 17.22** The twisted loop mattress suture. Putting the needle through the loop doubles the number of sutures across the defect and halves the tension in the suture. The twist avoids a large loop which may result in necrosis of the oral mucosa within the loop

## Postoperative Management

### Airway

The airway should be carefully monitored in the postoperative period. Care in a relatively high-dependency setting with monitoring of oxygen saturation is essential. If necessary, airway obstruction can be managed temporarily with a nasopharyngeal airway, inserted in a unilateral cleft on the non-cleft side. Positioning of the tube is critical. The use of a tongue stitch can be life-saving in some cases. It must be inserted deeply through the posterior tongue at the end of palate repair.

### Analgesia

Analgesia needs to be titrated against sedation. The use of opioids should be minimised as they can depress respiration and discourage the commencement of feeding. As soon as possible, analgesia with a combination of paracetamol and ibuprofen is desirable.

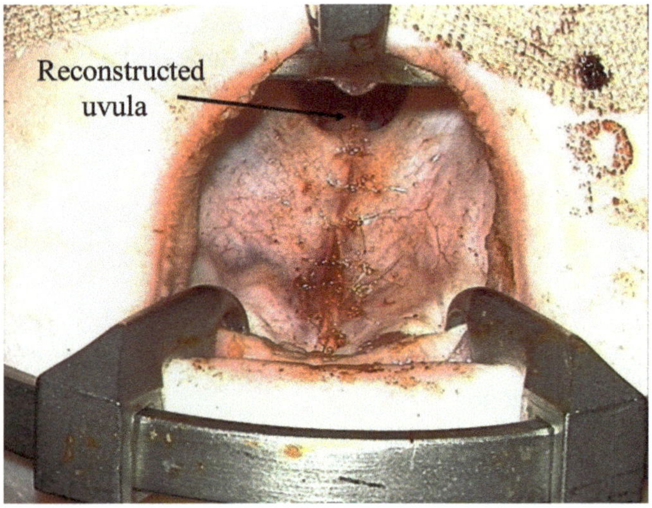


Fig. 17.23 Closure – in this case without lateral releasing incisions

## Antibiotics

Prophylactic antibiotics are controversial. The author prefers to use Penicillin V in infants under 12 months (as prophylaxis primarily against beta-haemolytic streptococcus) and broader spectrum antibiotics in older patients for 5 days. The evidence for benefit is not strong.

## Feeding

Oral feeding is commenced as soon as the child awakes from anaesthesia. Clear fluids are given for the first feed and then milk feeding can begin – usually using whichever feeding technique was used prior to repair. In some low-resource countries, breast milk has been the mainstay of feeding before surgery and can be continued afterward, often with manual expression of milk.

## Arm Splints

Arm splints have been shown not to be necessary and have been abandoned [12].

## Complications and Follow-Up

### Complications

The most important early complications are airway obstruction and bleeding. Measures to reduce these risks and to manage them have been described above.

Later complications include fistula formation and more major dehiscence. These are mostly related to tension in the repair, with major breakdowns probably resulting from poor dissection and/or haematoma and infection.

### Follow-Up

Follow-up of patients in many countries is very difficult but every effort should be made to do so – for the benefit of both the patient and the surgeon. A surgeon who is not following up his or her own patients is not going to learn from mistakes. Ideally, follow-up care should be undertaken by a multi-disciplinary cleft team as described in Chap. 37.

The final outcome of cleft surgery is not known until full maturity at the age of 20 years. However, much of this outcome has been determined by the primary surgery and especially primary palate repair.

## References

1. Pichler H. Zur operation der doppeltenlippen-gaumenspalten. Dtsch Z Cir. 1926;195:104.
2. Veau V, Ruppie C. Anatomiechirurgicale de la division palatine. J Chir (Paris). 1992;20:1.
3. Wardill WEM. Technique of operation for cleft lip and palate. Br J Surg. 1937;25:97.
4. Kilner TP. Cleft lip and palate repair technique. In: Maingot R, editor. Postgraduate surgery, vol. 3. London: Medical Publishers; 1937.
5. Sommerlad BC. A technique for palate repair. Plast Reconstr Surg. 2003;112:1542–8.
6. von Langenbeck B. Weitere Erfahrungenim Gebiete der Uranoplastic mittels Ablusung des mucosperriostealen Gaumenüberzuges. Arch Klin Chir. 1861;5:170.
7. von Langenbeck B. Die Uranoplastikmittles Ablosung des microsperiostalen Gaumenüberzuges. Arch Klin Chir. 1862;2:205.
8. Sommerlad BC. The use of the operating microscope in cleft palate repair and pharyngoplasty. Plast Reconstr Surg. 2003;112:1540–1.
9. Sommerlad BC, Mehendale FV. A modified gag for cleft palate repair. Br J Plast Surg. 2000;53:63–4.
10. Rees LS, Sommerlad BC. Twisted loop mattress suture. Ann R Coll Surg Engl. 2012;94(4):274.
11. Sommerlad BC, Fenn C, Harland K, Sell D, et al. Submucous cleft palate - a system of grading and a review of a consecutive series of 40 submucous cleft palate repairs. Cleft Palate-Craniofac J. 2004;41:114–23.
12. Jigjinni V, Kangesu T, Sommerlad BC. Do babies require arm splints after cleft palate repair? Br J Plast Surg. 1993;46:681–5.

# Cleft Palate repair: Double-Opposing Z-plasty Technique

18

Craig Birgfeld and Solomon Obiri-Yeboah

**Key Points**

- There are five reasons for performing Furlow palatoplasty:
  1. It effectively closes soft palate cleft.
  2. It inherently includes intervelar veloplasty (IVVP).
  3. Z-plasty lengthens the palate.
  4. Double-opposing z-plasty reduces overlap of nasal and oral incisions.
  5. Z-plasty resists cicatricial shortening of the palate.
- The technique can be used in primary palate repair or as a secondary treatment for velopharyngeal insufficiency (VPI).
- The technique may improve speech outcomes.
- While some surgeons have avoided Furlow palatoplasty for perceived increased fistula rate, recent studies show similar rates to other palatoplasty techniques.

## Introduction

The goal of palatoplasty is to separate the oral cavity from the nasal cavity and to normalize palatal anatomy such that dynamic, complete closure of the nasopharynx can produce normal speech. Surgical techniques have evolved over the past centuries and outcomes have improved. One evolution of soft palate closure is the Furlow palatoplasty, first described by Dr. Leonard Furlow in 1978 [1, 2] and later popularized by Dr. Randall and his lineage at the Children's Hospital of Philadelphia [3, 4]. This technique utilizes a double-opposing z-plasty to lengthen the palate while simultaneously creating an intervelar veloplasty with the goal of reducing velopharyngeal inadequacy. While this technique has gained popularity among American cleft surgeons, debate remains over its advantages or weaknesses compared to other techniques, and it has not become universally accepted. In developing countries, additional obstacles exist to performing any palatoplasty, much less a Furlow palatoplasty.

## Patient Selection and Clinical Planning

### Timing of Surgery

Timing of palatoplasty balances the improvement in speech seen with early surgery [5, 6] with the negative effects on facial growth attributed to early surgery [7]. For most American cleft centers, the cleft palate is repaired around 9–12 months of age to balance these competing forces. But, there are centers that perform concomitant lip and palate surgeries [8, 9] and others who perform two-stage repairs with soft palate repair early and hard palate repair closer to age 6 [10–12]. In most developing countries, due to lack of institutional comprehensive cleft care (multidisciplinary cleft teams), postoperative follow-up is very poor. Hence there may be pressure to combine lip and palate repair, combined with the fear that patient may not return after the cheiloplasty has been done. Also, due to lack of expertise, financial difficulties, and strong traditional belief systems, patients may not present until later in life if at all [13].

At whatever age the palatoplasty is performed, the patient's health should be optimized. Because of the risk of

C. Birgfeld (✉)
Division of Plastic Surgery, Department of Surgery, University of Washington and Seattle Children's Hospital, Seattle, WA, USA
e-mail: craig.birgfeld@seattlechildrens.org

S. Obiri-Yeboah
Department of Oral and Maxillofacial Sciences, Kwame Nkrumah University of Science and Technology, Kumasi, Ghana

School of Medicine and Dentistry and Komfo Anokye Teaching Hospital, Kumasi, Ghana

© Springer Nature Switzerland AG 2021
J. W. Swanson, D. W. Low (eds.), *Global Cleft Care in Low-Resource Settings*, https://doi.org/10.1007/978-3-030-59105-2_18

airway compromise, surgery for any patient with upper respiratory infection (URI) symptoms should be postponed until at least 2 weeks after resolution of symptoms. Additionally, malnourished patients may have an increased risk of dehiscence and fistula formation.

Poor nutrition can be worsened by feeding difficulties inherent with cleft palate. In developing countries where access to formula, food and feeding apparatus, such as Haberman nipples is limited, this malnutrition can be further exacerbated. Through the collaboration between Seattle Children's and Komfo Anokye Teaching Hospital multidisciplinary cleft team Kumasi, Ghana, a cheaper flexible cup (NIFTY cup) was developed (see Chap. 7 "Nutrition"). Many mothers find it easy to feed their babies with cleft palate breast milk with this device, thereby reducing the challenge of feeding. For patients who present later in life, oral hygiene can be a factor in success of palatoplasty, and ideally the patient will have all oral health issues addressed prior to palatoplasty. Developing countries depend on mission trips, and the few institutionally based teams are surgery biased, and therefore patients that present late in life may not have the luxury of seeing a dentist before palatoplasty.

## Operative Planning

Successful palatoplasty begins with optimal communication between the surgeon and anesthesiologist. Intraoperative extubation and endotracheal tube malposition and/or occlusion can occur due to use of a mouth gag. In developing countries where pediatric ventilators and CO2 monitors may not be available, over- or under-ventilation may go undetected until the patient becomes acidotic or alkalotic. Preferably, a cuffed oral RAE tube taped down the middle of the lip to the chin is used, if available. If kinking at the tongue retractor component of the Dingman occurs, the tube can be reinforced with a slightly larger ET tube cuffed around the smaller ET tube (Fig. 18.1). The communication should continue throughout the surgery and especially upon extubation. Every cleft surgeon strives to avoid reintubation by an inexperienced anesthesiologist along a freshly repaired palate.

## Relevant Anatomy

Normal palatal anatomy includes a hard palate comprised of oral mucosa, bone, and nasal mucosa; a soft palate comprised of oral mucosa, muscle, and nasal lining; and the uvula. Muscular contributions include the levator veli palatini, the tensor veli palatini, the palatoglossus and palatopharyngeus muscles, and the superior constrictors of the pharynx (Fig. 18.2). In the cleft palate, these components are disrupted to varying degrees (Fig. 18.3). With soft palate clefts, the levator muscles are sagittally oriented rather than transverse and are abnormally attached to the posterior hard palate (Fig. 18.4). The tensor veli palatini muscles course around the hamulus and may require release to allow oral mucosal closure.

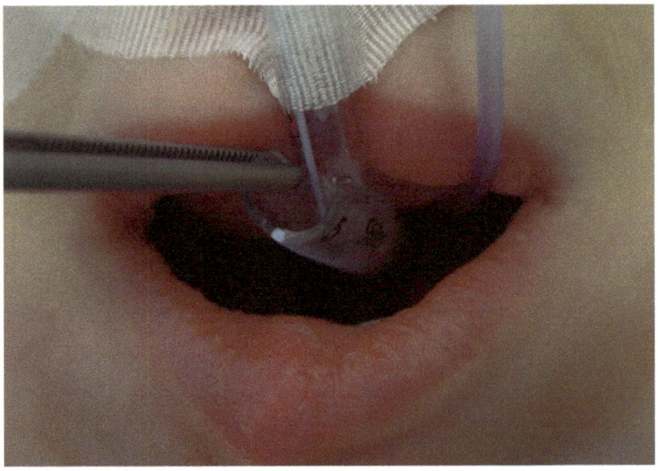

Fig. 18.1 Reinforcing the curve of the oral RAE tube with a larger endotracheal tube beneath the Dingman mouth gag tongue retractor

## Key Equipment (Fig. 18.5)

- Dingman mouth gag.
- 8 French soft tip suction catheter passed through the nose into the nasopharynx and attached to suction in lieu of a throat pack.
- Several elevators – Freer, Molt #9 periosteal dental, Woodson, and Blair ("hockey stick") elevators.
- Angled beaver blade or crescent blade.
- Kerrison punch rongeur can aid in release of greater palatine vessels from foramina.
- 4-0 and 5-0 Vicryl sutures on tapered needle for mucosal closure.
  - *While numerous suture material and needle types may be useful for palatoplasty, in developing countries, the options may be limited to one or two.

## Procedural Technique

Proper positioning and lighting is crucial for successful palatoplasty. A shoulder roll for neck extension can aid exposure of the posterior palate and pharynx. In addition to adequate OR lights, a headlamp can improve visualization, but may not be available in developing countries. A Dingman mouth gag is carefully placed with an adequately sized tongue blade to retract the tongue without constricting it upon the teeth.

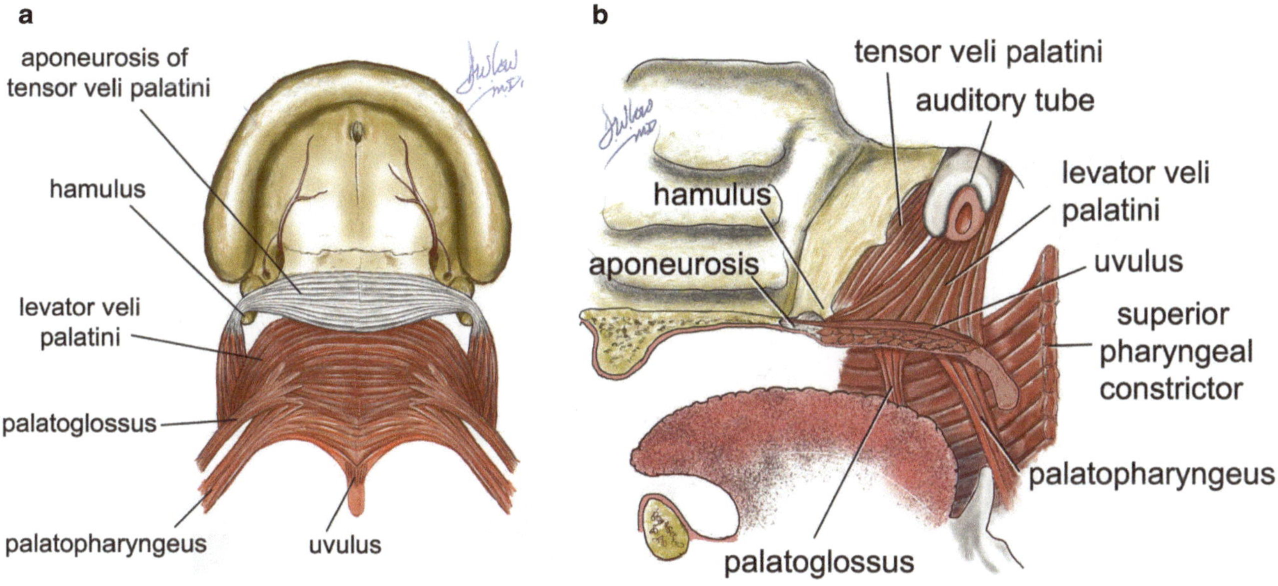


**Fig. 18.2** Muscular anatomy of the soft palate

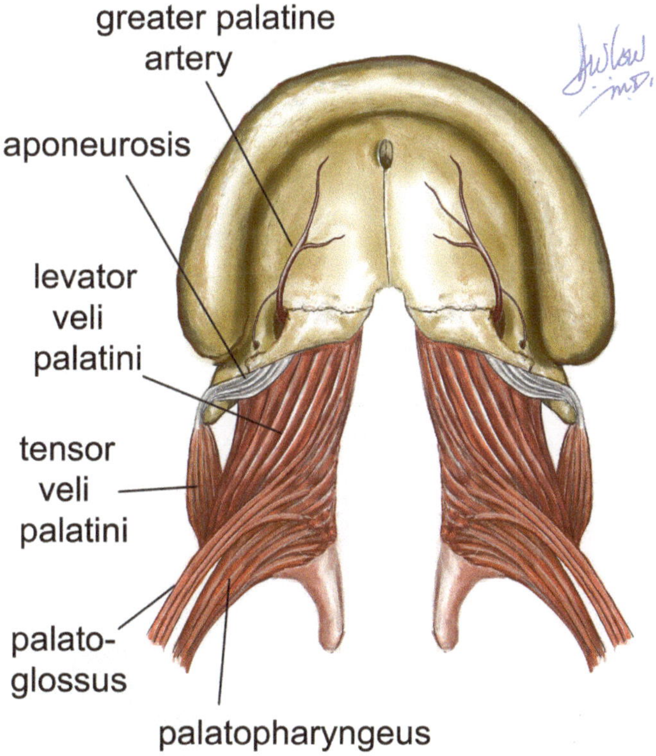


**Fig. 18.3** Veau classification of cleft palates

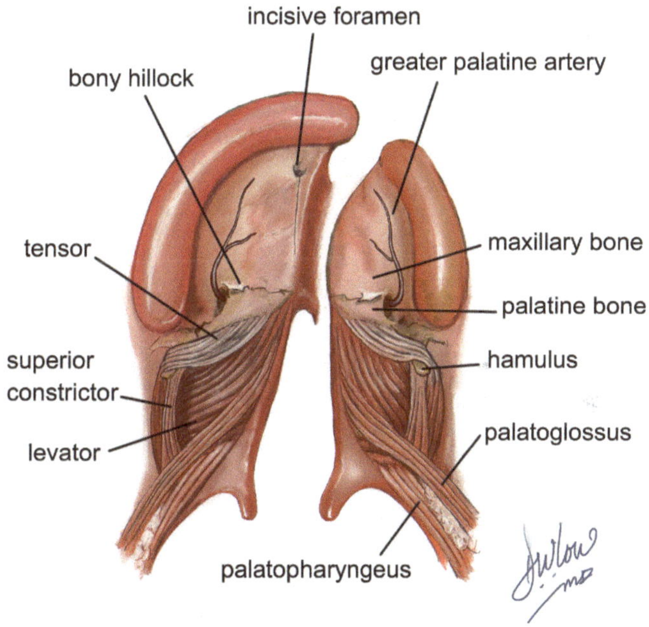


**Fig. 18.4** Anatomy of the levator veli palatini and tensor veli palatini muscles in cleft palates

After carefully padding all pressure points, check to insure the mouth gag does not impinge the lips or tongue or kinks the ET tube. Proceed then with precise injection of local anesthetic with hydrodissection of the palatal mucosa to aid in dissection. In many centers in developing countries, cleft palates are left undone due to the lack of Dingman mouth retractor for adequate mouth opening. Due to cost, most centers depend on foreign donations and mission trips to provide this crucial equipment, and maintaining that equipment can be cost prohibitive.

Before designing the Furlow palatoplasty for soft palate closure, consider the planned technique for hard palate closure. For submucous cleft palates (SMCP) and Veau I clefts, no hard palate work may be necessary. For Veau II palates, some elevation of hard palate mucosa will be necessary, and lateral relaxing incisions may be helpful to provide a tension-free closure. For Veau III cleft palates, one may consider a

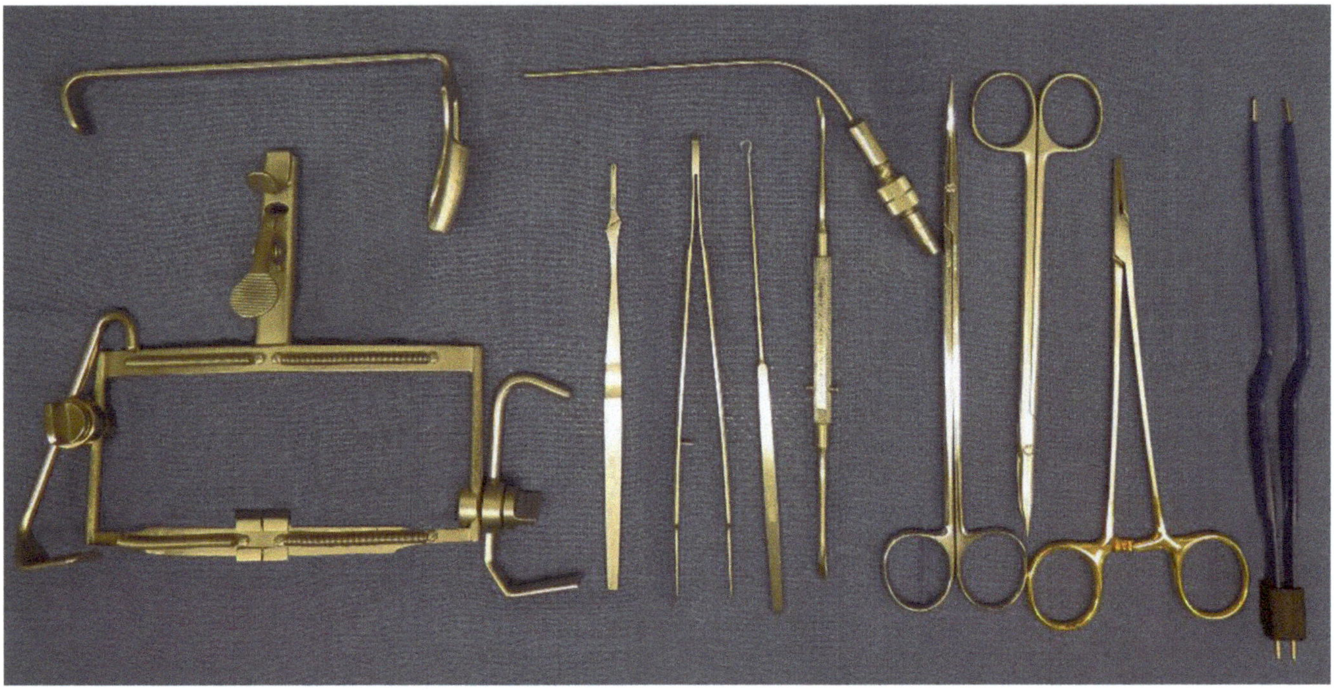

Fig. 18.5 Array of surgical instruments which can be helpful when performing a Furlow palatoplasty

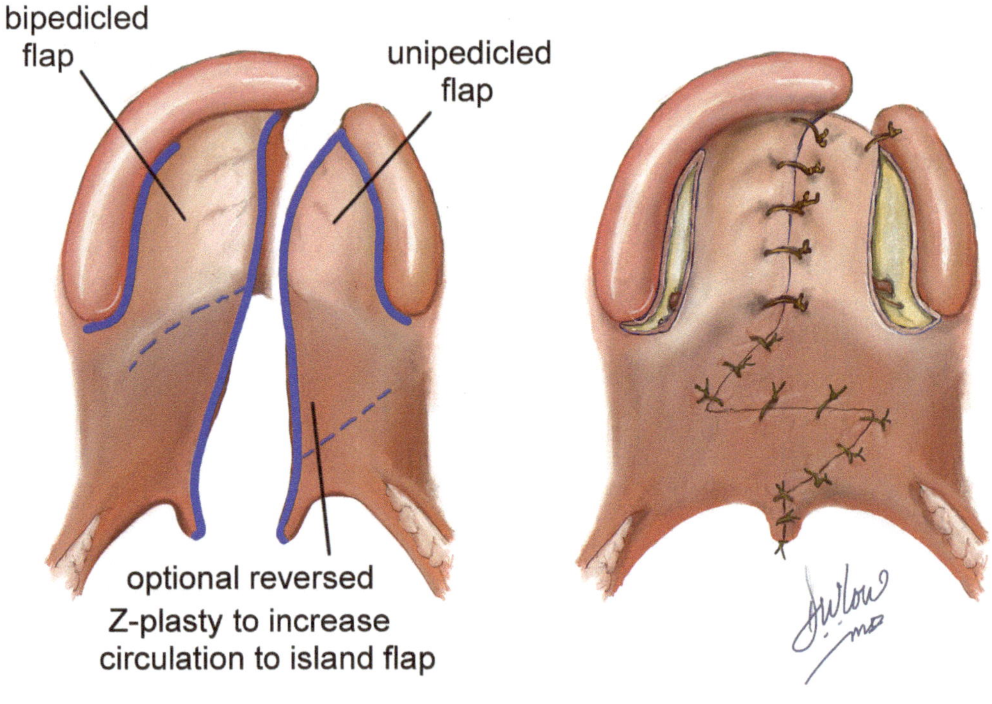


Fig. 18.6 Design of a "hybrid" hard palate repair utilizing a bipedicled flap on the greater segment and a unipedicled flap on the lesser segment

hybrid repair of the hard palate with which the mucosa of the greater segment is elevated as a bipedicled flap, whereas the lesser segment is elevated as a unipedicled flap based on the greater palatine vessel (Fig. 18.6). In this case, the surgeon may alter the design of the Furlow oral mucosa z-plasty to optimize blood supply to the unipedicled flap.

By convention, when designing the Furlow z-plasty flaps for soft palate closure of the oral mucosa, the posteriorly based myomucosal flap is on the patient's left to better accommodate a right-handed surgeon (Fig. 18.7). However, the z-plasty can be reversed for surgeon's preference or to optimize blood supply to a unipedicled hard palate flap as

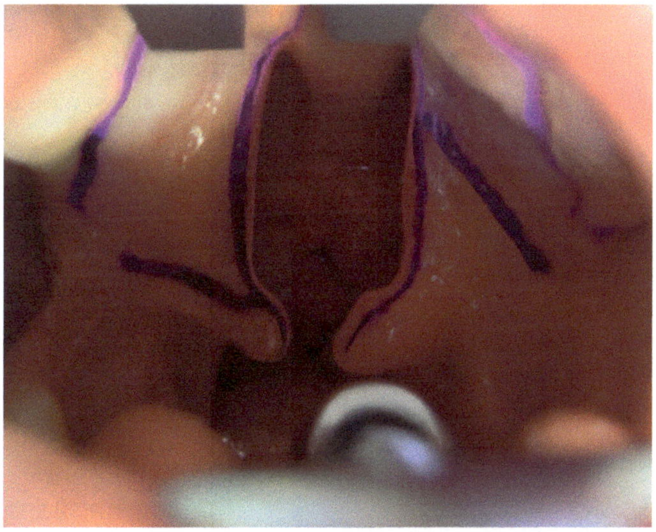

Fig. 18.7 Design of incisions for performing a Furlow palatoplasty

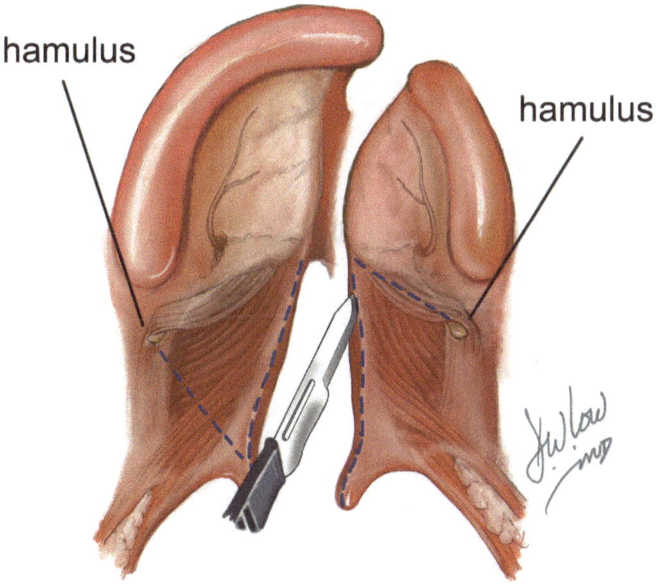


Fig. 18.8 Incisions of the soft palate oral mucosa

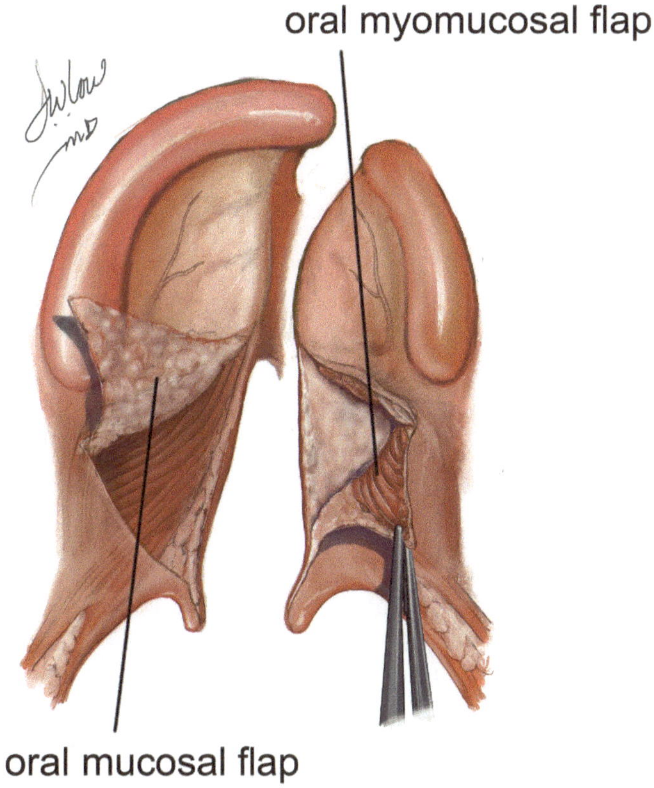


Fig. 18.9 Elevation of soft palate oral mucosal flaps

long *as the posteriorly based flap is the myomucosal flap*. First, identify the hamulus on the right and left. The z-plasty flap on the left extends from the hamulus to the hard palate/soft palate junction. On the right, it extends from the hamulus to the base of the uvula.

Begin by incising along the edge of the cleft separating the oral from the nasal mucosa. By starting with the soft palate, the surgeon can perform the delicate dissection with a sharp knife, and any bleeding will not obstruct the field (Fig. 18.8). Next, incise the oral mucosa z-plasty flaps. On the left, the incision can be carried through the levator musculature separating it from its abnormal attachment to the posterior hard palate. On the right, the incision must stop in the submucosal plane as this flap is anteriorly based and mucosal only. Carefully dissect the nasal lining from the levator musculature on the left. Dissect laterally into the space of Ernst, and then bluntly dissect onto the pterygoid plate to further mobilize the nasal lining flap and enable it to transpose to the opposite side (Fig. 18.9). Once dissection is complete, perform the left double-opposing z-plasty cut through the nasal lining from the base of the uvula toward the hamulus, thereby creating an anteriorly based flap of nasal lining alone. On the right side, elevate the oral mucosa flap in the submucosal plane taking care to maintain adequate thickness of the flap while avoiding injury to the underlying musculature. Lateral dissection extends to the space of Ernst when the opposing z-plasty cut can be made creating a posteriorly based flap of nasal lining and levator musculature (Fig. 18.10). Care should be taken to leave a cuff of nasal lining attached to the posterior hard palate to allow inset of the opposite z-plasty flap. Additionally, a posteriorly based flap of vomer mucosa can be turned back to aid in closure of the nasal lining at the hard palate/soft palate junction which can be a challenging area to close in wide clefts and is known to be a frequent location of post-op fistulas.

Once soft palate dissection is complete, proceed with hard palate dissection if indicated (Fig. 18.11). Begin with lateral relaxing incisions on the lingual side of the alveolus. Take care to hug the alveolus in the region of the greater

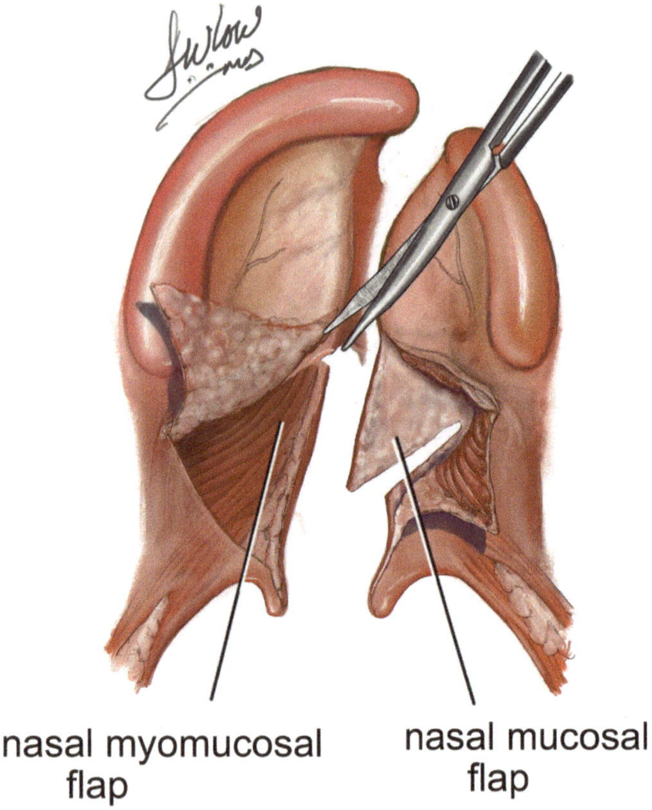


**Fig. 18.10** Double-opposing z-plasty cuts of the soft palate nasal mucosa

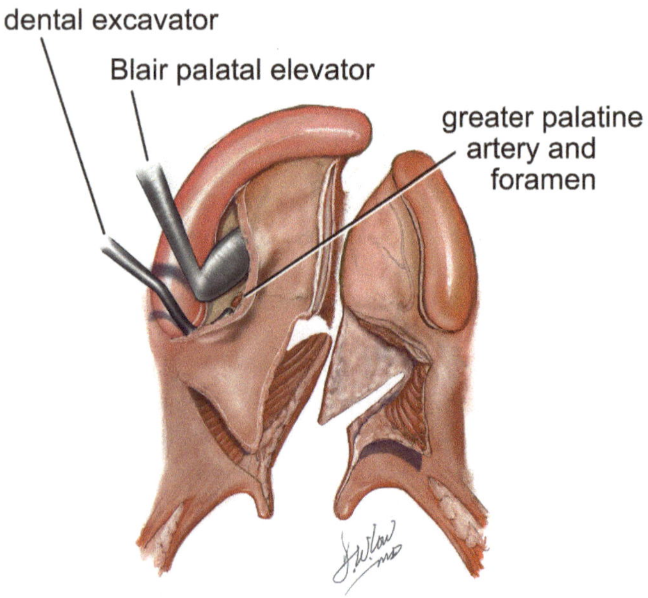


**Fig. 18.11** Elevation of hard palate mucoperiosteal flaps from lateral relaxing incisions

palatine vessel to avoid injury. More anteriorly, care must be taken to avoid injury to developing tooth buds which can be present on the palatal side of the alveolus. Then, elevate the hard palate mucoperiosteal flaps from the relaxing incisions toward the cleft edge using an elevator. Elevating the mucosa first allows better visualization of the oral-nasal mucosa junction at the cleft to avoid incising too far on the nasal side and short-changing the nasal mucosa available for closure. Carefully dissect from anterior to posterior beneath the flaps sequentially past three bony spicules indicating gradual proximity to the greater palatine vessels. Under direct visualization, release the fascial sleeve around the palatine vessel as it exists the foramina to allow medial transposition of the oral mucosal flap. If kinking of the vessel is seen upon this transposition, then remove the bone around the medial aspect of the foramina with a Kerrison punch or fine-tipped rongeur.

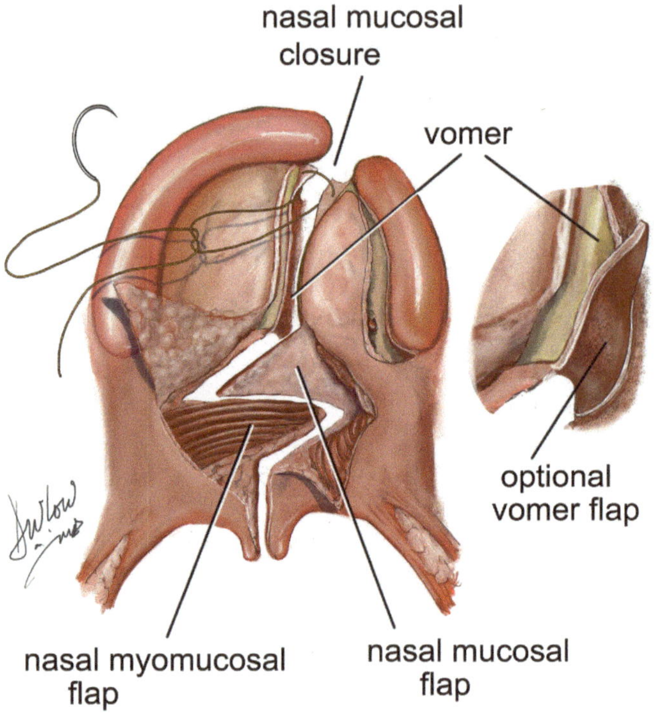


**Fig. 18.12** Elevation and suturing of hard palate nasal lining flaps to optional (if necessary) vomer flap and transposition of soft palate nasal lining flaps

After complete elevation of the hard palate oral mucosa, carefully elevate the nasal lining from the nasal side of the hard palate with an elevator until it can reach the vomer flap similarly elevated from the vomer (Fig. 18.12). After complete mucosal and muscular dissection, begin closing the nasal lining of the hard palate from anterior to posterior. At the hard palate/soft palate junction, transpose the nasal lining flaps of the soft palate z-plasty and inset. If tension exists, further dissection along the skull base to the lateral pharynx can provide greater mobilization. After inset, complete soft palate nasal lining closure from anterior to posterior out to the tip of the uvula and then around to the oral side. Horizontal mattress sutures for the uvula closure can provide mucosal

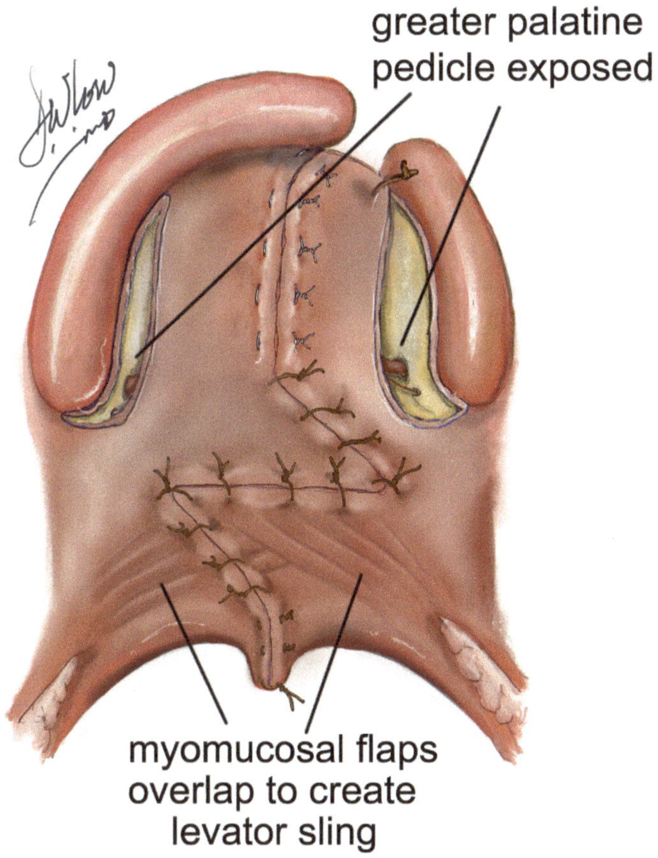


**Fig. 18.13** Completed Furlow palatoplasty repair

edge eversion to help prevent a bifid uvula postoperatively which tends to draw the parents' eye.

Next, transpose and inset the soft palate oral mucosal z-plasty flaps. If too much tension exists, releasing the tensor veli palatini tendon as it courses around the hamulus can be helpful. This can be done with careful dissection or by fracturing the hamulus. If tension still exists, the lateral relaxing incisions can be extended posteriorly, although at the risk of forming posterior scar bands. If too much tension still exists, consider partially closing the back-cuts in a V to Y fashion, so the z-plasty flaps have less distance to travel.

Final closure involves suturing the hard palate oral mucosal flaps together at the midline from posterior to anterior (Fig. 18.13). Again, mattress sutures can aid with mucosal eversion both to reduce fistulas and to prevent indented mucosa which is prone to catching food postoperatively. Care should be taken to completely and securely inset the anterior hard palate flap to the premaxilla and alveolar cleft. Fistulas at the incisive foramen or U-shaped fistulas behind the premaxilla in Veau IV clefts can be very challenging to deal with when it comes time to perform the alveolar bone graft.

After closure, the lateral relaxing incisions can be packed with Surgicel to reduce bleeding. Resist the urge to close these incisions as this will increase the tension along the midline repair and may compromise the vascularity of the flaps. Carefully suction out the pharynx to avoid aspiration of clot, and maintain the position of the ET tube when removing the mouth gag as accidental extubation can occur. Lastly, consider use of a soft nasal trumpet airway or a tongue stitch to protect the airway after extubation and reduce the risk of a traumatic reintubation.

## Follow-Up and Complication Management

The patient should be closely monitored in the recovery room with adequate positioning and pulse oximetry since airway obstruction is a common result of palatoplasty. One should consider a prolonged stay in the recovery room before transferring to the ward as the nurse to patient ratio is more conducive to safety in the PACU. Typically, an overnight stay for observation is planned although longer stays may be necessary if oral intake is not adequate post-op. Arm restraints and the avoidance of pacifiers are used to reduce trauma to the suture line and are frequently continued until healing is verified. Minimization of narcotics can not only reduce the associated respiratory depression which intensifies airway obstruction but also improve the patient's appetite and ability to feed.

Early complications of palatoplasty include airway obstruction, bleeding, palatal hematoma, and palatal dehiscence. At times, airway obstruction can be managed with a nasal or soft oral airway or with steroids or racemic epinephrine. But, patients with these unusual requirements should receive greater levels of post-op care in either the ICU or step-down unit. Some patients require reintubation which should be done with the surgeon present to reduce the risk of traumatic injury to a fresh palate repair. Excessive bleeding and/or palatal hematoma can exacerbate airway obstruction and may require a prompt return to the OR for evacuation and hemostasis. Early palatal dehiscence is rare but, if recognized, should be repaired acutely.

Late complications of palatoplasty include oronasal fistula formation and velopharyngeal inadequacy (VPI). The first treatment of an oronasal fistula is detection. Patient's palates should be carefully inspected for such on every post-op visit, and the patient should be asked about the presence of nasal regurgitation at every visit. Once a fistula is detected, it should be classified [14] to plan reconstruction. Speech should be assessed by the surgeon and, ideally, a speech and language pathologist each year to detect nasal air escape. If present, further workup is warranted, and a surgical correction may be indicated. Of note, in patients who have undergone primary Furlow palatoplasty, surgical treatment of VPI usually involves either a sphincter pharyngoplasty [15] or posterior pharyngeal flap [16]. However, some surgeons have recently reported success "re-Furlowing" a Furlow [17]. Treatments of oronasal fistulas are varied and depend on size and location and are beyond the scope of this chapter.

## Challenges to Performing Furlow Palatoplasty in Developing Countries

Surgery, like other vocations, is an apprenticeship: transfer of skills from mentor to mentee. Most often, surgeons use the technique they are comfortable with and which produces the best results. Unlike the developed world where cleft palate and craniofacial surgery is part of fellowship program and a subspecialty with additional training, in developing countries, the story is different. Many surgeons in developing countries are not specially trained cleft surgeons. Most learned from mission partners and short attachments and observations in centers in developed countries and therefore are comfortable with techniques that are simple and produce equally good results. A short and quick survey on the AFAOMS (African Association of Oral and Maxillofacial Surgeons) WhatsApp reveals the following responses:

1. "Don't use Furlow palatoplasty because have never really understood it and think there are other simpler techniques that work perfectly."
2. "Don't use Furlow palatoplasty because it's more technical than practical."
3. "Don't use Furlow palatoplasty because is difficult to transfer unlike other simple technique that are easy to teach."
4. "Do not use Furlow because, think muscle dissection is inadequate for optimum function."
5. "Do use it but not often. Think it should be used as a secondary procedure for short palate."

Although the Furlow palatoplasty may have its advantages over other cleft palate repair techniques, it has not yet become popularized in sub-Saharan Africa as noted by the brief survey above.

## Advantages of the Furlow Palatoplasty

As stated previously, the goal of palatoplasty is to separate the mouth from the nose and to optimize speech. While many techniques exist, there is evidence that a Furlow palatoplasty is more likely to attain this goal. Large series of patients who underwent Furlow palatoplasty find fistula rates that are comparable to or lower than other techniques [4, 18] and speech outcomes demonstrate lower rates of VPI [19]. In the end, the best palatal repair technique is the one with which the surgeon has the most comfort and experience and is most likely to deliver safe, effective, reproducible results. Depending on the surgeon's training and access to necessary equipment and supplies, the Furlow palatoplasty may or may not be the appropriate palatoplasty technique in developing countries.

## References


1. Furlow LT Jr. Cleft palate repair by double opposing Z-plasty. Plast Reconstr Surg. 1986;78:724–38.
2. Furlow, L. T., Jr. Annual Meeting of the Southeastern Society of Plastic and Reconstructive Surgeons. Boca Raton, FL. 1978).
3. Randall P, LaRossa D, Solomon M, Cohen M. Experience with the Furlow double-reversing Z-plasty for cleft palate repair. Plast Reconstr Surg. 1986;77:569–76.
4. Jackson O, et al. The Children's Hospital of Philadelphia modification of the Furlow double-opposing Z-palatoplasty: 30-year experience and long-term speech outcomes. Plast Reconstr Surg. 2013;132:613–22. https://doi.org/10.1097/PRS.0b013e31829ad109.
5. Dorf DS, Curtin JW. Early cleft palate repair and speech outcome. Plast Reconstr Surg. 1982;70:74–81.
6. Ysunza A, et al. Speech outcome and maxillary growth in patients with unilateral complete cleft lip/palate operated on at 6 versus 12 months of age. Plast Reconstr Surg. 1998;102:675–9.
7. Friede H, Enemark H. Long-term evidence for favorable midfacial growth after delayed hard palate repair in UCLP patients. Cleft Palate Craniofac J. 2001;38:323–9. https://doi.org/10.1597/1545-1569_2001_038_0323_lteffm_2.0.co_2.
8. Farina R. Total unilateral harelip: correction of severe deformity of the palate & lips in a single operation; Le Mesurier's cheiloplasty & Veau-Ernst's gnatho-urano-staphyloplasty. Ann Chir Plast. 1958;3:199–205.
9. Kantar RS, et al. Single-stage primary cleft lip and palate repair: a review of the literature. Ann Plast Surg. 2018;81:619–23. https://doi.org/10.1097/SAP.0000000000001543.
10. Schweckendiek H. The problem of early and late surgery in congenital fissure of the of the lips and palate. Z Laryngol Rhinol Otol. 1951;30:51–6.

11. Schweckendiek W, Doz P. Primary veloplasty: long-term results without maxillary deformity. A twenty-five year report. Cleft Palate J. 1978;15:268–74.
12. Friede H, et al. Comparisons of facial growth in patients with unilateral cleft lip and palate treated by different regimens for two-stage palatal repair. Scand J Plast Reconstr Surg Hand Surg. 1999;33:73–81.
13. Olasoji HO, Hassan A, Ligali TO. Challenges of cleft care in Africa. Afr J Med Med Sci. 2009;38:303–10.
14. Smith DM, et al. The Pittsburgh Fistula classification system: a standardized scheme for the description of palatal fistulas. Cleft Palate Craniofac J. 2007;44:590–4. https://doi.org/10.1597/06-204.1.
15. Sie KC, et al. Sphincter pharyngoplasty: speech outcome and complications. Laryngoscope. 1998;108:1211–7.
16. Armour A, Fischbach S, Klaiman P, Fisher DM. Does velopharyngeal closure pattern affect the success of pharyngeal flap pharyngoplasty? Plast Reconstr Surg. 2005;115:45–52; discussion 53.
17. Gosain AK, Chim H, Sweeney WM. Double-opposing Z-Plasty for secondary surgical management of velopharyngeal insufficiency following primary furlow palatoplasty. Cleft Palate Craniofac J. 2018;55:706–10. https://doi.org/10.1177/1055665618756072.
18. Yamaguchi K, Lonic D, Lee CH, Yun C, Lo LJ. Modified furlow palatoplasty using small double-opposing Z-Plasty: surgical technique and outcome. Plast Reconstr Surg. 2016;137:1825–31. https://doi.org/10.1097/PRS.0000000000002181.
19. Timbang MR, et al. A systematic review comparing Furlow double-opposing Z-plasty and straight-line intravelar veloplasty methods of cleft palate repair. Plast Reconstr Surg. 2014;134:1014–22. https://doi.org/10.1097/PRS.0000000000000637.

# Palatal Fistulas and Repair

# 19

Ghulam Qadir Fayyaz and Muhammad Ashraf Ganatra

**Key Points**

- The two main goals of cleft palate repair are to create a barrier between nasal & oral cavities, and good speech production. Palatal fistula is an abnormal communication after cleft palate repair) between nasal and oral cavities.
- There are two problems with palatal fistula: nasal emission with distortion of voice and nasal regurgitation of liquids and food both of which can lead to social embarrassment and bad smell.
- Multiple fistula classifications exist. We favor a classification that incorporates location, size, and velopharyngeal competence.
- Effective fistula repair is based on separate reconstruction of the nasal mucosa as well as the oral mucosa, as well as reconstruction and retropositioning of the levator musculature, when possible.
- Key techniques include nasal turn-in flaps, mucoperiosteal flaps +/– radical palatine vessel dissection for increased reach, cheek mucosal or FAMM flaps, and tongue flap.
- For symptomatic fistulae, the goal should be not only to close the fistula but enable production of adequate speech.

## Introduction

The main objective of cleft palate repair is twofold: to create a barrier preventing secretions between nasal and oral cavities, and to create an airtight seal to facilitate speech production. Although a fairly rare complication in designated cleft centers in high-income countries, palatal fistulas are reported in up to 60% of palate repairs in low-resource settings [1, 5]. Type of cleft palate, width of the cleft, method of cleft palate repair, patient nutritional status, and expertise of the operating surgeon may be contributing factors [2]. Bilateral complete cleft palate is associated with greatest fistula risk [3]. Assessment and treatment of palatal fistulae is critical to attain good palatal structure and function [4]. Several classification systems have been described, each with advantages but limitations in elaborating the nature of the fistula, its impact on the function of the palate, the number of fistulae, fistula position, and the complexity of reconstruction required. In low-resource settings, because of the lack of proper facilities and resources, the variety of fistula types can be encountered [6]. Adequate fistula evaluation requires thorough symptom assessment including speech hypernasality, defining the extent of the fistula, assessment of palatal length and motion, and identifying reliable and well-vascularized options for tissue transposition. Repair of the nasal fistula should always be done by reconstructing both the nasal and oral mucosal layers, to reduce the chance of recurrence. Key techniques for fistula treatment include nasal mucosa turnover flaps (including vomer flap), mucoperiosteal flaps, local/random flaps, buccal myomucosal or FAMM flap, and tongue flap.

## Causes and Prevention of Fistulas

Fistula formation may relate to patient factors (type and width of palate, nutritional status), surgeon factors (method of repair, experience), and contextual factors (meticulousness of repair, lack of care continuity). Fistulas may be caused by a variety of factors (Table 19.1), but inadequate palatal tissue dissection and mobilization, coupled with closure under tension are often responsible. Patients at greatest risk for fistulae have bilateral complete cleft palate and wide

G. Q. Fayyaz (✉)
Plastic Surgery Services Institute of Medical Sciences, & CLAPP Hospital, Lahore, Pakistan

M. A. Ganatra
Department of Plastic Surgery, Dow University of Health Sciences, Karachi, Pakistan

© Springer Nature Switzerland AG 2021

J. W. Swanson, D. W. Low (eds.), *Global Cleft Care in Low-Resource Settings*, https://doi.org/10.1007/978-3-030-59105-2_19

**Table 19.1** Common procedures for fistula repair

| Tissue layer/ deficiency | Technique |
|---|---|
| Oral mucosa | Mucoperiosteal flap (ipsilateral or contralateral)<br>Buccal myomucosal flap<br>FAMM flap<br>Gingivobuccal sulcus flap (passed through alveolar cleft)<br>Tongue flap |
| Nasal mucosa | Turnover flap<br>Vomer flap |
| VP insufficiency | Palatal revision with intravelar veloplasty (levator muscle reconstruction and retropositioning)<br>Furlow's double opposing Z-plasty<br>Pharyngeal flap or pharyngoplasty |

(bilateral incomplete) cleft palates [3]. Most fistulae develop in first 7 days; however, sometimes due to doubtful blood supply, fistula may develop as late as 10–14 days.

**Potential Causes of Palatal Fistula**

1. Single-layer closure in the hard palate; no nasal layer closure, only oral layer closure done.
2. Difficulty in adequate dissection of nasal layer under the hard palate bone, which may lead to insufficient release and tight nasal layer closure.
3. Inadequate dissection of the mucoperiosteal flap on one or both sides, resulting in difficulty to bring the mucoperiosteal flaps comfortably in the midline.
4. Rough tissue handling especially to the medial edges.
5. Excessive use of cautery at the medial edges of mucoperiosteal flaps and near the pedicle.
6. Tight closure in the midline.
7. Suture knots are tied too tight; even if the tissues have been adequately released and the medial edges of the mucoperiosteal flaps are opposed to each other without any tension but the sutures knots are tied too tight, leading to exsanguination and later necrosis of the tissues in between the knots.
8. Postoperative severe infection.
9. If the child is a finger sucker, postoperative finger suction can lead to damage to the suture line and fistula formation.

There are several consequences of a fistula, including: nasal regurgitation, hypernasal speech, compromised dentition, and halting further cleft reconstruction (e.g., unable to tolerate alveolar bone grafting when a large fistula is present).

Both the problems can be very embarrassing, so a thorough examination needs to be carried out and an appropriate solution/plan is devised to close the fistula/improve the speech. Sometimes the fistula is there but may be asymptomatic, in that case it can be left as such.

Several perioperative measures may prevent a palatal fistula:

- Gentle tissue handling.
- Adequate dissection of the nasal layer and mucoperiosteal flaps on both sides, loose enough to bring both edges in the midline without any tension.
- Hand restraints postoperatively if the child is finger sucker.
- Use of natural honey postoperatively three times daily by a soft plastic spoon (avoiding water drinking for 15 minutes after each honey intake) may improve healing or decrease the size of small fistula, based on several small studies from Indonesia [12].

## Fistula Evaluation

### Symptoms and Examination

It is important to perform a thorough examination of the fistula. A simple illumination test using a nasopharyngoscope can be helpful for inspection of the fistula. The nasopharyngoscope also helps to evaluate soft palate mobility and the competency of the velopharyngeal (VP) closure.

To examine possible influences during speech, the fistula may be temporarily plugged, using a palatal plate, chewing gum, or dental wax. Speech samples can be recorded before and after plugging the fistula. If hypernasality decreases after plugging, the nasality is mainly caused by the fistula. However, in addition to fistula repair a period of speech therapy may be needed to unlearn VP dysfunction. On the other hand, if the hypernasality persists even after plugging, then an additional VP surgery should be considered. This simple method makes decision-making more algorithmic and effective.

The critical limit of fistula size that has an adverse effect on speech has been discussed by many authors. Many of them suggest that an area exceeding 4.5–5 mm$^2$ can badly affect the speech, which correlates to a diameter of 2–3 mm. Symptoms include hypernasality, audible nasal escape, and weakness of pressure consonants. Even a small fistula may also cause VP dysfunction or regurgitation, which is an embarrassing problem during socialization. Leakage of fluids and lodging of food particles can be troublesome for patients.

Fistula should be treated conservatively during early stages after the primary palate repair. No attempt should be made to repair it surgically as the tissues are edematous and friable and the stitches will not hold the tissue and it will cut through. Minimum time to wait for the fistula closure is 6–9 months after the previous surgery. Conservative management is advised for an asymptomatic fistula.

## Indications for and Timing of Fistula Repair

The two main symptoms that are indications for fistula repair are speech disturbance or nasal regurgitation. A third reason is when the fistula will interfere with needed surgery, such as alveolar bone grafting.

Some would argue that fistulas causing disturbance in speech should undergo early repair, whereas the closure of fistulas without any speech problems may be delayed, if possible, until completion of orthodontic maxillary arch expansion, and be combined with secondary alveolar bone grafting. Some authors have reported that orthodontic treatment can cause disruption of the repaired fistula, thus repair after palatal expansion may be optimal to prevent recurrence [10]. However, the psychological and social impact of the symptomatic palatal fistula calls for early surgical treatment. We usually opt for an early closure for a symptomatic fistula, at least 6–9 months after palatal repair.

If a patient with palatal fistula is aged between 12 and 15 months, it is difficult to make any objective assessment about speech outcome. Our policy is to close the fistula 6–9 months after previous surgery so that there is no more nasal regurgitation. Then at 4 years of age, an objective nasopharyngoscope or videofluoroscope examination can be performed to evaluate speech.

## Fistula Classification

Ohsumi classifies three sizes of fistula (A: <2 mm, B: 2–5 mm, and C: >5 mm); however, we find in practice most fistula seen in low-resource settings are larger than 5 mm. Another classification described by Richardson and Agni [13] distinguishes small (area < 50 mm$^2$) from medium (area 50–100 mm$^2$) size and hard from soft palate in location. Building on work by Cohen [1] and Folk [8] to classify fistulae based on location, the Pittsburgh Classification system [9] categorizes fistulae at seven different zones starting from the uvula to the alveolus (Fig. 19.1). While this is perhaps the most widely used and comprehensive classification system used today, limitations include its orientation to palatal midline, relation of the incisive foramen (which is difficult to visualize when a large cleft is present with no bone) and the abbreviated incorporation of palatal function to a suffix, +/−.

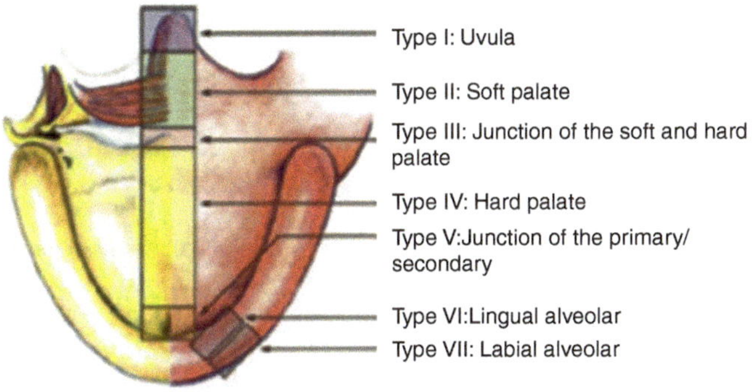


**Fig. 19.1** Pittsburgh Palatal Fistula Classification System

Despite these advances, consistently classifying the exact nature of the fistula, the number of fistulae (single or multiple), fistula location, its impact on the function of the palate and speech, and the complexity of reconstruction required is an ongoing challenge [4]. A classification is important to communicate among the interdisciplinary team and other surgeon colleagues, as well as to track outcomes to refine treatment schemes.

## Pakistan Comprehensive Fistula Classification

Given these challenges, based on an assessment of over 2500 fistula repairs by the author's team, a comprehensive fistula classification has been developed and reported (14) (Fig. 19.2). It includes four components:

- Location (L): Distinguishing location along the palate, laterality, multiple, and extent
- Size (S)
- Velopharyngeal competency (V)
- Dehiscence (D), if present

### Location (L)

A fistula present under the lip, going into the nose(it is usually due to failure to close the nasal floor during cleft lip repair) should never be called as oro-nasal fistula to avoid confusion. We better call it as labio-nasal fistula which clearly means that it starts under the lip and goes into the nose.

During repair of the complete cleft palate, some surgeons usually close the nasal layer up to the anterior end of the hard palate but leave the cleft of the alveolus as an intended fistula. However, we better call it as palato-alveolar communication (Fig. 19.3).

Fistulas are characterized by location—from anteriorly (alveolus) to posteriorly (uvula) in six zones along the palate, including laterality (Fig. 19.3). Subtotal or multiple fistulas are denoted as such. A fistula is called a midline fistula if

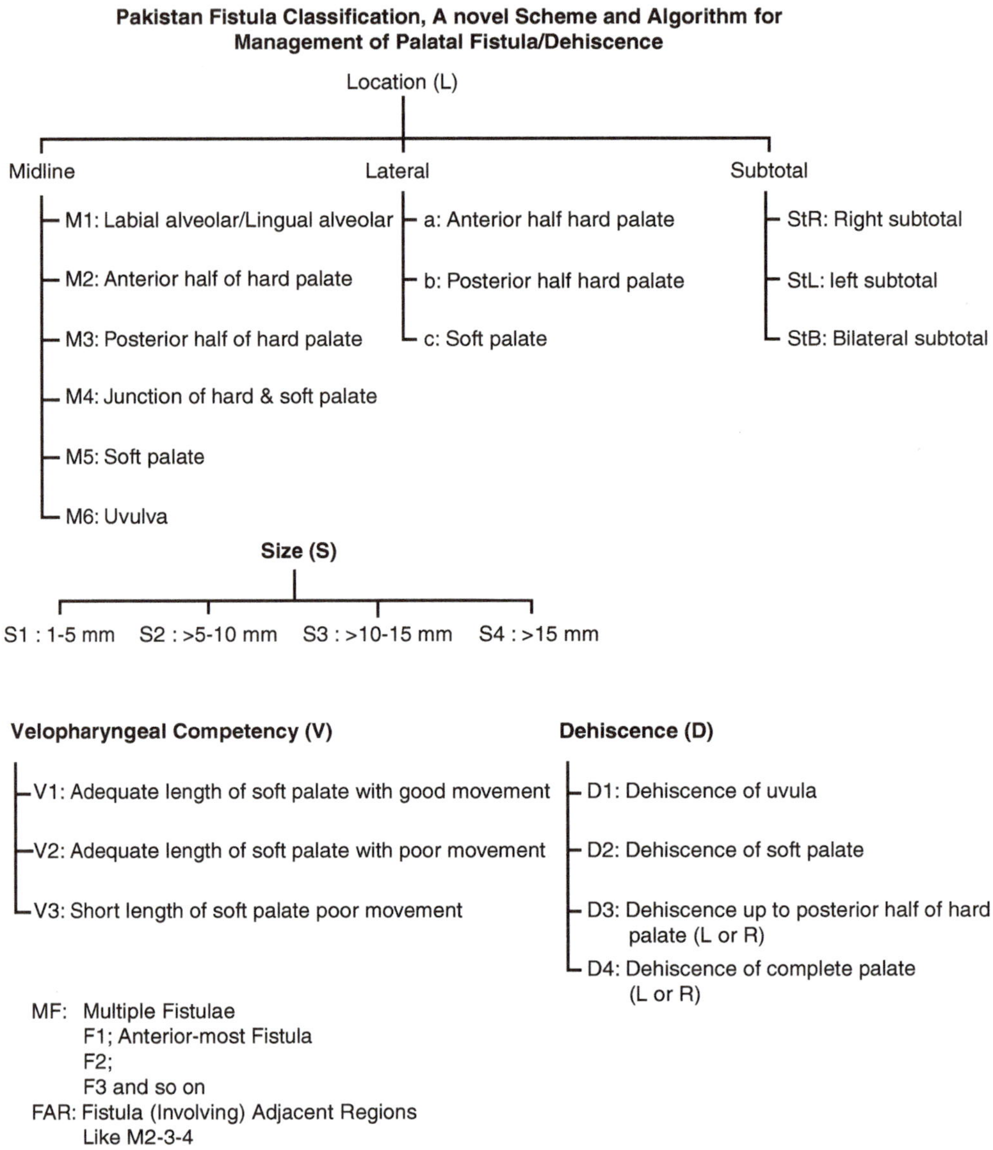


**Fig. 19.2** Description of different types of fistula and dehiscence as per Pakistan Comprehensive Fistula Classification System

more than 50% of its transverse diameter is within 10 mm of the midline (5 mm on either side).

Fistulas around the alveolus (M1) warrant clarification. Inadequate closure of the nasal or oral mucosa between the alveolar segments may leave an *unrepaired alveolar cleft* or a *naso-alveolar* or *palate-alveolar* fistula, which can be closed at the time of alveolar bone grafting. However, if the patient is symptomatic (nasal regurgitation, hypernasal speech), it can be repaired earlier. Further, inadequate closure of the nasal floor anterior to the alveolus at the time of cleft lip repair can leave a *naso-labial* fistula. Because these involve the alveolus, they are distinguished from palatal (oro-nasal) fistulas.

Sometimes the midline fistula is longer, involving two or more midline zones, it is then called FAR (fistula adjacent regions), connoted for instance as M2–3 if involving the posterior hard palate and hard-soft junction.

If an anterior fistula extends from the midline to the lateral side and involves 50% or more of the hard palate, it is called a subtotal fistula, and can be unilateral or bilateral. These fistulae indicate damage to either one or both greater palatine arteries (during previous surgery), resulting in loss of anterior palatal tissues (Fig. 19.4).

Figures 19.5, 19.6, 19.7, 19.8, 19.9, 19.10, 19.11, 19.12, 19.13, 19.14, 19.15, 19.16, and 19.17 show different patients having different types of midline fistula, FAR (fistula adjacent regions), lateral fistula, and subtotal fistula.

## Size

Largest fistula diameter is used to classify size, with increasing size generally indicating more difficult repair.

- *S1* = 1–5 mm
- *S2* = >5–10 mm

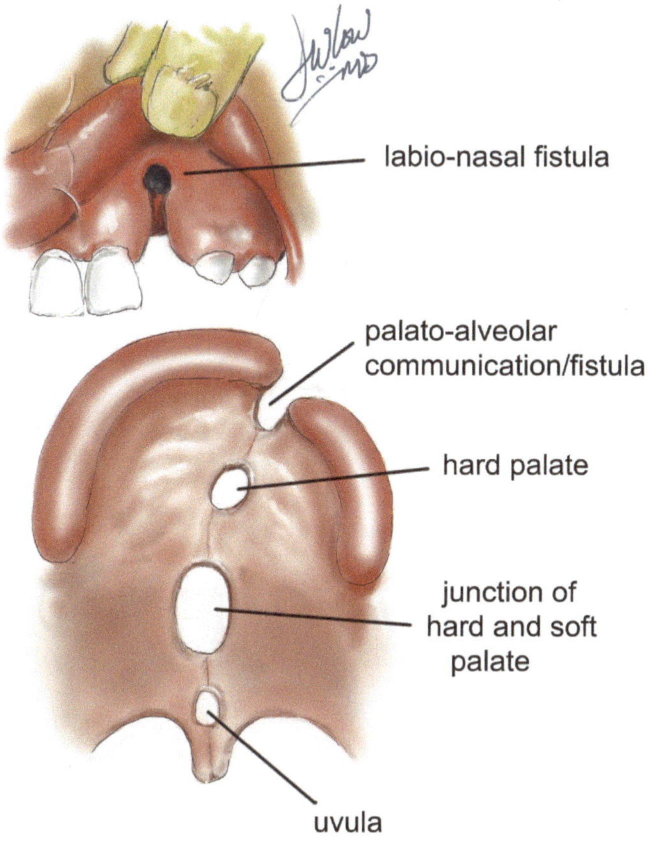


**Fig. 19.3** Location of different fistulae in the palate and under the lip

- *S3* = > 10–15 mm
- *S4* = > 15 mm to any large size

## Velopharyngeal Competence

The most important function of the palate is good speech production. If the speech is good in the presence of a symptomatic fistula, closing the hole in the palate is all that needs to be done. But if we close the hole in the palate without knowing the functional status of the palate, the patient's speech may still not improve. Thus evaluation by a speech language pathologist should always be performed and only then is the management plan finalized so that not only the fistula is closed but the speech improves as well.

Function of the palate is categorized into three types:

- *V1* = Palate length is adequate and there is velopharyngeal competence
- *V2* = Palate length is adequate but there is velopharyngeal incompetence
- *V3* = Palate length is inadequate and there is velopharyngeal incompetence

## Multiple Fistulae

MF (multiple fistulae) are written as F1(anterior-most) and then F2 or F3 posteriorly. The location and size of each fistula is described uniquely, although velopharyngeal

**Fig. 19.4** Schematic diagram showing location of different fistulae as per Pakistan Comprehensive Fistula Classification System

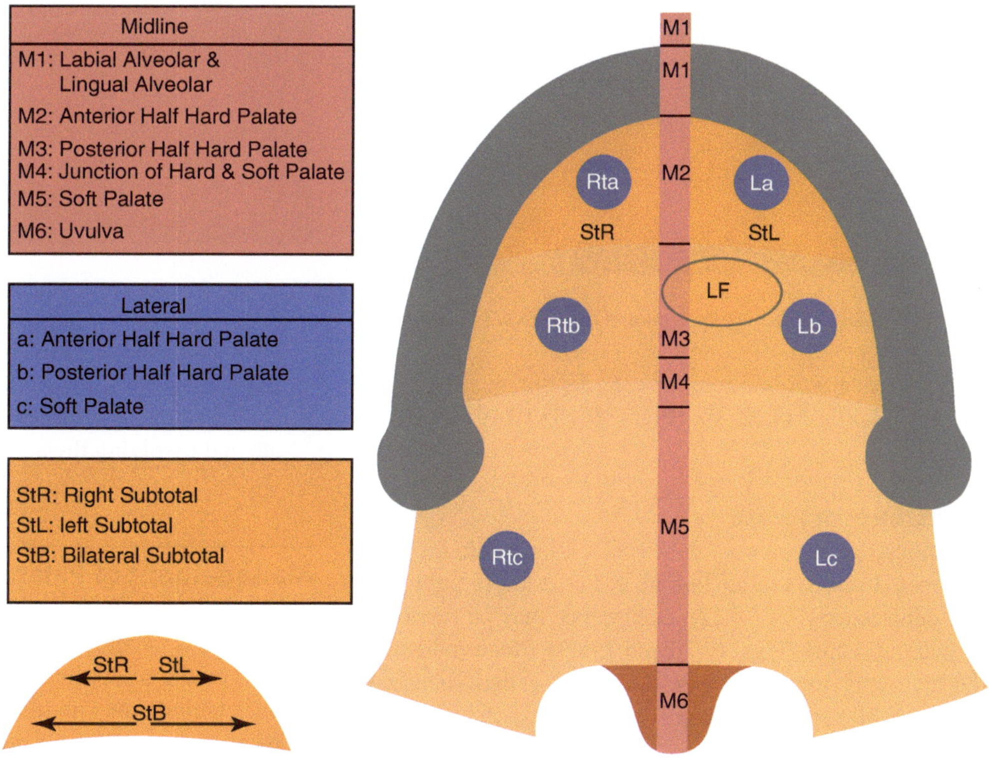


**LF:** A fidtula involving the midline as well as lateral side of the palate and if more than 50% of the transverse width of the fistula is away from the midline, it will be labeled as lateral fistula (LF).

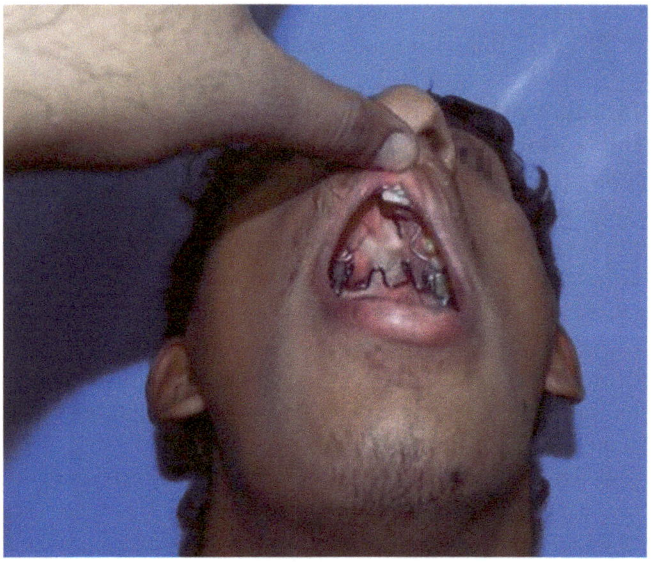

**Fig. 19.5** A young patient showing palatal fistula at M1 and M2 location

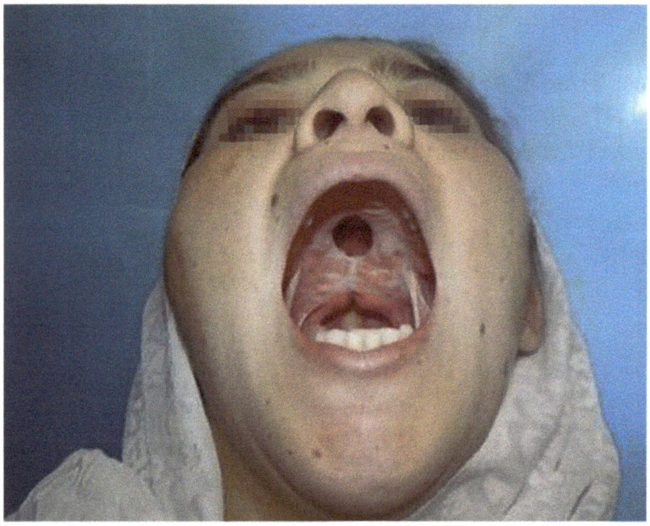

**Fig. 19.6** *Young girl having large palatal fistula at M3 location*

incompetence will be same for each fistula, e.g., MF: - F1; M3 S2 V3, F2; M4 S1 V3 (Figs. 19.18, 19.19, 19.20, and 19.21).

### Dehiscence of Palate

Classification of extent of dehiscence after palate repair has not been described in the literature, but is important to classify dehiscence (Fig. 19.22). Dehiscence may be found with or without fistula (Figs. 19.20 and 19.23). Please note that if the uvula is intact, it should not be called dehiscence (Figs. 19.24, 19.25, 19.26, and 19.27).

- D1 = Dehiscence of uvula
- D2 = Dehiscence of uvula and extending into soft palate

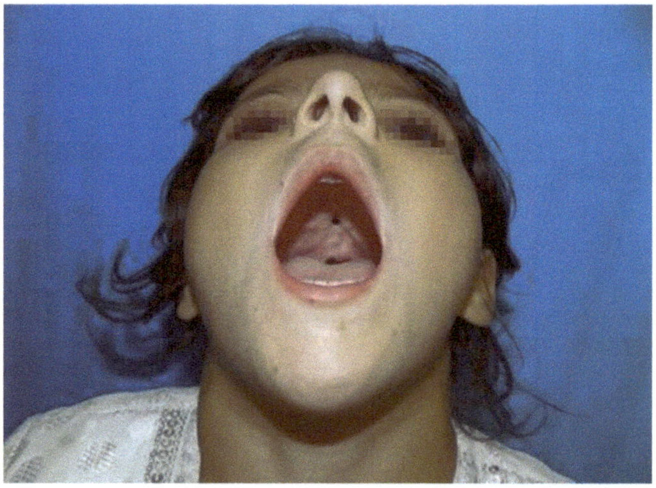

**Fig. 19.7** *A young girl having palatal fistula at M4 location*

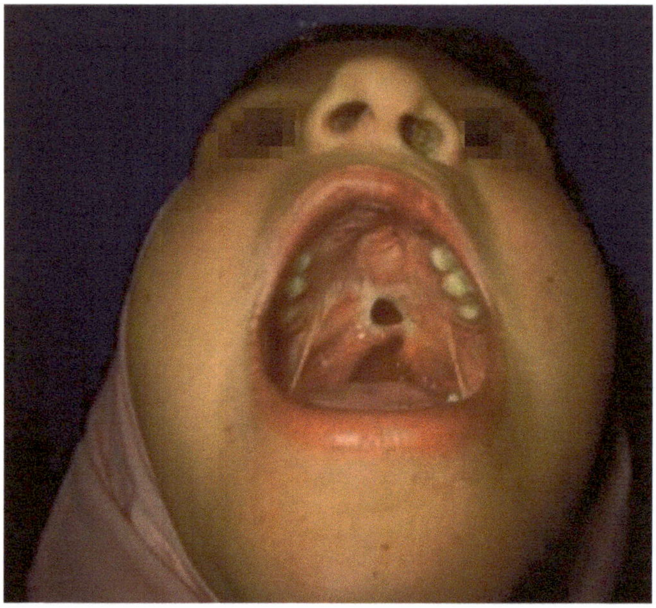

**Fig. 19.8** *A young girl having palatal fistula at M5 location*

- D3 = Dehiscence of uvula, soft palate and extending into hard palate (posterior half only)
- D4 = Complete dehiscence of uvula, soft palate, hard palate and involving the alveolus as well.

## Management of Palatal Fistula

Most fistulae occur in the midline and are the result of excess tension on the suture line. Factors affecting success of fistula closure include the site of fistula, size of fistula, and degree of palate scarring (due to previous surgeries). The difficulty index is greater for transversely placed fistula, those in anterior hard palate area, after bilateral complete cleft palate

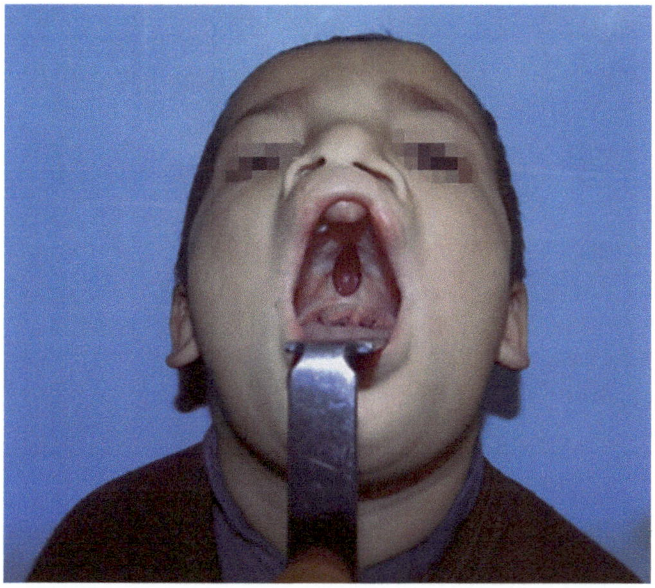

Fig. 19.9 *Patient having FAR (fistula adjacent regions) M2–3-4*

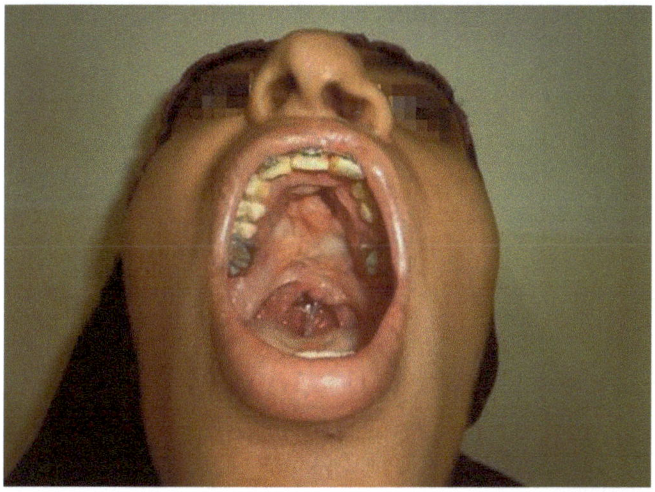

Fig. 19.10 *A young girl having lateral palatal fistula at La, in anterior half of the hard palate on left side*

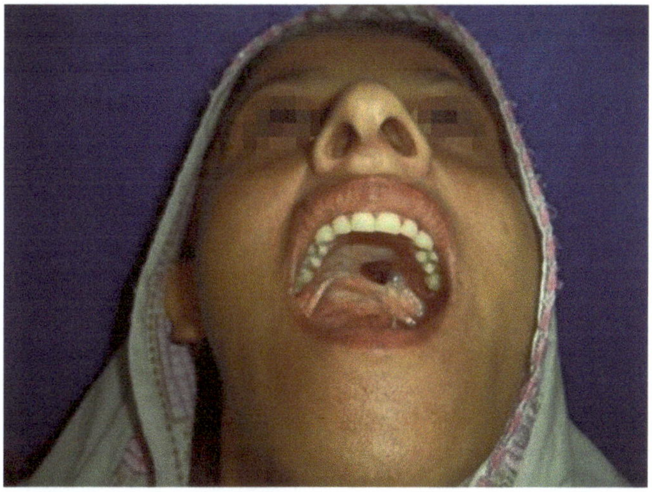

Fig. 19.11 *A young girl having lateral palatal fistula at Lb, in posterior half of the hard palate on left side*

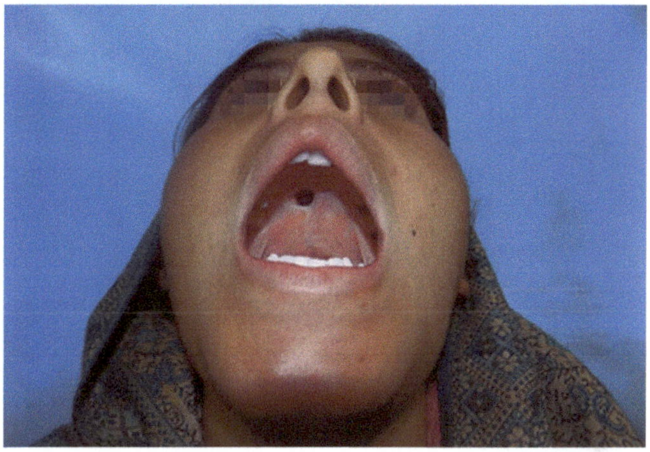

Fig. 19.12 *A young girl having lateral palatal fistula at Rb, in posterior half of the hard palate on right side*

repair, and previously failed attempt to close the fistula. Even after fistula repair, recurrence rates can be as high as 96% c.When well planned and executed, surgical management is generally the optimal treatment for oro-nasal fistulas. Though in very difficult cases or patients with severe cardiac abnormalities, good obturators (if needed with speech bulbs) can be made to plug the fistula very effectively.The principle of fistula surgery is to perform multiple-layered closure so as to minimize tension on any single layer and provide redundancy if there is inadequate healing of one layer. In the hard palate, this is generally two layers (oral and nasal mucosa), and in the soft palate, three layers (oral mucosa, levator muscle, and nasal mucosa). Extensive dissection and undermining are often needed to enable tension-free closure, given previous surgical scar.There are several appropriate techniques depending on fistula characteristics, from local flaps to free tissue transfer (Table 19.1). Emphasis should always be on good speech production and not just closing the hole in the palate. A turn-in flap for nasal layer closure and oral layer cover provided by mucoperiosteal flaps or transposition flap from buccal, vestibular, or facial regions can be used, or tissues from the nasal cavity, septum, or turbinate. One should be aware of growth disturbance, donor site morbidity, or visible scars. Our practice is to use local palatal mucosa or mucoperiosteal flap tissue to cover the defect (as replacing like tissue with like tissue) in most of the cases. With an extremely large fistula, heavily scarred palate, and contracted dentoalveolar arch, orthodontic palatal expansion may be required first, followed by a large tongue flap or free tissue

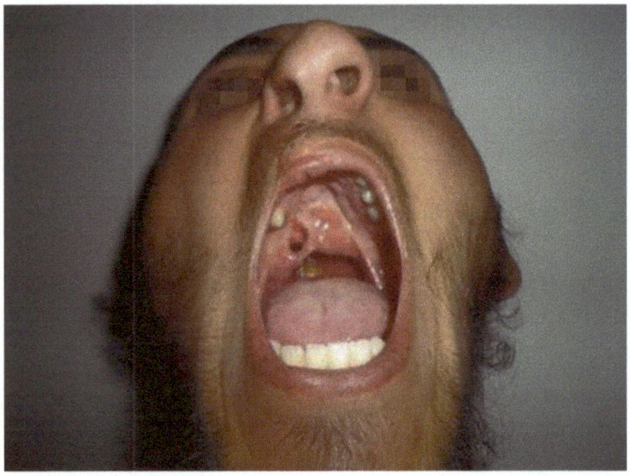

**Fig. 19.13** *A young man having lateral palatal fistula at Rc, in lateral portion of soft palate on right side*

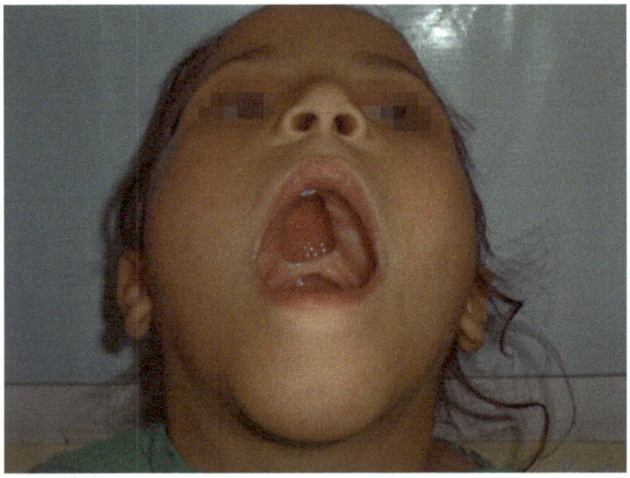

**Fig. 19.14** Patient having StR (subtotal right) fistula. This is due to damage to the greater palatine artery on right side during previous surgery

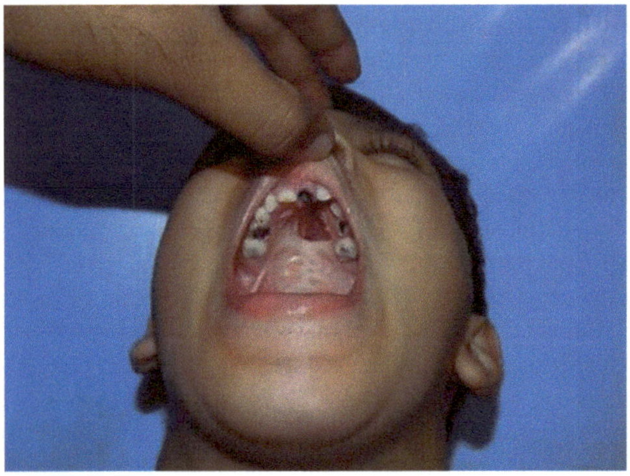

**Fig. 19.15** Patient having StL (subtotal left) fistula. This is due to damage to the greater palatine artery on left side during previous surgery

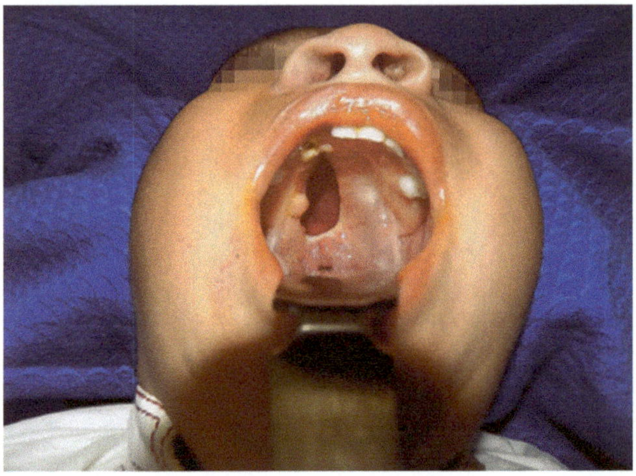

**Fig. 19.16** Patient having StR (subtotal right) fistula. This is due to damage to the greater palatine artery on right side during previous surgery

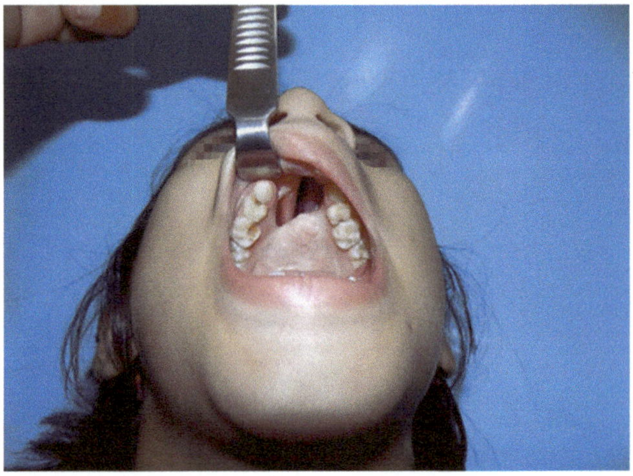

**Fig. 19.17** A young girl having StB (subtotal bilateral) fistula. This is due to damage to the greater palatine artery on both sides during previous surgery

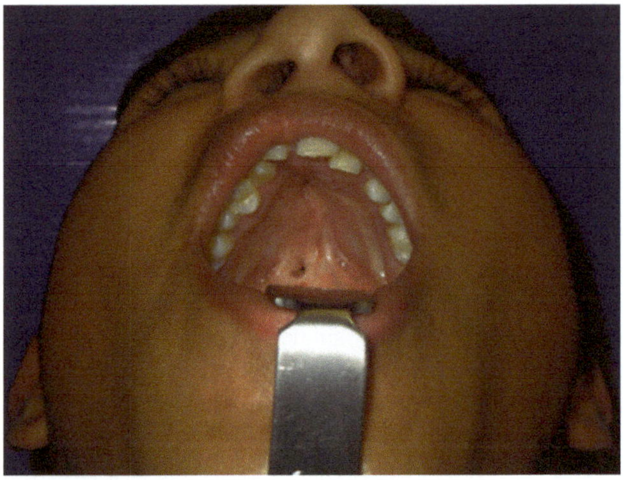

**Fig. 19.18** A patient with multiple fistulae, MF: F1 is the anterior-most fistula which is M2, F2 is the fistula at the junction of the hard and soft palate M4

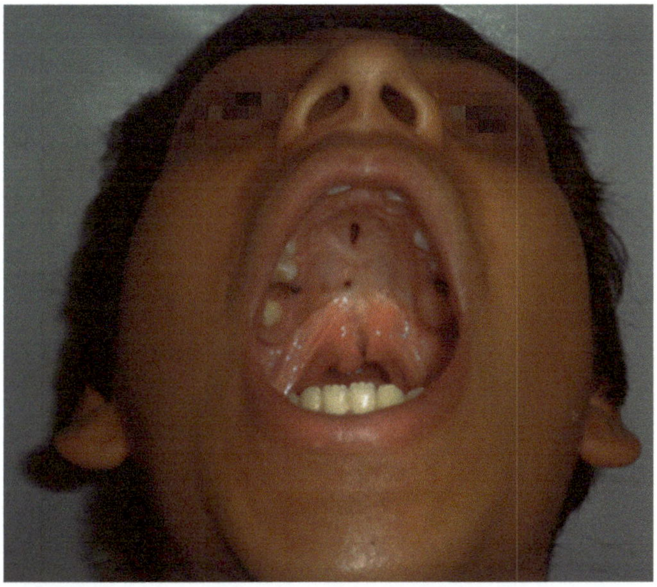

Fig. 19.19 A patient with multiple fistulae, MF: F1 is the anterior-most fistula which is M2, F2 is the fistula at the posterior half of the hard palate in the midline which is M3

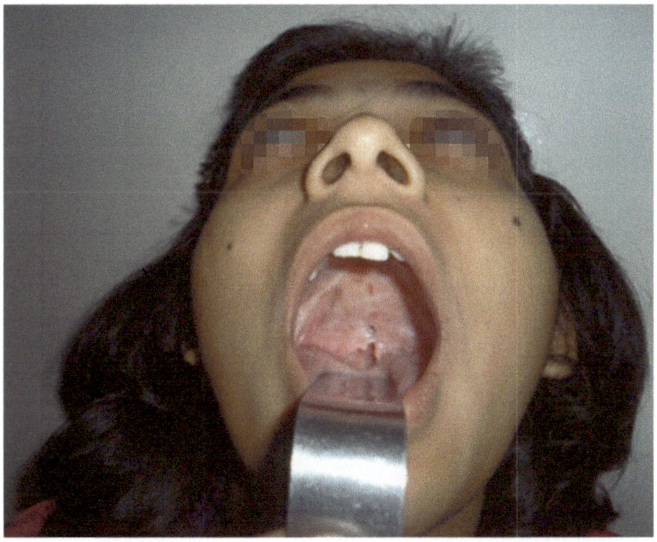

Fig. 19.20 A patient with multiple fistulae, MF: F1 is the anterior-most fistula which is M2, F2 is the fistula in the soft palate area which is M5 and there is dehiscence of the uvula which is D1

transfer. Radial forearm free flap has been used commonly for large palatal fistula.

## Turnover Flap

Also called a "turn-in flaps," are primarily used to approximate or reconstruct nasal mucosa.

These are developed as 3–5 mm (or sometimes more) margins of tissue around the edges of the fistula (Fig. 19.28).

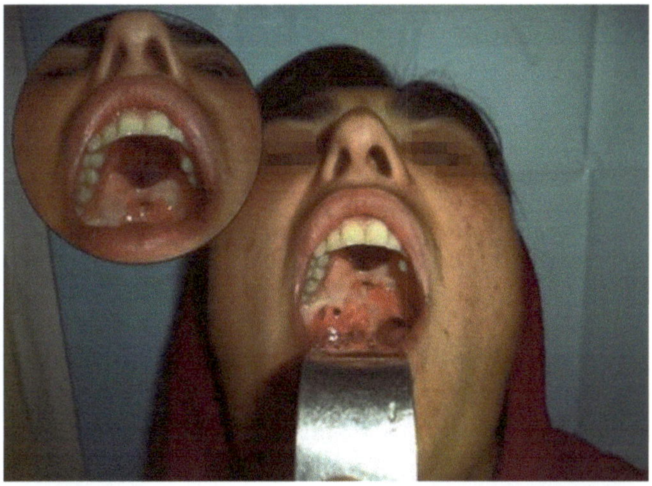

Fig. 19.21 A patient with multiple fistulae, MF: F1 is StB (subtotal bilateral) involving the anterior portion of hard palate on both sides. F2 is the fistula at the posterior half of the hard palate in the midline which is M3. F3 is the fistula in the lateral part of the soft palate on the right side which is Rc

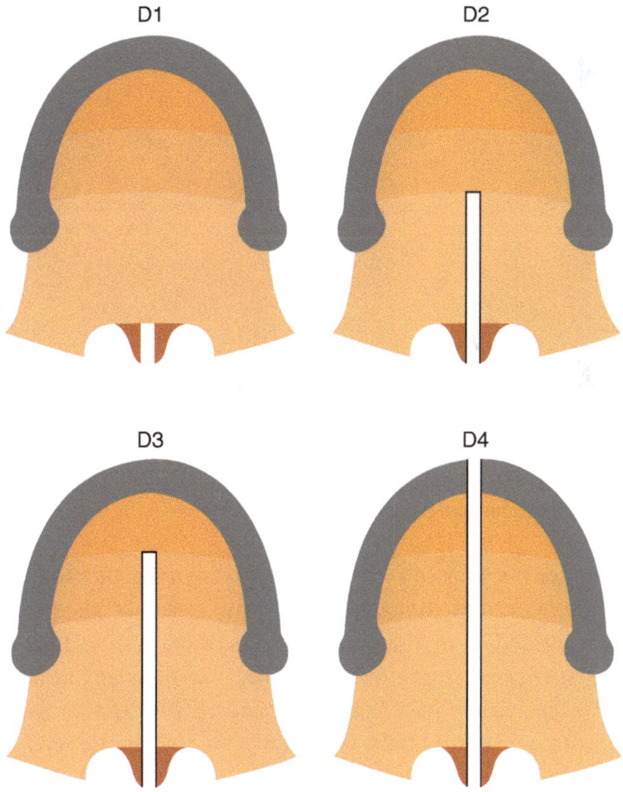


Fig. 19.22 Schematic diagram showing the different types of dehiscence; from D1 to D4

Extreme care should be taken to ensure that dissection at the outer margins of the turn-in flaps is on the bone/cartilage, so that the periosteum or perichondrium is raised with the flaps. One can use the tip of a needle, pressed against

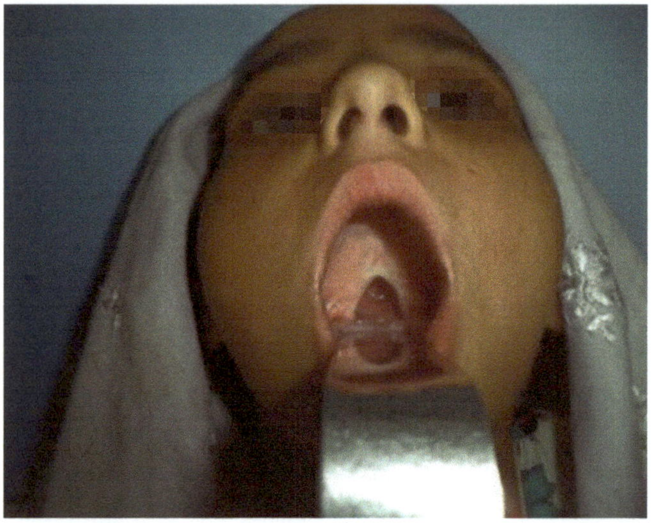

**Fig. 19.23** Patient having dehiscence of the uvula and soft palate, D2

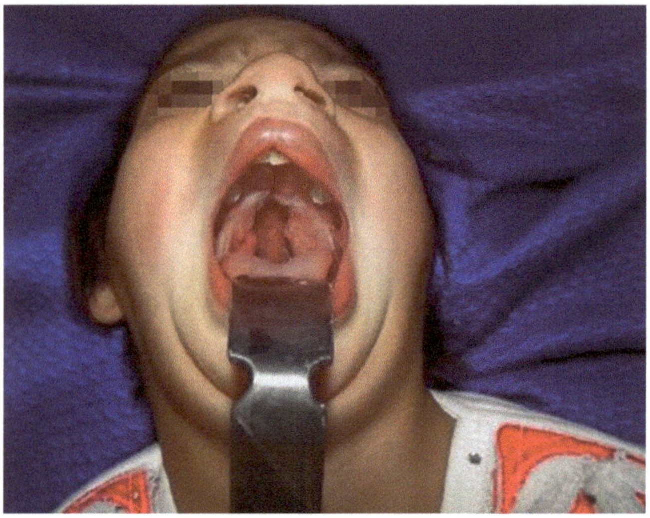

**Fig. 19.24** Patient having dehiscence of the uvula, soft palate and posterior half of the hard palate, D3

the outer margins of the turn-in flaps, to make sure that the needle is onto the bone. Otherwise more tissues need to be incorporated along the outer margins of the turn-in flaps to give sufficient strength. Mobilizing the flaps in the sub-periosteal or sub-perichondrial space enables robust tissue recruitment, and should continue until the tissues can be brought medially and approximated to one another with minimal tension. Nasal layer closure is by polyglactin sutures, interrupted or continuous, though our preference is always continuous sutures as it saves both time and sutures (Fayyaz GQ, 2018). Nasal layer closure suture line should be covered by an oral mucosal flap/s, such as mucoperiosteal flaps, buccal sulcus mucosal flap, buccinator flap, tongue flap, or a free flap (Figs. 19.29, 19.30, 19.31, and 19.32).

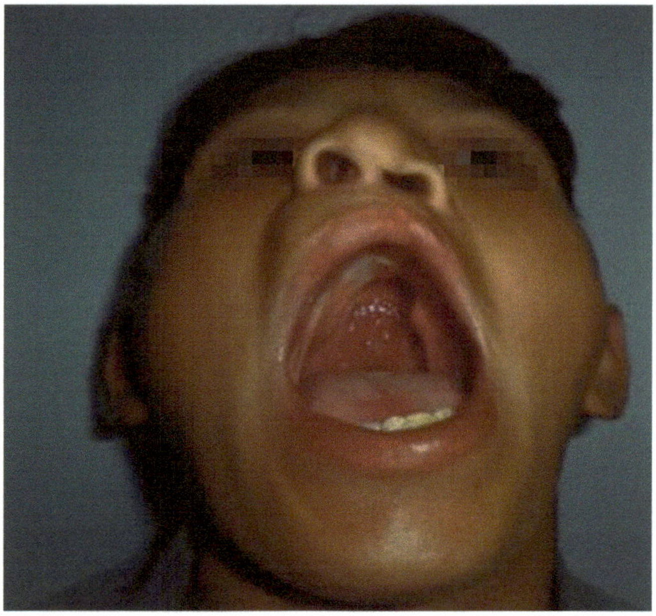

**Fig. 19.25** Patient having dehiscence of the uvula, soft palate and posterior half of the hard palate, D3 as there is more damage to the palatal tissues on the left side, so we label it as D3-L

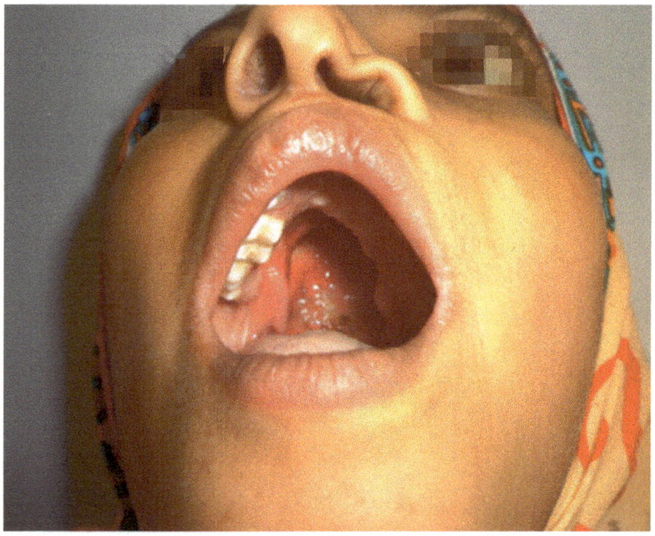

**Fig. 19.26** Patient having dehiscence of the uvula, soft palate and posterior half of the hard palate, D3 as there is more damage to the palatal tissues on the right side, so we label it as D3-R

## Mucoperiosteal Flap

This flap is composed of palatal mucosal tissue and the underlying periosteum, and is the workhorse of primary palate repair, during which it is reflected away from the palatine process of the maxilla.

Mucoperiosteal flaps can be bipedicled (on the ascending palatine branch of facial artery, lesser palatine artery and greater palatine vessels) or unipedicled (on the greater palatine vessels). In incomplete cleft palate, mucoperiosteal flaps are often bipedicled, while in complete cleft palate cases, the mucoperiosteal flap most of the times is cut anteriorly and based mainly on greater palatine vessels (Fig. 19.33).

*Radical dissection of greater palatine vessels* increases mobility of the mucoperiosteal flaps, so that both the flaps can be approximated in the midline without any tension. This procedure is beneficial in wider palates and is crucial in all secondary (previously operated) palatal repairs [11].

When the mucoperiosteal flap is elevated away from the hard palate, attention is given to the release of greater palatine vessels, which are located just anterolateral to the posterior end of the bony palate. We use a 15-number blade to separate the greater palatine vessels from the undersurface of the lateral portion of the mucoperiosteal flap (Figs. 19.31 and 19.32). There is no stringent minimum or maximum extent of the radical dissection away from the mucoperiosteal flap, rather, the idea is to make the mucoperiosteal flap mobile enough to be moved medially to gently approximate the opposite flap. So, in very young kids, 10 mm dissection may be quite enough; however in adult palates or wide palates, sometimes 20 mm or more dissection may be needed. Now if the mucoperiosteal flaps still cannot be brought to midline without tensions, one can incise the soft tissues medial to the pedicle, using surgical blade no.11. This will result in complete release of the pedicle, and so the mucoperiosteal flaps can be moved further medially. Although it has been described by many authors, to do osteotomy of the palatine bone at the greater palatine foramen to enhance the movement of the greater palatine vessels, we did not have to fracture the bone at the greater palatine foramen to further release the vessels (if we follow the above steps), in the last 15 years.

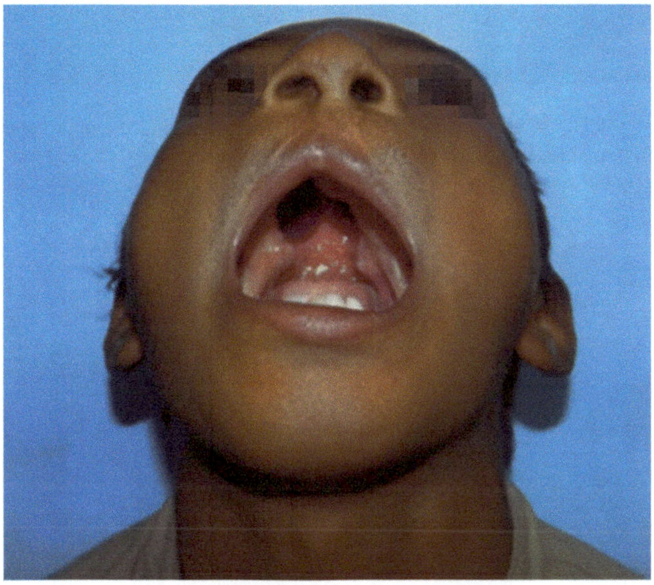

Fig. 19.27 Patient having dehiscence of the uvula, soft palate and posterior half of the hard palate, D3 as there is more extensive damage to the palatal tissues on the right side, so we label it as D3-R

Radical dissection of the greater palatine vessels should be done under direct visualization (by elevating a unipedicled mucoperiosteal flap, Fig. 19.34) by those inexperienced in these maneuvers. With more and more experience, this procedure can be employed in Langenbeck procedure as well.

**Levator Retropositioning** In a normal Palate, levator veli palatini muscles lie horizontally, with the right& left sides joining each other to make a levator sling. This levator sling has a key role in the speech production.

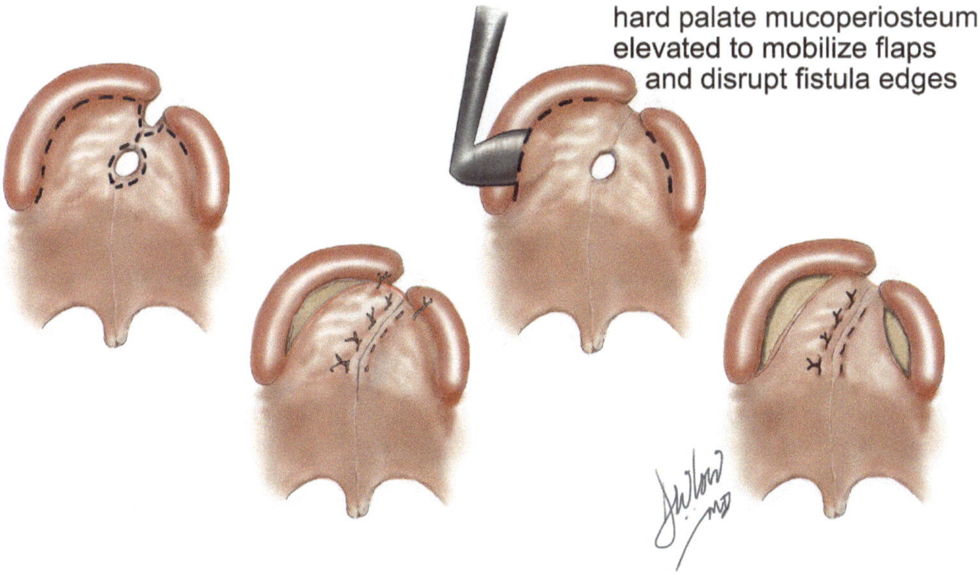


Fig. 19.28 Turn-in flaps for nasal layer closure and mucoperiosteal flaps for oral layer closure

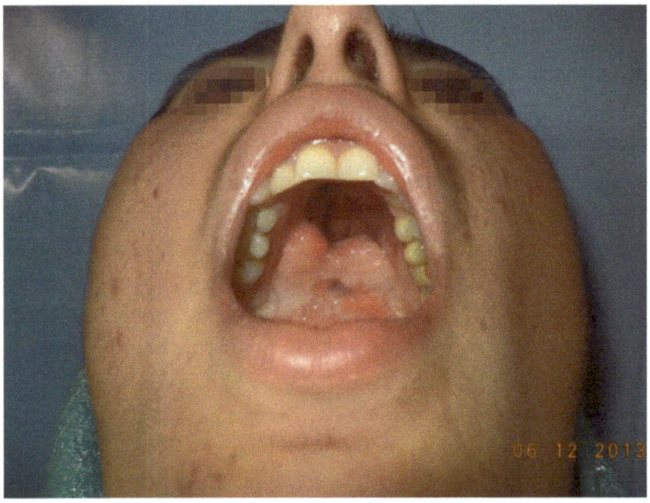


**Fig. 19.29** Subtotal bilateral fistula & S4, Vomer can be seen in the midlinf

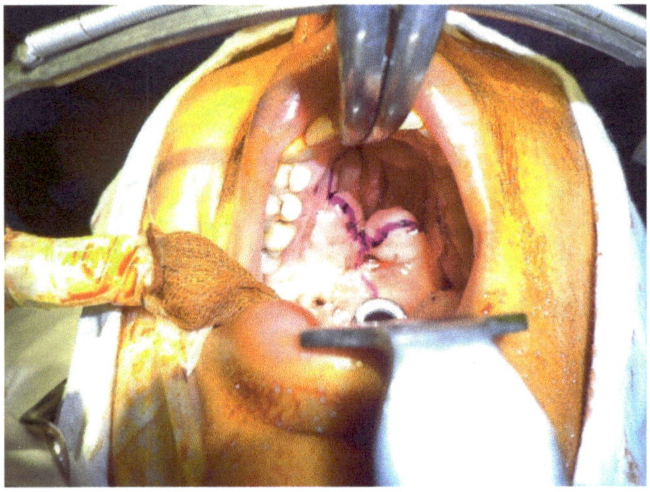

**Fig. 19.30** Marking for turn-in flaps

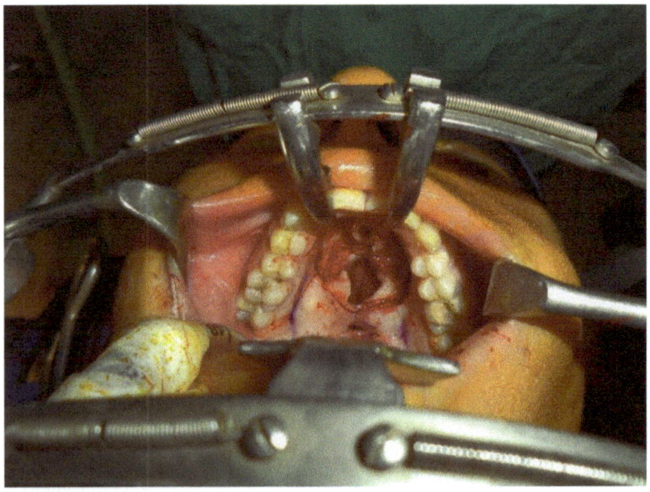

**Fig. 19.31** Turn-in flaps being mobilized away from the bone (anteriorly and bilaterally) and posteriorly, from the palate, to the midline for nasal layer closure

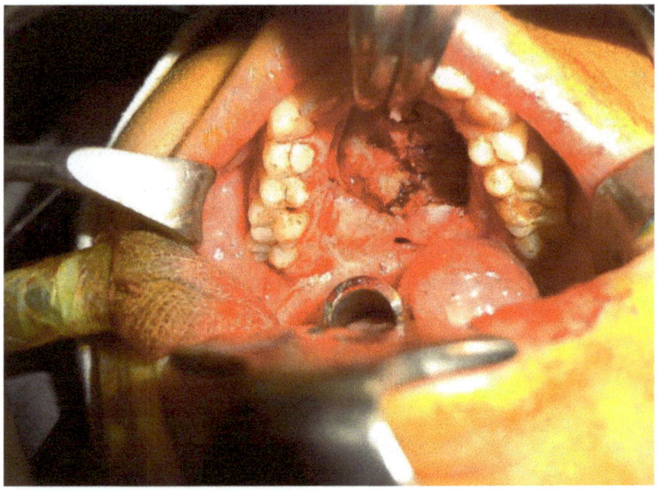

**Fig. 19.32** Turn-in flaps have been adequately mobilized and brought in the midline to be sutured together. Nasal layer has been closed properly but comfortably

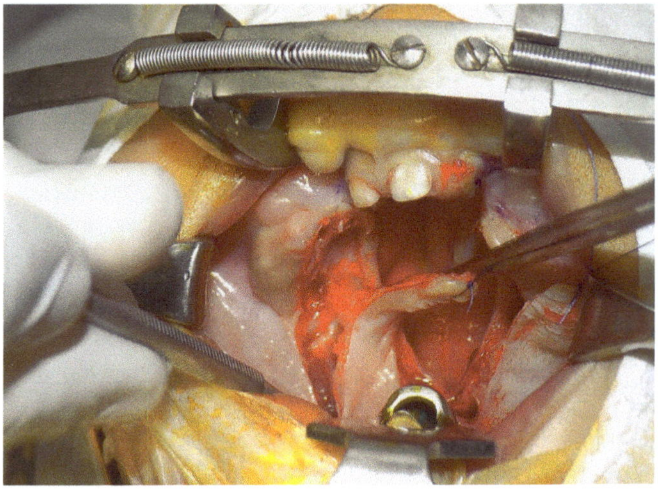

**Fig. 19.33** A patient with bilateral cleft palate, right mucoperiosteal flap is elevated off the palatine shelf

In a cleft palate patient, levators do not lie horizontally to make a levator sling. Rather the levators are directed obliquely upwards (anteriorly) to the palatine aponeurosis on both sides of the cleft (Fig. 19.33). This abnormal attachment of the levators is responsible for faulty speech production. Unless the levators are dissected away from the palatine aponeurosis and then shifted from oblique to transverse direction to reconstruct the levator sling, speech will not be normal (Figs. 19.35 and 19.36).

We always use three sutures to approximate the levators. First of all, we pass a stitch from the middle of the right levator complex and then take the bite of the right nasal mucosa near the uvula and then left nasal mucosa near the uvula. Lastly, the needle passes through the middle of the left levator complex and so the knot is tied. The idea is to change the orientation of Levators from oblique(Abnormal) to transverse(Normal)

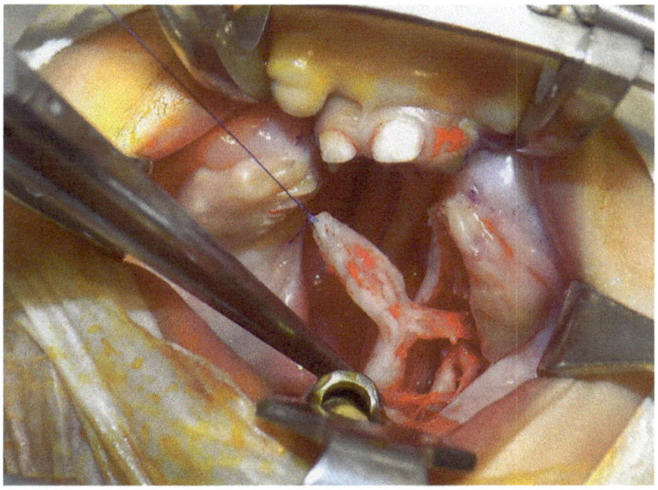

Fig. 19.34 Left mucoperiosteal flap elevated off the palatine shelf and radical dissection of the pedicle in a bilateral complete cleft palate patient

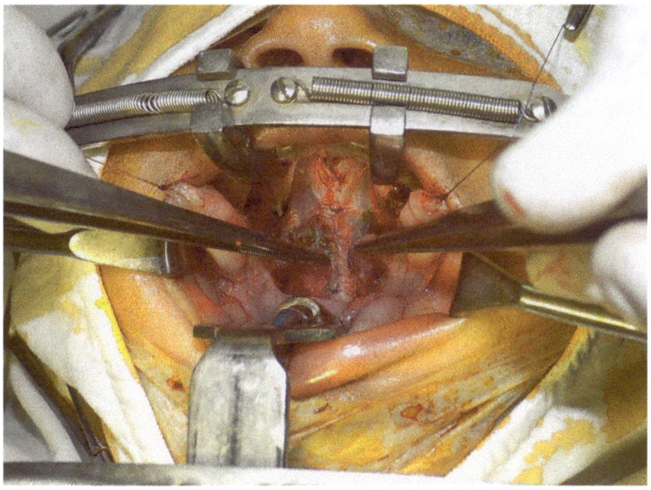

Fig. 19.36 Levators have been dissected away from the nasal layer on both sides

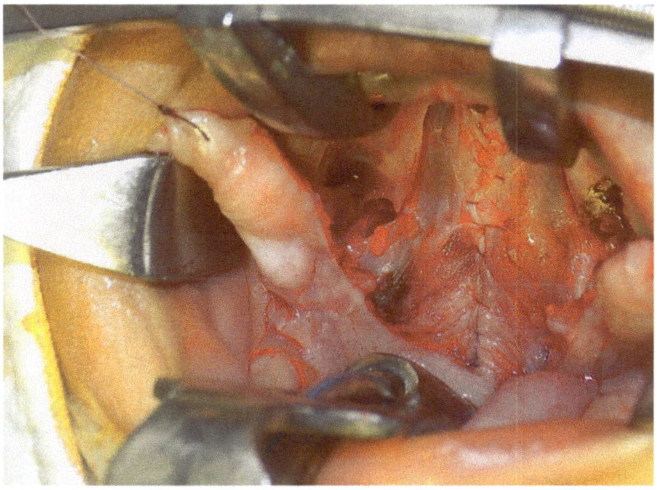

Fig. 19.35 Palatal muscles lying obliquely and going upwards, anteriorly

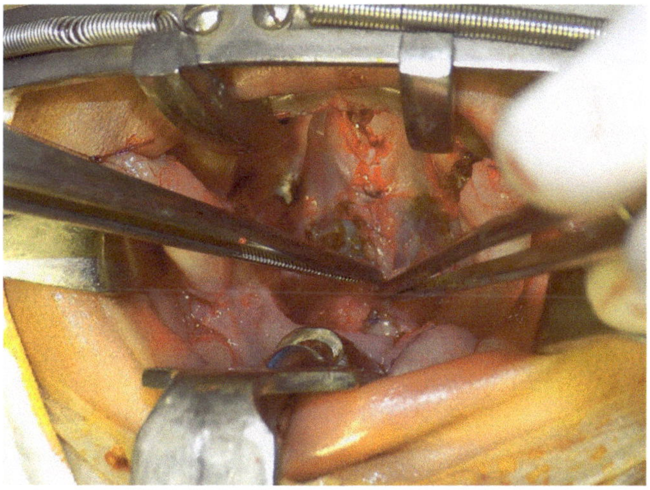

Fig. 19.37 Levators can be approximated comfortably to each other after dissection

(Fig. 19.37). Two more sutures (mattress) are applied: one anterior and another posterior to the first suture (Fig. 19.38).

## Ginvigobuccal Sulcus Flap

Repair of the anterior palate/nasal floor in the alveolar cleft can be performed directly during primary lip/palate repair with tissue of the nasal floor and/or vomer. However, in previously operated lip/palate patients in whom this is not reconstructed, a naso-alveolar fistula is present and the tissues are tight and scarce. If an alveolar cleft is present, nasal layer closure can use local tissues on both sides of the alveolus (vomer flap medially and lateral nasal flap laterally) (Fig. 19.37). Oral layer cover can be provided in two ways: by advancing the mucoperiosteal flap anteriorly (which may not be possible in many of the cases) and by gingivobuccal sulcus mucosal flap (Fig. 19.38). This flap can be raised from left or right side but will be based superior to the alveolus so that it can be turned comfortably into the alveolus defect. Buccal sulcus mucosal flap is taken from the lateral portion of the buccal sulcus and then turned postero-medially to the cover the nasal layer suture line at the alveolus and most anterior palate (Figs. 19.39, 19.40, and 19.41).

## Premaxilla Gingival Flap

A defect adjacent to the premaxilla in a bilateral cleft can similarly be reconstructed with a premaxillary gingival lining flaps and then by bilateral mucoperiosteal flaps (Fig. 19.42) or buccal sulcus mucosal flaps.

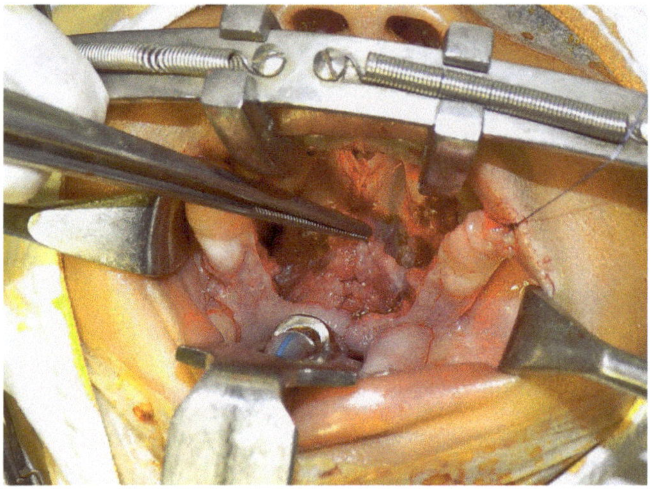

Fig. 19.38 The repositioning of the levator sling from an oblique to transverse orientation not only serves to create a dynamic velopharyngeal sphincter for nasopharyngeal closure and speech production but also serves to lengthen the soft palate

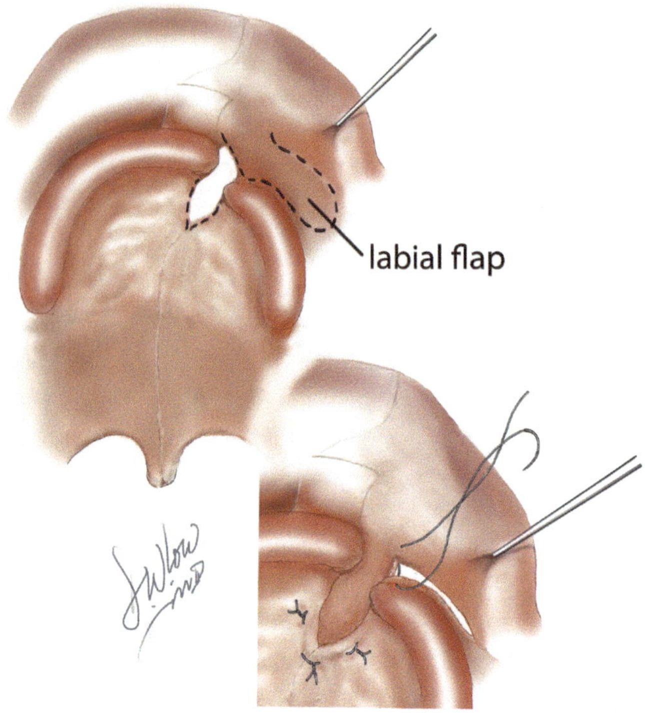


Fig. 19.39 Turn-in flap for nasal layer closure and buccal sulcus mucosal flap for oral layer closure

## Tongue Flap

Large anterior palatal defects are usually the result of trauma, cancer ablation, or failed cleft palate repair. Majority of these defects can be covered by re-repair of the palate; by elevation and approximation of both mucoperisteal flaps after nasal layer closure has been closed by turn-in flaps.

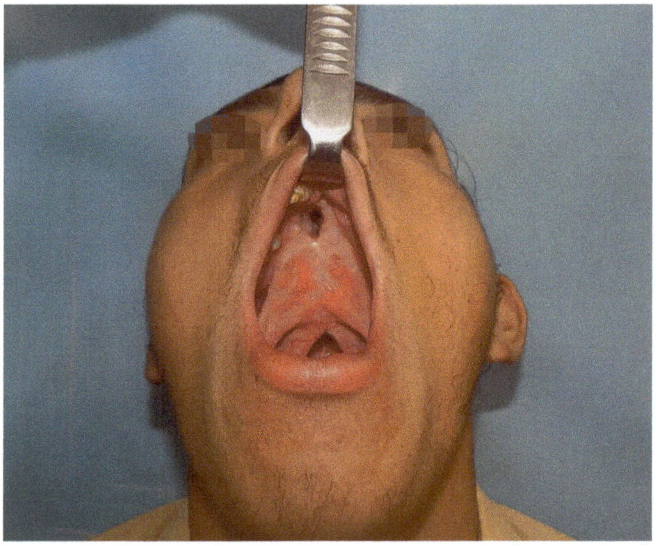

Fig. 19.40 Anterior fistula associated with alveolar gap. (M2, S3, V1). Plan of management: nasal layer closure by turn-in flaps and oral layer closure by buccal sulcus mucosal flap (BSMF)

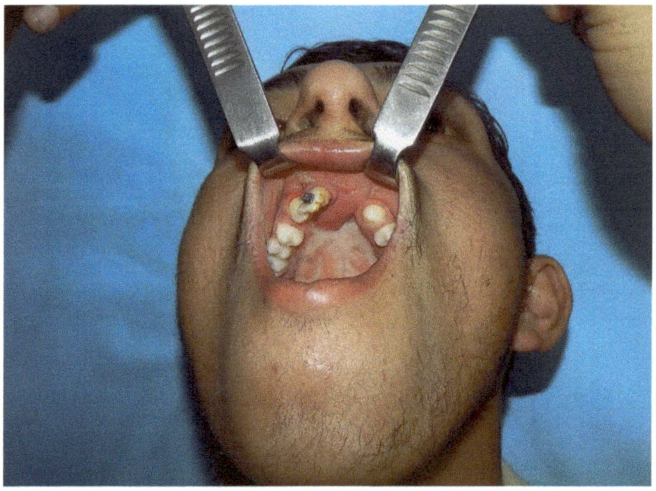

Fig. 19.41 BSMF has adequately covered the defect, with complete healing

However, if the defects are too large or more anteriorly placed to be covered by the mucoperiosteal flaps, or when one or both mucoperiosteal flaps have been damaged during previous surgery, then tissues from tongue or buccinator muscle flap (Fig. 19.43) are transferred to cover the palatal defect.

Tongue flap can be used in two ways: anteriorly based tongue flap from dorsal surface and anteriorly based tongue flap from ventral surface. Most surgeons use the dorsal tongue flap. Nasal layer of the defect is closed by the remainder of the palatal tissues (Figs. 19.30, 19.31, and 19.32) and oral cover is provided by the tongue flap. Tongue flap is detached after 2–3 weeks (Figs. 19.44, 19.45, 19.46, 19.47, and 19.48).

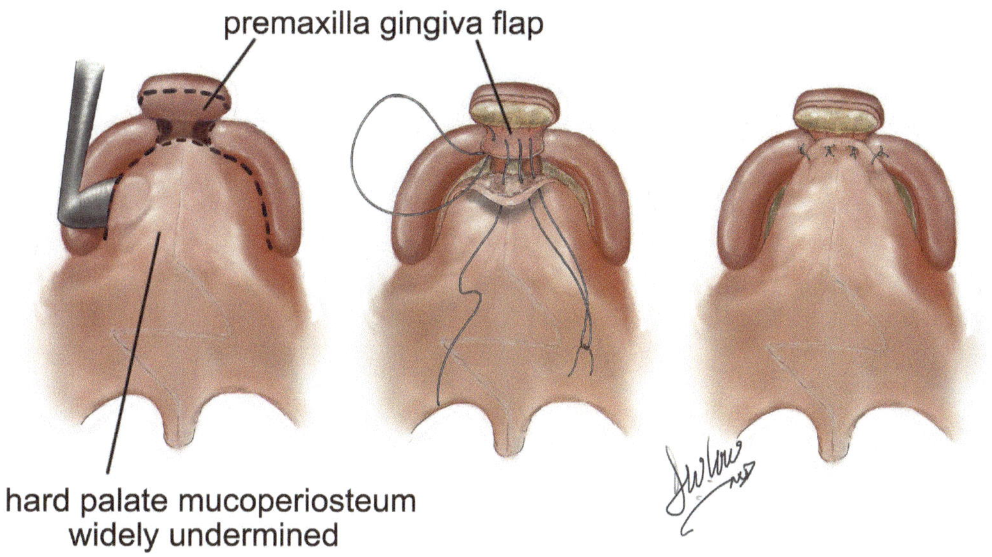


Fig. 19.42 Use of premaxilla gingival flap for closure of bilateral fistula after bilateral lip repair

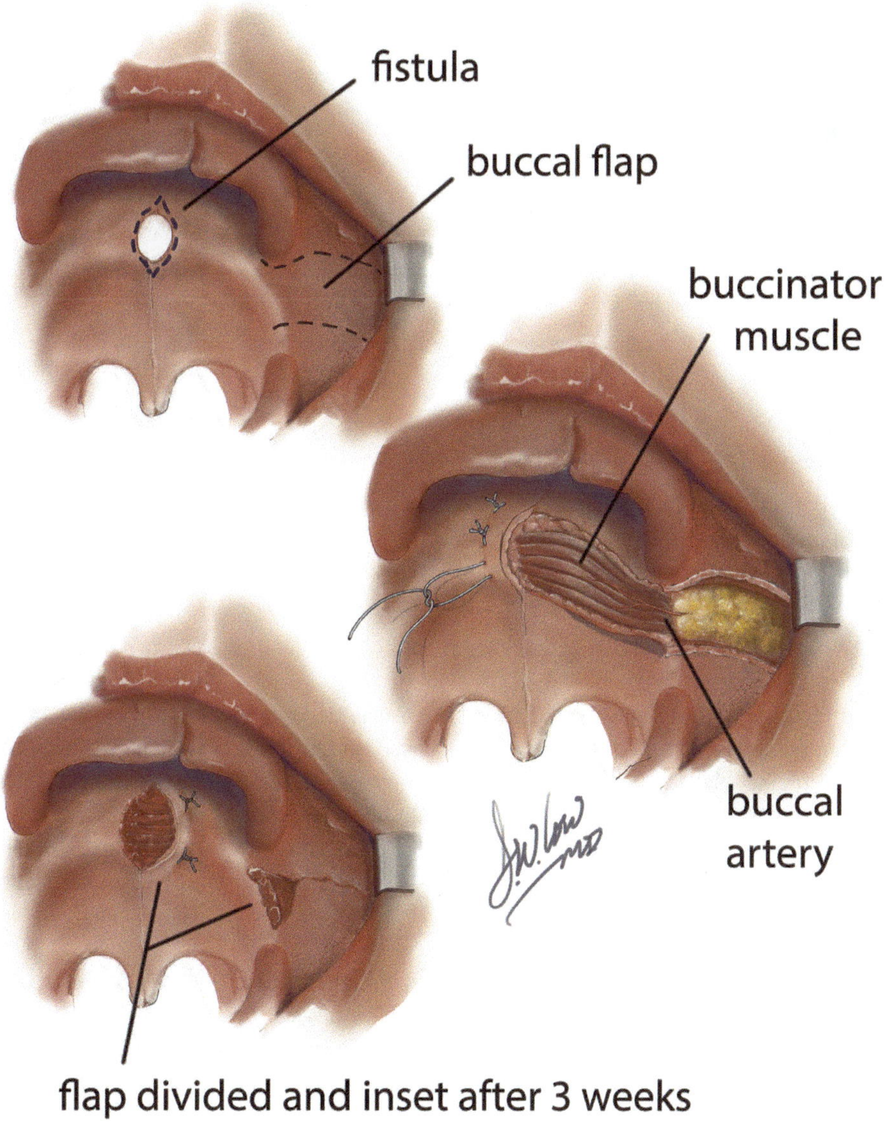


Fig. 19.43 Use of buccinator flap to cover the anterior fistula

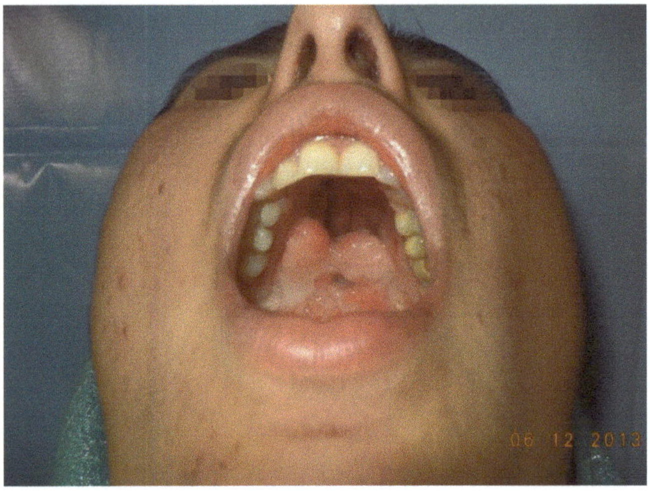


Fig. 19.44 Preoperative picture

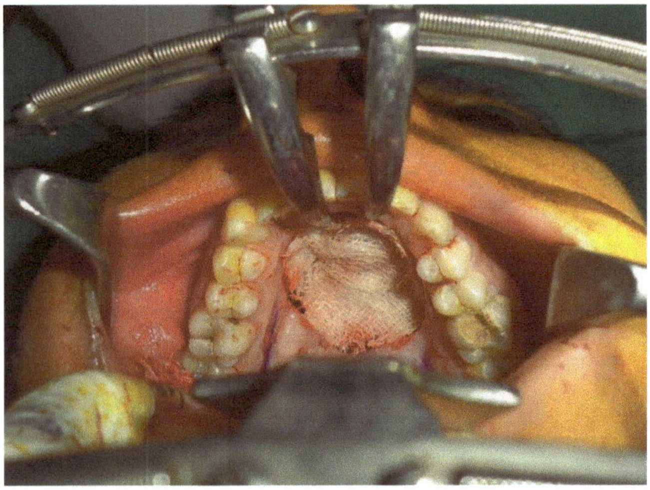

Fig. 19.45 Measurement of the defect and its exact pattern is to be transferred onto the tongue to raise a large tongue flap

## FAMM or Buccal Myomucosal Flap

The facial artery myomucosal (FAMM) flap was described by Dr. Julian Pribaz in 1992. This flap is based on branches of the facial artery and it can be raised basing it superiorly or inferiorly depending on retrograde or antegrade blood supply. Superiorly based flap can be used for defects in the anterior hard palate, alveolus, upper lip, nasal floor, and septum. Inferiorly based flap can cover the defects of the floor of the mouth, lower lip, soft palate, posterior hard palate area, and tonsillar fossa and cheek. Ian Jackson and Robert Mann have subsequently described a buccal mucosal or myomucosal flap based on the buccinator muscle (Fig. 19.43), but which does not require dissection of a specific arterial pedicle. This can be transferred as a myomucosal or axial muscular flap.

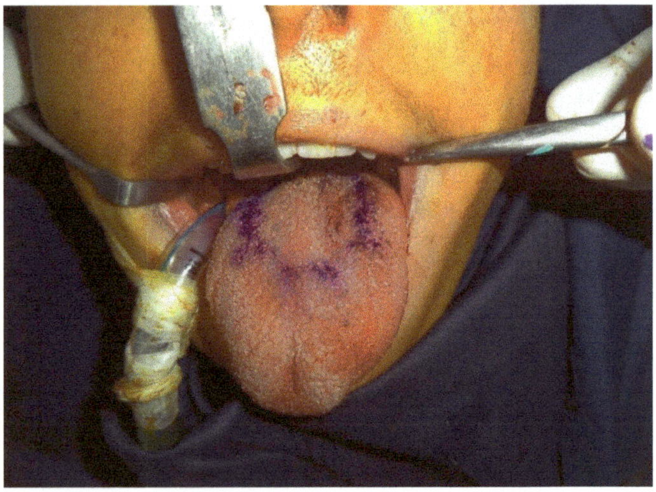

Fig. 19.46 Pattern of the defect is transferred onto the tongue, 4–5 mm of extra tissue was included on all sides. Tongue flap was raised with some thin portion of muscles to maintain good vascularity. After the tongue flap was raised, the donor defect on the tongue was closed primarily. Tongue flap was then attached to the margins of the fistula all around. We use Vicryl 3/0 suture for such attachment

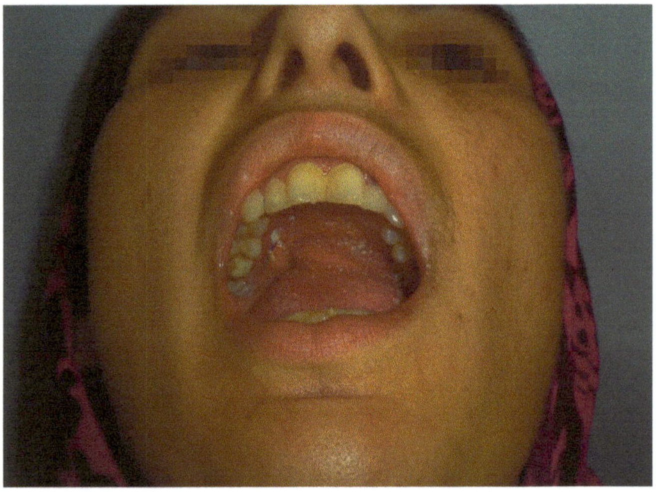

Fig. 19.47 Tongue flap attached to the anterior palate to cover the StB fistula. Picture taken after three weeks of surgery. Tongue flap is ready to be detached now

## Algorithmic Approach to Procedure Selection

Based on fistula location, certain fistula repair techniques may be more appropriate (Fig. 19.49).

### Midline Fistulae; M1 to M6

#### Management of M1

Anterior-most fistulae in the midline (M1-labial-alveolar or lingual-alveolar) are usually small. Management requires closure in two layers.

## M2 or M3

Midline fistulae in the region of the hard palate (M2 or M3) may vary from small to large size. In these cases, nasal layer is closed by turn-in flaps, taken from around the margins of the fistula, a flap can be raised from the buccal sulcus and then transposed through the alveolar defect, into the defect (Fig. 19.50). In case the alveolus is not cleft, then mucoperiosteal flap/s(one or both) can be raised on one or both sides and mobilized medially to provide oral layer cover.

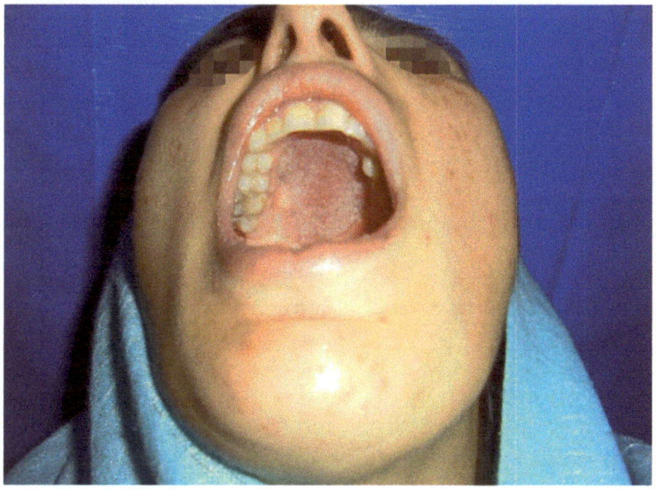

**Fig. 19.48** Complete view of the extended tongue flap closing the three palatal fistulae successfully

## Management of M3 (Fig. 19.51)

If the function of the soft palate is inadequate (V2) as reported by the speech pathologist, complete re-repair of the palate has to be done so that proper retropositioning of the levators can be carried out to improve the function of the soft palate. However, when the length of the soft palate is short as well (V3), pharyngeal flap may have to be added to increase the length of the soft palate in addition to palate re-repair.

## M4

The area of M4 (junction of hard and soft palate), re-repair of the palate with radical dissection of the greater palatine vessels (to increase the mobility of the mucoperiosteal flap), along with dissection of the levator muscle and retropositioning should be done (Fig. 19.52).

If the length of the soft palate is short (V3), a pharyngeal flap is to be added.

## Management of M5

In the region of the soft palate (M5), closure of a fistula is relatively easy. The nasal layer can be closed with a turn-in

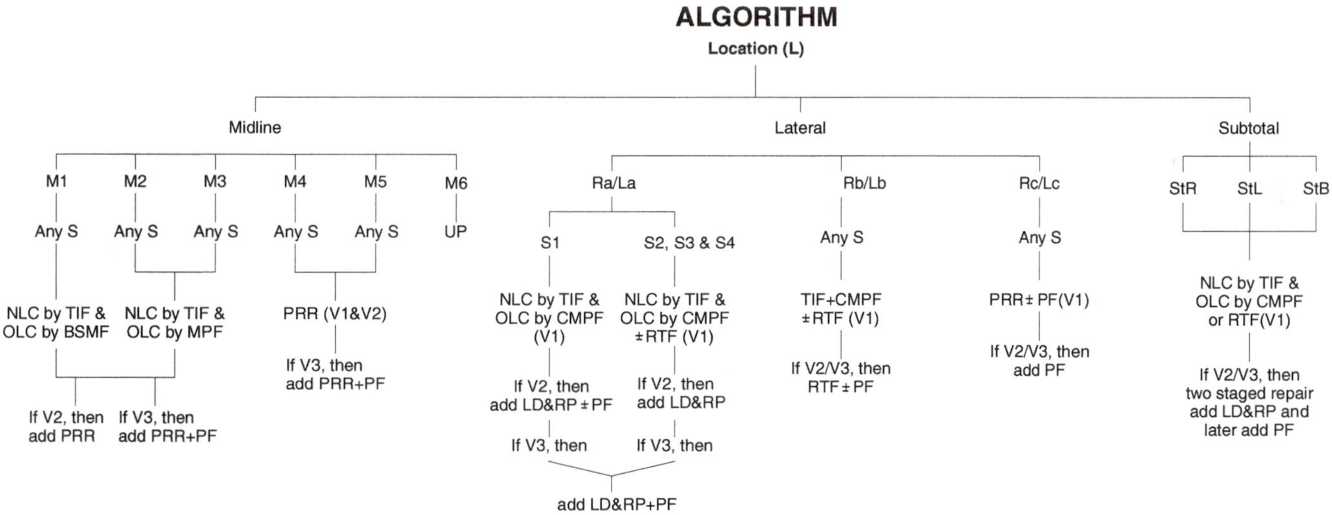


NLC: Nasal Layer Closure
OLC: Oral Layer Closure
TIF: Turn-in Flap
BSMF: Buccal Sulcus Mucosal Flap
MPF: Muco-Periosteal Flap

CMPF: Contralateral Muco-Periosteal Flap
PRR: Palate Re-Repair
LD&RP: Levator Dissection & Retro-Position
PF: Pharyngeal Flap
RTF: Regional Tissue Flap (Tongue Flap, FAMM Flap)
UP: Uvulo Plasty

**Fig. 19.49** Algorithm for management of different types of palatal fistulae

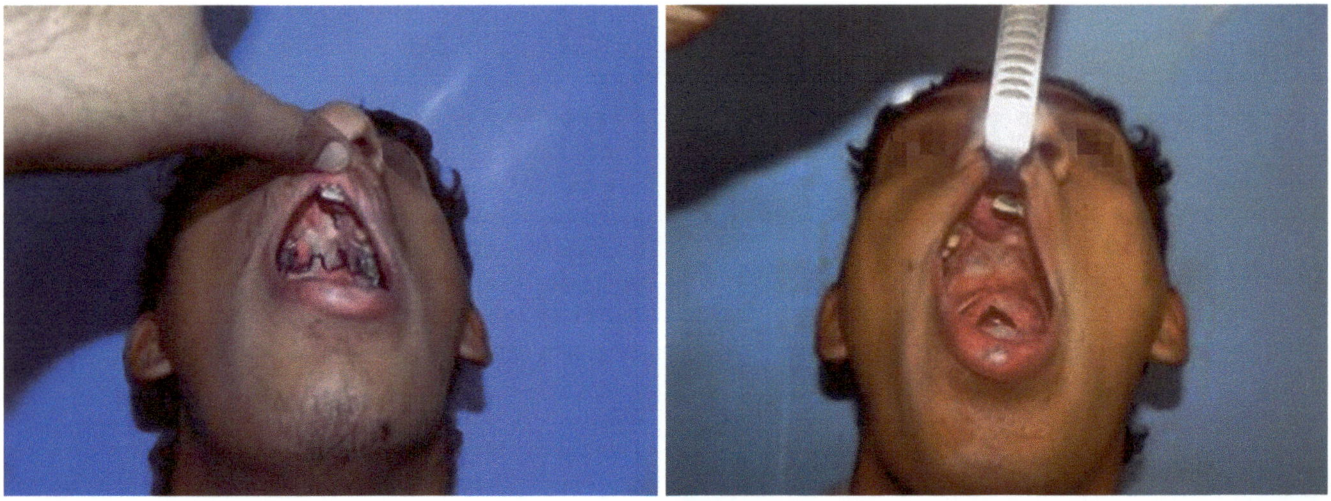

**Fig. 19.50** (*Left*) A 20-year-old man with a fistula involving M1 and M2, 13 mm in longitudinal dimension with good palatal movement (M1,2 S3 V1). (*Right*) Repair of the fistula with nasal layer closure by turn-in flap and oral layer closure by buccal sulcus mucosal flap

flap and oral layer closure can be performed using adjacent palatal tissues (Fig. 19.53).

### M6

Fistula in the uvula (M6) can be managed by closure in two layers.

## *FAR* (Fistula Adjacent Regions)

Many a times the fistula is longer than usual and it extends from one zone to the other adjacent or even into the next zone (spanning two or three or rarely four zones in the midline) in the midline. The management will depend on the examination of the functional status of the soft palate by Speech Language Pathologist.

We may need closure in two layers, palate re-repair (Fig. 19.54) or pharyngeal flap in V1, V2, or V3 (Fig. 19.55) respectively.

## Management of Lateral Fistulae

### Ra or La, S1 & S2

Regarding the management of lateral fistulae, fistulae of the anterior hard palate (Ra or La) can be treated with nasal layer closure by turn-in flaps and oral layer closure by contralateral mucoperiosteal flap.

One may need cClosure in two layers (Fig. 19.56), palate re-repair or pharyngeal flap in V1, V2, or V3 respectively. Furlow's palatoplasty or Orticochea pharyngoplasty may be the procedures of choice by some surgeons.

### Ra or La, S3–4

For larger fistulae of this region (S3 or S4), after the nasal layer closure by turn-in flaps, we may need to provide oral layer cover with contralateral mucoperiosteal flap or regional tissue flaps such as facial artery myomucosal, tongue, cheek mucosa, and other flaps. The management of cases with V2 or V3 is by palate re-repair or/and pharyngeal flap. One may opt for Furlow's palatoplasty or Orticochea pharyngoplasty as well.

### Rb or Lb

**Lb Fistula**

Lateral palatal fistulae in the posterior half of the hard palate are usually rare, but their management is even more difficult. A large turn-in flap is required for nasal layer closure. Oral layer closure can be achieved with a contralateral mucoperiosteal flap (Fig. 19.57) or regional tissue flaps such as a facial artery myomucosal flap or a tongue flap.

If function of the soft palate is inadequate (V2 or V3), palate re-repair with or without a pharyngeal flap may have to be added or Furlow's palatoplasty or Orticochea pharyngoplasty may be more helpful.

### Rb

Lateral palatal fistulae in the posterior half of the hard palate on the right side are even more rare, and their management is always difficult. A large turn-in flap is required for nasal layer closure. Oral layer closure can be achieved with a contralateral (left) mucoperiosteal flap (Figs. 19.58, 19.59, and 19.60) or regional tissue flaps such as a facial artery myomucosal flap or a tongue flap.

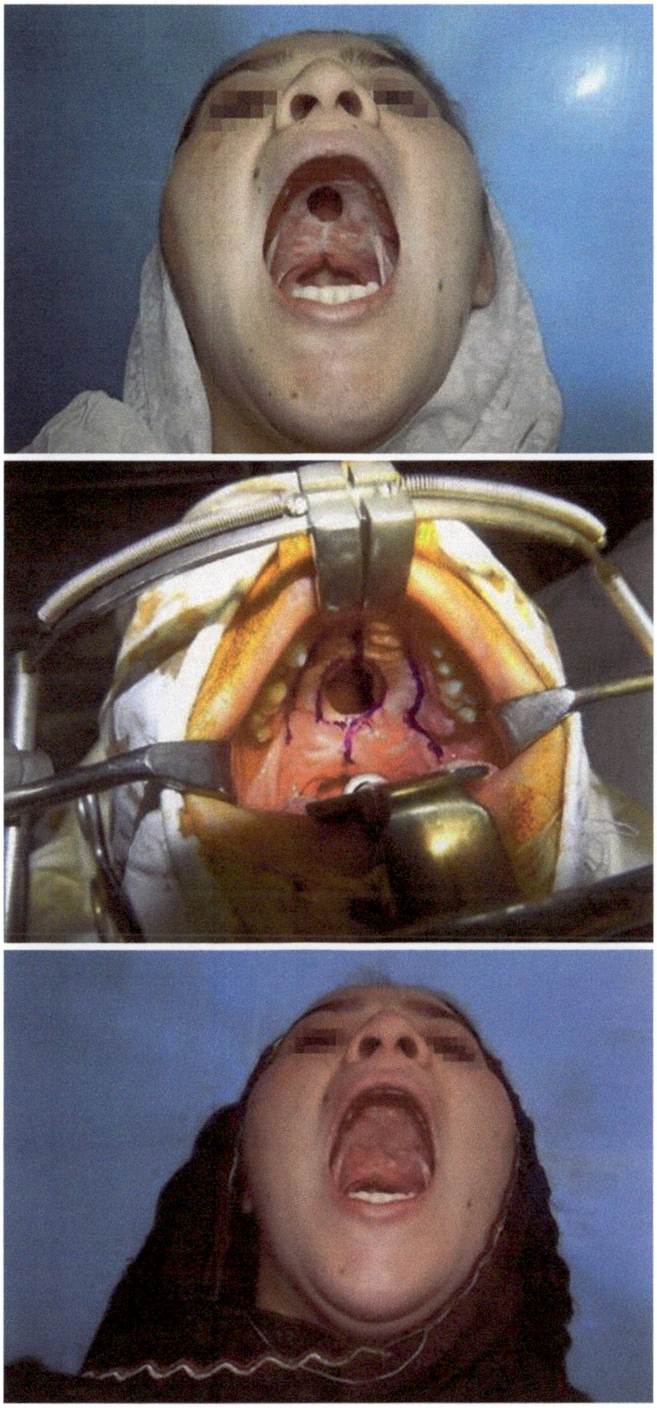

**Fig. 19.51** *(Above)* A 15-year-old girl with a large fistula in the posterior half of the hard palate, 12 × 8 mm, with poor palatal movement (M3 S3 V2). *(middle)* Marking of the turn-in flap for closure of the nasal layer. *(Below)*. Oral layer closure with bilateral mucoperiosteal flaps. Release of the greater palatine artery and retropositioning of the levator muscles results in comfortable closure of the oral layer in addition to lengthening of the palate

### Rc or Lc

Lateral palatal fistulae in the region of the soft palate (Rc or Lc are the most rarest) of any size indicate soft- tissue deficiency in the region of the soft palate, and this requires palate re-repair with or without the addition of the pharyngeal flap depending upon the available tissues (Fig. 19.61).

### Subtotal Fistulae

The most difficult fistulae are subtotal fistulae that involve the midline as well as the lateral regions of the anterior hard palate. The main reason behind unilateral or bilateral subtotal fistula/e is damage to the greater palatine artery on one or both sides during initial surgery for two flap palatoplasty.

Management depends upon the size of the fistula and functional status of the soft palate. In case of unilateral StL or StR fistula, with V1, nasal layer will be closed by turn-in flaps and oral layer cover will be provided by contralateral mucoperiosteal flap after radical dissection of greater palatine artery, which increases the mobility of mucoperiosteal flap (Figs. 19.62 and 19.63) to reach the opposite side to cover the suture line of nasal layer closure. In case of subtotal bilateral cases, nasal layer closure is by large turn-in flaps and oral layer closure is by tongue flap (Fig. 19.64) or free flap.

### Subtotal Bilateral Fistula

In case of V2, palate re-repair has to be done as well in addition to the procedure employed above. In case of V3, palate re-repair with addition of pharyngeal flap, or Furlow's palatoplasty is the procedure of choice.

### Multiple Fistulae

Multiple fistulae will be described as MF and then the anterior-most fistula will be mentioned as F1 with location, size, and status of the soft palate function, then the next fistula will be mentioned as F2 with its features and so on. Management plans will be made which will cater to all the fistulae for a particular patient.

If these fistulae are located in the midline, the management would be easier like in FAR (fistula adjacent regions). Most of the cases can be managed with palate re-repair with dissection of the greater palatine artery and dissection & retropositioning of levators (Fig. 19.65). If velopharyngeal sta-

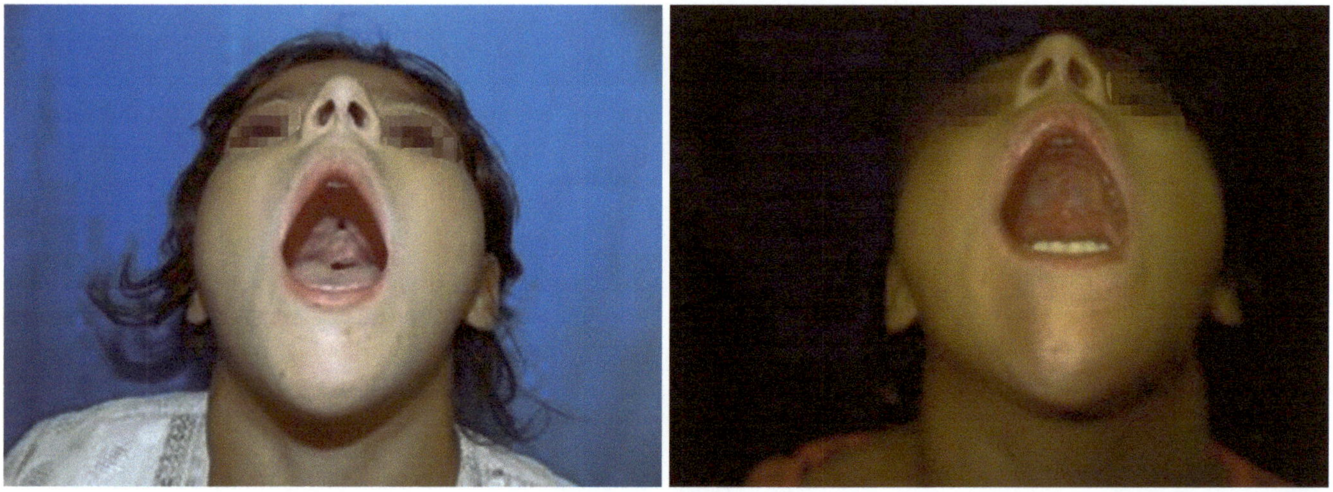

**Fig. 19.52** (*Above, left*) A young girl with a fistula at the junction of hard & soft palate, 6 x 4 mm, with good palatal movement (M4 S1 V1). (*Above, right*) Repair of the fistula with a turn-in flap for nasal layer closure and oral layer closure with approximation of both mucoperiosteal flaps

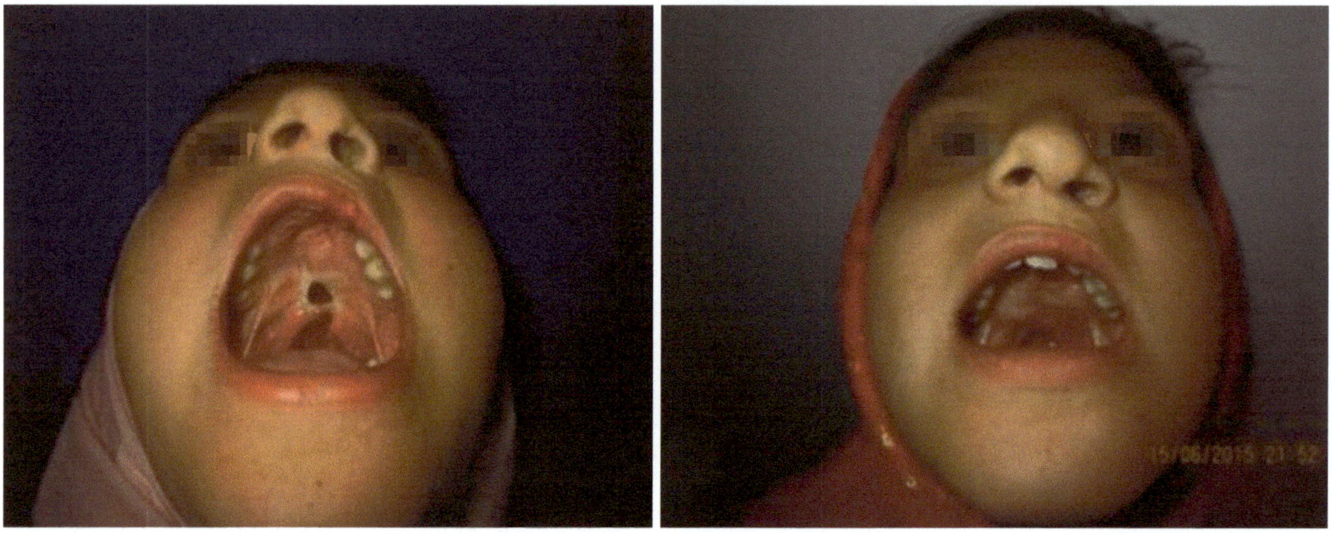

**Fig. 19.53** (*Left*) A 6-year-old girl with a fistula in the soft palate, 9 x 10 mm in the largest dimension, with poor palatal movement (M5 S2 V2). (*Right*) Repair of the fistula with palate re-repair

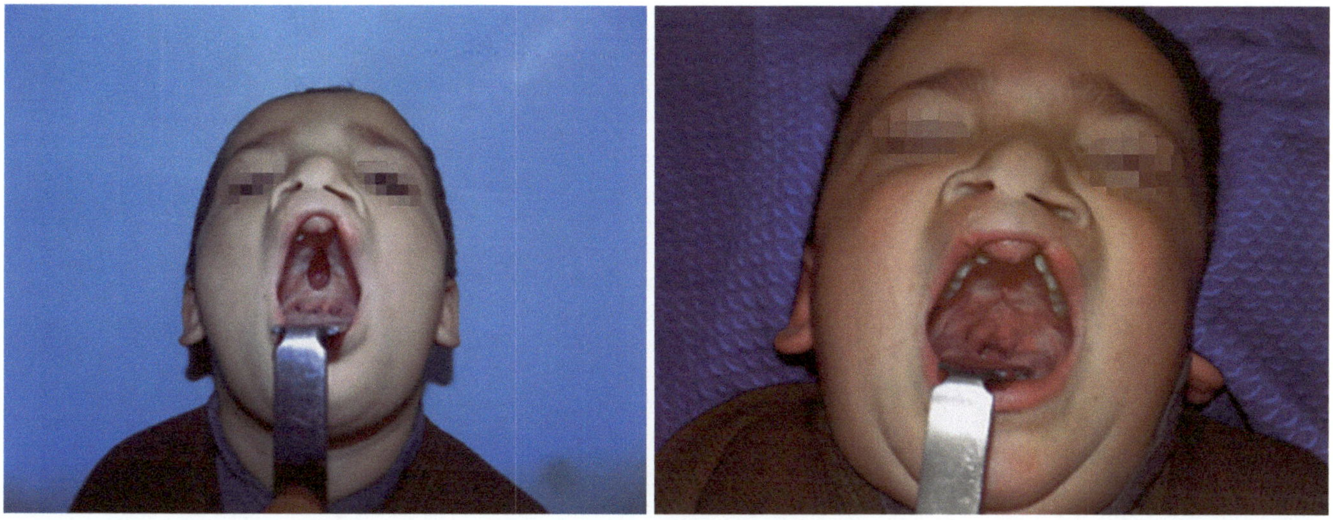

**Fig. 19.54** Patient having FAR (fistula adjacent regions) M2-3-4. The management as per our algorithm is closure of the nasal layer by turn-in flaps and oral layer cover provided by both mucoperiosteal flaps moved medially to cover the nasal layer closure

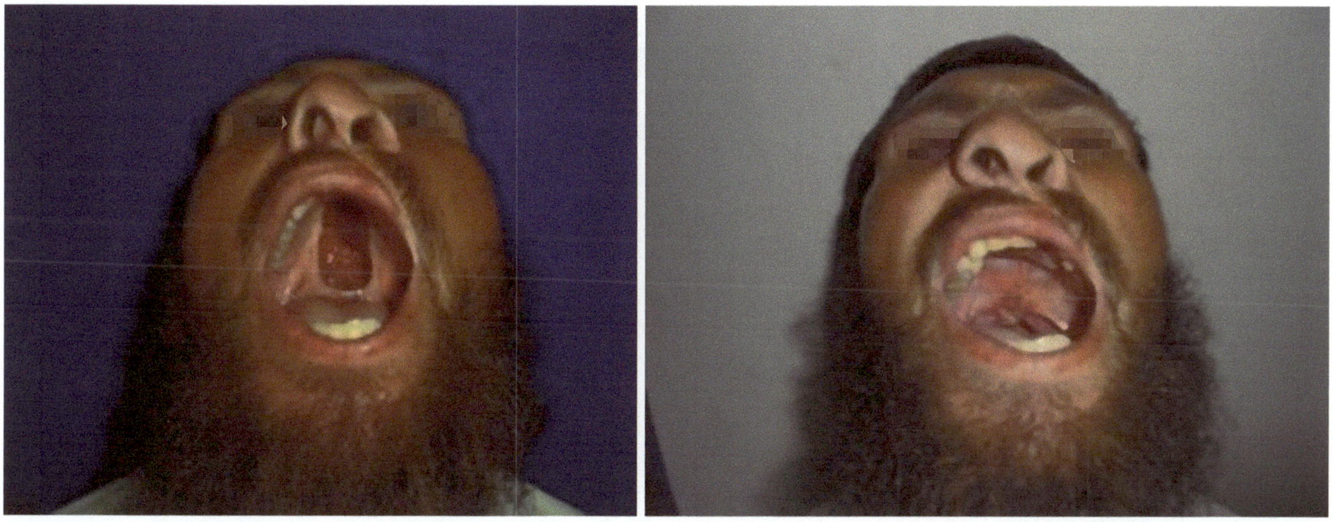

**Fig. 19.55** A 26-year-old man with a very large midline fistula involving M2, M3, M4, and M5, approximately 32 × 12 mm, with poor movement of the soft palate (M2-3-4-5, S4 V3). Repair of the palate with palate re-repair and addition of the pharyngeal flap. Levator muscle retropositioning was done along with a pharyngeal flap to lengthen the palate

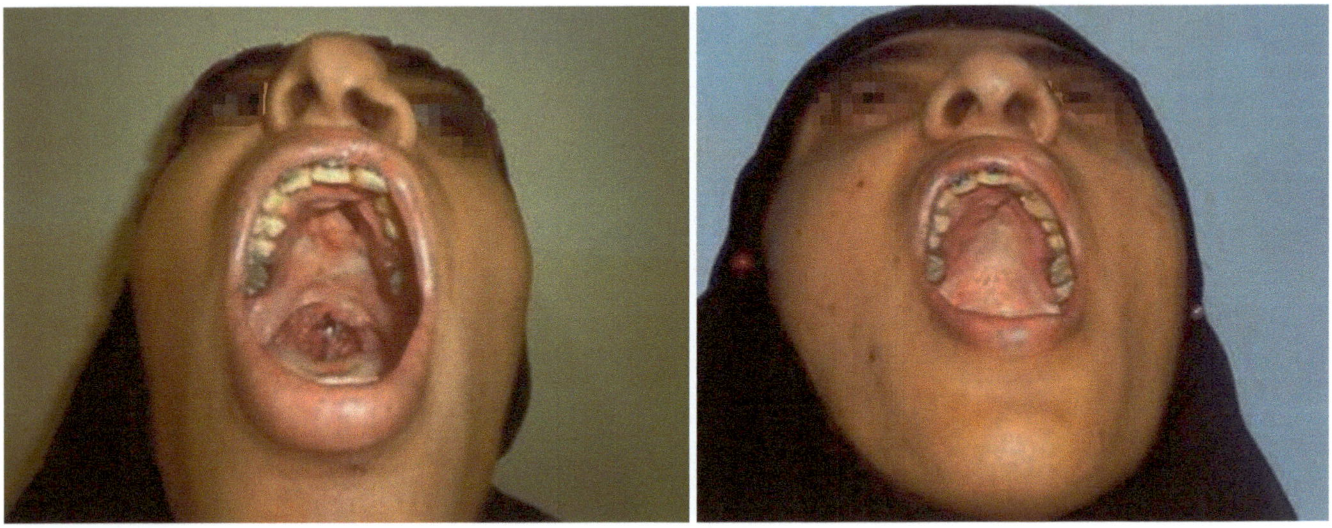

**Fig. 19.56** (*Left*) An 18-year-old female patient with a lateral fistula involving the anterior half of the hard palate on the left side (La), 14 × 4 mm, with good movement of the palate (La S3 V1). (*Right*) Repair of the fistula with nasal layer closure by turn-in flaps and oral layer closure by contralateral mucoperiosteal flap

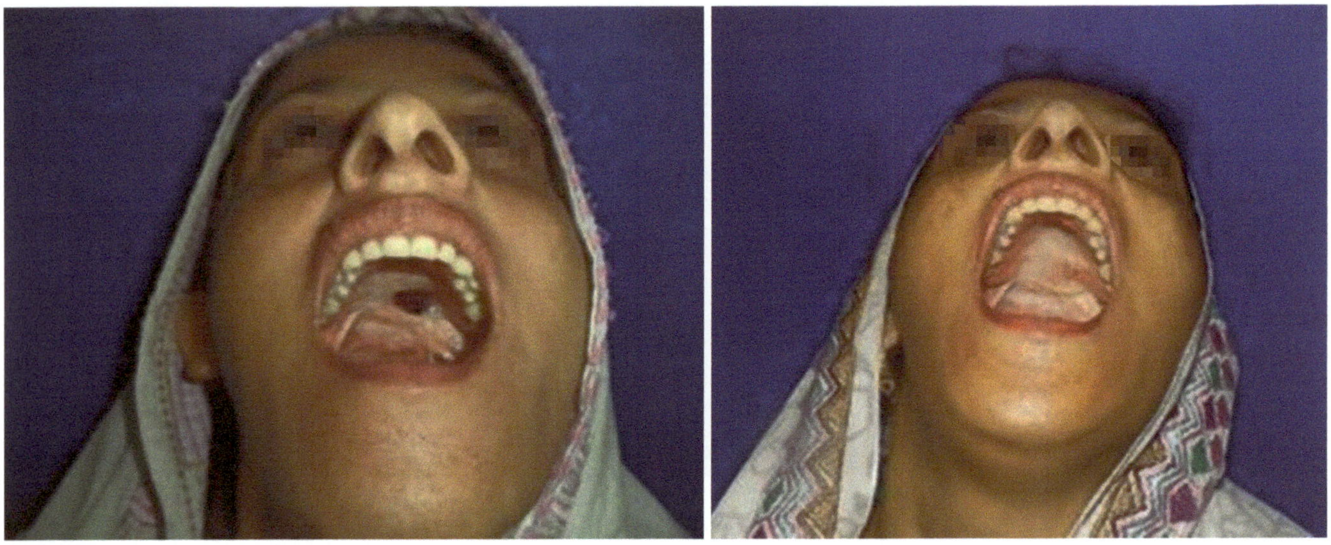

**Fig. 19.57** (*Left*) A 23-year-old woman with a lateral fistula in the posterior half of the hard palate on the left side (Lb), 12 × 8 mm, with good movement of the palate (Lb S3 V1). (*Right*) Repair of the fistula with nasal layer closure by turn-in flaps and oral layer closure by a contralateral mucoperiosteal flap

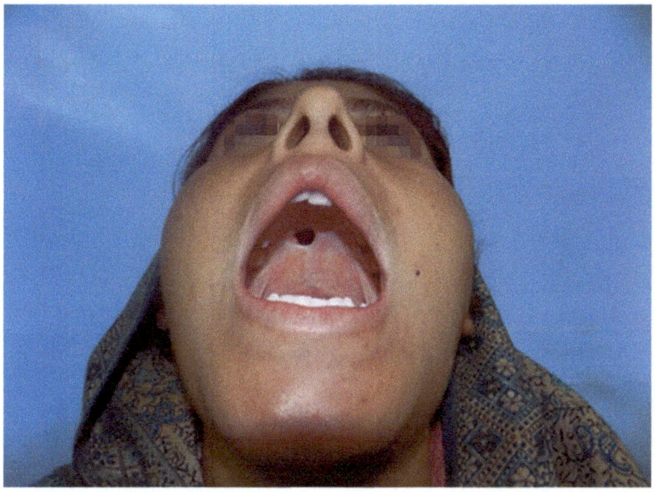

Fig. 19.58 A 21-year-old girl with a lateral fistula in the posterior half of the hard palate on the right side (Rb), 11 × 8 mm, with poor movements of the palate (Rb S3 V3)

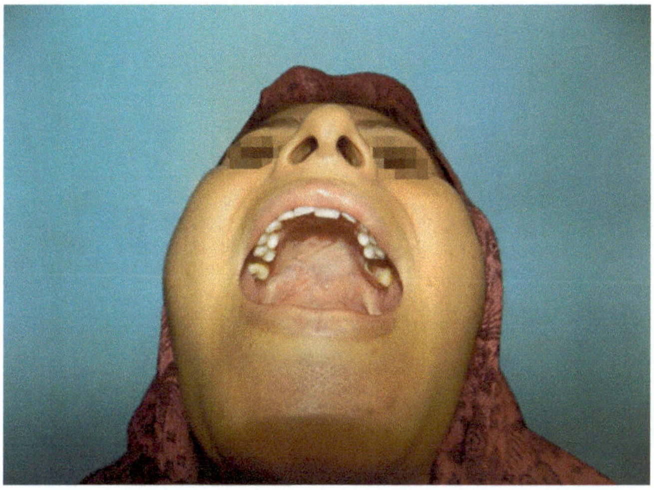

Fig. 19.59 (*Below*) Repair of the fistula is with nasal layer closure by turn-in flaps and oral layer closure by a left contralateral mucoperiosteal flap

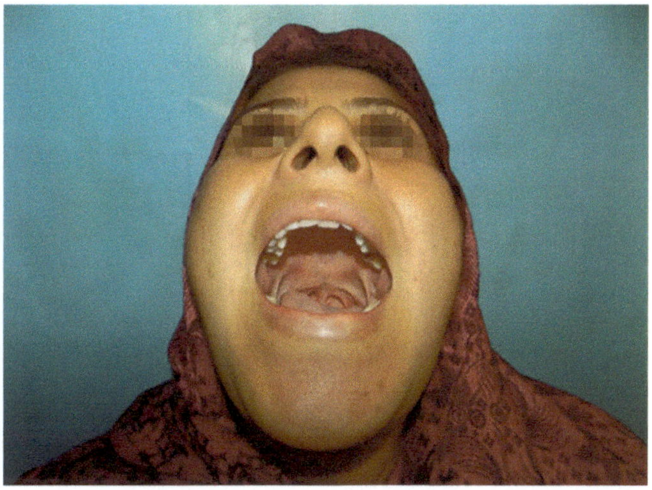

Fig. 19.60 Pharyngeal flap was added at the same stage to lengthen the palate while levators were attached to each other and at the base of the pharyngeal flap to improve the speech outcome

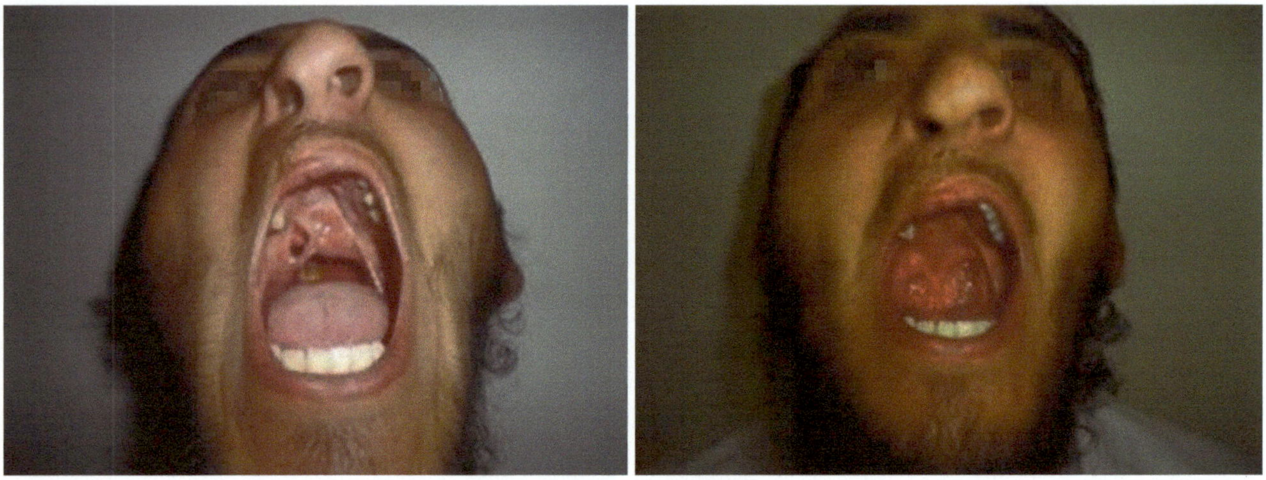

**Fig. 19.61** (*Left*) A 28-year-old man with a lateral fistula of soft palate on the right side (Rc), 7 × 6 mm, with reduced movement of the palate (Rc S2 V3). (*Right*) Repair of the fistula with palate re-repair and a pharyngeal flap

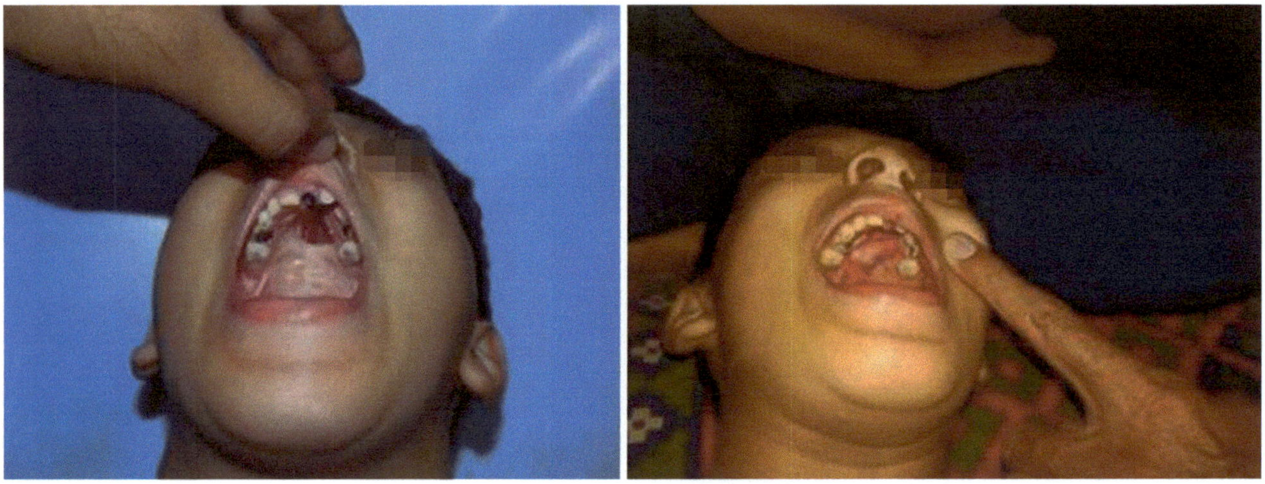

**Fig. 19.62** Subtotal left fistula, StL: nasal layer was closed by turn-in flaps and oral layer cover was provided by right contralateral mucoperiosteal flap (left). One year postoperative view shows excellent healing with complete closure of the subtotal left fistula(right)

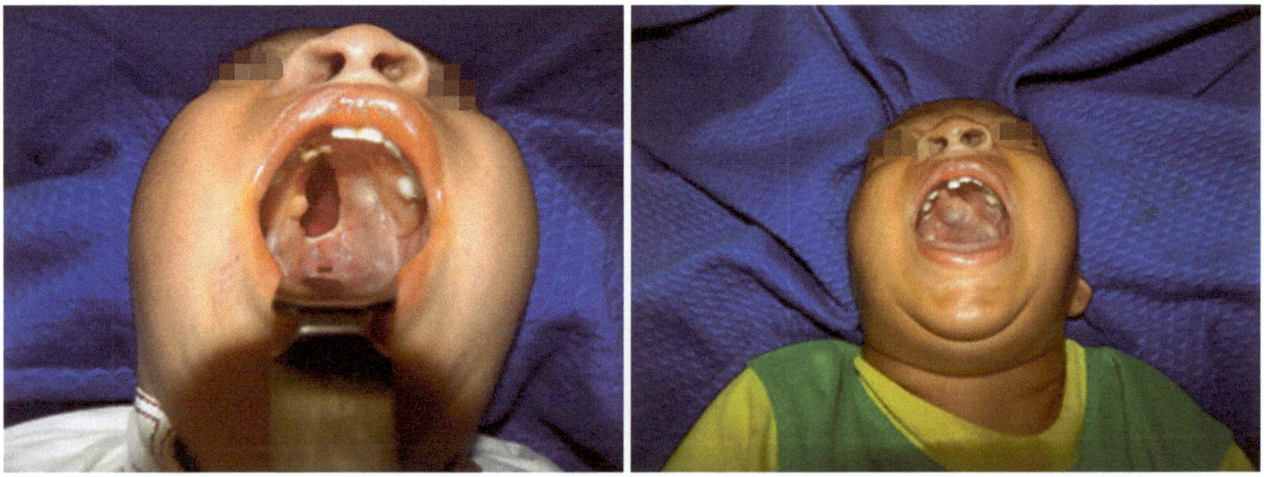

**Fig. 19.63** Subtotal fistula, right StR: nasal layer was closed by turn-in flaps and oral layer cover was provided by left contralateral mucoperiosteal flap (*left*). One year postoperative view shows excellent healing with complete closure of the subtotal right fistula (right)

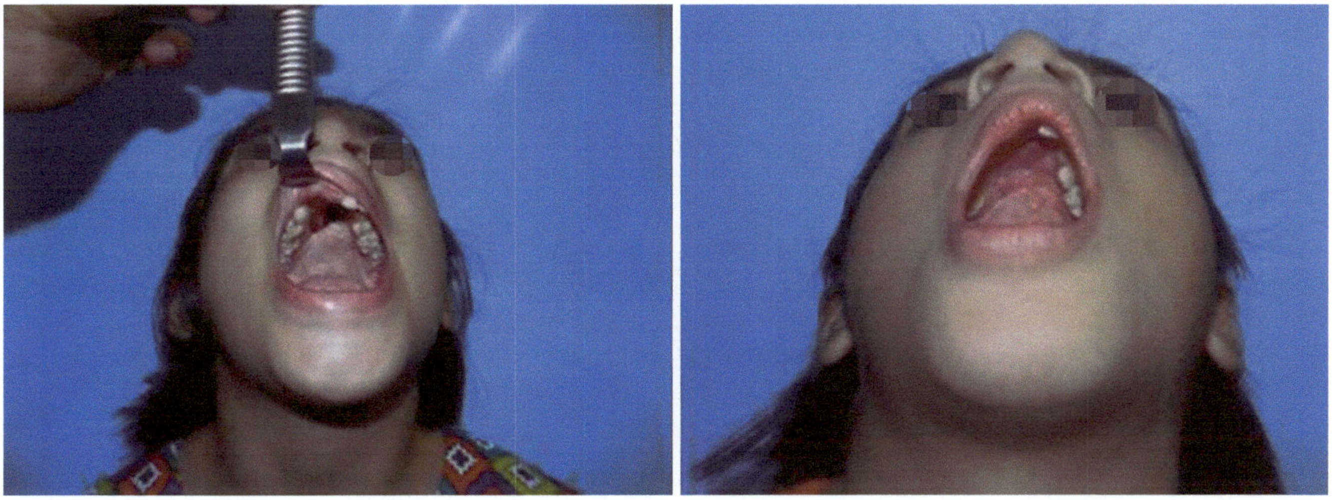

Fig. 19.64 An 8-year-old girl with a subtotal bilateral (StB) fistula involving both sides of the hard palate, 25 × 12 mm, with good palatal movement (StB S4 V1) (left). The nasal layer was closed by large turn-in flaps, and the oral layer cover was provided with a tongue flap. Six months postoperative view shows complete healing of the large subtotal bilateral fistula (right)

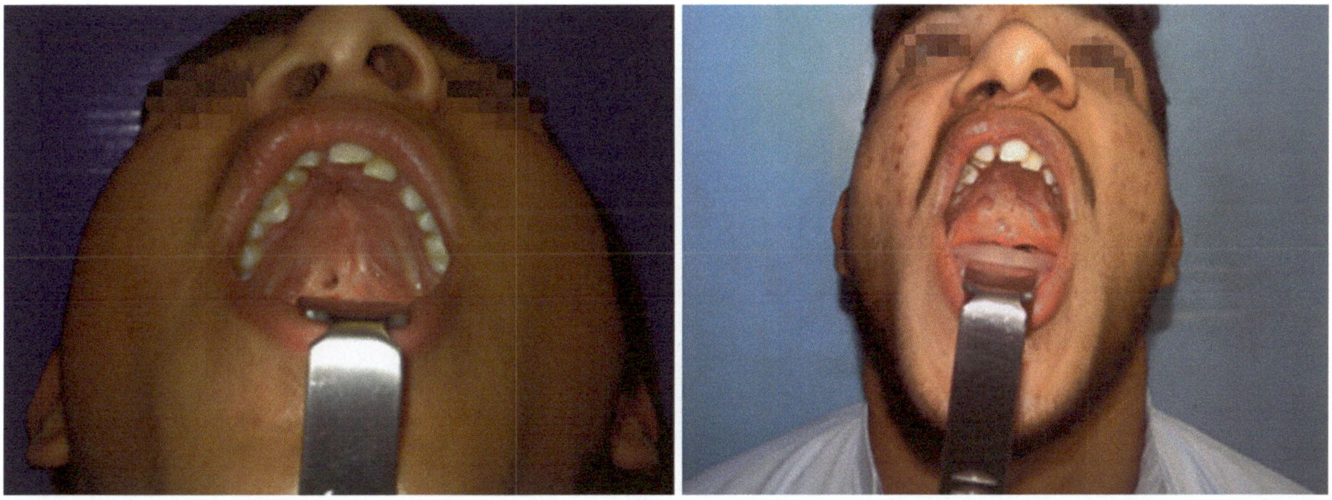

Fig. 19.65 Multiple fistulae; F1:- M2, S1 V2 & F2:- M4,S1,V2 (left); As per our algorithm, nasal layer will be closed by turn-in flaps while oral layer cover will be provided by both mucoperiosteal flaps. As the velum function status is V2, palate re-repair has to be done, so levator dissection and retropositioning will be done to improve the good speech production. Late postoperative view shows very good healing of the palate, with successful closure of both the fistula (right)

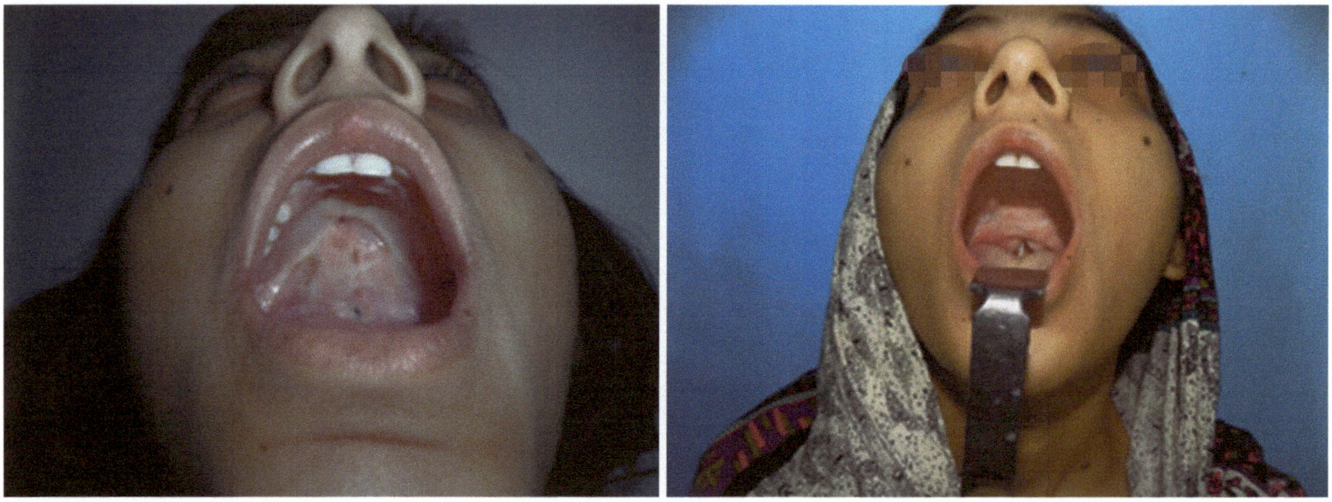

Fig. 19.66 Multiple fistula patient with dehiscence; F1: - M2, S1, V3; F2: - M5, S1, V3 & D1. (Left) As per our algorithm, this patient has two fistulae in the midline zone, while there is dehiscence of the uvula, while the velum function status is V3. (Right) Palate was Re-repaired with the addition of pharyngeal flap to improve the speech outcome. Levators were dissected on both sides, superiorly based pharyngeal flap was raised and then turned 180 degrees to be attached to the anterior-most limit of the nasal layer of the soft palate. Lateral sides of the pharyngeal flap were sutured to the nasal layers of the soft palate. Levators from both sides were sutured to each other and at the base of the pharyngeal flap. This results in better excursion of the pharyngeal flap and hence the speech improved in this patient just like speech in a normal person

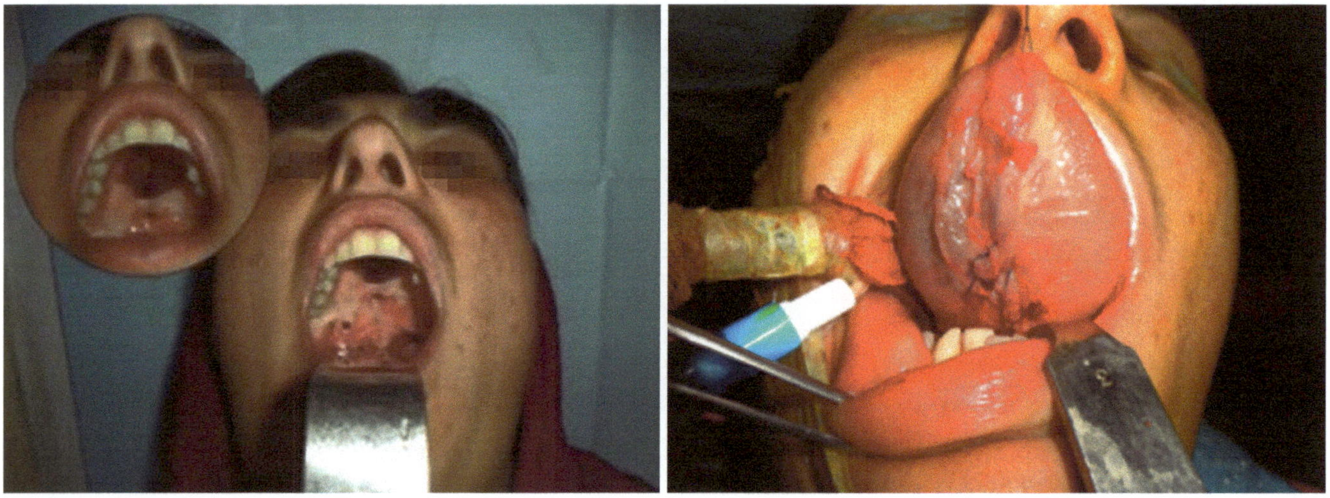

Fig. 19.67 (Left) This patient has a subtotal bilateral fistula (StB) and other fistulae in midline and lateral regions (M3&Rc), StB can be covered by tongue flap or large bilateral FAMM flaps or a large cheek mucosal flap, while those in the midline or lateral part of the soft palate can be managed with palate re-repair or a pharyngeal flap may be added for oral layer cover. (Right) Initially the tongue was not mobile enough to allow use of tongue flap. So, the tongue was released ventrally by making a transverse incision and the resultant defect was closed longitudinally. Defect over the tongue was closed primarily and a small defect at the base of the oral cavity was left as such for spontaneous epithelialization

tus is V3, then pharyngeal flap should be added as well (Figs. 19.66, 19.67, 19.68, 19.69, and 19.70).

In cases where there is a lateral fistula in the anterior hard palate (La) and a midline fistula in the soft palate (M5) with V2 status of the soft palate function, the management for La will be nasal layer closure by turn-in flaps and oral layer cover by contralateral mucoperiosteal flap. Management of M5 will be nasal layer closure by turn-in flaps and palate re-repair.

## A Unique Combination of All Three Types of Fistulae

Subtotal bilateral fistula(*StB*), with midline fistula(*M3*) and a lateral fistula(*Rc*).

Multiple fistula patient: F1:-StB, S4,V2, F2:- M3, S2, V2, F3:- Rc, S1, V2.

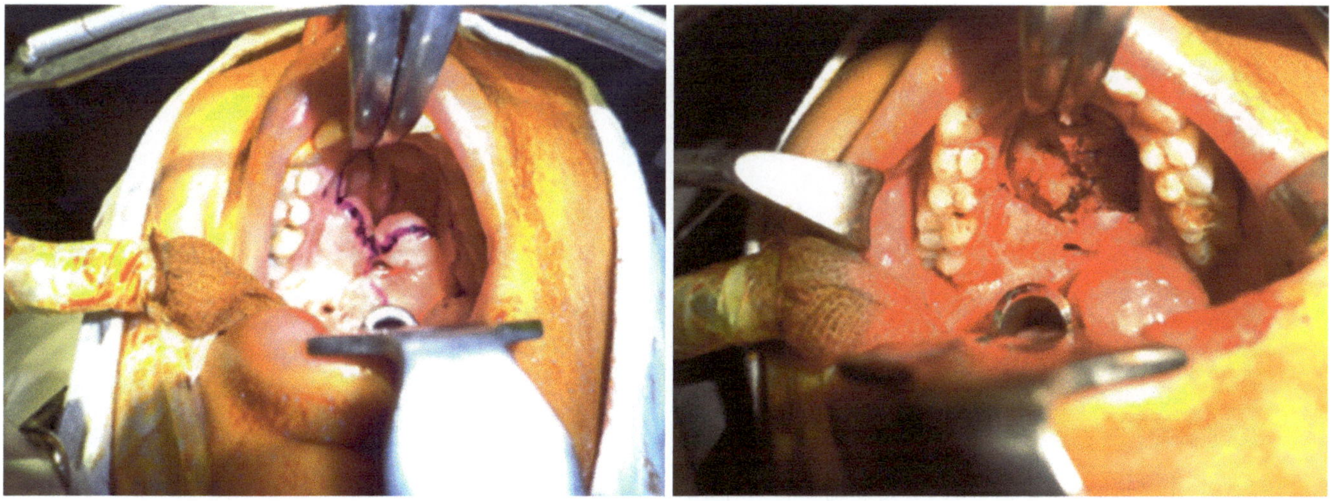

**Fig. 19.68** (Left) Marking of the large turn-in flap, all around the margins of the StB fistula to mobilize the tissues to close the nasal layer. The incision is made deep down to the bone anteriorly and bilaterally while posteriorly palatal tissues are incised to be turned-in anteriorly. (Right) Turn-in flaps have been adequately mobilized and brought in the midline to be sutured together. Nasal layer has been closed properly but comfortably

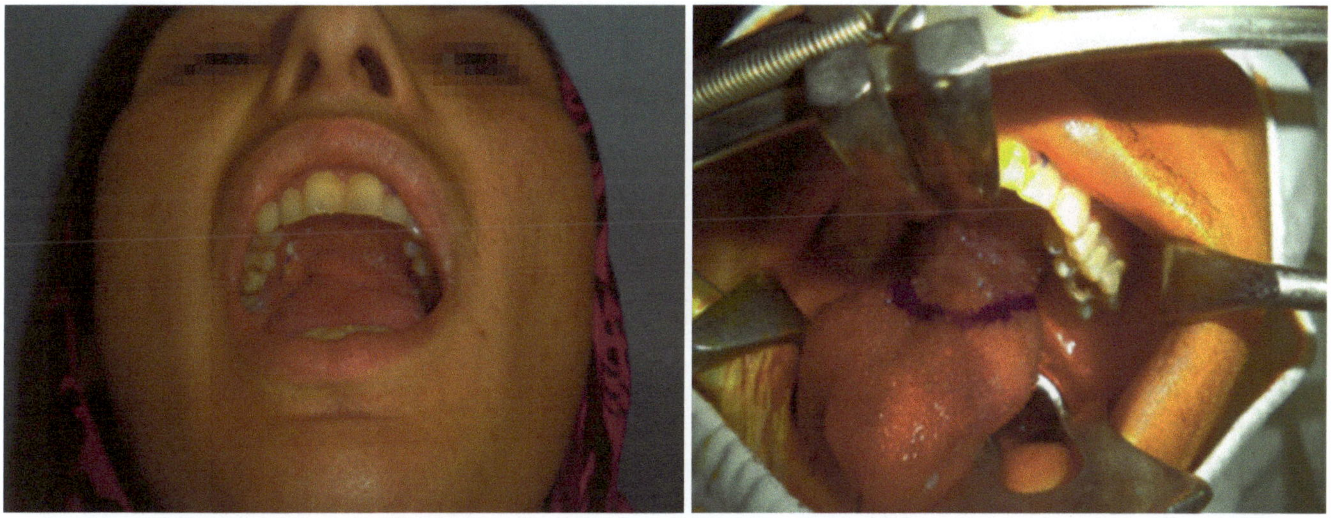

**Fig. 19.69** (Left) Tongue flap attached to the anterior palate to cover the StB fistula

So the next step is to bring a flap from the tongue which will cover this defect adequately.

After three weeks, a decision was taken to detach the tongue flap. But what about the two fistulae still left (M3 and Rc) to be closed? After much thought processing, a new plan was made to cover both the fistulae by taking some extra tissue from the anterior portion of the tongue and using that extra tissue to cover both the fistulae. (Right) Marking to raise the extra tissue from the tongue to be used to cover F2 & F3 (M3&Rc) fistulae.

Other surgeons may opt for a free flap to cover such large and multiple fistulae in the palate.

## Dehiscence

Certain situations may arise when there is dehiscence of the palate with or without fistula in the palate.

If there is only dehiscence of the uvula *(D1)*, uvuloplasty along with fistula closure can suffice.

If there is dehiscence of the soft palate (*D2*) and velopharyngeal status is V2, re-repair of the soft palate with retropositioning of the levator muscles should be done (Fig. 19.71).

Dehiscence of uvula, soft palate and posterior hard of the hard palate, *D3* (Fig. 19.72).

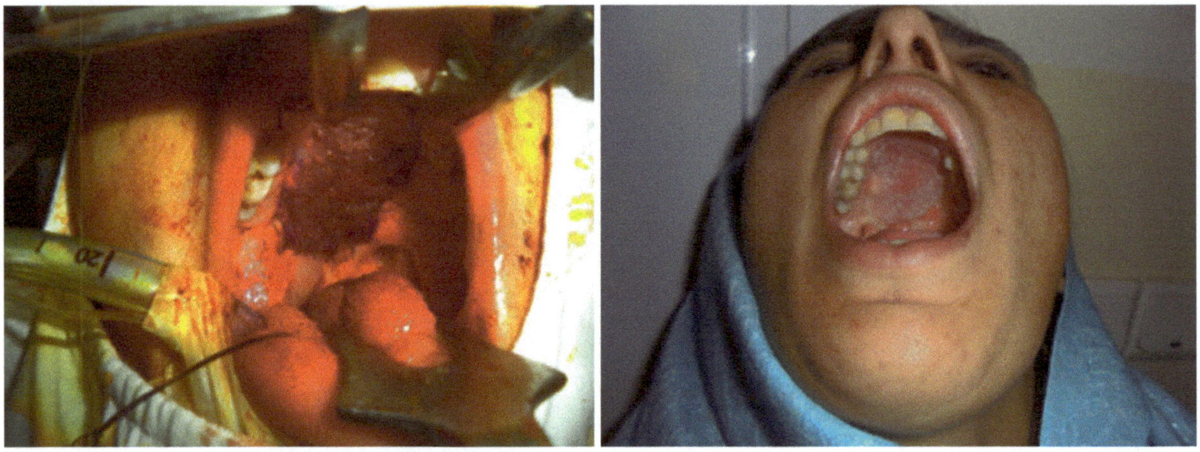

**Fig. 19.70** (Left) Tongue flap has covered completely both M3 &Rc fistulae. The portion of the flap appeared dusky for 2–3 days. However, ultimately it healed uneventfully. (Right) Complete closure of the three fistulae (StB, M3, & Rc) by an extended tongue flap with excellent healing of the area

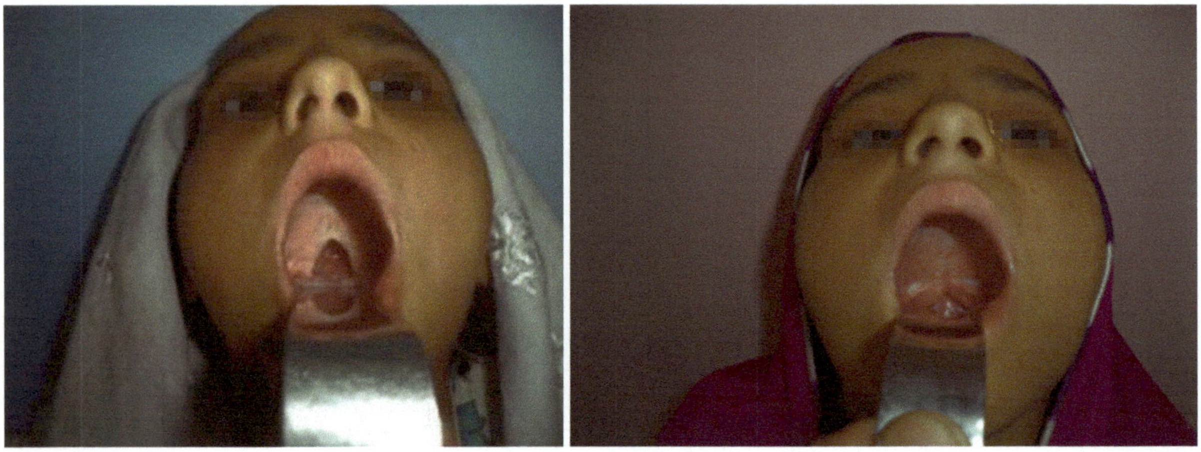

**Fig. 19.71** D2: A patient having dehiscence of uvula and soft palate, our algorithm shows the management as palate re-repair with dissection and retropositioning of levators

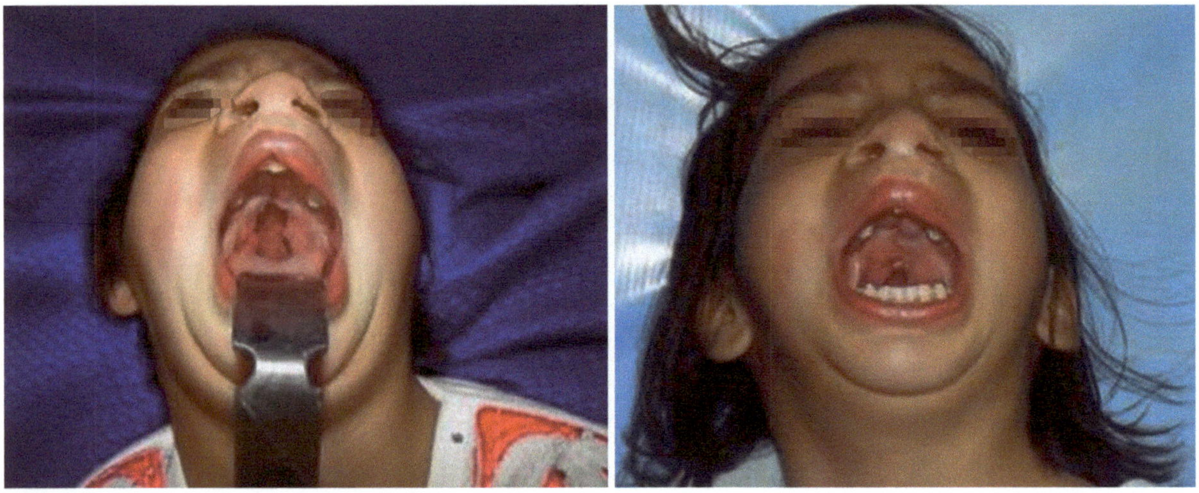

**Fig. 19.72** D3: (Left) A patient having dehiscence of uvula, soft palate and posterior half of the hard palate, (Right) Our algorithm shows the management as palate re-repair with dissection and retropositioning of levators. This patient may need a pharyngeal flap to lengthen the palate to improve the speech outcome

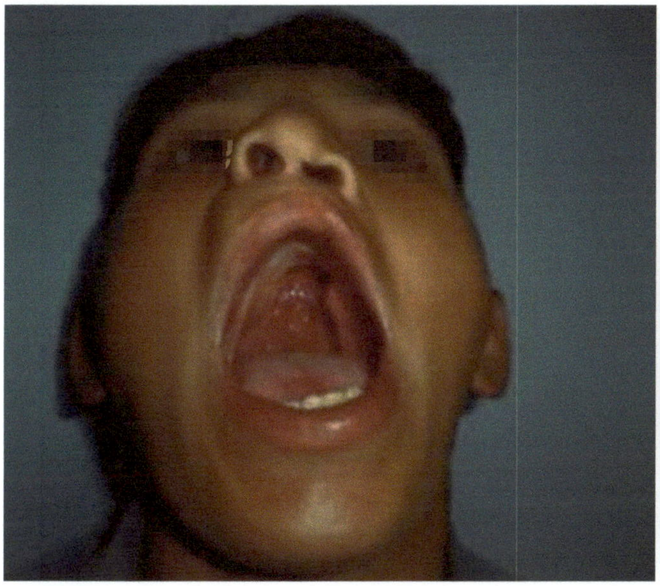
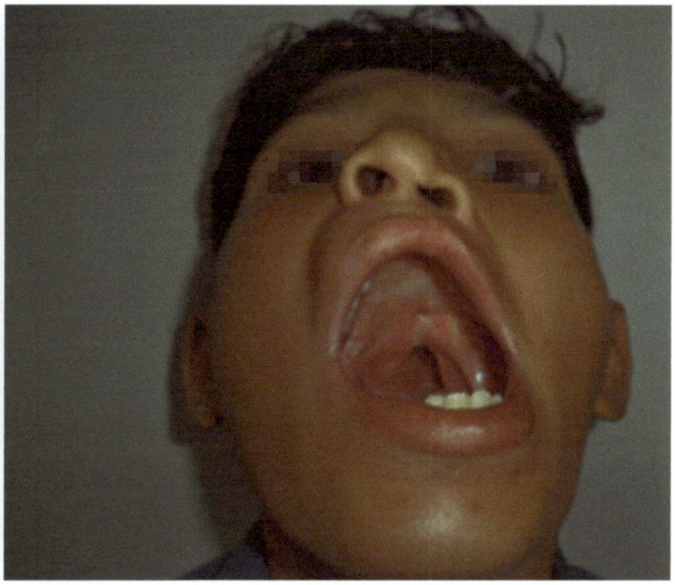

**Fig. 19.73** D3-L: (Left)A patient having dehiscence of uvula, soft palate and posterior half of the hard palate, there is loss of tissues on left side after previous surgery so it is called as D3-L. (Right) Management is nasal layer closure by turn-in flaps and oral layer cover is provided by right contralateral mucoperiosteal flap. This patient will need a pharyngeal flap (Fig. 19.74) in the next stage to lengthen the palate to improve the speech outcome

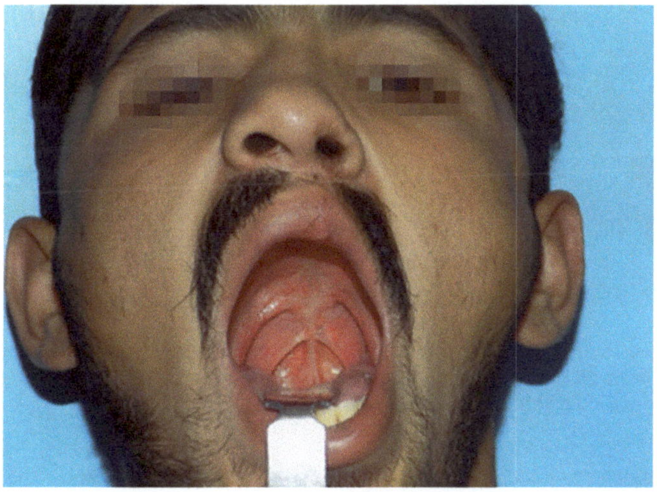

**Fig. 19.74** Same patient after pharyngeal flap has been added and it has lengthened the palate and reduced nasal air emission. Patient's speech has improved considerably

## Complicated Dehiscence

When there is extensive damage to the palatal tissues on one or other side in addition to dehiscence, we call it complicated dehiscence.

### D3-L

The patient below was operated for left unilateral cleft palate repair but developed complete dehiscence of the palate with loss of anterior two–thirds of the hard palate mucosa & portion of the soft palate on the left side and partial damage to the right side. The pedicle on left side was damaged that is why the left side of the palate has been lost almost in total (Fig. 19.73).

### D3-R after Unilateral Cleft Palate repair

The patient below was operated for left unilateral cleft palate repair but developed complete dehiscence of the palate with loss of anterior two–thirds of the hard palate mucosa & portion of the soft palate on the right side and partial damage to the left side. The pedicle on right side was damaged that is why the right side of the palate has been lost almost in total (Fig. 19.75).

### D3-R after Bilateral Cleft Palate repair

The patient below was operated for bilateral cleft palate repair but developed complete dehiscence of the palate with loss of anterior two-thirds of the hard palate mucosa & portion of the soft palate on the right side and medial one-fourth of the hard palate mucosa on left side. The pedicle on right side was damaged that is why the right side of the palate has been lost almost in total. The damage on the left side is due probably to the tight sutures, resulting in necrosis of the medial portion of the left flap (Fig. 19.76). Velopharyngeal status is V3.

Such patients need a pharyngeal flap in the next stage to lengthen the palate to improve the speech outcome (Fig. 19.77).

If the whole palate is dehisced (*D4*), re-repair of the palate with or without addition of some local or regional tissues (pharyngeal flap) may be needed.

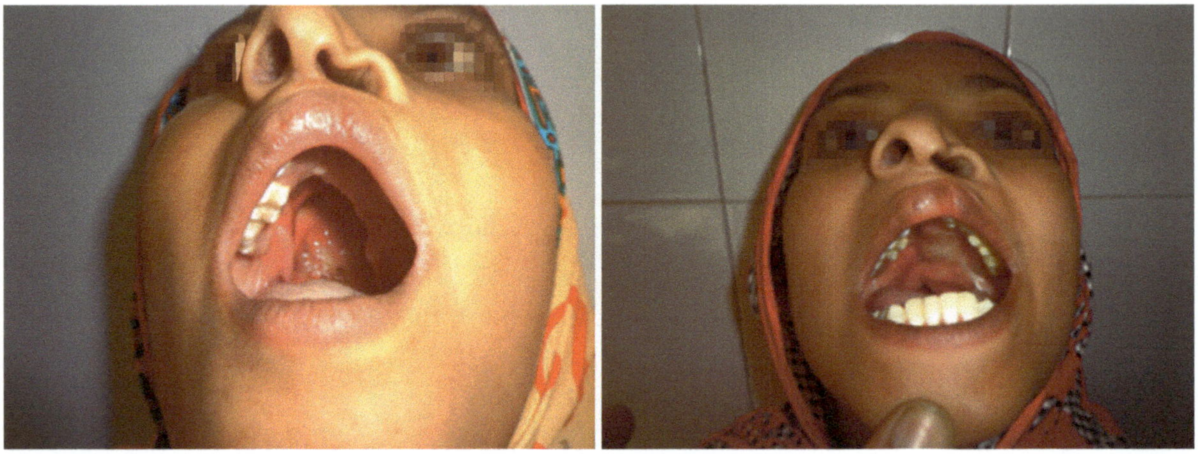

**Fig. 19.75** D3-R: (Left) A patient having dehiscence of uvula, soft palate and posterior half of the hard palate, there is extensive loss of tissues on right side after previous surgery, so it is called D3-R. Management is nasal layer closure by turn-in flaps and oral layer cover is provided by left contralateral mucoperiosteal flap. Pharyngeal flap (in the next stage) can lengthen the palate to improve the speech outcome

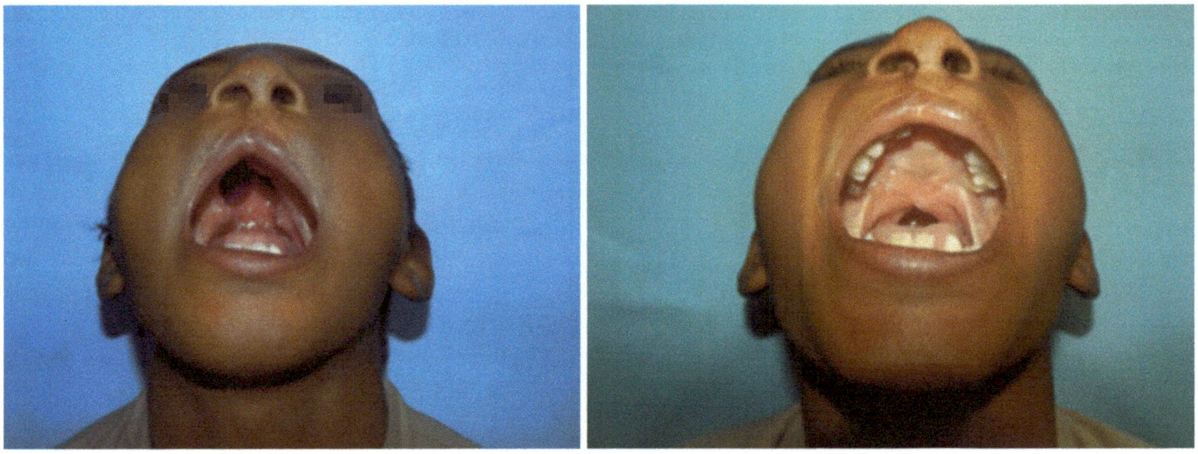

**Fig. 19.76** D3-R: (Left) A patient having dehiscence of uvula, soft palate and posterior half of the hard palate, but there is even more extensive loss of tissues on right side (D3-R) as well as some partial damage on the left side after previous surgery. (Right) Management is nasal layer closure by turn-in flaps and oral layer cover is provided by left contralateral mucoperiosteal flap

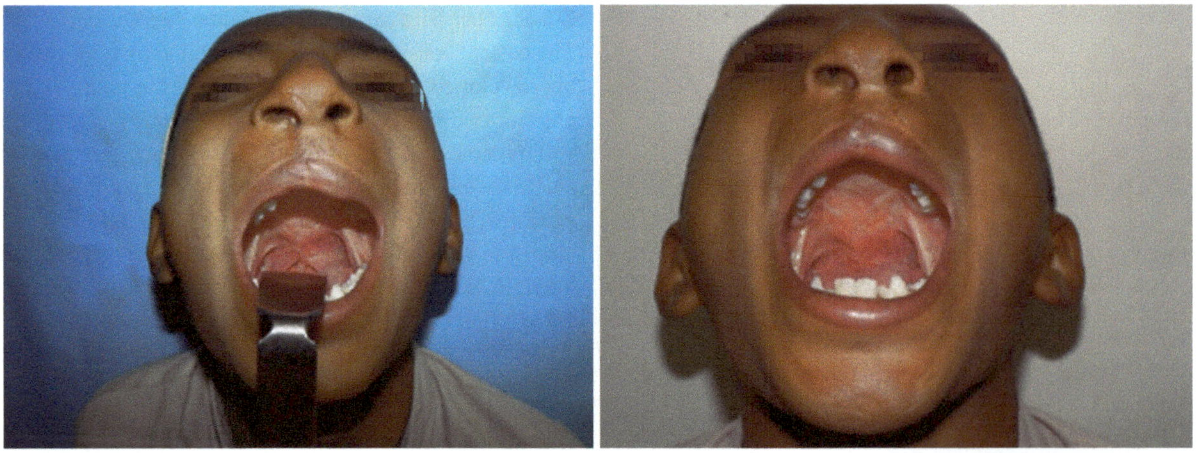

**Fig. 19.77** Picture shows pharyngeal flap was added to the palate in the above patient. The palate has been lengthened and nasal air emission has been reduced considerably

**Important Precaution to Avoid a Disaster**

In case of secondary palatal surgery, when originally the patient had incomplete cleft palate and the surgery performed was Langenbeck procedure, there may have been inadvertent damage to the greater palatine artery on one or both sides, though it may go unnoticed with no bad consequences. The reason is that the anterior half of the mucoperiosteal flap still continues to get good blood supply from its anterior attachment with the alveolus. Now if this patient has a fistula in the midline and during closure of that fistula, the surgeon decides to raise the mucoperiosteal flap cutting it anteriorly at the alveolus, from anterior to posterior side, it will lead to a disaster as there is no greater palatine artery and so the anterior half of the mucoperiosteal flap will get necrosed. In all such we usually make lateral incision first and look for the presence or absence of the pedicle, if the pedicle is present, we will raise the mucoperiosteal flap from anterior to posterior direction. If the pedicle is not present, then we will repair the fistula by Langenbeck procedure only.

## Conclusion

If this algorithm is followed in letter and spirit, the recurrence rate after palatal fistula repair is very low. However, it depends upon the expertise of the surgeon, meticulous execution of the surgical plan, and thoughtful postoperative care. The fistula recurrence rate is highest in subtotal bilateral fistula, then lateral fistula, with lowest in the midline fistula. The focus should always be on the function of the palate and not just closing the hole in the palate. Speech always improves when the surgery is performed according to the algorithm. Patient compliance and support of the family are very important determinants of speech improvement.

Index items:- Cleft palate, Palatal fistula, Pittsburgh Fistula Classification, Midline fistula, Lateral fistula, Subtotal fistula, Multiple fistulae, FAR (fistula adjacent regions), Turn-in flaps, Mucoperiosteal flap, Greater palatine vessels, Radical dissection of pedicle, FAMM flap, Tongue flap, Uvula, Levator dissection, La, Lb, Lc, Ra, Rb, Rc, StR, StL, StB, MF, Dehiscence, D1, D2, D3, D4, Buccal sulcus mucosal flap (BSMF), Pharyngeal flap, VPI, Bardach palatoplasty, Langenbeck palatoplasty, Pakistan Comprehensive fistula classification, Causes of palatal fistula

## References


1. Cohen SR, Kalinowski J, LaRossa D, Randall P. Cleft palate fistulas: a multivariate statistical analysis of prevalence, etiology, and surgical management. Plast Reconstr Surg. 1991;87:1041–7.
2. Amaratunga NA. Occurrence of oronasal fistulas in operated cleft palate patients. J Oral Maxillofac Surg. 1988;46:834–8.
3. Muzaffar AR, Byrd HS, Rohrich RJ, et al. Incidence of cleft palate fistula: an institutional experience with two-stage palatal repair. Plast Reconstr Surg. 2001;108:1515–8.
4. Diah E, Lo LJ, Yun C, Wang R, Wahyuni LK, Chen YR. Cleft oronasal fistula: a review of treatment results and a surgical management algorithm proposal. Chang Gung Med J. 2007;30:529–37.
5. Sommerlad BC. A technique for cleft palate repair. Plast Reconstr Surg. 2003;112:1542–8.
6. Fayyaz GQ, Gill NA, Ishaq I, et al. A model humanitarian cleft mission: 312 cleft surgeries in 7 days. Plast Reconstr Surg Glob Open. 2015;3:e313.
7. Bardach J, Morris H, Olin W, McDermott-Murray J, Mooney M, Bardach E. Late results of multidisciplinary management of unilateral cleft lip and palate. Ann Plast Surg. 1984;12:235–42.
8. Folk SN, D'Antonio LL, Hardesty RA. Secondary cleft deformities. Clin Plast Surg. 1997;24:599–611.
9. Smith DM, Vecchione L, Jiang S, et al. The Pittsburgh fistula classification system: a standardized scheme for the description of palatal fistulas. Cleft Palate Craniofac J. 2007;44:590–4.
10. Richardson S, Agni NA. Palatal fistulae: a comprehensive classification and difficulty index. J Maxillofac Oral Surg. 2014;13:305–9.
11. Fayyaz GQ, Gill NA, Chaudry A, et al. Radical dissection of greater palatine artery and dynamic reconstruction of cleft palate. Plast Reconstr Surg Glob Open. 2017;5:e1235.
12. Kreshanti P, Sudjatmiko G, Bangun K. The effect of honey give as oral drops in precipitating epithelialization of lateral palatal defects post two flap palatoplasty. Jurnal Plastik Rekonstruksi. 2012;1:5.
13. Fayyaz GQ, Gill NA, et al. Pakistan comprehensive fistula classification: a novel scheme and algorithm for Management of Palatal Fistula/dehiscence. Plast Reconstr Surg. 2019;143:140e.

## Cleft Palate Revision, Case 1

### Case Study: Soft Palate Reconstruction in a Bilateral Cleft Lip and Palate Patient

Percy Rossell-Perry

#### Case Analysis

This 3-year-old boy with congenital bilateral cleft lip and palate has undergone previous cleft palate repair. The mother explains that the boy had a severe hemorrhage during early postoperatory bleeding requiring surgical revision in operating room.

After cleft palate revision (based on the physical exam), the patient develops an extended palatal flap necrosis with consequent loss of palatal tissue from hard and soft palate as in below figure. The hard palate has been repaired using one flap (the left one), but the soft palate in the affected side remains severely affected. The remainder soft palate is retracted and short in size.

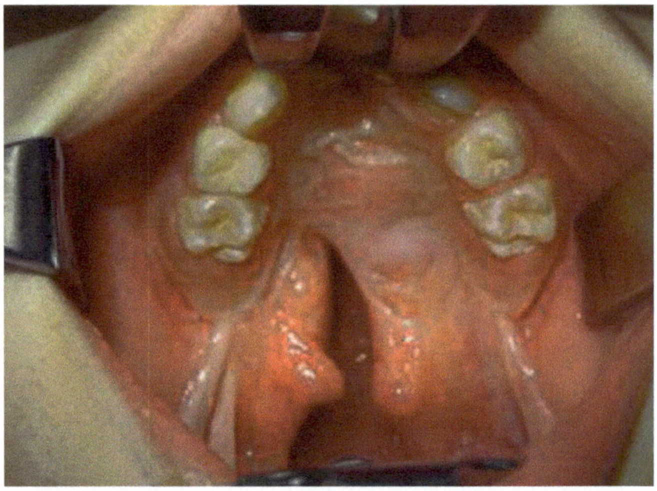

Goals of reconstruction are to create a competent soft palate improving length and function.

#### Treatment Considerations

Different alternatives could be considered for this case, but we basically consider a re-repair or use of regional flap. Even when a re-repair is possible in some palatal sequelae, this is mostly limited to palatal fistula repair. Palatal tissue necrosis leaves a scar as well as retracted tissue that is difficult to be reused and with higher rate of a new necrosis. This is the reason why a regional flap was chosen in this case.

In this case, an axial buccinator flap was designed based on the facial artery to provide enough tissue to the soft palate. Conventional non-axial buccinator flap is contraindicated because of the lateral relaxing incisions performed during primary repair.

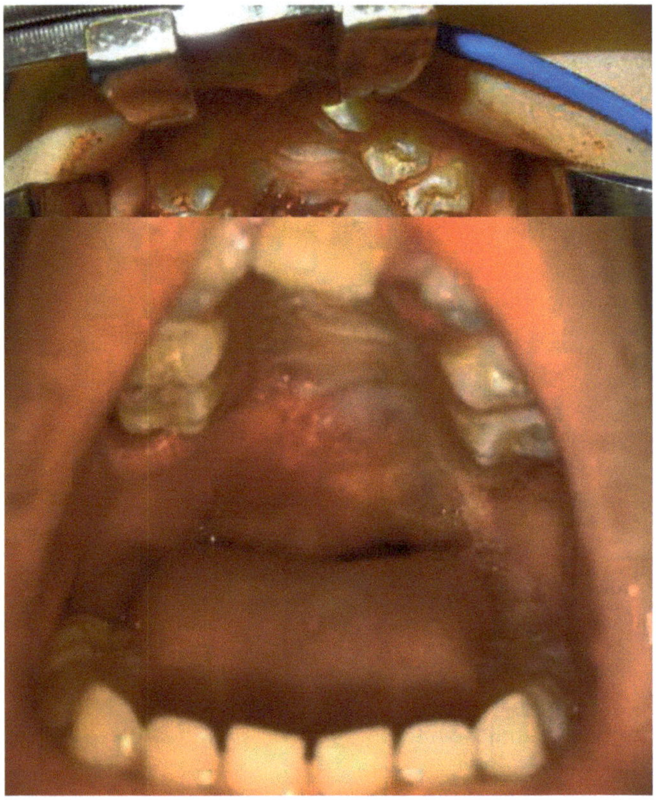

Eight months after this reconstruction, the soft palate is increased in length and function. However, speech therapy should be provided and an interdisciplinary evaluation must be done at 5 years to evaluate competence of the velopharyngeal sphincter and possible requirement of VPI surgery.

## Cleft Palate Principles, Case 2

### Case Study: Large Anterior Oronasal Fistula Reconstruction in a Bilateral Cleft Lip and Palate Patient

Percy Rossell-Perry

### Case Analysis

This 18-year-old boy with congenital bilateral cleft lip and palate has undergone previous cleft lip and palate repair and presents with a severe lip and palate sequelae. After primary palatoplasty, the patient develops a severe palatal defect consisting of a large anterior oronasal fistula which essentially occupies the full space of the hard palate, due to bilateral distal flap necrosis. This fistula is affecting speech and feeding with poor quality of life.

Goals of reconstruction are to close the fistula and restore palatal integrity, as well as to facilitate competent soft palatal length and function.

### Treatment Considerations

Anterior bilateral cleft palate fistulas are challenging for any reconstructive surgeon. Different strategies have been proposed for their correction. Local tissues are limited to use only in smaller fistula cases (generally less than 1 cm of diameter), and most moderate to severe defects are a good indication for regional or distant flaps. I like to use the FAMM (Facial Artery Myo-Mucosal) flap because it is well vascularized, although there are some limitations as it has a difficult surgical dissection with risk of injuring facial nerve branches and parotid duct sectioning.

In this case, I designed a posteriorly based FAMM flap to provide enough healthy tissue to repair the defect. Donor site was closed primarily and there were few associated complications. The nasal layer is closed using advancement mucosal flaps from nasal mucosa. The oral mucosal defect is reconstructed fully by insetting the posteriorly based FAMM flap. The pedicle does not require later division when this is properly positioned. One year after reconstruction, flap viability is evident and the defect is closed.

Velopharyngeal insufficiency is often associated with these cases with significant loss of palatal tissue and scar retraction, and it is important that this is assessed preoperatively and incorporated into the plan. One could consider further posterior/soft palatal mobilization, interposition of a contralateral tissue flap, or if needed, intravelar veloplasty at the same time as the FAMM flap. However, given the large anterior defect, I planned to stage subsequent velopharyngeal insufficiency surgery. Alternatives techniques for this case would include a tongue flap, but which is two stages. The patient will require future orthodontics, and surgery for alveolar clefts closure.

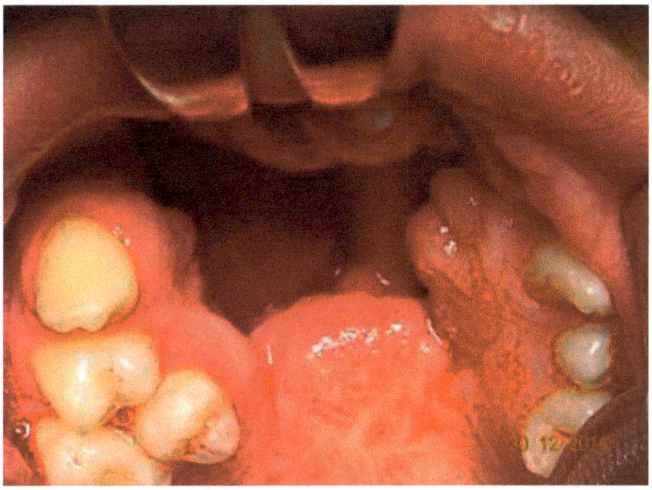

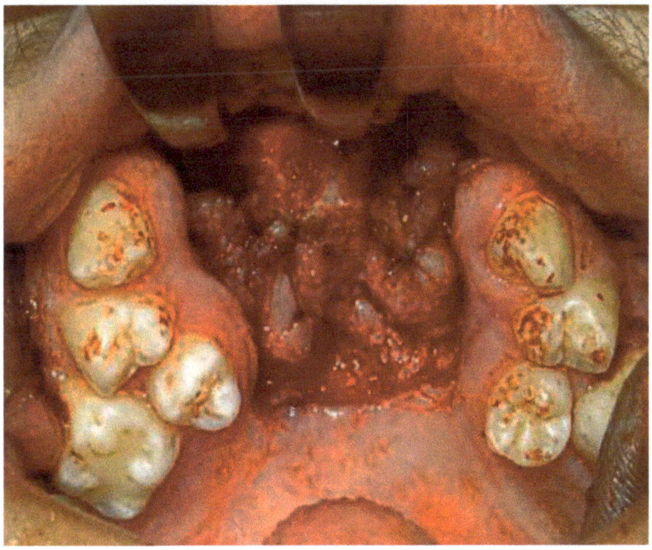

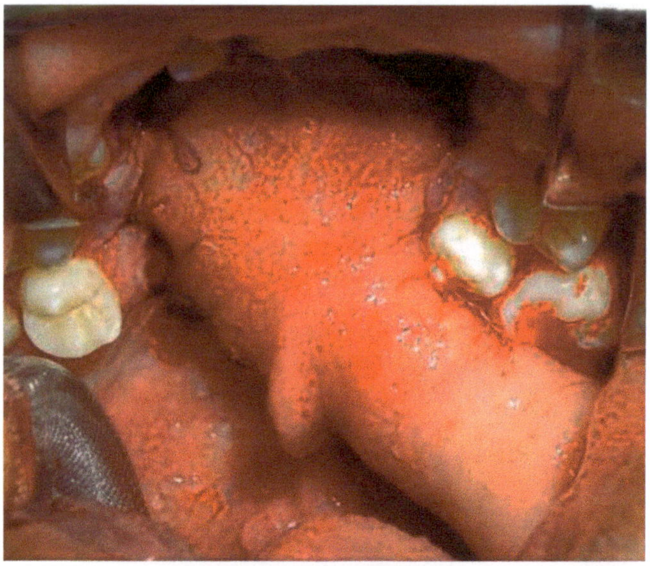

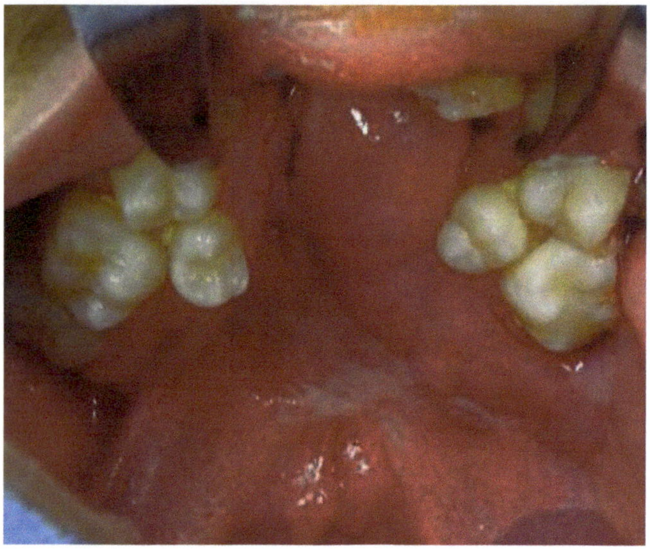

# Speech Surgery and Treatment of Velopharyngeal Insufficiency

20

Oksana A. Jackson and Felicity V. Mehendale

**Key Points**

- A good primary repair is essential for minimizing velopharyngeal dysfunction after palatoplasty.
- Speech assessment and velopharyngeal imaging are critical to identifying which patients are proper candidates for speech surgery and to guide procedure selection.
- Oronasal fistulas of the hard palate and large nasoalveolar fistulas should be closed before proceeding with speech surgery.
- Optimizing function of the soft palate is the first goal of speech surgery.
- Pharyngoplasty should only be performed in settings where appropriate postoperative recovery and blood transfusion facilities exist, and long-term follow-up is possible to monitor for and treat obstructive sleep apnea.

## Introduction

For normal speech production, the palate and pharyngeal walls must achieve complete closure, thus separating the oropharynx and nasopharynx and allowing for the proper direction of airflow during speech. The inability to achieve this closure adequately during speech is termed velopharyngeal insufficiency, incompetence, or dysfunction. Velopharyngeal dysfunction (VPD) manifests as hypernasal speech and audible nasal emission of air, and can be accompanied by compensatory articulation errors, all of which can make speech difficult to understand and unpleasing to the ear.

Normal velopharyngeal function relies on proper anatomic proportions, function, and coordination of the soft palate and pharyngeal musculature [1–4]. Velopharyngeal dysfunction can be congenital or acquired, and the most common type worldwide occurs post-palatoplasty. Cleft width and severity, as well as the type of palatoplasty repair performed, may influence postoperative palatal function, but above all a good primary palate repair with careful tissue handling and proper muscle repositioning is essential to preventing VPD.

Other causes of VPD include an unrecognized submucous cleft palate (Figs. 20.1 and 20.2). Velopharyngeal dysfunc-

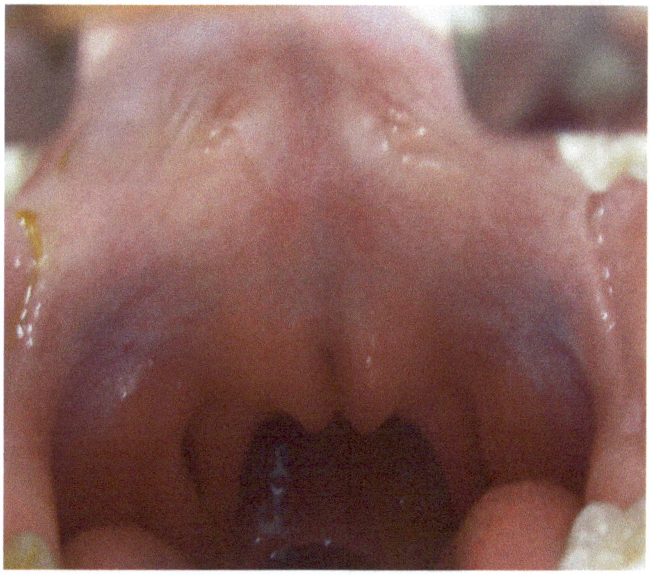

Fig. 20.1 Photo of classic overt submucous cleft palate with complete bifid uvula, zona pellucida, and severe palpable notching of the posterior border of the hard palate

**Electronic Supplementary Material** The online version of this chapter (https://doi.org/10.1007/978-3-030-59105-2_20) contains supplementary material, which is available to authorized users.

O. A. Jackson (✉)
Division of Plastic Surgery, Children's Hospital of Philadelphia and University of Pennsylvania, Philadelphia, PA, USA
e-mail: jacksono@email.chop.edu

F. V. Mehendale
University of Edinburgh, Edinburgh, Scotland, UK
e-mail: felicity.mehendale@ed.ac.uk

© Springer Nature Switzerland AG 2021

J. W. Swanson, D. W. Low (eds.), *Global Cleft Care in Low-Resource Settings*, https://doi.org/10.1007/978-3-030-59105-2_20

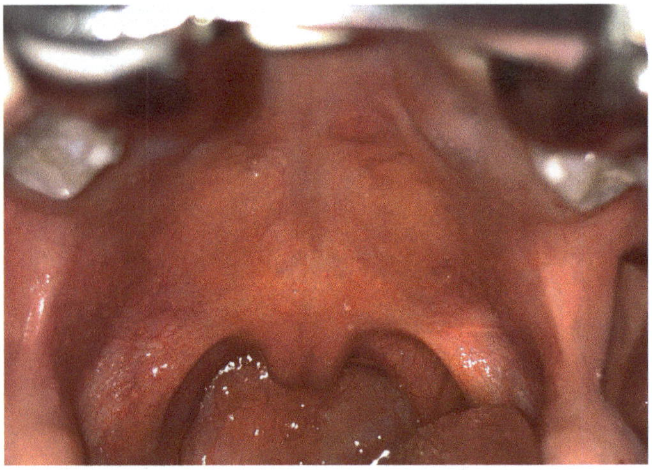

**Fig. 20.2** Photograph of occult submucous cleft palate with lesser form of a bifid uvula. This patient also had a flattened posterior nasal spine

tion may also occur in syndromic conditions in the presence or absence of clefting of the palate, the most common of which is 22q11.2DS. Patients with 22q11.2DS are medically complex, often present with severe VPD that is multifactorial in origin, and should be evaluated for systemic comorbidities prior to surgical intervention [5, 6]. Velopharyngeal mislearning is a lesser-known variant of VPD and is an articulation disorder where symptoms of VPD are present despite normal anatomy and a physiologically normal mechanism. The most common type is phoneme-specific VPD where air is volitionally pushed through the nose on certain sounds, giving the perception of VPD without true hypernasality [7, 8]. The treatment is limited to speech therapy and will not improve with surgery.

**Causes of Velopharyngeal Dysfunction**

- Submucous cleft palate
- Post-palatoplasty
  - Incomplete velar muscle repositioning
  - Velar muscle injury
  - Oronasal fistulae
  - Scarring of the velum
  - Short velum
- Non-cleft velopharyngeal disorders
  - Palatopharyngeal disproportion
  - Neuromuscular disorders
  - Post adenotonsillectomy
  - Palatal tumors
- VP mislearning

**Most Common Multisystem Features of 22q11.2 Deletion Syndrome.** [5, 9–11]

- Dysmorphic facial features (Fig. 20.3)
- Congenital cardiovascular disease—conotruncal anomalies
- Palatal features
  - VPD, often severe with compensatory articulation and poor intelligibility
  - SMCP, classic or occult forms
  - Velopharyngeal disproportion with wide and deep pharynx
  - Overt cleft palate or cleft lip and palate (less common)
  - Neuromuscular disorders of the palate
- Learning disability/developmental delay including motor and speech
- Endocrine disorders—hypocalcemia, hypoparathyroidism
- Immune disorders—recurrent infections, autoimmune diseases
- Neuropsychiatric disorders—autism spectrum and attention disorders, schizophrenia
- Gastrointestinal disorders—gastroesophageal reflux, dysmotility/dysphagia, constipation

## Patient Selection and Clinical Planning

Speech assessment, complemented by velopharyngeal imaging, is necessary to properly identify patients who would benefit from surgery and to select the appropriate surgical intervention. Nasoendoscopy and videofluoroscopy can provide complementary information about velopharyngeal anatomy and function. The details of speech assessment and velopharyngeal imaging are covered in Chap. 29 on Speech and Language Disorders. Significant information can be gathered from oral examination and speech assessment alone, and palate surgeries such as fistula closure, revision palatoplasty, and palatal lengthening can be performed in the absence of imaging if unavailable. However, imaging is critical to accomplishing safe and effective surgical treatments in the following clinical situations: in cases of congenital VPD, in cases where palatal motion appears minimal, and in planning secondary pharyngoplasty after palate function has been optimized. Joint evaluation by the surgeon and speech pathologist is essential to diagnose correctly whether speech problems require surgical treatment, or speech therapy, or a combination of both. This is important in communication of the treatment prognosis and in managing patients' expectations.

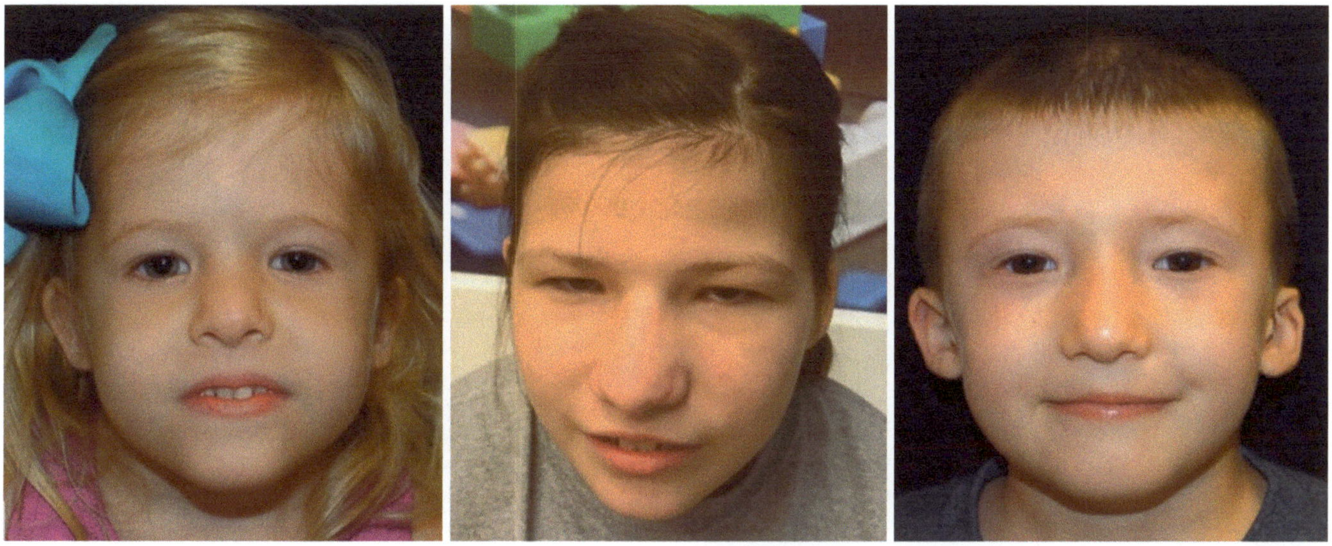

Fig. 20.3 Composite facial photographs of children with 22q11.2 deletion syndrome demonstrating distinct but variable facial features including hooded eyelids, broad nasal bridge, bulbous nasal tip, low set ears and ear anomalies, hypoplastic nasal ala, small mouth, flattened philtral column

**Steps in Preoperative Evaluation**

1. Speech assessment—Diagnose VPD, characterize severity and articulation disorders
2. Oral examination—Assess for SMCP, fistulae, palatal scarring, levator muscle malposition
3. Clinical history—Recognize medical comorbidities or syndromic diagnosis
4. Velopharyngeal imaging—Surgical planning based on closure pattern, gap size, and motion

## Procedure Selection and Timing of Surgery

Surgical treatment for velopharyngeal dysfunction should follow a step-wise algorithm to optimize long-term speech outcome and minimize complications. The first and most important goal of speech surgery is to optimize velar function. This requires an intact palate with proper muscle position and length. Only after velar integrity and function have been optimized, should more aggressive procedures such as pharyngoplasty be considered.

**Algorithm for Procedure Selection for VPD**

1. Palate exam
   - SMCP → Palatoplasty
   - Oronasal fistulae → Repair fistulae, Palate revision
   - Evidence of levator muscle malposition → Palate re-repair with intravelar veloplasty, Furlow re-repair
   - Palate intact with good motion → Palatal lengthening
   - Palate intact with poor motion → Pharyngoplasty*
   - Persistent VPD after palate repair/lengthening → Pharyngoplasty*
   - Significant velopharyngeal disproportion → Pharyngoplasty*

*Choice and tailoring of pharyngoplasty technique guided by velopharyngeal imaging

- Coronal pattern (palatal motion > > lateral wall motion) → Sphincter pharyngoplasty
- Circular pattern (palatal motion = lateral wall motion) → Posterior pharyngeal flap

Palatal integrity should be restored early by closure of any significant oronasal fistulae. Palate re-repair can be performed at any age once language is present and VPD is diagnosed. After the velar muscles have been properly retropositioned and there is evidence of decent velar motion on examination, palatal lengthening with buccal myomucosal flaps can be successful [12, 13]. This technique can allow the soft palate to achieve closure without adding scar to the velum or incurring significant risk of airway obstruction.

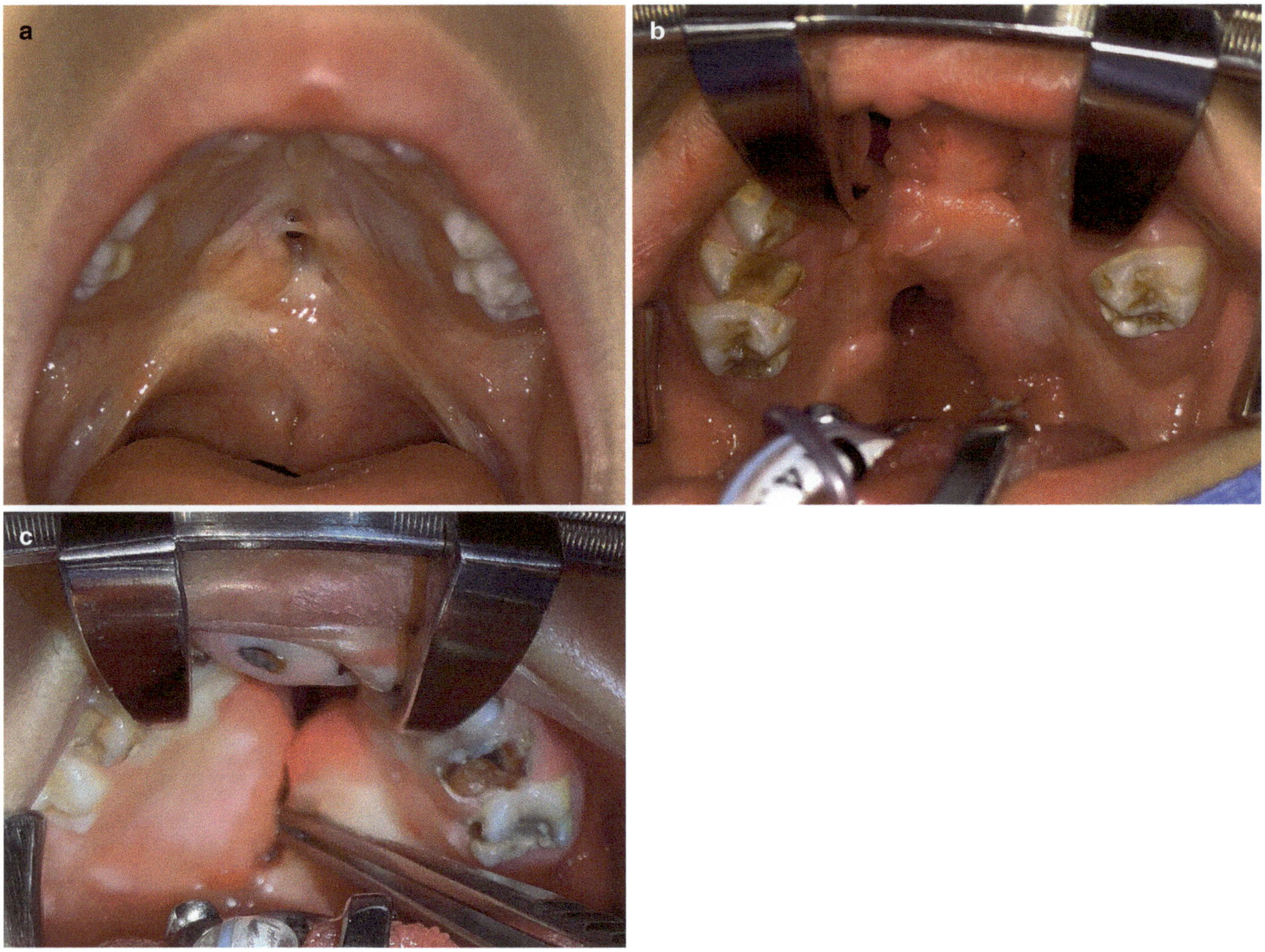

Fig. 20.4 (a–c) Palates with significant scar, dehiscence, and oronasal fistulae

The multiply operated and heavily scarred palate is a difficult challenge (Fig. 20.4a–c). Often, dense scar tissue is limited to the midline and hard-soft palate junction at the sites of previous incisions or areas of delayed healing, but the laterally displaced muscle bundles have been minimally manipulated and are healthy. In these situations, palate re-repair with muscle repositioning by any technique may be successful. In addition, re-repair by the Furlow technique can lengthen the palate and break up the restrictive midline scar [14]. In other cases, new healthy tissue must be added during re-repair due to the severity of the palatal stiffness and shortness. Buccal myomucosal flaps will stretch over time with repetitive velar excursion, and improvements in VPD may continue over several years in this situation [13].

If soft palatal length and function have been optimized, and VPD persists, pharyngoplasty is the next step. Various surgical techniques have been described including posterior pharyngeal flap, Hynes pharyngoplasty, and Orticochea sphincter pharyngoplasty [15–21]. These procedures rearrange the local tissues of the palate and pharynx to narrowing the velopharyngeal port, and should be tailored to each patient's unique anatomy to optimize results and minimize complications. More obstructive procedures are typically performed when motion is limited, although under-correction in these challenging cases may be intentional to avoid the complication of obstructive sleep apnea. Patient factors linked to less successful outcomes include increased preoperative severity of speech and the poorly dynamic mechanism [22].

The pediatric airway has a small area, and tonsillar and adenoid hypertrophy are more common in younger children, therefore pharyngoplasty techniques are not recommended before the age of 4 years due to concerns for obstructive sleep apnea. Because they significantly alter the nasopharyngeal airway, these procedures should not be done in settings where regular long-term follow-up and proper screening for obstructive sleep apnea are not available.

**Pitfalls**

- Enlarged tonsils and adenoids may interfere with proper placement of a posterior pharyngeal flap or sphincter pharyngoplasty inset.
- Adenotonsillectomy performed a minimum of 4 months prior to pharyngoplasty can improve surgical outcomes and minimize the risk of postoperative obstructive sleep apnea. Patients and parents should be warned that VPD may increase after adenoidectomy.

In the absence of palatal motion due to neuromuscular causes or secondary to damage from multiple repairs, treatment options are limited to prosthetic devices such as palatal lifts or speech bulbs, described further in Chap. 29. In addition, patients with advanced age and VPD complicated by compensatory misarticulation may not benefit from surgical intervention despite repairable anatomic differences due to deeply established patterns of speech. Surgical interventions should be coupled with appropriate speech therapy for optimal outcomes.

## Relevant Anatomy

The velopharyngeal space extends from the posterior border of the hard palate to the posterior pharyngeal wall and includes seven muscles (Fig. 20.5). The levator veli palatini is the primary muscle responsible for elevation and retraction of the velum against the pharyngeal walls, but the superior pharyngeal constrictor, musculus uvulae, and palatopharyngeus also contribute to velopharyngeal closure. The palatopharyngeus has a transverse component which courses from the velum to the lateral pharyngeal walls, and a vertical component. These vertically oriented fibers of the palatopharyngeus constitute the posterior tonsillar pillars and are used in sphincter pharyngoplasty. The superior pharyngeal constrictor is a thin muscle that forms the upper and lateral walls of the pharynx and produces inward movement of the pharyngeal walls during speech and swallowing. The upper segment likely influences velopharyngeal closure patterns [23]. Posterior pharyngeal flaps are random flaps and are raised to include the oral mucosa as well as superior pharyngeal constrictor muscle for a more robust and vascularized flap.

The buccinator is a thin muscle that forms the lateral wall of the oral cavity and whose function is to pull back the angle of the mouth and flatten the cheek (Fig. 20.6). It arises from the outer surfaces of the alveolar processes of the maxilla and mandible at the region of the first and second molar teeth and from the pterygomandibular raphe. Its fibers converge toward the angle of the mouth and insert into the orbicular oris. The orientation of these fibers allows for easy identification of the muscle during buccal flap surgery. It is supplied by branches of the facial artery and the buccal branch of the maxillary artery, and innervated by the buccal branch of the facial nerve on its superficial surface. The buccal fat pad is also superficial to the muscle and can be visualized during dissection; penetration of the fascia can lead to the nuisance

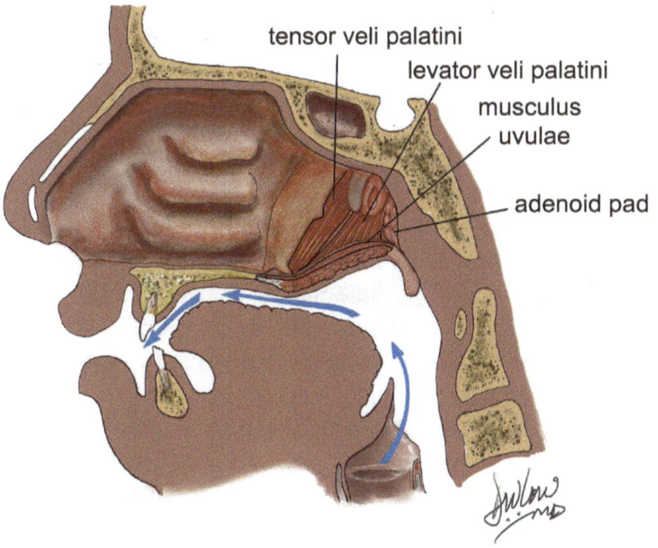


Fig. 20.5 Illustration of activated velopharyngeal mechanism showing soft palate musculature in detail and elevation of velum with contact to adenoid pad of posterior nasopharynx

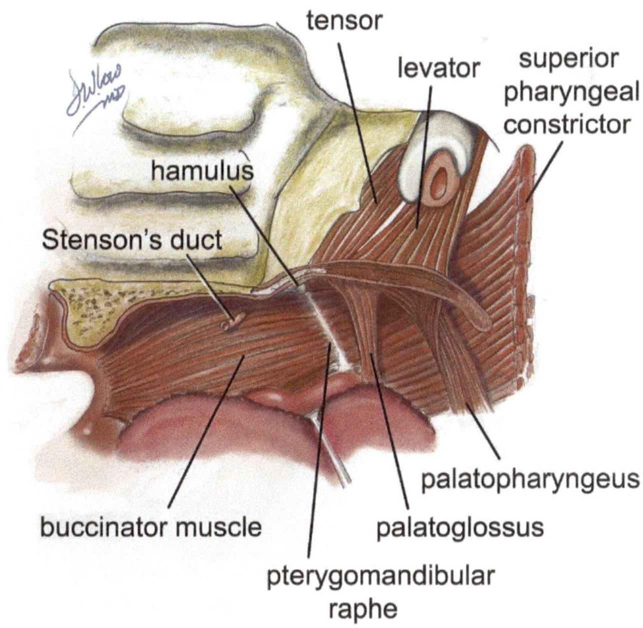


Fig. 20.6 Buccinator muscle anatomy showing muscle fibers running in an anterior direction to the oral commissure where they insert and blend with fibers of the orbicularis oris muscle. Note interrupted by Stenson's duct at the position of the maxillary second molar

of buccal fat herniation during harvest. The parotid duct penetrates the muscle and opens into the mouth in the vicinity of the maxillary second molar, and should be noted and excluded during flap design.

## **Key Equipment** (Fig. 20.7)

- Oral mouth prop or "Dingman" retractor allows access to the palate and oropharynx.
- Several elevators—Freer and angled dental excavator are useful in elevating the mucoperiosteum off the hard palate and for dissection around the greater palatine pedicle.
- Oral curved or angled retractors allow superior retraction of the velum for access to the posterior pharynx.
- Palate hooks can be used to retract tissues with minimal trauma.
- Rubber catheters can be used to retract the uvula and soft palate and expose the posterior pharynx either by encircling the velum or being sewn directly to the nasal surface and retracted through the nose (Fig. 20.8a–c).
- A needlepoint cautery used on a very low power setting can be used to score the mucosal lining and elevate flaps in the posterior pharynx with minimal blood loss.
- 4–0 Chromic or Vicryl suture on tapered needles for mucosal closure of the palate, buccal surface, and donor site areas of the nasopharynx. Double-armed sutures (4–0 Monocryl) are particularly useful for posterior pharyngeal flap inset.

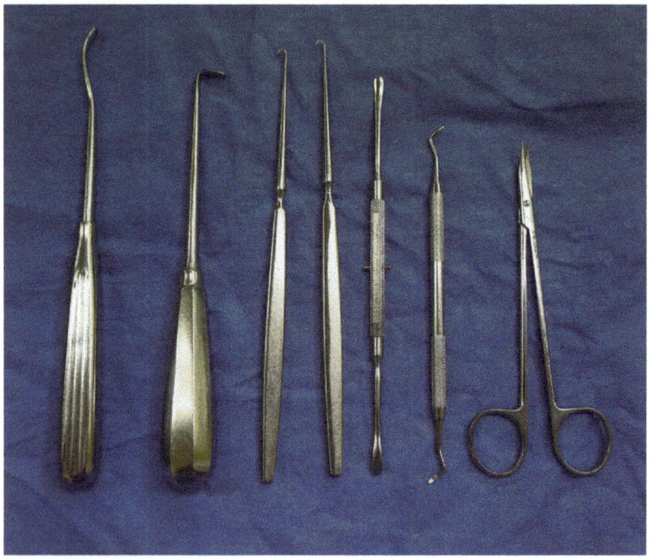

**Fig. 20.7** Helpful instruments for VPD surgery

## Anesthesia

General orotracheal anesthesia is employed during surgery. Locoregional anesthesia is an important adjunct to manage postoperative pain. Long-acting local anesthetic solutions such as bupivacaine or ropivacaine can be injected into the local tissues at the completion of the procedure, or in the case of palatal surgery, the suprazygomatic maxillary nerve block can be effective. It is important to respect dosing guidelines which are covered in Table 3 in Chap. 10.

## Patient Preparation

The patient should be positioned supine on the table with the neck extended. A shoulder roll is helpful to achieve neck extension or the bed may be placed in Trendelenburg position. An oral rinse with chlorhexidine solution or commercial mouthwash can be used to cleanse the oral cavity. Use of epinephrine containing solutions is critical to optimize visualization particularly during palate dissection. 1% Lidocaine with epinephrine 1:100,000 (maximum dosing of 7 mg/kg) can be used for infiltration of the tissues; in addition, pledgets soaked in epinephrine solution without lidocaine (by mixing 1:1000 epinephrine solution with 100 cc of saline to a final dilution of 1:100,000) can be applied liberally to the tissues and can be very helpful in achieving optimal hemostasis. A Dingman retractor or similar mouth prop is placed for visualization of the oral cavity and posterior pharynx. With the neck extended, a throat pack is not necessary, however, it may be required if oxygen concentrations through the anesthesia circuit are high in order to minimize risk of airway fire during the use of cautery.

## Procedural Techniques

### **Furlow Cleft Palate Re-repair** (Fig. 20.9)

Palate re-repair by the Furlow double opposing z-plasty technique is indicated when there is suspicion of sagittally oriented levator veli palatine muscle fibers. This can occur due to incomplete levator muscle repositioning during the primary repair or due to secondary velar scarring in the midline tethering the musculature to the hard palate. Levator muscle malposition often can be observed intraorally and with velopharyngeal imaging. In other cases, muscle position may be hard to determine, but may be suspected if the

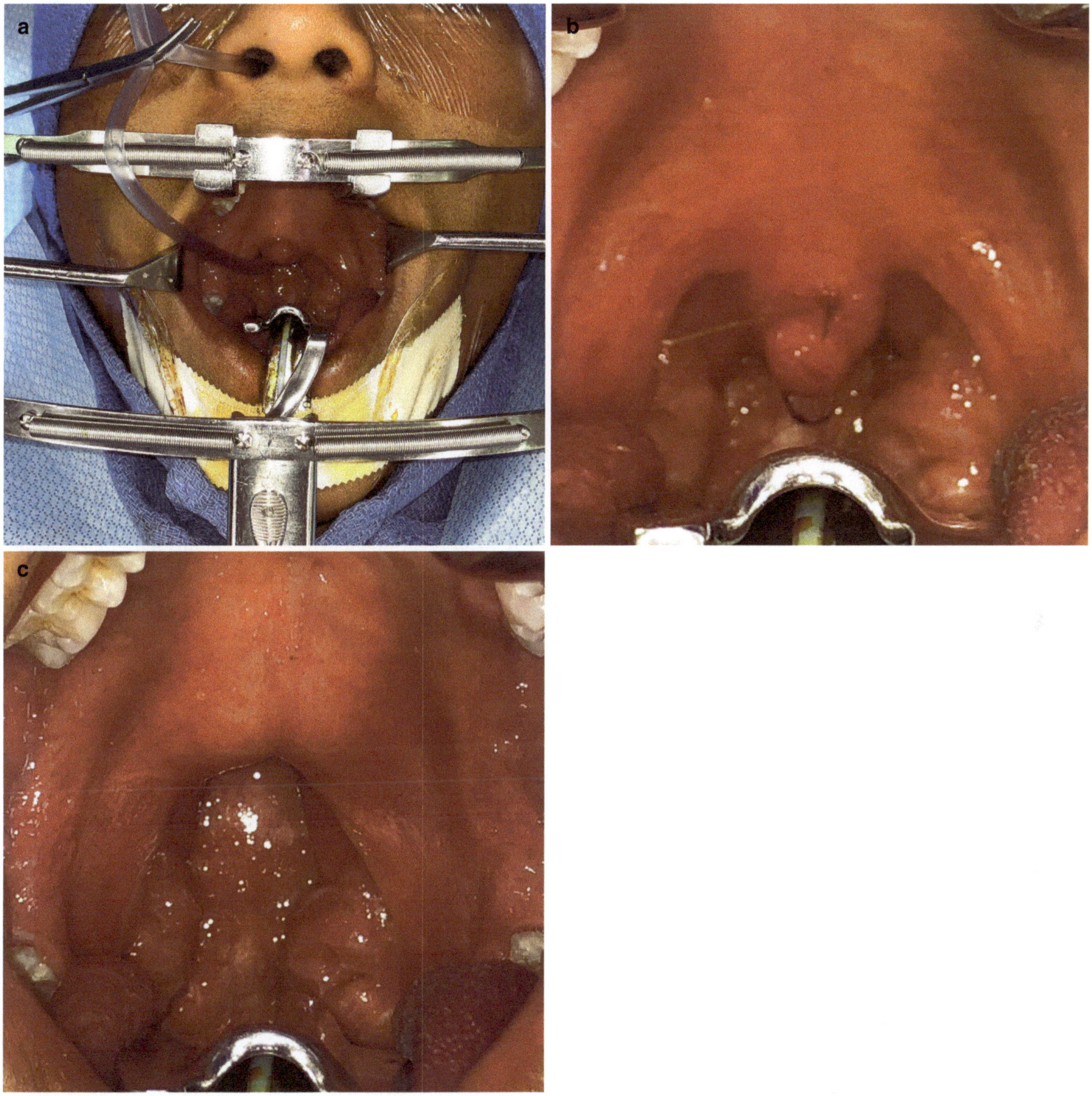


Fig. 20.8 (**a–c**) Retraction of the velum for exposure of the posterior pharynx can be accomplished with a plastic catheter looped around the velum (**a**) or sewn to the nasal surface of the uvula (**b**) and retracted superiorly through the nose (**c**)

palate is short with limited motion and a midline scar is present. Numerous published reports describe the success of this technique for correction of post-palatoplasty VPD [14, 24, 25]. Advantages include re-orienting the velar muscle into a transverse position, potentially lengthening the palate, z-scar pattern in the velum which prevents secondary longitudinal contracture during healing, and minimal risk of incurring obstructive sleep apnea. The technique is similar to primary Furlow palatoplasty that is described in greater detail in Chap. 18.

## Surgical Steps

- An incision is made through the midline of the velum in the old sagittal scar. This incision extends from the hard palate through the uvula. Typical z-plasty incisions are planned as described in Chap. 18 (Fig. 20.10a–c).
- The soft palate flaps are raised with tenotomy or fine-tipped scissors. Often dense scar tissue is present in the midline and at the posterior border of the hard palate centrally and this is sharply divided with fine scissors as the flaps are raised.

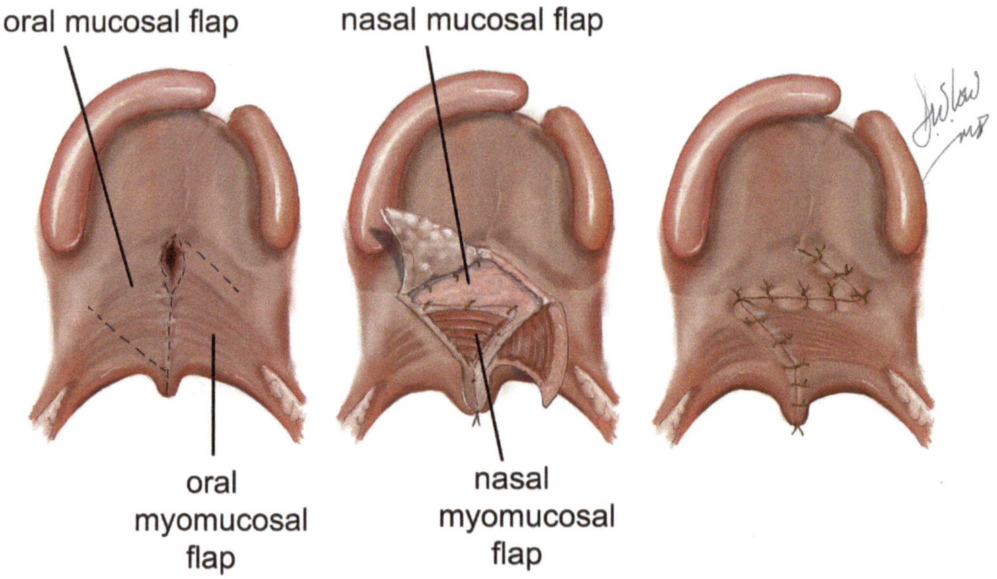


**Fig. 20.9** Furlow re-repair technique illustrating incisions in the midline of the soft palate incision around an oronasal fistula and traditional z-plasty; elevation of flaps and inset of nasal sided flap; final closure with inset of oral sided flaps and levator muscle overlap and retropositioning

- Care is taken to identify the levator muscle bundles within the soft palatal flaps. Often the muscles are scarred medially but laterally can be identified and traced back to the levator tunnels. With flap rotation and inset, these muscles are transversely repositioned and often can be overlapped greater than 10 mm. No additional suture placement in the muscles themselves is typically performed (Fig. 20.10b).
- Posterolateral relaxing incisions are usually required for this procedure to obtain adequate advancement of the anteriorly based oral mucosal flap and tension-free closure. Through the lateral releases and/or through a central extension of the sagittal incision onto the hard palate, the vascular pedicles can be identified and the surrounding fibrous attachments and scar tissue released.
- Closure is performed with absorbable sutures on both nasal and oral layers in an interrupted fashion (Fig. 20.10c)

## Sommerlad Palate Re-repair with Radical Muscle Dissection and Retropositioning

In patients with levator veli palatini muscles that are in a suboptimal position (too anterior), a Sommerlad palate re-repair with radical muscle dissection and retropositioning has been shown to be effective in improving velopharyngeal function, both in patients who have had little to no muscle dissection at their original palate repair and in patients who have had some degree of muscle dissection (often referred to as intravelar veloplasty) during their primary palate repair [26, 27]. This procedure aims to release the anteriorly tethered velar muscles and place them more posteriorly in the velum (retroposition), thus achieving reconstruction of the levator sling in a more posterior and functionally effective position. It is important to note that the more dissection that has been done previously in the velum, the more scarring there is likely to be, thus making this revision operation more challenging. The advantage of a palate re-repair with radical muscle dissection and retropositioning is that it can improve velar function and increase the functional length of the velum (distance from the back of the hard palate to the levator knee). Moreover, unlike a pharyngoplasty, it does not distort the anatomy of the pharynx and does not rely on the creation of a permanent obstruction in the pharynx to achieve velopharyngeal competence [27].

Sommerlad advocates the use of the operating microscope, not only to enable a more precise dissection, but also to facilitate teaching, training, and an adequate view for all theatre staff [28]. The operating microscope also allows for a more comfortable position for the surgeon. The procedure is similar to the muscle dissection performed in a primary palate repair and detailed in Chap. 17 [27, 29].

**Tips and Tricks**

- Secondary surgery of the scarred palate is often difficult and dissection can be bloody.
- Bipolar cautery is useful in controlling bleeding while minimizing thermal damage.
- Infiltration with a solution of epinephrine along with local anesthetic as well as pledgets soaked with epinephrine solution or Afrin can control oozing enough to allow for better visualization. It is important to wait to give the epinephrine time to achieve vasoconstriction.
- Small rolls of gauze can also be used to apply point pressure to bleeding sites.

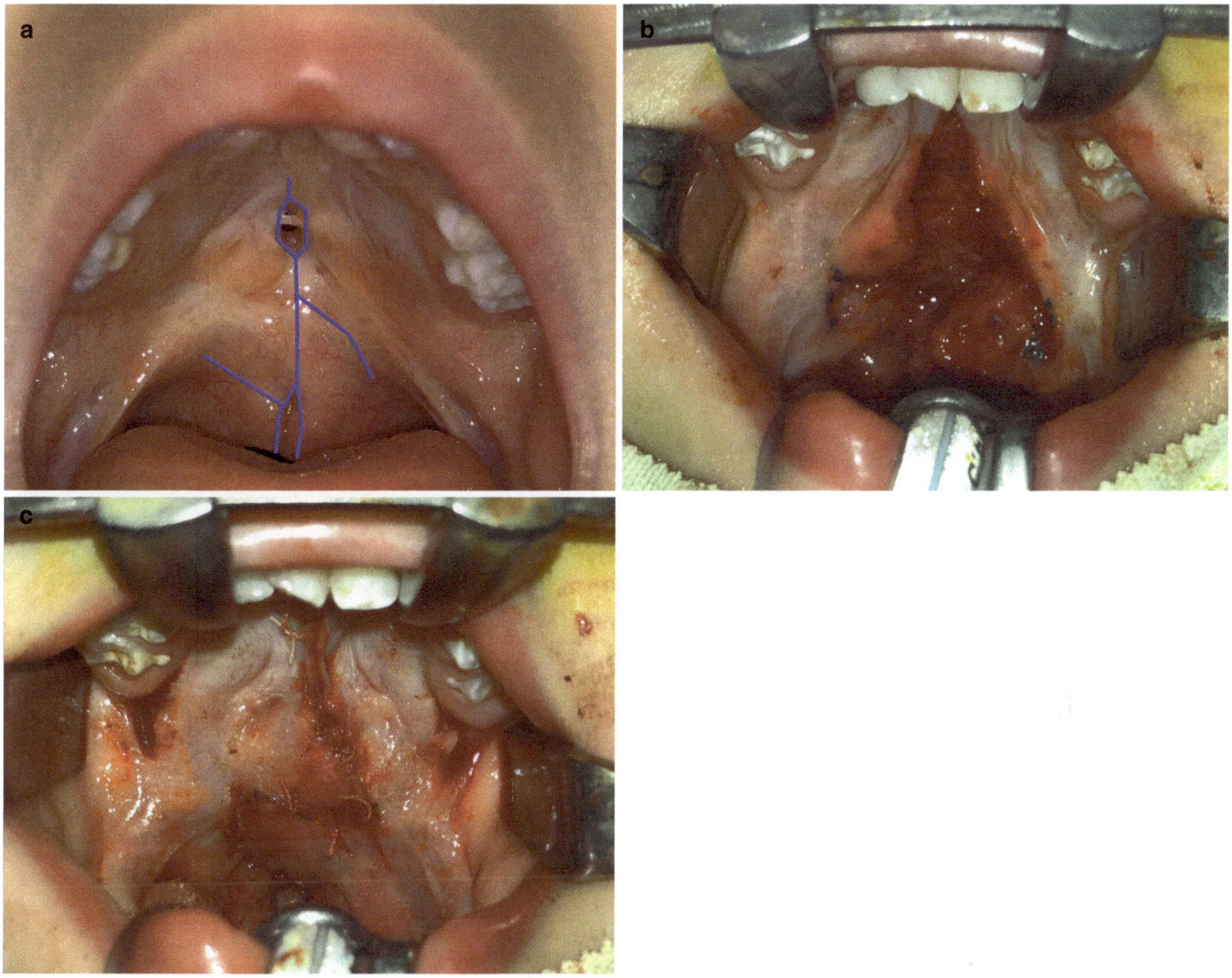


**Fig. 20.10** (**a–c**) Furlow palate re-repair with oronasal fistula closure demonstrating incisional design (**a**), dissected soft palate z-flaps with right-sided anteriorly based oral mucosa flap, and left-sided posteriorly based oral myomucosal flaps, ready for inset in rotated position (**b**). Posterolateral releases were needed to accomplish final closure without tension. These are left open to heal secondarily (**c**)

## Palatal Lengthening with Bilateral Double Opposing Buccal Myomucosal Flaps (Fig. 20.11)

This procedure introduces healthy tissue into the velum at the hard-soft palate junction, thus allowing for retropositioning of the velar musculature and lengthening of the palate without compromising the upper airway. Scar tissue at this junction limiting velar excursion is released and the healthy tissue of the buccal flaps can then stretch to accommodate velar closure. The buccal flaps are random flaps and thus it is important to harvest the flaps near full thickness of the buccinator muscle and maintain a minimum of 1.5 cm of width of the flap for viability [12, 13, 30].

### Surgical Steps

**Palate dissection**

- A transverse incision is made across the soft palate through the oral mucosa approximately 2–3 mm behind the hard-soft palate junction (Fig. 20.12a).
- The abnormal muscle attachments and scar tissue are released from the posterior border of the hard palate with tenotomy or similar fine-tipped scissors.
- The incision is completed through the nasal mucosa leaving a cuff of nasal mucosa attached to the hard palate to allow for suturing during flap inset.

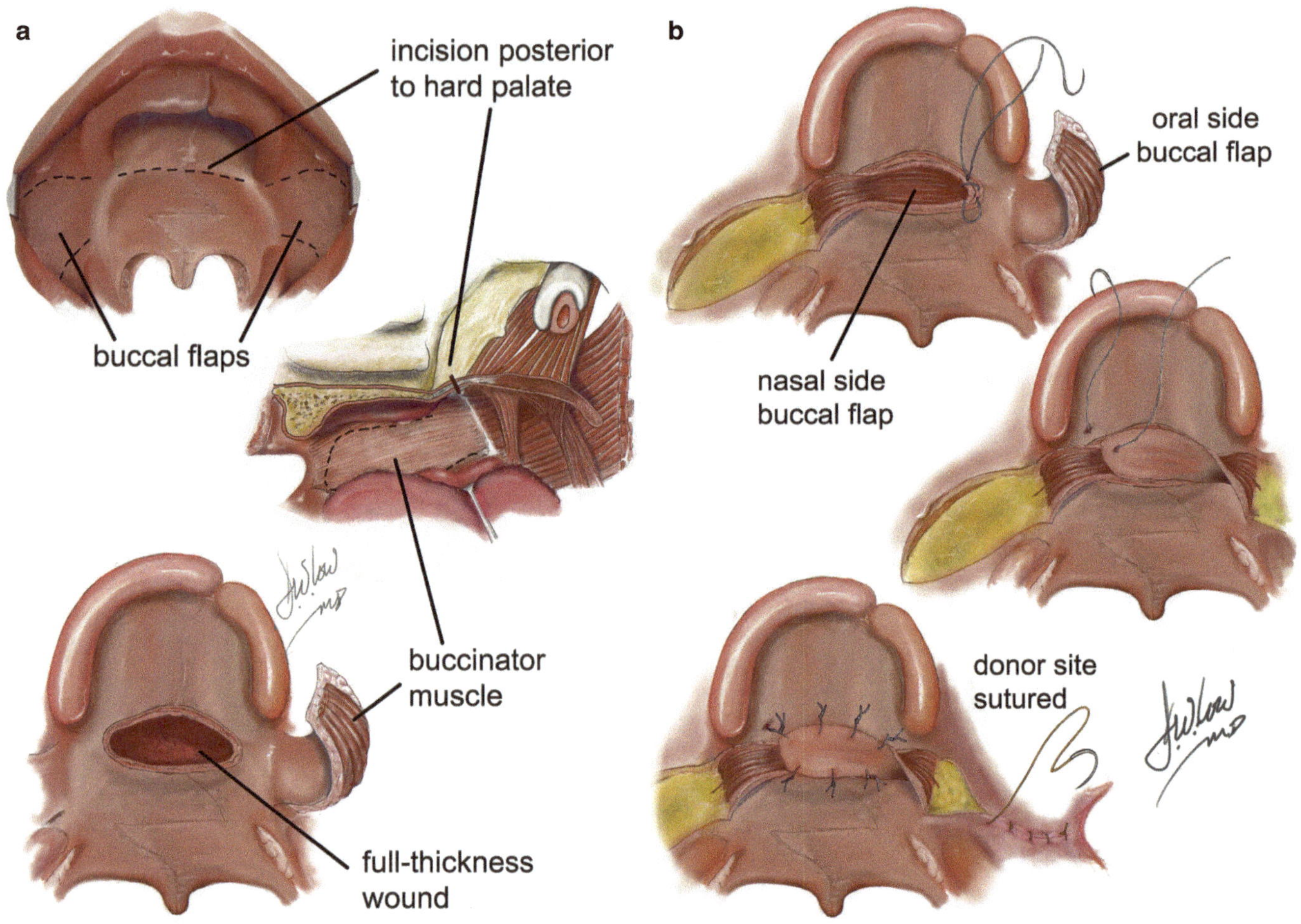


**Fig. 20.11** (**a**, **b**) Illustration of palatal lengthening technique with bilateral buccal myomucosal flaps (**a**) Buccal flap incision design and palatal incision at the hard-soft palate junction which is deepened full-thickness through the velum. (**b**) Inset of the buccal flaps in an overlapping fashion and closure of the buccal donor site with a running dissolvable suture

- Once completely released from the hard palate, the soft palate moves posteriorly leaving a large full-thickness gap (Fig. 20.12b).

**Flap design and elevation**

- Bilateral buccal flaps are outlined with their base at the retromolar trigone extending toward the oral commissure (Fig. 20.12c).
- The width of the flap is 15–18 mm at its base and tapers slightly as it approaches the oral commissure.
- The opening of Stenson's duct near the maxillary second molar should be identified and avoided.
- The flap is elevated with fine-tipped scissors from the commissure to the trigone incorporating approximately 90% thickness of the buccinator muscle. A stitch placed near the oral commissure for superior retraction facilitates this harvest.

**Flap inset and closure**

- One flap is interposed in the palatal opening with the buccal mucosal surface nasal to close the nasal side and interrupted absorbable sutures used to secure it in place.
- The second flap is overlapped to close the oral surface and similarly sutured in place (Fig. 20.12d).
- The buccal flap donor sites are closed with absorbable sutures leaving space open at the base to prevent compression of the flap pedicles (Fig. 20.12e).
- The buccal flap pedicles can be divided and the small intentional lateral palatal fistulas closed at a later date if bothersome to the patient due to impingement by the posterior molars. This should be done a minimal of one month from the initial surgery to allow for local vascular ingrowth to the flaps.

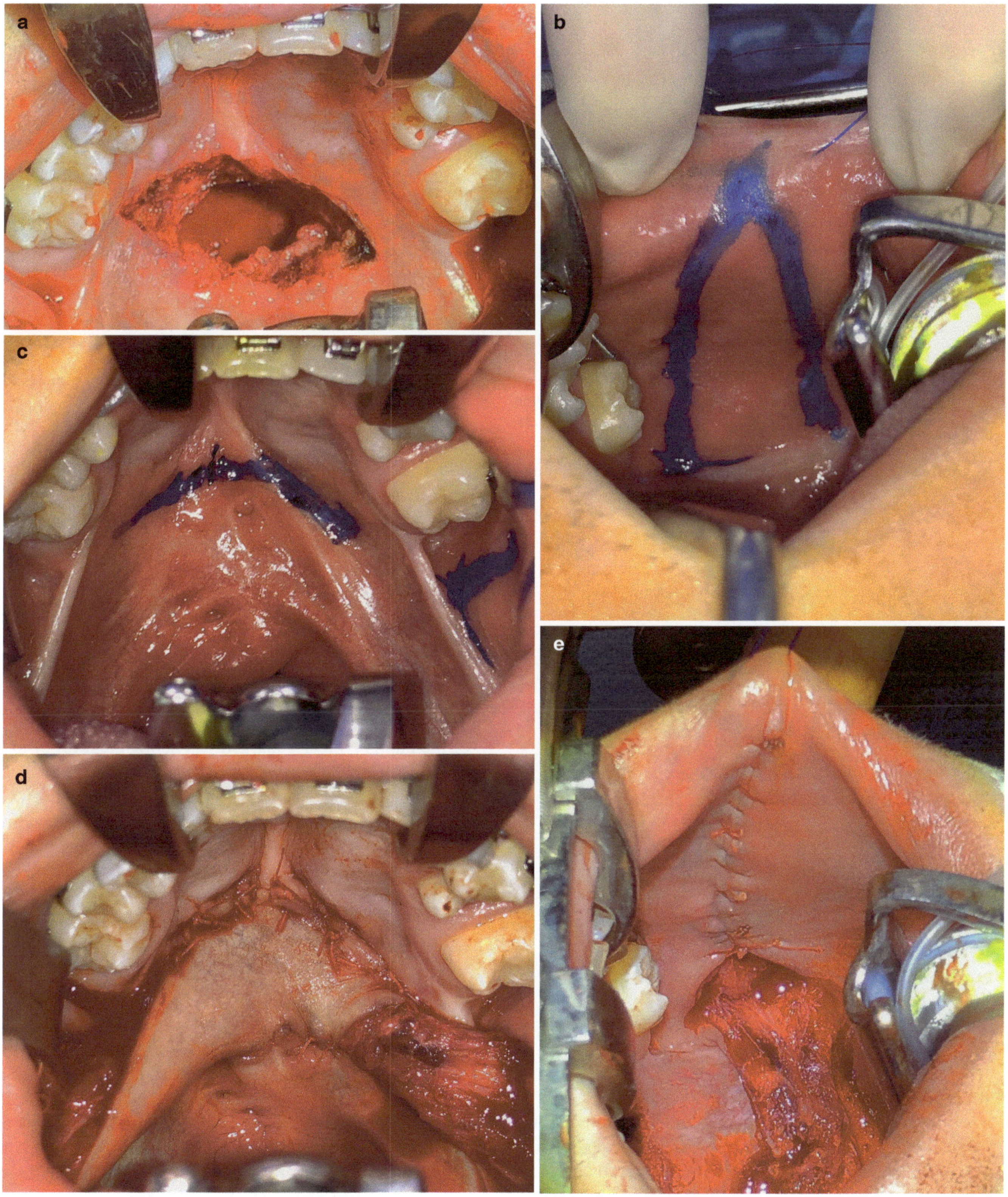

Fig. 20.12 (**a**–**d**) Operative photographs of palatal lengthening with bilateral opposing buccal myomucosal flaps demonstrating: palate incision at hard-soft palate junction (**a**) and full-thickness dissection (**b**), buccal flap design (**c**), inset of buccal flaps (**d**), and closure buccal donor site (**e**)

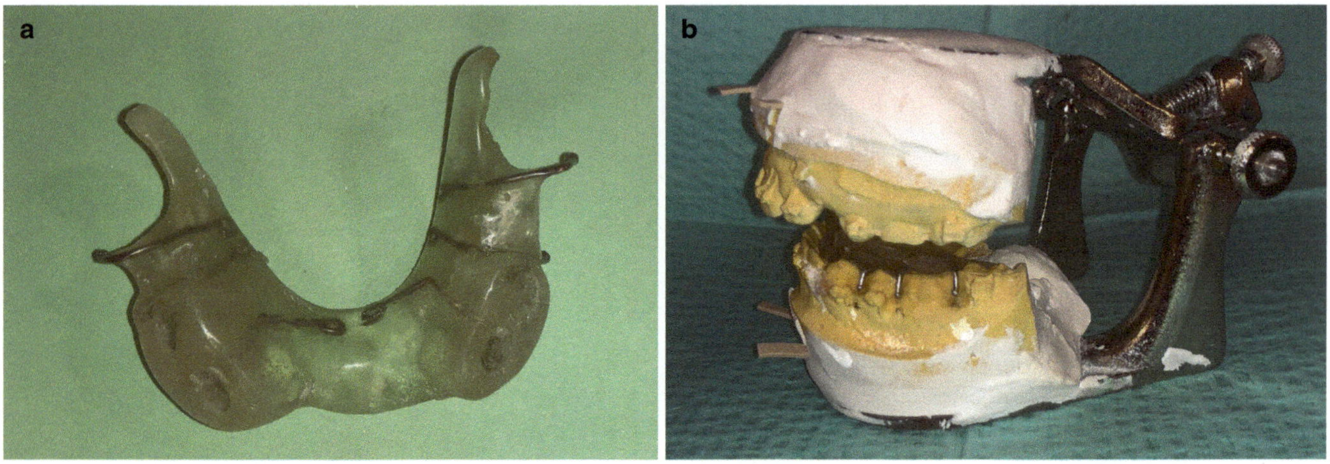


**Fig. 20.13** (**a**, **b**) Photographs of oral bite block splint. Splint is made of acrylic and custom fitted to mandibular teeth with clasps (**a**). Splint shown on model (**b**), demonstrating how it prevents posterior molars from contacting, thus protecting buccal myomucosal flap pedicles in older patients

Video 20.1 Oral examination after palatal lengthening surgery

**Pitfalls**

- Older children with erupted second and third molars can bite the pedicles of the buccal myomucosal flaps postoperatively leading to necrosis of the flaps.
- Ranging the jaw at the completion of the procedure can visualize compression of the flaps.
- An oral bite block splint worn for 2 weeks can protect the pedicles during the critical phase of healing and local vascular ingrowth (Fig. 20.13a, b).
- Bite block splint for palatal lengthening can be fabricated on the table and sewn or wired to the upper or lower teeth with materials such as moldable nasal splints (aquaplast) and silicone tubing. Within a dental hospital setting, glass ionomer cement can also be effective in creating customized bite blocks that are built up on the teeth. The ionomer comes off spontaneously after a few weeks.

## Posterior Pharyngeal Flap (Fig. 20.14)

Posterior pharyngeal flap surgery uses tissue from the posterior pharyngeal wall to occlude the central nasopharyngeal area. A rectangular flap of tissue is raised consisting of mucosa and the underlying superior pharyngeal constrictor muscle, and this flap is attached to the soft palate. The technique can vary widely: the flap can be based cranially or caudally, the donor site can be closed or left open to heal secondarily, the flap can be lined or left unlined, and the dimensions of the flap can vary considerably [16, 31–34]. The authors' preferred approach follows the technique originally described by Argamaso and detailed by Kirschner and consists of a wide unlined superiorly based flap without closure of the donor site and is detailed below [16, 31].

### Surgical Steps

**Flap design** (Fig. 20.15a)

- The flap is outlined with a marking pen on the posterior pharyngeal wall.
- The transverse incision corresponding to the lower border of the flap is typically marked just below the level of the uvula.
- The flap width is tailored to the degree of lateral pharyngeal wall motion seen on preoperative studies. The width of the flap should ideally exceed the width of the visualized velopharyngeal gap as there will be some degree of flap contracture and remodeling. In patients with minimal motion, this may span near the entire width of the posterior pharynx.

**Flap elevation** (Fig. 20.15b, d)

- A fine needlepoint cautery on low power is used to score the mucosal borders of the flap.
- The incision is deepened with the cautery through the muscular layer to the prevertebral fascia.
- The flap is raised superiorly in this avascular plane by a combination of blunt dissection and cautery.
- The flap is raised to the adenoid bed and its length is designed to inset without tension or redundancy.

**Velar pocket creation** (Fig. 20.15c)

- A wide transverse pocket of 6–8 mm in depth is created along the posterior border of the soft palate behind the uvula.

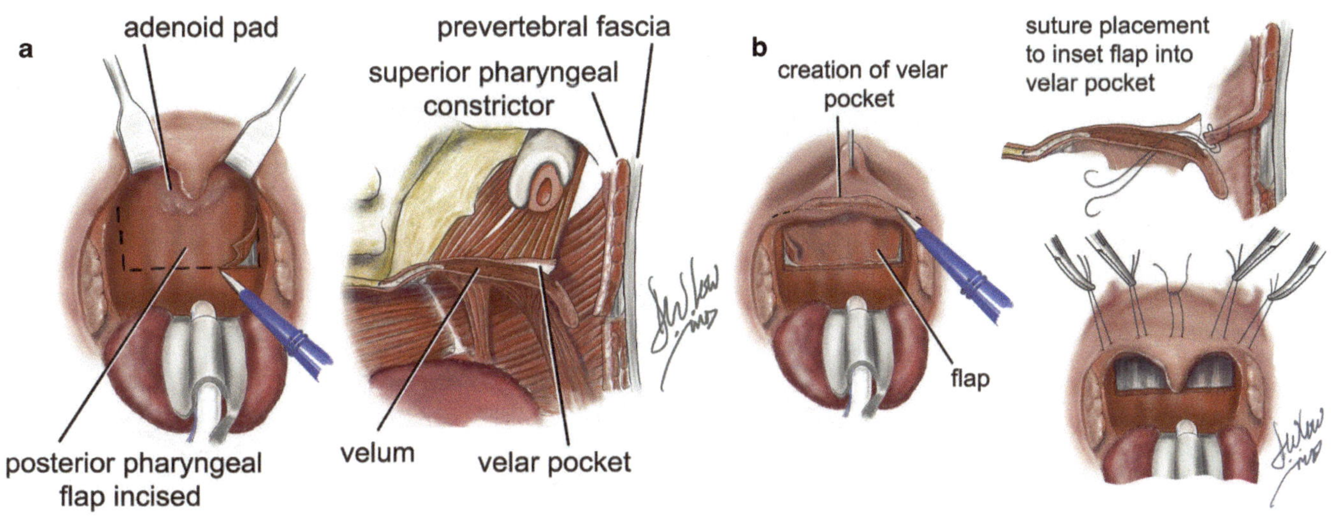


**Fig. 20.14** (**a**, **b**) Illustration of posterior pharyngeal flap procedure: (**a**) design and cautery elevation of wide rectangular flap from posterior pharyngeal wall and lateral view of velum showing location of pocket between nasal mucosa and velar musculature, (**b**) creation of velar pocket on posterior border of velum and mattress suture inset into velar pocket

- With retraction on the uvula and velar border, a semicircular mucosal incision is scored with the cautery.
- Tenotomy scissors are then used to spread the tissues laterally and create a pocket between the nasal mucosa and velar musculature.
- The two lateral pockets are joined centrally with sharp dissection in the central velum.

**Flap inset** (Fig. 20.15d–f)

- The flap is inset into this pocket with a series of absorbable sutures that are tied on the oral surface of the palate.
- The width of inset is dictated by the degree of preoperative lateral wall motion. The most lateral flap inset points should always exceed the flap width to stretch the flap and prevent tubing. If there is very little or no lateral wall motion, the inset can span laterally into the tonsillar fossa.
- A double-armed suture facilitates this inset if available. Typically, five evenly spaced sutures are placed along the inferior border of the flap, brought through the pocket and tied on the oral surface.

## Sphincter Pharyngoplasty (Fig. 20.16)

Sphincter pharyngoplasty techniques use tissue from the lateral pharynx to circumferentially narrow the nasopharyngeal area and augment the posterior pharyngeal wall. As described by Orticochea, the tissue of the bilateral posterior pharyngeal pillars consisting of the palatopharyngeus muscles is utilized to create a sling just below the adenoid pad [35]. This technique narrows the nasopharynx at the level of inset and in theory is a dynamic structure.

### Surgical Steps

**Flap creation:**

- Two superiorly based rectangular flaps are designed over the posterior tonsillar pillars (Fig. 20.17a).
- The lateral borders of the flaps are scored with a fine cautery.
- The tenotomy or other fine-tipped scissors are used to deepen the incisions and separate the palatopharyngeus muscle from the tonsillar bed.
- A curved instrument such as a right-angle clamp or elevator is then used to encircle the palatopharyngeus muscle, and the plane is dissected bluntly superiorly and inferiorly by advancing this instrument (Fig. 20.17b).
- The inferior border of the flap is then released with the cautery facilitated by superior traction on the curved retractor.
- The donor sites are closed with interrupted resorbable suture such as 4–0 Chromic. The inferior aspect remains open to allow for drainage.

**Flap inset:**

- A transverse incision is made in the posterior pharyngeal wall just below the adenoid pad. This incision is deepened through mucosa with the cautery but should not be deepened through the muscle as this may cause inferior migration of the sphincter flaps.
- The flaps are rotated 90 degrees and inset into the transverse incision either end to end or in an overlapping fashion (Fig. 20.17c).
- The level of inset of these flaps and the degree of overlap can vary widely, and again are tailored to the patient's

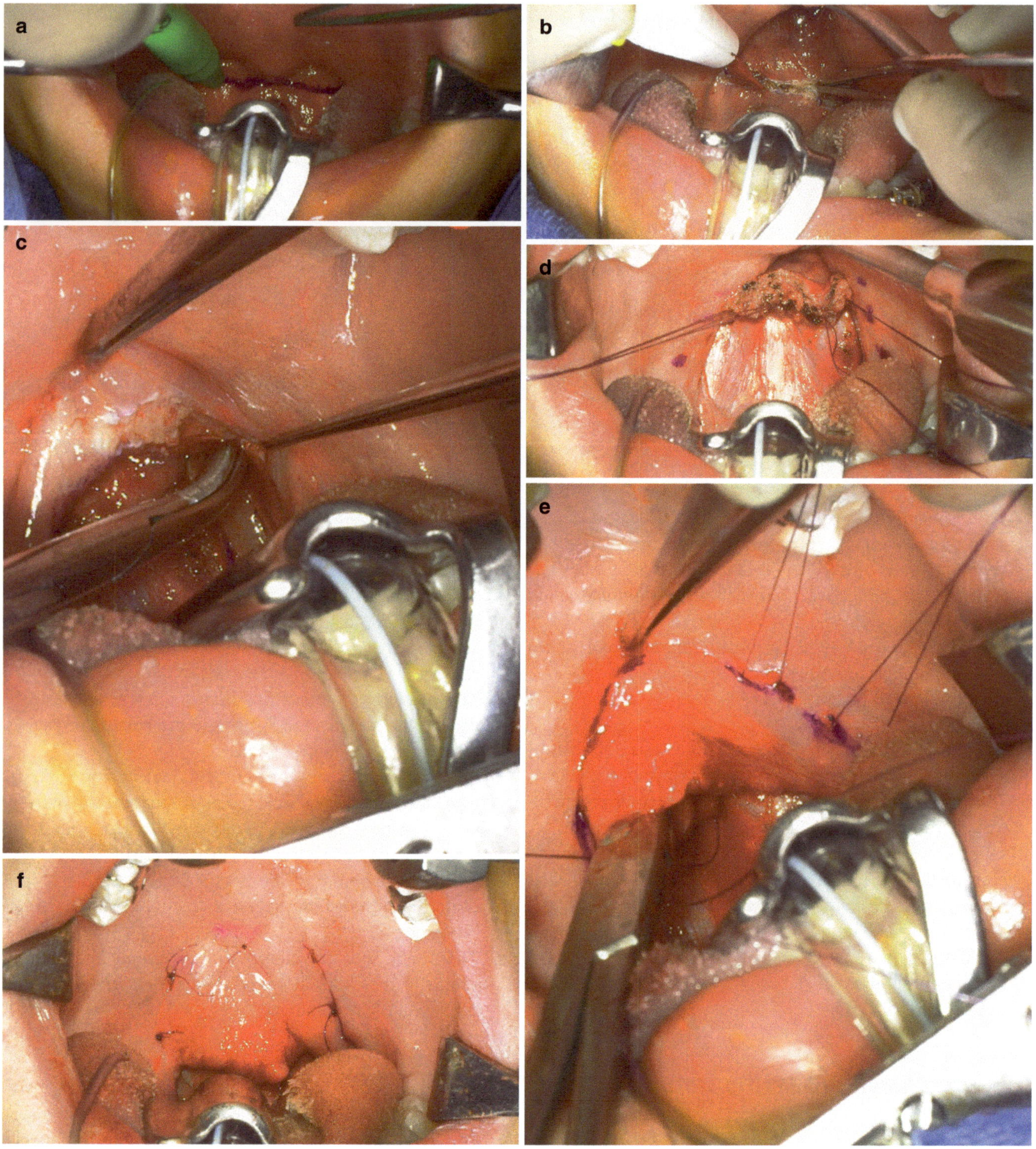


Fig. 20.15 (**a**–**f**) Posterior pharyngeal flap surgery demonstrating flap design (**a**), flap incision and elevation (**b**, **d**), velar pocket creation (**c**), and flap inset into the velar pocket (**d**–**f**)

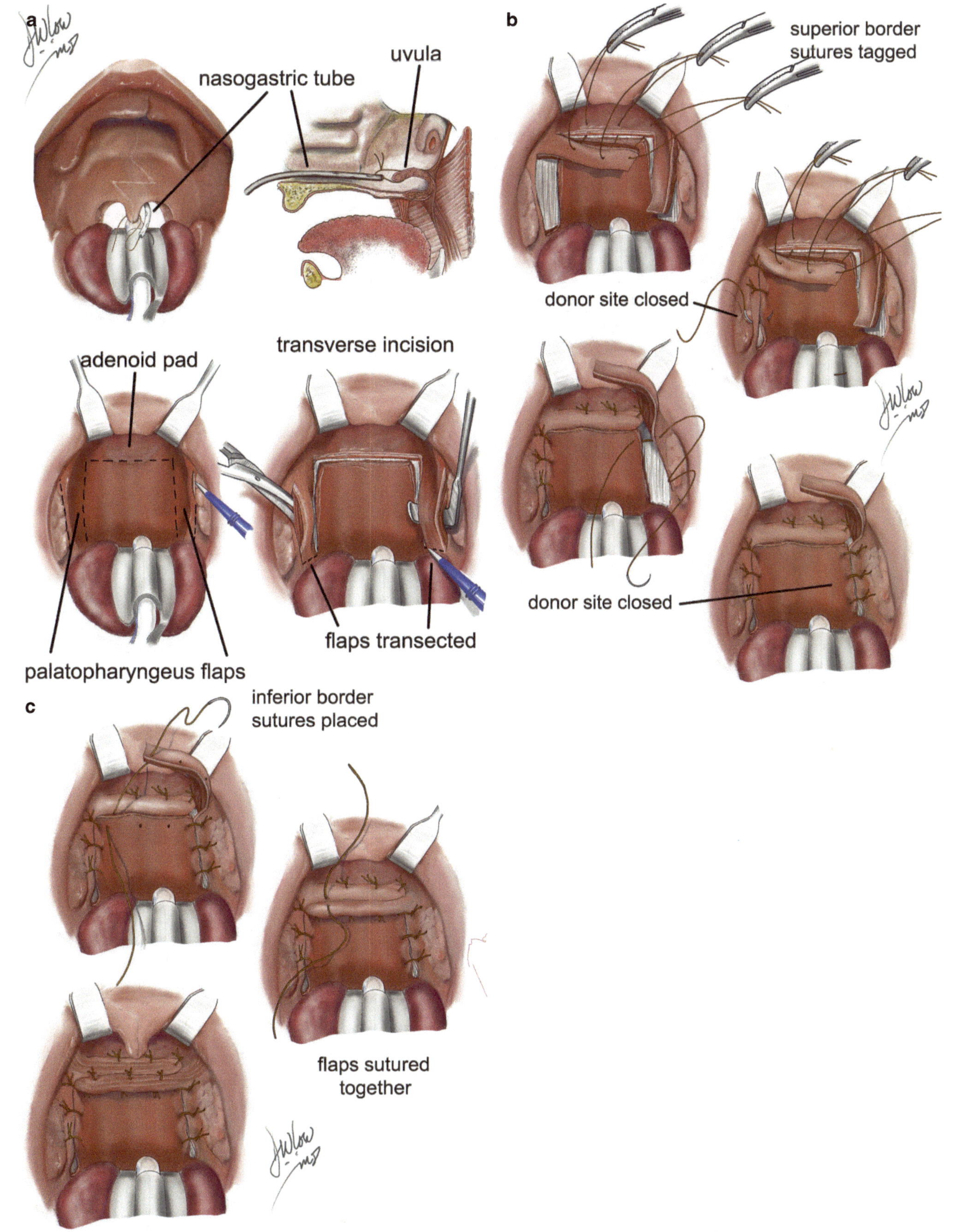


**Fig. 20.16** (**a**–**c**) Illustration sphincter pharyngoplasty: (**a**) retraction of uvula and bilateral sphincter flap design overlying posterior tonsillar pillar, incision of flaps and blunt undermining, (**b**, **c**) suturing of flaps and interrupted closure of donor site

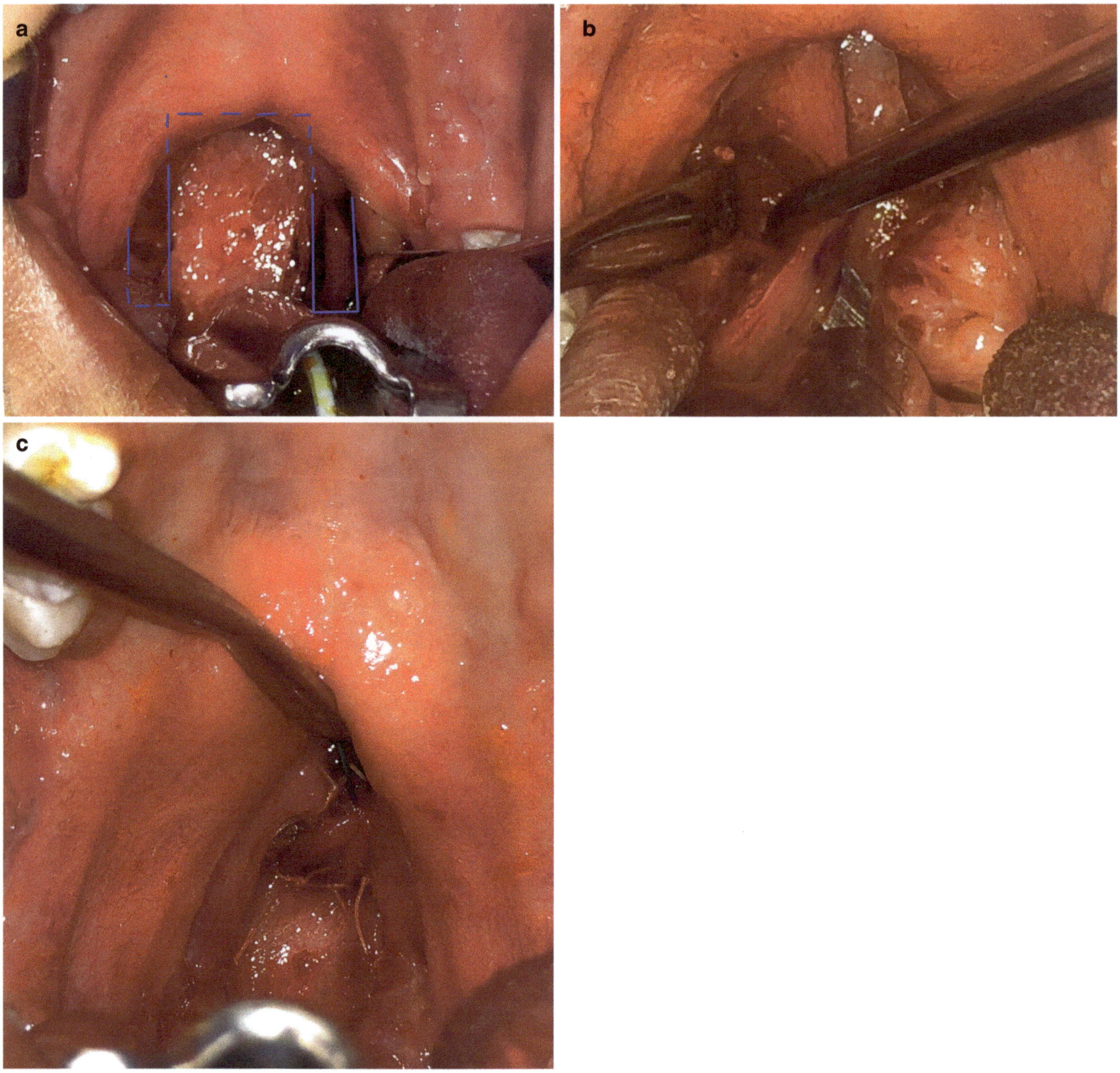

**Fig. 20.17** (**a–d**) Sphincter pharyngoplasty: (**a**) Design of superiorly based flaps incorporating vertical fibers of palatopharyngeus muscle in posterior tonsillar pillar, anterior pillar, and tonsil are retracted forward on the patients left side with a palate hook. Dotted lines show location on non-visualized incisions. (**b**) Dissection of the flaps with a curved elevator encircling the palatopharyngeus muscle fibers and used to dissect bluntly superiorly and inferiorly. (**c**) Flap inset with absorbable sutures

preoperative anatomy. The level of inset should be at the site of attempted velopharyngeal closure. The larger the velopharyngeal gap, the greater the flaps should overlap with minimal overcorrection to minimize risks of obstructive sleep apnea.

## Hynes Pharyngoplasty (Fig. 20.18a–c)

Hynes wrote two slightly different descriptions of a pharyngoplasty which has contributed to some of the lack of clarity around types of pharyngoplasties [36, 37]. However, a Hynes differs from a traditional sphincter pharyngoplasty in that Hynes flaps are based, and inset, higher than is the case with an Orticochea-type pharyngoplasty. Flaps that are inset adequately cranially should not be visible postoperatively on intra-oral examination. The Hynes flaps are overlapped along their entire length and inset at the point of attempted velopharyngeal closure, thus reducing the size of the space that the velum needs to close [17]. The level at which the flaps should be inserted is determined from a lateral videofluoroscopy, by identifying the level of attempted velopharyngeal

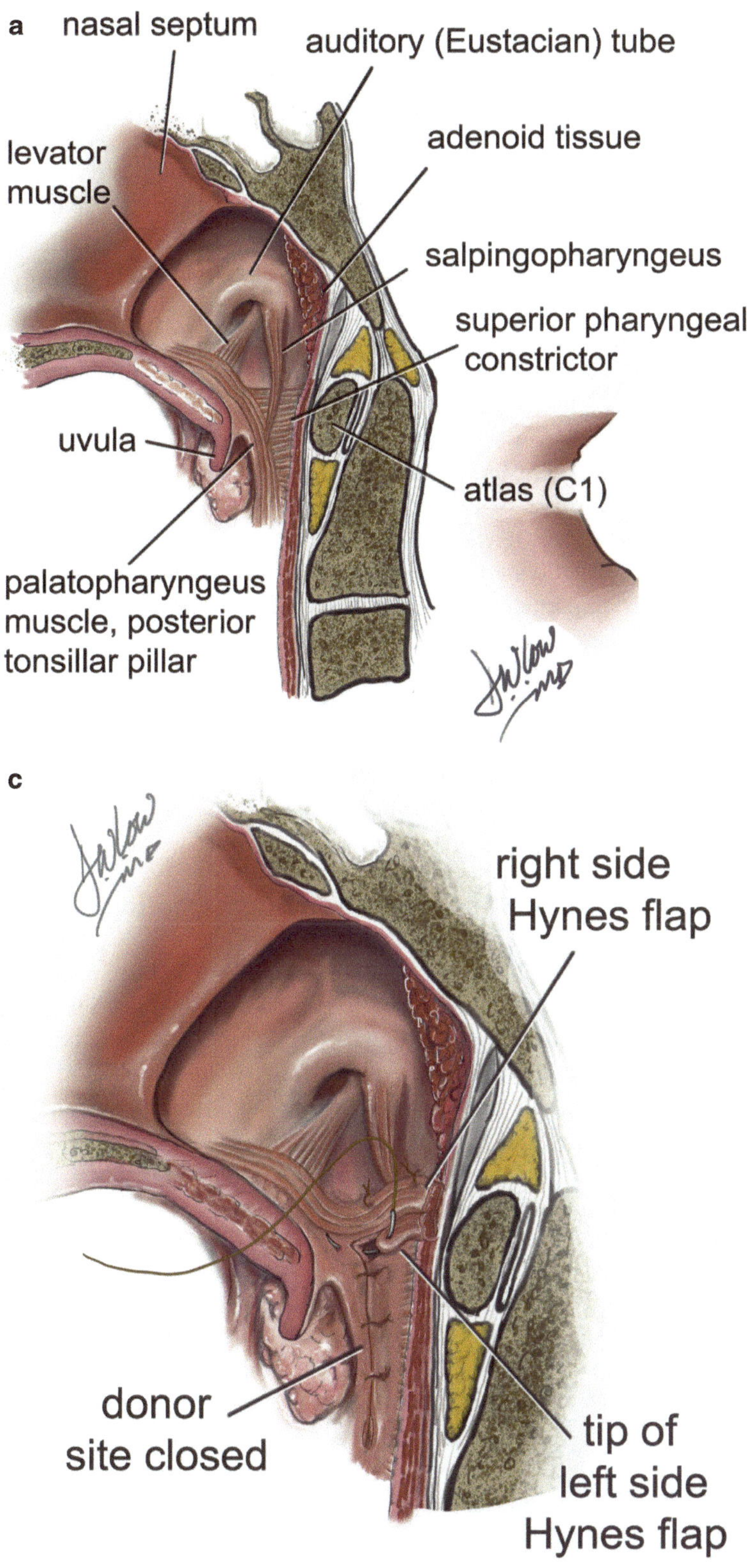


**Fig. 20.18** (**a–c**) Illustration of Hynes pharyngoplasty: (**a**) Nasopharyngeal anatomy in mid-sagittal plane demonstrating relationship of adenoid pad, Eustachian tube, and velum. (**b**) Outline of Hynes flap. The flaps' width and length are determined by the size of the VP gap as well as the ability to close the donor defects. In the above two-dimensional representation of the posterolateral pharyngeal wall, the flap width appears narrower than is actually the case. (**c**) Flaps are transposed 90 degrees and inset at the level of anticipated velopharyngeal closure

closure, relative to the position of the arch of the atlas vertebra. This boney landmark is then palpated intraoperatively, and the level of inset is marked by a transverse line on the posterior pharyngeal wall. The higher level of insertion of the Hynes flaps does make surgical access more difficult and it may be necessary to split the velum to achieve adequate access. However, an advantage of this more cranial flap design and inset is that the pharyngoplasty does not tether the velum allowing a greater range of movement. All pharyngoplasties narrow the oro and nasopharynx to some degree, thus screening and monitoring for obstructive sleep apnea is critical. The Hynes pharyngoplasty should only be considered after velar function has been optimized and it should not be performed in cases where velar function is poor [38].

### Surgical Steps

- Patient positioned supine with neck extended.
- Inspect and palpate for abnormal internal carotid arteries.
- Identify level of attempted velopharyngeal closure and draw flap inset incision (usually close to the level of the Eustachian tubes) (Fig. 20.18a–b).
- Two rectangular flaps are designed along the posterolateral pharyngeal walls, avoiding extension into the posterior tonsillar pillars. The medial edges of the flaps are continuous with, and at right angles, to the inset incision. The flaps contract after elevation and often need to be bigger than might be expected. The inset incision serves simply to provide two raw edges to which to suture the medial edges of both flaps. It should not be dissected widely, because this will cause flattening of the soft tissue bulge created by the Hynes flaps.
- The caudal edges of the flaps are tapered to ease closure of the donor defect.
- Local solution is infiltrated and time is allowed for the epinephrine to achieve adequate vasoconstriction.
- The flaps are elevated including palatopharyngeus, superior constrictor, and salpingopharyngeus (which is a small muscle that is usually not separately identified).
- The flaps are then transposed through 90 degrees and their medial edge is sutured to the edge of the inset incision and their lateral edges are sutured to the flap from the opposite side. Either the right or the left flap may be inset first and the contralateral flap is inset caudal to this (Fig. 20.18c).

### Tips

- A Hynes pharyngoplasty should not be carried out in settings where there is no facility for adequate postoperative airway monitoring and blood transfusion.
- Superficial tattooing of the key points can be done with a hypodermic needle and surgical ink after flap planning. Using a hypodermic is helpful because the ink is often smudged after local infiltration. This is particularly helpful during the Hynes procedure, because it is usually not possible to visualize the entire surgical field and flap outline while operating and loss of these bearings can lead to flaps that are too narrow or too broad.
- Gentle pressure from a pledget on an artery forceps can be very useful to stabilize the pharyngeal mucosa when making the initial incisions.
- Closure of the first donor defect before elevating the second flap can help in stabilizing the pharyngeal mucosa and in evaluating the degree of tension that will result from closure of the second donor defect.
- Closure of the donor defects before insetting the flaps reduces tension on the flaps.
- The divided superior constrictor muscle retracts and it is important to ensure that sutures include both the muscle and mucosa.
- The elevated flaps contract and can easily become twisted so it is important to make sure they are not twisted before insetting the flaps.
- Suturing the apex of the flap into the right angle of the incision before placing other sutures.

## Posterior Pharyngeal Wall Augmentation

Posterior pharyngeal wall augmentation has been attempted using a variety of synthetic and autologous materials, most recently, fat grafting. In most reports this was used for small VP gaps, which affect only quality, not intelligibility of speech and there is insufficient high-quality evidence to demonstrate effectiveness for significant VPI. There is anecdotal evidence of severe complications of fat embolism following fat grafting, thus, the authors do not recommend this approach.

**Field Solutions**

- Nasal stent, NP airways, and tongue stitches can be placed at the completion of the procedure for prophylactic airway protection during emergence from anesthesia and initial postoperative swelling.
- Nasal stents can be fashioned from any soft tubing material including rub rubbers, feeding tubes, pediatric silicone suction tubing, and nasogastric suction tubes (Fig. 20.19).

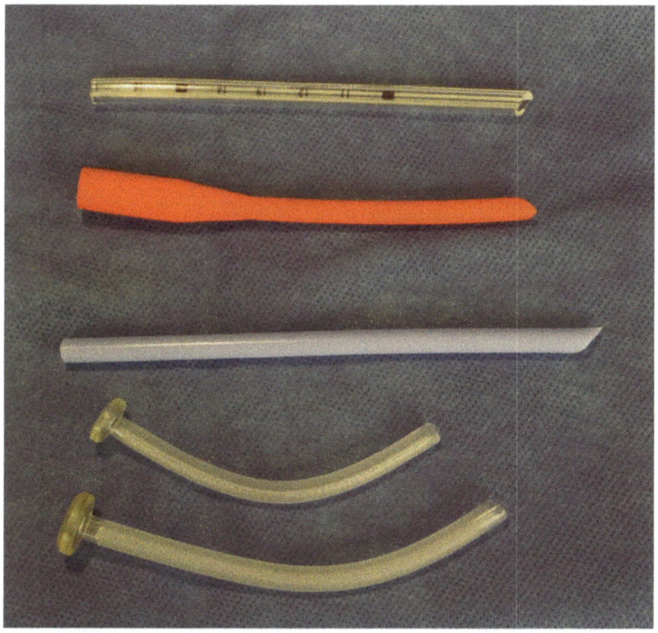

**Fig. 20.19** Nasopharyngeal airways can be used to stent the nasal airway after pharyngoplasty or these stents can be created from any type of silicone or soft plastic tubing such as nasogastric suction and feeding tubes

**Pitfalls**

- Patients with 22q11.2 can have medial deviation of the internal carotid arteries placing them at risk of injury during pharyngoplasty. The position of the internal carotid arteries varies depending on the degree of neck extension [39]; therefore, re-inspection and palpation after the patient is positioned for surgery and immediately prior to injection of local anesthetic and incision are essential.
- Visible or palpable pulsations in the oropharynx may indicate vascular anomalies and surgeons should proceed cautiously.
- Preoperative imaging studies such as MRI or CTA can diagnose anomalies. Intraoperative hand-held Doppler mapping can also be of assistance.

## Prosthetic Management

In some patients, surgery for VPD is not recommended due to medical risk, surgical difficulty, or anticipated failure. In these cases, prosthetics can offer the advantage of reducing the VP gap when the patient is awake and speaking but importantly, the prosthetic can be removed at night to preserve an adequate airway.

**Contraindications to VPD Surgery**

- High anesthetic risk
- Limited mouth opening/difficult access
- Previous radiotherapy in the velopharyngeal region
- Bleeding disorders
- Multiple failed previous velopharyngeal surgery
- Preexisting airway obstruction
- Extremely large velopharyngeal gaps, when any surgery for VPD is likely to cause excessive airway narrowing
- Very prominent and medially displaced internal carotid arteries
- Complete velar palsy

Broadly, two types of prosthetics address different pathology; both are extensions of a removable appliance attached to the teeth.

- Palatal lift—for immobile velums of adequate length (e.g., neurological or coordination disorders).
- Speech bulb—for very short velums that will not achieve closure or following extensive tumor resection.

**Disadvantages of Prosthetics**

- May require multiple visits to dental services (and in the case of a speech bulb, requires repeated nasoendoscopy to tailor the size and shape of the bulb).
- Needs appropriate dental expertise.
- Patient compliance needed and may not be suitable for all patients.
- Difficult for younger children to tolerate.

## Follow-up and Complication Management

Palatal repair and VPD surgery are overall low-risk procedures. Complications, although infrequent, can be life-threatening, particularly in the case of pharyngoplasties, which should not be performed without adequate perioperative monitoring and blood transfusion facilities. Overnight admission for pain control is typical, as well as to ensure proper hydration after surgery. Parental education on the importance of oral hygiene and a pureed-soft diet for several weeks after surgery is essential. Immediate complications may include oral bleeding, adverse airway events such as desaturation or airway obstruction, reduced oral intake, or problems with healing resulting from flap dehiscence, flap necrosis, or subsequent oronasal fistulae. Secondary palatal surgery is unlikely to cause sleep apnea but this is the main long-term complication of concern following pharyngoplasties and pharyngeal flaps. Other reported unwanted effects include swallowing dysfunction, reduced nasal drainage, difficulty clearing secretions, and hyponasal speech [40]. Patients undergoing pharyngoplasty should be monitored long term for symptoms of apnea, which can include heavy snoring, gasping, or choking at night, and daytime drowsiness, although it is important to note that children may also present with hyperactivity and poor concentration. If these are noted, formal sleep studies should be performed, followed by supportive respiratory treatments such as continuous positive airway pressure (CPAP) or flap reversal if indicated.

## References


1. Kummer AW. Anatomy and physiology: the orofacial structures and velopharyngeal valve. In: Kummer AW, editor. Cleft palate and craniofacial anomalies: effects on speech and resonance. Clifton Park: Delmar Cengage; 2008. p. 3–33.
2. Moon JB, Kuehn D. Anatomy and physiology of normal and disordered velopharyngeal function for speech. In: Bzoch KR, editor. *Communicative disorders related to cleft lip and palate*. Austin: Pro-Ed; 2004. p. 67–98.
3. Perry JL. Anatomy and physiology of the velopharyngeal mechanism. Semin Speech Lang. 2011;32(2):83–92.
4. Raol N, Hartnick CJ. Anatomy and physiology of velopharyngeal closure and insufficiency. Adv Otorhinolaryngol. 2015;76:1–6.
5. Bassett AS, et al. Practical guidelines for managing patients with 22q11.2 deletion syndrome. J Pediatr. 2011;159(2):332–9 e1.
6. Jackson O, et al. Palatal evaluation and treatment in 22q11.2 deletion syndrome. Am J Med Genet. 2019;179(7):1184–95.
7. Baylis A. Noncleft velopharyngeal disorders. In: Losee JE, Kirschner R, editors. Comprehensive cleft care. Boca Raton: Taylor and Francis Group; 2016. p. 581–9.
8. Trost-Cardamone J. Classification of velopharyngeal inadequacies. Cleft Palate J. 1989;26:68–70.
9. McDonald-McGinn DM, Sullivan KE. Chromosome 22q11.2 deletion syndrome (DiGeorge syndrome/velocardiofacial syndrome). Medicine (Baltimore). 2011;90(1):1–18.
10. McDonald-McGinn DM, et al. 22q11.2 deletion syndrome. Nat Rev Dis Primers. 2015;1:15071.
11. Fung WL, et al. Practical guidelines for managing adults with 22q11.2 deletion syndrome. Genet Med. 2015;17(8):599–609.
12. Hens G, et al. Palate lengthening by buccinator myomucosal flaps for velopharyngeal insufficiency. Cleft Palate Craniofac J. 2013;50(5):e84–91.
13. Mann RJ, et al. The double-opposing buccal flap procedure for palatal lengthening. Plast Reconstr Surg. 2011;127(6):2413–8.
14. Perkins JA, et al. Furlow palatoplasty for management of velopharyngeal insufficiency: a prospective study of 148 consecutive patients. Plast Reconstr Surg. 2005;116(1):72–80; discussion 81-4
15. Gart MS, Gosain AK. Surgical management of velopharyngeal insufficiency. Clin Plast Surg. 2014;41(2):253–70.
16. Kirschner RE, Baylis AL. Surgical considerations in 22Q11.2 deletion syndrome. Clin Plast Surg. 2014;41(2):271–82.
17. Mehendale FV, et al. Surgical management of velopharyngeal incompetence in velocardiofacial syndrome. Cleft Palate Craniofac J. 2004;41(2):124–35.
18. Spruijt NE, et al. In search of the optimal surgical treatment for velopharyngeal dysfunction in 22q11.2 deletion syndrome: a systematic review. PLoS One. 2012;7(3):e34332.
19. Swanson EW, et al. Speech outcomes following pharyngeal flap in patients with velocardiofacial syndrome. Plast Reconstr Surg. 2011;127(5):2045–53.
20. Ysunza A, et al. Surgical treatment of submucous cleft palate: a comparative trial of two modalities for palatal closure. Plast Reconstr Surg. 2001;107(1):9–14.
21. Moss AL, Pigott RW, Albery EH. Hynes pharyngoplasty revisited. Plast Reconstr Surg. 1987;79(3):346–55.
22. Jiramongkolchai P, et al. Speech outcomes in children with 22q11.2 deletion syndrome following surgery for velopharyngeal insufficiency. Int J Pediatr Otorhinolaryngol. 2016;88:34–7.
23. Perry JL, Kuehn D. Anatomy and physiology of the velopharynx. In: Kirschner R, Losee JE, editors. Comprehensive cleft care. Boca Raton: CRC Press; 2016. p. 475–91.
24. Chen PK, et al. Correction of secondary velopharyngeal insufficiency in cleft palate patients with the Furlow palatoplasty. Plast Reconstr Surg. 1994;94(7):933–41; discussion 942–3
25. Noorchashm N, et al. Conversion Furlow palatoplasty: salvage of speech after straight-line palatoplasty and "incomplete intravelar veloplasty". Ann Plast Surg. 2006;56(5):505–10.
26. Sommerlad BC, et al. Cleft palate re-repair – a clinical and radiographic study of 32 consecutive cases. Br J Plast Surg. 1994;47(6):406–10.
27. Sommerlad BC, et al. Palate re-repair revisited. Cleft Palate Craniofac J. 2002;39(3):295–307.
28. Sommerlad BC. The use of the operating microscope for cleft palate repair and pharyngoplasty. Plast Reconstr Surg. 2003;112(6):1540–1.
29. Sommerlad BC. A technique for cleft palate repair. Plast Reconstr Surg. 2003;112(6):1542–8.
30. Hill C, et al. Buccinator sandwich pushback: a new technique for treatment of secondary velopharyngeal incompetence. Cleft Palate Craniofac J. 2004;41(3):230–7.
31. Argamaso RV. Pharyngeal flap surgery for velopharyngeal insufficiency. Oper Tech Plast Surg. 1995;2:233–8.
32. Karling J, et al. Comparison between two types of pharyngeal flap with regard to configuration at rest and function and speech outcome. Cleft Palate Craniofac J. 1999;36(2):154–65.
33. Sie KC, et al. Sphincter pharyngoplasty: speech outcome and complications. Laryngoscope. 1998;108(8) Pt 1:1211–7.
34. Sullivan SR, Marrinan EM, Mulliken JB. Pharyngeal flap outcomes in nonsyndromic children with repaired cleft palate and velopharyngeal insufficiency. Plast Reconstr Surg. 2010;125(1):290–8.
35. Orticochea M. Construction of a dynamic muscle sphincter in cleft palates. Plast Reconstr Surg. 1968;41(4):323–7.
36. Hynes W. Observations on pharyngoplasty. Br J Plast Surg. 1967;20(3):244–56.
37. Hynes W. Pharyngoplasty by muscle transplantation. Br J Plast Surg. 1950;3(2):128–35.
38. Mehendale FV, et al. Effect of palate re-repairs and hynes pharyngoplasties on pediatric airways: an analysis of preoperative and postoperative cardiorespiratory sleep studies. Cleft Palate Craniofac J. 2013;50(3):257–67.
39. Mitnick RJ, et al. The use of magnetic resonance angiography prior to pharyngeal flap surgery in patients with velocardiofacial syndrome. Plast Reconstr Surg. 1996;97(5):908–19.
40. Wells MD, Vu TA, Luce EA. Incidence and sequelae of nocturnal respiratory obstruction following posterior pharyngeal flap operation. Ann Plast Surg. 1999;43(3):252–7.

# Alveolar Bone Graft

21

Jordan W. Swanson, David W. Low, Allan Porras, and Armando Siu

**Key Points**

- Six reasons for performing alveolar bone graft (ABG):
  1. Facilitate canine and lateral incisor tooth eruption
  2. Stabilize the alveolar arch to prevent collapse and anterior crossbite and to restore physiologic continuity of the dental arch
  3. Provide bony foundation for the nasal base and ala
  4. Close the nasal floor, including vestibular or oronasal fistula if present
  5. Provide bone stock to enable maxillary advancement to correct midface retrusion as well as support dental implants if needed
  6. Allow for proper orthodontic alignment of the teeth
- Secondary bone grafting using cancellous bone from the iliac crest in the age of mixed dentition (7–9 years) is the gold standard of treatment.
- Orthodontic-surgical joint planning is optimal, and generally the maxilla is widened transversely with a palatal expander shortly before bone grafting.
- Autologous graft is reliable. Recombinant human bone morphogenic protein-2 (BMP-2) with potential use of a demineralized bone matrix carrier may be used to reduce donor site morbidity with early evidence of similar graft outcomes.

## Introduction

The alveolus or alveolar bone is the tooth-bearing portion of the maxilla (upper jaw). In a complete cleft of the lip and palate, the alveolus is generally clefted as well (Fig. 21.1). There are five potential consequences of an unrepaired bony cleft: (1) lack of canine and/or lateral incisor tooth eruption, (2) discontinuity of the alveolar arch leading to collapse of the segments and maxillary crossbite, (3) inadequate bony support of the overlying nasal ala and lip causing nasal base asymmetry, (4) persistence of a nasolabial fistula and regurgitation or speech incompetence, and (5) unstable maxilla that cannot be repositioned in orthognathic surgery (Fig. 21.2). Alveolar bone grafting (ABG) is performed to facilitate canine and lateral incisor tooth eruption, stabilize the alveolar arch to prevent collapse and anterior crossbite, provide bony foundation for the nasal base and ala, close the nasal floor, and provide bone stock to enable maxillary advancement to correct midface retrusion as well as support dental implants if needed.

## Patient Selection and Clinical Planning

### Timing of Surgery

To comprehend better the various ideologies concerning the timing of the alveolar cleft grafting, one first should have a firm grasp of its classification:

J. W. Swanson (✉) · D. W. Low
Division of Plastic Surgery, Children's Hospital of Philadelphia and University of Pennsylvania, Philadelphia, PA, USA
e-mail: swansonj@email.chop.edu; david.low@uphs.upenn.edu

A. Porras
Oral and Maxillofacial Surgery, Proactive Dental Solutions and Operation Smile Nicaragua, Managua, Nicaragua
e-mail: aporras@proactivedentalsolutions.com

A. Siu
Operation Smile Nicaragua, Managua, Nicaragua

© Springer Nature Switzerland AG 2021
J. W. Swanson, D. W. Low (eds.), *Global Cleft Care in Low-Resource Settings*, https://doi.org/10.1007/978-3-030-59105-2_21

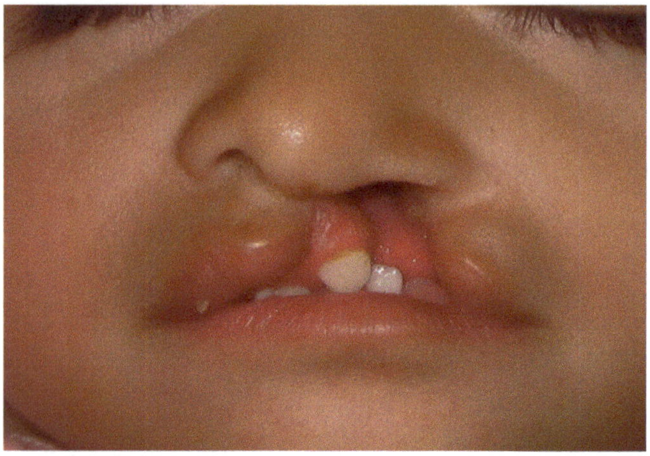

Fig. 21.1 Left unilateral alveolar cleft

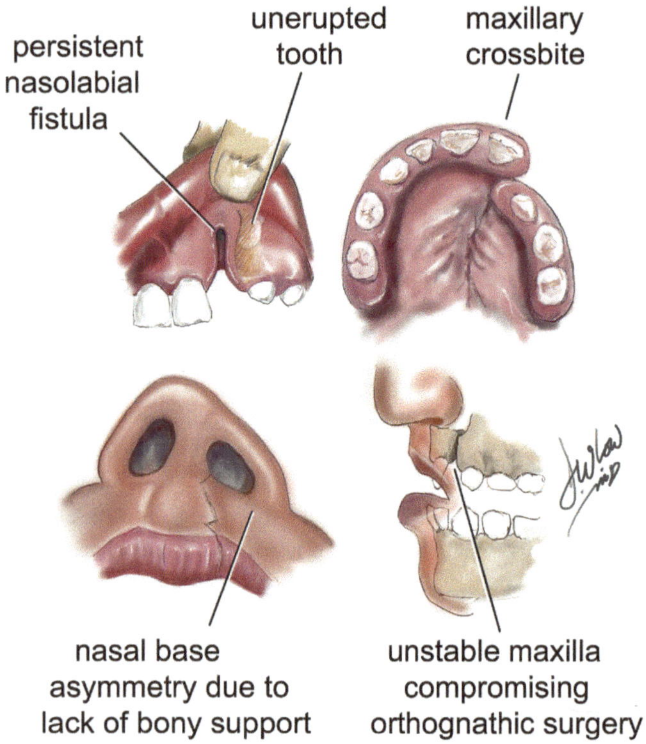


Fig. 21.2 The consequences of an unrepaired alveolar cleft

- Primary (0–2.5 years, usually at the time of lip repair)
- Early secondary (2–5 years, before the eruption of permanent incisors)
- Secondary (6–13 years, before the eruption of the permanent canines)
- Late (>13 years, after the eruption of the permanent canines)

## Secondary Bone Grafting

Alveolar grafts, like all bone, require mechanical stimulation to avoid resorption. Timing the bone graft to the natural eruption of permanent teeth into the graft provides this stimulation, as do orthodontic dental movements. Grafting at time of mixed dentition (7–9 years of age, but up to 6–11 years in some patients) coincides with this mechanical stimulation and avoids consequences of impaired midfacial growth from surgery and associated scarring prior to that time.

A panoramic radiograph is typically obtained to visualize the alveolar cleft preoperatively (Fig. 21.3). This can also be used to evaluate the eruption of the canine crown to verify canine descent [7].

A joint orthodontic-surgical plan is essential, in order to correct premorbid maxillary segmental collapse and crossbite through the grafting process. An appropriately widened maxilla has increased transverse diameter to match the lower dental arch, with rounded alignment of the two or three alveolar segments. Preoperative orthodontic preparation is usually preferred, because the alveolar segments have increased mobility for manipulation prior to locking them together with graft. However, disadvantages of presurgical expansion can include widening of the alveolar cleft to a size that makes gingival flap closure difficult. This is particularly of concern for patients with a large existing oronasal fistula; in this patient group, postoperative arch expansion may be advisable at least in part. This is further discussed in Chap. 23.

Additional considerations must be taken into account for older patients (12+). First, while some benefits of bone grafting are still available and even critical (stabilizing the maxilla in advance of orthognathic surgery, providing continuity and stability of the maxillary arch, achieving oronasal fistula closure, for instance), spontaneous eruption of canine or lateral incisor teeth is no longer possible. Second, the bony maxilla tends not to be amenable to expansion by a palatal expander to correct arch collapse much above this age. Thus, a surgically assisted rapid palatal expansion (SARPE) is generally performed, in which a maxillary osteotomy immediately precedes the expansion. Other benefits may be to provide nasal support and placement of dental implants if necessary.

Displaced primary teeth adjacent to the graft site can be extracted at the time of bone grafting in most cases, but if there is concern for maintaining a viable mucosal cuff, these can be extracted 3–6 weeks prior to ABG.

## Gingivoperiosteoplasty (GPP)

Gingivoperiosteoplasty (GPP) can be performed during primary lip repair. Flaps of gingival and periosteal tissue

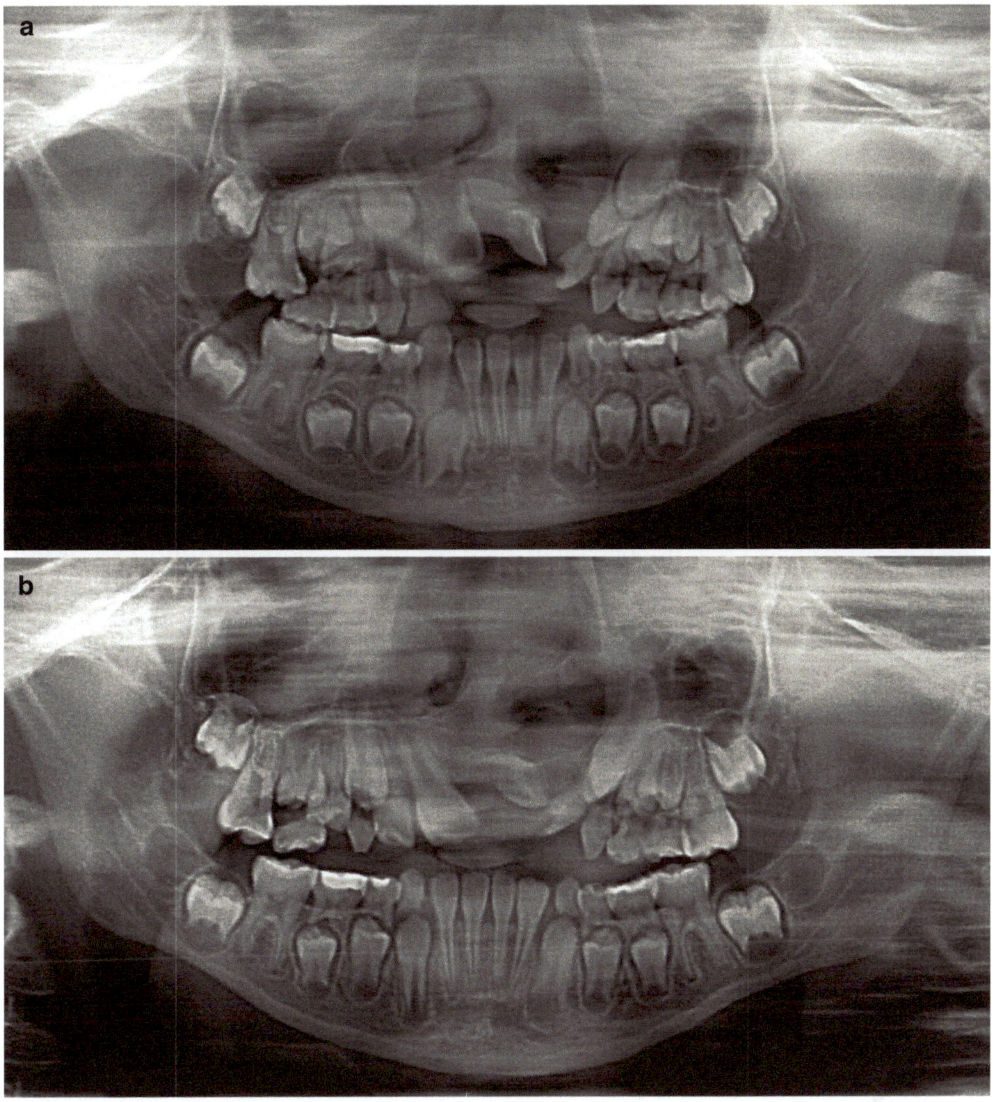


**Fig. 21.3** Panorex of a 6-year-old patient with left alveolar cleft, prior to (**a**) and following (**b**) bone graft

are dissected from facing alveolar cleft borders and used to construct “roof, floor, and walls” that can generate bone across a small gap. Modest success rates (50–70%) are reported but only when Latham appliance or nasoalveolar molding (NAM) is used adjunctively to narrow the alveolar gap to approximately 2 mm at the time of GPP [4, 5]. No negative effects on facial growth have been reported. In our experience it is quite rare to encounter patients with well-aligned alveolar segments separated by only a 2 mm gap in low-resource settings. The likelihood of successful bone formation over a larger gap is small. Primary bone grafting in infancy (for example with rib graft) is not shown to be effective and major has donor site morbidity [1–3].

## Grafting Material and Donor Sites

### Autologous Bone Graft

Autologous bone has been the conventional graft substrate, and historical use of cortical iliac/rib bone blocks has given way to cancellous bone with its superior integration, incorporation, and facilitation of tooth eruption [8]. Cancellous bone is rapidly revascularized over 3 weeks, unlike cortical bone which maintains volume by creeping substitution.

Published success rates of autologous ABG are typically 80–90% [6]. A canine can be expected to erupt in all patients though in a minority may erupt palatally rather than on the dental arch, and approximately half will show lateral incisor eruption.

### Donor Site Selection

The iliac crest is generally preferred, due to its high density of bone marrow and endochondral cancellous bone volume [9]. Its location permits a two-team approach of simultaneous graft harvest during alveolar site preparation, which minimizes anesthetic and operative time. The primary drawback is postoperative pain, although newer modalities improve its management (see Anesthesia). Long-term donor site disability or deformity is rare, and minimizing muscle and periosteal dissection reduces these consequences. Reapproximating the cartilage cap may minimize anterior iliac contour irregularity. Cranial bone graft, although described, is primarily cortical bone [10].

### Bone Graft Substitutes

An off-the-shelf grafting substitute to autologous bone could eliminate the pain and scar of donor graft sites, the added operative and anesthetic time, small risk of donor site disability, and heterogeneity and limited volume of graft material. Recombinant human bone morphogenetic protein-2 (rhBMP-2) was approved by the FDA for maxillofacial use in 2007 and is the best studied substitute to date [12]. Many teams use cadaveric demineralized bone matrix (DMB), which consists of organic collagen, as a three-dimensional "carrier" of the liquid BMP. Early data suggest similar dental eruption and stability, but further insight into clinical and dental outcomes is needed [11, 13]. The complication profile also appears similar, with consistently increased rates of transient alveolar edema but without greater dehiscence rates. Although associated with shorter operating room (OR) time and inpatient stays, at a material cost of $300–3000 per patient, rhBMP/DMB is not yet cost-effective in most low-resource settings. Finally, although early- to short-term mitogenic risks of carcinoma do not appear formidable in the growing facial skeleton, parents need to be advised of this risk.

## Operative Staging of Fistulas and Bilateral Clefts

In cases of larger nasolabial or oronasal fistula or less experienced surgeons, it is often preferable to perform a staged approach with first fistula closure (see Chap. 20) followed by alveolar cleft graft. If both are done in combination and a watertight closure is not achieved or too much tissue tension is present, risk of fistula recurrence and loss of graft is high.

Unilateral alveolar clefts are grafted in a single stage. Bilateral alveolar clefts introduce two particular concerns: volume of defect and perfusion of premaxillary tissue. The volume of cancellous bone graft required to fill a bilateral alveolar defect may exceed what is readily available in the iliac wing of the appropriately aged patient. Thus, the surgeon may need to consider harvesting from the contralateral hip or consider staging the procedure. Typically, following a 6-month interval, abundant cancellous bone has regenerated in the original site which can be reharvested. Additionally, single-stage bilateral alveolar cleft reconstruction creates additional challenge in sufficiently mobilizing gingival mucosal flaps, while limiting premaxillary dissection and consequent risk to blood supply. Therefore, most surgeons perform two-staged reconstruction of bilateral alveolar clefts with an interval 6-month period.

## Operative Planning

### Radiographic Evaluation

A preoperative panoramic X-ray (panorex) is important to assess the extent of bony bridging, which can be difficult to clinically assess beneath the mucosa (Fig. 21.3). A cone beam 3D CT offers higher-fidelity bone image, where available (Fig. 21.4). Other radiographic evaluation may include occlusal and periapical films of the cleft region for a more detailed evaluation.

### Orthodontic Expansion

Preoperative orthodontic preparation is usually necessary to expand the anterior maxillary crossbite, due to inward collapse of the mobile alveolar segments, and to align the anterior teeth. This process often takes at least 4 weeks and may utilize a palatal expander such as a Hyrax to gradually widen the anterior palate to restore appropriate maxillary width (see Chap. 23). This preoperative expansion is important because an ABG "locks in" the palatal segments into fixed position.

## Relevant Anatomy

The three-dimensional alveolar cleft is best thought of as the shape of a tornado or a pyramid placed upside down on its point. Viewed frontally (coronal plane), the width of the cleft is greater at the piriform margin of the alveolus (superior) than the dental margin (inferiorly) (Fig. 21.5). A more critical visualization is laterally (sagittal plane), again showing a much larger defect superiorly, where the alveolus tends to have considerable posterior projection, than inferiorly.

Incisional design depends on whether a nasolabial or oronasal fistula is present. In either case, attached alveolar gingiva, which lines the alveolar process portion of the cleft, must be maintained in proximity to the anticipated site of dental eruption to ensure viability of adult teeth. When the

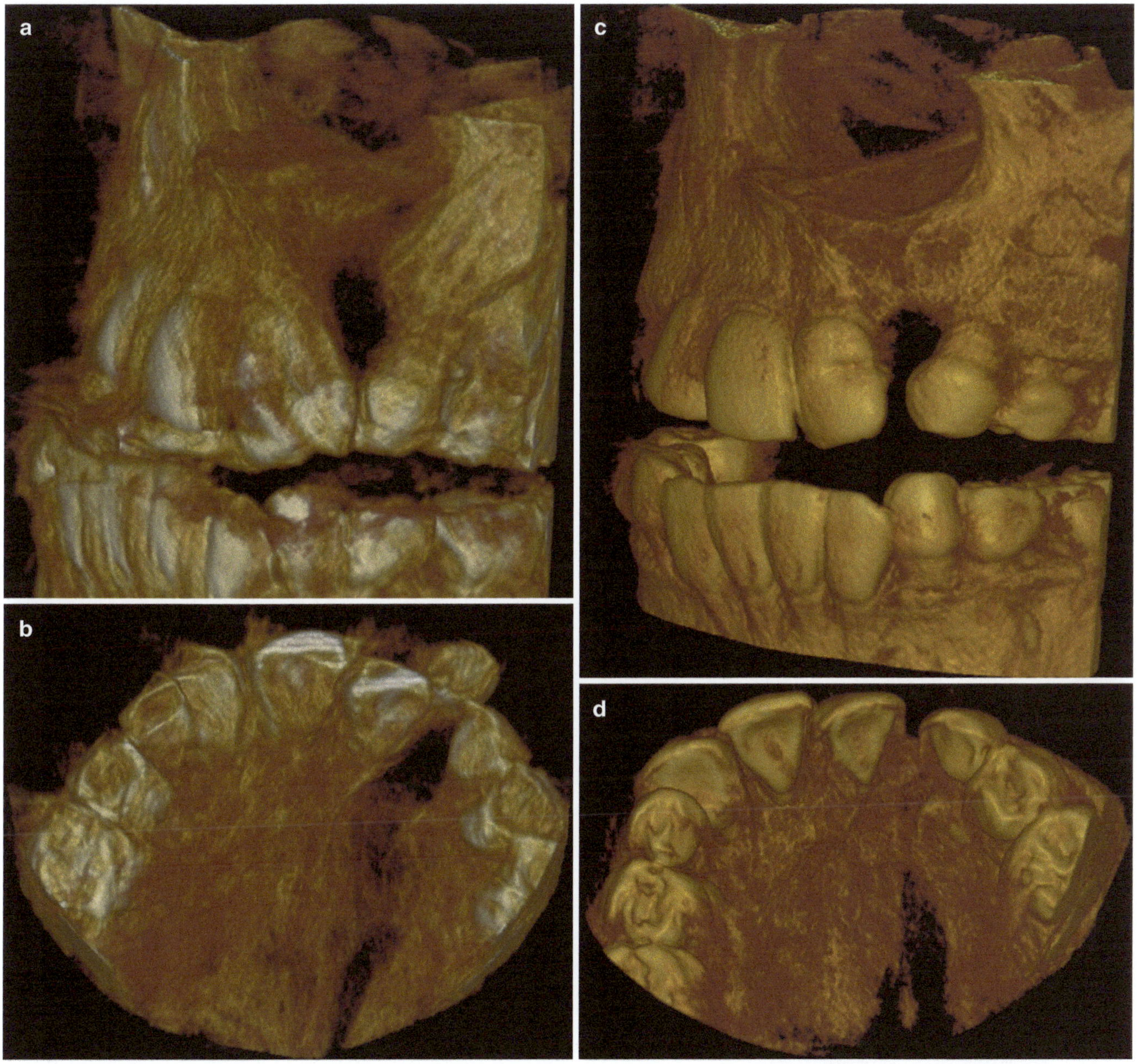


**Fig. 21.4** Cone beam 3D CT scan of a 6-year-old patient with left alveolar cleft, prior to (**a**, **b**) and following (**c**, **d**) repair

nasal floor has been appropriately repaired at time of lip repair, and a fistula is not present, incisions are typically designed parallel to the incisors through the gingival mucosa. The incision is typically positioned anteriorly of the midsagittal plane, preserving more tissue to transpose posteriorly, because additional anterior gingiva can be transposed through lateral dissection, release, and advance to a greater degree than posterior gingiva.

In the presence of a fistula, simultaneous closure of multiple tissue layers must be planned, in addition to the gingival reconstruction of the alveolus, the nasal floor-alveolar interface, as well as the oral roof-alveolar interface (Fig. 21.6). The nasal floor is generally best closed with the use of a vomer flap raised in the subperichondrial plane medially and a lateral nasal wall flap raised in the subperiosteal plane laterally. The oral roof, which is the posterior extension of the alveolar gingiva into the palate, can generally be closed with subperiosteal dissection over the bony palatal shelves and medial tissue rotation with a lateral back cut as needed.

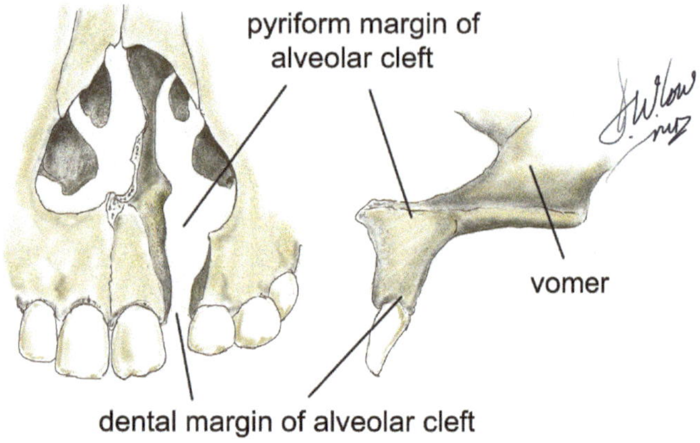


**Fig. 21.5** Coronal and sagittal views of the 3D alveolar cleft deformity, resembling a "tornado"

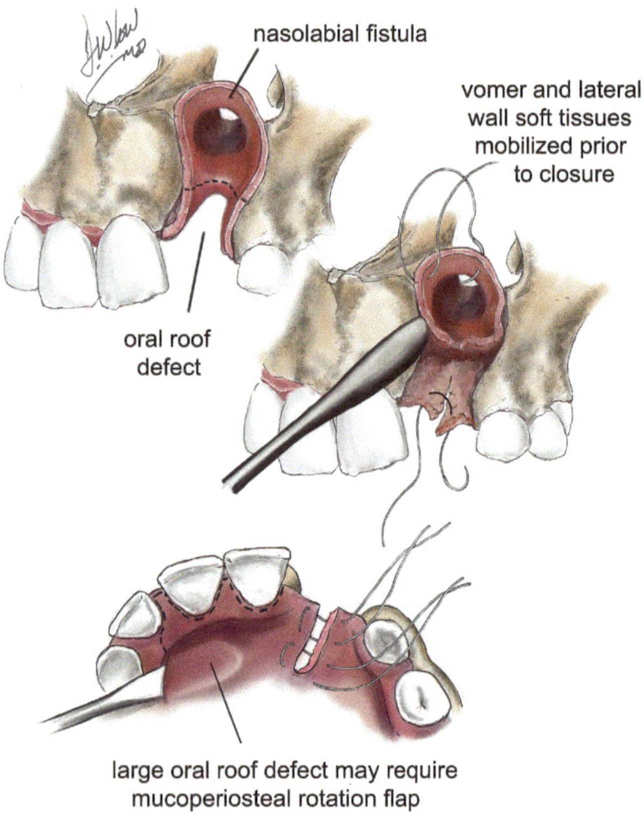


**Fig. 21.6** Incisions and closure pattern of a nasolabial fistula at time of alveolar bone grafting

Failure to completely close all mucosal surfaces over the bone graft will result in salivary contamination and graft resorption. Repeat of the procedure is then necessary and often more difficult due to the presence of scars.

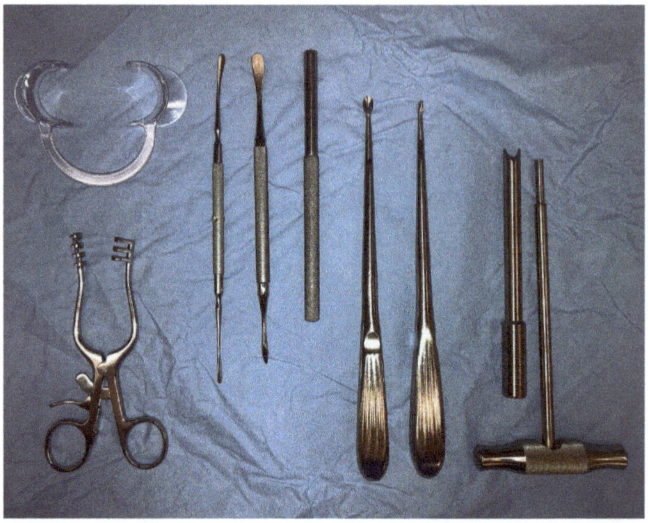

**Fig. 21.7** Helpful instruments for alveolar bone graft. (**a**) "Plastic smile" lip retractor, (**b**) Weitlaner self-retaining retractor for iliac exposure, (**c**) Freer and (**d**) Molt #9 periosteal elevators, (**e**) bone tamp, (**f**) McElroy-type curettes, (**g**) trephine for percutaneous graft harvest

## **Key Equipment** (Fig. 21.7)

### Mouth Field

- Plastic "smile" lip retractor allows the surgeon to operate, while an assistant harvests bone graft.
- Several elevators – Freer, Molt #9 periosteal dental, Woodson, and angled pharyngoplastic dental – can each be helpful for subperiosteal gingival cuff elevation.
- A bone tamp enables solid graft packing.
- 4-0 and 5-0 Vicryl suture on tapered needle for mucosal closure.

### Hip Field

- A Weitlaner sharp self-retaining retractor allows one surgeon to harvest graft while the assistant prepares the recipient site.
- An Obwegeser periosteal elevator facilitates elevation of the cartilaginous cap.
- McElroy-type curettes, especially 8–12 mm cup diameter, are the mainstay of cancellous bone harvest.
- Alexander-type gouges, 8–12 mm diameter, are also helpful for harvesting bone.
- A trephine, such as the Spine-Tech grinding harvester, can be used for percutaneous graft harvest.
- 2-0, 3-0, and 4-0 Vicryl suture for muscular, superficial fascia, and dermal reapproximation; 4-0 Monocryl subcuticular closure.

## Splint

A stabilization dental splint provides two functions postoperatively. First, it stabilizes the alveolar segments, preventing collapse and assuring rigidity to enable bony healing. This is particularly important in a bilateral cleft, in which the mobile premaxillary would otherwise prevent graft take. Second, it provides mechanical protection to the healing mucosa. This can be fabricated from acrylic by an orthodontist preoperatively and bonded at time of surgery. Alternatively, it can be made intraoperatively (see Field Hack box).

**Field Hack: Intraoperative Splint Fabrication**

A postoperative acrylic dental splint can be fabricated in the operating room by the surgeon. The acrylic polymer powder is mixed 1:1 with liquid monomer on the back table to make a cylinder 12 cm in length and 1 cm in diameter. This is molded to the maxillary dentition, bringing mandibular dentition into occlusion and then removing the excess with a high-speed burr.

## Anesthesia

General orotracheal anesthesia is employed during surgery. Locoregional anesthesia is an important adjunct, particularly for the hip donor site which causes the majority of postoperative pain.

### Hip Donor Site

#### Transverse Abdominis Plane (TAP) Block

Injection of long-acting local anesthesia in the plane between the internal oblique and transversus abdominis muscles of the lateral abdomen blocks the intercostal nerves (T7–12) and iliohypogastric nerve (T12-L1) that provide sensation of the iliac crest region [14]. This offers superior pain control and shorter length of stay than field anesthesia or systemic narcotics and is similar to a long-acting analgesia infusion catheter [15]. An 18 gauge needle is inserted into the ipsilateral inferior lumbar triangle, which is bordered by the iliac crest inferiorly, latissimus dorsi muscle posteriorly, the external oblique muscle anteriorly, and the costal margin superiorly (Fig. 21.8). This can be performed with a blunted needle using the "double pop" technique – representing the needle traversing the fascial extensions of the external oblique followed by internal oblique muscles. Bupivacaine (0.4 mL/kg of 0.5% or 0.8 mL/kg of 0.25%) is infiltrated; this reserves 20% of maximal local anesthesia dose to be used in the alveolar region. If available, ultrasound guidance enables visualization of this plane as well as appropriate hydrodissection with infiltration (Fig. 21.9).

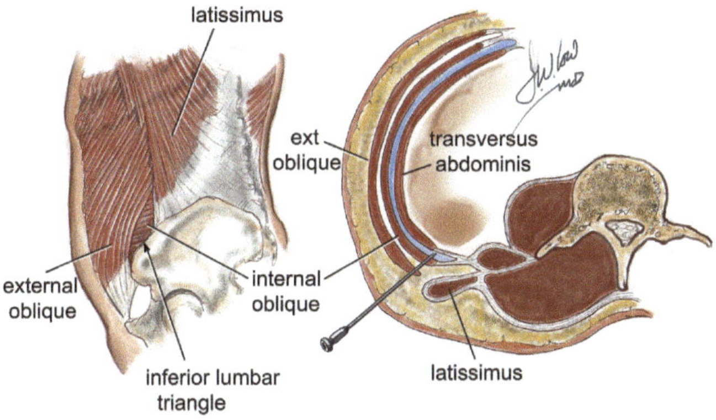


Fig. 21.8 Inferior lumbar triangle formed by the iliac crest, latissimus dorsi, and external oblique muscles which is accessed for a posterior transverse abdominis plane (TAP) block

#### Bupivacaine-Soaked Sponge

Alternatively, an absorbable gelatin sponge (Gelfoam) can be infiltrated with bupivacaine and placed inside the iliac crest harvest site prior to closing the cartilage cap. Additional dose can be infiltrated as a field block. Again, a dose of 0.4 mL/kg of 0.5% or 0.8 mL/kg of 0.25% is used, reserving 20% of maximal local anesthesia dose to be used in the alveolar region.

### Alveolar Recipient Site

Bilateral infraorbital nerve blocks are placed and partially reduce innervation to the superior dental plexus. Superior alveolar nerve branches are not addressed by the infraorbital nerve block and are best addressed with field infiltration (ordinarily a mixture of lidocaine, bupivacaine, and epinephrine; for instance, equal parts lidocaine 1% with epinephrine 1:100,000 and bupivacaine 0.25%). This should include the alveolar cleft, anterior palate, nasal floor, and lateral gingival tissue to be advanced.

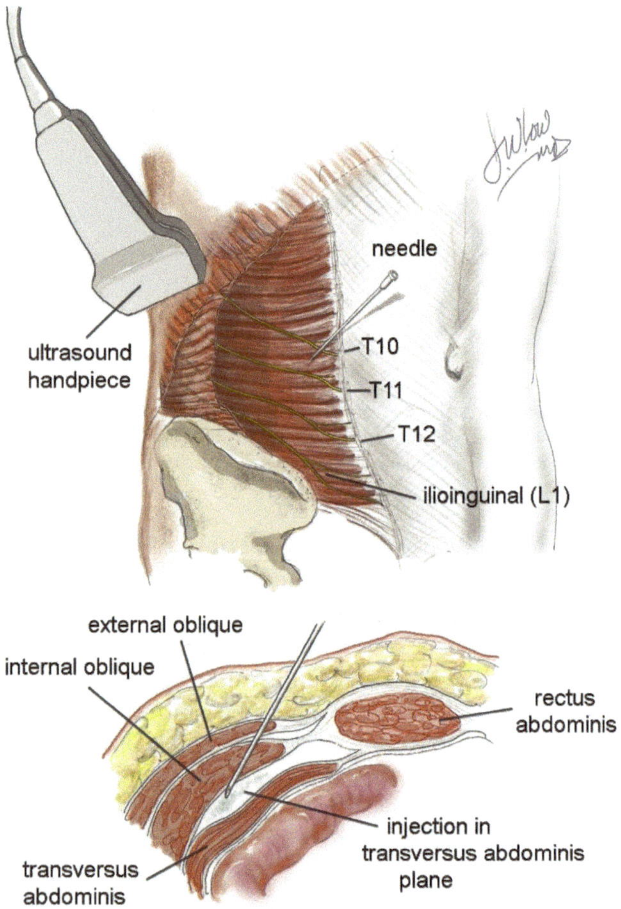


**Fig. 21.9** Transverse abdominis plane (TAP) block. Ultrasound can give visual guidance and the "double pop" technique through the fascial extensions of the external followed by internal oblique muscles to give palpable guidance, to correct positioning in the transversus abdominis plane. Here showing an anterior approach

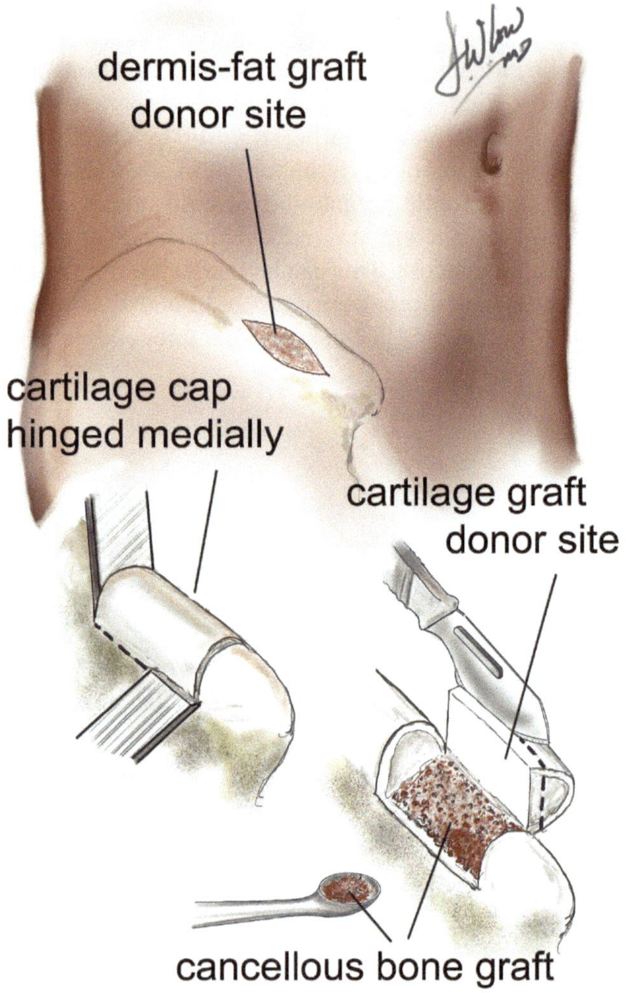


**Fig. 21.10** The anterior superior iliac crest is exposed, and the cartilage cap is hinged medially, to access cancellous bone for graft harvest. Placing the iliac crest incision 2 cm lateral to the anterior iliac prominence reduces visibility of scar and avoids the lateral femoral cutaneous nerve. Soft tissues are retracted medially during bone graft harvest. The anterior superior iliac crest incision can also be used for harvesting an elliptical dermis-fat graft

## Procedural Technique

Separate sterile fields and instruments are used at the hip donor site and mouth, to prevent cross contamination of oral flora to the clean hip. When possible, use a two-team approach for simultaneous graft harvest during recipient preparation.

### Iliac Crest Graft Harvest

A 30-degree bump is placed under the hip, and a 3-cm-long incision is designed parallel to and 2 cm lateral to the anterior superior iliac crest (ASIC) (Fig. 21.10) [16]. This incision design both hides the scar in the shadow lateral to the iliac crest prominence and prevents iatrogenic damage to the more medial lateral femoral cutaneous nerve [6]. The nondominant hand is used to place traction over the soft tissue to align the incision directly over the ASIC, and subcutaneous tissue and muscle fascia are incised down to the cartilage cap, and the Weitlaner retractor is inserted. Wide access can be facilitated through a small incision by sliding the soft tissue superiorly and inferiorly along the ASIC. A "treasure chest" pattern is incised with a scalpel through the cartilage cap, leaving the cap "hinged" medially like the lid of a treasure chest (Fig. 21.10).

This exposes the trilaminar iliac crest, with cortical bone medially and laterally and cancellous bone centrally. Cancellous bone is then harvested with a curette or gouge, with care to avoid including the cortical bone or cartilage. Volume needed is determined by recipient defect, generally 4–6 cc for a unilateral cleft. A cortical bone graft can be harvested from the lateral crest if needed for stability but will have less osteoinductive attributes. Following harvest, the cartilage cap is replaced anatomically to prevent hip contour irregularity and overlying tissue closed in three layers.

## Alveolar Cleft

After a throat pack is placed, the mouth and nose are cleaned thoroughly with chlorhexidine rinse to decrease bacterial load. In a technique similar to that first reported by Abyholm [9], incisions are designed along the medial and lateral alveolar cleft gingiva (Fig. 21.11a). The incision is carried up superiorly at the transition point from buccal to palatal mucosa, taking care to aim toward the lip and not the nasal floor. Next, medial and lateral mucoperiosteal flaps are designed with the incision through interdental papillae to enable anterior gingival closure. In a bilateral cleft, the entirety of mobilization must be done from the lesser segment (laterally); this is also generally our practice in unilateral clefts. The lesser segment flap is raised in a subperiosteal plane, with lateral periosteal release to enable medial transposition.

Additionally, the periosteum can be scored horizontally 2 cm above the inferior border to enable unfurling inferomedially. Sufficient mobilization allows the gingival flap to be shifted one tooth width toward the cleft. Medially, the gingival tissue is raised approximately 1 cm in width to enable cleft exposure and flap inset.

Posterior gingival flaps are then elevated in the subperiosteal plane, which are contiguous with palatal mucosa posteriorly (Fig. 21.11b). Ample elevation is critical in this posterior space, as the bone deficit is primarily posteriorly. A rasp can be used gently along the cortical bone surface staying superficial to prevent tooth root exposure, which may facilitate graft take. Finally, dissection proceeds superiorly toward the nasal floor. If a fistula is not present, wide dissection creates space beneath the intact nasal floor to enable graft positioning and can be performed with scissors or needle-point electrocautery. If a fistula is present, subperichondrial dissection of a vomer flap is performed medially, and subperiosteal dissection of lateral nasal wall flap is performed inferior to the inferior turbinate laterally. In bilateral clefts, a V-shaped fistula between the premaxilla and palatal mucosa is often encountered. An angled scalpel blade is helpful to incise horizontally at the nasal-oral mucosal junction, with ample submucosal elevation to enable closure of the nasal mucosa and oral mucosa as separate layers. Endpoint of dissection is reached once there is sufficient graft space, corresponding to the inverted pyramid shape up to the level of the piriformis, with volume of approximately 4–6 cm$^3$.

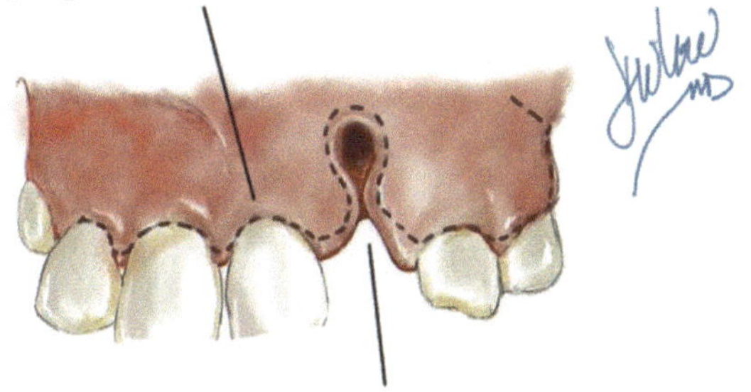


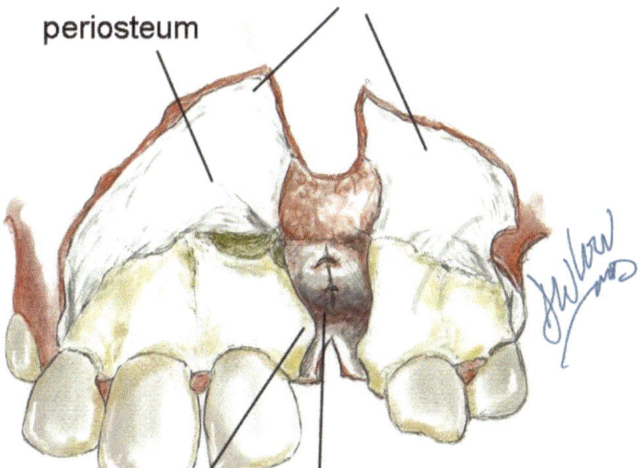


**Fig. 21.11** Marginal incisions along the alveolar cleft gingiva are extended up into the buccal mucosa, as is a vertical lateral releasing incision (**a**, upper). After elevating anterior gingival flaps, subperiosteal dissection is carried posteriorly to create a space for graft behind the alveolar bone, followed by closure of the nasal mucosa (**b**, lower)

Closure is then performed of the nasal floor and mobilized fistula tissue as needed, using 4-0 or 5-0 Vicryl suture (Fig. 21.11b). The posterior gingival flaps are then approximated in everted fashion to close the oral mucosa. Generally, inserting a Dingman mouth gag and placing these sutures and tying knots down on the palatal surface are advantageous. Cancellous graft is brought from the clean (hip) to contaminated (mouth) field and any large pieces or morselized with a rongeur to ease packing (Fig. 21.12). Pressure is placed sequentially as each piece is added using a tamp or Freer elevator to ensure tight packing. A cortical fragment (strut) can be placed on the roof of the defect prior to placement of cancellous bone; however, we find that this does not necessarily facilitate better bone take and can increase risk of extrusion. Careful attention is paid to the placement of early

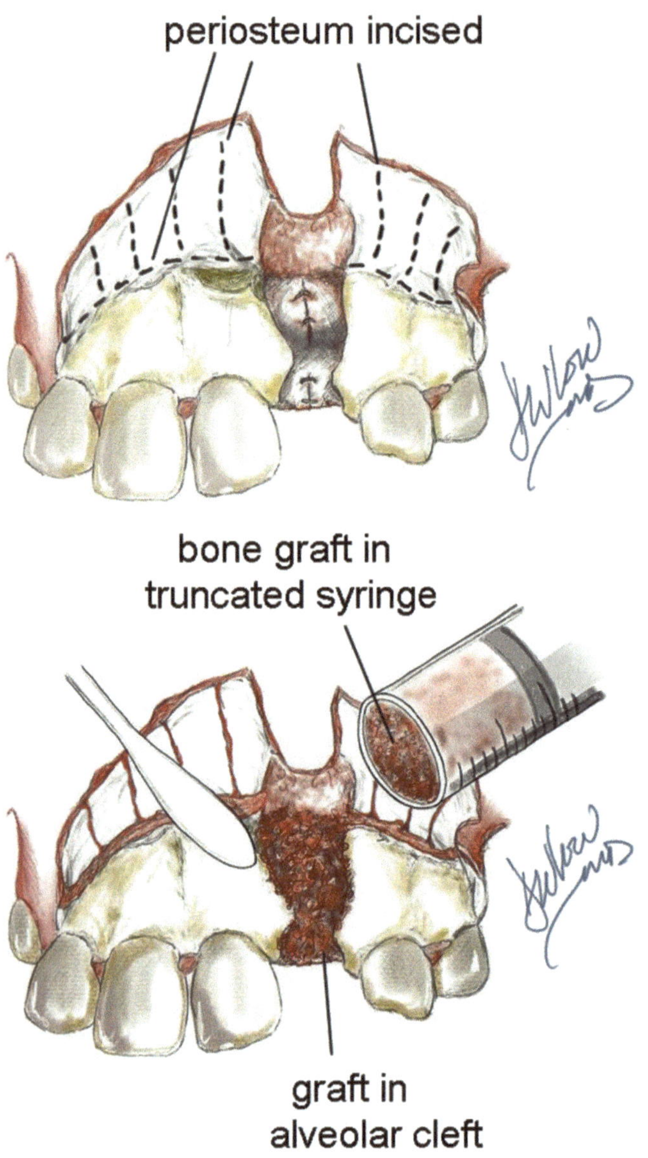


**Fig. 21.12** Cancellous bone graft delivered into alveolar cleft. Scoring of the periosteum in multiple planes enables expansion of gingivoperiosteal flaps to cover graft with minimal tension

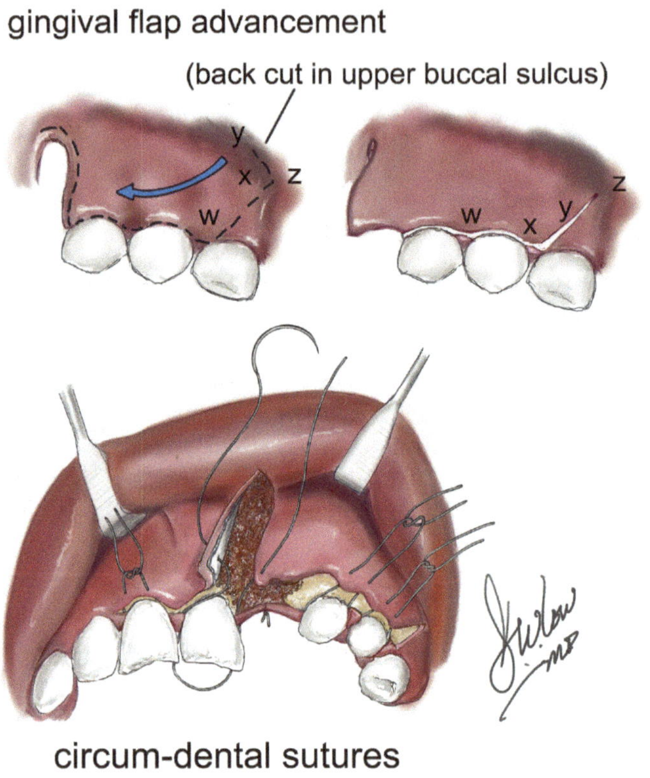


**Fig. 21.13** Gingival flaps are rotated and advanced toward the alveolar cleft, which is facilitated by a back cut. Circum-dental sutures provide secure, watertight approximation of the advanced flap

graft pieces superoposteriorly to fill beneath the nasal floor and behind the alveolar segments bilaterally to ensure tooth root support. The anterior gingival flaps are closed in interrupted fashion, thus medializing the lateral gingival-periosteal flap (Figs. 21.13 and 21.14). The flap is also secured along the dental margin using interrupted or circum-dental sutures. Finally, the dental splint is placed and secured. It can be bonded using dental adhesive or wired to the teeth or brackets and is usually kept in place for 6 weeks.

**Tips and Tricks: Alveolar Bone Graft**

- Inserting a Dingman mouth gag to enable suture placement and tie down on the palatal surface often facilitates a more robust closure.
- After the nasal layer closure, injecting saline into the nostril with a 10 cc syringe can ensure a watertight closure with no leaks.
- Horizontal scoring of the maxillary periosteum is critical to enable the flap to be advanced inferiorly and medially advanced without tension. Vertical scoring of the maxillary periosteum may also be helpful for medial mobilization of the advancement flap.
- Good hygiene is essential – preoperative chlorhexidine mouth cleanse, postoperative antibiotics, and separate instrumentation for the donor site – to preserve graft viability and prevent cross contamination.

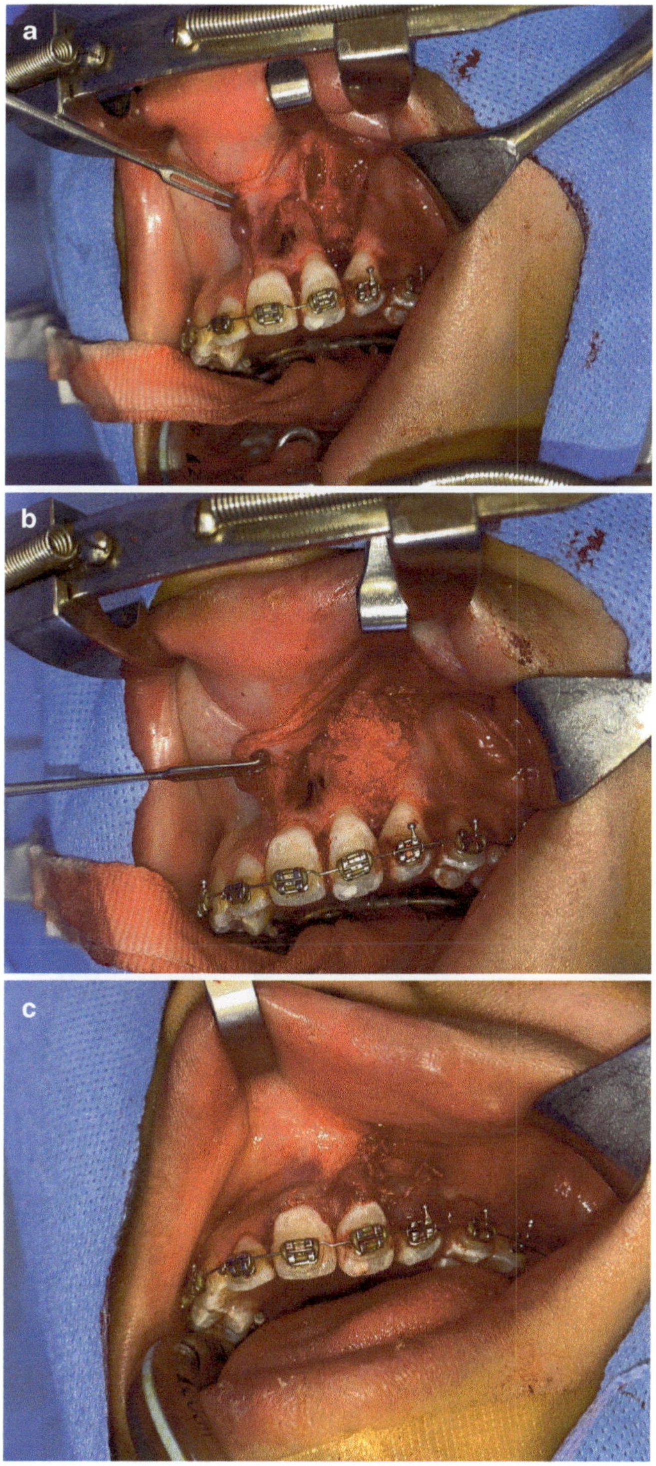


Fig. 21.14 Subperiosteal exposure of a left alveolar cleft (**a**), completion of cancellous bone grafting (**b**), and gingival flap closure (**c**). V to Y mucosal advancement flap combined with the dermis-fat graft provides additional bulk and mucosa to correct upper lip deficiency

## Simultaneous Tip Rhinoplasty and Lip Augmentation

Iliac crest bone grafting provides the opportunity to harvest cartilage and dermis-fat grafts from the same donor site to be used for tip rhinoplasty and lip augmentation. For lip augmentation, an ellipse can be superficially incised and de-epithelialized just below the iliac crest to provide a suitable dermis-fat graft to correct a volume deficiency such as a whistle deformity along the vermilion margin. For minor deficiencies, a vertical incision in the vermilion provides enough exposure to create a submucosal pocket. The graft can be stabilized with absorbable sutures at the corners. For larger deficiencies, a V to Y mucosal advancement flap combined with the dermis-fat graft provides additional bulk and mucosa to correct the deficiency (Fig. 21.15).

In the unilateral cleft, augmentation of the typically hypoplastic lower lateral crus with a thin iliac crest cartilage graft can provide useful support after centralizing the alar domes with permanent monofilament suture. Excision of a crescent of skin along the alar rim with a small transverse extension in the columella provides adequate exposure, and complete and meticulous dissection of the lateral crus permits easy splicing to the cartilage graft and mobilizes the alar web. The shape of the crescent is created using a template of the contralateral alar rim (Fig. 21.15). The most challenging part of the dissection is separation of the surprisingly adherent intranasal skin from the cartilage. A block of cartilage can be harvested from the cartilage cap for augmentation of the deficient ala in a unilateral cleft (Figs. 21.16 and 21.17). Extending the length of the lateral crus helps to prevent recurrent collapse of the tip and helps to support the external nasal valve. Chromic quilting sutures help to stabilize the intranasal skin and prevent recurrent webbing after placement of the cartilage graft in the pocket.

Iliac cartilage can also be used for a columella strut graft in a bilateral cleft nasal deformity. The graft can be placed in a precise pocket using either the lip scar, if one is also revising the cleft lip scars, or through the upper buccal sulcus after raising the premaxillary gingiva flap. Long-lasting but absorbable monofilament mattress sutures can be placed through the skin, medial crura, and cartilage graft to stabilize the columella construct.

## Follow-Up and Complication Management

Overnight admission for pain control is typical; same-day discharge may be considered when a TAP block, trephine harvest, or bone graft substitute is used. There are no hip

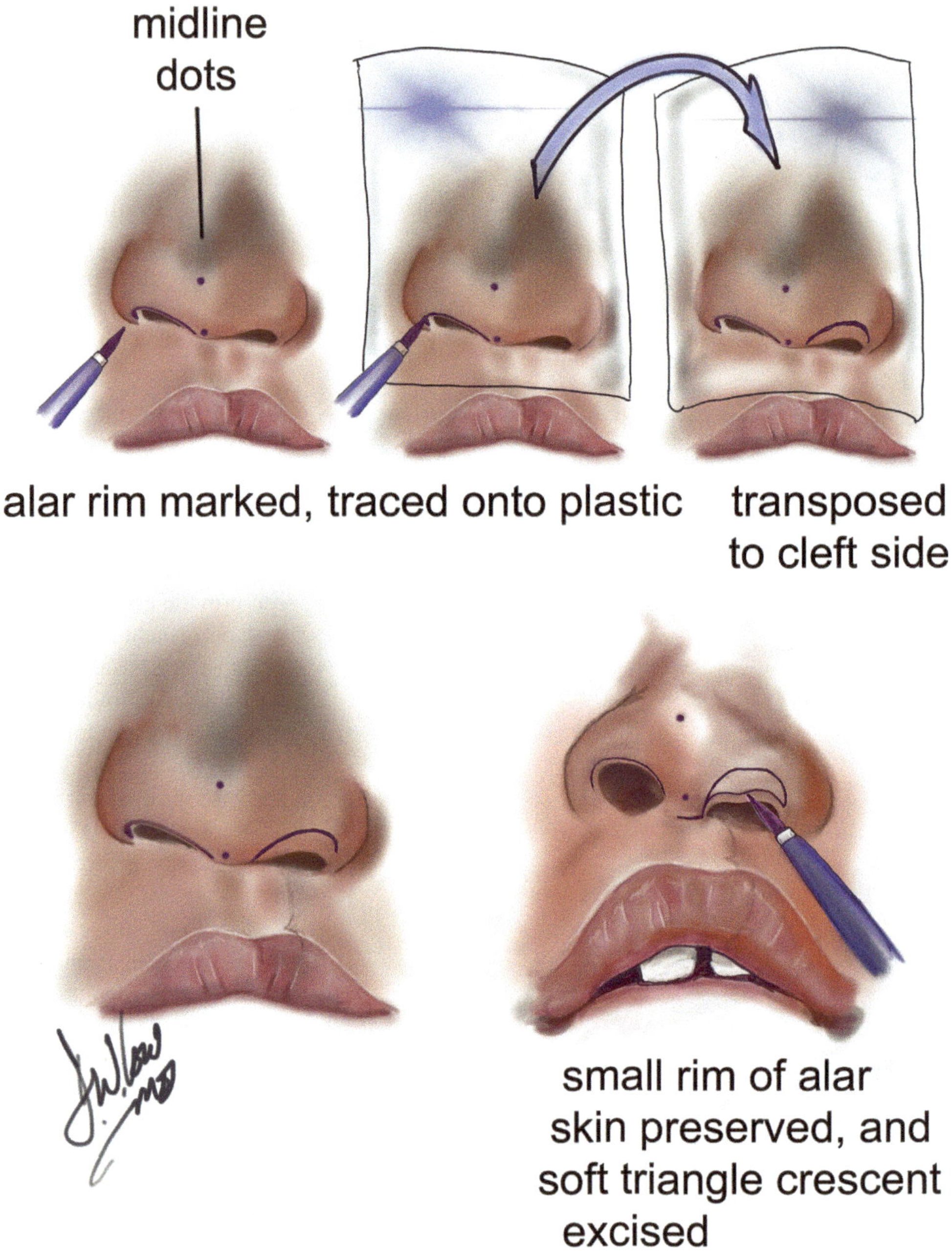


**Fig. 21.15** Template guidance for excising a crescent of alar rim skin to provide exposure and address soft triangle collapse

donor site precautions or ambulation limitations. Postoperative antibiotic prophylaxis is employed (oral amoxicillin-clavulanic acid, 7–14 days) to prevent graft infection and resorption, although there is little evidence to guide antibiotic selection or duration. Parental education on the importance of pureed ("soft" or "no chew") diet for 6 weeks and oral hygiene is essential and aided by three times daily chlorhexidine or saline mouthwash. Elixir non-steroidal anti-inflammatory agents (e.g., ibuprofen) and/or acetaminophen for 4–7 days are issued for pain control.

A panoramic radiograph is repeated 6 months postoperatively to assess for bony calcification across the alveolar cleft. The most common complication is graft resorption, which requires repeat grafting in approximately 10% of cases, and is typically associated with partial mucosal incisional dehiscence. Dehiscence and partial graft exposure can sometimes be salvaged by debriding the exposed piece(s) of cancellous graft.

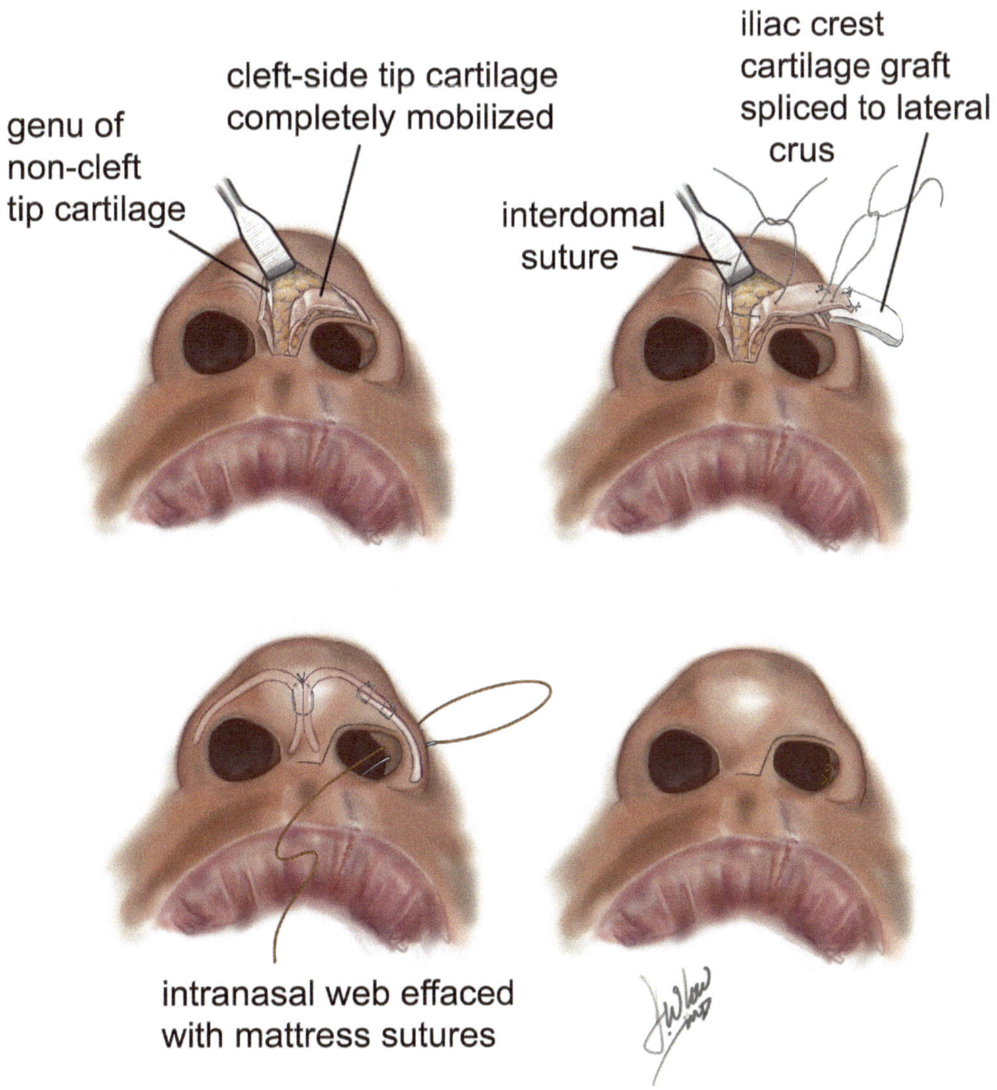


**Figs. 21.16 and 21.17** Tip rhinoplasty at time of alveolar bone graft utilizing iliac cartilage graft

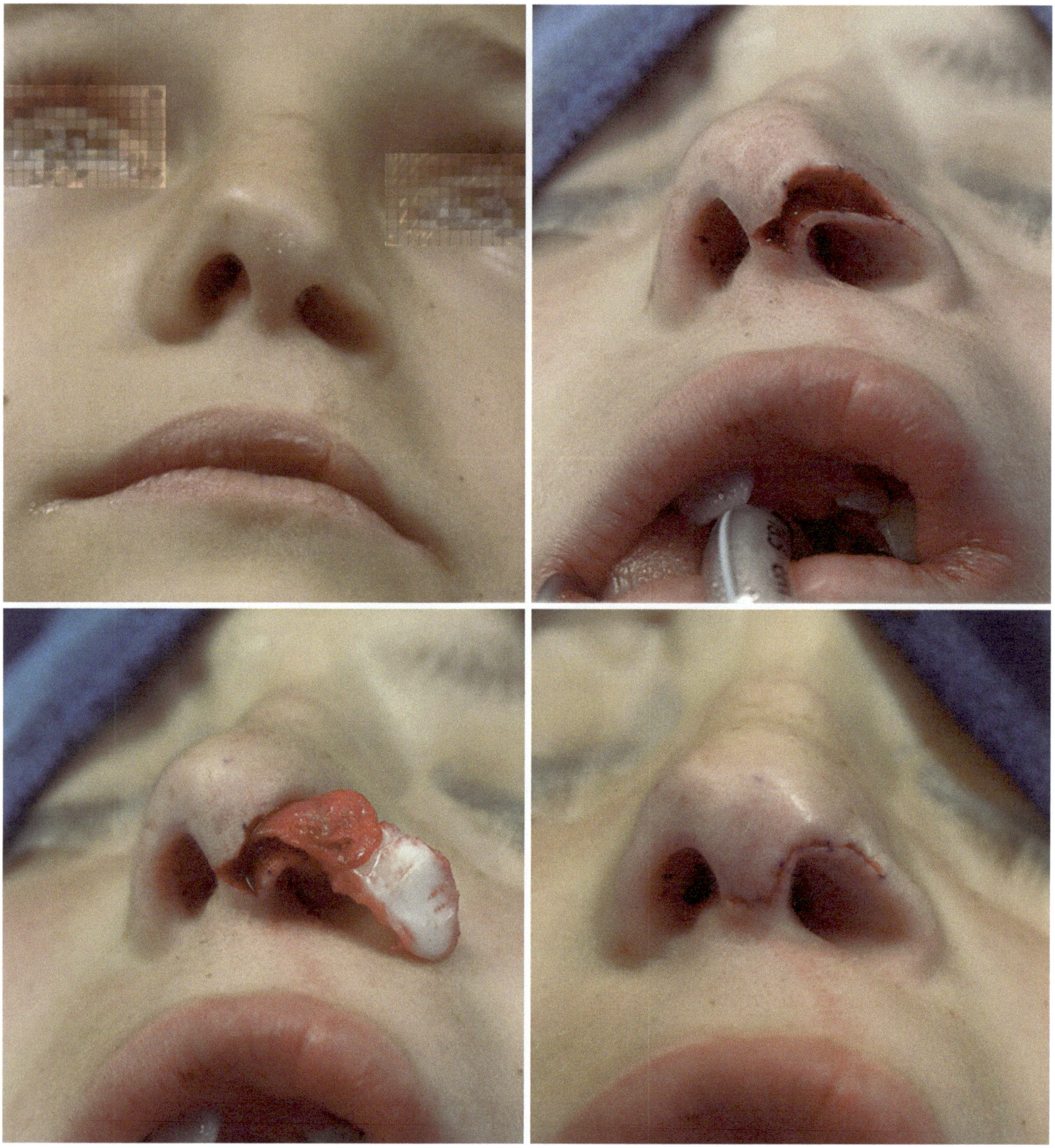

Fig. 21.16 (continued)

## References


1. Eppley BL, Sadove AM. Management of alveolar cleft bone grafting – state of the art. Cleft Palate Craniofac J. 2000;37(3):229–33.
2. Jolleys A, Robertson NR. A study of the effects of early bone-grafting in complete clefts of the lip and palate – five year study. Br J Plast Surg. 1972;25(3):229–37.
3. Denadai R, Raposo-Amaral CE. An overview of protocols and outcomes in cleft care. In: Alonso N, Raposo-Amaral CE, editors. Cleft lip and palate treatment. Cham: Springer; 2018.
4. Sato Y, Grayson BH, Garfinkle JS, Barillas I, Maki K, Cutting CB. Success rate of gingivoperiosteoplasty with and without secondary bone grafts compared with secondary alveolar bone grafts alone. Plast Reconstr Surg. 2008;121(4):1356–67.
5. Power SM, Matic DB. Gingivoperiosteoplasty following alveolar molding with a Latham appliance versus secondary bone grafting: the effects on bone production and midfacial growth in patients with bilateral clefts. Plast Reconstr Surg. 2009;124:573–82.
6. Hopper RA. Alveolar clefts. In: Neligan P, editor. Plastic surgery. 3rd ed. London: Elsevier; 2011.
7. Long RE Jr, Paterno M, Vinson B. Effect of cuspid positioning in the cleft at the time of secondary alveolar bone grafting on eventual graft success. Cleft Palate Craniofac J. 1996;33:225–30.
8. Boyne PJ, Sands NR. Secondary bone grafting of residual alveolar and palatal clefts. J Oral Surg. 1972;30(2):87–92.
9. Abyholm FE, Bergland O, Semb G. Secondary bone grafting of alveolar clefts. A surgical/orthodontic treatment enabling a non-prosthodontic rehabilitation in cleft lip and palate patients. Scand J Plast Reconstr Surg. 1981;15(2):127–40.
10. Rawashdeh MA, Telfah H. Secondary alveolar bone grafting: the dilemma of donor site selection and morbidity. Br J Oral Maxillofac Surg. 2008;46:665–70.
11. Hammoudeh JA, Fahradyan A, Gould DJ, et al. A comparative analysis of recombinant human bone morphogenetic protein-2 with a demineralized bone matrix versus iliac crest bone graft for secondary alveolar bone grafts in patients with cleft lip and palate: review of 501 cases. Plast Reconstr Surg. 2017;140:318e–25e.
12. Liang F, Leland H, Jedrzejewski B, et al. Alternatives to autologous bone graft in alveolar cleft reconstruction: the state of alveolar tissue engineering. J Craniofac Surg. 2018;29:584–93.
13. Alonso N, Risso GH, Denadai R, Raposo-Amaral CE. Effect of maxillary alveolar reconstruction on nasal symmetry of cleft lip and palate patients: a study comparing iliac crest bone graft and recombinant human bone morphogenetic protein-2. J Plast Reconstr Aesthet Surg. 2014;67(9):1201–8.
14. Rafi AN. Abdominal field block: a new approach via the lumbar triangle. Anaesthesia. 2001;56:1024–6.
15. Punekar IRA, Koltz PF, Smith DI, et al. The evolution of iliac bone graft donor site analgesia in cleft patients: transversus abdominis plane block is safe and efficacious. Ann Plast Surg. 2018;81:441–3.
16. de la Torre JI, Tenenhaus M, Gallagher PM, et al. Harvesting iliac bone graft: decreasing the morbidity. Cleft Palate Craniofac J. 1999;36:388–90.


## Alveolar Bone Grafts, Case 1

### Case Study: Extruded Premaxilla in an 8-Year-Old Male with Bilateral Cleft Lip/Palate

Vilma Arteaga and Edwar Alvarez

#### Case Analysis

This 8-year-old boy with bilateral cleft lip, palate, and alveolus has undergone previous lip and palate repair, but his premaxilla is anteriorly and inferiorly displaced. His posterior maxillary segments are collapsed and he has small nasolabial fistulas in line with the unrepaired alveolar segments, and a small anterior palatal fistula near the incisive foramen. He is entering age of mixed dentition, although retains primary dentition.

Goals of care are to level his premaxilla with his maxillary arch, create an arch with bony contiguity and appropriate width, and achieve mucosal patency.

#### Treatment Considerations

*When orthodontic care is available*, planning should be made jointly by orthodontist and surgeon and begins with obtaining orthopantogram X-ray (OPG). This patient's dental age appears delayed, and OPG is not likely to yet show canine root development. Orthodontic preparation can involve: (1) elevation of premaxilla (for instance, using Plana's tracks; 6–12 month process), (2) transverse maxillary expansion (hyrax, hass, or quad-helix expanders; 1–3 months), (3) gradual repositioning of premaxilla into middle third space created after expansion, or (4) use of a myofunctional appliance (made from acrylic or prefabricated device, such as Myobrace). Following orthodontic repositioning, alveolar bone grafting can be performed. Given the fistula presence, bone grafting is likely to be more durable if each side is grafted in staged procedures. A small fistula can be closed at the time of bone graft placement; however, larger fistulas are better closed in a staged fashion 6 months prior to bone grafting.

*When orthodontic care is not available*, consideration could be made for a surgical premaxillary setback (see Chap. 23). However, in this case, because of the collapsed posterior maxillary segments, there is no space in which to reposition the premaxilla. Thus it would not be beneficial.

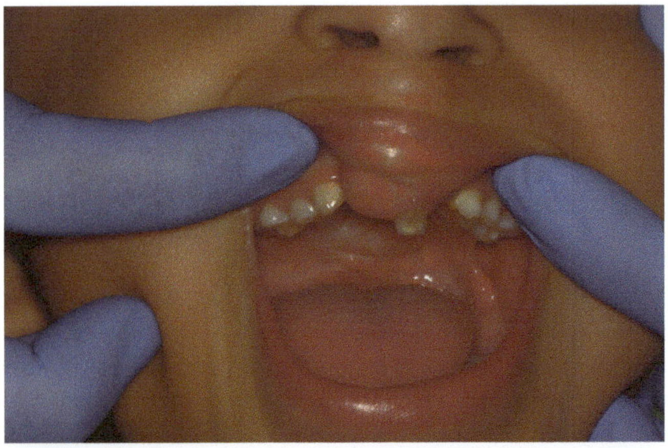

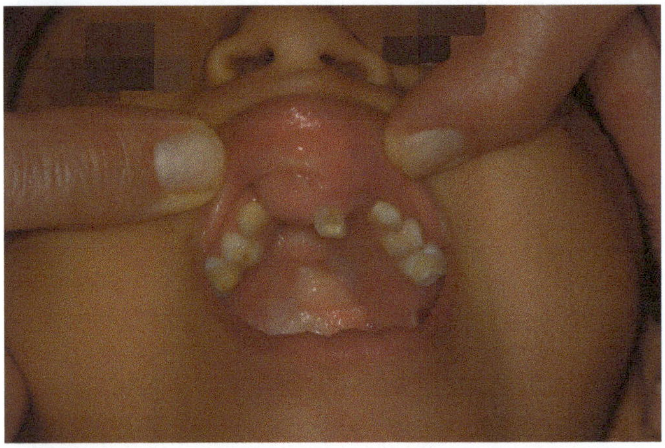

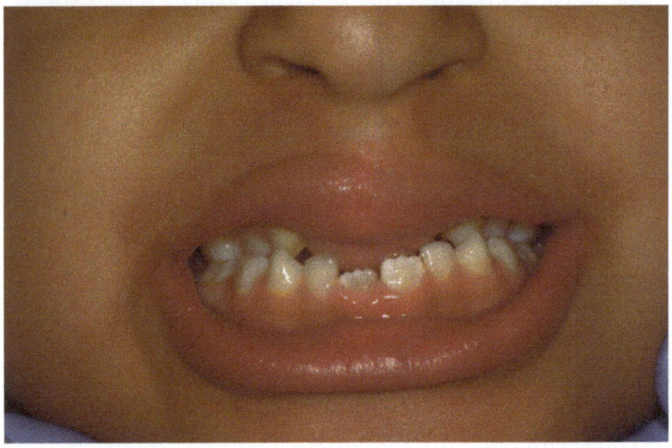

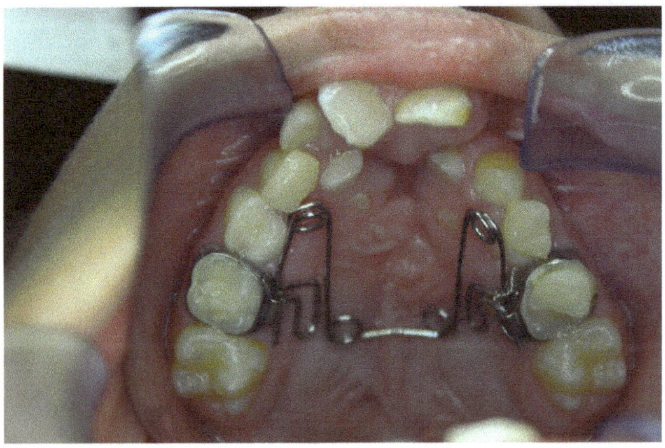

## Alveolar Bone Grafts, Case 2

### Case Study: Extruded Premaxilla in a 4-Year-Old Male with Bilateral Cleft Lip/Palate

Edwar Alvarez and David Alvarez

#### Case Analysis

This young boy with bilateral cleft lip, palate, and alveolus has undergone previous lip and palate repair, but his premaxilla is more severely exposed with anterior and inferior displacement. The upper lip rests behind the premaxilla, retracting it away from the alveolar arc.

Goals of care are to level his premaxilla with his maxillary arch, create an arch with bony contiguity and appropriate width, and achieve mucosal patency.

#### Treatment Considerations

This patient is too young for orthodontic manipulation or bone grafting, and given the gap between his alveolar segments, options could include a premaxillary setback or sulcoplasty.

In this case, a sulcoplasty was performed with T-shaped division of the premaxillary gingiva, advancement of the gingivobuccal mucosa, and relocation of the lip to recreate a sulcus. This has improved the premaxillary-upper lip relation, which with time may enable the band-like effect of the orbicularis oris muscle to retract the premaxilla into the alveolar arc.

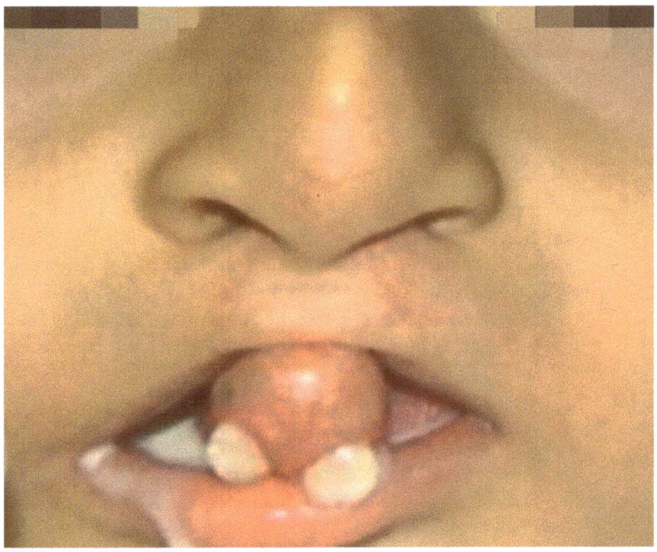

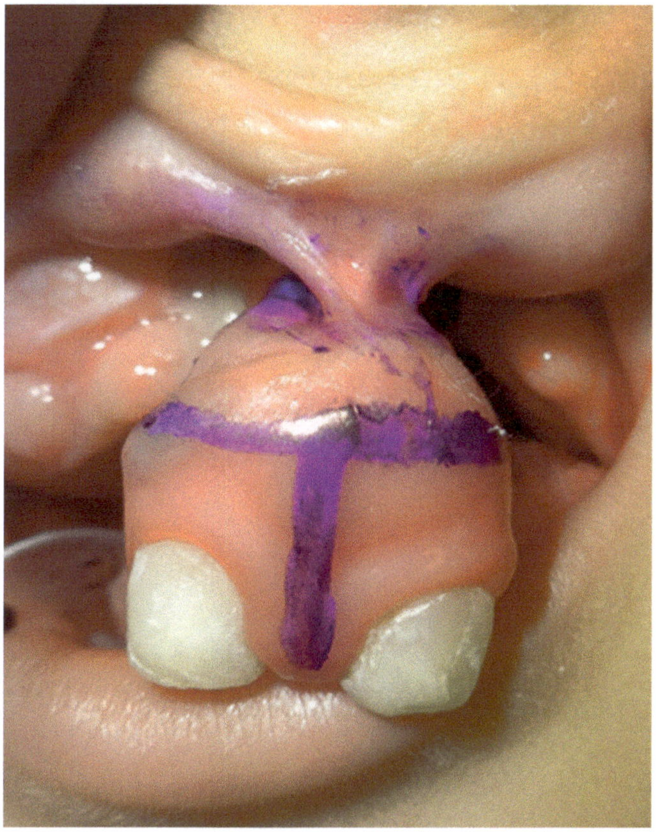

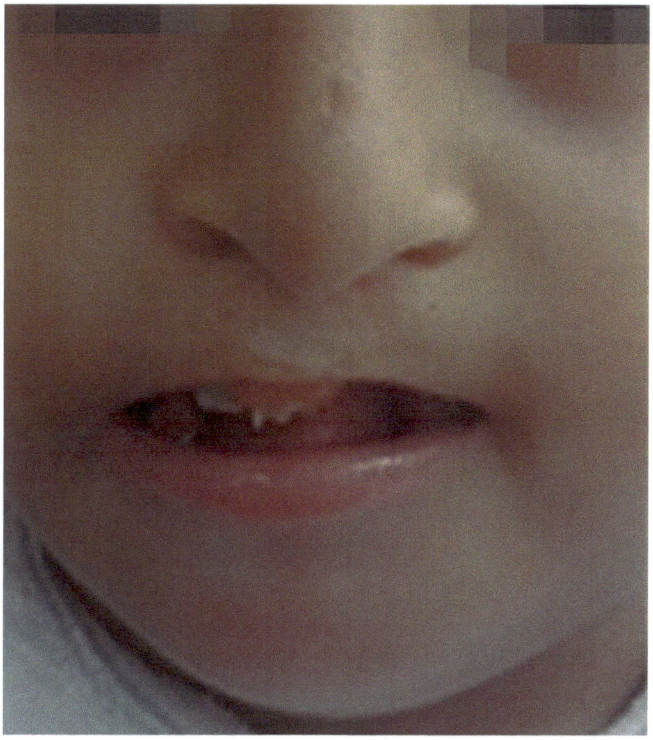

# Cleft Rhinoplasty

# 22

Jesse A. Taylor and Robin Yang

**Key Points**

- The cleft nasal deformity associated with the primary cleft lip/nose for both unilateral and bilateral clefts represents a complex spectrum of deformity for the cleft reconstructive surgeon.
- The central location of the nose and lip makes them among the most notable facets of a person's appearance.
- In addition, there is a considerable functional airway component to the nose and nasopharynx that evolves throughout childhood.
- The spectrum of the cleft nasal deformity involves all tissue layers of the nose including the mucosal lining, osseo-cartilaginous vault, and external skin.
- Adequately treating the cleft nasal deformity requires understanding (a) the anatomical differences in the cleft nose, (b) diagnostic maneuvers to assess nasal functional compromise, (c) timing of surgical intervention, and (d) technical elements of definitive rhinoplasty at the culmination of facial growth.

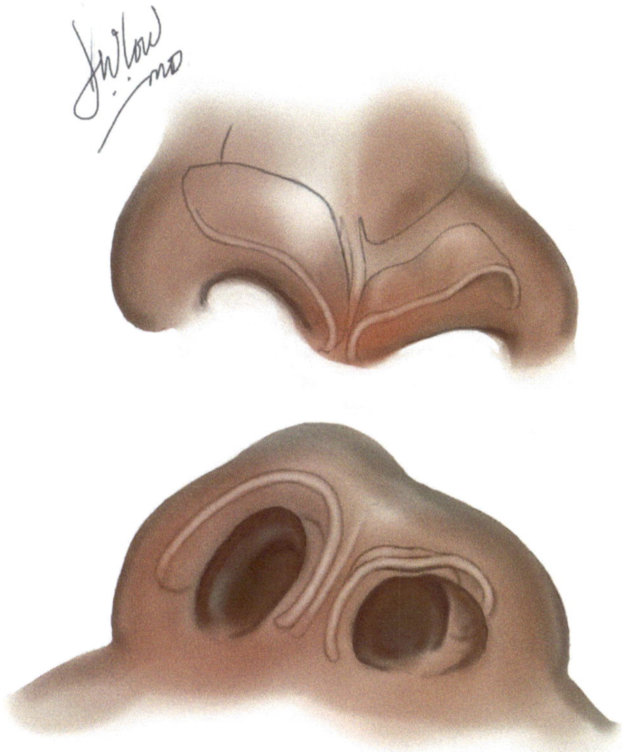

**Fig. 22.1** Characteristic unilateral cleft nasal deformity. Note the deviation of the columella and caudal nasal septum to the noncleft side with a lateral, inferior, and posterior retraction of the alar base

## Introduction

The unilateral cleft nasal deformity is an imbalance of aberrant soft tissue structures as well as hypoplasia of the underlying skeletal foundation (Fig. 22.1: Unilateral cleft nasal deformity). There is deviation of the columella and caudal nasal septum to the noncleft side with a lateral, inferior, and posterior retraction of the nasal and alar base. In addition, the cephalad nasal septum is deviated toward the cleft side. The asymmetric nasal tip results from the irregular lower lateral cartilages on the cleft side. The introverted lower lateral cartilages also contribute to the depressed cleft-sided vestibular webbing and thickened ala.

Bilateral cleft nasal deformities are characterized by a lack of nasal tip projection rather than the asymmetry that is seen in the unilateral deformity (Fig. 22.2: Bilateral cleft nasal deformity). There is a shortening and lack of soft tissue of the columella and upper lip. Widening of the interdomal distance in the nasal tip and cephalic rotation of the nasal tip,

J. A. Taylor (✉)
Department of Plastic Surgery, The Children's Hospital of Philadelphia, Philadelphia, PA, USA

R. Yang
Department of Plastic Surgery, Johns Hopkins Hospital, Baltimore, MD, USA

© Springer Nature Switzerland AG 2021



J. W. Swanson, D. W. Low (eds.), *Global Cleft Care in Low-Resource Settings*, https://doi.org/10.1007/978-3-030-59105-2_22

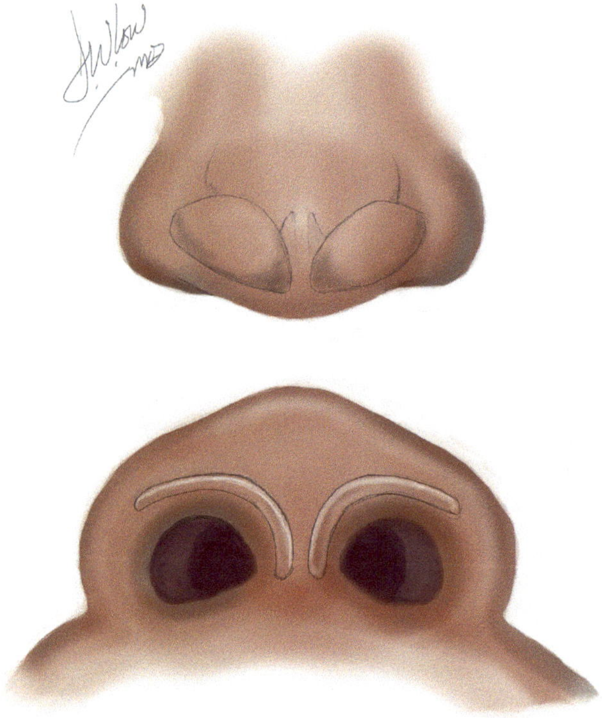


Fig. 22.2 Characteristic bilateral cleft nasal deformity. Note the lack of nasal tip projection with shortened columella, widening of the interdomal distance in the nasal tip with cephalic rotation

Table 22.1 Characteristic features of unilateral and bilateral cleft nasal deformities

| Anatomical Feature | Unilateral CLND | Bilateral CLND |
|---|---|---|
| Upper two-thirds | | |
| Nasal Root | Widened and deviated | Moderate widening and deviation |
| Dorsum | Deviated toward the CL side | Midline |
| Lower Thirds | | |
| Alar base | Inferior/posterior displaced on CL side with increased width. | Inferior/posterior displacement BL, Wide BL |
| Nasal Tip | Asymmetric | Flat, broad with weak projection |
| Alar Rim/ nostril shape | Flattened nostril on CL side. Obliquely oriented on the CL side. Contralateral side usually more vertical | Obliquely oriented BL |
| Intranasal | | |
| Vestibule | Vestibular web on CL side | Vestibular webs BL |
| Septum | Caudal septum deviated to non CL side | Variable position of the septum |
| Turbinates | Hypertrophied bilaterally variable | Hypertrophy bilaterally variable |
| Midface | | |
| Maxilla | Variable maxillary hypoplasia and malar flattening | Variable maxillary hypoplasia and malar flattening |

all of which combine to de-project the nasal tip. The nasal septum usually remains in the midline, though it may be deviated in cases in which the clefting is asymmetric—for instance, a complete cleft on one side and incomplete on the other. Proper correction of the cleft lip nasal deformity requires a fundamental knowledge of the bony, cartilaginous, and soft tissue anatomy that defines the initial deformity at infancy (Table 22.1: Comparison of bilateral and unilateral cleft nasal deformity).

An understanding of the effects of surgery on the growth and development of the nose and iatrogenic contributions to a secondary deformity are also important factors. Early or primary nasal correction at the time of cleft lip repair can provide a good foundation that may minimize the degree of deformity but does not necessarily obviate the need for subsequent surgery for both functional and aesthetic reasons [1]. As with all congenital deformities, there are psychosocial factors that the cleft reconstructive surgeon must consider [2] which may translate to balancing nasal growth potential and "normalizing" the deformity to allow for emotional growth. Because primary rhinoplasty, that is, rhinoplasty accompanying cleft lip repair, is covered elsewhere in this text, the focus of this chapter will involve the techniques of secondary cleft rhinoplasty during the school-aged years and definitive rhinoplasty when facial growth is complete.

## Nasal Assessment

Preoperative evaluation should start with a complete history and physical examination of prior operative records. The evaluation should take into account the skin integrity as well as the overall facial harmony, proportions, and relations to adjacent structures such as the forehead, midface, and chin [3]. This is particularly poignant in patients with a history of cleft lip/nasal deformities. Dentofacial deformities that warrant skeletal surgery in the noncleft population are approximately 2%. Maxillary hypoplasia is reported to be up to 30% in the congenital cleft/lip patient population [4]. Other cleft-related procedures such as alveolar bone grafting and orthognathic surgery can have profound effects on the nasal architecture. For example, a Le Fort I advancement generally increases the columellar angle and elevates the nasal tip and

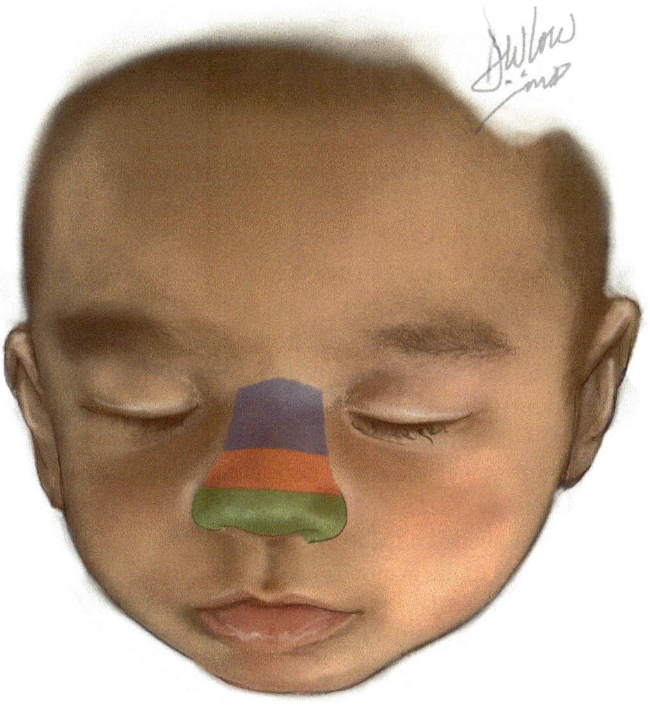

Fig. 22.3 The “nasal thirds” classification. The upper third consists of paired nasal bones and the midline bony septum, the middle third is composed of the midline dorsal septum and upper lateral cartilages, and the lower third includes the nasal tip composed of the caudal septum, the lower lateral cartilages, and the alar regions

widens the nasal base [5, 6]. An alveolar bone graft can correct the posterior displacement of the alar base. Functional disturbances of the nasal airway are found in 60% of patients with a history of a cleft [7, 8].

Nasal form is traditionally described in nasal thirds (Fig. 22.3: Nasal thirds). The upper third or the bony vault consists of paired nasal bones and the midline bony septum (vertical plate of the ethmoid bone). The middle third of the nose is composed of the midline dorsal septum and the right and left upper lateral cartilages. The lower third is composed of the nasal tip composed of the caudal septum, lower lateral cartilages, and the alar regions. A proper intranasal exam can reveal septal deviations, bone spurs, turbinate hypertrophy, vestibular webbing, and internal/external nasal valve collapse. A Cottle maneuver, modified Cottle maneuver, and endoscopic examination should be performed to rule out all potential causes of obstruction. This is important in the cleft population as most patients are accustomed to obstructive breathing and they may not be able to detail their symptoms [9]. Preoperative photography should be utilized in a systematic fashion to help document and detail the extent of deformity that may have been missed from a clinical exam alone. Lastly, a facial CT scan, if available, may help diagnose sinus disease and posterior nasal deformities such as bone spurs and septal deformities.

## Timing of Surgery

Traditional teaching and dogma are such that invasive procedures for nasal correction at the primary correction are ineffective and can cause irreparable harm to the nasal cartilage and soft tissues [10]. However, more recent studies with good long-term results demonstrated that synchronous correction of some of the nasal deformities during the primary cleft lip repair can result in better appearance and function during childhood and reduce the complexity of secondary rhinoplasty, with better outcomes [8, 11]. Thus, nowadays, many children in developed countries will have undergone some form of primary nasal correction at the time of their initial cleft lip repair. Such correction can be highly variable, from simply dissecting the tip and placing McComb sutures to radical “semi-open” nasal tip dissection and direct repositioning of the lower lateral cartilages. Regardless, some children will still exhibit obvious residual and/or iatrogenic deformities, and an understanding of prior operative maneuvers may be helpful. Opportunities to correct these deformities in conjunction with other surgeries include (1) pre-school age (4–5 years of age) if cleft lip revisions are advised or if there are sleep-related surgeries planned and (2) school age (5–10 years of age) if an alveolar bone graft procedure is indicated. In general, most intermediate corrective surgeries during childhood are focused on the lower third of the nose. Definitive rhinoplasty is most often indicated when there is maturity of the craniofacial skeleton (males 16–18 and females around 15–17). This timing may also be delayed if there is a maxilla-mandibular discrepancy requiring orthognathic surgery which would change the anatomical positioning of the nose.

## Intermediate Correction Techniques/School-Aged Rhinoplasty

As discussed previously, most techniques utilized for secondary rhinoplasty during the developmental years of life are focused on the lower third of the nose. This involves techniques to level the alar bases, reposition the caudal septum, and improve the position of the lower lateral cartilages.

## Repositioning of the Caudal Septum

In our practice, the caudal septal displacement is addressed during the primary cleft lip repair. This is approached through the incisions utilized for repair of the lip. When encountered as a secondary revision, an intranasal septal incision can be utilized. The abnormal caudal septal attachments can be released from the anterior nasal spine and vomer. Additional septal scoring can be performed on the concave side to correct any buckling or collapse. The corrected positioning of the septum can be secured with a more permanent suture to the periosteum of the maxilla. Alternatively, the caudal septum is easily reached from incisions for alveolar bone grafting, and most caudal septal repositioning and scoring can be done from intraoral incisions if no additional rhinoplasty maneuvers are planned.

## Leveling of the Alar Base

The secondary cleft nasal deformity and alar base can be displaced in all planes (inferior, lateral, and posterior). Occasionally a posterior displacement can be corrected by an alveolar bone graft [6]. Vertical and horizontal repositioning can be accomplished by a V-Y advancement flap of the abnormal alar base positioning. Horizontal narrowing can be achieved with advancement of the Y segment. The vertical position can be changed by altering the angle of the same Y segment. There should be some form of overcorrection to compensate for growth and relapse.

## Correction of the Lower Lateral Cartilages

The goals of correction should be focused on the dysmorphic lower lateral cartilage and the short vertical columella. A semi-open approach can be utilized with intranasal rim incisions. This incision can be performed as traditionally described by Tajima and Maryyama [12]. A reverse U-shaped incision across the abnormal plica or webbing of the affected cleft nasal side is placed in the inner aspect of the intranasal rim. From this incision, the inferior two-thirds of the nose are undermined bilaterally in the subcutaneous plane. The composite U-shaped flap including the lower lateral cartilage is then sutured to the alar cartilage of the normal side as well as to the lateral cartilages bilaterally till symmetry is achieved (Fig. 22.4: Tajima drawing).

When alar bases are in reasonable position, Potter's technique or the Tajima technique can be utilized, involving a conventional open rhinoplasty approach. The superomedial-based V-Y chondromucosal composite flap on the cleft side can elevate and advance the nasal tip. This flap encompasses the lateral crura of the lower lateral cartilage and the attached nasal mucosa. An interdomal suture is used to suspend and advance

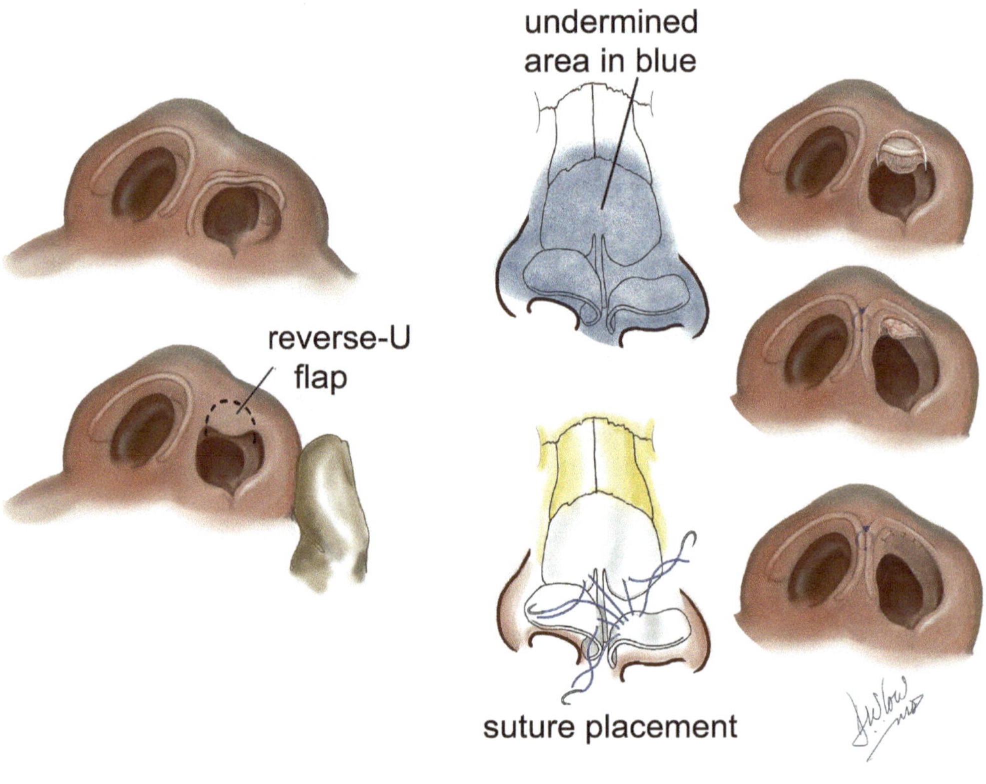


**Fig. 22.4** Tajima technique for lower lateral cartilage and soft tissue repositioning

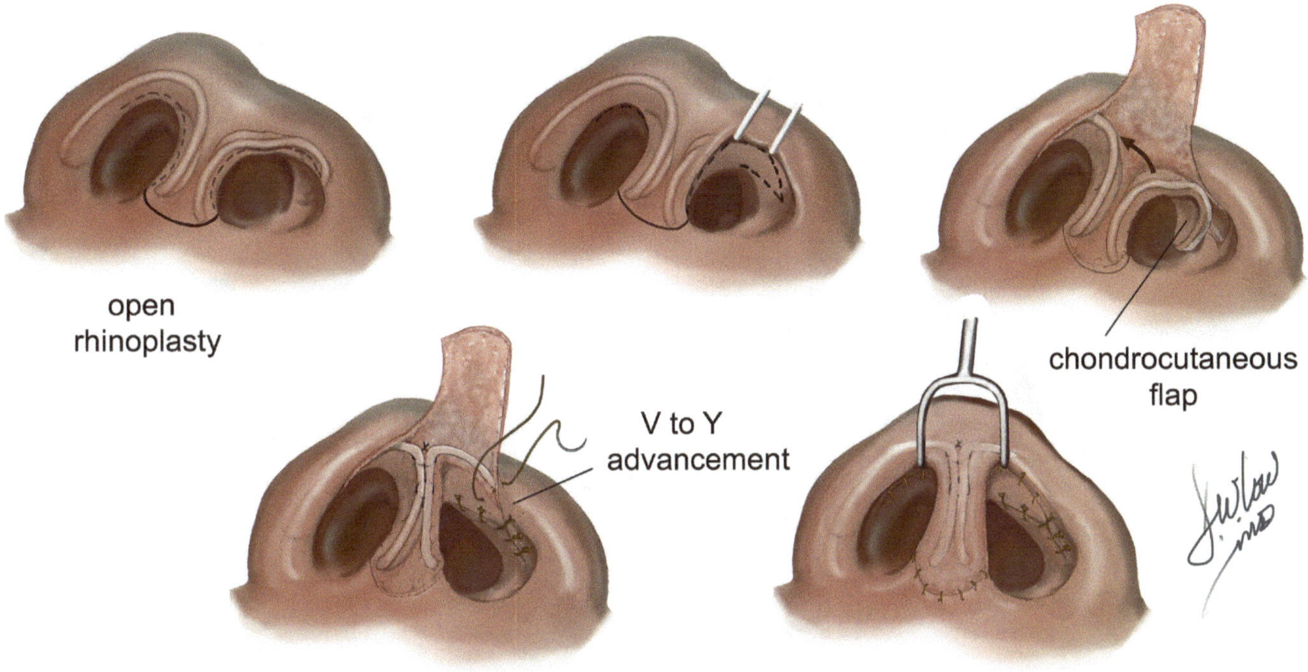


**Fig. 22.5** Potter technique of superomedially based V-Y chondromucosal composite flap on the cleft side to elevate and advance the nasal tip

the newly created composite flap to the contralateral side to achieve symmetry of the tip and improve projection (Fig. 22.5: Potter's technique). The dorsal soft tissue is often defatted prior to closure in order to allow for improved tip definition.

## Definitive Rhinoplasty

Definitive septorhinoplasty is performed once the patient has reached skeletal maturity and is the final intervention for many cleft patients. The goals of definitive rhinoplasty should be creation of symmetry and harmony at all levels of the nose, relief of any nasal obstruction, and long-term stability. Definitive cleft rhinoplasty usually entails common rhinoplasty maneuvers—nasal bone osteotomies, septoplasty, dorsal reduction/augmentation, spreader grafts, lower lateral cartilage refinement, and repositioning—but often these must be done in a more radical fashion than typical for aesthetic rhinoplasty.

### Approach

The senior author prefers an open or external approach to the nose via stair-step trans-columellar or inverted V incision. An open approach allows maximal access to reconstruct and reshape under direct visualization as well as obtain graft material from the septum or the alar cartilages. Typical rhinoplasty sequencing is described in Table 22.2. Pre- and postoperative photos of a patient with unilateral cleft lip nasal deformity are shown (Fig. 22.6).

**Table 22.2** Typical sequencing for definitive rhinoplasty

| |
|---|
| 1. Dorsal reduction |
| 2. Medial nasal osteotomies |
| 3. Septal reconstruction (including spreader grafting) |
| 4. Dorsal augmentation |
| 5. Nasal tip refinement (including columellar strut grafting and tip grafting) |
| 6. Lateral nasal osteotomies |

Each maneuver is only performed when needed

### Nasal Dorsal Augmentation

Dorsal augmentation techniques for a definitive rhinoplasty in a cleft patient should be performed akin to techniques for functional and aesthetic rhinoplasty. Reduction techniques as well as conservative osteotomies should be utilized for asymmetry correction and contouring. In cases that require dorsal augmentation, various different grafting materials have been described. Diced septal cartilage can be used for moderate nasal dorsum deformities and has been shown to

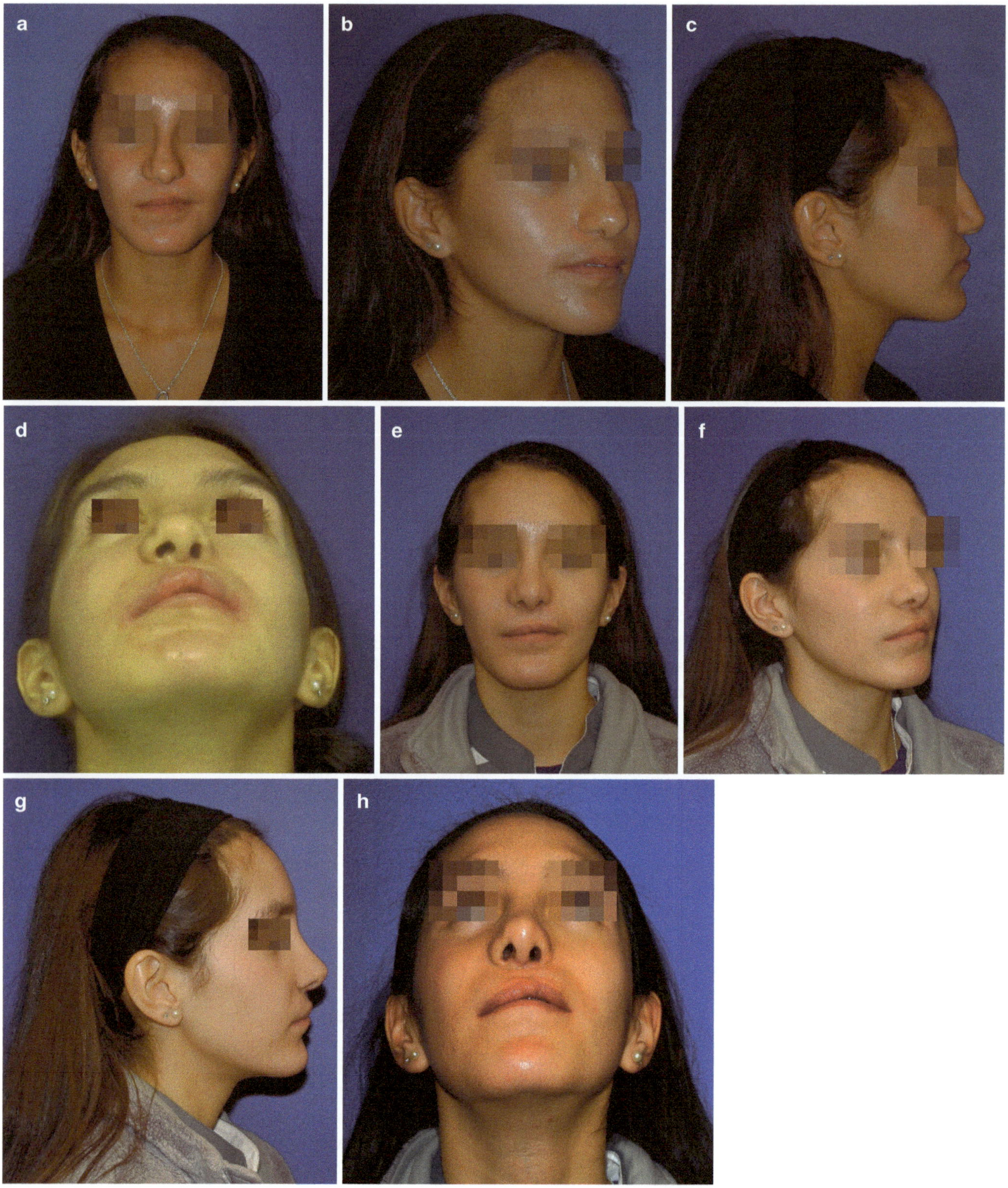


**Fig. 22.6** A 16-year-old female with left unilateral cleft nasal deformity, prior to (**a–d**) and following (**e–h**) septorhinoplasty including submucosal septal resection, dorsal recontouring, internal spreader grafts, tip resuspension and cartilaginous augmentation, and bony osteotomies and repositioning

be an easy, safe, and predictable technique to augment the nasal dorsum [13]. For more significant deformities, autologous costal cartilage is preferred for structure and definition. Care must be taken in carving and fixating costal cartilage so as to avoid long-term warping. Other graft materials such allografts, homografts, and alloplastic materials (silicone, porous polyethylene) have been described. The senior author prefers the utilization of autologous material for reconstruction of significant dorsal collapse.

## Septal Reconstruction

The septum is the foundation for a stable reconstruction of the cleft nose. Complete separation of the medial crura of the lower lateral cartilages to the septum should be performed as well as any ligamentous attachments that can contribute to the septal displacement. In most cases, the septum will be harvested for graft material. Special care is taken to leave a minimum of 1 cm L-shaped septal strut for tip and dorsal nasal support. Full mobilization of the septum may also require securing the caudal septum to the maxillary crest or anterior nasal spine. Occasionally a burr hole can be made in the nasal spine in order to facilitate repositioning and suturing the septum. The authors prefer a 5-0 clear permanent monofilament suture to secure the caudal septum to the nasal spine, when necessary. It is important to identify an asymmetric nasal spine prior to securing the nasal septum in unilateral cleft cases.

## Internal Nasal Valve

Patients with a cleft nasal deformity will often require rehabilitation of their internal nasal valve. Spreader grafts, usually harvested from the septum or conchal bowls of the ears, are placed between the dorsal septum and the upper lateral cartilages (Fig. 22.7: Spreader grafts). They typically span the inferior edge of the bony pyramid to the inferior edge of the upper lateral cartilage, though they can be extended as "nasal extension grafts" and mimic true extension grafts that are typically separate from the spreader grafts. Spreader grafts create a widened superior angle of the internal nasal valve, resulting in increased nasal airflow [14]. The senior author utilizes spreader grafts in approximately 90% of definitive cleft rhinoplasty cases given their ability to straighten the nasal dorsum and septum while increasing nasal airflow.

## Nasal Tip/Alar Appearance

The nostril is a three-dimensional ovoid structure, and contracture and scarring of the nostril can cause a decrease in the diameter and lead to stenosis and collapse of the external nasal valve. In addition, alar rim notching and lateral vestibular webbing are common problems seen in secondary cleft nasal deformities. Micro-nostril deformities are a very difficult problem to correct, and an increase in size often requires recruitment of new soft tissue to the nostril/alar apparatus in

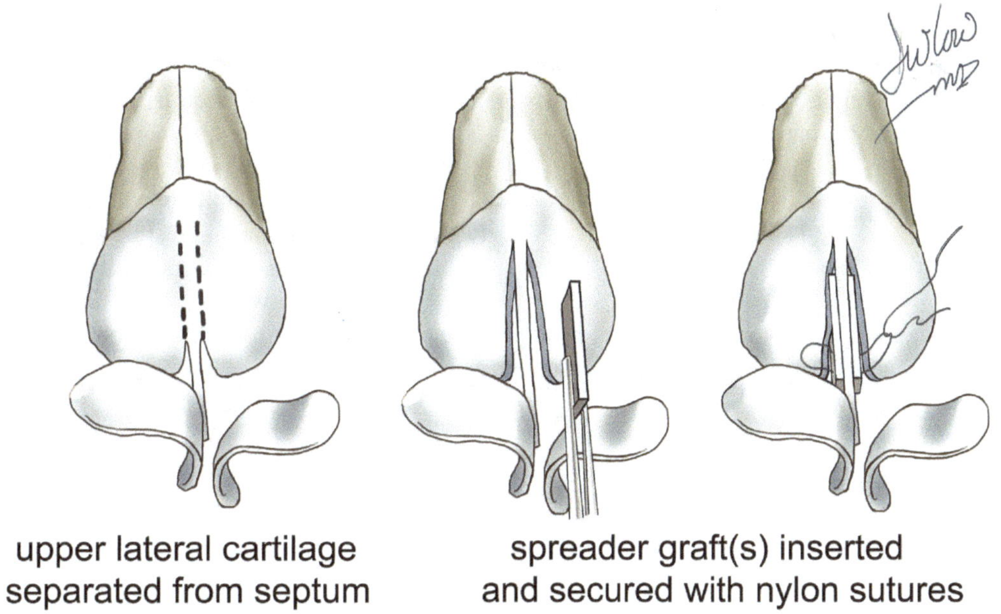


Fig. 22.7 Spreader grafts, placed unilaterally or bilateral between septum and upper lateral cartilage, expand the internal valve

the form of a composite graft (skin and cartilage) from the ear.

Nasal tip correction should focus on improving symmetry, definition, and projection. Cleft nasal deformities often lack structural support. In most cases, the tip needs projection and rotation. Columellar strut grafts are particularly helpful in supporting the nasal tip and are often utilized with tip modifying suture techniques. A columellar strut graft is often placed in between the existing medial crura of the lower lateral cartilages, increasing tip projection and reinforcing the strength of the medial crura. It can be left as a free-floating piece or affixed to the basal premaxilla/anterior nasal spine. Other grafts such as septal extension grafts and tip shield grafts can also be utilized for nasal tip. Cleft rhinoplasty is one of the rare exceptions to the current moratorium on tip grafting, and as with other aspects of cleft rhinoplasty, tip grafting may need to be done in a more radical fashion than typically performed in aesthetic rhinoplasty.

In addition to graft placement for augmentation, the reconstructive surgeon can utilize any combination of lateral crus resection/cephalic trim, transdomal sutures, interdomal sutures, lateral crural mattress sutures, and columellar septal sutures. The lateral crus of the clefted lower lateral cartilage may be concave, causing weakness of the alar region and collapse of the external nasal valve. Utilization of an alar rim graft can offer support to the lower lateral cartilages and the alar rim. A lateral crural strut graft can be placed deep to the existing lower lateral crura. The lateral edge is placed in a pocket developed at the pyriform aperture. This can elevate and reshape the nasal alar region. Importantly, the nasal tip skin must be defatted aggressively to allow the nasal skin to redrape over the new cartilaginous structure. Otherwise, both fat and scar that may exist in the tip will camouflage the improved definition and symmetry that have been achieved with surgery. Characteristic cleft rhinoplasty is shown in Fig. 22.8.

## Complications

Although a relatively safe procedure, postoperative complications and deformities should be considered. It is prudent that any clinician performing rhinoplasties should keep the functional sequela in the forefront of their treatment algorithms. Common problems associated with postoperative functional disturbances can be related with residual septal deviations, internal and external nasal valve problems, or inferior turbinate irregularities. A common problem of the internal valve can be caused by inappropriate separation of the upper lateral cartilages from the septum causing collapse. In addition, deep nasal osteotomies can narrow the pyriform aperture, or over-resection of the alar cartilage can all cause external nasal valve collapse. Utilization of autografts such as rib grafts or ear cartilage can augment areas of nasal deficiency or collapse. Any graft has the potential for displacement, resorption, infection, distortion, warping, or undesired cartilage overgrowth. With adequate technique the risks for resorption or distortion are minimal. Overcorrection is often utilized to anticipate the amount of graft resorption or warping. Occasionally wrapping of larger grafts from the rib which can be wrapped with autologous fascia can limit the amount of warping or unwanted growth of cartilage.

## Postoperative Care

Surgical technique, philosophy, and management of cleft care vary from institution to institution as well as from practitioner to practitioner. This also holds true for postoperative protocols after cleft-related procedures. The senior author prefers the utilization of intranasal splints after any manipulation of the nose in infants and school-aged patients (Fig. 22.9: Intranasal splint). These nasal splints are secured into the septum and left in place between 2 weeks to 2 months. Occasionally if there is some collapse of the alar rim or soft triangle, a removable splint can be placed. Definitive rhinoplasty in the skeletally mature cleft patient usually involves nasal osteotomies. The authors feel it important to utilize external nasal splinting in conjunction with internal nasal splinting. The external splint is typically worn for 1–2 weeks, while the internal splints stay in position for 3–4 weeks.

An adult male before and after cleft rhinoplasty is shown in Fig. 22.10.

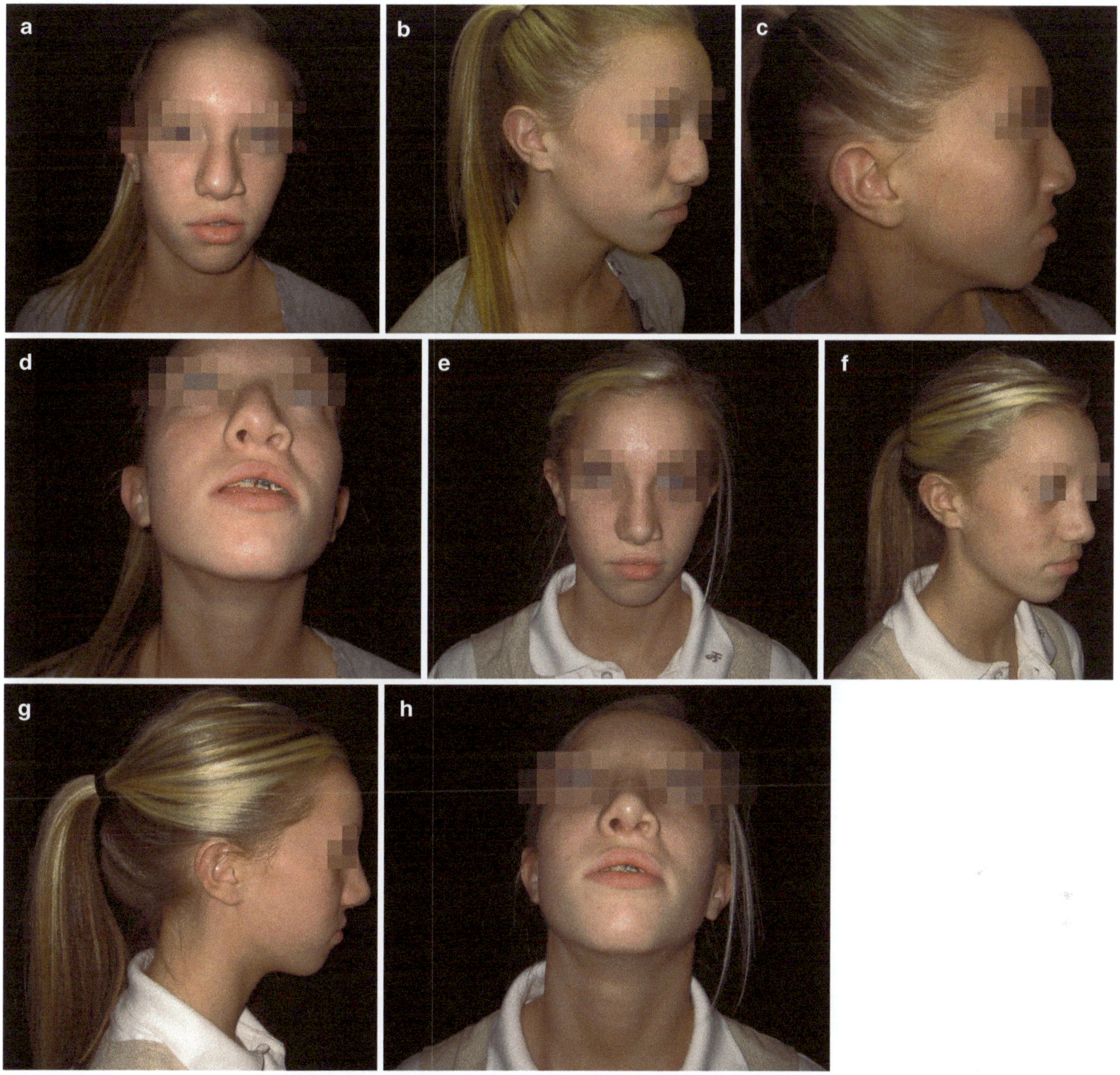


**Fig. 22.8** A 15-year-old female with left unilateral cleft nasal deformity, prior to (**a–d**) and following (**e–h**) septorhinoplasty including submucosal septal resection, dorsal recontouring, internal spreader grafts, tip resuspension and cartilaginous augmentation, and bony osteotomies and repositioning

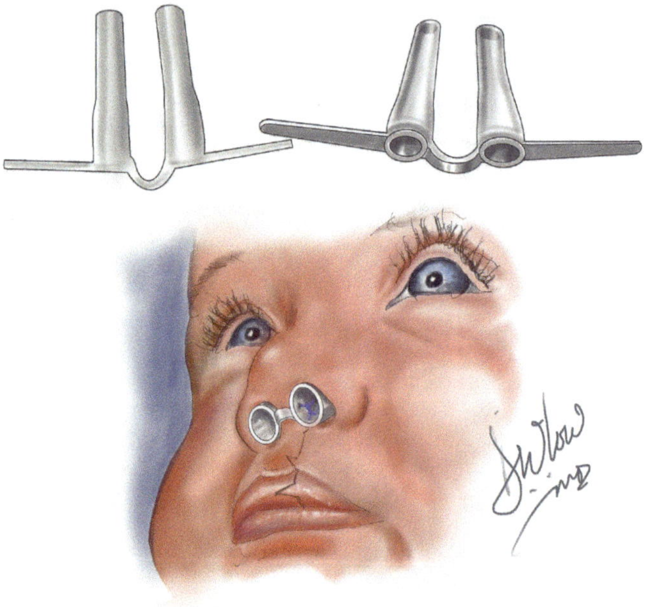

**Fig 22.9** Intranasal silicone splint

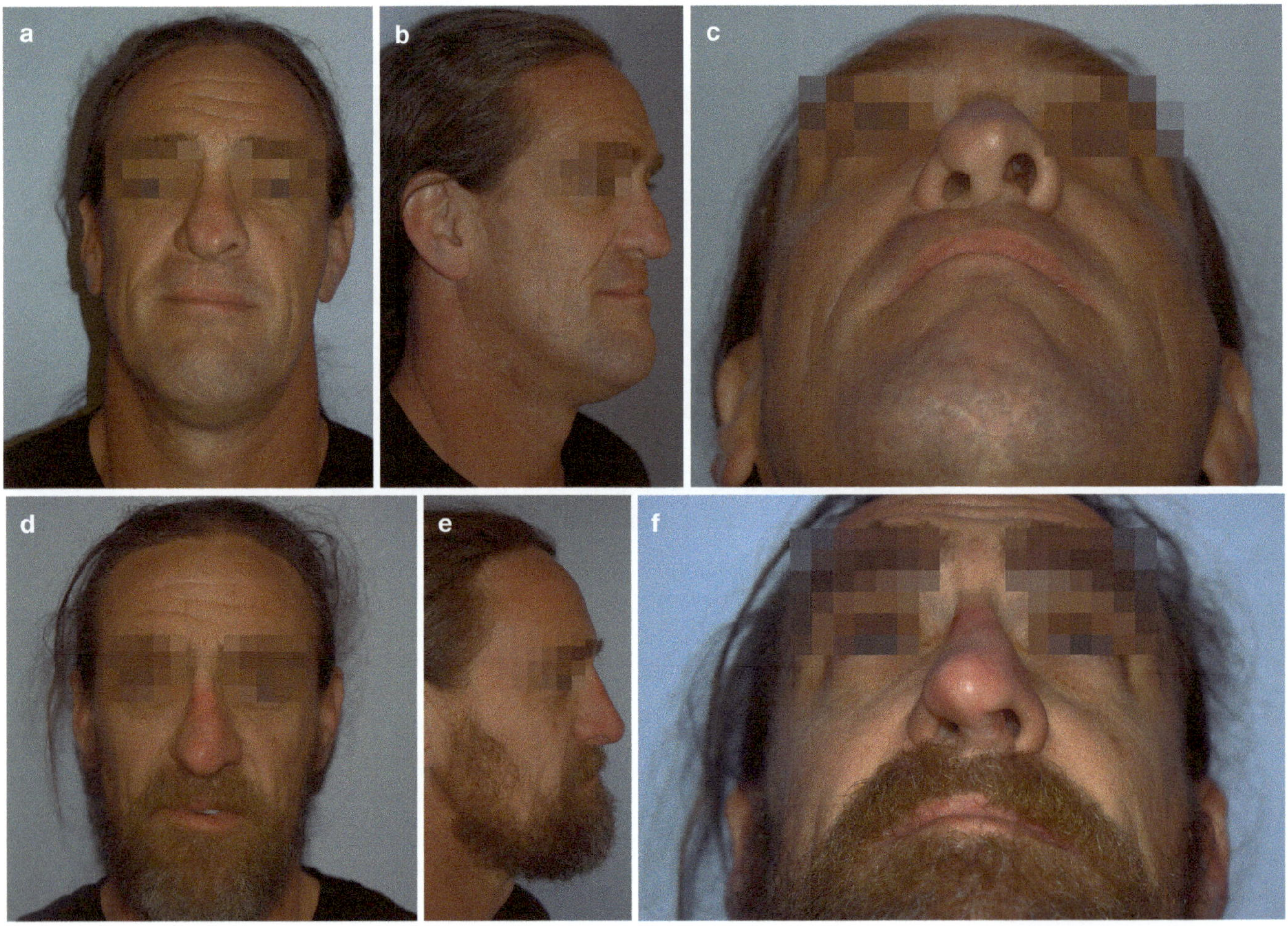


**Fig. 22.10** Adult male with right unilateral cleft nasal deformity, prior to (**a–c**) and following (**d–f**) septorhinoplasty including submucosal septal resection, dorsal recontouring, internal spreader graft, tip resuspension and cartilaginous augmentation, and bony osteotomies and repositioning

## References


1. Henry C, Samson T, Mackay D. Evidence-based medicine: the cleft lip nasal deformity. Plast Reconstr Surg. 2014;133(5):1276–88.
2. Zeraatkar M, Ajami S, Nadjmi N, Faghihi SA, Golkari A. A qualitative study of children's quality of life in the context of living with cleft lip and palate. Pediatr Health Med Ther. 2019;10:13–20.
3. Woodard CR, Park SS. Nasal and facial analysis. Clin Plast Surg. 2010;37(2):181–9.
4. DeLuke DM, Marchand A, Robles EC, Fox P. Facial growth and the need for orthognathic surgery after cleft palate repair: literature review and report of 28 cases. J Oral Maxillofac Surg. 1997;55(7):694–7.
5. Vasudavan S, Jayaratne YSN, Padwa BL. Nasolabial soft tissue changes after Le Fort I advancement. J Oral Maxillofac Surg. 2012;70(4):e277.
6. Krimmel M, Schuck N, Bacher M, Reinert S. Facial surface changes after cleft alveolar bone grafting. J Oral Maxillofac Surg. 2011;69(1):80–3.
7. Drake AF, Davis JU, Warren DW. Nasal airway size in cleft and noncleft children. Laryngoscope. 1993;103(8):915–7.
8. Warren DW, Drake AF. Cleft nose. Form and function. Clin Plast Surg. 1993;20(4):769.
9. Stewart MG, Witsell DL, Smith TL, Weaver EM, Yueh B, Hannley MT. Development and validation of the nasal obstruction symptom evaluation (NOSE) scale. Otolaryngol Head Neck Surg. 2004;130(2):157–63.
10. Ortiz-Monasterio F, Olmedo A. Corrective rhinoplasty before puberty: a long-term follow-up. Plast Reconstr Surg. 1981;68(3):381.
11. Mulliken J, Kim D. Repair of bilateral incomplete cleft lip: techniques and outcomes. Plast Reconstr Surg. 2013;132(4):923–32.
12. Tajima S, Maruyama M. Reverse-u incision for secondary repair of cleft lip nose. Plast Reconstr Surg. 1977;60(2):256–61.
13. Rohrich RJ, Hollier LH. Use of spreader grafts in the external approach to rhinoplasty. Clin Plast Surg. 1996;23(2):255.
14. Baker SR. Diced cartilage augmentation: early experience with the Tasman technique. Arch Facial Plast Surg. 2012;14(6):451–5.


## Septorhinoplasty, Case 1

### Case Study: Alar Deformity Reconstruction in a Unilateral Cleft Lip and Palate Patient

Percy Rossell-Perry

A 12-year-old female patient with a right unilateral cleft lip initially treated using conventional Millard technique. The right alar base has been partially amputated probably due to the subnasal incision or alar necrosis. This severe deformity is affecting the patient functionally and aesthetically.

This complication is not rare after use of Millard technique. Sometimes use of the subnasal incision across the alar base causes consequent amputation of the ala.

Goals of repair are to create a more symmetric nose and improve the nasal function.

### Treatment Considerations

The nasal ala is difficult to repair well due to the specific characteristics of the alar tissues, which are convex and distinct from adjacent subunits. Local and regional flaps provide tissue that is often of poor match, obliterate subunit borders, and leave a donor site scar. Composite grafts are a good option since the donor site scar is often not visible. Main disadvantages are the risk of scar contracture, patch-like appearance, and different color of the graft. Considering the importance of the donor site scar, a composite graft was selected in this case.

The upper portion of the auricular helix was selected, utilizing a composite of auricular cartilage, anterior and posterior skin, and subcutaneous fat. The recipient ala tissue was released from its insertion and the scar tissue was removed. The composite graft (cartilage and skin) was designed slightly bigger than the size of the defect considering the graft retraction. Then the graft was placed filling the defect and fixed using absorbable sutures.

One year after alar reconstruction, the symmetry of the nose was improved and the patient reported improved breathing with less nasal obstruction. The donor site has a well-developed scar cosmetically acceptable.

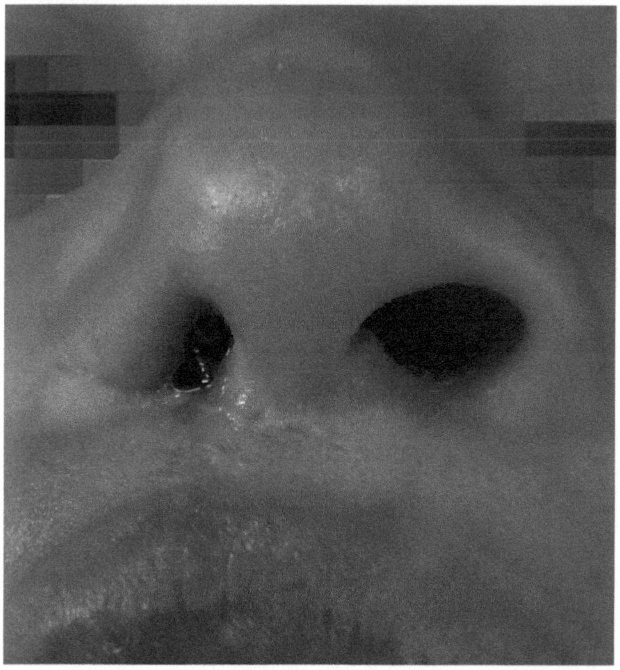

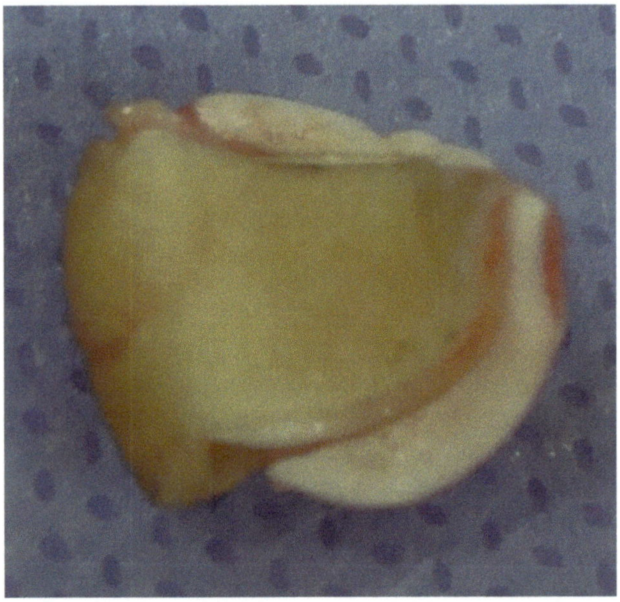

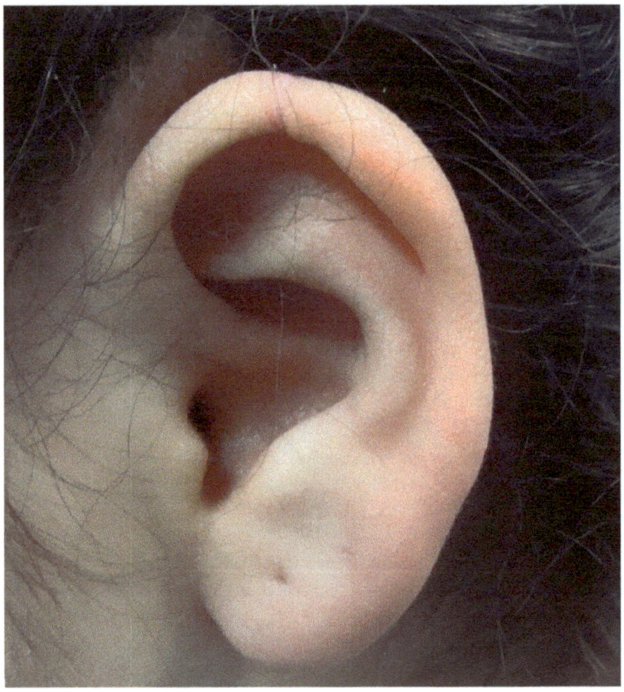

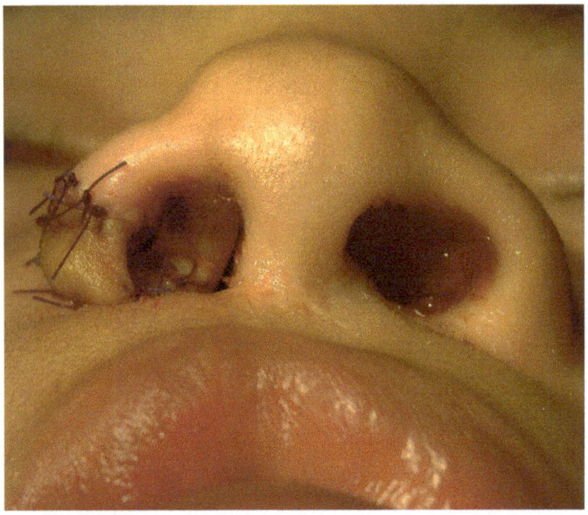

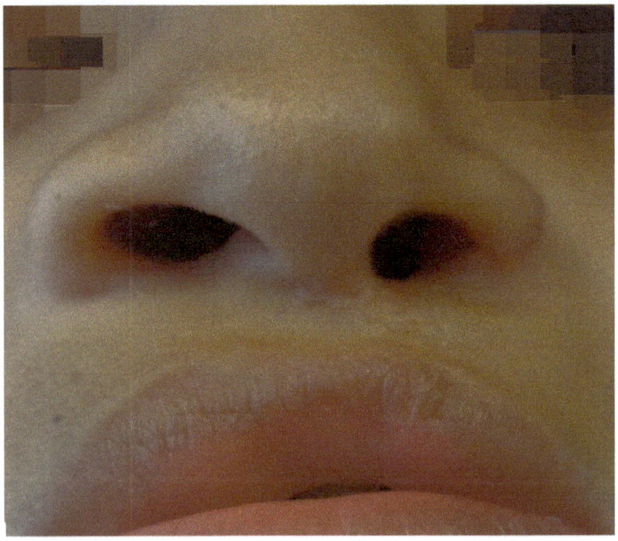

## Septorhinoplasty, Case 2

### Case Study: Secondary Cleft Nasal Repair in a Unilateral Cleft Lip and Palate Patient

Percy Rossell-Perry

Secondary cleft nose is a common deformity in patients with cleft lip and palate, typically associated with deficient or absent primary repair, or progression of the nasal deformity with growth. Associated aesthetic and functional problems affect the quality of life of these patients. Deviation of the septum and columella, distortion of alar cartilage position, nostril asymmetry, and loss of nasal tip projection are common findings in these cases. Different strategies have been described for its reconstruction with different levels of efficacy.

This is a 16-year-old male patient who comes to the office requesting improvement of the nasal deformity. There is a significant asymmetry of the nostril and loss of nasal tip projection on the left. In addition, septal deviation and lower turbinate hyperplasia is associated with functional impairment.

Goals of repair are to create a more symmetric nose and reduce nasal obstruction.

#### Treatment Considerations

Many surgeons seek in a secondary cleft rhinoplasty to create a Caucasian nose aesthetically (changing tip projection using tip cartilage grafts and performing nasal osteotomies). However, I see the main objective being to create a symmetric nose.

I like to use the V-Y-Z method (a combination of Potter's and Berkeley's techniques). This is a V composite advancement flap combined with a lateral Z plasty. This method lets the surgeon obtain improvement of nasal tip projection, nasal vestibule lengthening, and symmetry of the nostrils. I believe the symmetry of the nostril is the most difficult objective to be achieved by the surgeons, and that this technique most maximizes the projection of the alar cartilage.

In addition, the reposition of the nasal base and functional treatment (septoplasty and turbinectomy) are often required. Sometimes a small piece of cartilage graft may be necessary to prevent pinched nose after alar cartilage displacement.

Postoperatively, the symmetry of the nose is achieved and there is an improvement of the nasal tip projection as you may see in below figures.

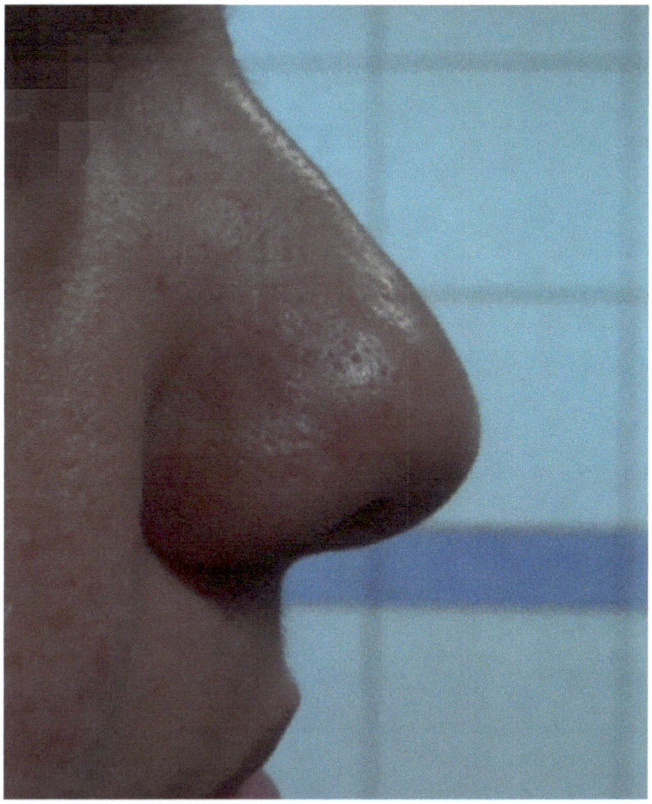

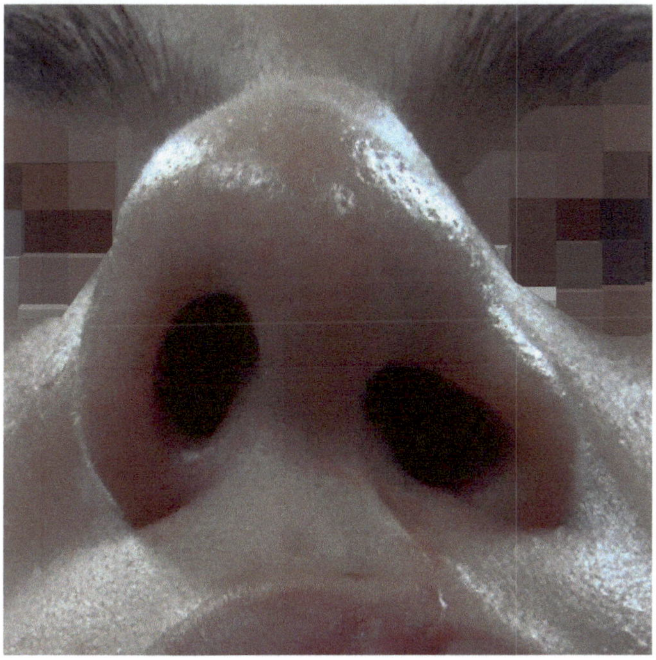

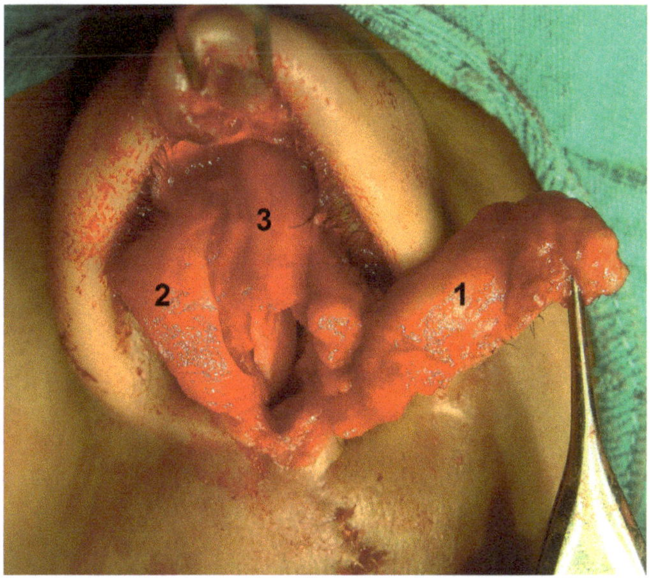


Intraoperative view using the V-Y-Z technique. 1. Alar composite flap. 2. Alar cartilage non-cleft side. 3. Dorsum

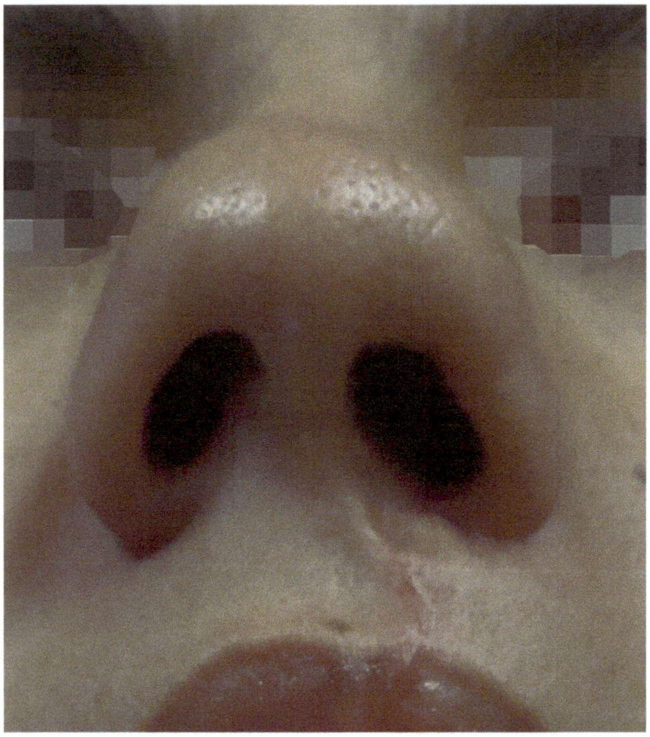

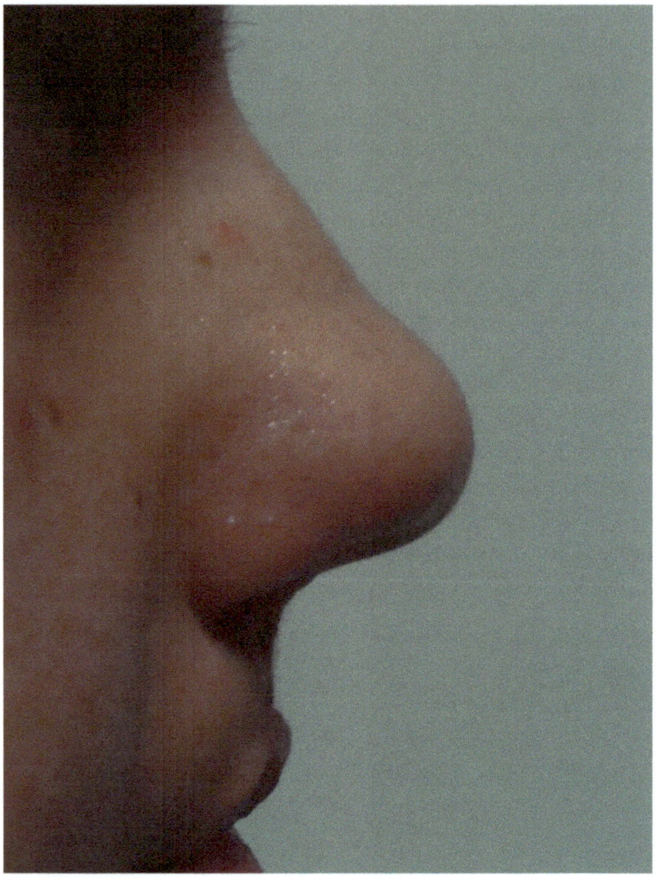

# Orthognathic Surgery

# 23

Nicolas E. Sierra, Adriana Agell-Sogbe, Jorge Pamias, Scott P. Bartlett, and Nivaldo Alonso

**Key Points**

- CLP deformities, as well as primary reconstructive surgery, can lead to restriction of midfacial growth.
- Up to 30% of adult CLP patients display secondary dentofacial deformities (DFDs) with three-dimensional maxillary hypoplasia.
- Orthognathic surgical procedures reposition maxillary and/or mandibular bones to restore dentofacial function and aesthetics.
- Orthognathic surgery preparation demands the coordinated approach of the orthodontic, speech pathology, and surgical specialists.
- Adequate preparation, planning, surgical technique, and postoperative follow-up are necessary to reduce the risk of postoperative skeletal and dental relapse.

## Introduction

The underlying cleft deformity, and primary surgery to correct it, can affect the physiological development of the facial skeleton and soft tissue. The typical dentofacial deformity (DFD) displayed by patients with cleft lip/palate (CLP) includes degrees of midfacial retrusion and three-dimensional (3D) malposition of the maxillary segments. Orthognathic ("ortho," to shape, and "gnathic," the jaw) surgery (OS) is a powerful set of procedures to reposition the facial skeleton and correct both aesthetics and function. OS preparation demands the coordinated approach of the orthodontic, speech pathology, and surgical specialists. Maxillary advancement with 3D reposition is the procedure of choice, sometimes in combination with mandibular setback and/or rotation of the occlusal plane. Adequate orthodontic preparation, surgical planning, and postoperative follow-up reduce the risk of relapse.

OS is typically the most invasive type of surgery performed in patients with clefts, with greater risks of blood loss and airway compromise than in other procedures. The technical competency demanded and need for equipment and special supplies make OS a greater challenge for low-resources countries. Patient involvement with the decision-making to undertake OS is essential, because of the preparation required and magnitude of the procedure. But, like septorhinoplasty, it is often among the most life-changing surgeries experienced by patients as they complete comprehensive cleft care.

## The Cleft Dentofacial Deformity

CLP primary surgery in early childhood could lead to skeletal growth restriction caused by surgical scarring. The typical DFD associated with the CLP adult patient is a Class III malocclusion caused by degrees of maxillary 3D hypoplasia. Although most CLP patients have essentially normal man-

N. E. Sierra
Pediatric Oral and Maxillofacial Surgery Unit, Oral and Maxilofacial Surgery Department, Vall d´Hebrón University Hospital, Barcelona, Spain

A. Agell-Sogbe
Orthodontics and Maxillary Orthopedics Unit, Oral and Maxilofacial Surgery Department, Vall d´Hebrón University Hospital, Barcelona, Spain

J. Pamias
Orthognatic Surgery Unit, Oral and Maxilofacial Surgery Department, Vall d´Hebrón University Hospital, Barcelona, Spain

S. P. Bartlett
University of Pennsylvania, Children's Hospital of Philadelphia, Philadelphia, PA, USA
e-mail: BARTLETTS@email.chop.edu

N. Alonso (✉)
Faculty of Medicine of the University of São Paulo, Hospital das Clinicas at the University of São Paulo, São Paulo, Brazil
e-mail: nivalonso@usp.br

© Springer Nature Switzerland AG 2021

J. W. Swanson, D. W. Low (eds.), *Global Cleft Care in Low-Resource Settings*, https://doi.org/10.1007/978-3-030-59105-2_23

dibular growth, some patients with maxillary retrusion may also develop anterior open bite with open mandibular angle, steep mandibular occlusal plane, or lateral mandibular cant [1–3].

The indication for OS in adult CLP patients has been reported to be around 20–50% [4]. However, adequate dental follow-up by the orthopedic/orthodontic team during infancy improves dentofacial form, function, and growth, which might reduce the incidence and severity of secondary DFDs. Conversely, the incidence of DFDs increases with the absence of lateral incisors, the severity of the cleft type, the number of previous surgical interventions, and earlier timing of primary surgeries. In addition, the more traumatic the operation, the more severe are the modifications in skeletal growth. Furthermore, adult CLP patients with poor dentistry follow-up may display severe maxillary arch misalignment/misleveling, associated oronasal fistulas, cleft bony defects, soft tissue scarring, and degrees of dental and periodontal decay (Figs. 23.1 and 23.2).

## Orthognathic Surgery: Team Approach

A coordinated approach of the CLP orthognathic patient by the cleft surgery, orthodontic, and speech pathology teams is necessary to achieve optimal and stable aesthetics and function.

## Intermediate Procedures and Alveolar Bone Grafting

### Surgical Reposition of the Premaxilla (SRP) for BCLP Patients [5]

The growing BCLP patient may develop 3D premaxillary malposition (PM) causing disruption of maxillary arch leveling and alignment. Sagittal protrusion of the premaxilla is physiological and tends to spontaneously decrease during growth as lateral maxillary segments catch up; therefore, it is not advisable to surgically correct it in growing patients. In the other hand, vertical excess of the premaxilla severely impairs occlusion and is a cosmetic problem that does not improve with growth and therefore should be prevented or corrected [6]. Likewise, clockwise rotation of the premaxilla is seldom restored by orthodontic treatment alone.

The SRP could be considered when PM makes alveolar bone grafting (ABG) difficult or impossible to perform. Ideally, SRP should be performed during mixed dentition, according to the developmental stage of the upper canines and the planned ABG (8–12 years old). However, in patients displaying severe vertical excess with social-psychological implications, the procedure could be considered in earlier stages of development. Orthopedic/orthodontic preparation should achieve maxillary arch alignment with slight overexpansion of the lateral segments to allow the repositioned premaxilla to fit between them and, also, to facilitate maneuvers throughout the procedure.

SRP must be planned to achieve maxillary arch leveling and alignment. The extent of premaxillary upward reposition, setback, or rotation can be aided by a preoperative CT imaging analysis and/or conventional model surgery, if available. A surgical splint will guide the bone resection intraoperatively and will stabilize the premaxilla postoperatively. Currently, modern 3D virtually generated splints are a potentially feasible alternative in the mission/outreach setting when accurate data collection is available (Fig. 23.3a, b, c).

The SRP can be performed with or without simultaneous ABG. The surgical team should weigh the risks and benefits of either choice, especially in the outreach/mission setting. From our perspective, and considering the risk of premaxillary necrosis and its severe consequences for midfacial development, we prefer to avoid simultaneous procedures. Instead, we recommend a staged approach; first addressing the SRP and later the oronasal fistulas and ABG [4, 5].

### (Secondary) Alveolar Bone Grafting Prior to Orthognathic Surgery [7, 8]

ABG must be performed to level and unite maxillary segments prior to or during orthognathic surgery and is ideally performed at time of mixed dentition (6–12 years old) following palatal expansion. The procedure will offer the biomechanical support for adequate eruption of the lateral incisor and the canine. In addition, the restoration of the dentoalveolar continuity will facilitate the movement of the maxilla en bloc while reducing the risk of transverse relapse, if a maxillary advancement is later performed [9] (Fig. 23.4a–d).

### Tertiary Alveolar Bone Grafting

Under adequate dental, orthopedic, and ortho-surgical follow-up, simultaneous ABG with OS is safe and cost-effective. The procedure enables correction of the oronasal fistula, alveolar cleft, and maxillary malposition in a single procedure. However, higher risks of bone graft exposure, transverse relapse, and periodontal decay are of great concern in patients without adequate dental/orthodontic follow-up.

The adult CLP patient without access to dental/orthodontic care through growth is a common clinical scenario in the mission/outreach setting. These patients usually display oronasal fistulas, severe scarring of the oral mucosa, and a combination of dental/periodontal decay, partial anodontia/

edentulism, dental malpositions (rotations/crowding), and maxillary arch misleveling and misalignment. In such cases we prefer to address the clinical challenges in a staged approach:

- First, provide restorative dentistry while educating on oral health care.
- Second, start orthodontic preparation to achieve maxillary arch expansion, leveling, and alignment (surgically assisted as necessary).
- Third, oronasal fistula closure +/− ABG (when watertight closure of mucoperiosteal flaps is warranted).
- Fourth, ABG.
- Fifth Orthognathic surgery.

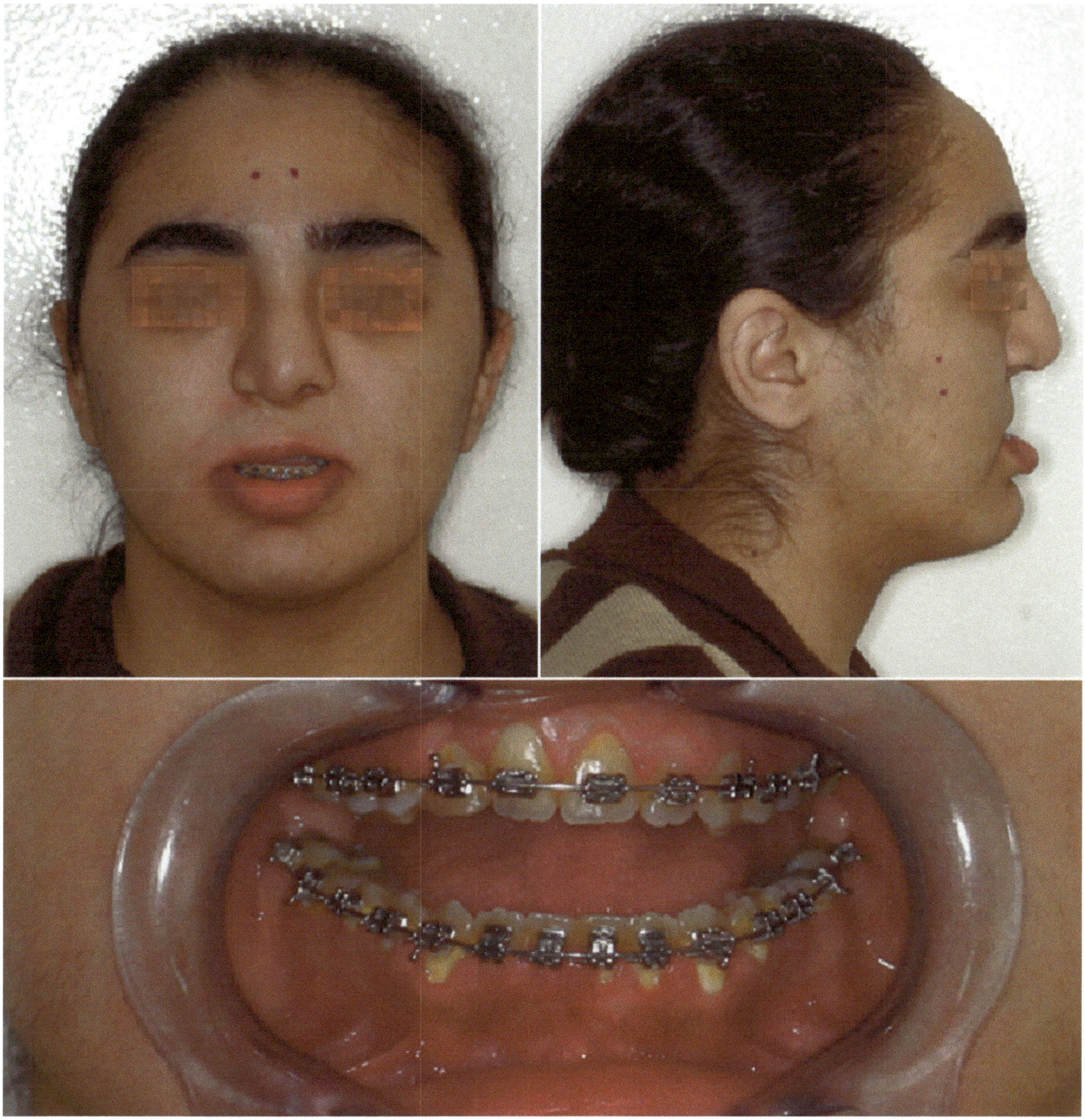

**Fig. 23.1** Showing the common secondary dentofacial deformities (DFDs) of a unilateral CLP secondary DFD

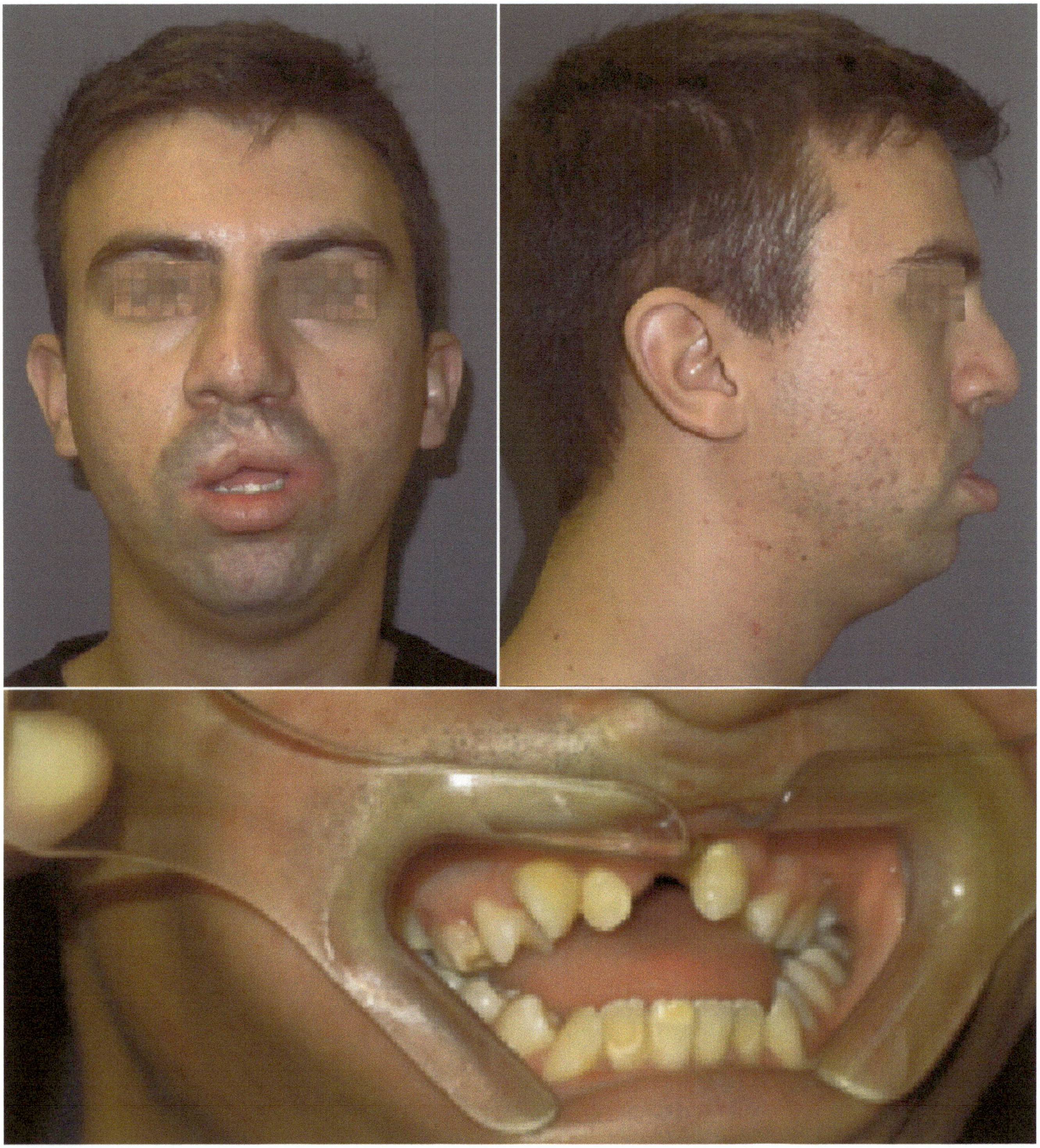

Fig. 23.2 Showing the common anatomical features of the bilateral CLP

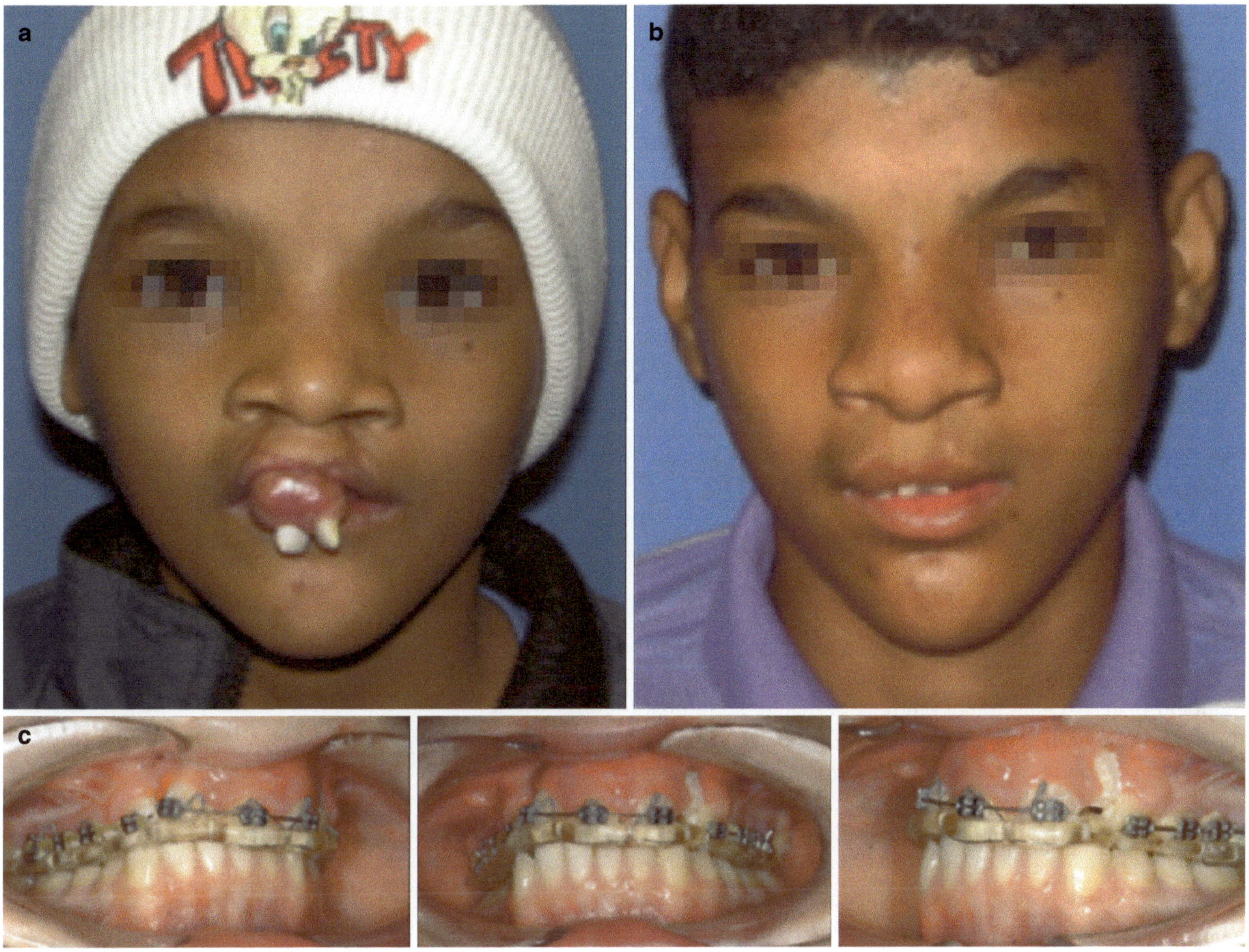


**Fig. 23.3** Surgically-assisted premaxillary repositioning. (**a**) (upper left) Premaxillary malposition (PM). (**b**) (upper right) Same patient after SRP. (**c**): (lower) The premaxilla is stabilized using the surgical splint

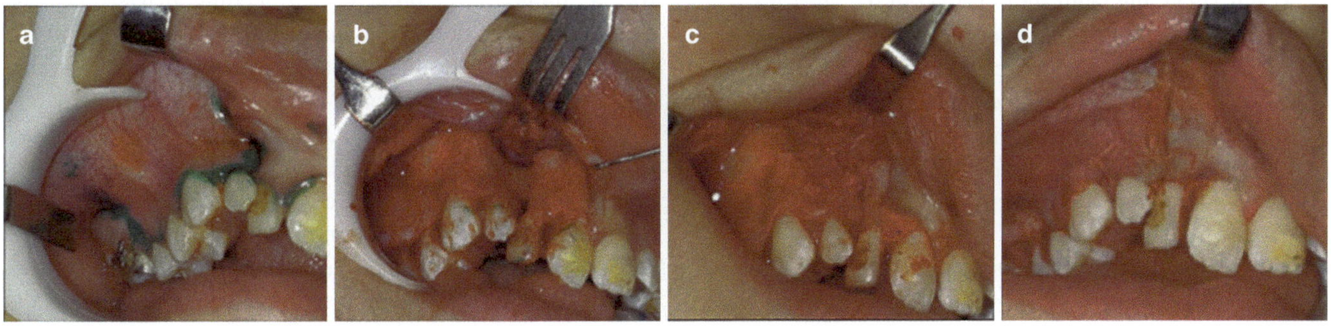


**Fig. 23.4** Secondary alveolar bone grafting. From left to right. (**a**): Detail of the incisions. (**b**): Closure of the fistula/nasal floor. (**c**): Cancellous bone graft filling the alveolar defect. (**d**): Mucoperiosteal flaps are sutured to cover the graft

## Treatment Planning

### Timing for Definitive Orthognathic Surgery

OS should ideally be performed in a patient with complete maxillomandibular growth. However, in patients with definitive dentition displaying DFDs causing severe psychological and/or functional disability, the interdisciplinary team could consider an earlier intervention. In such cases, the potential need for additional surgical intervention at completion of growth should be clearly stressed with the patient and the family.

### The Pre-orthodontic Stage: Setting the Surgical-Orthodontic Treatment Plan [10]

Dentofacial analysis is similar to non-cleft patients and includes detailed data collection of the facial anatomy, the arches and the teeth. The clinical assessment should be supported by radiographic analysis. The panoramic and lateral cephalometric X-rays provide enough information to set a treatment plan. If facial tomography is available, additional information about the periodontal bony support and the cleft bony bridging could better guide the orthodontic planning (Fig. 23.5).

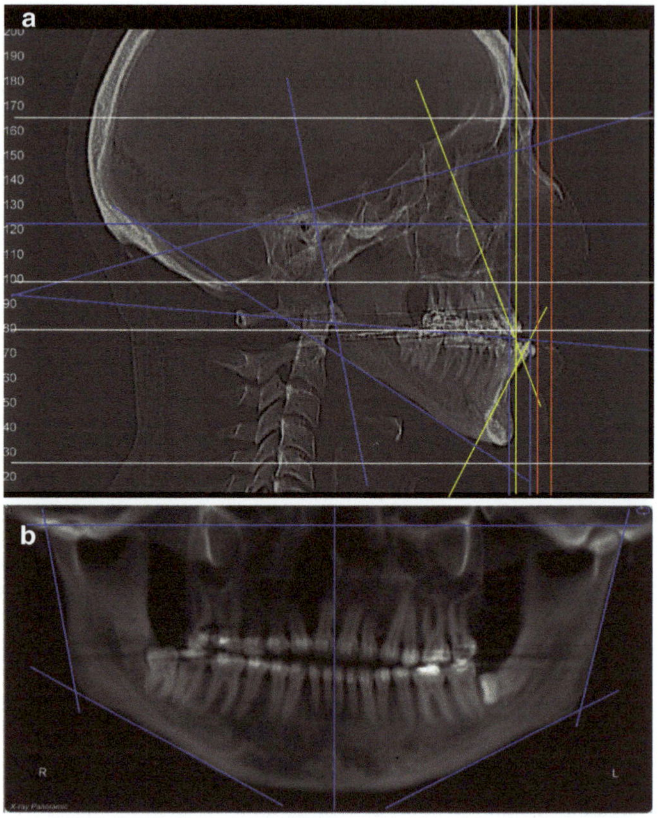

Fig. 23.5 (**a**) (above): The lateral facial Tele X-ray (2D cephalometry) provides information about facial proportions, facial projections, incisor inclination, occlusal planes, anteroposterior discrepancy, etc. (**b**) (below): The panoramic X-ray provides information about mandibular symmetry and third molars

The orthodontic preparation will provide maxillary arch leveling and alignment for a stable postoperative dental occlusion. Dental rotations and compensations should be corrected to warrant postoperative functionality, aesthetics, and long-term stability. The incisors positioning should be planned to achieve ideal angulation; however, mild compensations could provide adequate outcomes for a surgical plan with maxillary advancement only.

At this stage, the team should rule out the need for intermediate surgical procedures, such as surgically assisted rapid palatal expansion (SARPE), segmental maxillary distractions, subapical osteotomies, etc. which might accelerate and facilitate orthodontic preparation but demand more sophisticated orthodontic assessment and surgical experience.

### Considering a Bimaxillary Approach

Although most patients with a cleft palate have primarily a maxillary abnormality, at the pre-orthodontic stage, a key decision is whether to perform only maxillary advancement or bimaxillary treatment of the maxilla and mandible.

Relative indications for bimaxillary surgery include:

1. Mandibular (skeletal) asymmetry – especially of severity to cause poor occlusion
2. Steep mandibular/occlusal plane – causing anterior open bite
3. Major maxillary advancements – exceeding 10–14 mm

In lower-resource settings, teams should weight the risks for a bimaxillary procedure (bleeding/airway) against accepting a functional and stable surgical outcomes with a shorter and more straightforward surgery even if sacrificing the best possible aesthetics.

Most teams consider that CLP patients with anteroposterior discrepancies greater of 10–14 mm are beyond the limits of a maxillary advancement-only approach. In such cases, the team could consider a combined mandibular setback to reduce the amount of maxillary advancement. The setback should be kept to the minimum to reduce the risk of soft tissue ptosis and major changes of oropharyngeal volume. A sliding advancement genioplasty can be performed with mandibular setback to preserve chin projection.

In cases with extreme anteroposterior discrepancy >25 mm, the team should decide between performing a staged maxillary advancement and using distraction osteogenesis, if devices are available and adequate follow-up can be provided by the local team [11].

## Surgical Treatment Plan [12]

The LeFort I and its modifications are the most common type of osteotomy used for the majority of CLP patients with secondary DFDs. Wide alveolar clefts can be closed by differential segmental advancement. A detailed three-dimensional surgical plan can be addressed later according to the achievements and limits of orthodontic preparation.

The overall surgical plan should be driven by the analysis of facial proportions, occlusal relationships, intra-arch features, and radiological analysis (Figs. 23.6 and 23.7).

## Preoperative Orthodontic: Surgical Planning

OS procedures have been traditionally planned using 2D cephalometry (Fig. 23.8); however, 3D virtual planning provides advantages when available (Fig. 23.9):

- Improved planning accuracy for intraoperative performance and final surgical outcome; for example, yaw and mid-line adjustments according to the skull base and bony collisions, especially in cases with maxillomandibular asymmetries.

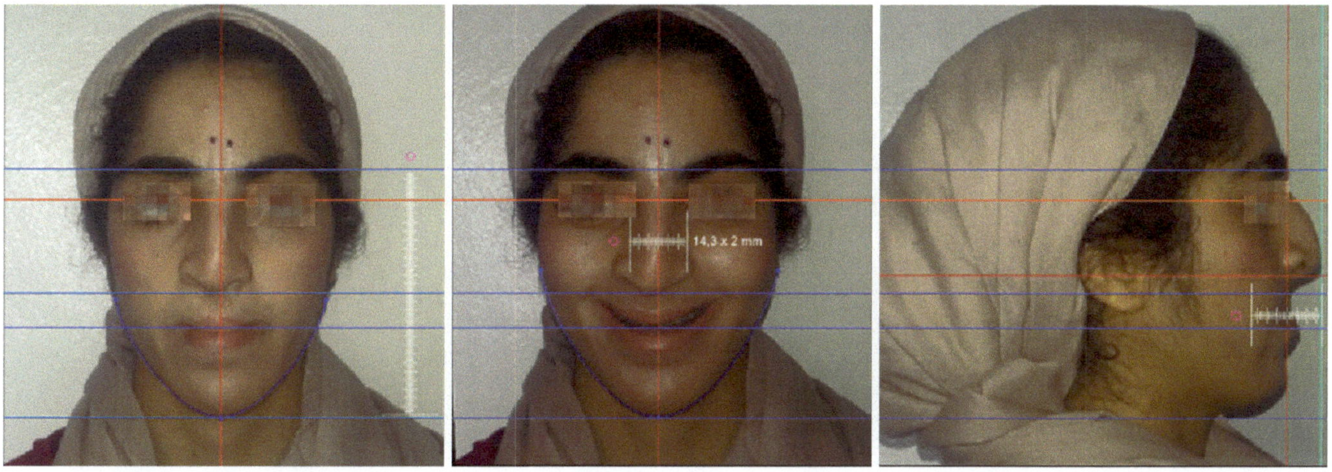


Fig. 23.6 Clinical facial analysis; facial symmetry, facial proportions, facial projections, maxillary height – incisor show – gingival show

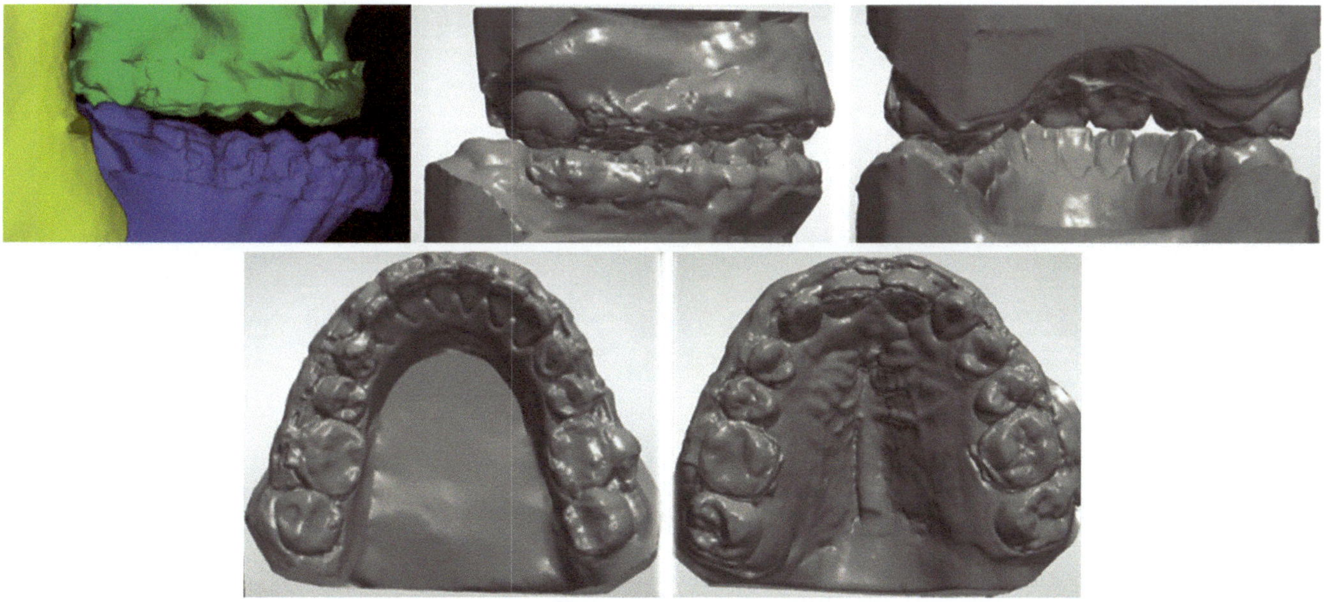

Fig. 23.7 Above left: Preoperative occlusal relationships. Occlusal relationships corrected into class I with stone models including: Above center: Lateral. Above right: Transverse relationships. Below left: Lower arch. Below right: Upper arch

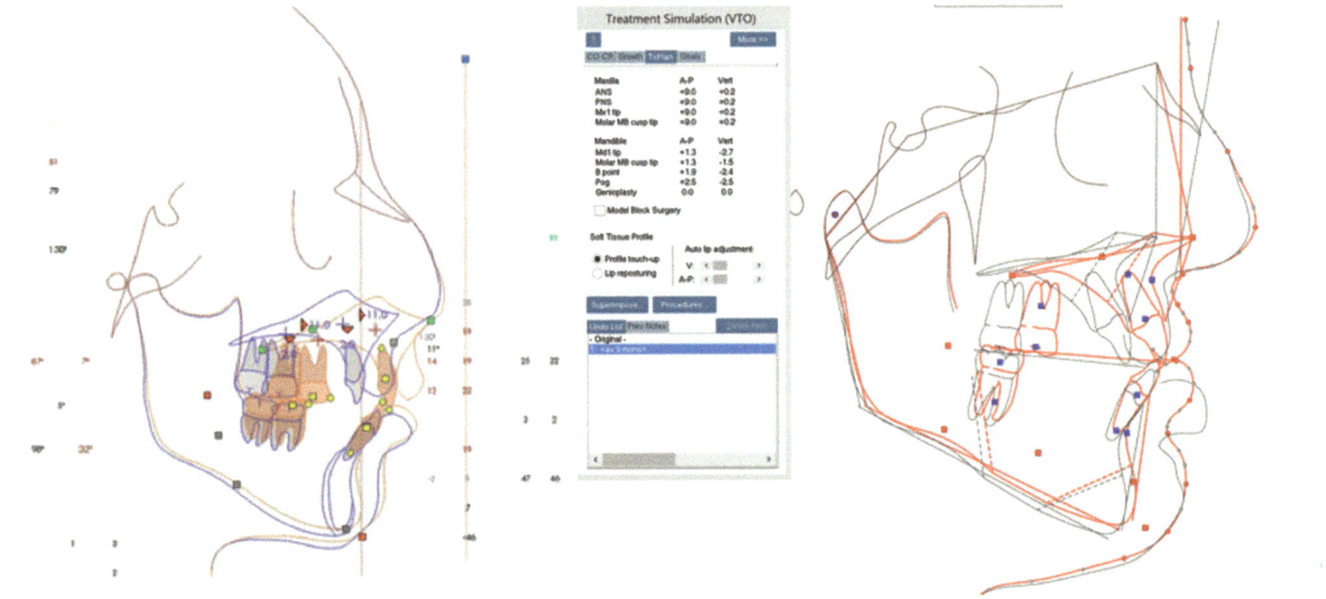


**Fig. 23.8** Examples of 2D cephalometric analysis and surgical treatment plan

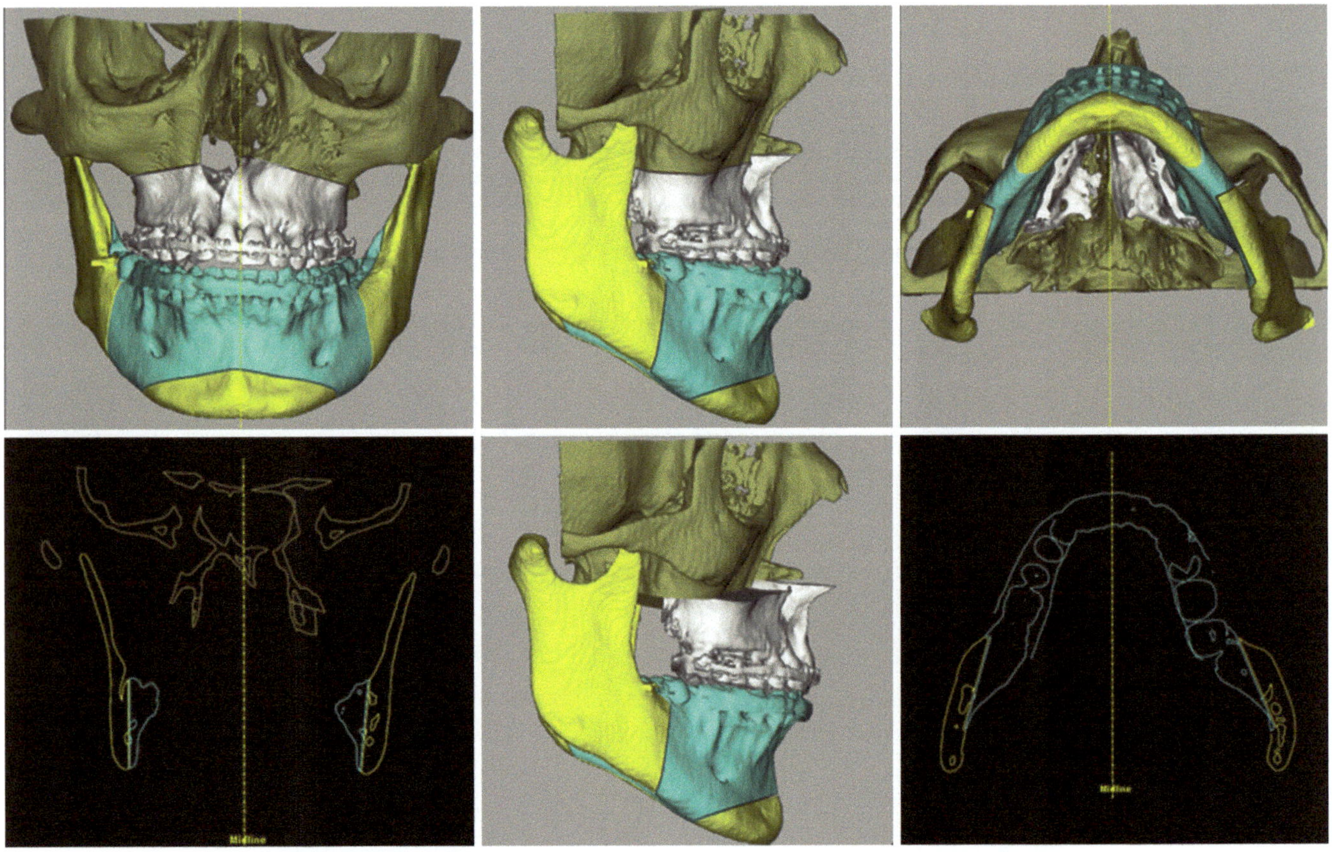


**Fig. 23.9** (Below): 3D surgical treatment plan. Above: 3D volumes displaying preoperative anatomy with osteotomies. Below: Surgical simulation. LeFort I maxillary advancement taking occlusion to class I. Details of potential bony collisions predict intraoperative difficulties and required adjustments

**Table 23.1** Comparative table: Key elements for data collection and analysis during orthognathic surgery planning

| Data element | Conventional | Virtual |
|---|---|---|
| Standard and calibrated clinical pictures (Fig.23.6)<br>With calibration point and using a ring flash to avoid back shadow | x | x |
| Arch impressions(Fig. 23.7)<br>High-definition impressions, with accurate definition of the cusps | x | x |
| Lateral cephalogram | x | |
| Facial CT scan (Fig. 23.9):<br>The facial CT scan must be performed with the use of a premanufactured waxbite. The waxbite provides a guide of the centric relation of the condyle and creates space between the dental cusps to avoid superimposition | | x |
| Bite registration for stone model | Optional | |

- Intraoperative modifications can be planned, while others can be avoided due to lack of technical feasibility.
- Improved definition of overall facial harmony and soft tissue envelope.
- When operative splints can be produced virtually (using 3D printing), it prevents the need for stone model surgery (and associated technique and material cost).
- A treatment consensus is much easier to achieve with a 3D simulation that is based on more overall information.

## Data Collection [13]

Different essential data is needed depending on whether conventional or virtual surgical planning is utilized (Table 23.1).

## Surgical Planning

For conventional planning, or when splints are generated from plaster "stone" models, "model surgery" is necessary. For virtual planning, digital data is imported into the virtual planning platform, which allows the orthodontic/surgical team members to discuss and plan, through software directly or with a third party provider using web meetings.

Either conventional or virtual planning enables the surgeon to plan and then simulate the surgery before entering the operating room and to create splints to guide movements. Assessing and modifying the intended plan for factors such as impactions, descents, yaw/pitch/roll maxillomandibular movements, collisions, and soft tissue modifications is more facile with virtual planning and image segmentation (Fig. 23.9).

## Surgical Sequence for Bimaxillary Procedures: Maxilla vs Mandible First

*Maxilla First:* Cleft orthognathic surgery is highly influenced by palatal scarring and soft tissue limited compliance. Accordingly, the surgical team could be unable to set the maxilla in the pre-planned position [14–16]. In major maxillary advancements, we find a maxilla-first approach optimal for two different surgical plans:

1. Maxilla advancement to class I occlusion using a single final splint
2. Maxillary advancement combined with a mild mandibular set back using both intermediate and final splint

*Mandible First:* This approach would be recommended in those cases planned for the simultaneous correction of oronasal fistulas with alveolar bone grafting and orthognathic surgery. In such cases, it is common to perform differential advancement/reposition of maxillary segments. The accuracy of the procedure might be facilitated using a mandible-first approach, because it is the more stable jaw.

### Strategies in Major Maxillary Advancements (>12–15 mm)

1. Set a bimaxillary procedure: Major maxillary advancement of the maxilla with a minimal mandibular set back.
2. Plan for maxillary advancement using distraction osteogenesis. Indicated in extreme maxillary advancements. Adequate devices and close postoperative orthodontic/surgical follow-up should be available. The use of virtual planning and stereolithographic skull models offer advantages such as [11]:
   - Planning/performing osteotomies
   - Select and custom bend the distraction device
   - Adjustment of vectors
   - Reduction of operative time
3. Set a staged maxillary advancement. The first stage will advance the maxilla as far as possible, followed by a second stage 3–6 months later to complete the advancement (with or without a combined mandibular procedure).

## Orthodontic and Oral Surgical Preparation

Orthodontic preparation prior to surgery should include:

- Banded molars
- Rectangular arch wires
- Adequate surgical lugs
- Strongly bonded brackets
- Final splint with palatal arch reinforcement

If a mandibular repositioning (bilateral split sagittal osteotomy) is planned, the osteotomy will cut through the third molars ("8 s"). Several studies have shown in HICs that removing third molars at time of BSSO is safe and does not compromise stability of result. However, to prevent an added technical element and acknowledging potentially greater risk in low-resource settings, this can also be performed 6 months prior to orthognathic surgery.

## Surgical Techniques

### Maxillary Advancement

The technical modifications of the standard LeFort I in cleft patients might include the following:

- Incision: Vertical incisions and subperiosteal tunneling preserve vestibular mucoperiosteal flaps on the anterior premaxilla/maxilla to maintain as much blood supply as possible.
- Elevation of nasal floor: Severe adhesions should be expected. The complete release of the scar tissue at the level of the cleft can be addressed after an initial downfracture mobilization of the maxilla. Repair of nasal floor lacerations should be carried out after the release.
- Osteotomies: Thick cortical bone might cause the osteotomies to be more difficult. The standard LF1 osteotomy can be modified according to the clinical features of each patient, i.e., high quadrangular LF1 osteotomy for patients with high midface deficiency and normal nasal projection.
- Maxillary downfracture: It should be achieved without excessive force. If mobilization is difficult, posterior attachments are often the cause.
- Maxillary release and advancement: Strong soft tissue attachments caused by scarring should be expected. Gentle stretching with controlled traction using the Rowe forceps, bone hook, or transosseous wires will achieve progressive mobilization. Blunt dissection with a molt curette or even the finger can help to release the scar tissue.
- Fixation: The use of interpositional blocks of corticocancellous bone grafts are often used to increase bone contact and reduce the risk of relapse.
- Ancillary surgical procedures: Lip V-Y lengthening, lip lipofilling, cheek lipofilling, nasal alar cinch stitch to prevent widening, bichectomy, etc. can be added to the surgical plan according to the facial aesthetic needs of every patient.

### Mandibular Repositioning

- For mandibular osteotomies, the BSSO is commonly done with an intraoral incision.
- The cuts can be made either by first making perforating holes through the cortex with a drill and then connecting the holes with a fissure burr, or with a reciprocating saw. Osteotomes aid in completion through the inferior cortex.
- Separation is facilitated with Smith forceps.
- Rotation, advancement, and set back could be planned to adjust to the final position of the maxilla or even for just small correction of facial asymmetries.
- The fixation is usually done by three bicortical screws on each side, either placed in straight line or triangular pattern, or can use a thick plate and monocortical screws (Figs. 23.10 and 23.11).

### Key Equipment

When performing orthognathic surgery procedures in outreach/mission settings, the team must warrant the availability of adequate and sufficient surgical equipment, including:

- Osteotomy instruments set
- Bone graft harvesting set
- Rotational gear (burrs and drills)
- Cutting gear (reciprocating +/− oscillating saws)
- Fixation devices for osteosynthesis (plates, screws, wires)
- Wire cutters that remain at patient's side whenever jaw is wired shut, for airway emergency

### Splint and Bony Fixation Alternatives for Low-Resource Setting

Fixation of the maxillary segment is most important at the four vertical buttresses: the paired nasomaxillary buttresses medially and zygomaticomaxillary buttresses laterally. Standard fixation in higher-resource settings utilizes titanium plates, typically "L-shaped," each 0.8 mm in thickness, and secured by 2–3 screws on each side of the osteotomy. In lower-resource settings, they may not be available. One option is to use other internal fixation plates for hand or extremity trauma. Another option, used historically in many settings, is to use wires, often 22–24 gauge in thickness, at the same four buttress sites (Fig. 23.12). Interposition bone graft, including notched cortical segments, is important to prevent compression. Rigid maxillomandibular fixation for a full 6–8 weeks is critical to prevent relapse.

If a preoperative splint is not available, one can be fashioned intraoperatively with methylmethacrylate to assist postoperative stability. Similarly, and particularly for a maxillary advancement with reasonable match in arch, MMF without a splint can be used. If brackets/arch bars are not available, a combination of Ernst ligatures and ivy loops or any other type of dental ligature could be used in order to

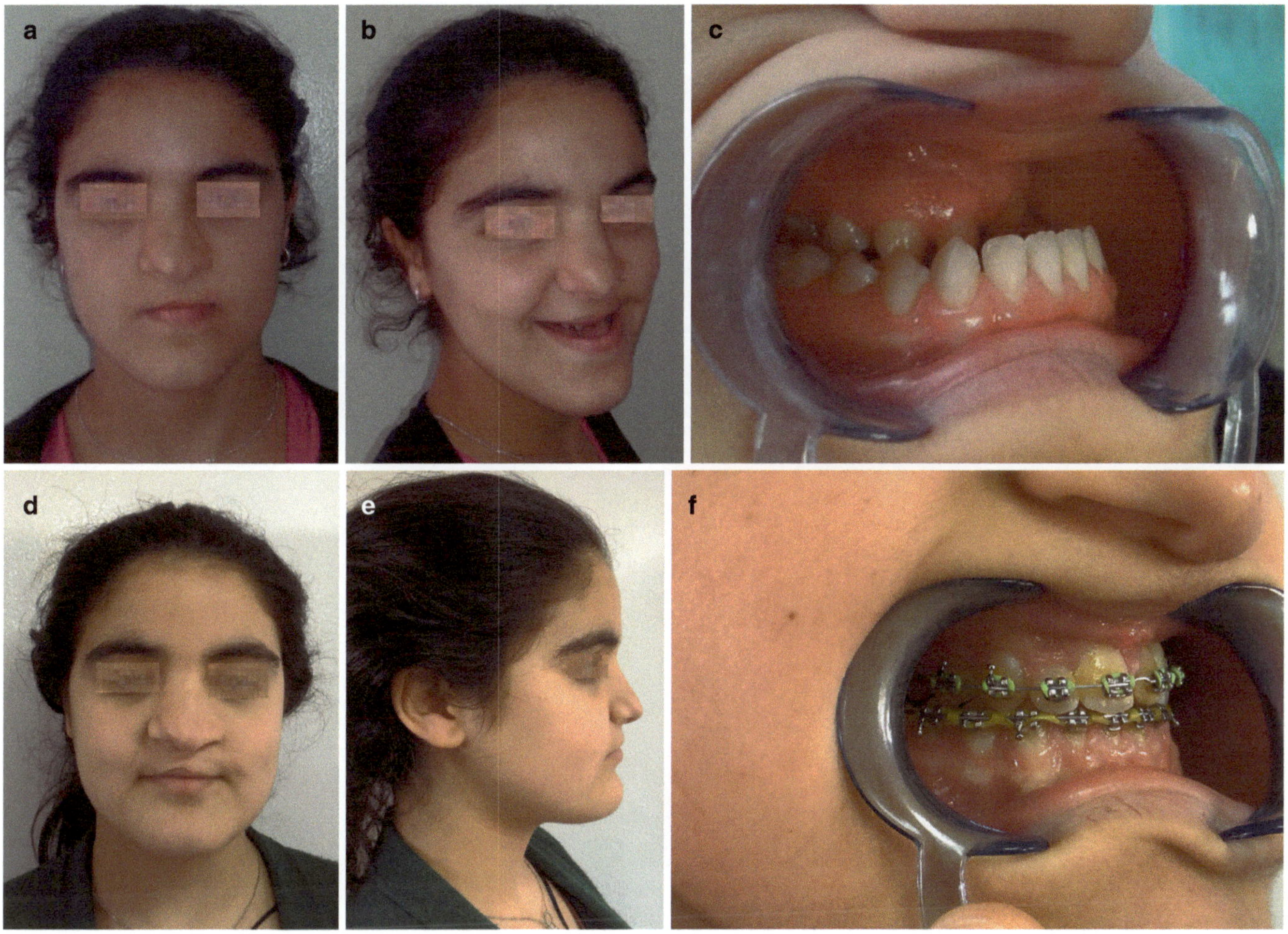

**Fig. 23.10** (**a**,**b**,**c**) Unilateral cleft patient with important midface retrusion. (**d**,**e**,**f**) Postoperative view after maxillary advancement and mandibular adjustment

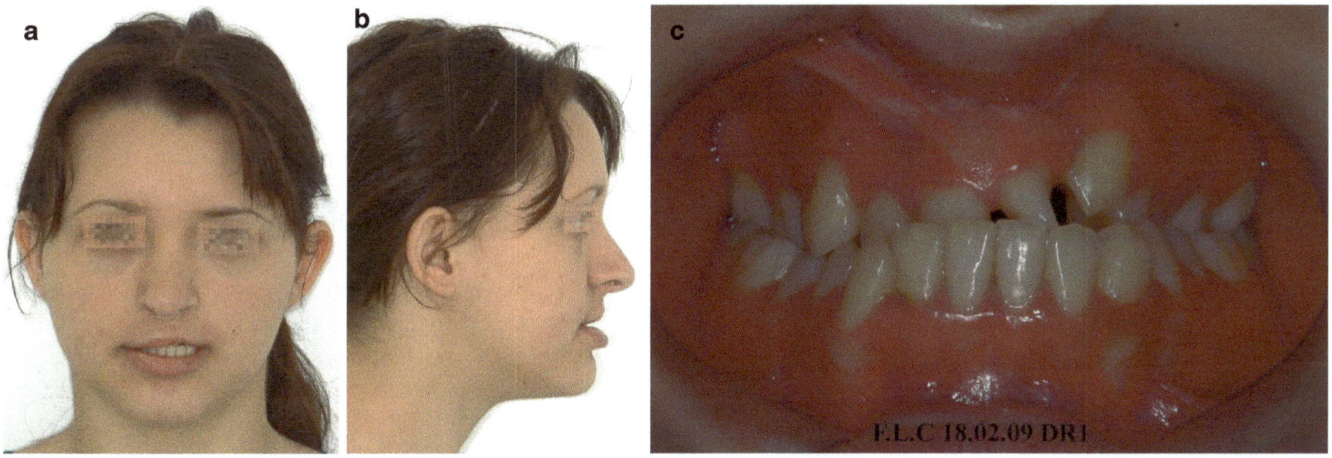

**Fig. 23.11** (**a**) UCP frontal view pre-op, (**b**) profile view, (**c**) initial occlusion before orthodontic, (**d**) occlusion after orthodontic preparation, g)final occlusion after surgery and orthodontic treatment (**e**) frontal view after maxillary advancement and mandibular repositioning, (**f**) profile view post-op

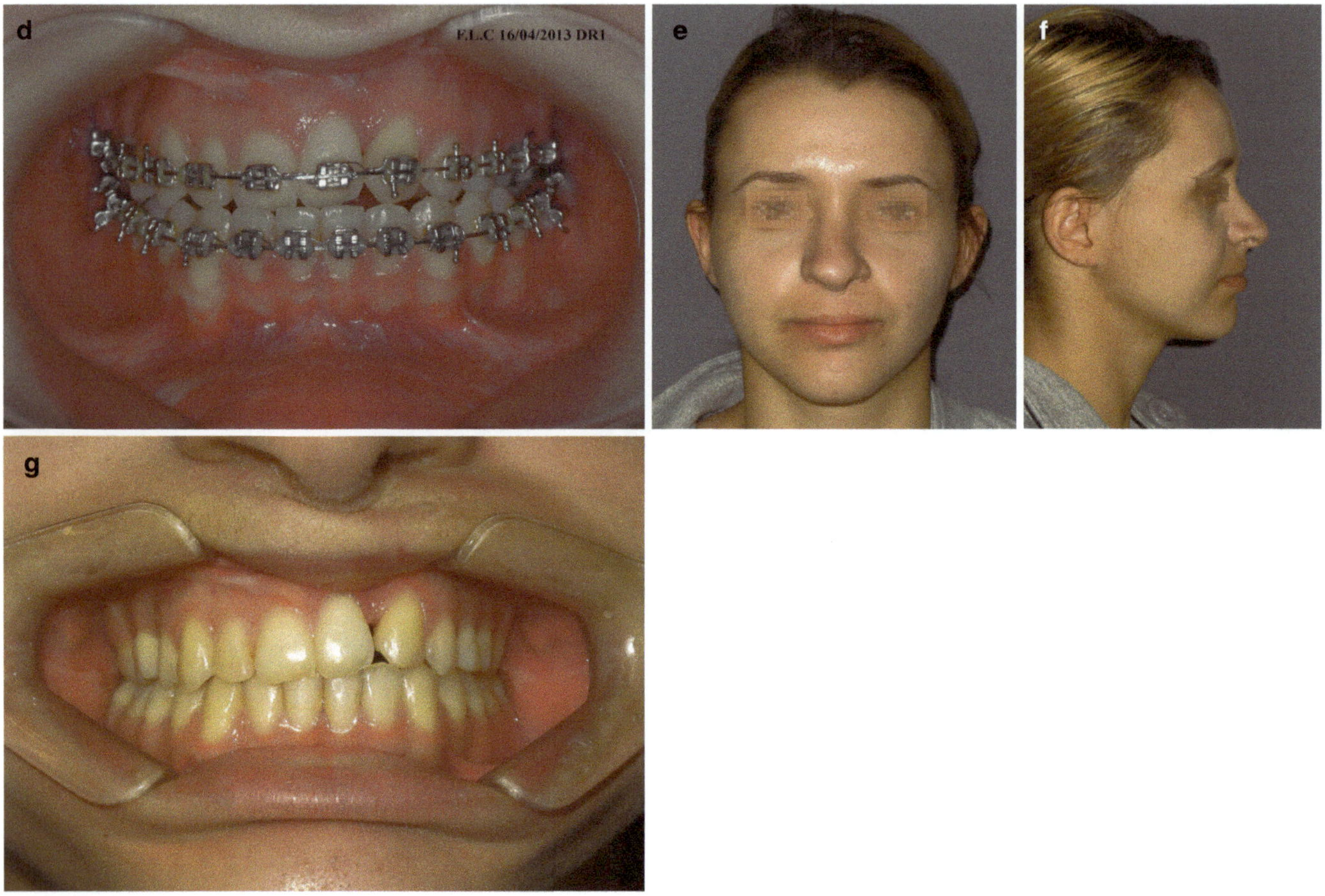


Fig. 23.11 (continued)

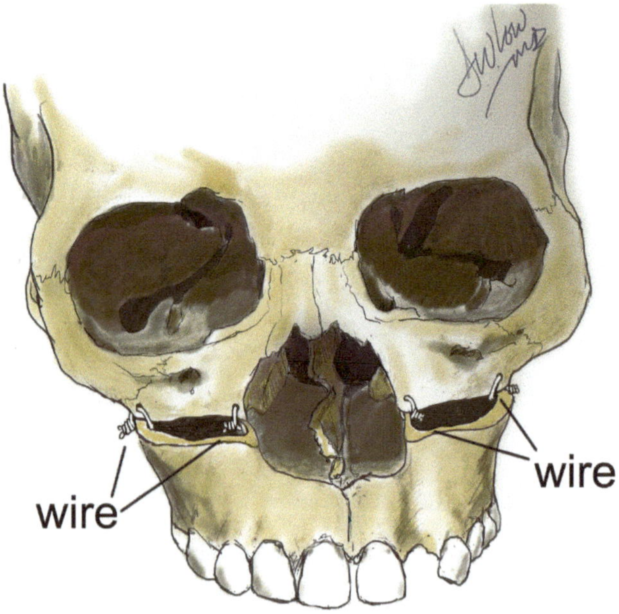


Fig. 23.12 Figure depiction displaying the use wires for internal fixation of the maxilla

place the patient in MMF at the end of the procedure (Fig. 23.13).

## Anesthetic Considerations

- Nasotracheal intubation is performed, secured with a permanent suture to the nasal septum intraoperatiely. Preoperative evaluation should assess for presence of a pharyngeal flap.
- The suprazygomatic nerve block using a combination of bupivacaine and lidocaine controls the perioperative pain, blocks the hemodynamic response during the osteotomies, and reduces the risk of trigemino-cardiac reflex.
- General anesthesia can be balanced with alfa2 agonists (dexmedetomidine and clonidine) offers:
  - Reduced sympathetic system responses
  - Reduced needs of hypnotics and narcotics
  - Decreased mid-blood pressure and bleeding

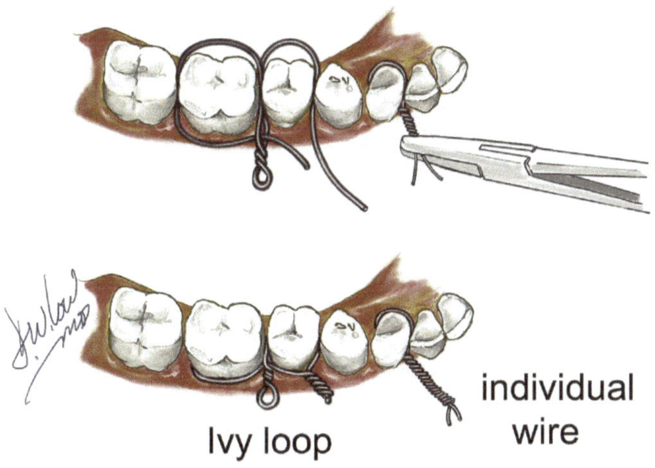


Fig. 23.13 Figure depiction displaying the use of wires for intermaxillary fixation. A combination of Ivy loops and Ernst ligatures can be used to achieve bite fixation

  - Increased analgesic effects of narcotics and analgesics
  - Decreased postoperative agitation and delirium of awakening
- The use of tranexamic acid might reduce the intraoperative and postoperative bleeding.
- The use of high dose dexamethasone reduces postoperative edema and nausea.

### Postoperative Orthodontic: Surgical Care

- Soft diet for 8 weeks.
- Swelling control measures: Ice packs and head elevation.
- Strict oral hygiene: Soft brushing and chlorhexidine rinses.
- Occlusal splint: Might be maintained for 8 weeks in cases of segmented maxillary advancement +/− alveolar bone grafts.
- Elastics: Clear instructions should be provided to the patient using class I anteriorly and class III laterally.

## Postoperative Stage [17]

### Long-Term Stability

Relapse following orthognathic surgery in cleft patients is significantly more frequent than in non-cleft patients. In most cases, relapse would occur during the first 6 postoperative months. Several factors can reduce the risk of relapse after maxillary advancements in cleft patients;

- Optimal orthodontic preparation with stable occlusal relationships (intercuspidation).
- Maxillary advancement with adequate release of soft tissue.
- Mild overcorrection whenever possible.
- Rigid fixation with high-profile titanium plates.
- Interposed cortico-cancelous bone grafts at the osteotomy.
- The surgical splint should be maintained in situ for 3–6 weeks postoperatively.
- Close postoperative orthodontic follow-up with adequate use and modification of elastics therapy throughout the consolidation process.

### Postoperative Velopharyngeal Insufficiency [18]

- A preoperative speech assessment by an experienced speech-language pathologist should be systematically performed at start of orthodontic preparation. Potential voice changes and to a greater extent postoperative VPI should be discussed with the patient. It has been shown that there is no relationship between the amount of maxillary advancement and postoperative velopharyngeal function. Those patients exhibiting borderline insufficiency preoperatively may display velopharyngeal deterioration; however, for most cases, maxillary advancement is not likely to affect vellum function. In the other hand, surgical correction of skeletal relationships and occlusion may translate into improvements in certain aspects of speech disorders (articulation) [15, 16]. Finally, those CLP patients with pharyngeal flaps should ideally be intubated with nasoendoscopic assistance. Sectioning of the flap is sometimes needed to achieve adequate maxillary advancement.

### Final Considerations for Context

Although orthognathic surgery is considered "beyond reach" in many low-resource settings, there are a growing number of settings in which orthognathic procedures can be done in modified fashion and obtain the desired results. Investments in dental, orthodontic, and anesthesia platforms are likely to make subsequent orthognathic endeavors more effective. Practitioners in low-resource settings must consider the overall resources that the institution and health system have and whether or not it justifies doing the outlined procedure in this patient population.

It is possible to do certain types of cleft orthognathic surgery with a minimum of materials. For example, common resources in middle-income countries include an orthopantogram and cephalometrogram, dental study models, and an articulator to do model surgery and to make an intermediate and/or final splint. In low-income settings, if these are not available, then it is certainly possible to use X-rays and stone models alone to determine if a surgical procedure might be the best option for a patient. In some cases, a straightforward maxillary advancement, wired into place after achieving occlusion with the mandible and wired MMF, can achieve a stable result without a splint or fixation plates. It is also possible that certain patients in these settings may have recycled materials such as midfacial distractors available to them that might be used in concert with a basic LeFort I procedure, particularly to bring more severe cases into a more functional position. This can avert true disability for patients in terms of form and function, the latter including speech, chewing, eating, and swallowing. Similarly, bimaxillary surgery should be avoided in the most constrained environments if a less complicated LeFort I can achieve reasonable improvement. Again we would stress that in these low-income settings one has to very much analyze risk and benefit to determine if surgery of this nature should be done. If the surgical team is comfortable and the hospital has the resources with regard to anesthesia, nursing, and postoperative care, then it can be considered.

**Tips and Tricks**

- OS preparation, planning, performance, and follow-up demand the coordinated approach by the surgical, orthodontic, and speech therapy team.
- Inclusion of patient (young adult!) in decision-making and may find helpful to speak with patients who have been through procedure before.
- Avoid simultaneous ABG and OS in the mission/outreach setting.
- When considering a bimaxillary procedure, any mandibular set back should be kept to the minimum.
- CLP patients with pharyngeal flaps should ideally be intubated with nasoendoscopic assistance. Sectioning of the flap is sometimes needed to achieve adequate maxillary advancement.
- When considering major maxillary advancements, there are different alternatives: staged maxillary advancement, bimaxillary procedure, and distraction osteogenesis.
- Consider the use of a protective palatal splint during maxillary downfracture and mobilization to prevent splitting of maxilla across the cleft.
- The use of interposed corticocancellous bone grafts, rigid internal fixation, and also close postoperative orthodontic and surgical follow-up reduces the risk of skeletal relapse.

## References


1. Semb G. A study of facial growth in patients with bilateral cleft lip and palate treated by the Oslo CLP team. Cleft Palate Craniofac J. 1991;28(1):22–39; discussion 46-8
2. Semb G. A study of facial growth in patients with unilateral cleft lip and palate treated by the Oslo CLP team. Cleft Palate Craniofac J. 1991;28(1):1–21; discussion 46-8
3. Shetye PR. Facial growth of adults with unoperated clefts. Clin Plast Surg. 2004;31(2):361–71.
4. Good PM, Mulliken JB, Padwa BL. Frequency of Le Fort I osteotomy after repaired cleft lip and palate or cleft palate. Cleft Palate Craniofac J. 2007;44(4):396–401.
5. Backdahl M, Nordinke. Replacement of the maxillary bone defect in cleft palate. A new procedure. Acta Chir Scand. 1961;122:131–7.
6. Sierra NE, Ferrer-Fuertes A, Salazar-Perez B, Cho-Lee GY, Marti-Pages C, Rivera-Baro A, et al. Surgical repositioning of the Premaxilla using a minimally invasive endonasal approach. Cleft Palate Craniofac J. 2018;55(6):830–6.
7. Abyholm FE, Bergland O, Semb G. Secondary bone grafting of alveolar clefts. A surgical/orthodontic treatment enabling a non-prosthodontic rehabilitation in cleft lip and palate patients. Scand J Plast Reconstr Surg. 1981;15(2):127–40.
8. da Silva Filho OG, Ozawa TO, Bachega C, Bachega MA. Reconstruction of alveolar cleft with allogenous bone graft: clinical considerations. Dent Press J Orthod. 2013;18(6):138–47.
9. Alonso N, Freitas RS, Amundson J, Raposo-Amaral C. Bone graft in alveolar cleft lip and palate. In: Alonso N, Raposo-Amaral C, editors. Cleft lip and palate treatment: a comprehensive guide, vol. 1. Cham: Springer International Publising AG; 2018. p. 247–61.
10. Camara PR, Bastos EO, Curi D, Alonso N. Orthodontic treatment of patients with orofacial cleft. In: Alonso N, Raposo-Amaral CA, editors. Cleft lip and palate treatment: a comprehensive guide, vol. 1. Cham: Springer International Publising AG; 2018. p. 269–77.
11. Chua HD, Hagg MB, Cheung LK. Cleft maxillary distraction versus orthognathic surgery--which one is more stable in 5 years? Oral Surg Oral Med Oral Pathol Oral Radiol Endod. 2010;109(6):803–14.
12. Posnick JC, Ricalde P. Cleft-orthognathic surgery. Clin Plast Surg. 2004;31(2):315–30.
13. Schendel SA. Computer simulation in the daily practice of orthognathic surgery. Int J Oral Maxillofac Surg. 2015;44(12):1451–6.
14. Alonso N, Bastos EO, Capuchino G Jr. Orthognathic surgery in cleft patients. In: Alonso N, Raposo-Amaral CA, editors. Cleft lip and palate treatment: a comprehensive guide, vol. 1. Cham: Springer International Publising GA; 2018. p. 279–95.
15. Rosenstein S, Kernahan D, Dado D, Grasseschi M, Griffith BH. Orthognathic surgery in cleft patients treated by early bone grafting. Plast Reconstr Surg. 1991;87(5):835–92; discussion 40-2
16. Eskenazi LB, Schendel SA. An analysis of Le Fort I maxillary advancement in cleft lip and palate patients. Plast Reconstr Surg. 1992;90(5):779–86.
17. Wolford LM. Effects of orthognathic surgery on nasal form and function in the cleft patient. Cleft Palate Craniofac J. 1992;29(6):546–55.
18. Phillips JH, Klaiman P, Delorey R, MacDonald DB. Predictors of velopharyngeal insufficiency in cleft palate orthognathic surgery. Plast Reconstr Surg. 2005;115(3):681–6.

# Lateral and Rare Craniofacial Clefts

# 24

Anil Madaree and Phuong D. Nguyen

**Key Points**

- Craniofacial clefts occur spontaneously.
- Tessier description of clefts (0–14) by using counter clockwise rotation is useful to group patterns and determine reconstructive strategies.
- Reconstruction is aimed at oral and nasal patency, protection of globes and restoration of anatomic subunits.

**Tips and Tricks**

1. The surgeon should have a clear understanding of the anatomy, extent, and pathway of the cleft. This allows for better preparation and planning of the repair.
2. A decision must be made whether the surgical correction is done in a single procedure or in a staged fashion. If staged, one needs to plan the sequence of correction of bone and soft tissue and the anticipated appropriate age for these procedures.
3. The placement of scars should be prioritized and carefully considered. These should be in natural anatomical lines as far as possible respecting the facial subunits. Sometimes a large flap adhering to the facial units results in a better outcome than multiple small flaps.
4. One must be aware of the status and anatomy of the dentition. Any procedure that is planned must ensure that the dentition is preserved as much as possible. Orthodontic assessment and manipulation may be necessary.
5. If there is a significant deficit of tissue, one must consider the use of tissue expanders, regional flaps, or free tissue transfer.
6. Minor touch-up procedures are often necessary to optimize the result. These include the use of fat transfer to correct minor deformities, symmetry, volume deficits, and contour irregularities.

## Introduction

Rare craniofacial clefts are a particularly challenging entity faced by reconstructive surgeons. The spectrum of clinical presentation is tremendous. However, as Dr. Henry Kawamoto eloquently stated: within the kaleidoscopic world of these rare clefts, order is made out of chaos to the trained plastic surgeon [1].

As such, reconstruction is carefully planned and may be performed in stages. These major facial clefts can be comprised of a defect in the bone, soft tissues, or both in the head and neck. The etiology is not completely ascertained and may be a mix of genetic, environmental, and idiopathic contributors. Implicating factors include radiation, infectious agents, metabolic imbalances, and many drugs and chemicals. Dr. Kawamoto described the incidence as 1.43–4.84 per 100,000 live births, though because of the rarity and variability, the true epidemiology is not known [1].

A. Madaree
Department of Plastic and Reconstructive Surgery, Inkosi Albert Luthuli Central Hospital; University of Kwazulu-Natal, Durban, South Africa
e-mail: MADAREE@ukzn.ac.za

P. D. Nguyen (✉)
Division of Plastic Surgery, Department of Surgery, Children's Memorial Hermann Hospital, University of Texas Health Science Center, Houston, TX, USA

© Springer Nature Switzerland AG 2021

J. W. Swanson, D. W. Low (eds.), *Global Cleft Care in Low-Resource Settings*, https://doi.org/10.1007/978-3-030-59105-2_24

Many attempts at classification have been presented, but the most enduring and logical is that of Dr. Tessier. This classification is created as a numerical system that runs counterclockwise, circumferentially around the orbit, in defined planes. The clefts are numbered from 0 to 14 and follow defined zones of the face and orbit which correlate with embryologic formation (Fig. 24.1). These numbered clefts incorporate both soft tissue and bony defects. The orbits define the horizontal axis dividing the face into upper and lower halves and, thus, separate the cranial clefts from the facial clefts. The clefts may have a single number or reflect a pairing of cleft numbers, usually one facial and one cranial. Clinically, the following combinations of clefts are often identified: 0 and 14, 1 and 13, 2 and 12, 3 and 11, 4 and 10, 5 and 9, and 6 and 8, adding up to 14. Cleft numbers 5–9 are considered lateral/facial clefts as they pass lateral to the infraorbital foramen. There is a large variability of clinical severity and expression in craniofacial clefts, and unusual combinations are seen. The value in Tessier's classification is that it directs the clinician to search for malformations in line along the entire axis. Skeletal landmarks are more consistent and reliable than soft tissue landmarks. In a review of 495 rare clefts treated over a 41-year period, Ortiz-Monasterio and Taylor described 65% had multiple clefts vs. 35% with a single cleft and 33% unilateral vs. 67% bilateral [2].

Formulating a reconstructive plan that addresses staging and prioritizes the placement of scars is very important. Scars should be in natural anatomical lines as far as possible respecting the facial subunits. Sometimes a large flap adhering to the facial units results in a better outcome than multiple small flaps (Fig. 24.2a,b).

## Facial Clefts

### Facial Cleft 0

A number 0 cleft lies within the umbrella of a median cerebrofacial malformation. These are developmental anomalies of the midline brain and facial structures. These median malformations are unique in that there may be deficient, normal, or excess tissue. The correlation between the severity of malformation between the brain and the face is variable.

A number 0 cleft is a midline clefting of the lip bisecting the philtral columns and nose through the columella. It has also been called frontonasal dysplasia, holoprosencephaly, median craniofacial dysgraphia, and centrofacial microsomia. There may be a cranial extension, or a number 14 cleft. The lip cleft may vary from a minor vermillion notch to a full-thickness median cleft with extension through the upper lip and up into the nasal floor. The columella may be narrow or absent, and the philtral columns may be widened or absent. The nasal tip may be blunted from lack of septal support. There is often a duplicated frenulum with a diastema between the maxillary central incisors. A true median cleft can give rise to an encephalocele, a cystic congenital malformation in which the central nervous system structures herniate through a defect in the cranium in communication with cerebrospinal fluid pathways. This area of weakness permits parts of the brain to escape the cranial space. The 0 cleft is medial to the canthus and thus does not disrupt the orbit.

Skeletal abnormalities vary from separation of the upper central incisors, to the absence of the premaxilla and a cleft of the secondary palate. Nasal deficiency includes potential absence of septal cartilage and/or nasal bones. If the bone defect extends superiorly, there may be hypotelorism or even cyclopia.

This midline cleft of the upper lip, columella, and nose can be considered as one of three groups:

1. Normal interorbital distance: These patients are treated in the same time frame as a unilateral cleft lip and normally repaired at 3 months of age. There are two subcategories in this group. First, there may just be a cleft of the lip (Fig. 24.3), or second, there may be a significant excess of tissue (Fig. 24.7a).
2. Hypotelorism (Fig. 24.4): There is often an absence of the columella in these cases. These patients have deficiency or absence of midline structures and fall into the holoprosencephaly spectrum. The life expectancy for these patients is very poor with most demising within the first several years of life. Surgery on these patients is fraught with postoperative complications. These are mainly related to airway problems and central nervous issues. This is compounded by the fact that repair of the lip often results in a single nostril cavity as the columella is absent. Therefore these centrally challenged patients do not cope with the dramatic decrease in the nostril aperture. If the patient survives to 1 year of age, surgery may be offered to the parents after due counselling on the postoperative risks including death.
3. Hypertelorism (Fig. 24.5): These patients will be considered for correction of the hypertelorism at the appropriate age and by the chosen procedure. The repair of the lip will be sequenced into tmhe plan.

#### Surgical Considerations

The repair of the lip is performed with the goal of having a midline scar and a lip of adequate length. A Rose-Thompson or diamond excision is marked. After these incisions, the muscle is dissected from the mucosa and skin. The mucosa is repaired. The muscle is repaired preferably with a nylon suture. Regarding the vermilion and mucosa, these are

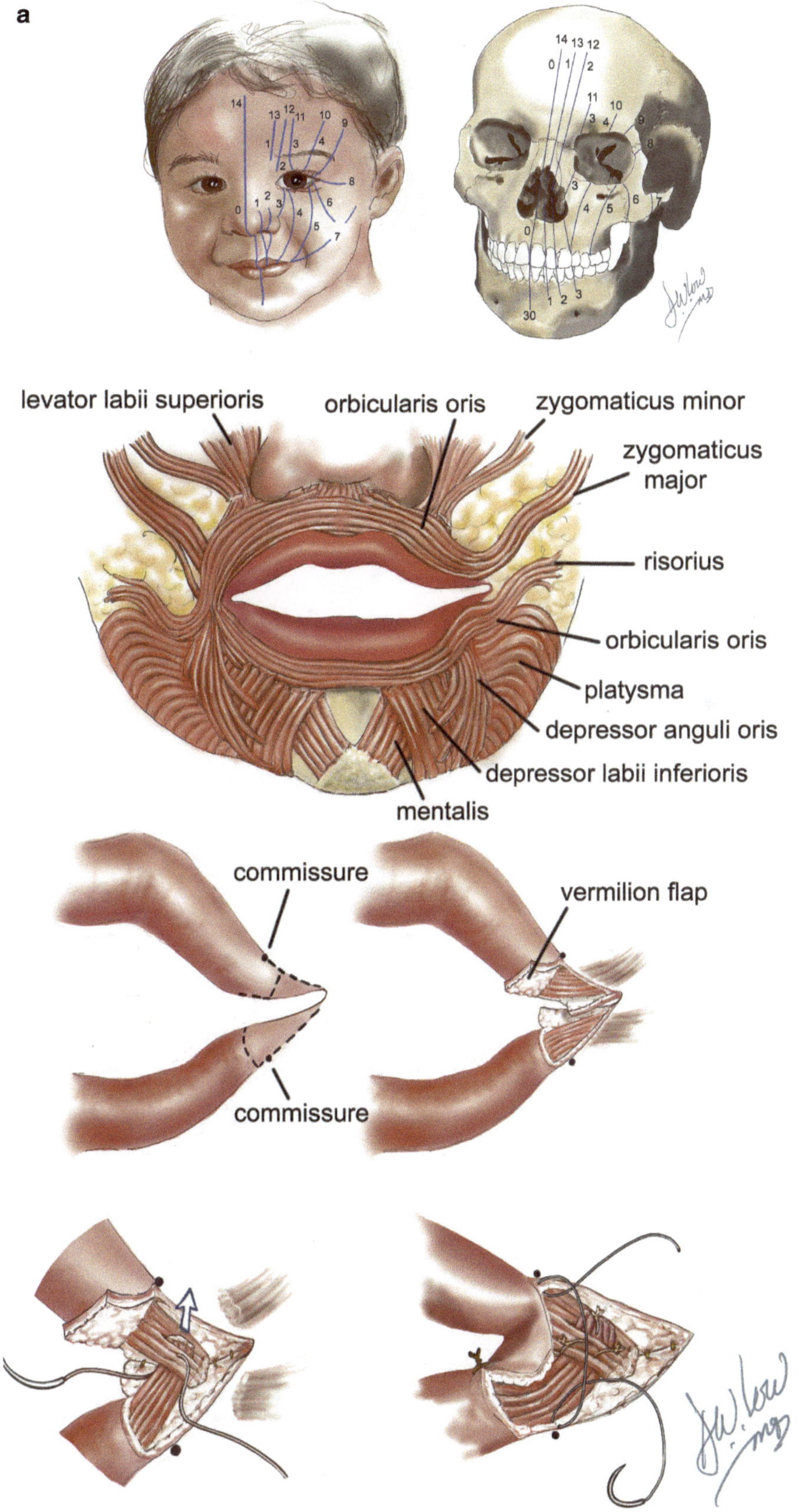


**Fig. 24.1** (**a**) Top: Soft tissue and bony landmarks of Tessier classification of clefts showing a counter clockwise format. Middle: Facial musculature. Bottom: Lateral cleft (Tessier 7) with interpolated orbicularis oris muscle flap and z-plasty repair. (**b**) Flap design and reconstruction for Tessier 3 cleft with scars placed in anatomic subunits and natural tension lines

Fig. 24.1 (continued)

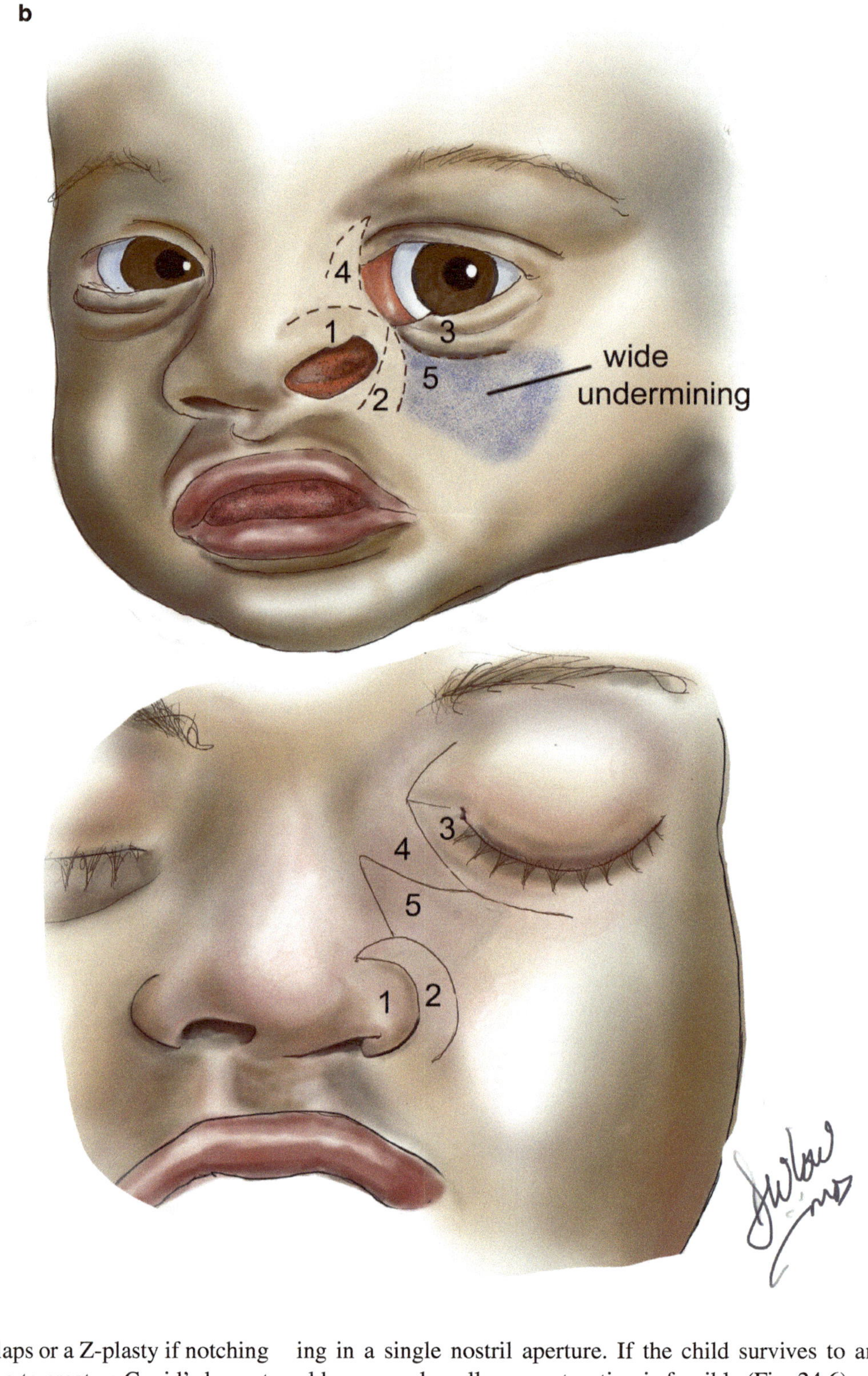


repaired in the midline or with flaps or a Z-plasty if notching is anticipated. No attempt is done to create a Cupid's bow at this stage. If the patient survives to an older age, this can be considered. If there are significant columella elements present, reconstruction of the columella is performed simultaneously. However, the columella is usually absent. In these cases, no attempt is made to reconstruct the columella resulting in a single nostril aperture. If the child survives to an older age, columella reconstruction is feasible (Fig. 24.6).

In the group with a normal interorbital distance, the type of repair is determined whether this is purely a cleft or if there is an excess of tissue. If it is purely a cleft, then the goal is to gain lip length and repair all facets of the lip elements. If there is an excess of tissue, the design incorporates excision of the

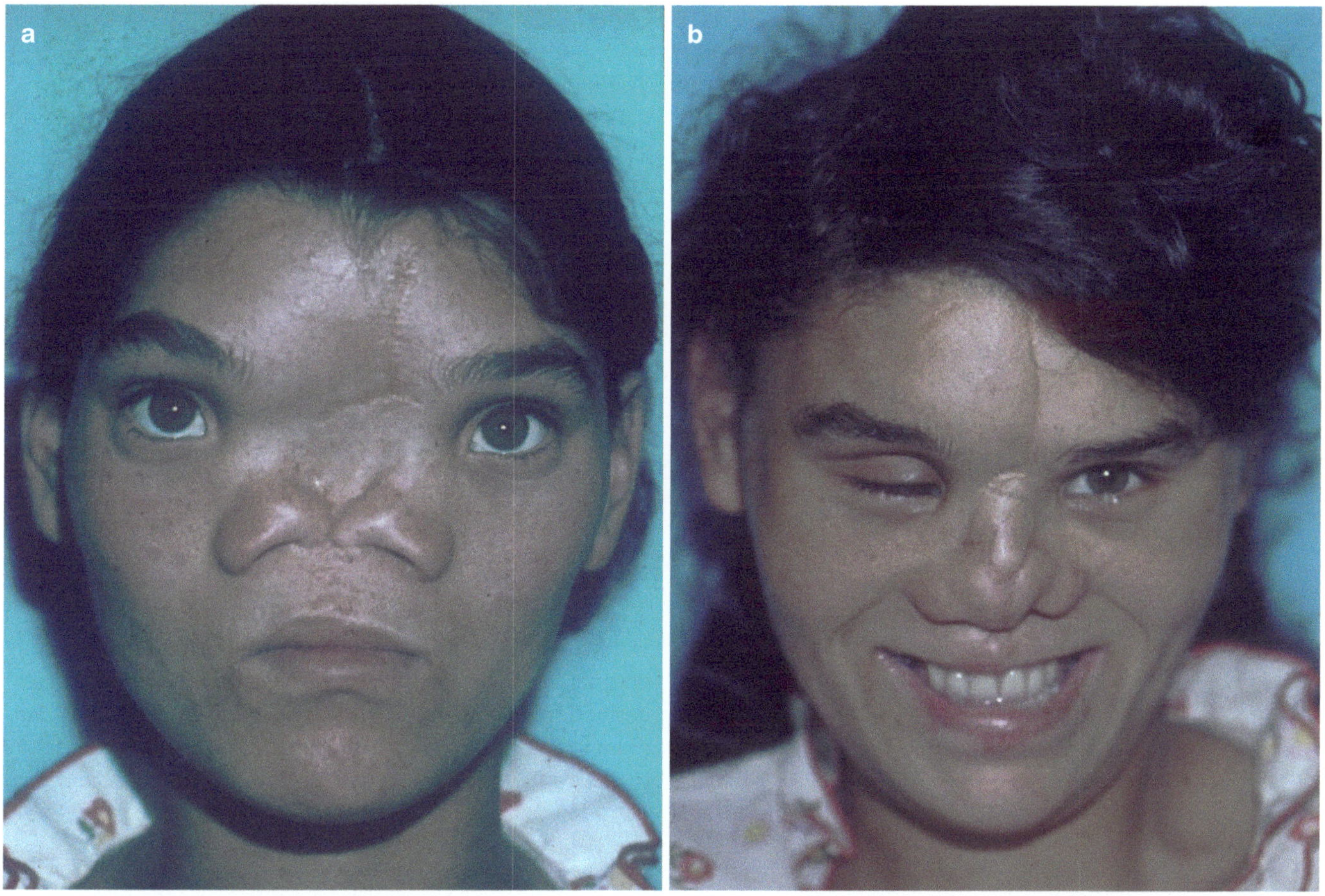


Fig. 24.2 (**a**) Facial cleft 0/14 with hypertelorism. (**b**) Undesirable patchwork appearance of soft tissue reconstruction

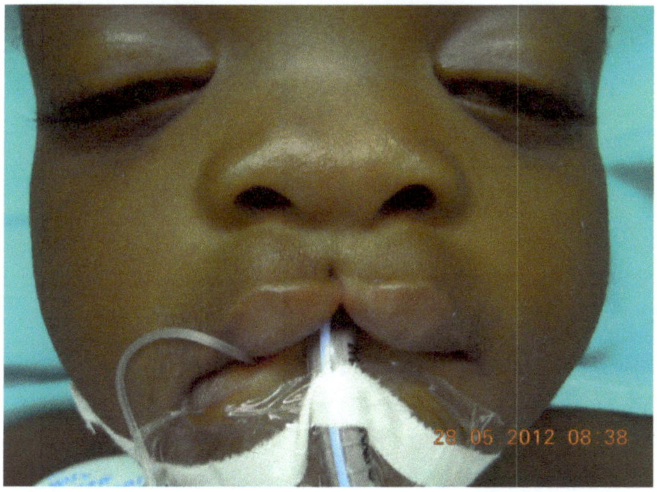

Fig. 24.3 Facial cleft 0

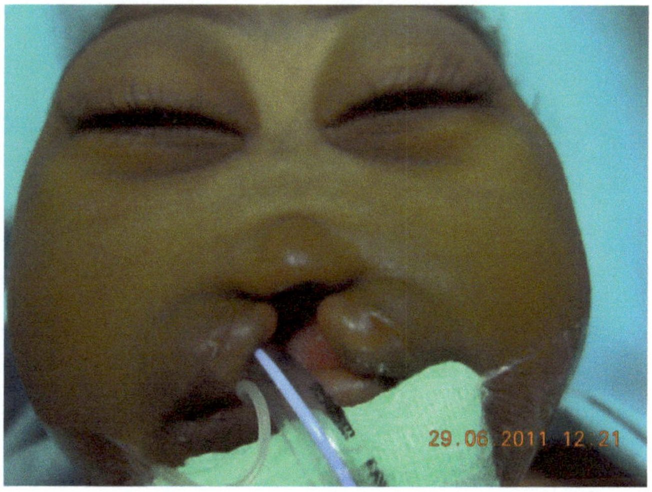

Fig. 24.4 Facial cleft 0 with hypotelorism and holoprosencephaly

excess tissue while also repairing the lip. Careful measurement and planning is required to determine what tissues can be sacrificed and how the tissues can be rearranged to get the best possible result. There is often a deformity of the nasal tip with excess tissue, bifid nose, fatty deposits between the domes, and a broad columella. These can be addressed via a rim incision, an open rhinoplasty, or a midline nasal tip incision depending on the reconstructive design (Fig. 24.7).

In facial cleft 0, there is sometimes a cleft of the columella and nasal tip. The nose may be bifid. Correction of these deformities is best done through a direct open approach with approximation of the medial crura and the ala domes (Fig. 24.8). Correction of the hypertelorism is performed after the age of 6 years.

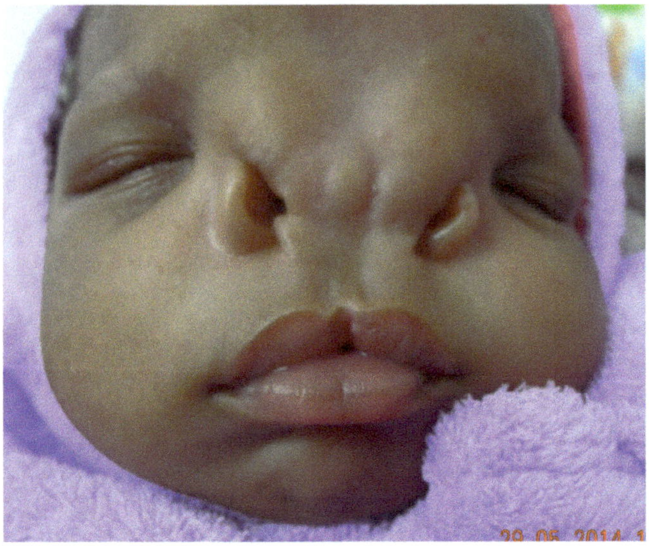

**Fig. 24.5** Facial cleft 0 with bilateral 13 components and hypertelorism

## Facial Cleft 1

The number 1 cleft is a paramedian facial cleft, similar to the common cleft lip, as it passes through Cupid's bow and through the alar cartilage. A pathognomonic feature is notching in the soft triangle of the nose (Fig. 24.9). The columella may be short and broad. The nasal tip and septum deviate away from the cleft. The overlying skin may have furrowing or wrinkles on the nasal dorsum. In the facial cleft 1, the cleft in the ala is just off the midline (Fig. 24.10).

The anterior incisors are oriented such that they face toward the cleft, creating an anterior open bite. There is a space between the nasal floor and the pyriform aperture. There may be extension posteriorly to create a complete cleft of the hard and soft palate.

### Surgical Considerations

There is no fixed method for correction of these clefts. This is due to the great variability in these deformities. There may be a deficiency or an excess of tissue. To plan the surgical correction, one must use the normal side as a guide and template to determine how best to rearrange the tissues and how to design the flaps. It is useful to pay attention to anatomical

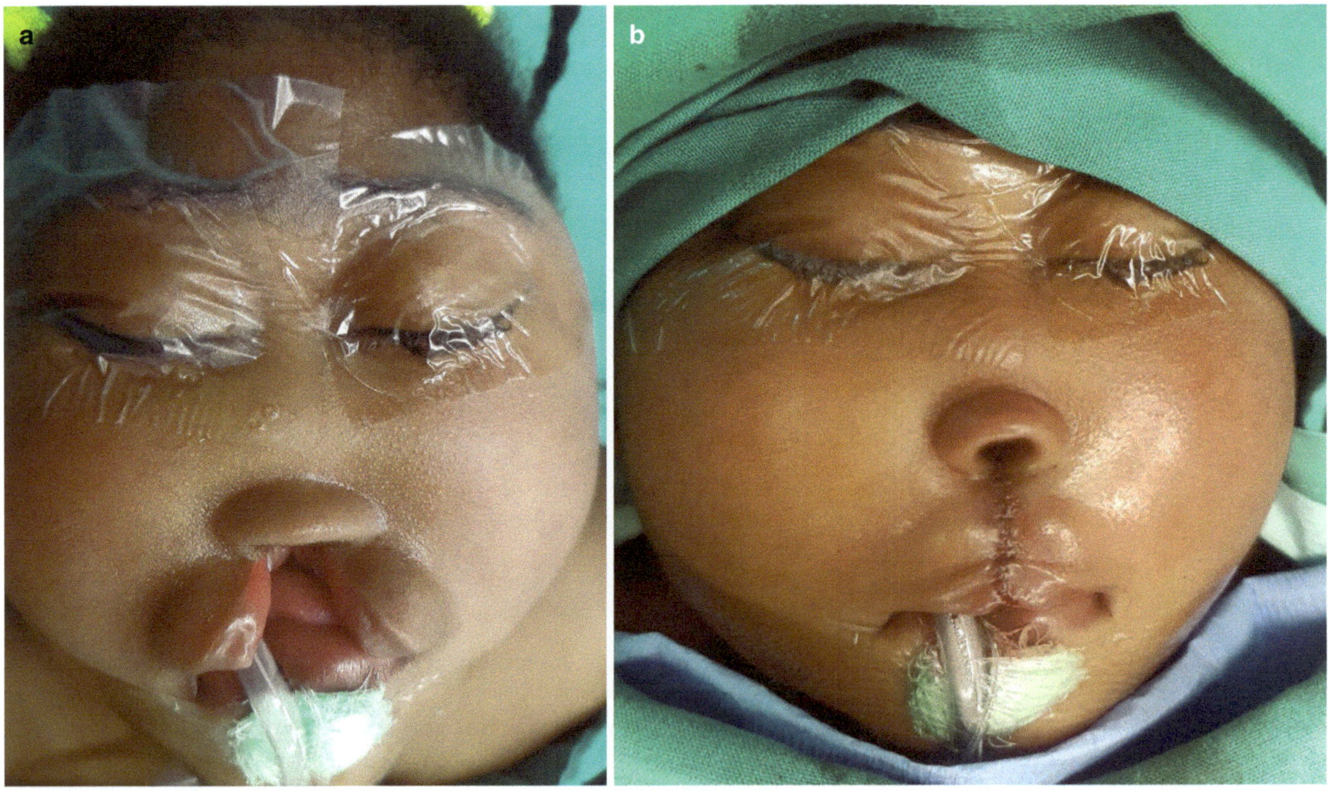


**Fig. 24.6** (**a**) Facial cleft 0 pre-op. (**b**) Immediate post-op

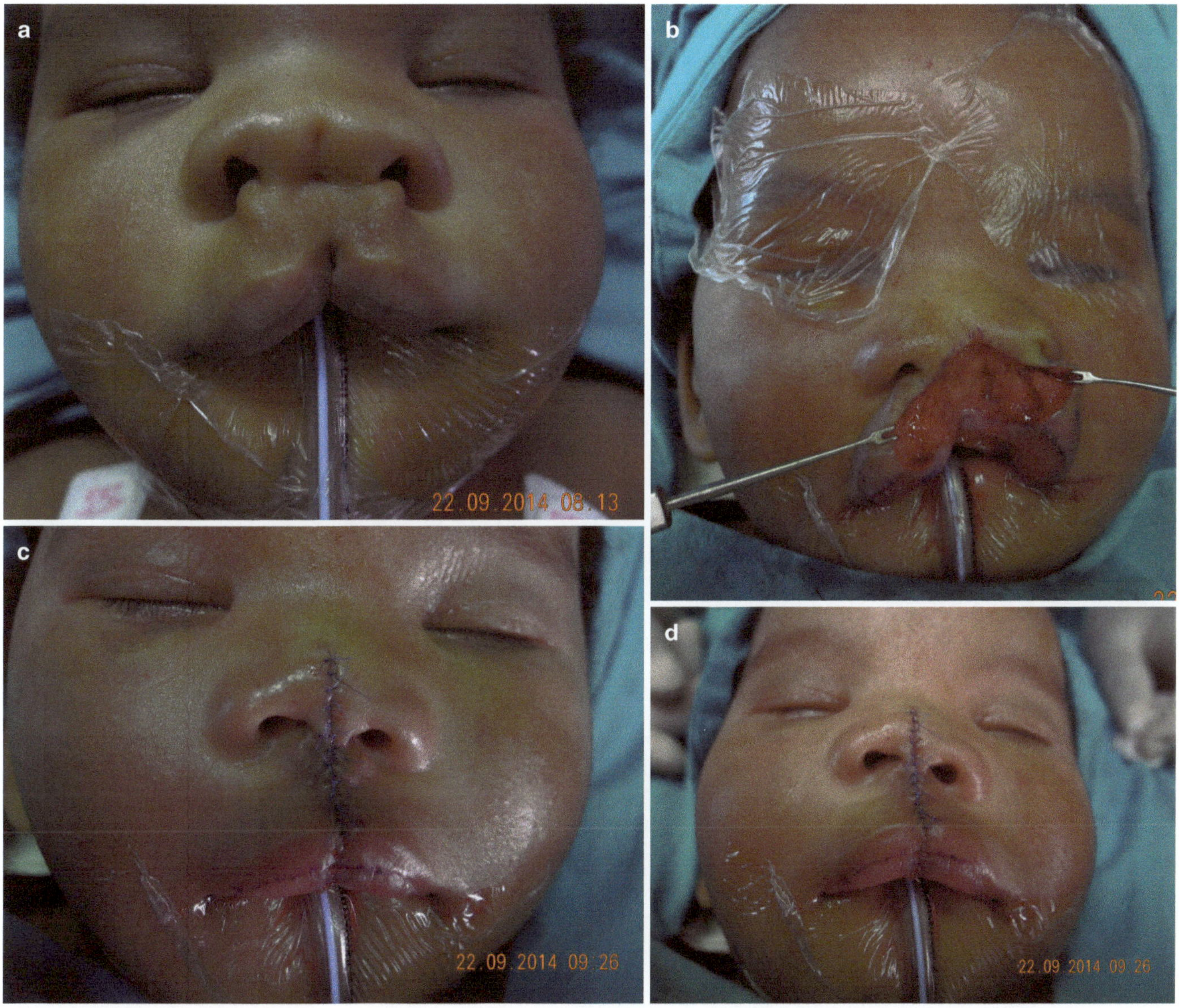


**Fig. 24.7** (**a**) Facial cleft 0 with excess tissue. (**b**) Intraoperative view showing dissected muscle. (**c,d**) Immediate post-op views

details such as the midline, alar base position, vertical length of ala, and circumference of the nostril. This will help to replicate as close as possible a mirror image of the normal side. If there is poor support, consideration must be given to the use of cartilage grafts. Figure 24.11 demonstrates a repaired facial cleft 1.

## Facial Cleft 2

This is also a paramedian facial cleft which may appear as a cleft lip; however, the nasal deformity is in the middle third of the alar rim, in contrast to the number 1 cleft. The ala is diminished and hypoplastic as opposed to a subtle notch. The lateral portion of the nose is flat, and the dorsum is broad. The eyelid is not involved. It may continue superiorly as a number 12 cleft, in which case one may observe distortion of the medial brow. Dentally, the cleft is between the lateral incisor and the canine. It continues into the pyriform aperture, lateral to the septum and medial to the maxillary sinus. Both a hard and soft palate cleft may be observed. The nasal septum is deviated away from the cleft.

### Surgical Considerations

Facial cleft 2 may be associated with excess and abnormal arrangement of tissue often with partial occlusion of the nostril on the affected side. One must be creative in addressing the nostril occlusion. Figures 24.12, 24.13, and 24.14

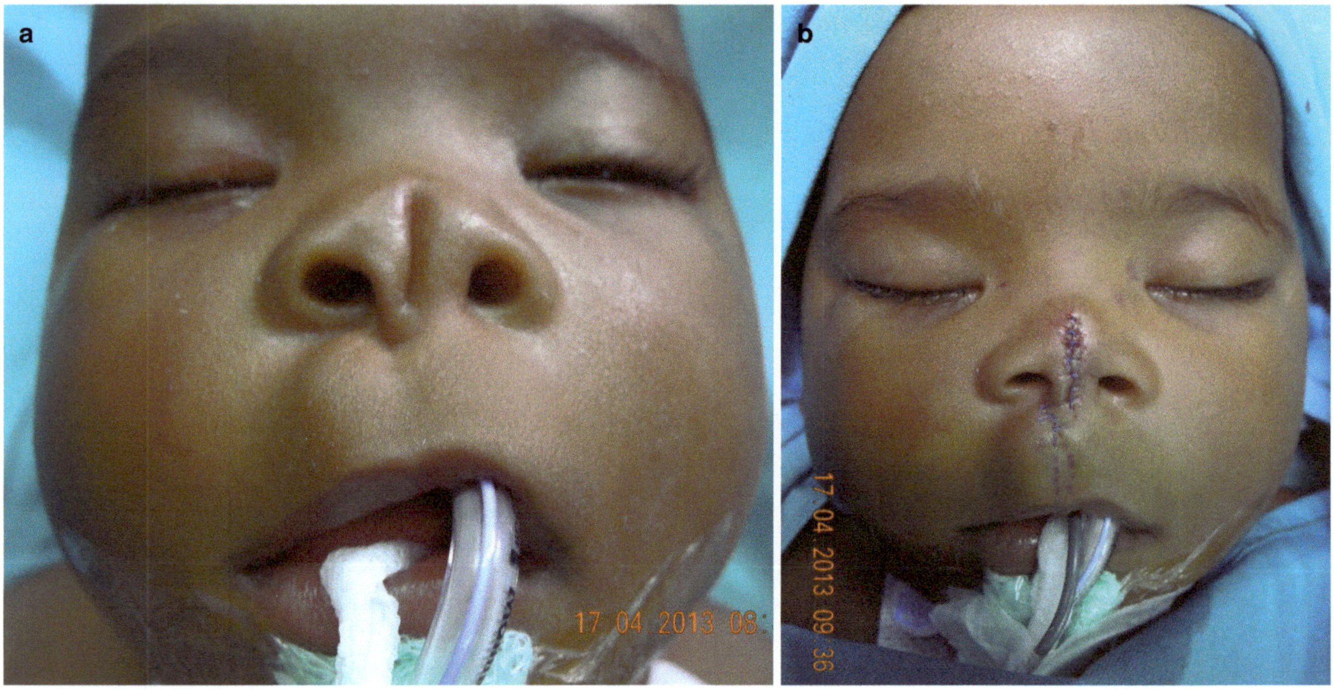


**Fig. 24.8** (**a**) Facial cleft 0 affecting columella and nasal tip. (**b**) Immediate post-op

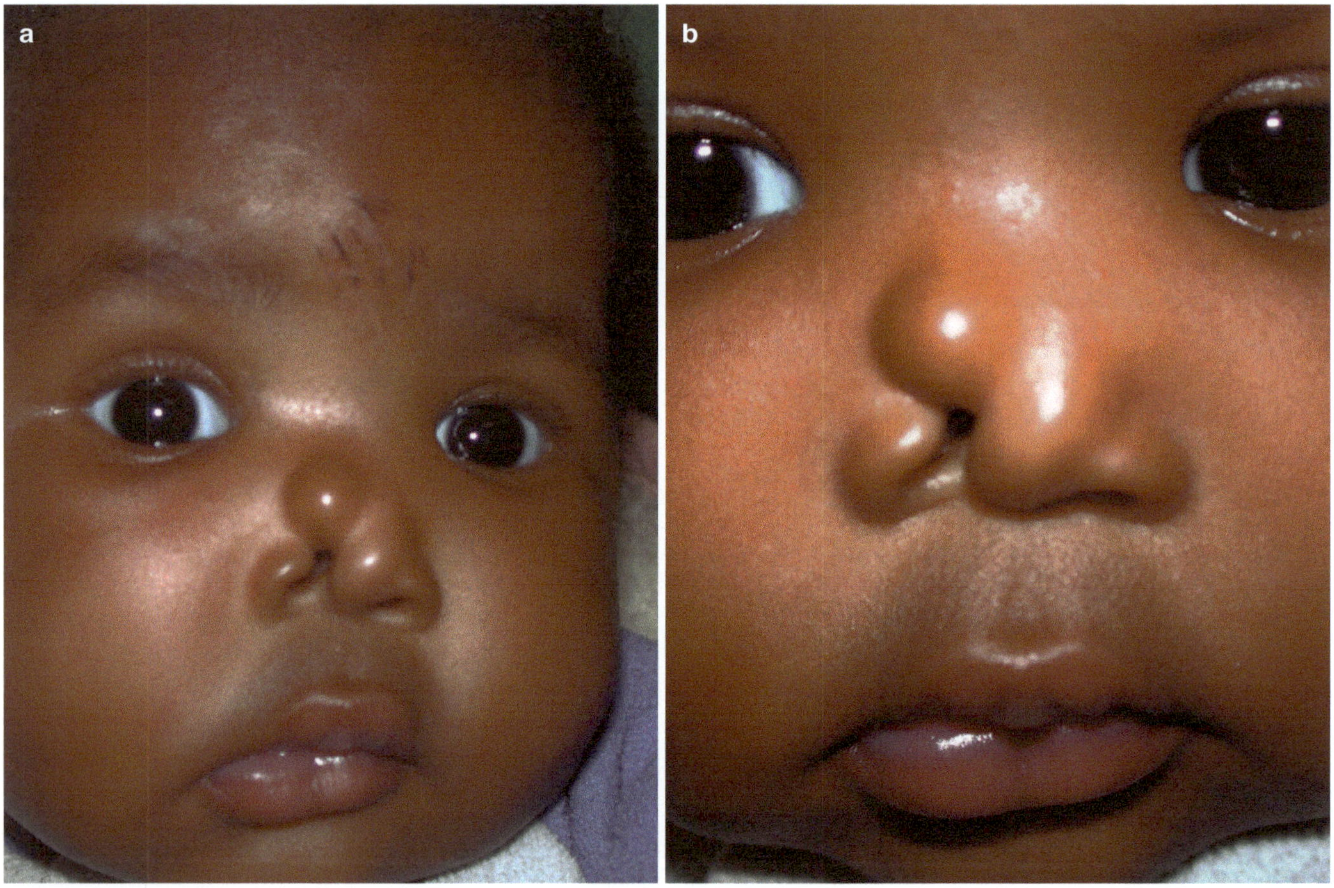


**Fig. 24.9** (**a**, **b**) Facial cleft 1

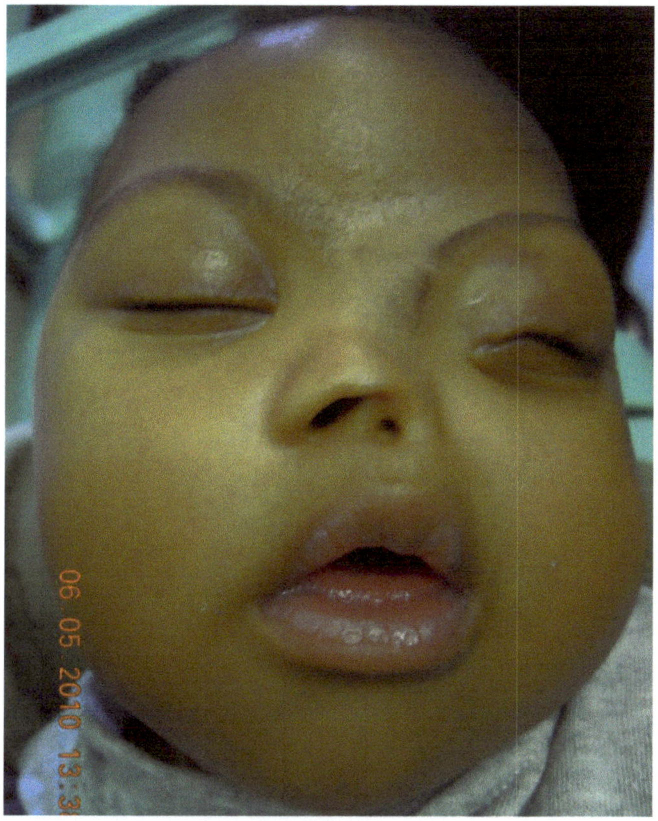

Fig. 24.10 Facial cleft 2

demonstrate facial cleft 2 with the design of repair and postoperative views. The facial cleft 2 spectrum includes various degrees of nasal hypoplasia and agenesis. This may present clinically as a proboscis, heminasal agenesis, or total arhinia (Figs. 24.15 and 24.18). If there is a substantial proboscis present, this can be repositioned and used to reconstruct the nose (Fig. 24.16). For heminasal agenesis, one could use a turnover skin flap of the normal ala to provide lining for the affected side. The skin cover for the entire tip is provided by a forehead flap in keeping with the nasal subunit principle of reconstruction (Fig. 24.17). In the rare case of total arhinia, the reconstruction is predicated on the intent to create patent nasal passages. The creation of nasal passages is challenging and involves drilling of the bone to create a tunnel which has to be lined by a flap or graft. Even if this is successful, stenosis of the neopassage is a frequent complication. The lining can be created by turnover flaps, while some authors prefer a free tissue transfer as the first stage. Costal cartilage and bone grafts are used to provide support for the nasal dorsum and the ala, nasal tip, and columella. The skin cover is best done with a forehead flap which may be pre-expanded to recruit more skin (Fig. 24.18). An alternative method for nasal reconstruction in these cases is prefabrication of a nose on the forehead or on the forearm as a free flap.

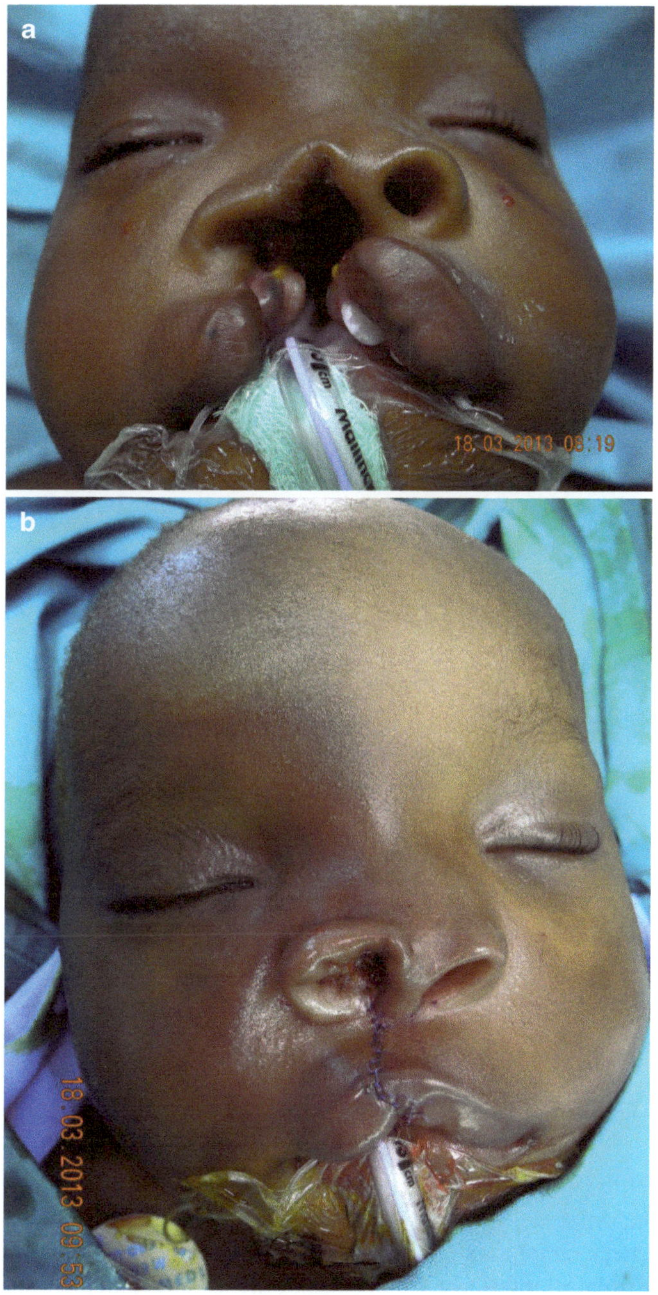


Fig. 24.11 (a) Facial cleft 1 and cleft lip pre-op. (b) Post-op

## Facial Cleft 3

Of the medial clefts, the number 3 cleft is the most common. In this cleft the alar base is affected and displaced in a cranial and lateral direction. The height of the ala cartilage is also deficient. The cleft continues into the lower eyelid. The cleft begins between the philtral column and the floor of the nose. There is deficiency of tissue between the alar base and the lower eyelid thereby shortening the nose on this side. It continues between the medial canthus and the inferior lacrimal punctum; the lacrimal system is disrupted. As such, blockage

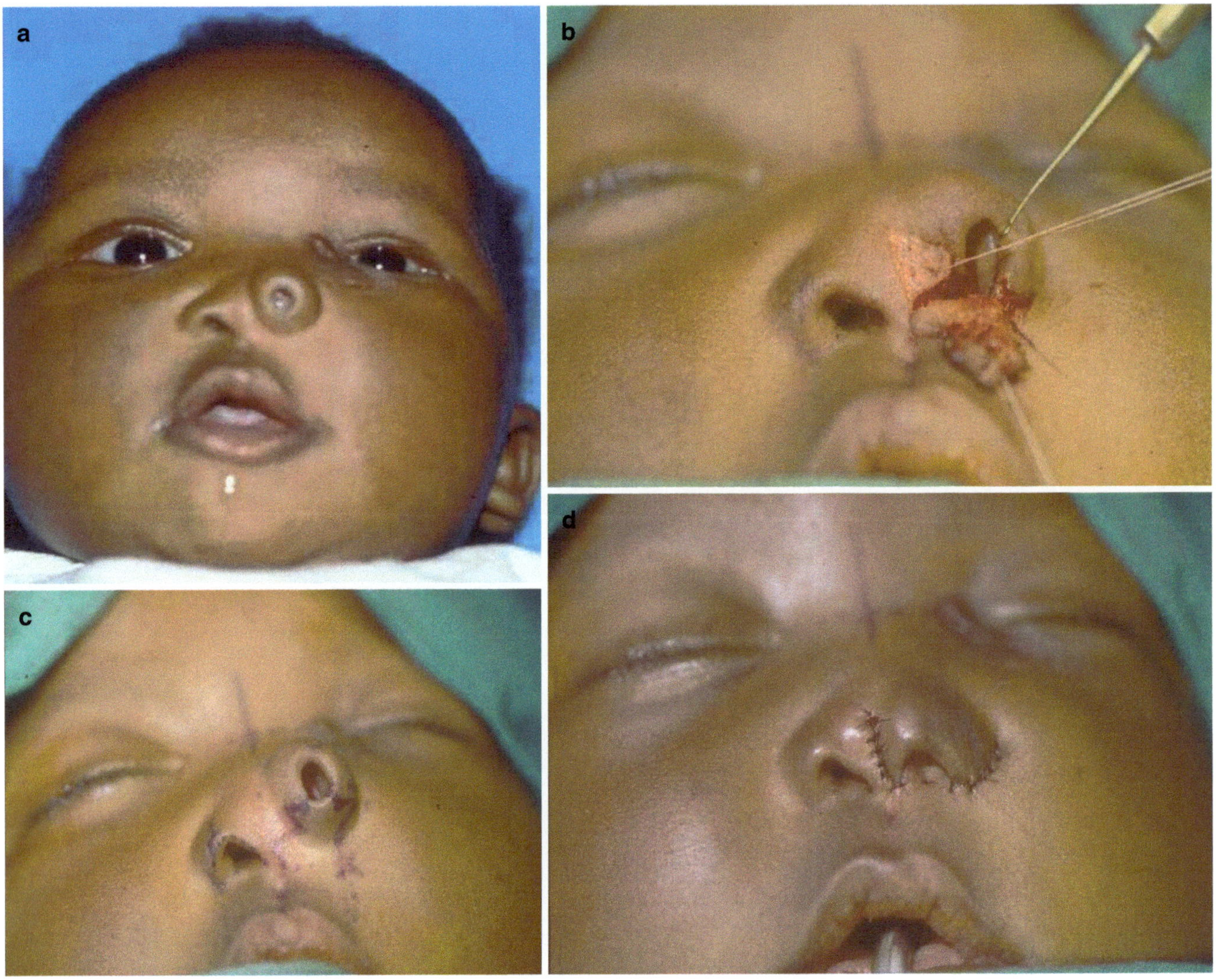


Fig. 24.12 (**a**) Facial cleft 2 pre-op. (**b**) Design of repair. (**c**) Intraoperative view. (**d**) Immediate post-op view

of the nasolacrimal duct results in recurrent infections of the lacrimal sac. The lower punctum may drain directly onto the cheek rather than into the nasal cavity. The medial canthus is displaced inferiorly. Colobomas of the lower eyelid are seen and are medial to the inferior punctum. The eye is malpositioned inferiorly and laterally. One must check for corneal erosions, ocular perforation, and loss of vision from corneal dessication. Globe protection is paramount.

Skeletally, there is direct communication between the oral, nasal, and orbital cavities. Dentally, it begins between the lateral incisor and canine. The anterior maxillary arch is flat as opposed to the keel-shape of the number 1 and 2 clefts.

### Surgical Considerations

The aim of surgery is to reconstruct the ala, the lower eyelid, and cheek and to perform a medial canthoplasty. The distance between the medial canthus and the ala base is significantly decreased compared to the normal side. One must aim to release and reposition the alar base to the level of the normal side. Flaps need to be designed to fit the anticipated resultant defect. Madaree et al. described a useful multi-flap technique to correct facial cleft 3 with camouflaging of scars in the lateral cheek/nasal junction and the superior ala groove (Figs. 24.1z and 24.19) [3]. Figure 24.20 demonstrates another patient with a long-term result. A cheek/cervicofacial flap (+/– tissue expander, if available) is an alternative technique that can be considered (Fig. 24.21).

## Facial Cleft 4

This cleft is lateral to the nose and median facial structures. The difference between facial cleft 4 and 3 is that here, the cleft in the lip commences lateral to the philtral column and the alar base is normal although it may be displaced. The orbicularis oris muscle is present in the lateral lip element, with no muscle medially. The cleft continues lateral to the nasal ala. There is no direct disfigurement of the nose or ala; however, the nose is displaced superiorly, particularly upon bilateral involvement. There may be a defect through the cheek and the lower eyelid. The medial canthus and nasolacrimal system are normal. Microphthalmia and anophthalmos may be seen.

Dentally, the cleft is between the lateral incisor and the canine. It continues through the facial skeleton extending lateral to the pyriform aperture into the maxillary sinus. There is direct connection between the oral cavity, maxillary sinus, and orbit, with an absence of the orbital floor. As such, the globe may be partially lying in the maxillary cavity (Fig. 24.22). The nasal cavity is not involved. The cleft is medial to the infraorbital foramen – this distinguishes the

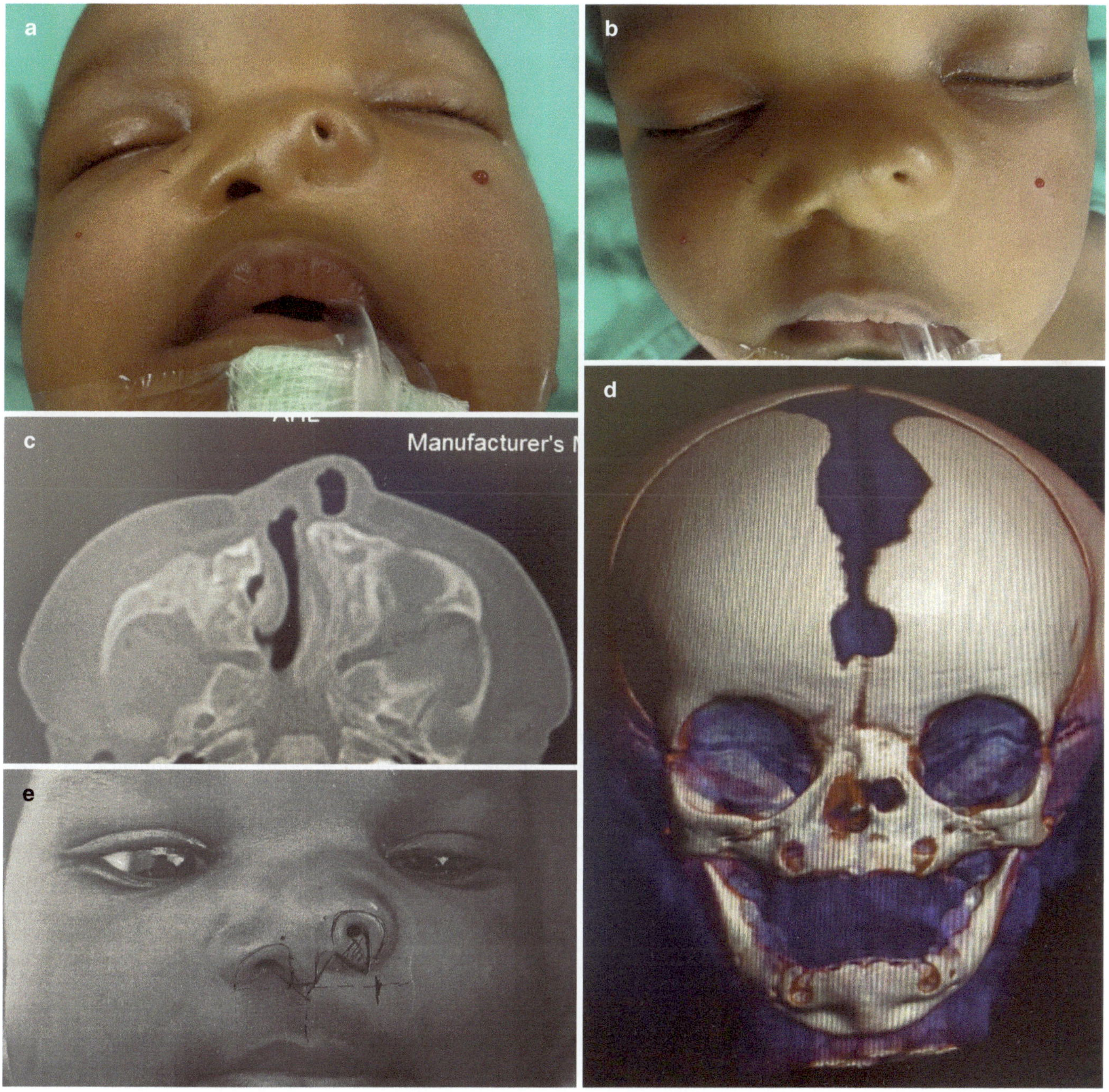


Fig. 24.13 (**a**,**b**)Facial cleft 2. (**c**,**d**) CT scan. (**e**) Planning of surgery on paper. (**f**) On table design of flap. (**g**) 2 week post-op view

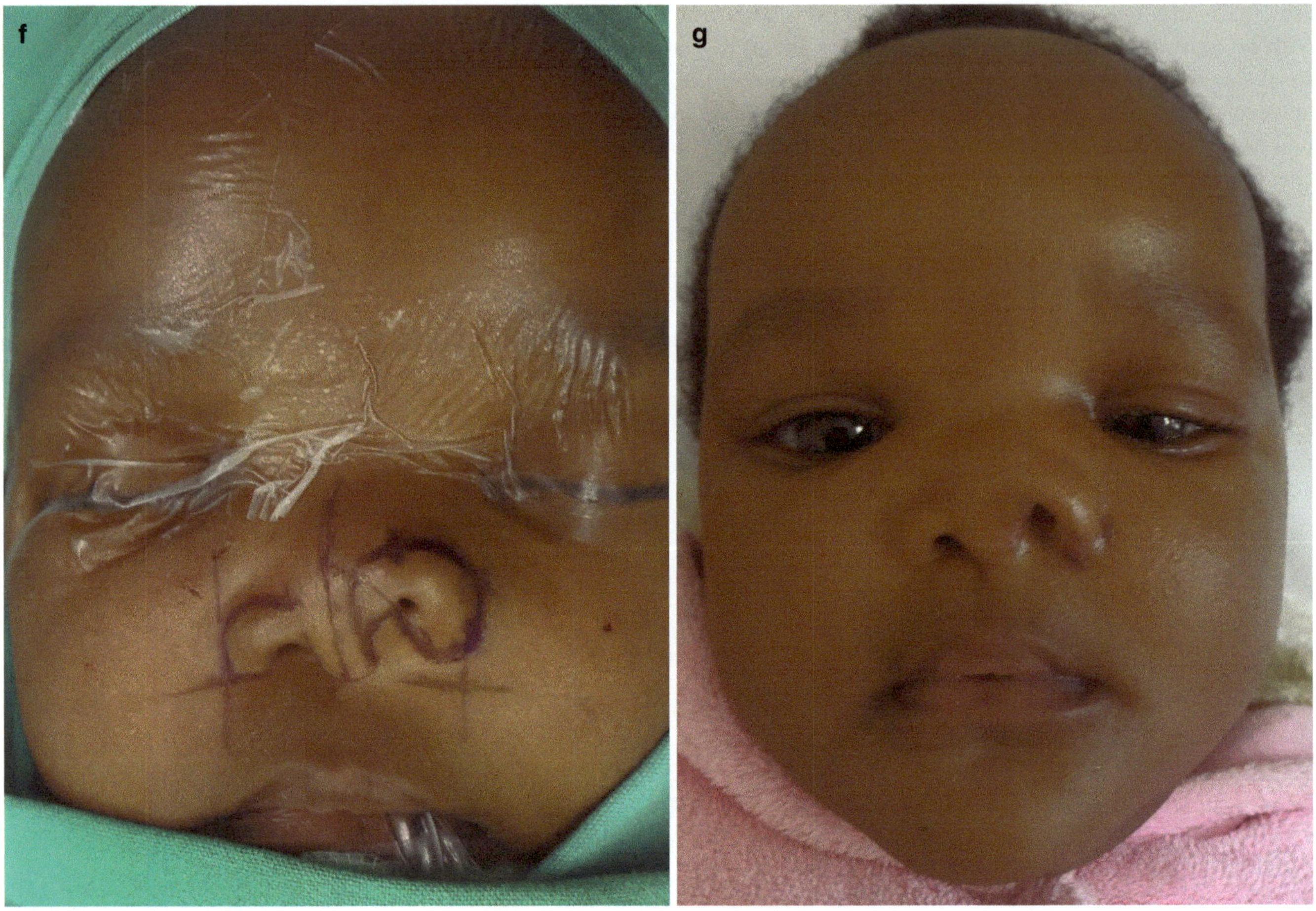


Fig. 24.13 (continued)

number 4 and number 5 clefts. The number 4 cleft terminates at the medial inferior orbital rim.

### Surgical Considerations

The surgical correction is similar to that of a facial cleft 3.However if there is a deficiency or absence of the orbital floor, one needs to design flaps that will separate the orbital and oral cavities. This may require the additional use of a bone or cartilage graft to provide support. Figure 24.22 demonstrates the reconstructive stages and the long-term result. Alonso et al. report on a large series of 21 cases of facial cleft 4 [4].

## Facial Cleft 5

The number 5 cleft is the rarest of the facial clefts. The cleft starts medial to the oral commissure and extends to the lower eyelid lateral to the inferior orbital nerve (Fig. 24.23). Racz et al. report on the phenotypic spectrum of this cleft, and da Silva Freitas et al. report on six cases of this rare cleft [5, 6].Skeletally, the cleft begins in the alveolus lateral to the canine in the region of the premolars. It then courses lateral to the infraorbital foramen and terminates in the lateral aspect of the orbital rim and floor. There may be prolapse of the orbital contents through the lateral orbital floor defect into the maxillary sinus, causing vertical orbit dystopia.

### Surgical Considerations

The soft tissue correction is aimed at reconstruction of the cheek. Although it may be relatively easy to close the skin defect, there is often a deficiency of soft tissue. After repair one may still be left with a furrow, and consideration must be given for a fat transfer as a secondary procedure.

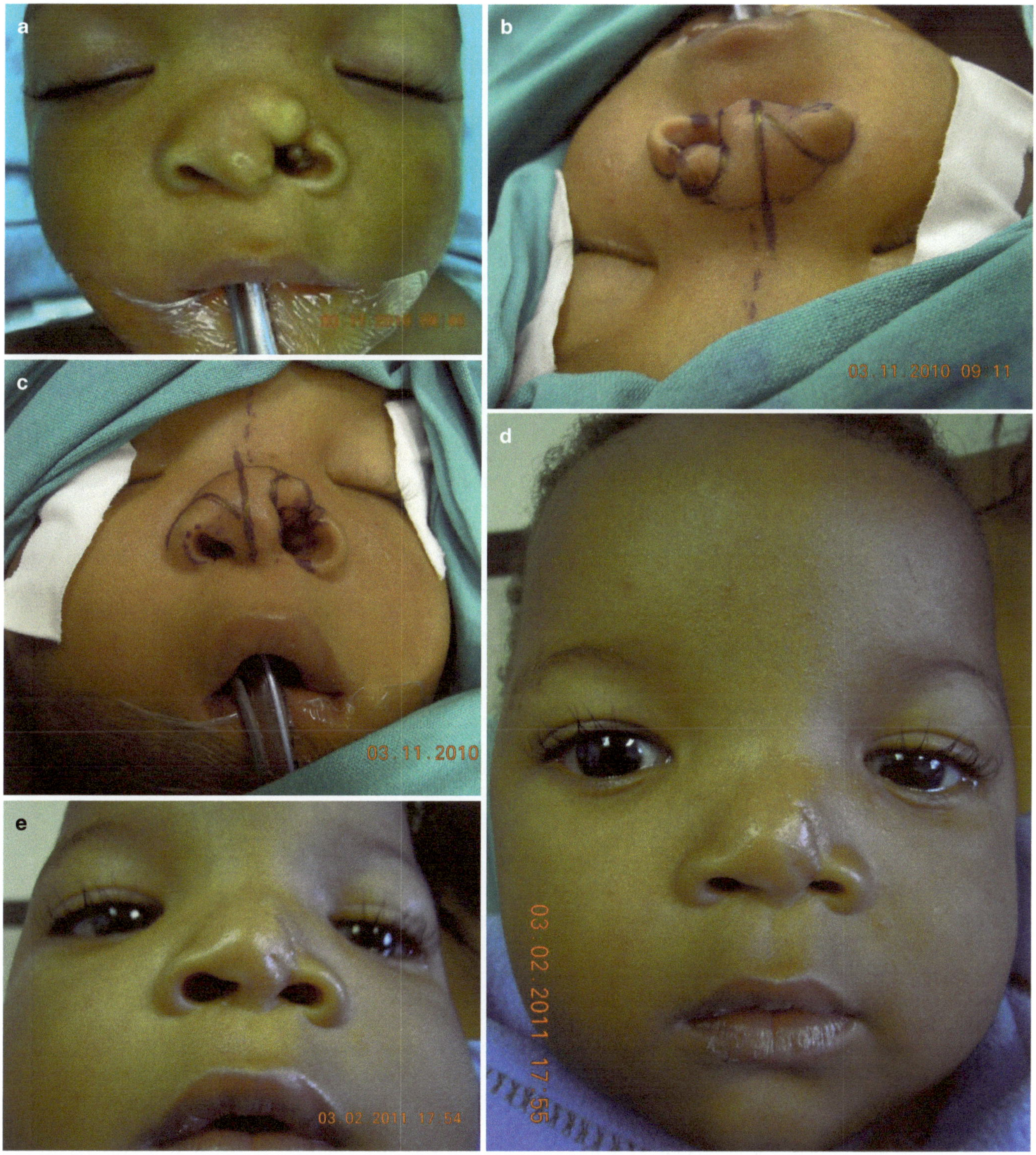


**Fig. 24.14** (**a**) Facial cleft 1. (**b**,**c**) Intraoperative design. (**d**,**e**) 3 month post-op

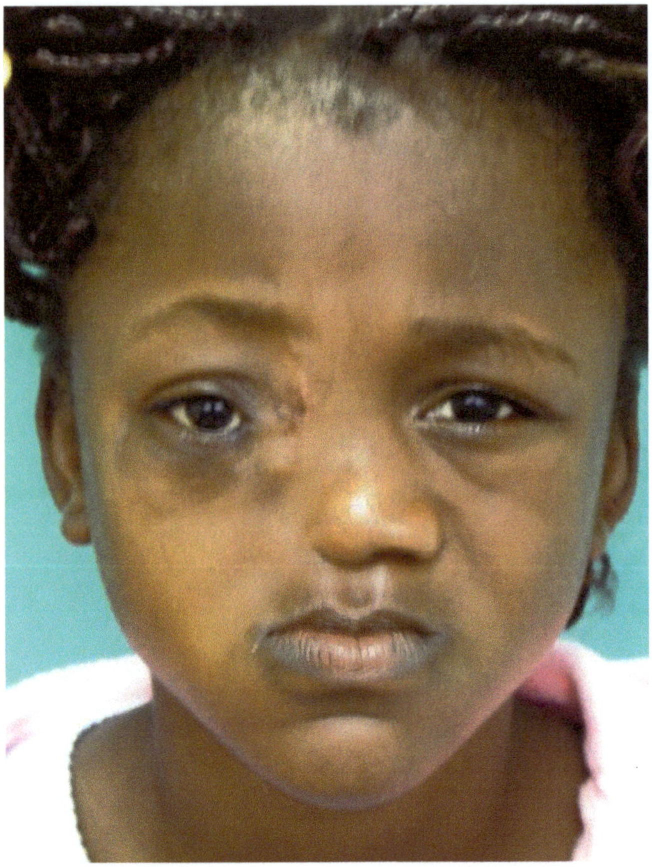

**Fig. 24.15** Facial cleft 2 with heminasal agenesis

## Facial Cleft 6

The number 6 cleft is a zygomaticomaxillary cleft and may represent an incomplete form of Treacher Collins syndrome. This is also a rare cleft in isolation. The soft tissue defect runs from the lateral lower eyelid toward the angle of the mandible. It is rare to have a defect in the skin.

The hallmark of this cleft is a vertical furrow from the oral commissure to the lateral lower eyelid. There may be a lower lid ectropion and antimongoloid slant due to the inferior displacement of the lateral canthus. There may also be a coloboma in the lateral lower eyelid.

Skeletally, the number 6 cleft penetrates the zygomaticomaxillary suture which separates the maxilla and zygoma. It does not involve the alveolus. The cleft connects to the inferior orbital fissure and terminates in the orbit at the lateral third of the orbital rim and floor. The zygoma is hypoplastic, though there is an intact zygomatic arch.

### Surgical Considerations

Reconstruction is aimed at correction of the soft tissue defect and may include the use of fat transfer. If there is a coloboma of the lower eyelid, this is repaired. Figure 24.20 demonstrates a facial cleft 6 on the left side and the long-term result after surgery is shown in Figs. 24.20 and 24.21.

## Facial Cleft 7

The number 7 cleft is the most common craniofacial cleft. It represents the temporozygomatic facial cleft and has had many other descriptive terms including craniofacial microsomia, hemifacial microsomia, otomandibular dysostosis, first and second branchial arch syndrome, Goldenhar syndrome, and macrostomia. This cleft is seen in Treacher Collins syndrome. There is an incidence of 1:5600 births. This cleft runs from the oral commissure in a lateral direction and may be unilateral or bilateral. Clinically this manifests as a macrostomia. In severe cases it can extend to the external auditory meatus (Fig. 24.24).

There is a variability of clinical expression, from a mild widening of the oral commissure with a preauricular skin tag, up to a complete fissure leading to a microtic ear. The parotid gland and duct may also be absent. There may also be facial nerve (cranial nerve VII) weakness. A range of external ear deformities may be seen from preauricular skin tabs to complete anotia [7].

From a skeletal standpoint, the posterior maxilla and mandibular ramus may be underdeveloped which creates a canted occlusal plane. The zygoma may be malformed, hypoplastic, and displaced. In the severe form, the zygomatic arch is malformed and may be a stump. Severe number 7 clefts can also cause orbital dystopia.

### Surgical Considerations

The goals of surgery:

1. Creation of a symmetrical oral aperture
2. Reconstruction of the commissures
3. Reconstruction of the modiolus
4. Correction of the vermilion and mucosa

In the case of a unilateral deformity, one should use the normal side as a template to design the reconstruction. A slight overcorrection is recommended. After the appropriate measurements and markings are made, key points are tattooed and a vasoconstrictor solution injected. An inci-

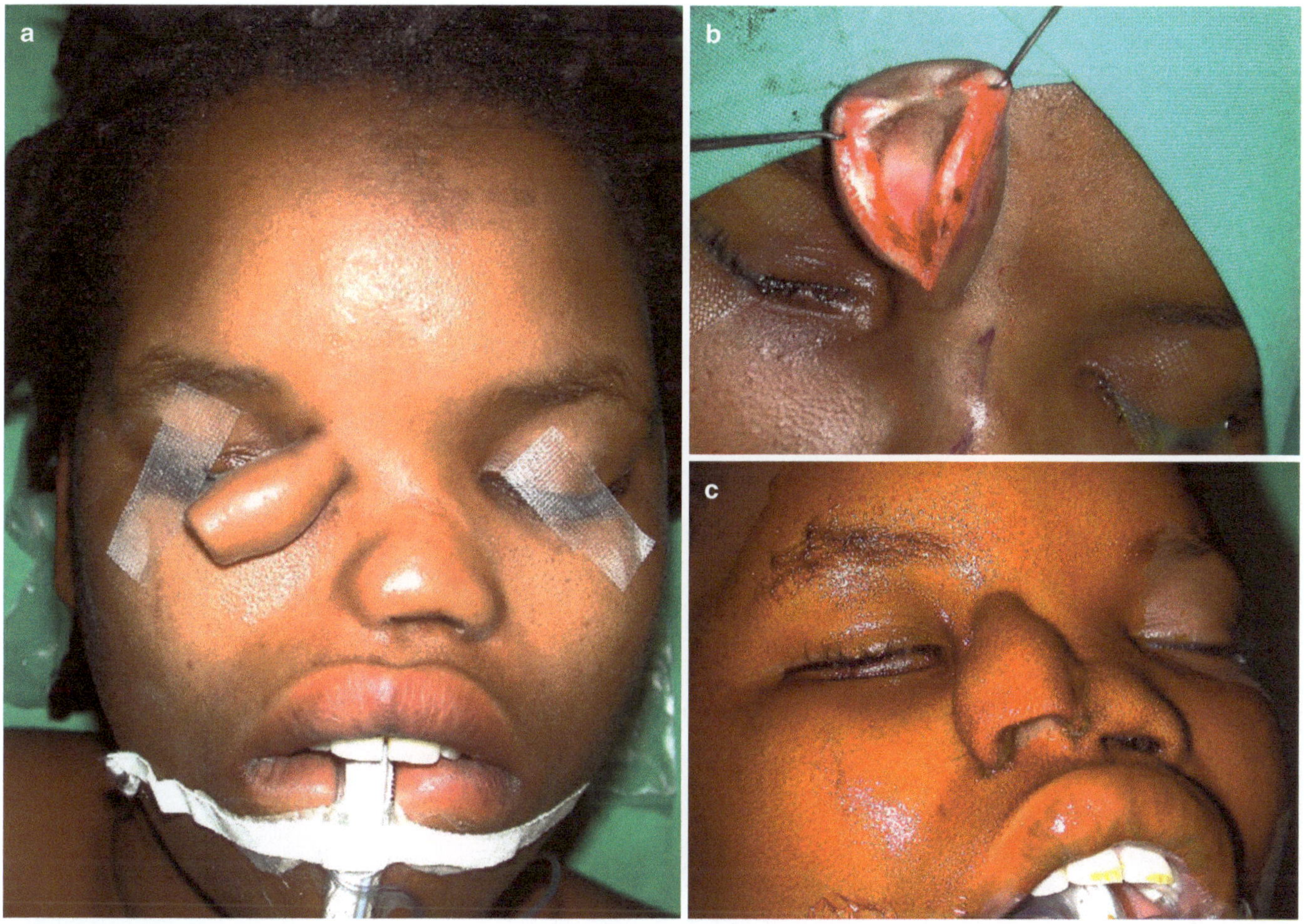

**Fig. 24.16** (**a**) Facial cleft 2 with proboscis. (**b**) Intraop view showing opening and advancement of proboscis. (**c**) Immediate post-op view

sion is made at the junction of the skin and vermilion border. Dissection proceeds to identify the orbicularis fibers in the upper and lower lips. The vermilion and mucosa is turned in and trimmed to close the mucosa. The modiolus is then reconstructed. The orbicularis of the lower lip is threaded through the fibers of the upper lip in a weave fashion. The skin is then closed in layers. A linear closure is preferable to that of a Z-plasty as this lies in a natural line and minimizes the extent of scars. In the unlikely event of a contracture forming, a Z-plasty may be considered as a revisional procedure (Fig. 24.24a,b,c). Tse et al. describe their method of repair with emphasis on subunit principle and meticulous muscle alignment [8].Rogers and Mulliken also emphasize the need to reconstruct the muscle with no need for a cutaneous Z-plasty [9].If there is a bilateral macrostomia, there is no normal side template to work from. In these cases, one has to use other landmarks such as the medial canthus. A vertical line dropped from this point is used to determine the position of the commissure (Fig. 24.25). Figure 24.1y shows incisional markings and reconstruction of the orbicularis oris sling, followed by lateral closure which can incorporate z-plasties to prevent contracture. Figure 24.26 demonstrates a 12-year follow-up of the patient in Fig. 24.27.

## Cranial Clefts

The cranial clefts are from 9 to 14. These may be associated with their facial counterparts adding up to 14. Thus the usual combination craniofacial clefts are 0/14, 1/13, 2/12, 3/11, 4/10, and 5/9. However one can also get unusual com-

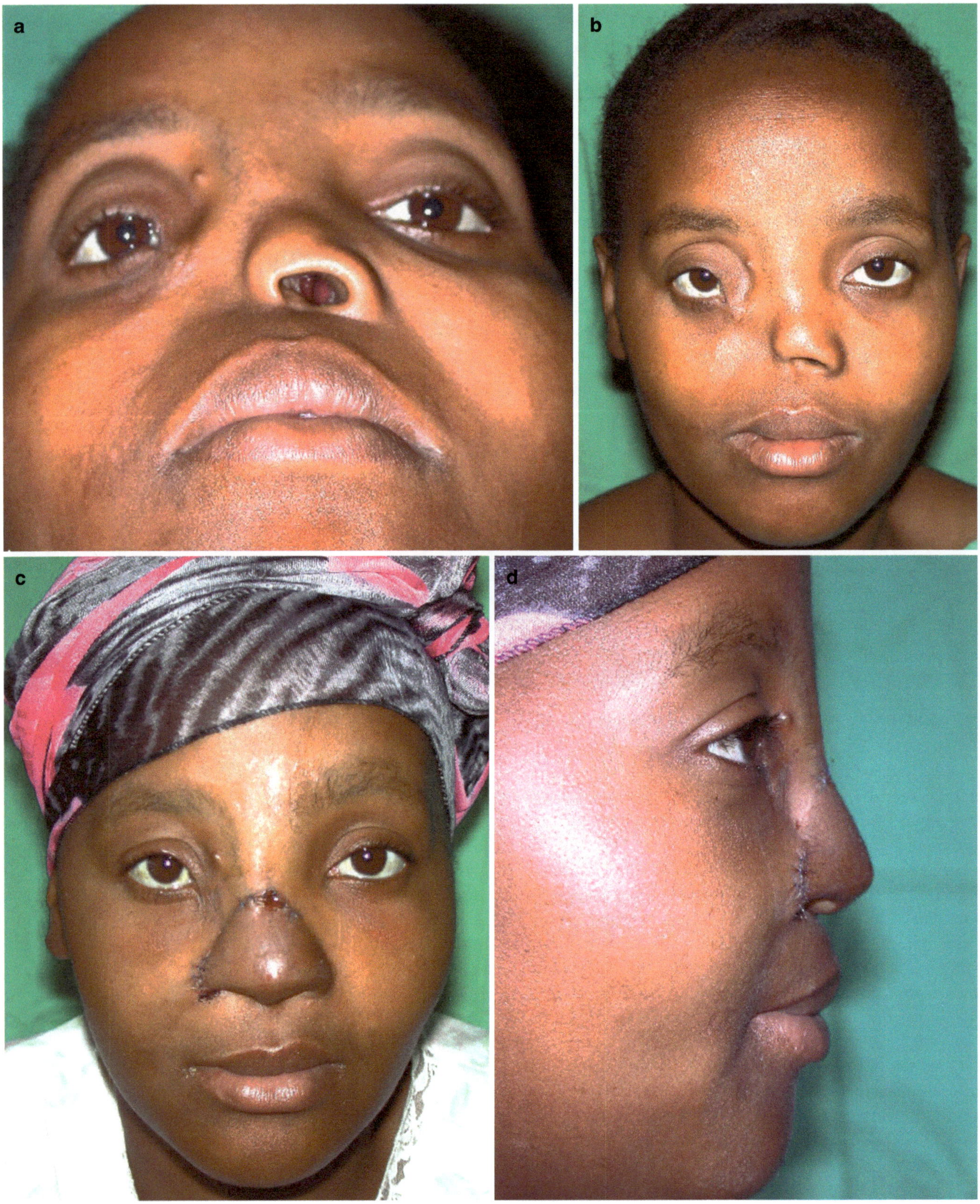


Fig. 24.17 (**a**,**b**) Facial cleft 2 with heminasal agenesis. (**c**,**d**) Forehead rhinoplasty after division

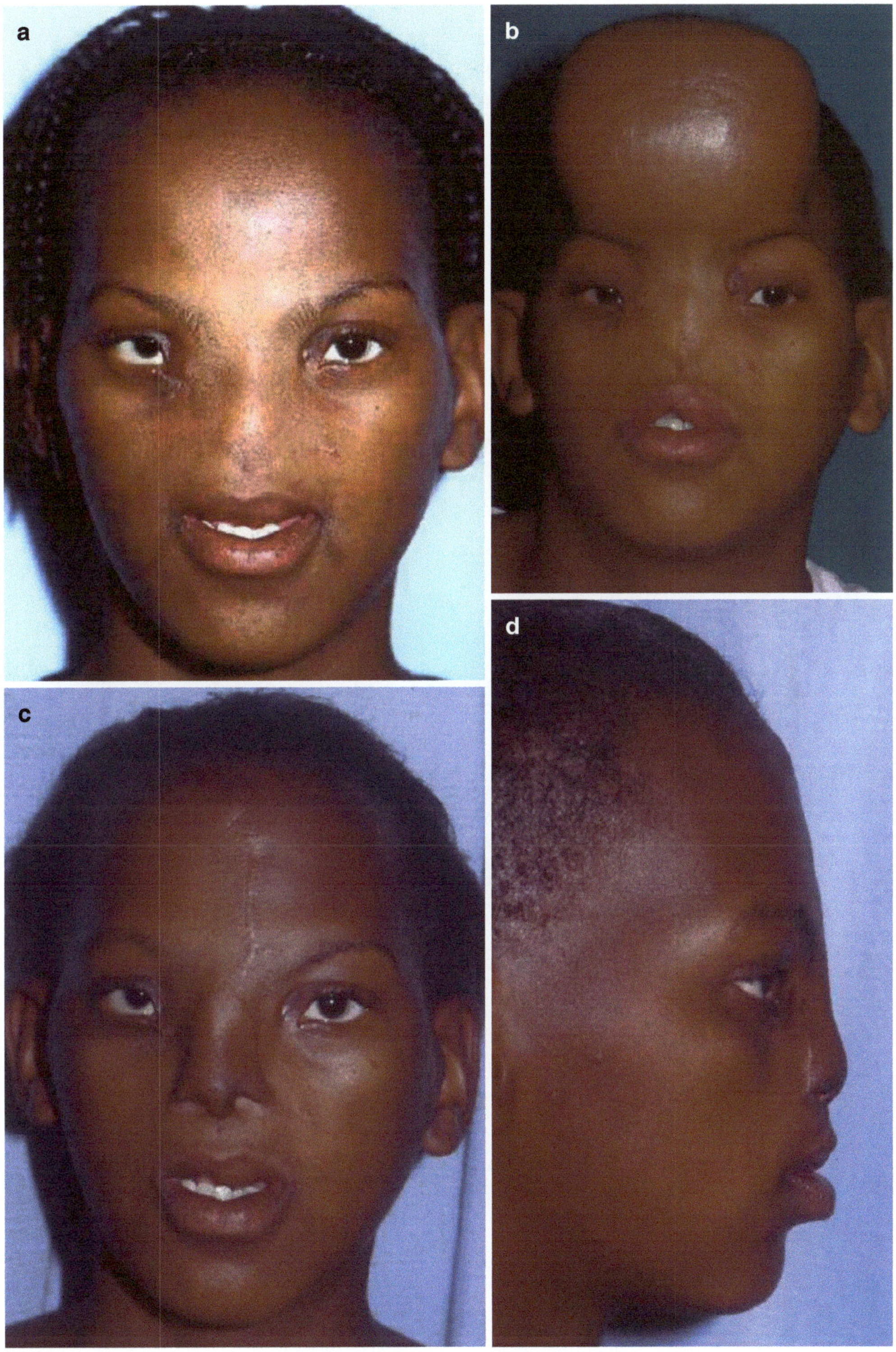


**Fig. 24.18** (**a**) Total arhinia. (**b**) Tissue expansion. (**c**,**d**) Post-op views

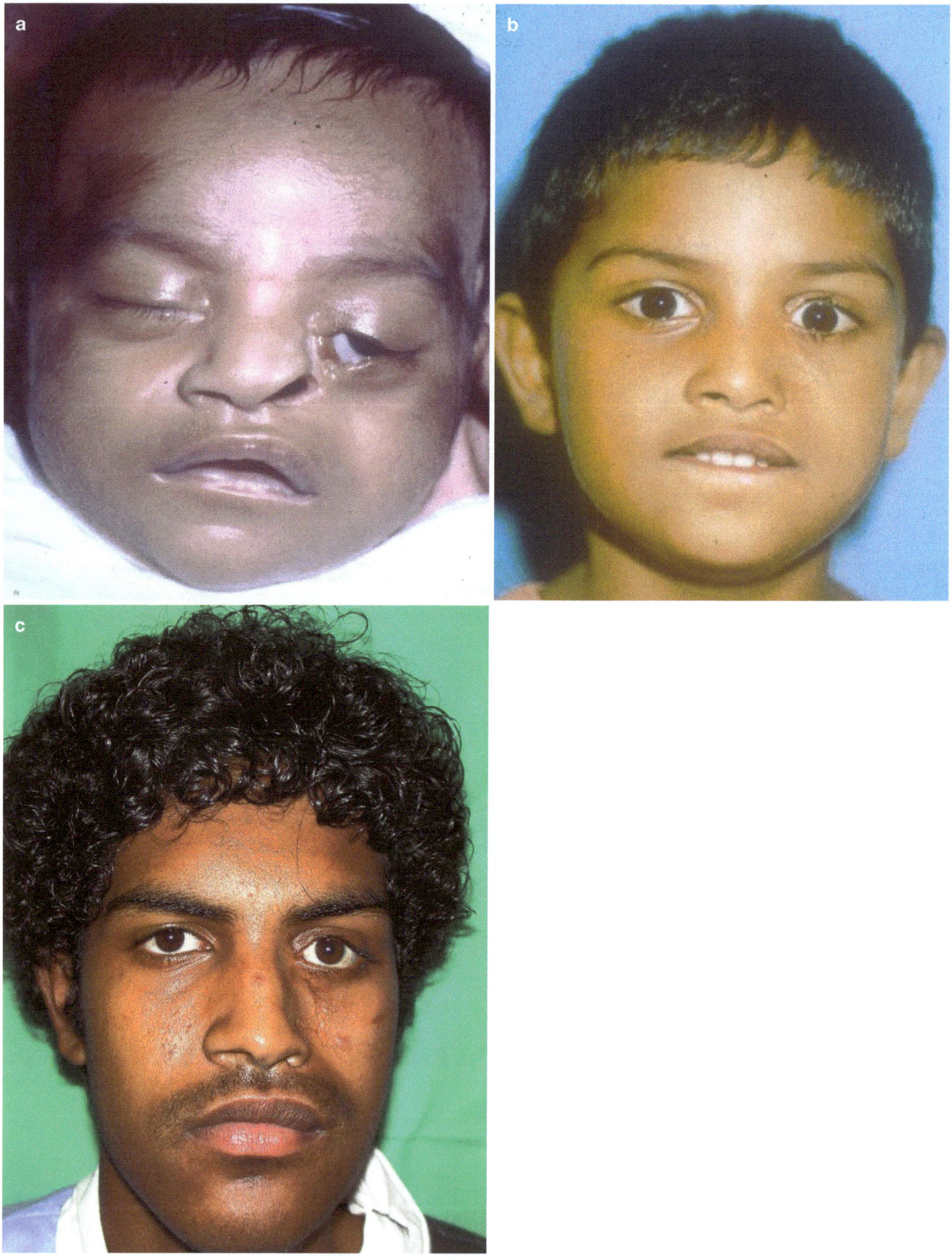


**Fig. 24.19** (**a**) Facial cleft 3. (**b**) 5-year post-op. (**c**) 20-year post-op

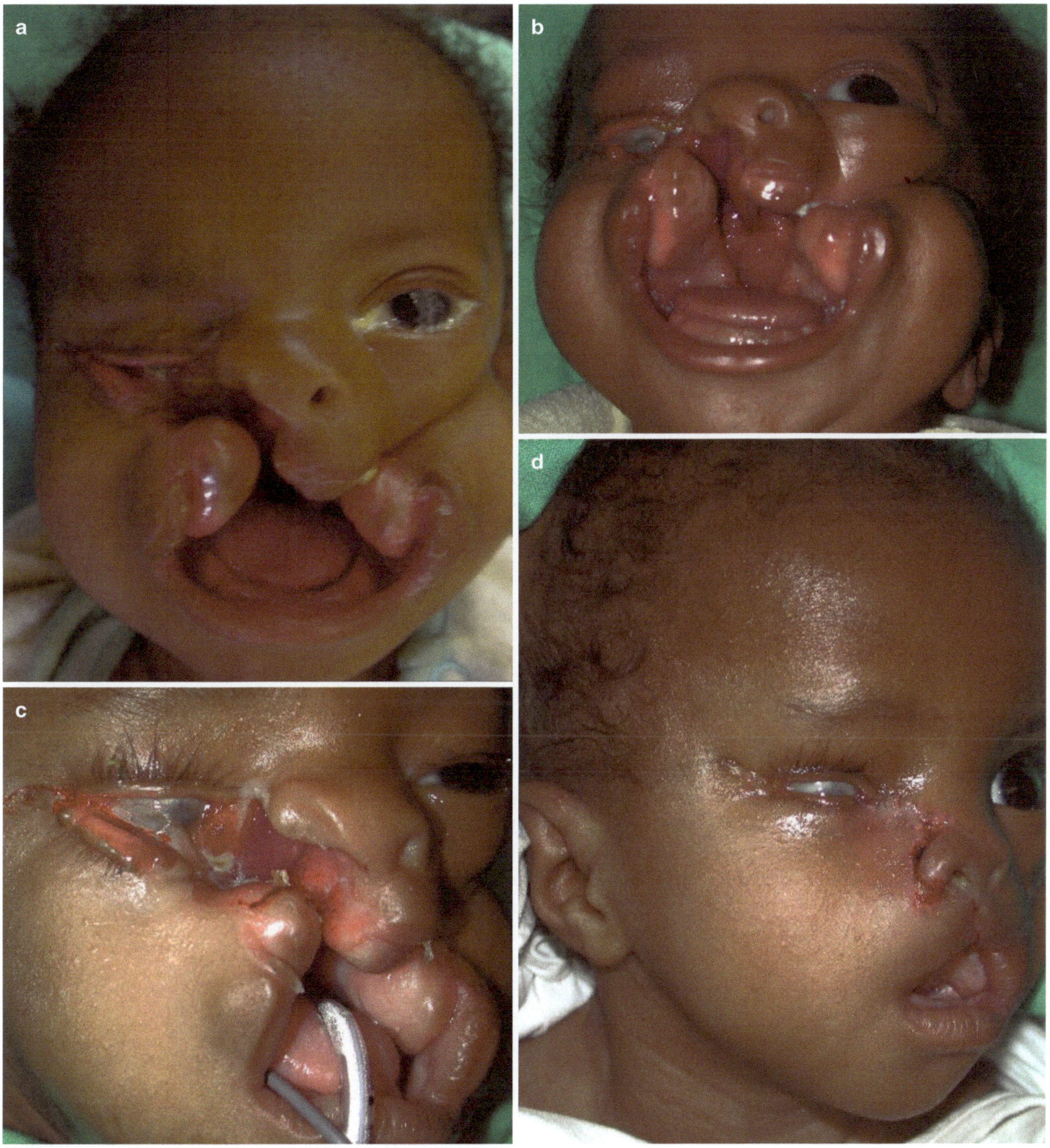


**Fig. 24.20** (**a**,**b**,**c**) Right side facial cleft 3. (**d**) 1-week post-op. (**e**) 10-year post-op

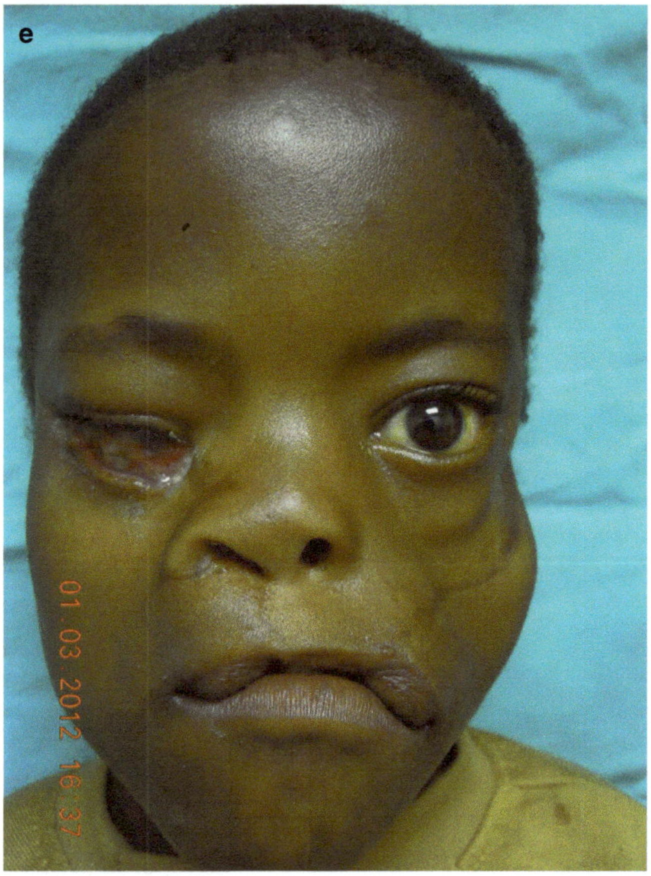


Fig. 24.20 (continued)

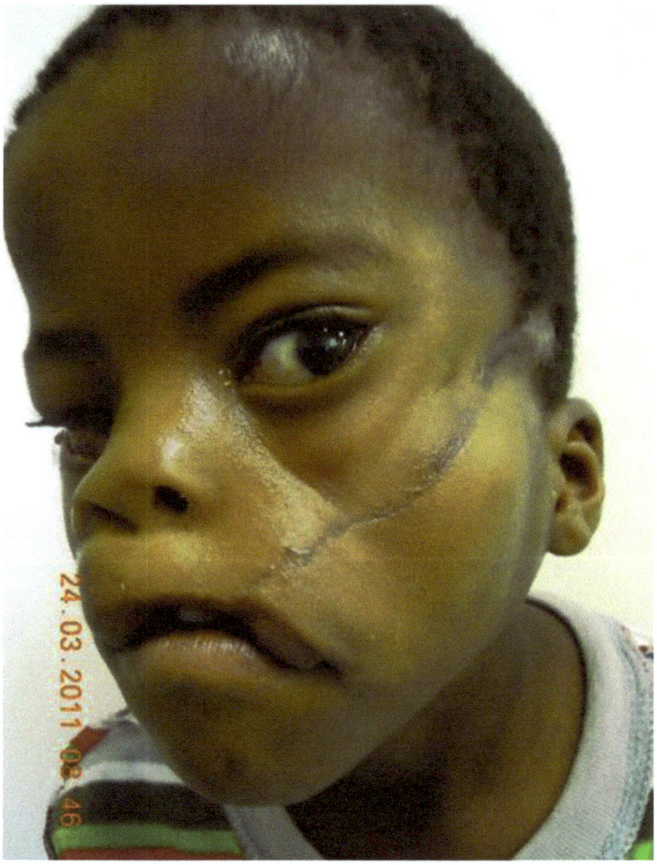

Fig. 24.21 Facial cleft 6 on left side 11 years post-op

binations which do not add up to 14. The cranial clefts may be associated with an encephalocoele. One often sees a deposit of fat on the dura underlying the defect in the bone. The appropriate surgery is performed to repair the encephalocoele and bone defect.

Cranial clefts can be unilateral or bilateral. They are often associated with hypertelorism. Correction of the soft tissue and bone may have to be staged. With regard to hypertelorism, the options for correction are orbital osteotomy (medial wall or box osteotomy) or facial bipartition (intracranial or subcranial).

## Facial Cleft 8

The number 8 cleft is a frontozygomatic cleft located at the lateral canthus. This cleft divides the facial clefts from the cranial clefts and is at the equator of Tessier clefts. It runs transversely from the lateral canthus to the temporal region. It rarely occurs as an isolated cleft (Fig. 24.28). There is a soft tissue malformation which presents as a true lateral commissure coloboma. Epibulbar dermoids are also often present, as in Goldenhar's syndrome.

### Surgical Considerations

This usually entails closure of the soft tissue and may require a lateral canthoplasty as well.

## Facial Cleft 6,7,8

These usually occur in combination and are invariably bilateral (Fig. 24.29). These are usually classified as Treacher Collins syndrome, and there is often a family history. Skeletally, the cleft is present at the zygomaticofrontal suture. In severe forms, the zygoma and lateral orbital wall may be missing.

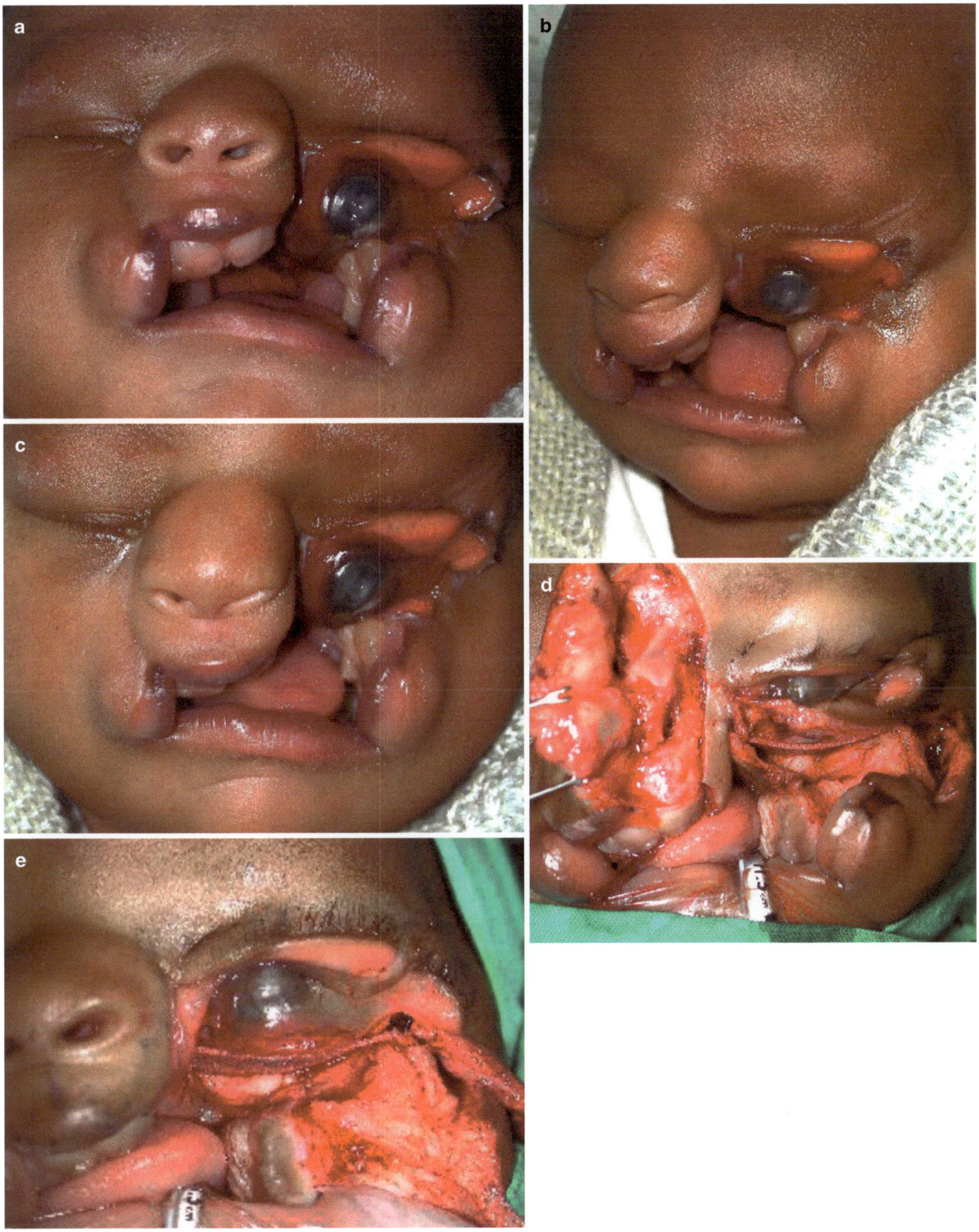


**Fig. 24.22** (**a**,**b**,**c**) Left facial cleft 4. (**d**,**e**) Intraop views. (**f**,**g**) Immediate post-op. (**h**) 10-year post-op

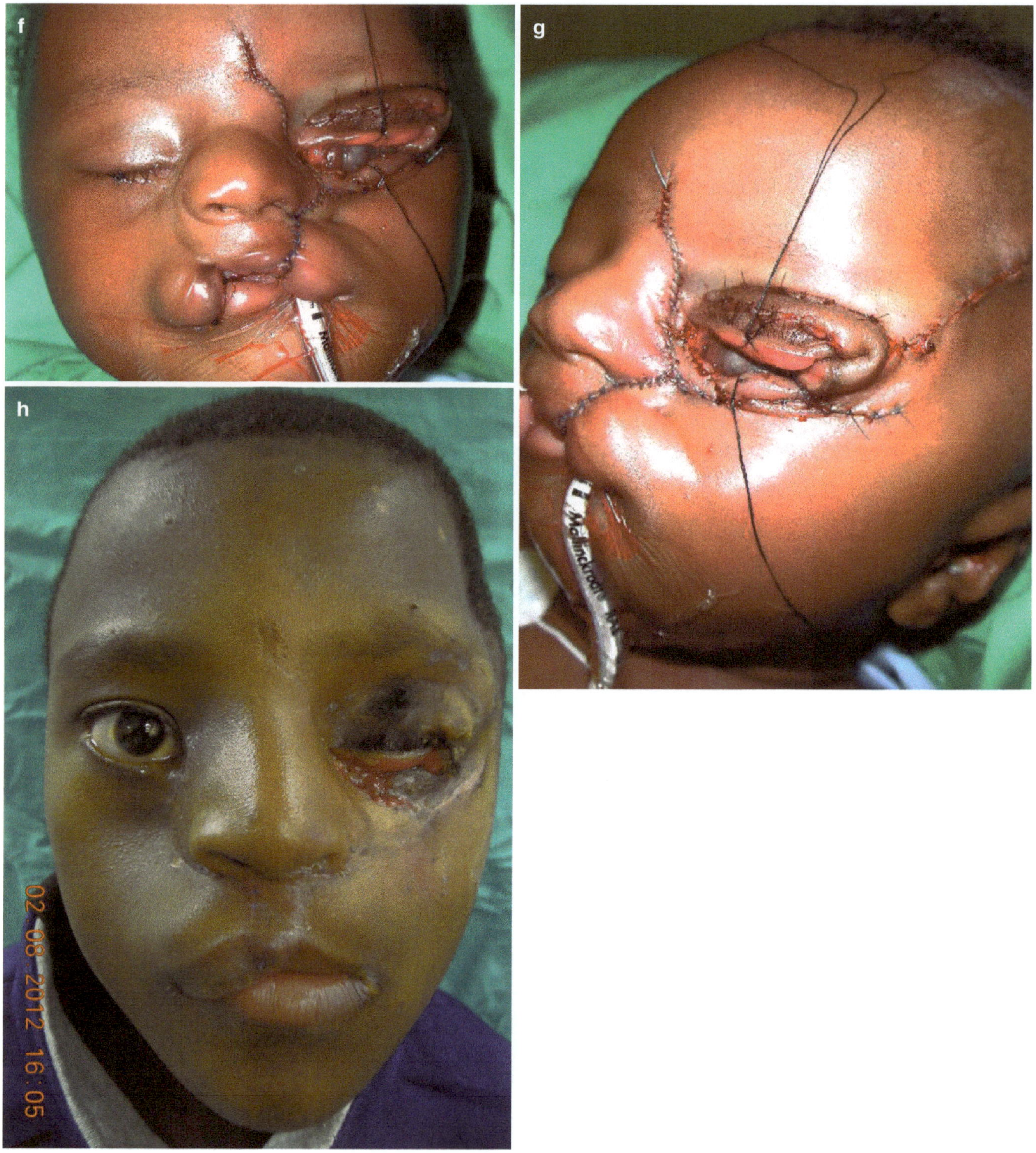


**Fig. 24.22** (continued)

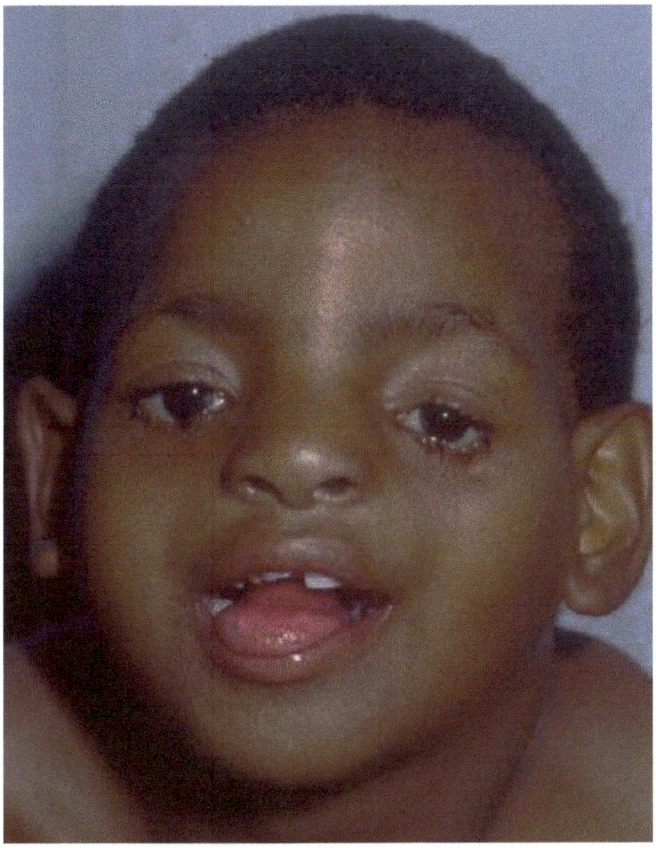

Fig. 24.23 Bilateral facial cleft 5

#### Surgical Considerations

The correction of these patients is not easy, and it is difficult to get predictable results. Repeat procedures may be needed. Options include:

1. Calvarial or rib grafts
2. Cartilage grafts
3. Pedicle temporal based flaps with or without calvarial bone or free tissue transfer
4. Distraction osteogenesis
5. Alloplastic augmentation
6. Fat transfer (Fig. 24.30)

### Facial Cleft 9

The number 9 cleft is quite rare and begins the medial movement through the cranial clefts. This is the first of the cranial clefts and runs obliquely in the lateral aspect of the upper eyelid. This may be just a coloboma or a full-thickness deficiency of the upper eyelid. There is lateral displacement of the globe due to orbital bony deficiency in the superolateral area. The lateral canthus is also displaced. The cleft extends into the temporoparietal hair-bearing scalp. There may be a palsy of the temporal branch of the facial nerve (cranial nerve VII).

#### Surgical Considerations

If there is a coloboma or a minor defect, a pentagonal wedge excision and reconstruction is indicated. If there is a more substantial defect, then other oculoplastic procedures may be indicated. These include tarsoconjunctival reconstruction with palatal mucosa or a nasal chondromucosal graft and a flap for skin coverage. A lid switch flap from the lower eyelid may also be used. Figure 24.31 demonstrates a patient after correction.

### Facial Cleft 10

The number 10 cleft is an upper central orbital cleft and is the cranial extension of a number 4 cleft. This cleft runs through the central part of the upper eyelid. There is often a deficiency of the eyelid with exposure of the globe (Fig. 24.32). The entire upper eyelid may be absent in its most severe form. Frontal hair projection may connect the temporoparietal region to the lateral brow.

Skeletally, the number 10 cranial cleft extends through the middle of the supraorbital rim, just lateral to the superior orbital foramen. This cleft is sometimes associated with an encephalocoele and bony defect in the mid-supraorbital region. There may be orbital hypertelorism in severe cases.

#### Surgical Considerations

The globe must be protected and an urgent procedure must be performed to reconstruct the upper eyelid. Depending on the extent and tissue laxity, this can be achieved by a lateral cantholysis and recruitment of tissue from tissue in the lateral canthal region. A semicircular flap designed in this region is usually successful to obtain closure. Figure 24.32 demonstrates the repair and result 20 years postoperatively.

### Facial Cleft 11

The number 11 cleft is an upper medial orbital cleft and is the cranial extension of the number 3 cleft. There may be

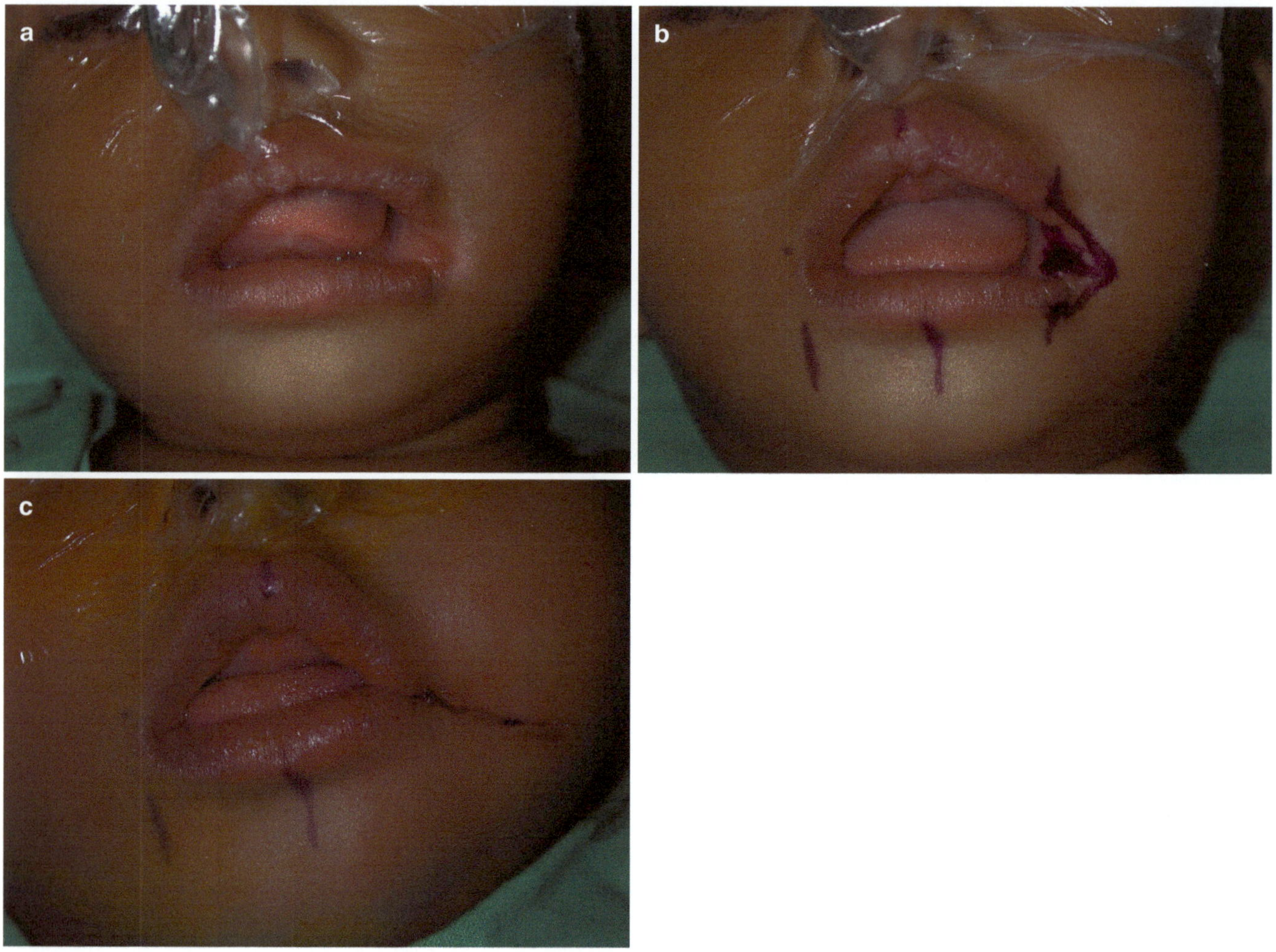

Fig. 24.24 (**a**) Facial cleft 7. (**b**) Intraop design. (**c**) Immediate post-op view

involvement of the medial third of the upper eyelid with a coloboma (Fig. 24.33). There may also be distortion of the upper eyebrow which extends up to the frontal hairline.

Skeletally, the cleft passes through the medial third of the supraorbital rim. Orbital hypertelorism may also be seen if the cleft passes through the ethmoid bone.

### Surgical Considerations

This is similar to the other upper lid facial clefts with the aim being reconstruction of the upper eyelid. Orbital bone surgery may be necessary.

## Facial Cleft 12

The number 12 cleft is medial to the medial canthus. Colobomas may extend to the medial aspect of the eyebrow. This cleft does not involve the upper eyelid. However it may result in a lateral and inferior displacement of the medial canthus (Fig. 24.34). The forehead skin is normal though there may be slight inferior displacement of the paramedian frontal hairline. From the skeletal aspect, the cleft ascends through the frontal process of the maxilla and travels superiorly to increase the size of the ethmoid sinus, producing orbital hypertelorism and telecanthus. The frontal and sphenoid sinuses are enlarged. Encephaloceles are not seen with this cleft.

### Surgical Considerations

This may include soft tissue correction, canthoplasty, or orbital bone surgery (Fig. 24.34).

## Facial Cleft 13

The number 13 cleft typically presents as a paramedian frontal encephalocele. This is located between the nasal bone and the frontal process of the maxilla. The eyelids and eyebrows

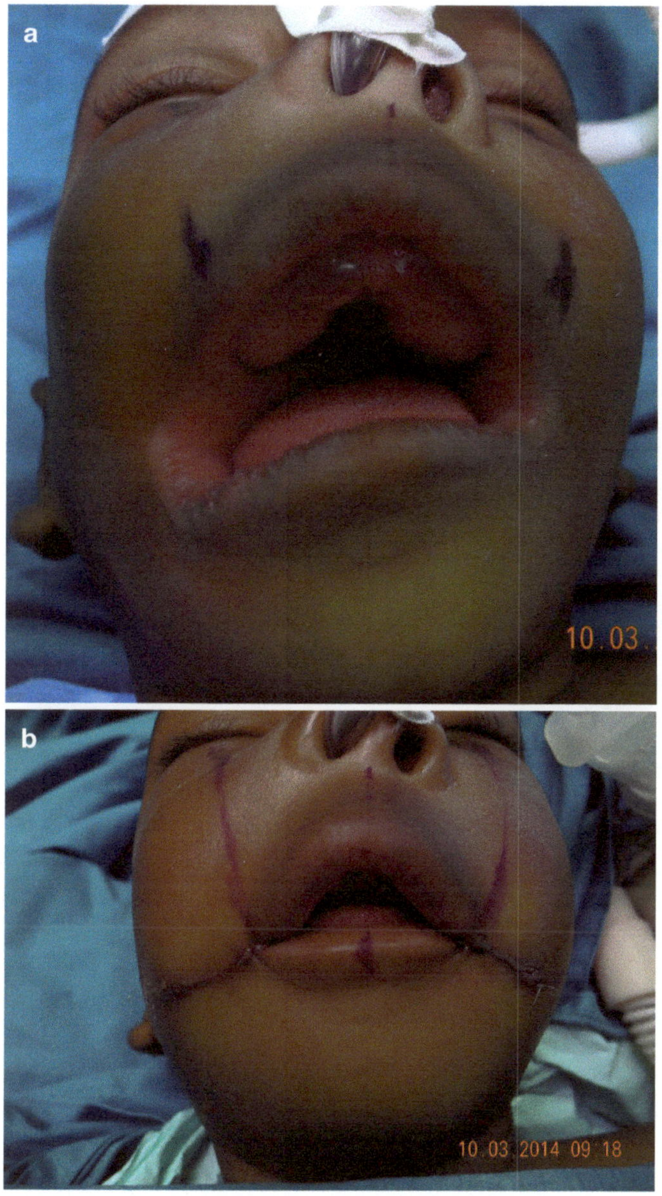


**Fig. 24.25** (**a**) Bilateral facial cleft 7. (**b**)Post-op views

are intact, and the cleft is located medial to this. This cleft is just off the midline (Fig. 24.35). Skeletally, the pathognomonic feature of this cleft is the effect on the cribriform plate. There is widening of the olfactory groove, the cribriform plate, and the ethmoid sinus, which results in hypertelorism.

### Surgical Considerations

This often entails bony orbital surgery. Figures 24.35, 24.36, and 24.37 demonstrate preoperative and postoperative cases of facial cleft 13.

## Facial Cleft 14

The number 14 cleft is present in the midline forehead and cranium and is thought of as an extension of number 0 clefts. Similarly, the soft tissue may be hypo- or hyper-plastic. A severe form of this cleft may be associated with severely limited life expectancy of hours to months. There may be orbital hypertelorism due to midline masses such as a frontonasal encephalocele (Fig. 24.38 and 24.39). There is often a bifid nose and poor dorsal nasal support. Skeletally, there is herniation of the intracranial contents through a medial frontal defect. The cribriform plate may be displaced caudally up to 20 mm [10]. The anterior cranial fossa slants upward, which is manifested in a harlequin eye deformity seen on x-ray.

### Surgical Considerations

Depending on the severity, the following procedures may be required:

1. Hypertelorism correction
2. Nasal reconstruction
3. Dorsal nasal augmentation with bone or cartilage grafts
4. Medial canthoplasty
5. Soft tissue reconstruction

Figures 24.40 and 24.41 illustrate preoperative, intraoperative, and postoperative results.

## Facial Cleft 30

Tessier made allowance for the discovery of new rare clefts that may occur in the lower face and lower lip. He described a facial cleft 30 as one that occurs in the midline of the lower lip. If other clefts are found in the lower face lateral to the midline presumably, they could be given a number between 15 and 29. Morritt et al. report on a case which may be a 28 or 29 [11].The facial cleft 30 may involve soft tissue, bone, or both. In its entirety, there is a midline cleft of the lower lip, a full-thickness defect of the mandible symphysis, a cleft or even duplication of the tongue, and a cleft of the floor of the mouth.

### Surgical Considerations

The repair can be undertaken at 3 months of age similar to a traditional cleft lip. The surgical plan is dependent on the severity and tissues involved. The cleft in the lower lip is repaired simply by paring the edges and suturing the lip elements in a transverse direction. If the vertical height of

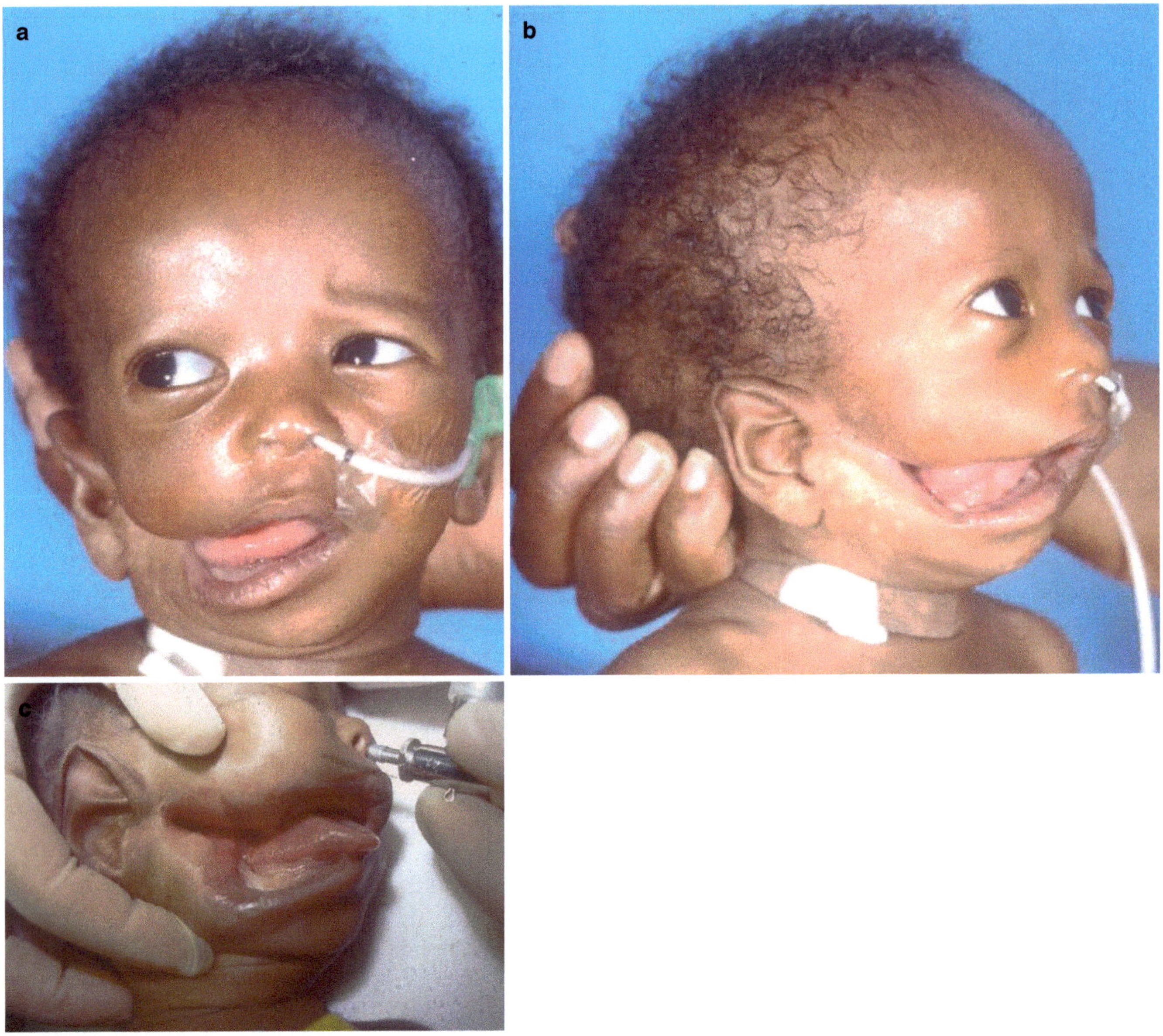

Fig. 24.26 (a–c) Facial cleft 7 with extension into middle ear - preoperative

the lip is short or if a contracture is anticipated, a Z-plasty is performed. If there is a defect in the mandible, the bone edges are freshened and fixed to each other with dental wire or a resorbable plate. If the tongue is duplicated, a longitudinal medial portion of each tongue is resected to allow reconstruction of a single tongue of adequate width. Figure 24.42 demonstrates a case of facial cleft 30 which was done in a mission setting with no power tools available. A hypodermic needle was used to make holes in the two halves of the mandible which was then fixed with dental wires.

## Anesthesia

Repair of rare craniofacial clefts routinely requires general anesthesia. There may be circumstances in older teenage or adult patients who have less extensive soft tissue deformity that may be amenable to repair under local anesthesia. Most often, orotracheal intubation is the mode of choice.

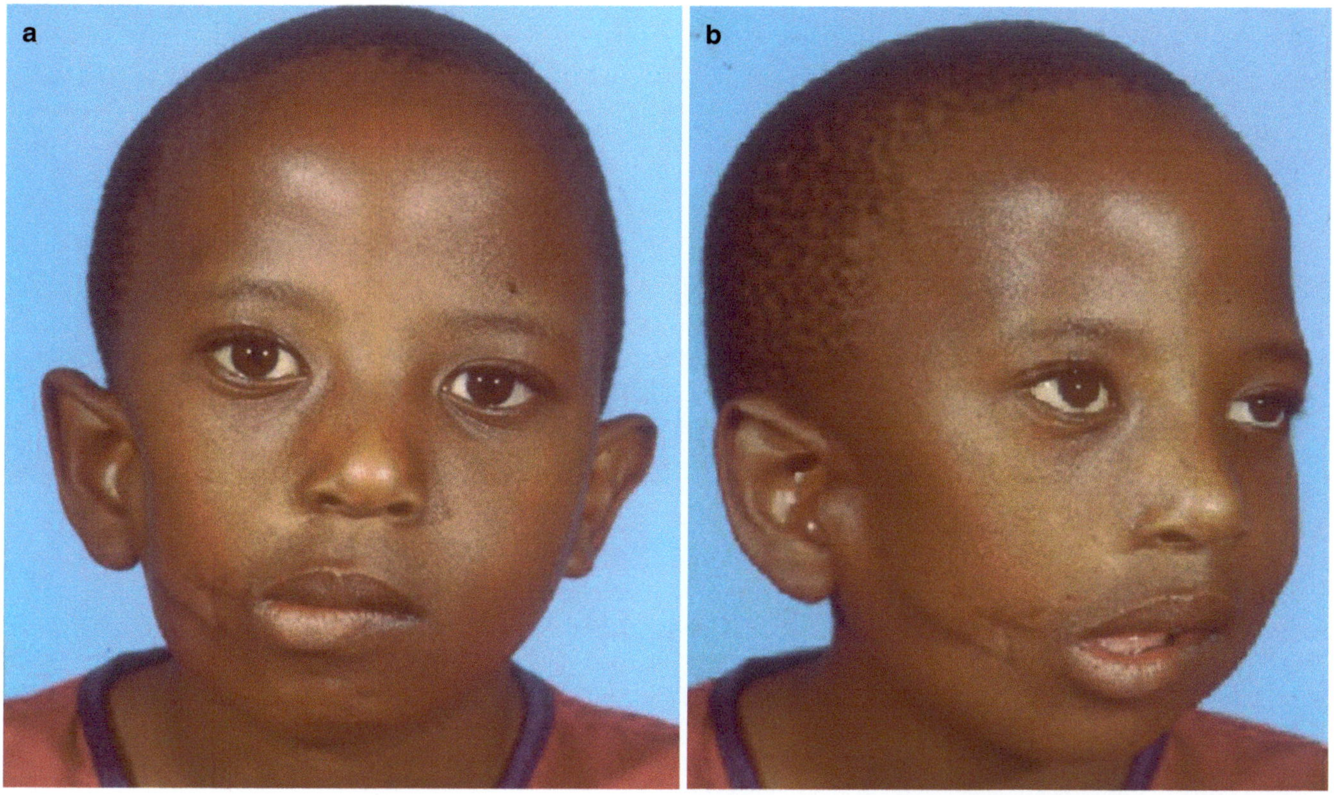


Fig. 24.27 (**a**, **b**) Long term post-operative result of repair of facial cleft 7

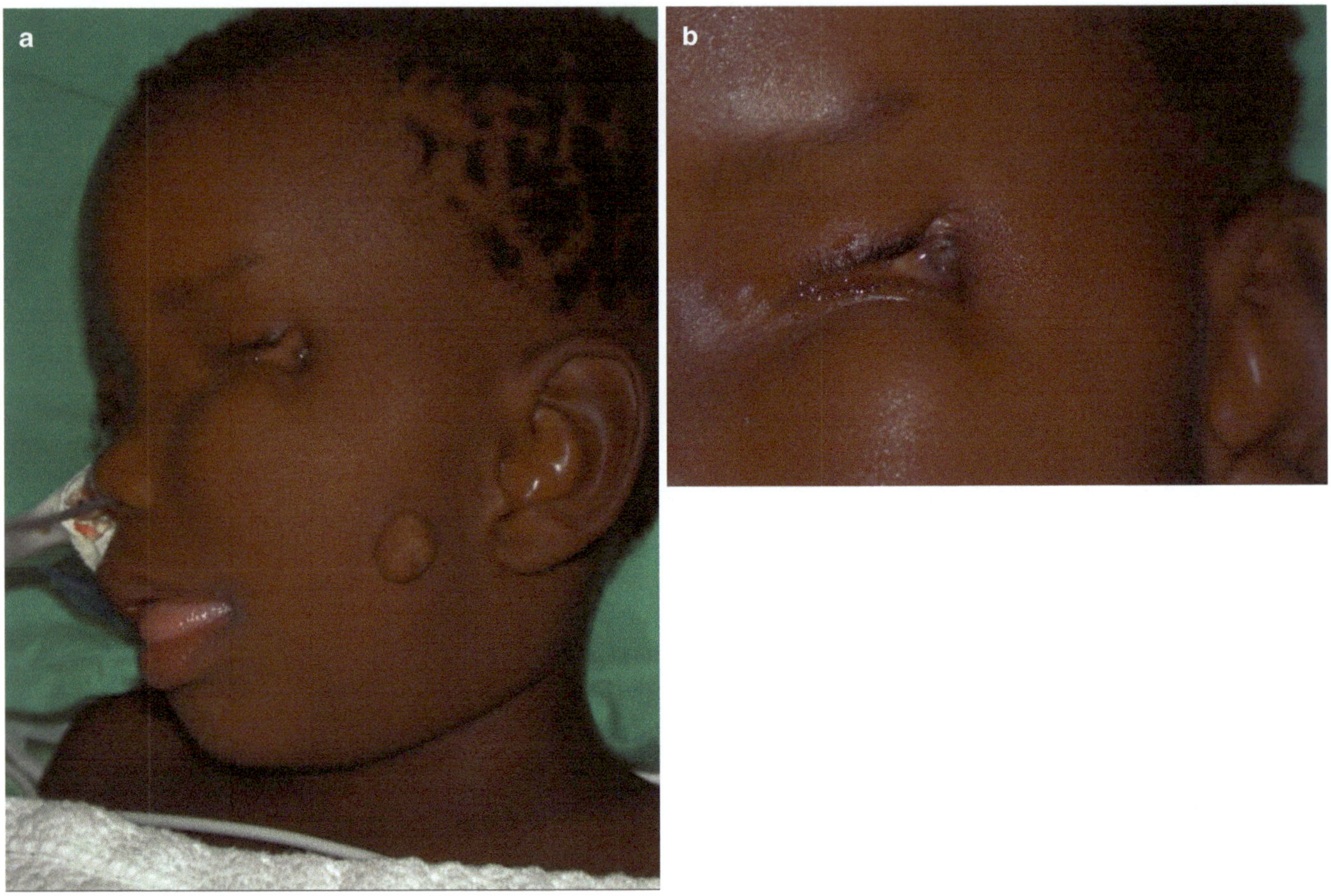

**Fig. 24.28** (**a**,**b**) Facial cleft 8

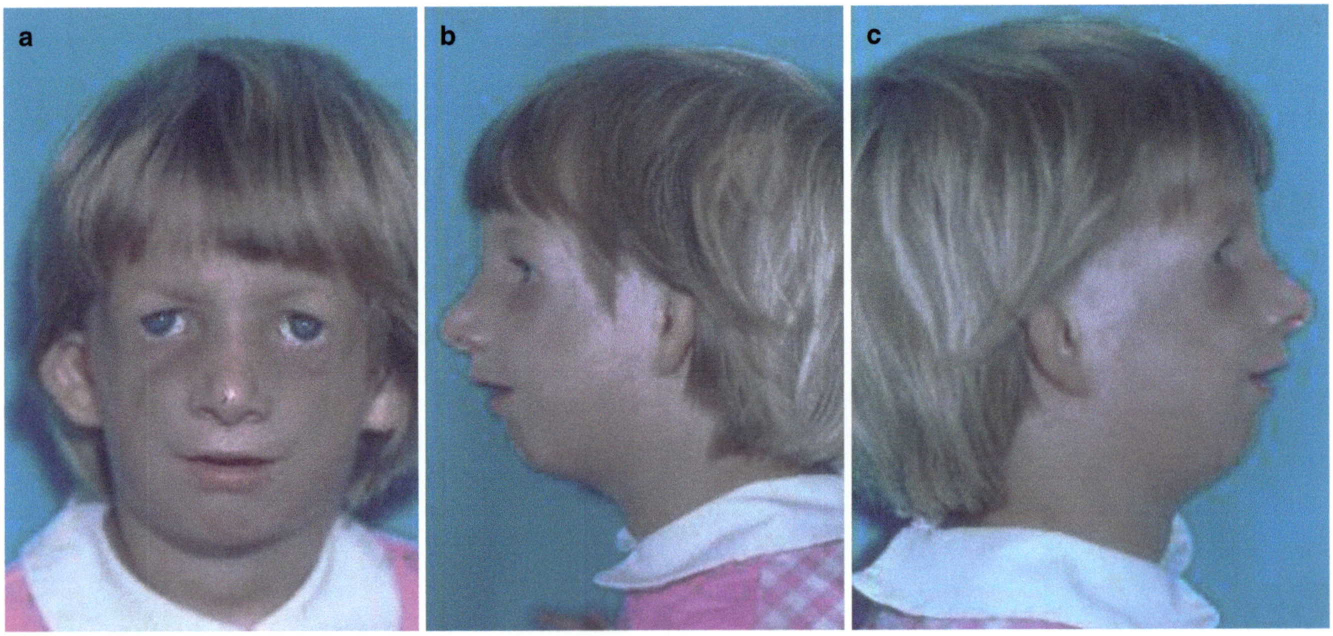

**Fig. 24.29** (**a**,**b**,**c**) Facial cleft 6,7,8 Treacher Collins syndrome

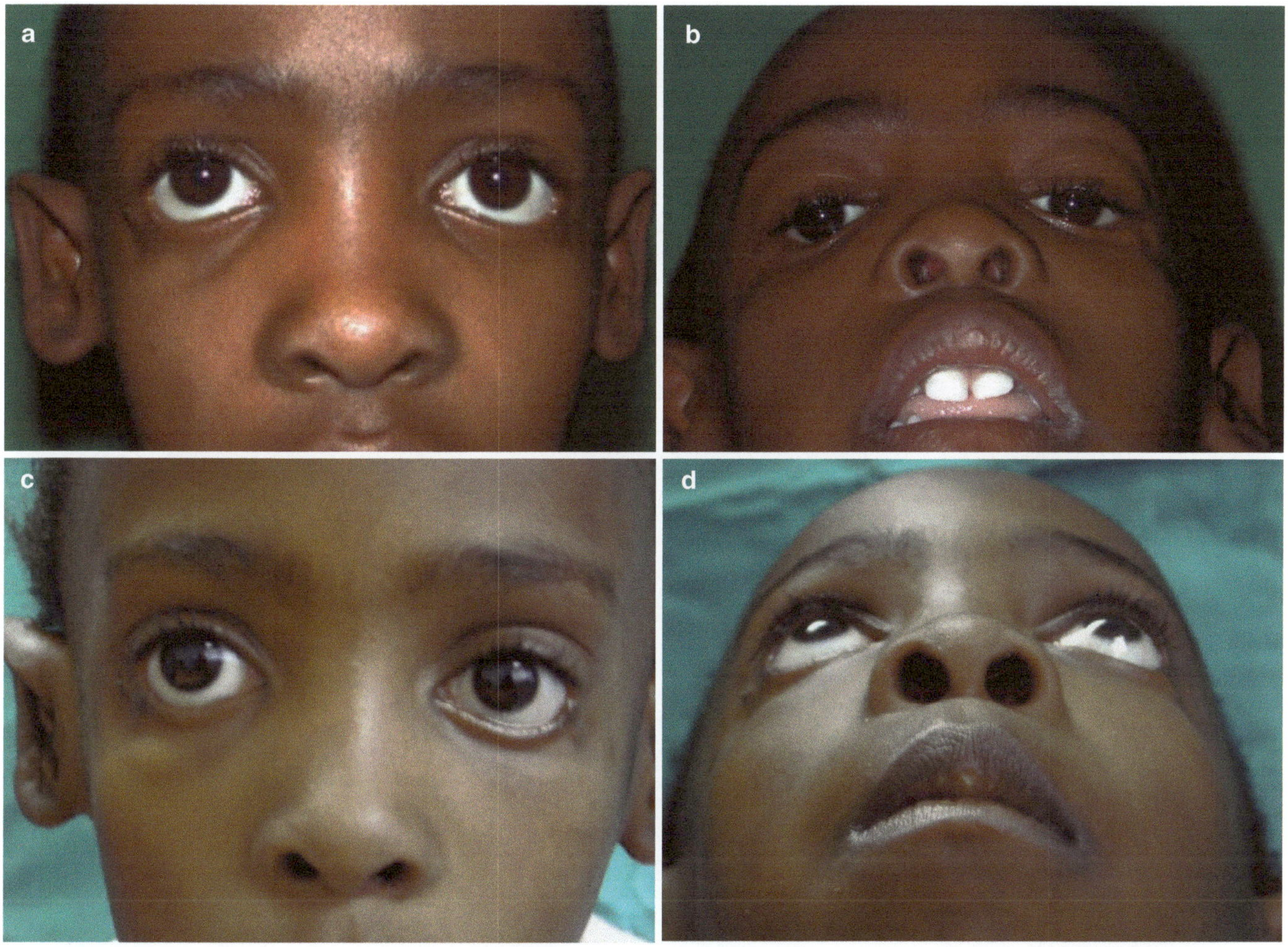


Fig. 24.30 (**a,b**) Treacher Collins pre-op. (**c,d**) 1-year post fat transfer

Fig. 24.31 (**a,b**) Facial cleft 9 post-op. Also repaired left unilateral cleft lip

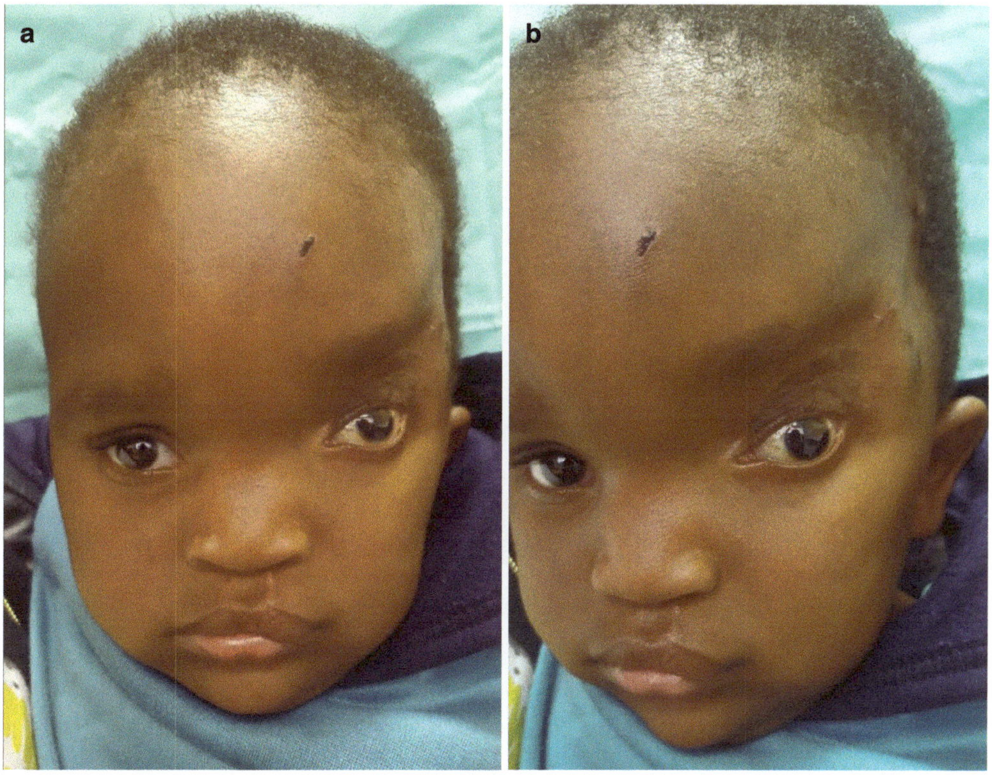

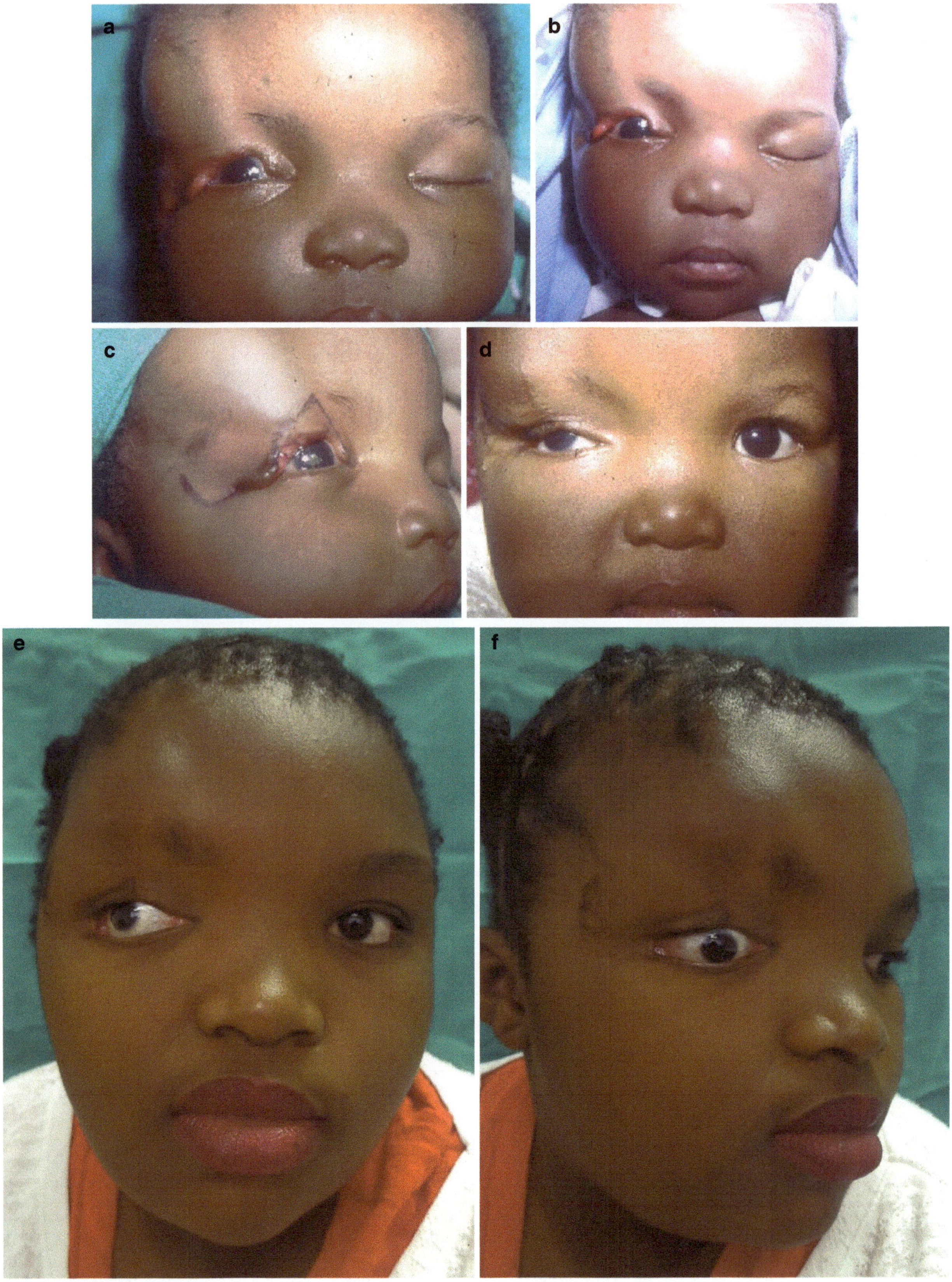


**Fig. 24.32** (**a,b**) Facial cleft 10. (**c**) Semicircular flap design. (**d**) 1-year post-op. (**e,f**) 26-year post-op

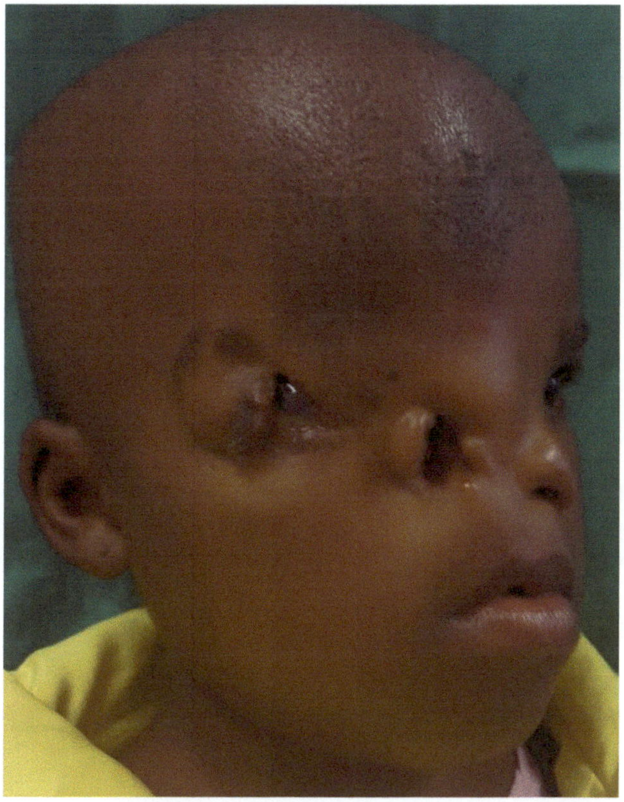

**Fig. 24.33** Facial cleft 11

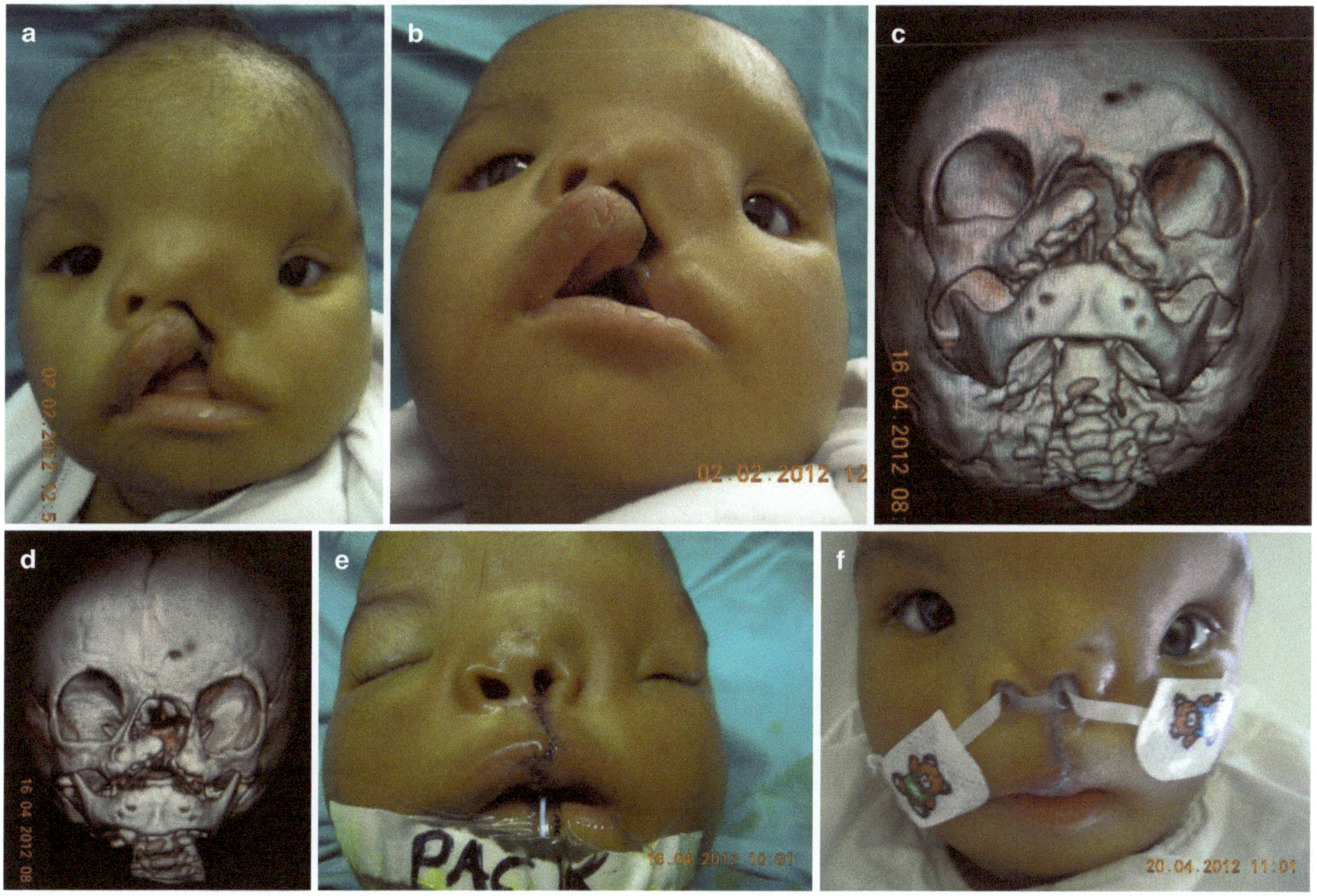


**Fig. 24.34** (**a,b**) Facial cleft 2,12 pre-op. (**c,d**) CT scan. (**e,f**) Post-op repair of lip and nose

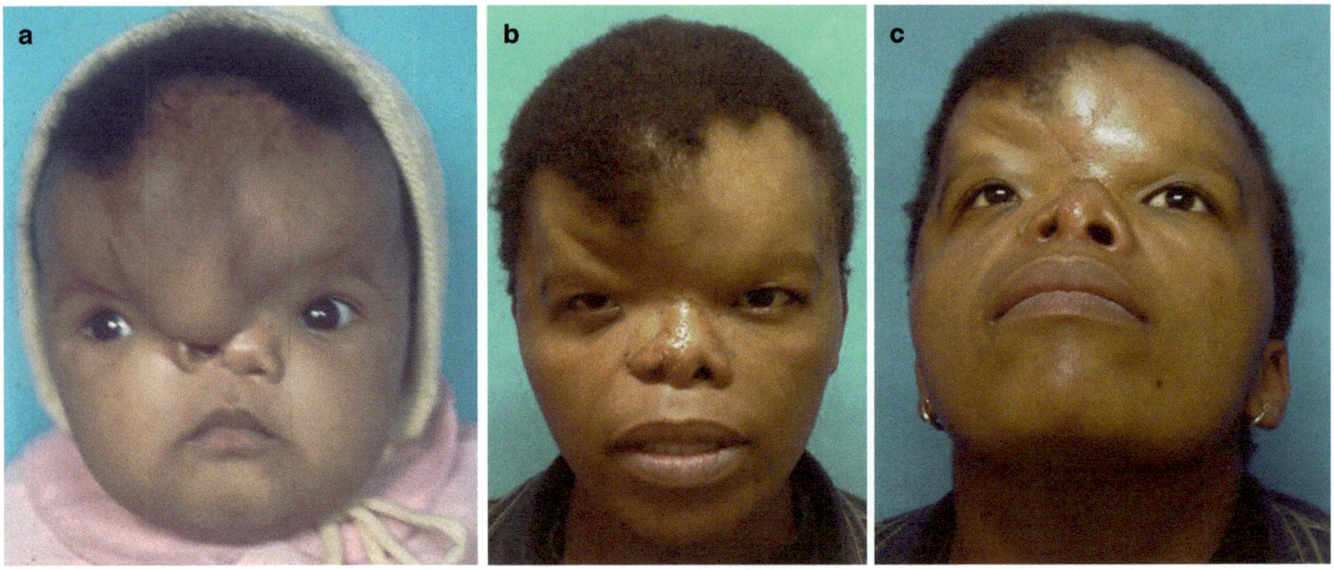

Fig. 24.35 (**a**) Facial cleft 1,13. (**b**,**c**) 20-year post-op

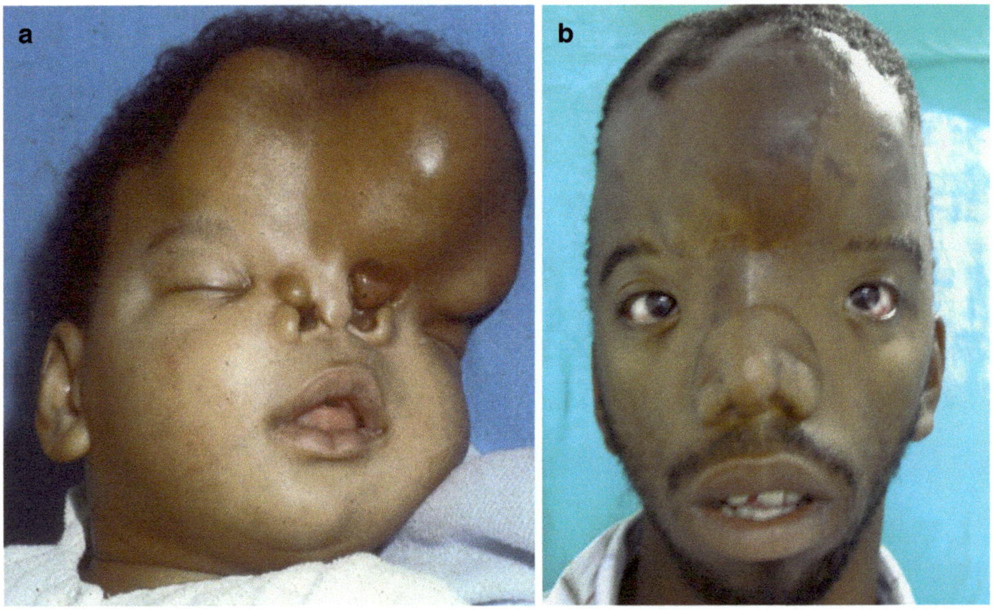

Fig. 24.36 (**a**) Facial cleft 1.13. (**b**) 22-year post-op

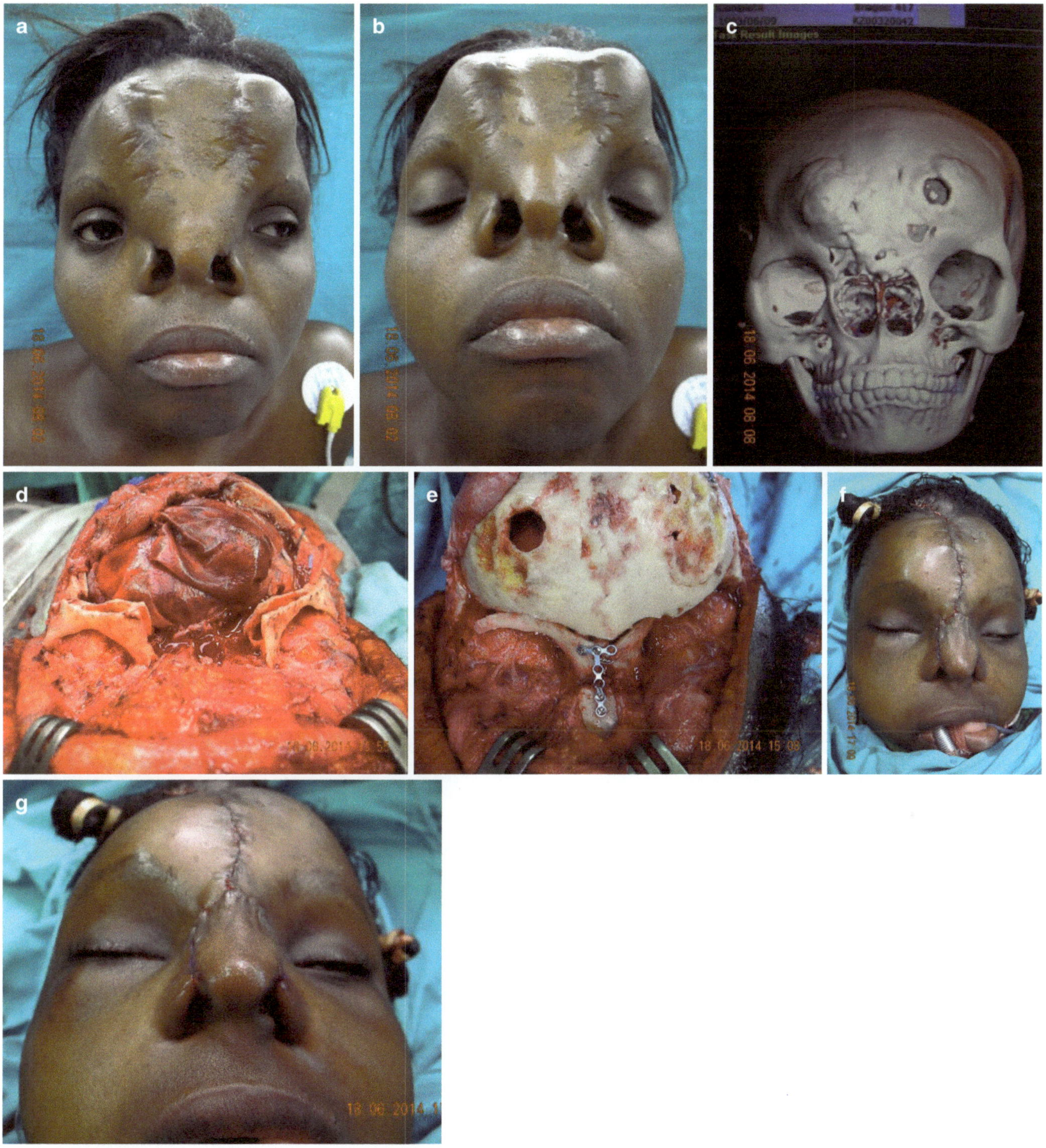

Fig. 24.37 (**a**,**b**) Facial cleft 1,13 post-surgery from another country. (**c**) CT scan. (**d**) Intraop showing resection of the bone for hypertelorism correction. (**e**) Intraop showing medial movement of orbits and nasal bone graft. (**f**,**g**) Immediate post-op view

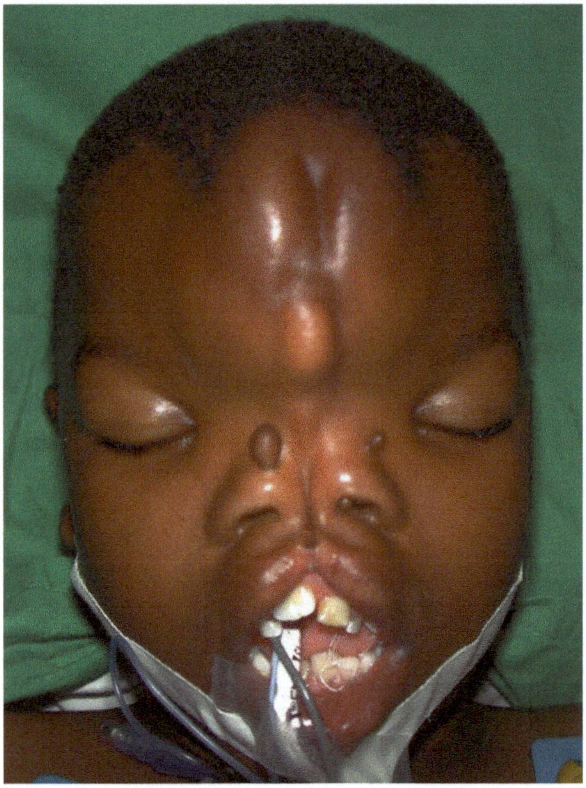

**Fig. 24.38** Facial cleft 0,14

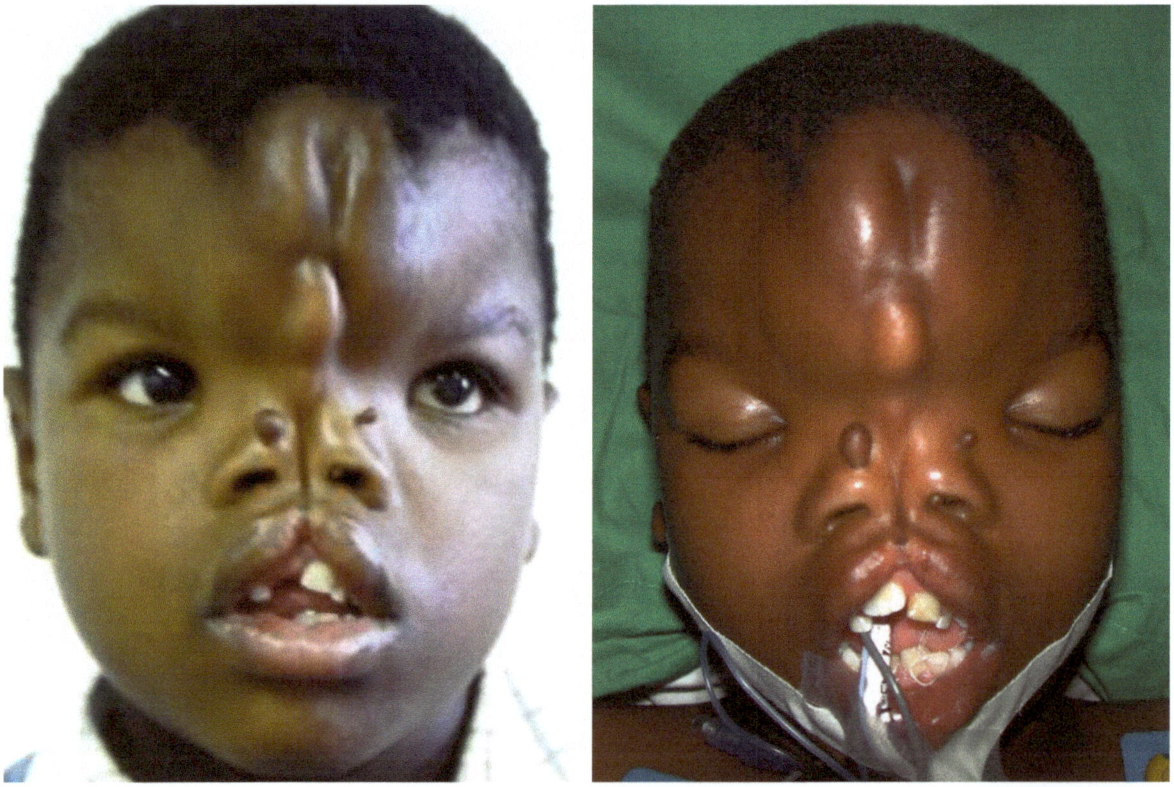

**Fig. 24.39** Two patients with midline Facial cleft 0–14.

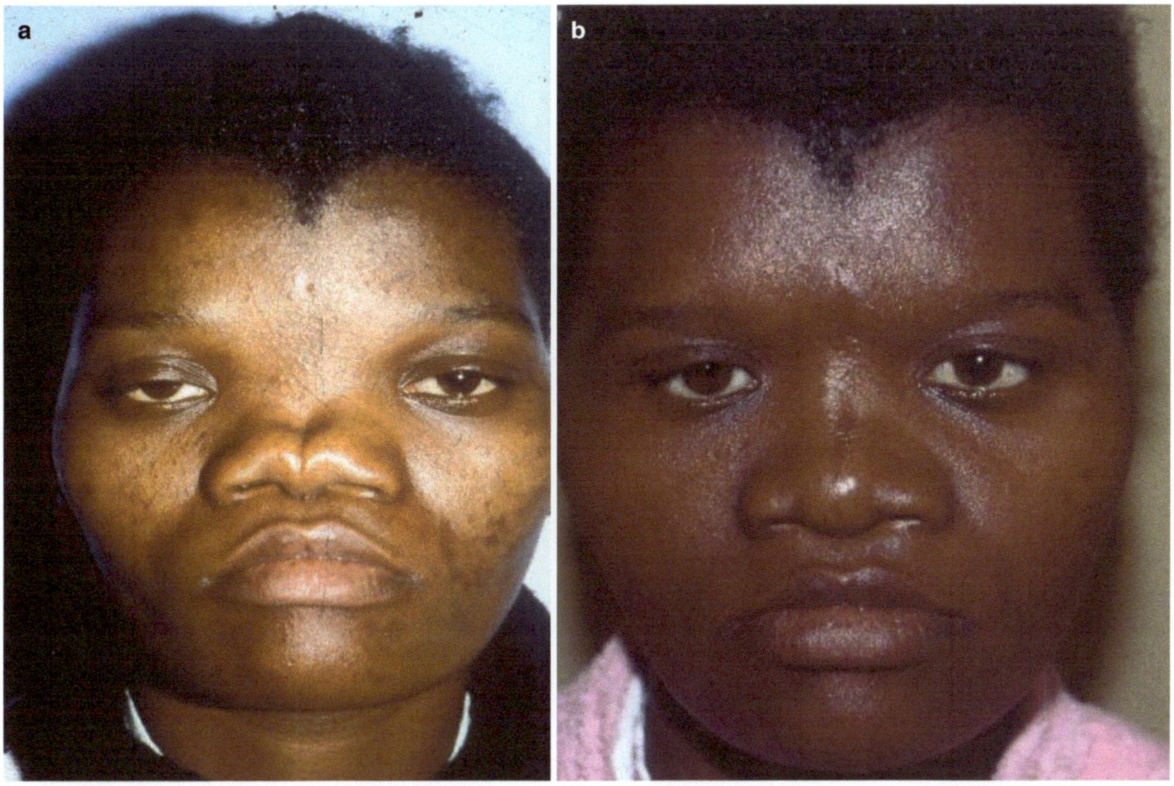

**Fig. 24.40** (**a**) Facial cleft 0,14 pre-op. (**b**) 18-month post-op

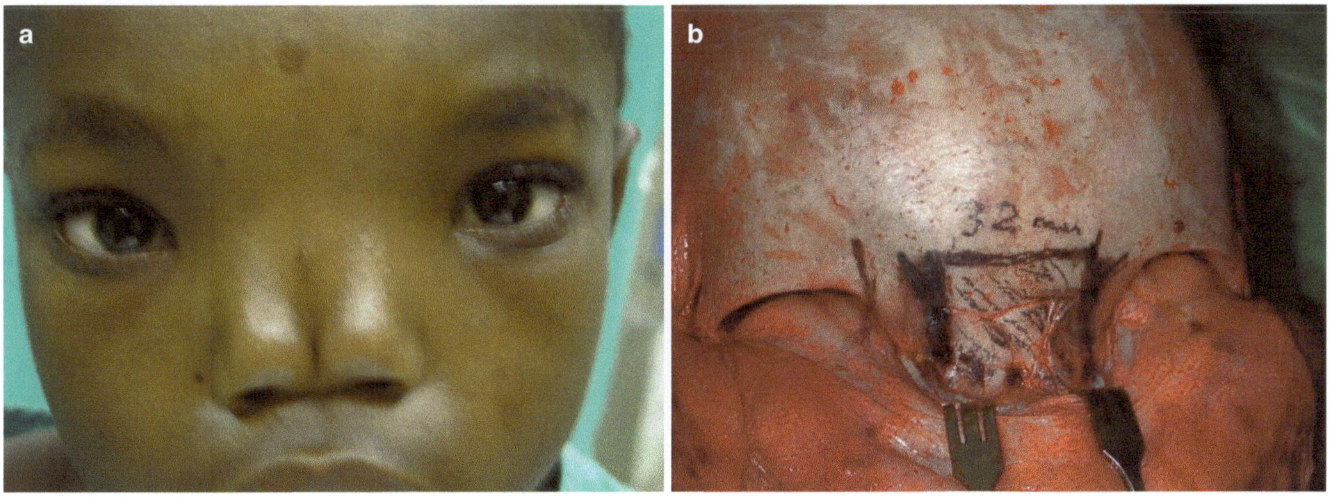

**Fig. 24.41** (**a**) Facial cleft 14. (**b**) Intraop showing planned resection for hypertelorism correction. (**c**) Intraop showing medial movement of orbits. (**d**) 2-week post-op

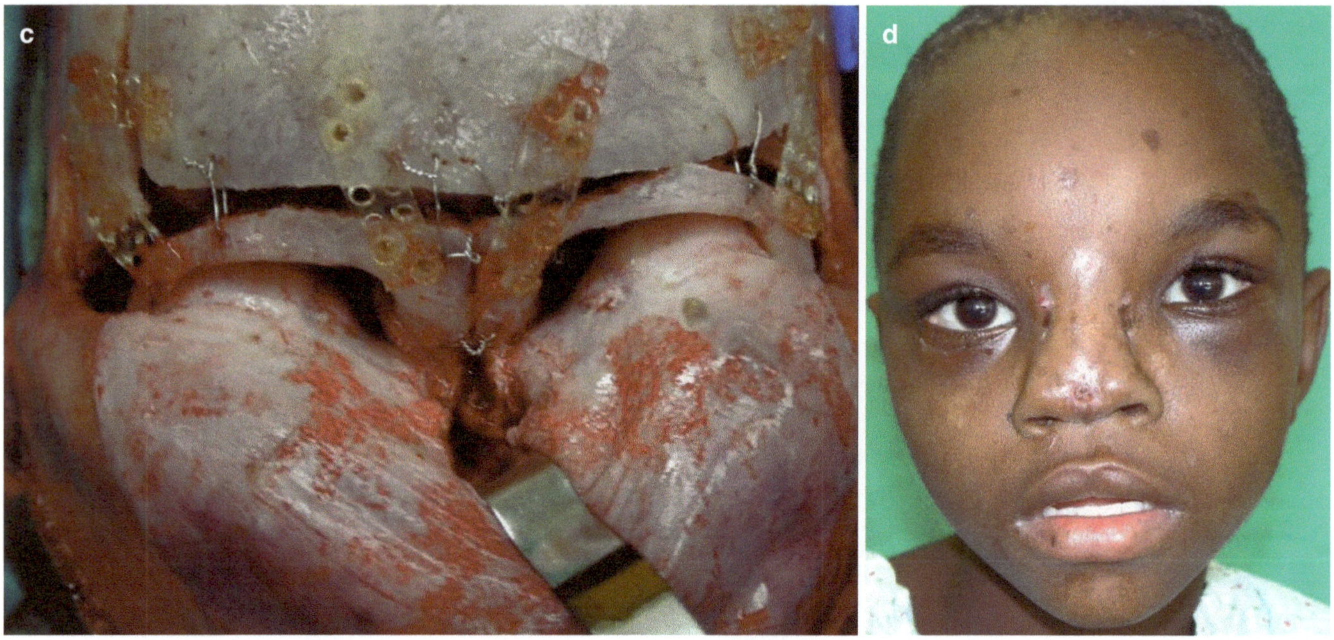


**Fig. 24.41** (continued)

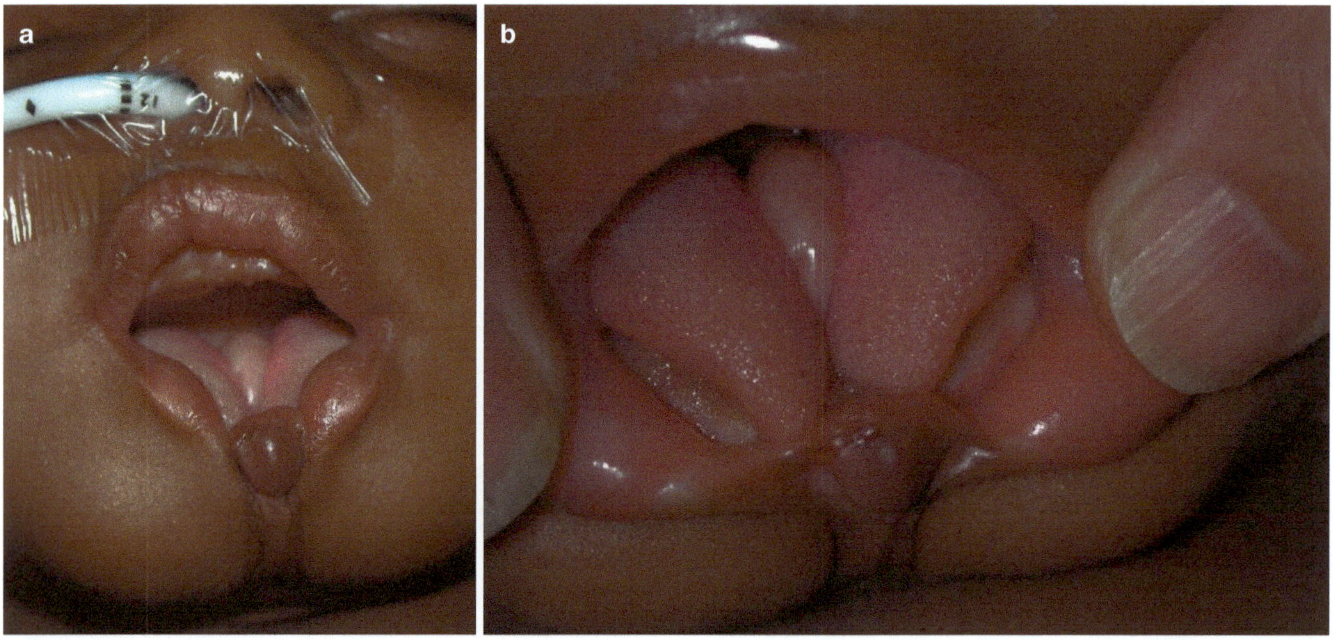


**Fig. 24.42** (**a**,**b**) Facial cleft 30 involving lower lip, mandible, and tongue. (**c**,**d**,**e**) 1-year post-op view

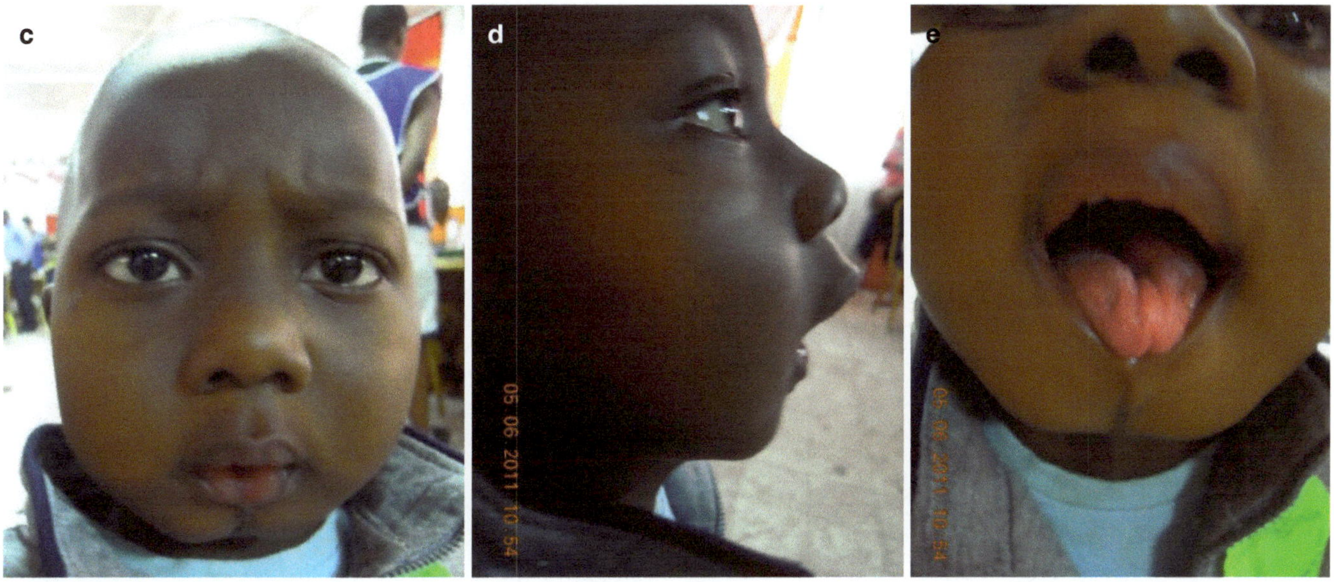

Fig. 24.42 (continued)

## References


1. Kawamoto HK Jr. The kaleidoscopic world of rare craniofacial clefts: order out of chaos (Tessier classification). Clin Plast Surg. 1976;3:529–72.
2. Monasterio FO, Taylor JA. Major craniofacial clefts: case series and treatment philosophy. Plast Reconstr Surg. 2008;122:534–43.
3. Madaree A, Morris WM, McGibbon IC. A method of repairing the no. 3 facial cleft. Br J Plast Surg. 1992;45:44–6.
4. Alonso N, Freitas Rda S, de Oliveira e Cruz GA, Goldenberg D, Dall'oglio Tolazzi AR. Tessier no. 4 facial cleft: evolution of surgical treatment in a large series of patients. Plast Reconstr Surg. 2008;122:1505–13.
5. da Silva Freitas R, Alonso N, Shin JH, Busato L, Dall'Oglio Tolazzi AR, de Oliveria e Cruz GA. The Tessier number 5 facial cleft: surgical strategies and outcomes in six patients. Cleft Palate Craniofac J. 2009;46:179–86.
6. Racz C, Dakpe S, Kadlub N, et al. Phenotypic spectrum of Tessier facial cleft number 5. J Craniomaxillofac Surg. 2018;46:22–7.
7. Converse JM, Coccaro PJ, Becker M, Wood-Smith D. On hemifacial microsomia. The first and second branchial arch syndrome. Plast Reconstr Surg. 1973;51:268–79.
8. Tse RW, Knight RJ, Fisher DM. Anatomic approximation approach to correction of transverse facial clefts. J Plast Reconstr Aesthet Surg. 2018;71:1600–8.
9. Rogers GF, Mulliken JB. Repair of transverse facial cleft in hemifacial microsomia: long-term anthropometric evaluation of commissural symmetry. Plast Reconstr Surg. 2007;120:728–37.
10. Tessier P. Orbital hypertelorism. I. Successive surgical attempts. Material and methods. Causes and mechanisms. Scand J Plast Reconstr Surg. 1972;6:135–55.
11. Morritt DG, Goodacre TE, Wall SA. A paramedian cleft of the lower lip. J Craniofac Surg. 2007;18:704–6.


## Craniofacial Clefts, Case 1

### Case Study: Persistent Lip, Nasal, and Eyebrow Deformities from a Tessier 3/11 Facial Cleft

Edwar Alvarez and David Alvarez

#### Case Analysis

This 19-year-old male presents with a bilateral cleft lip and facial cleft of Tessier type 3-11, with features of lip whistle deformity and lip asymmetry, retraction of the right nasal ala, bilateral nasoalveolar fistula, a tear duct fistula, and agenesis of the right eyebrow.

Goals of care are to improve lip continuity, reconstruct right nasal ala and bilateral nasal floor continuity, excise the tear duct fistula, and reconstruct his right eyebrow.

#### Treatment Considerations

Comprehensive secondary reconstruction was undertaken with bilateral cleft lip revision and orbicularis reconstruction and repair of bilateral nasolabial fistulas. A z-plasty flap interposition in the right nasal sidewall was designed to both extend the lateral nasal wall to reconstruct the right ala, as well as reconstruct the lacrimal duct fistula over a stent. Finally, eyebrow reconstruction was performed with transposition of a cutaneopilous flap from the right temporal scalp and pedicled on the temporal fascia with rotation to the right eyebrow region. Results at 1 year are shown.

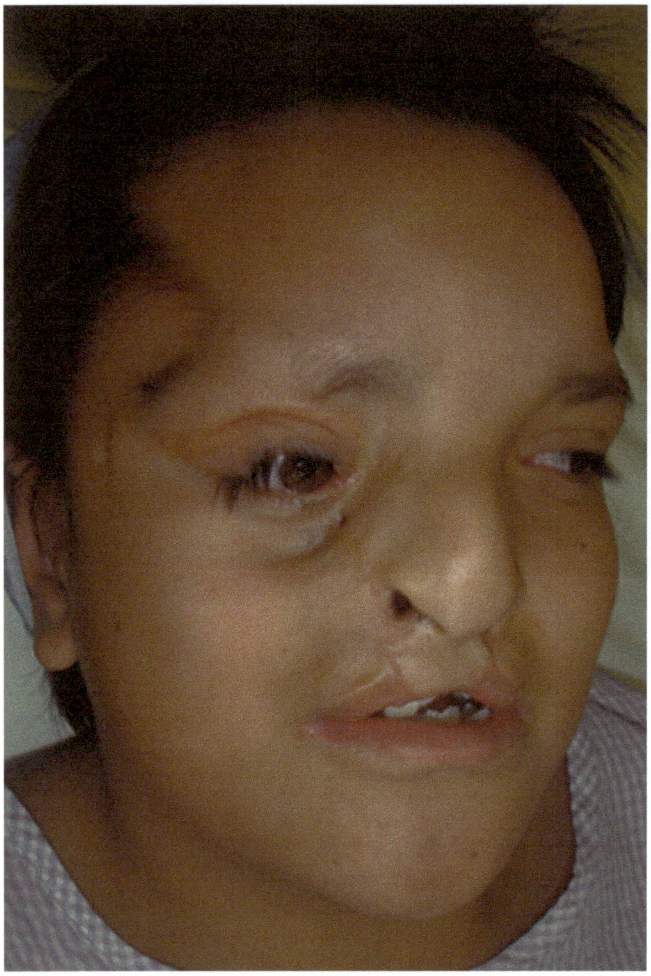

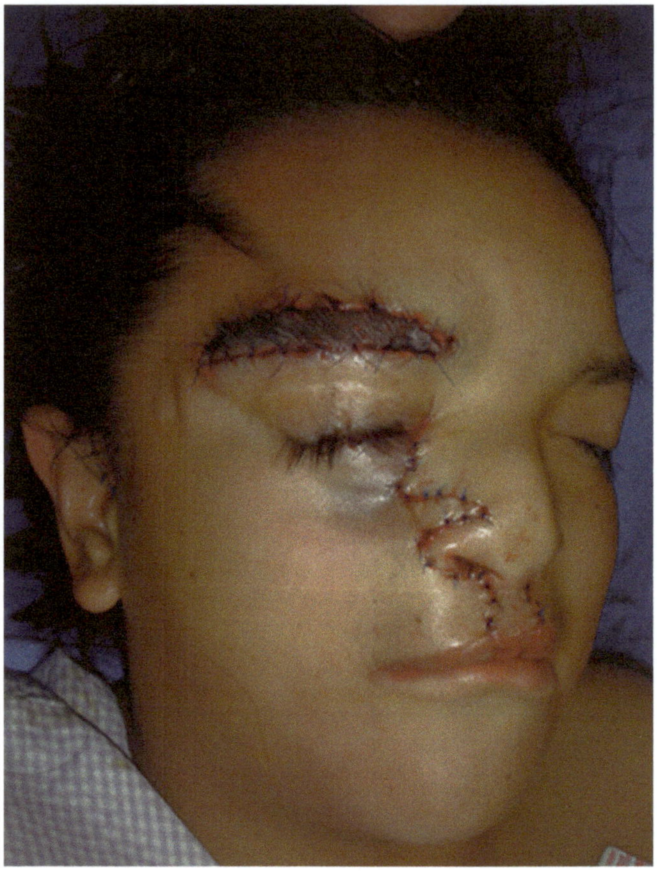

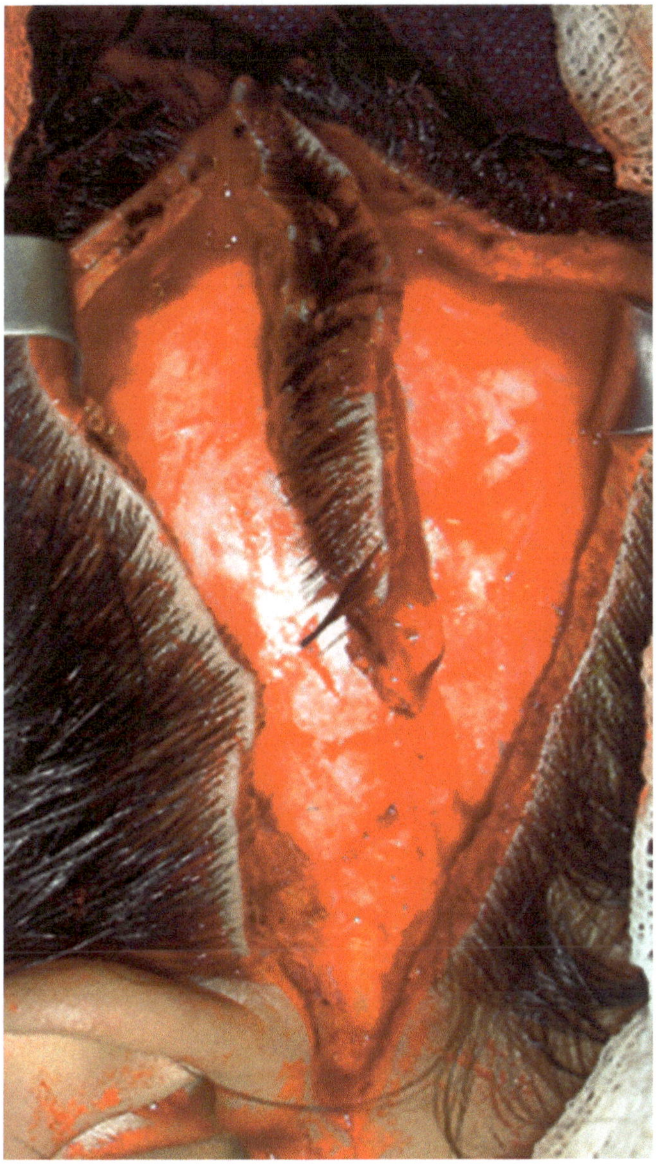

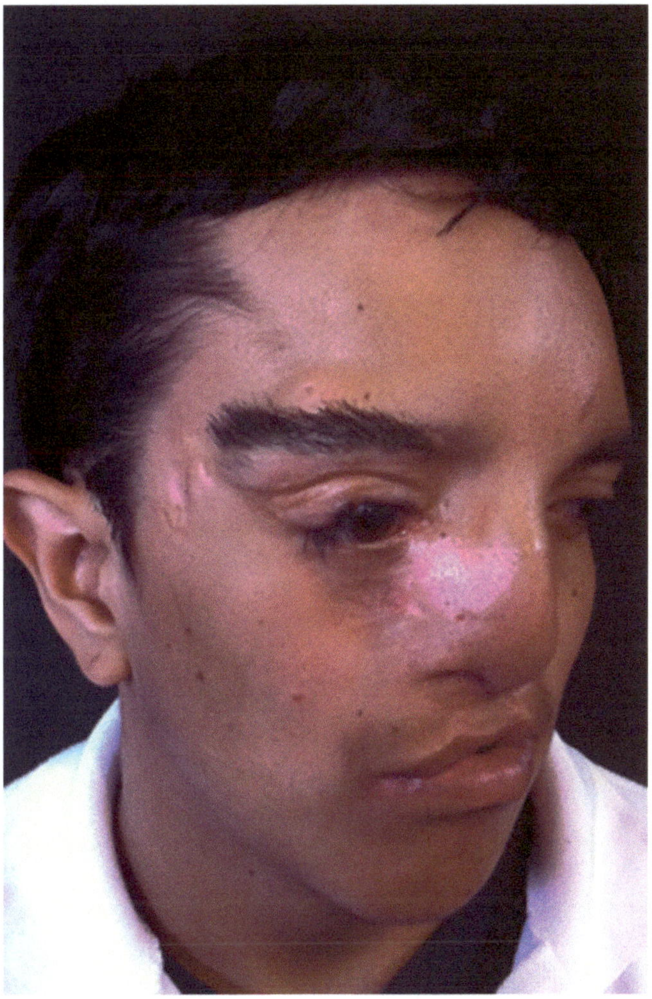

# Pierre Robin Sequence

# 25

Krishna Shama Rao and Chetana Kumar

**Key Points**

1. Pierre Robin sequence is a complex entity characterized by the triad of mandibular hypoplasia (small jaw), glossoptosis (hypotonic, retracted tongue) and respiratory obstruction.
2. Airway and feeding issues predominate early clinical management.
3. Techniques for establishing airway have temporary and/or long-term impacts.
4. Severity grading helps in clinical planning.
5. Management of PRS in neonates and infants requires specific skills.
6. Cleft palate, though incomplete, maybe difficult to close due to the cleft width.
7. Growth and speech need monitoring over a long period of time.
8. 100% catch-up growth is rarely achieved.

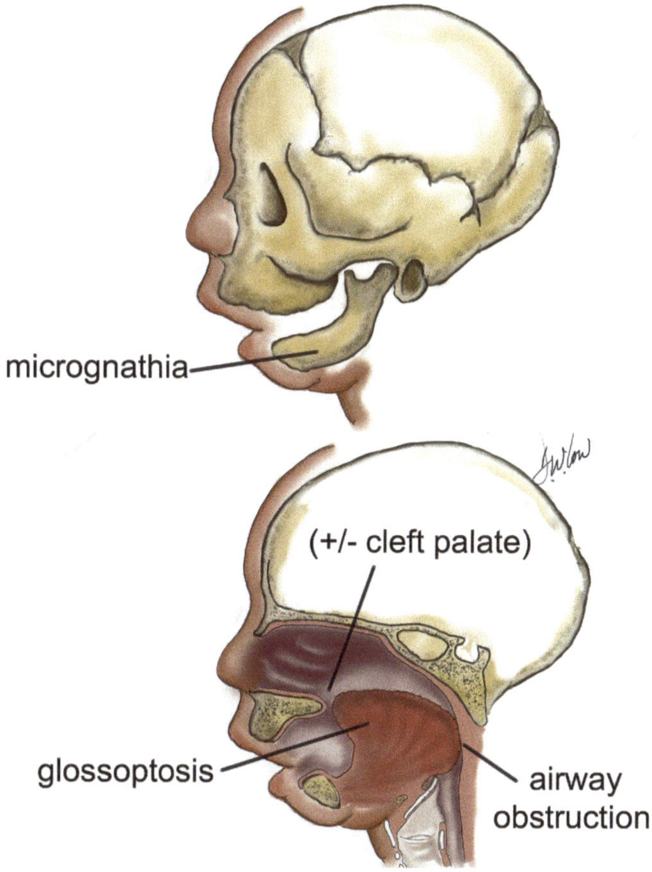


**Fig. 25.1** Classic feature of PRS

## Introduction

Pierre Robin sequence (PRS, or "Robin sequence, RS) is a clinical entity characterized by the triad of mandibular hypoplasia (small jaw), glossoptosis (hypotonic, retracted tongue), and respiratory obstruction. In addition, about half of patients have a posterior cleft palate [1] (Fig. 25.1). Originally classified as a syndrome, it is now considered a sequence. Current knowledge suggests that the sequence of events is as follows: in utero micrognathia, leading to glossoptosis, and due to the tongue blocking fusion of the palatal shelves, a cleft of the posterior palate. Clefts of the posterior palate may be isolated with a normal mandible and no glossoptosis. Isolated cleft palates tend to be narrower and V shaped in contrast to cleft palates in PRS, which tend to be wide and U shaped.

Patients with PRS are often non-syndromic. In a small number of cases, PRS is associated with known syndromes like Stickler syndrome, velocardiofacial syndrome, and rarely even Treacher Collins syndrome. These are classified

K. S. Rao (✉)
Inga Health Foundation, Bangalore, India

C. Kumar
Craniofacial Surgeon, Inga Health Foundation, Bangalore, India

© Springer Nature Switzerland AG 2021

J. W. Swanson, D. W. Low (eds.), *Global Cleft Care in Low-Resource Settings*, https://doi.org/10.1007/978-3-030-59105-2_25

as syndromic PRS. The incidence of PRS is generally estimated to be 1:8500 to 1:14,000 live births. There is no known sex preponderance. Genetic mutation has been implicated, but not confirmed, especially with reference to GAD 6, PVRL 1, and SOX 9 gene [2].

**Clinical Features**

- *Mandibular hypoplasia* of varying degrees, with elements of micrognathia (small jaw) or retrognathia (posteriorly positioned jaw). Often there is a large negative overjet of the mandibular alveolus relative to the maxillary alveolus.
- *Glossoptosis*. The tongue tends to occupy the oropharynx and, though small in size, may fall back toward the pharyngeal wall. Rudimentary tongue may be seen as well.
- *Respiratory obstruction* of varying severity. The obstruction is largely supra glottic in the oropharyngeal space, and the tongue is often implicated as the anatomical source of the obstruction; however, some reports suggest dysfunction in the pharyngeal wall movements as well. There may also be multilevel obstruction including subglottic, often due to laryngomalacia or tracheomalacia. Respiratory obstruction may be subtle to detect and related to patient position and sleeping or severe.
- *Cleft palate*, when present, is usually wide and U shaped. It may extend in to the hard palate (Veau class 2) or end at the hard-soft junction (Veau class 1.)
- *Feeding difficulty* due to increased respiratory effort as well as less than ideal swallowing mechanism.

**Severity Grading** [3] (Table 25.1):

**Table 25.1** Classification

| Severity | Exam | Feeding | Treatment |
|---|---|---|---|
| 1. Asymptomatic | Asymptomatic | Nursed in supine position | Careful observation, weight checks, supportive |
| 2. Mild | Possible desaturations, chest retractions in supine position | Nursed in prone position | Prone positioning, possible NP airway, possible CPAP ventilation |
| 3. Moderate | Desaturations, chest retractions | NG feeds may be necessary at least temporarily, possible PEG | NP airway, CPAP ventilation, TLA, or MDO |
| 4. Severe | Desaturations, hypoxemia, respiratory distress | NG feeds necessary at least temporarily, possible PEG | Definitive airway intervention (TLA, MDO, or tracheostomy) |

*PEG* percutaneous endoscopic gastrostomy, *NP* nasopharyngeal, *TLA* tongue = lip adhesion, *MDO* mandibular distraction osteogenesis, *CPAP* continuous positive airway pressure

**Evaluation**

Depending on equipment available, multidisciplinary workup should focus on four areas:

1. Oxygenation [4]
   - Physical exam should assess for chest retractions or gasping sounds, particularly while feeding.
   - Continuous *pulse oximetry* may detect desaturations but may be normal in infants even in the setting of moderate obstructive sleep apnea.
   - *Polysomnography* (PSG, a "sleep study") is the gold standard for detecting sleep apnea, including distinguishing obstructive from central sleep apnea and measuring severity with apnea-hypopnea index (AHI), $O_2$ nadir, and $ETCO_2$ nadir.
2. Jaw anatomy
   - A *skull radiograph or lateral cephalogram* can characterize the severity of micrognathia and jaw asymmetry such as in hemifacial microsomia. In addition, the absence of an airway stripe may indicate glossoptosis compressing the oropharynx.
   - A *CT scan* can give higher-fidelity anatomical detail and can enable a *3D skull model* to be printed for assessing anatomy and planning surgical intervention, such as by prepending mandibular distraction devices.
3. Airway anatomy
   - *Nasoendoscopy* [5] with availability of general anesthesia is the gold standard to assess (1) degree of glossoptosis and tongue-based airway obstruction, (2) potential improvement with jaw thrust which simulates mandibular distraction, and (3) other levels of obstructive airway disease that may be present, including laryngomalacia, tracheomalacia, or supra-/subglottic stenosis.
4. Feeding
   - Timed *feeding assessment* evaluates oxygenation while feeding, volume consumed, and possibility of breastfeeding which may be difficult in the presence of a cleft palate.

## Growth and Development

It is controversial when and to what degree "catch-up growth" may occur in patients born with RS. In most patients, future growth does occur. In asymptomatic or mild patients, the deficiency may remain subtle and require no intervention outside of the neonatal period. However, there is currently very little evidence to suggest catch-up growth *to normal* in patients with PRS. Growth spurts do lead to improvement in mandibular position, as well as airway availability. However, it is invariably less than normal for that age and often young adults present with a retruded chin (retrogenia) [6]. The first growth spurt happens by around 2 years of age, and subsequent growth spurts occur both preadolescence and postadolescence. Airway measurements too lag behind the normal right from birth into adulthood [7].

## Sequential Management of PRS

Breathing and feeding must both be managed in RS. The majority of interventions below improve both, but procedure choice is generally guided by need for airway support. A nasogastric (NG) or nasoduodenal (ND) feeding tube can be placed early after birth, as workup and any surgical intervention are planned or performed. In many cases this can be weaned, particularly following MDO; if tracheostomy is performed or wean is unsuccessful, a gastrostomy tube can be placed.

### Birth

The primary concern at delivery is maintenance of adequate airway to ensure 100% saturation. If the anomaly has been identified prenatally in a diagnostic scan, then a planned EXIT procedure (ex utero intrapartum treatment) can be performed. In an EXIT procedure, the cesarean section is paused after partial neonate delivery to enable an airway to be established such as through intubation or tracheostomy, prior to the umbilical cord being clamped and cut. Even in routine full-term normal delivery, it is important to have the presence of a pediatric anesthesiologist for intubation if necessary and a pediatric otolaryngologist or craniofacial surgeon to perform a tracheostomy, if absolutely needed. Subsequent management of the airway can proceed stepwise depending on the need or lack of active measures to keep the airway open. The craniofacial team and the airway team together assess further management and make a decision [8].

In the case of Grade 1 (asymptomatic), routine nursing in spine position can be initiated. A palatal plate may help assist feeding. In the case of Grade 2 or mild PRS, oxygen saturation may drop in supine position but pick up to normal once turned prone. Thus the management strategy would be nursing in prone position with oral feeds in head elevated posture or through an NG tube.

### CPAP or NP Airway

In the case of Grade 3 or moderate PRS, desaturation may be significant and need a nasopharyngeal (NP) airway continuous positive airway pressure (CPAP) device to keep the airway patent (Fig. 25.2). This might preclude oral feeds or NG feeds necessitating a percutaneous endoscopic gastrostomy (PEG). CPAP titration is critical and is best done in the hospital setting. Home CPAP devices are not recommended for infants with PRS. CPAP can either be a planned definitive intervention or a temporizing measure for a couple of weeks until definitive interventions such as tongue-lip adhesion (TLA) or mandibular distraction osteogenesis (MDO) are performed. With a CPAP or NP airway, continued monitoring should assess for adequate oxygenation while sleeping (via PSG) and adequate weight gain with the feeding regimen. Some evidence suggests that once the NP airway or CPAP is weaned between ages 6 and 12 months, moderate to severe OSA persists even if pulse oximetry is normal [8].

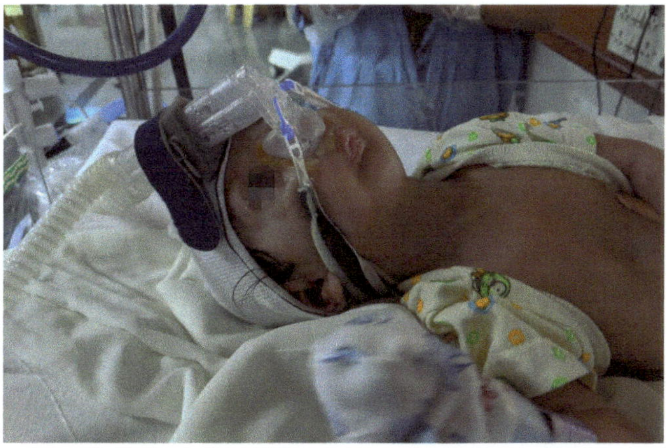

Fig. 25.2 Severe micrognathia CPAP with $O_2$

### Tongue-Lip Adhesion (TLA) [9]

Patients who fail prone positioning may be candidates for tongue-lip adhesion to maintain the tongue in an anterior position by temporarily suturing it to the inside of the lower lip. TLA is advantageous over MDO in that it requires very simple and inexpensive materials to perform; disadvantages include that reproducibility of the technique requires experience in tensioning the tongue sufficiently, early relapse can occur, and it limits the ability to feed.

During intubation, the surgeon can prepare the following items: 2 buttons, 30 gauge wire bent in half and crushed with a needle holder so the bend will pass through the lumen of a spinal needle, 3-0 Prolene suture tied to one button with the ends passed through the button holes, and 2-0 silk tie attached to the same button to retrieve it 3 weeks later.

An anteriorly based trapdoor flap is created on the inside of the lower lip and the underside of the tongue (Figs. 25.3 and 25.4). Chromic is used to suture the tongue flap to the posterior border of the lower lip mucosa. 4-0 Vicryl muscle layer sutures are placed but left untied until after placement

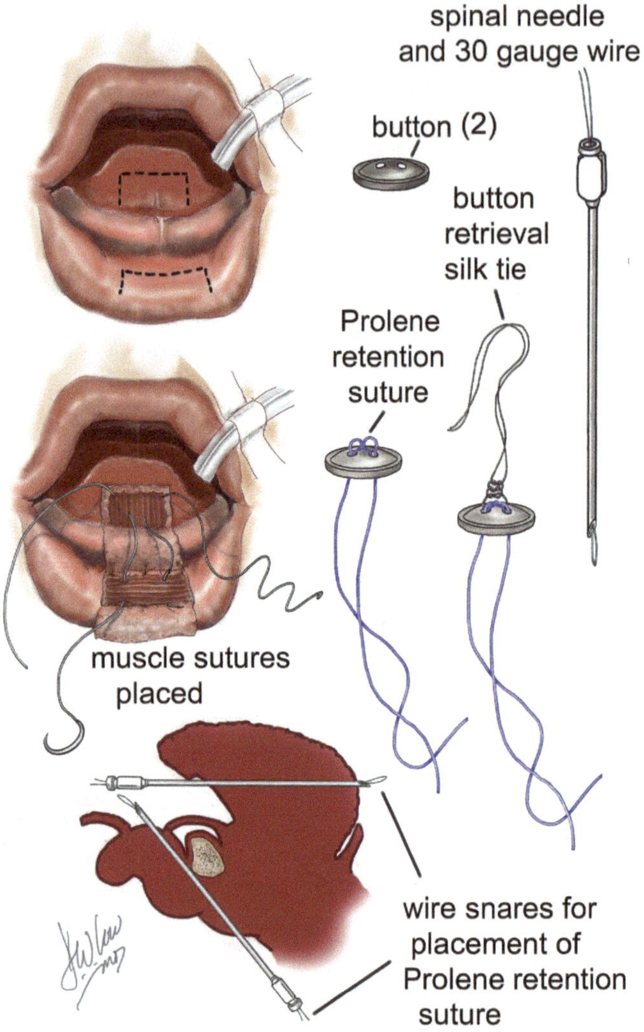


**Fig. 25.3** Principles of tongue-lip adhesion

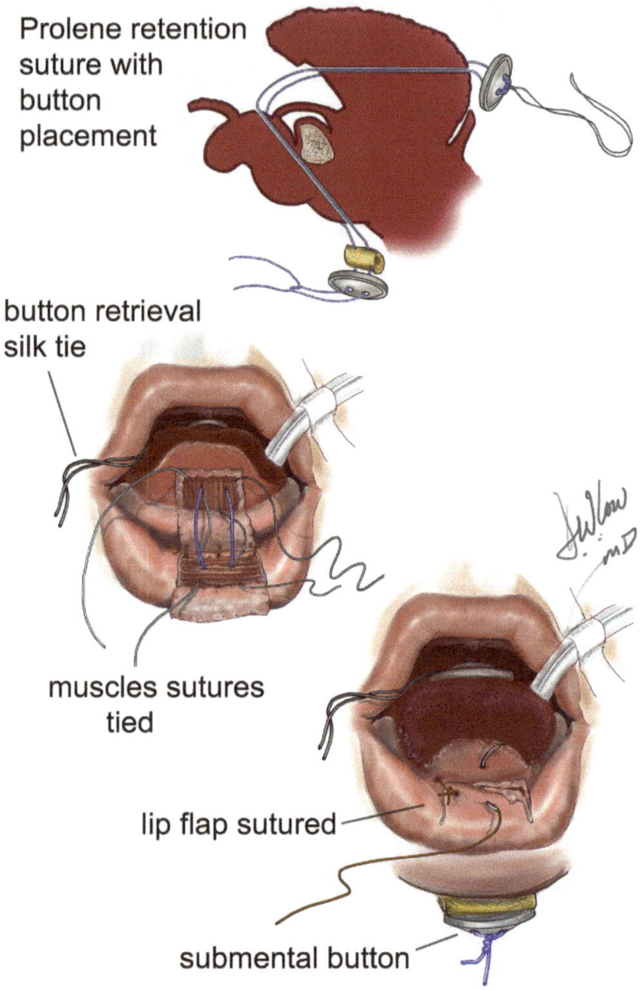


**Fig. 25.4** Completion of TLA

of the retention suture. A spinal needle with the wire snare is passed through the tongue wound to the posterior tongue to capture one of the Prolene ends. The needle and snare are again passed to capture the remaining Prolene end. The spinal needle or a hypodermic needle is then passed from a submental location through the lower lip wound, and the wire snare pulls the Prolene ends through the submental skin. Eventually the ends are passed through a Xeroform bolster and through a second button. The Vicryl muscle layer is approximated, and the lip mucosal flap is closure with additional interrupted chromic. The button retention suture is tied with sufficient tension to protect the soft tissue adhesion. It also helps to pull the tongue out of the oropharynx, decreasing the degree of glossoptosis. The silk suture is taped to the cheek.

In most cases the button remains for about 3 weeks. At that point the button should be fairly loose as the surgical closure gains tensile strength. The exposed chin button sutures are cut, and the silk suture retrieves the tongue button and residual Prolene suture.

Most surgeons will take down the adhesion prior to scheduling the palate repair, if a cleft palate is present. The patient should be approaching 1 year of age to allow for some mandibular growth and airway stability. The palate is repaired after 1 year of age. Although the lip adhesion takedown and the palate repair can be done simultaneously, the risk of airway obstruction is theoretically higher, and patients must be monitored carefully in the postoperative period.

## Mandibular Distraction Osteogenesis (MDO) [10]

Distraction of the mandible has become the primary procedure to definitively establish a patent airway in most children with PRS in many tertiary centers of higher resource countries. Compared to TLA, MDO has been found to more consistently and definitively normalize sleep apnea and prevent

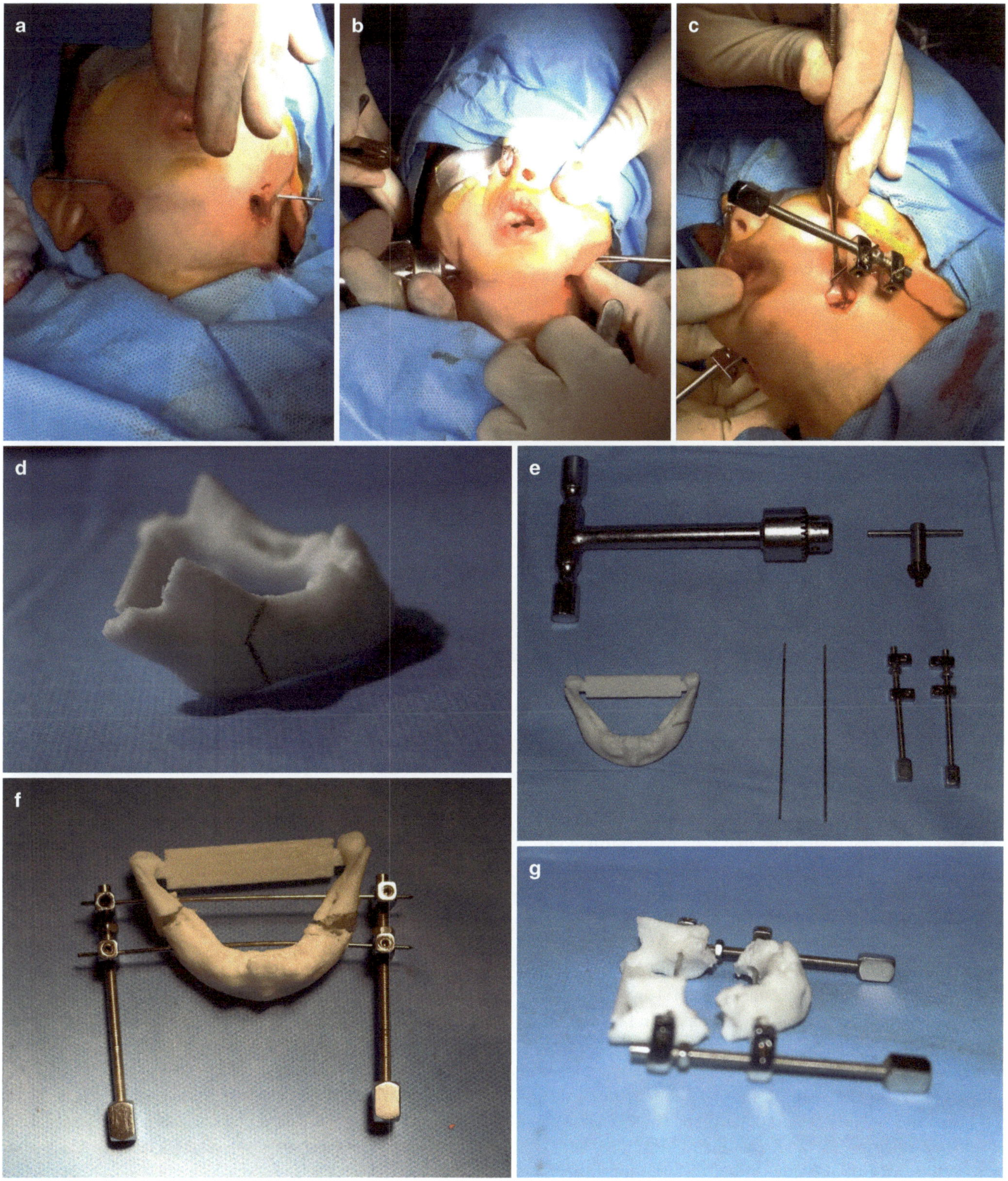


**Fig. 25.5** (**a–i**) Technique of mandibular external pin distraction. Postoperative view after MDO

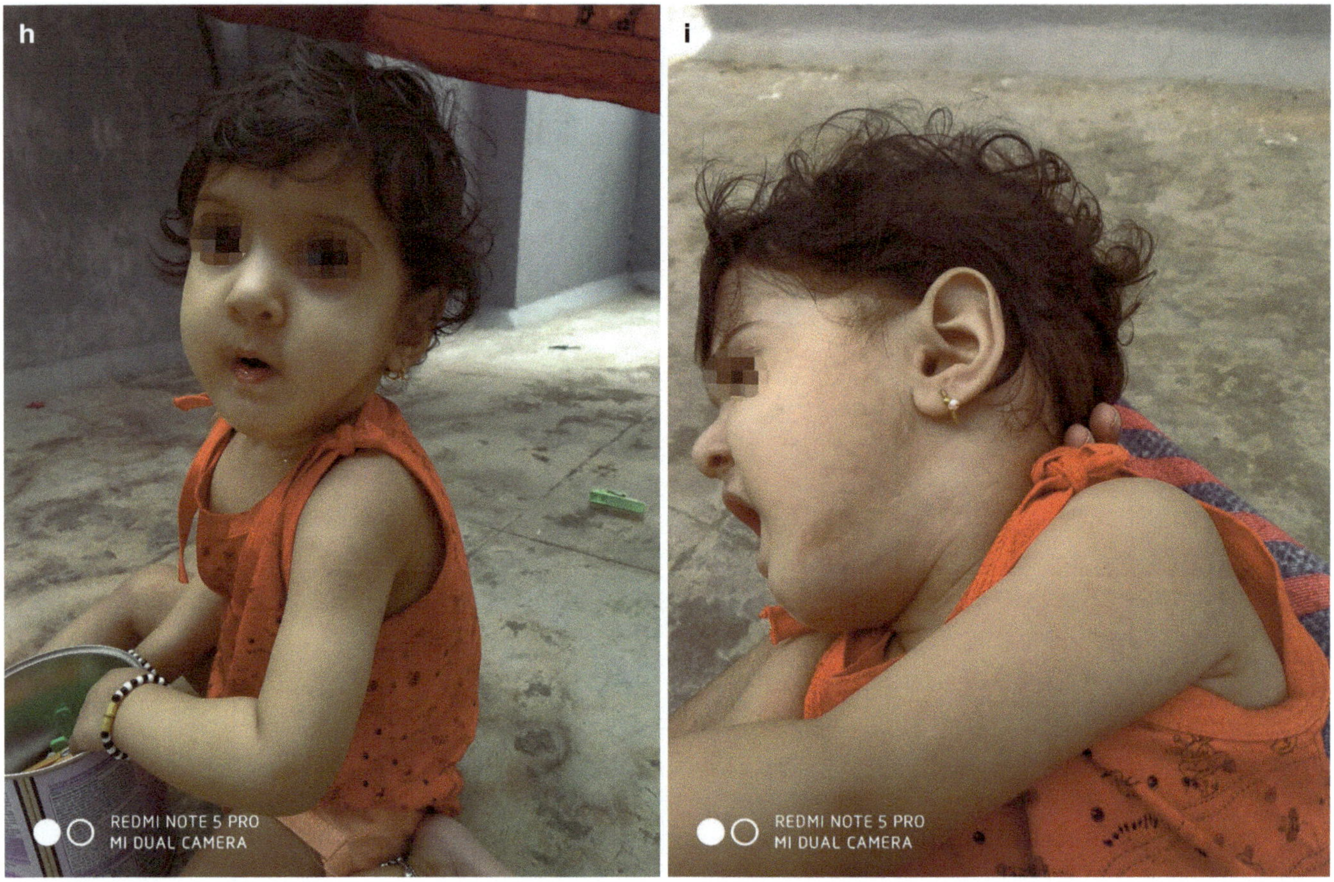


**Fig. 25.5** (continued)

the need for tracheostomy or gastrostomy tube feeding. However, it requires access to a mandibular distractor device and a bone cutting device (ultrasonic scalpel, reciprocating saw, or osteotome.) Surgeons in several low-resource settings reuse internal distractors that have been sterilized after previous use in high-resource countries. Locally sourced mandibular distractors are affordable costing around USD 70 per distractor.

### External Pin Mandibular Distraction [11]

The procedure is performed under general anesthesia using nasal or tracheal intubation. In neonates and infants up to the age of 1 year, the mandible is extremely small and soft. An external skin incision is used bilaterally to expose the mandible. With the help of the 3D model, the insertion points of the k-wires are predetermined. In this situation a k-wire is inserted through the mandible from one side across the floor of the mouth and through the other side ("kebab technique") (Fig. 25.5a–e). The second k-wire is passed anteriorly to the first wire at a distance pre-established based on the minimal distance between the distractor segments. Once the pins have been inserted, the distractor is connected. An osteotomy is then performed between the two pins on both sides.

The mandible is then distracted at the rate of two turns (1 mm) per day starting from day 2. Once significant distraction has been achieved and the airway becomes fully patent, then the process is stopped. This is followed by 2–3 months of consolidation period. The distractor is then removed under general anesthesia. The key element to recognize is that the k-wires are trans-mandibular and hence pass through the floor of the mouth. The posterior pin is placed at the highest point of the antegonial notch in order to avoid injuring deep structures. The procedure is done using a manual k-wire driver such that forces can be controlled. Rare complications can include floor of the mouth hematoma which can cause postoperative respiratory distress.

### Mandibular Internal Distractor [12]

This technique is performed under general anesthesia. A Risdon-type skin incision is made 1–2 cm inferior to the inferior border of the mandibular angle. The platysma is divided, and in the plane superficial to the submandibular gland, dissection proceeds superiorly to the pterygomasseteric sling encasing the mandible, which is divided longitudinally to enable subperiosteal exposure of the bone. Care is taken to avoid branches of the marginal mandibular nerve, which when approached cause twitching of the depressor labii muscle. A partial osteotomy is performed, usually using an inverted L shape to avoid molar tooth roots (Fig. 25.6a–f). The majority of the cortex is cut but sparing the cancellous bone encasing the inferior alveolar nerve. A piezoelectric saw, reciprocating saw, or osteotomes can be used to cut. The device is fixated using 3–4 screws in each of the footplates, each screw being 1.5–2 mm in width and 4–5 mm in length.

The distractor arms can either be directed posteriorly, behind the ears, or anteriorly, from the chin. In older children an intraoral device can also be used.

Once the distractor is placed, the osteotomy is completed, and the distractor opened to confirm completion then closed again. Activation is initiated from day 3, and distraction is completed based on the predetermined length of the device (2 cm or 2.5 cm) or to achieve an overcorrection of the mandible (usually about 5 mm mandibular overjet is sought.) Consolidation period is similar with time of 2 or 3 months. The device is removed at the end of the consolidation period under general anesthesia.

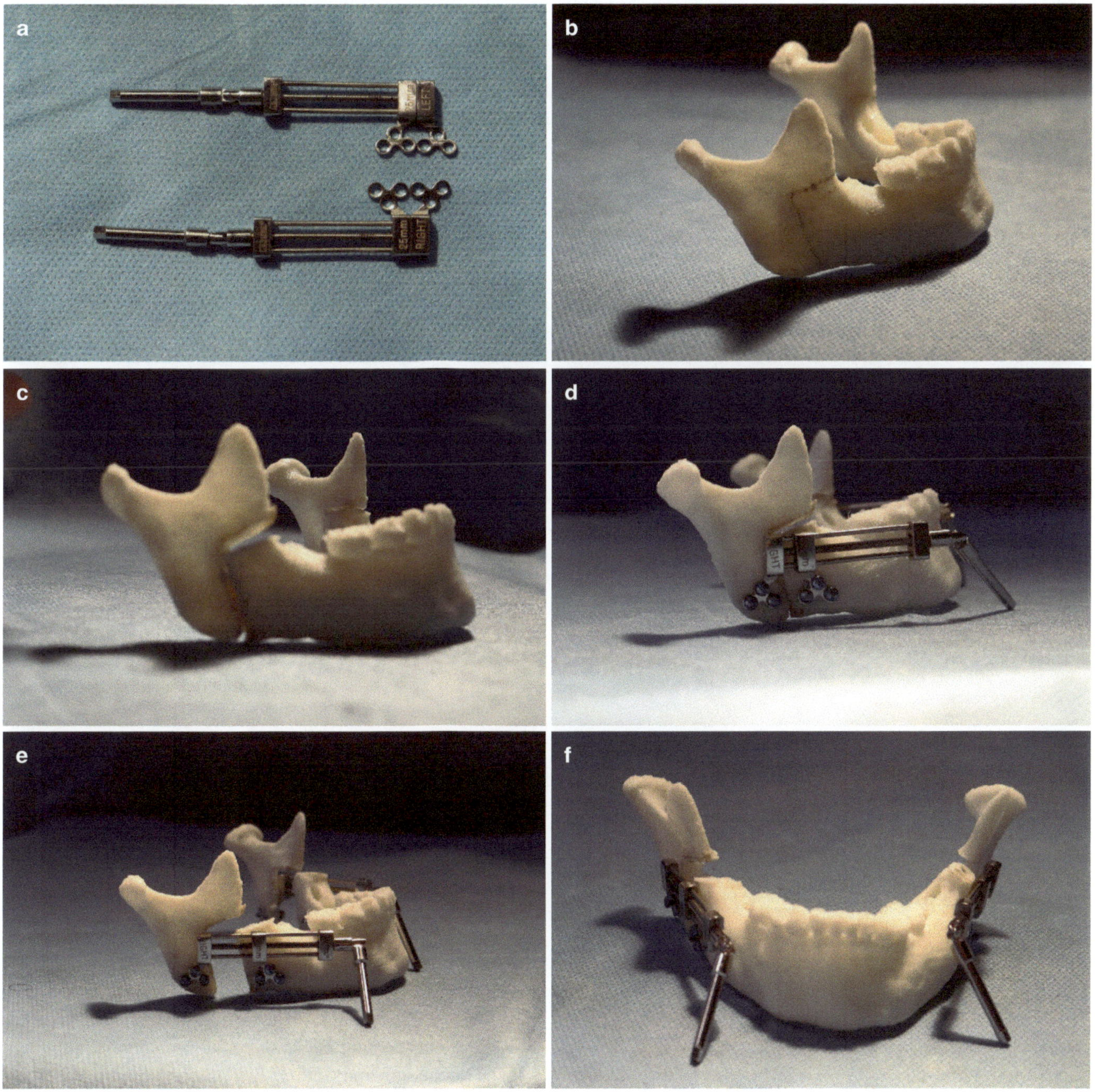


**Fig. 25.6** (**a–f**) MDO using internal distractor

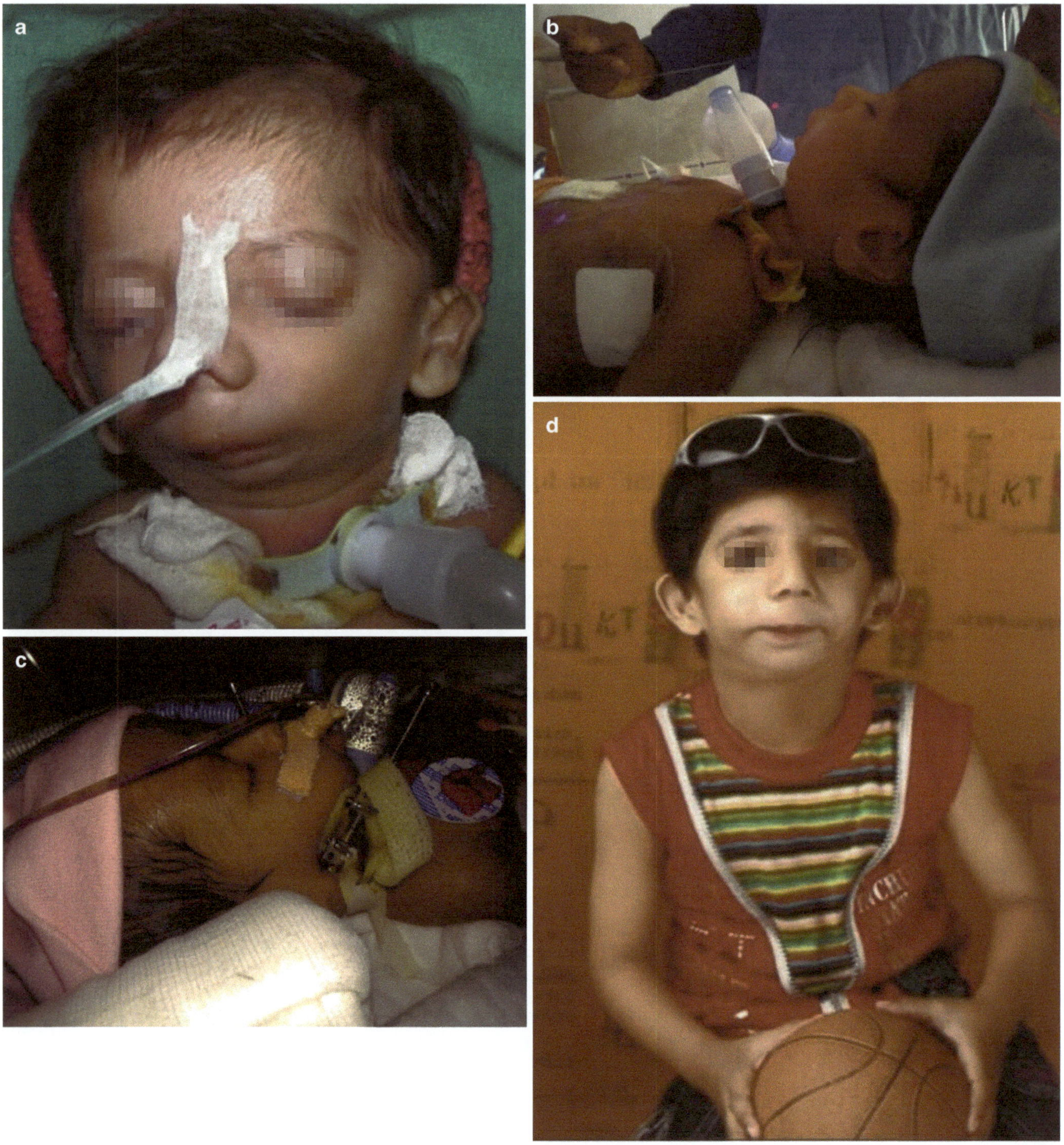

**Fig. 25.7** Tracheostomy at birth in syndromic PRS followed by MDO

## **Tracheostomy** [13]

A tracheostomy is usually reserved as a last option. Today the tracheostomy is used (1) for severe patients with multilevel airway disease (tracheomalacia, laryngomalacia) thought unamenable to TLA or MDO, (2) for patients who fail TLA or MDO, (3) where TLA or MDO are not available, or (4) as an interim procedure until TLA or MDO is performed at a later time (Fig. 25.7). Long-term complication includes granulation, stenosis, decannulation, and other problems.

The procedure may either have to be done as an emergency procedure or as a planned elective procedure. The technique involves cutting through skin and retracting the strap muscles and gaining access to the trachea. Maintenance of the tracheostomy requires skill and sometimes is difficult at home. Regular cleaning and tube change as required are necessary. The tracheostomy is usually maintained for at least several years until there is sufficient mandibular growth to allow normal breathing through the nose.

## Palatoplasty

[14] The classical cleft palate in PRS is described as U shaped, unlike a non-PRS isolated cleft palate which is usually narrow (Fig. 25.8). The isolated cleft of the posterior palate is usually closed between 6 months and 1 year, but in case a TLA or MDO is performed, then the palatoplasty is done after distractor removal or TLA release. For syndromic patients, usually palatoplasty is done after 1 year of age.

[15] Palatoplasty technique closes the gap and corrects the soft palate muscles, which are abnormally positioned and attached to the posterior margin of the hard palate, similar to a two flap palatoplasty. The soft palate muscles especially the levator palatini is dissected free of the nasal and palatal layers and positioned posteriorly and sutured. The palate is closed in three layers (Fig. 25.9).

## Follow-up

### Speech

There is evidence that isolated cleft of the palate has slightly poorer speech results compared to complete cleft lip and palate repairs. This is true even for PRS-related cleft palates. Adequate lengthening of the soft palate is of great importance. Speech therapy is initiated early and careful follow-up ensures a good outcome, and some patients may require additional surgery for velopharyngeal insufficiency.

### Growth [16]

There is evidence that facial growth and airway growth in PRS are sequential but reduced in absolute terms compared to normal children.

The growth pattern follows growth spurts but is invariably less than predicted for normal children. Thus catch up growth exists but is rarely 100% (Fig. 25.10).

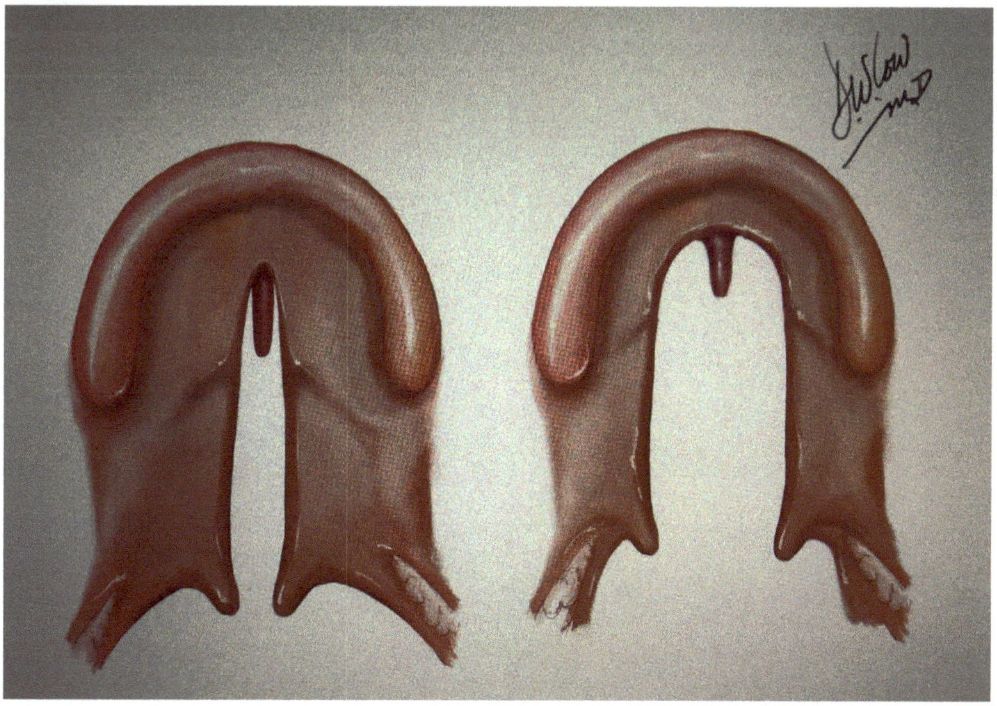

Fig. 25.8 (Left) isolated cleft palate – (right) palate in PRS

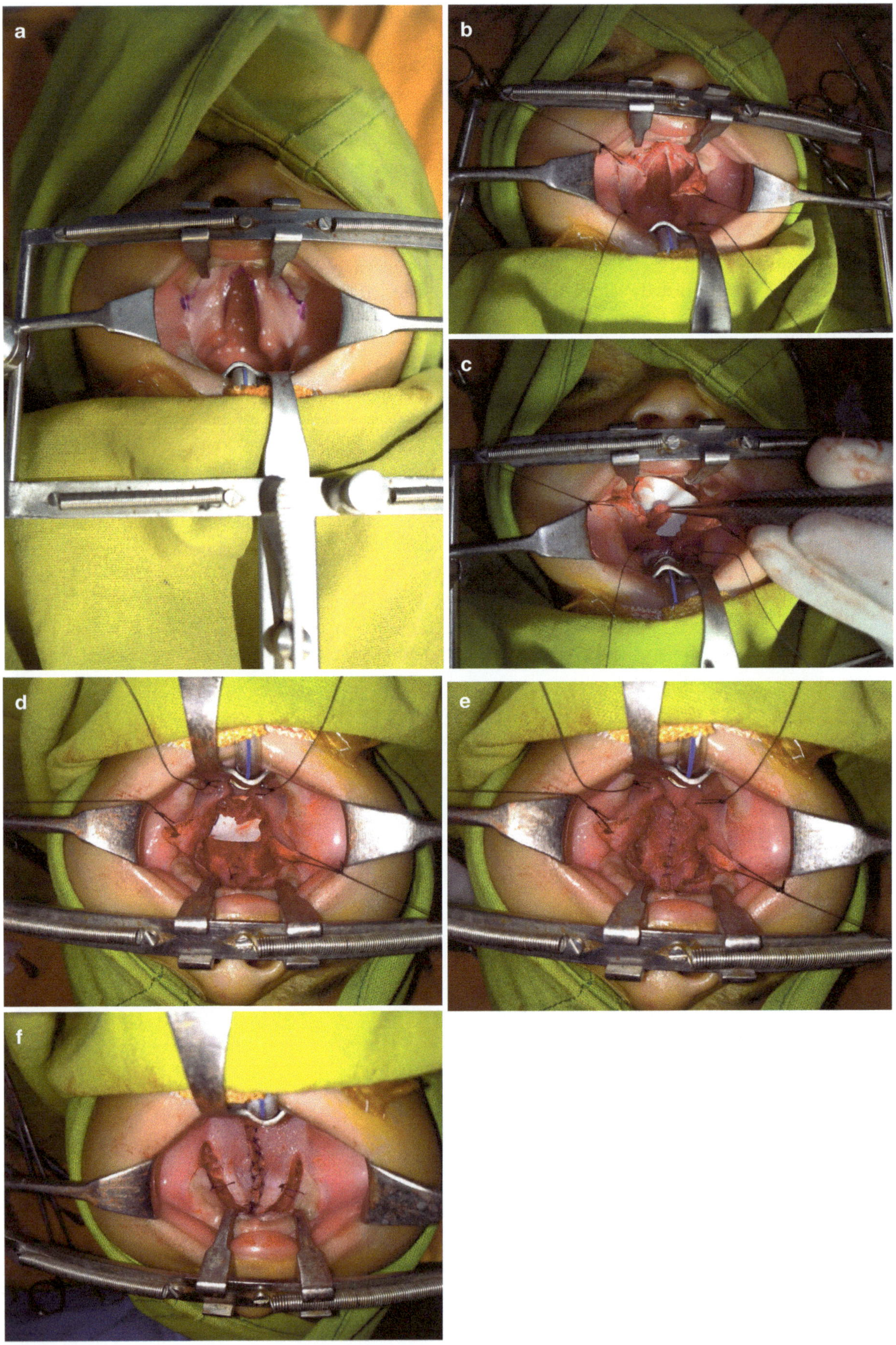


**Fig. 25.9** 3 Layer closer of cleft palate

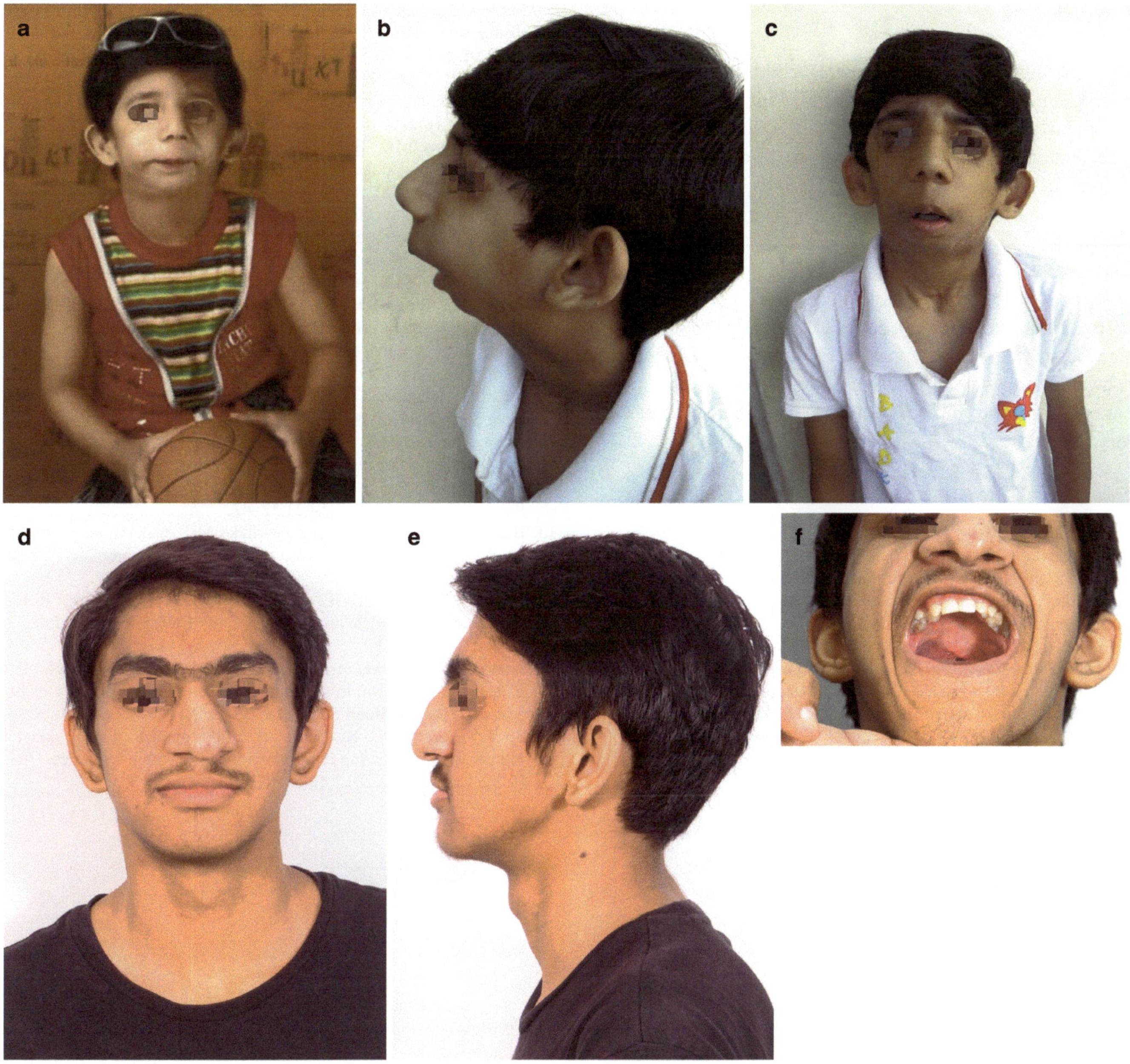

**Fig. 25.10** Some patients exhibit very little catch up growth (**a–c**), while others do tend to catch up (**d–f**). All must be followed closely until skeletal maturity

## Esthetics

On reaching adolescence several children have relative microgenia. This can be corrected with an advancement genioplasty. Rarely the mandible is severely retrognathic with malocclusion and may need traditional orthognathic surgery in adulthood.

## Conclusion

Pierre Robin sequence is a complex anomaly often requiring significant intervention prior to closure of the cleft palate. Airway management is critical to the well-being of the patient. Failure to thrive is common sequelae to the respiratory obstruction.

## Bibliography

1. https://ghr.nlm.nih.gov/condition/isolated-pierre-robin-sequence.
2. Linda P, Jakobsen MD, Knudsen A, et al. The genetic basis of the Pierre Robin sequence. Cleft Palate Craniofac J. 2006;43(2):155.
3. Cole A, Lynch P, Slator R. A new grading of Pierre Robin sequence. Cleft Palate Craniofac J. 2008;45(6):603.
4. Fahradyam A, Azadgoli B, et al. A single lab test to aid Pierre Robin sequence severity diagnosis. Cleft Palate Craniofac J. 2019;56(3):298–306.
5. Jake J, Lee MD, Matthew D, Ford MS, et al. Diagnosing tongue base obstruction in Pierre Robin sequence infants: sleep vs awake endoscopy. Cleft Palate Craniofac J. 2018;55(5):692–6.
6. Purnell CA, Janes LE, et al. Mandibular catch-up growth in Pierre Robin sequence: a systematic review. Cleft Palate Craniofac J. 2019;56(2):168–76.
7. Staudt CB, Gnoinski WM, et al. Upper airway changes in Pierre Robin sequence from childhood to adulthood. Orthod Craniofac Res. 2013;16:202.
8. Arlen Denny MD, Behrooz Kalantarian MD, et al. Mandibular distraction in neonates: a strategy to avoid tracheostomy. Plast Reconstr Surg. 2002;109:896–904.
9. Roberto L, Flores MD, Sunil S, Tholpady MD, et al. The surgical correction of Pierre Robin sequence: mandibular distraction osteogenesis versus tongue-lip adhesion. Plast Reconstr Surg. 2014;133(6):1433.
10. Jessica A, Ching MD, Justin D, Daggett MD, et al. A simple mandibular distraction protocol to avoid tracheostomy in patients with Pierre Robin sequence. Cleft Palate Craniofac J. 2017;54(2):210–5.
11. Andrew R, Scott MD, Robert J, Tibesar MD, et al. Mandibular distraction osteogenesis in infants younger than 3 months. Arch Facial Plast Surg. 2011;13(3):173.
12. AthariAlmajed MD, Alex Viezel-Mathieu MD, et al. Outcome following surgical interventions for micrognathia in infants with Pierre Robin sequence: a systematic review of the literature. Cleft Palate Craniofac J. 2017;54(1):32–42.
13. Benjamin Collins BS, Rosser Powitzky MD, et al. Airway management in Pierre Robin sequence: patterns of practice. Cleft Palate Craniofac J. 2014;51(3):283–9.
14. Godbout A, Leclerc JE, et al. Isolated versus Pierre Robin sequence cleft palates: are they different? Cleft Palate Craniofac J. 2014;51(4):406–11.
15. Andrews S, Sam M, et al. Surgical management of a large cleft palate in a Pierre Robin sequence: a case report and review of literature. J Pharm Bioall Sci. 2015;7(Suppl):2.
16. Shen YF, Vargervik K, Oberoi S, Chigurupati R. Facial skeletal morphology in growing children with Pierre Robin sequence. Cleft Palate Craniofac J. 2012;49(5):553–60.

# Part IV

# Comprehensive Cleft Care

# Cleft Dental Treatment and Naso-Alveolar Molding

26

Teresita Pannaci, Vilma L. Arteaga, Adriana Agell-Sogbe, Serena N. Kassam, and Michelle Scott

**Key Points**

- Dentists are among the first specialists to provide care to CLP patients and continue to help maintain oral health throughout life. For cleft patients, their dental home will be established earlier.
- Bone is preserved by primary teeth bordering the area of the alveolar cleft; they act as space maintainers (due to potential missing teeth), and they provide anchorage for early orthodontic intervention.
- Oral health not only affects quality of life, but for patients with cleft, prevention is even more important.
- Pre-surgical orthopedics, including nasoalveolar molding (NAM) and functional maxillary orthopedic (FMO) techniques, can be utilized to align the intraoral alveolar segments and contour nasal cartilages.
- When available, pre-surgical orthopedics can reduce the severity of the deformation and increase the likelihood of excellent aesthetic and functional results.
- Additional myofunctional treatment principles can be employed in patients from 2 to 6 years of age which may help promote normal facial growth and reduce stigmatizing deformities.

## Introduction

Dentists are among the first specialists to provide care to CLP patients and continue to help maintain oral health throughout life. The goal of dental treatments for cleft patients is to promote optimal dentofacial growth and reduce the invasiveness of surgical procedures which may compromise the development and shape of the maxillary arch. Some aspects of the cleft deformity such as the width of the fissure, the smaller segment size, the deviation and inclination of the premaxilla, and the morphology of the alar cartilage can be modified and improved before lip surgery applying pre-surgical orthopedics, including nasoalveolar molding (NAM)

**Electronic Supplementary Material** The online version of this chapter (https://doi.org/10.1007/978-3-030-59105-2_26) contains supplementary material, which is available to authorized users.

T. Pannaci (✉)
Vall d' Hebron Institute of Research, Barcelona, Spain

Operation Smile Venezuela, Virginia Beach, VA, USA

Operation Smile Morocco, Casablanca, Morocco

V. L. Arteaga
Maxillofacial Orthodontics and Orthopedics Ortodent, Guatemala City, Guatemala

Juan Pablo II Children Hospital, Operation Smile Guatemala, Guatemala City, Guatemala

A. Agell-Sogbe
Orthodontics and Maxillary Orthopedics Unit, Oral and Maxilofacial Surgery Department, Vall d´Hebrón University Hospital, Barcelona, Spain

S. N. Kassam
Pediatric Dentistry Department, New York University College of Dentistry, New York, NY, USA

Global Smile Foundation, Norwood, MA, USA

M. Scott
Department of Plastic and Reconstructive Surgery, Children's Hospital of Philadelphia, Philadelphia, PA, USA
e-mail: scottm9@email.chop.edu

© Springer Nature Switzerland AG 2021
J. W. Swanson, D. W. Low (eds.), *Global Cleft Care in Low-Resource Settings*, https://doi.org/10.1007/978-3-030-59105-2_26

and functional maxillary orthopedic (FMO) techniques. These are safe and effective treatment options even for low-resource settings, when available. The modalities can potentially alter vital functions of breathing, suction, and swallowing from the first day of treatment, potentially raising the life expectancy of the baby cleft patient and reducing the anxiety of the family environment.

## Dental Assessment, Oral Health, and Setting Expectations

### Prenatal Assessment: Treatment Course, Set Expectations, and Reduce Anxiety – Importance of Oral Health

Most centers have increased their prenatal diagnosis with the use of ultrasound.

Prenatal ultrasound will often detect cleft lip with/without cleft palate. When prenatal diagnosis is not possible or available, the next optimal time for first evaluation is within the first few days and at latest within the first few weeks of life.

An early diagnosis is important, as it can allow the family to establish cleft team care, while the child is in utero. This provides the opportunity for anticipatory guidance and to explain the stages, timeline, and treatment course of comprehensive cleft care. Also can help with psychosocial support for the caregivers, provide education, and alleviate anxiety. This is particularly helpful for specialty feeding and if any pre-surgical treatment is anticipated soon after birth [1, 2].

## Treatment Course and Timeline (Fig. 26.1a, b)

### Establishment of Dental Home

Dental home care refers to education given by the dentists to the parents in order to establish healthy oral care practices at home (Fig. 26.2).

Parents should establish a dental home for infants by 12 months or within 6 months of the eruption of the first tooth [3]. For patients with cleft, their dental home will be established earlier. This will happen upon diagnosis, which can be prenatal or latest at birth, establishing their "cleft dental home care" [4].

### Common Infant Oral Anomalies

There are common infant oral anomalies seen on the alveolar ridges and palatal raphe: Bohn's nodules, Epstein pearls, and dental lamina cysts. All are benign and self-limiting. The incidence of natal teeth (present immediately at birth) and neonatal teeth (present during the first 30 days of life) is higher in patients with cleft, in particular BCLP (Fig. 26.3a–c). Ninety percent are true primary teeth and should not be extracted unless mobility and aspiration risk are noted. Eruption hematoma can also be seen (cyst around the erupting tooth crown), which is self-limiting upon eruption. Vomer ulcer can be seen at birth. It is caused from the rough surface of the tongue in contact with the vomer (due to the palatal shelves being open). It is usually self-limiting (Fig. 26.4a, b).

The use of pre surgical appliances can accelerate the eruption of neonatal teeth and primary teeth. This is due to malpositioned tooth buds and/or pressure from the appliance. Eruption hematoma can also be seen (Table 26.1).

### Importance of Primary Teeth

Maintenance of primary teeth is imperative for several reasons: bone is preserved by primary teeth bordering the area of the alveolar cleft, they act as space maintainers (due to potential missing teeth), and they provide anchorage for early orthodontic intervention. Preservation of this bone is valuable. It is important to avoid extraction of primary teeth bordering the cleft (Fig. 26.6a, b).

### Prevention and Oral Health

Oral health not only affects quality of life, but for patients with cleft, prevention is even more important. Dental caries is the most common preventable disease. (Fig. 26.7a). Prevention tips include tooth brushing before bed, with the age-appropriate size of fluoridated toothpaste, if not available, wipe or rinse teeth and/or gums with water after feeding and before bed, not going to bed with bottle, switching to water in bottle and/or sippy cup, limiting sugar containing snacks or drinks in between meals, and minimizing juice intake and limit to meal time only.

Early and frequent interaction with the pediatric dentist can facilitate anticipatory guidance, parent education, caries prevention, oral hygiene instructions for the parent and child, dietary consultation, and other preventive measures [3, 6]. Parents should help brushing their children's teeth twice a day, once the first tooth erupts, with the appropriate amount of 1000 ppm fluoridated toothpaste [3] (Fig. 26.7b). Children with higher caries risk may require additional therapies such as fluoride varnish [3] (Fig. 26.7c).

Nutritional guidance and good oral hygiene are essential. High sugar drinks and food seem to be an increasingly large contributor to poor hygiene, even in low-resource settings. It is important to reduce not only the quantity, but even more so, the frequency the sugar is in contact with the teeth.

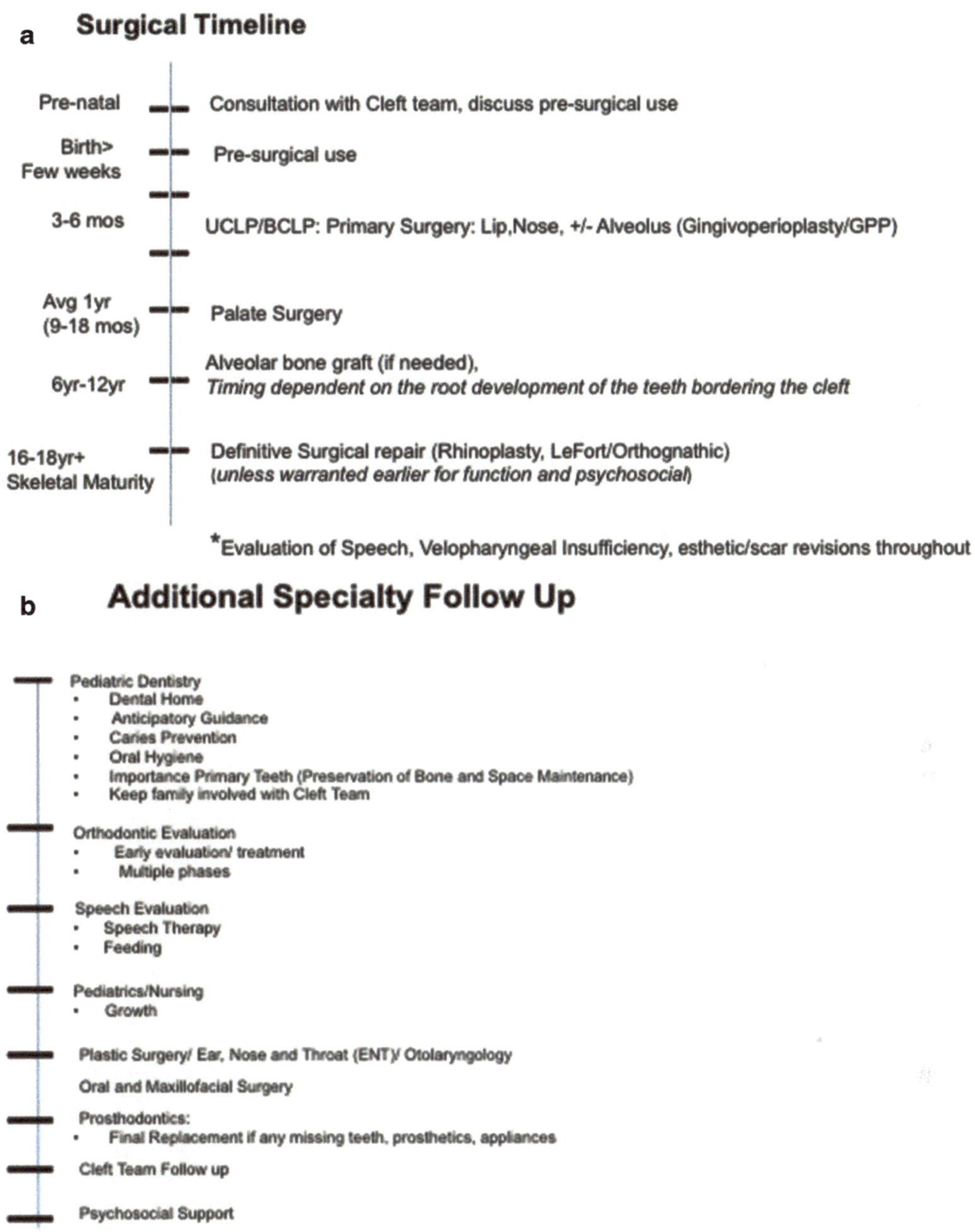


**Fig. 26.1** (**a**) *Dental home*. For patients with clefts, dental home care must be established by the time they start OFM-NAM treatment. (**b**) *Timeline caption*: it is important to note that each center may have their variations on surgical timing and type and/or use of pre-surgical therapy, based on research, training, cleft severity, any precluding medical conditions, and patient's access to care

## Pre-surgical Infant Orthopedics

The surgical repair of the infant with cleft lip and palate deformity can be a challenging and complex procedure. The cleft lip and palate deformity can present with varying degrees of severity. In general, the wider, more extensive clefts will present a more significant nasolabial deformity, which presents an even greater surgical challenge to obtain functional and esthetic success. Aesthetic outcomes tend to be poorer with more severe clefts. The basic goal of pre-surgical infant orthopedic management of the patient with cleft lip, alveolus, and palate is to normalize the deformed anatomy. By applying NAM or FMO techniques as pre-surgical treatment, the severity of the deformation can be reduced thus increasing the possibilities of better surgical and functional outcomes [7–11]. NAM and FMO techniques appear to be both safe and effective for both unilateral and bilateral clefts and applicable in low-resource settings.

NAM and FMO are two techniques currently in use that have similarities but also differences in philosophy and variations in their technique. The techniques are described here by two orthodontists who currently practice each technique in their respective locales. Dr. Scott was trained in the Grayson technique at University of California in Los Angeles

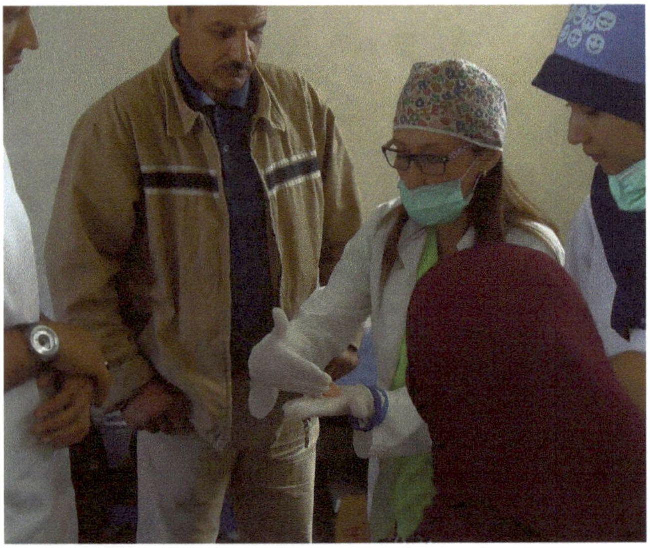

**Fig. 26.2** Dental care education for caregivers

and currently practices it at the Children's Hospital of Philadelphia. The NAM technique is used across many cleft centers in North America, and its use in large academic centers has landed to its extensive study and numerous publications to support its utility. Dr. Pannaci has a long-standing practice in Venezuela, and more recently in Spain, and has been one of the pioneers of the functional orthopedics concept. This concept has evolved over the past 25 years and spread particularly in Latin America among local volunteer Operation Smile dentists and orthodontists. There is accumulating positive clinical experience with this technique, however little formal published clinical research on outcomes to date. The Functional Orthopedics concept includes treatment prior to lip repair (FMO), which is similar to NAM, as well as treatment after lip repair including palatal activation and facial treatment. Although the superiority of one technique over the other is debated, it is also important to note controversy even about the benefits of infant orthopedics and that many centers do not advocate their use due to concerns for facial growth and added cost.

## Lip Taping

The simplest form of pre-surgical orthopedics is taping the cleft lip segments together with adhesive tape. This can be started within days of birth. It has several benefits including preventing retraction and separation of both the cleft lip soft tissue, as well as providing indirect traction on the maxillary segments from splaying. Different tape types can be used, including steri-strips and plastic medical adhesive tape. A width of about 1 cm seems to work best, with overlap of at least 5 cm on each cheek (Fig. 26.8a, b). Most practitioners recommend lip taping for nearly 24 hours per day if possible, being removed briefly every 2–4 days for bathing. To prevent inflammation on the cheeks from the adhesive, minimize the frequency of tape removal. If available, DuoDERM gel pads (approximately 3 × 4 cm in size) can be applied to the cheeks

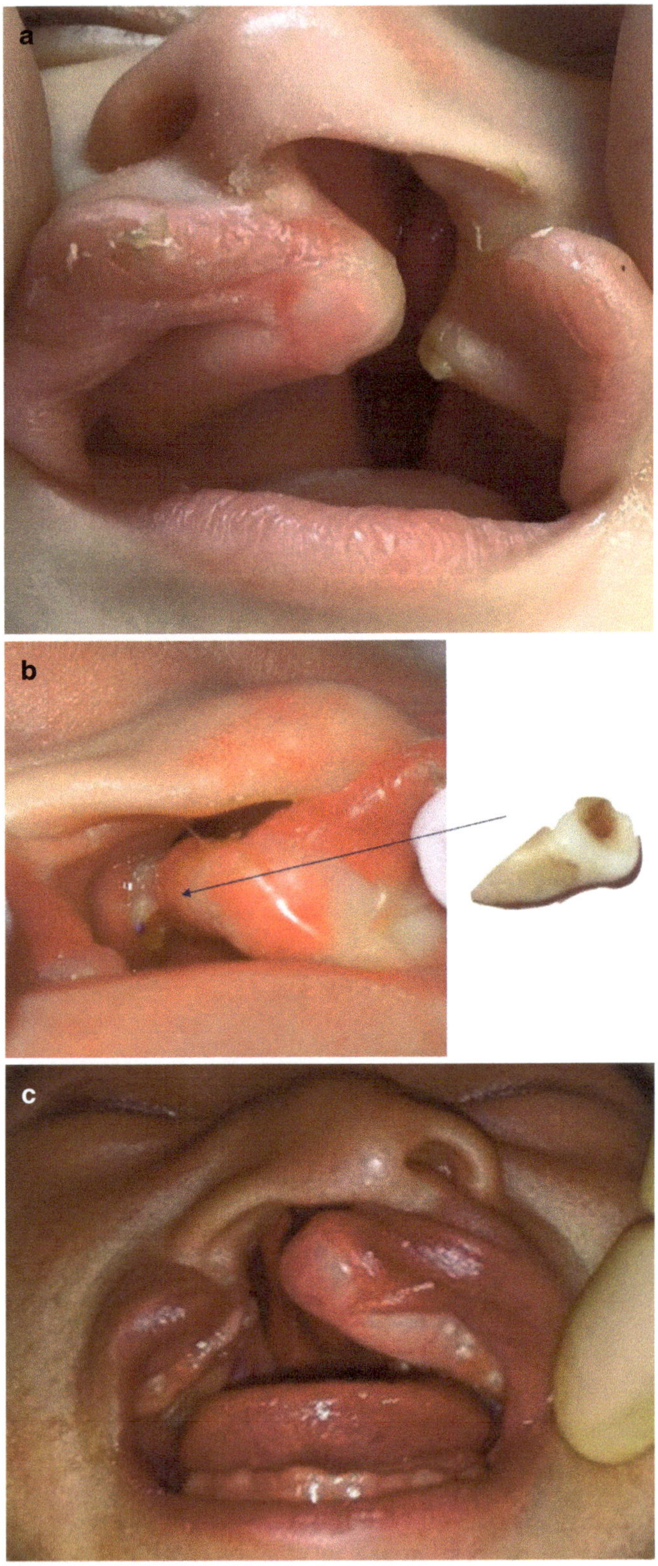

**Fig. 26.3** (**a**) *Natal teeth*. Present immediately at birth. (**b**) *Neonatal caption teeth*. Present during the first 30 days of life. (**c**) *Epstein pearls*

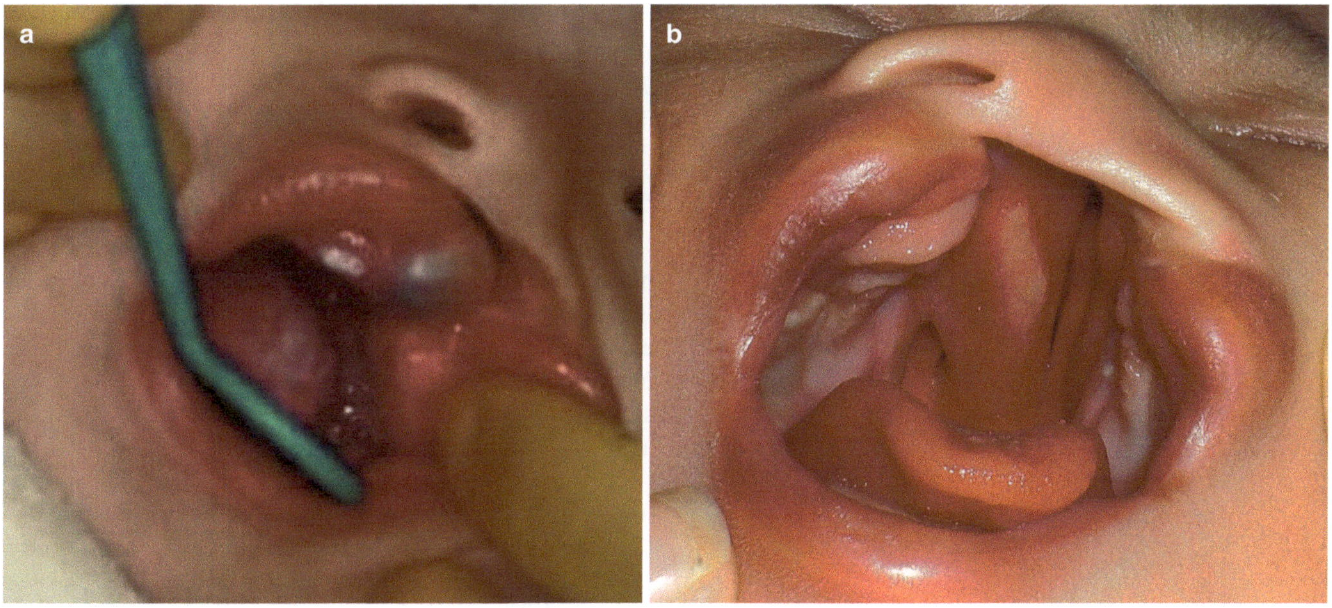

Fig. 26.4 (**a**) *Eruption hematoma*. (**b**) Vomer ulcer caused by the continuous contact of the tongue with the sensitive mucosa of the vomer. It's usually self-limiting

Table 26.1 Common dental anomalies and risk factors in cleft lip and palate (Fig. 26.5)

| Dental anomalies | Oral manifestations [5] | Risk factors in CLP contribute to [5] |
|---|---|---|
| • Agenesis (most commonly the maxillary primary or permanent lateral incisor followed by the second premolars)<br>• Supernumerary teeth<br>• Malformed/peg crown<br>• Enamel hypoplasia<br>• Impaction<br>• Dens invaginatus/ evaginatus<br>• Ectopic eruption<br>• Malpositioned teeth (most commonly the maxillary lateral incisor palatally placed) | • Higher caries risk and prevalence in both the primary and permanent dentition<br>• Poor oral hygiene<br>• Increased periodontal disease | • Malocclusion<br>• Malposition of the teeth in the area of the cleft<br>• Enamel hypoplasia<br>• Early orthodontic appliance wear<br>• Food impaction<br>• Fear of parents to brush surgical site<br>• Restricted access to the teeth in the area of the cleft, from resulting tension after lip repair/scar<br>• Excessive nursing, bottle, sippy cup<br>• Cariogenic diet and liquids |

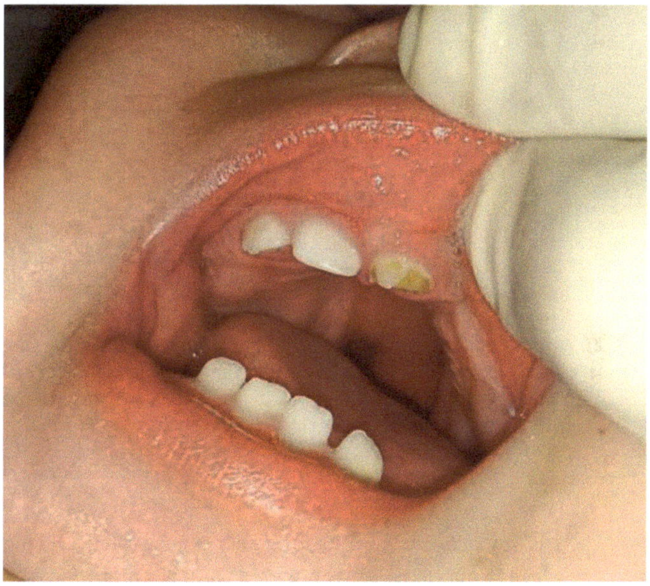

Fig. 26.5 *Dental anomalies*. Enamel hypoplasia

for 1–2 weeks at a time, with the lip tape applied over the top of the DuoDERM and changed more frequently. In settings where neither NAM or FMO is available, lip taping often reduces the severity of a cleft by the time of lip repair, primarily for bilateral repairs. It is also a component of NAM and can be combined with FMO (Fig. 26.8c).

## Nasoalveolar Molding (NAM)

Currently, nasoalveolar molding (NAM) is used in many major centers for preoperative orthopedic management of the cleft lip and palate patient. NAM was developed by Grayson in 1993 with a concept combining an intraoral molding device along with a nasal molding stent to address the alveolar deformity and the deformity of the nasal cartilages and the columella tissue deficiency in infants with both unilateral and bilateral cleft lip and palate [8]. The goal of NAM therapy is to align and approximate the intraoral alveolar segments and to achieve correction of the nasal cartilages, repositioning of the alar cartilages superior to toward the tip and address asymmetrical and or a deficient columella utilizing negative sculpting and passive molding of the alveolus and nasal tissues [8].

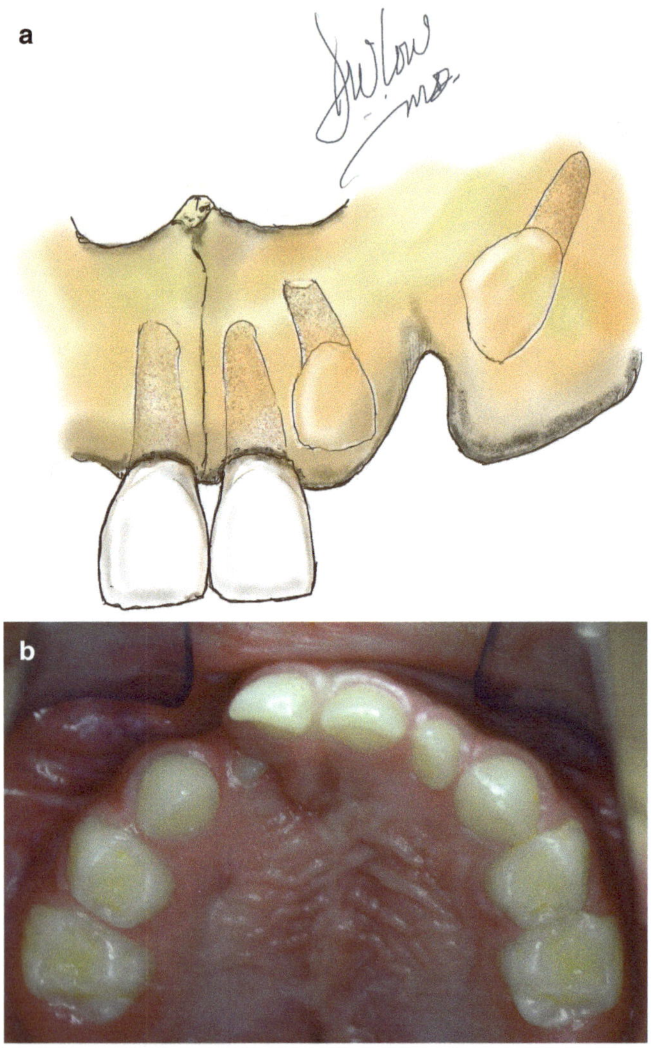


**Fig. 26.6** (**a**) Avoiding the extraction of the primary teeth bordering the cleft, the alveolar bone is preserved. (**b**) *Teeth bordering cleft caption*: importance of primary teeth – bone is preserved by primary teeth bordering the area of the alveolar cleft. Space maintenance (due to potential of missing teeth). Provide anchorage for early orthodontic intervention

NAM is initiated within the first few weeks of life. This early intervention takes advantage of the plasticity in the cartilages of the neonate caused by the high level of hyaluronic acid which allows for manipulation of the cartilaginous tissue [9].

## Technique

The impression of the intraoral cleft defect is ideally achieved in the first week of life to take advantage of the aforementioned cartilaginous plasticity [9]. It is recommended that the impression be performed in a hospital setting or in a facility that is able to manage a potential airway emergency [10]. The infant is held in an inverted position, while a custom tray is loaded with heavy-bodied polyvinyl siloxane impression material. The impression tray is placed into the infant's mouth. Careful attention to the tongue position and airway must be executed until the impression material is set. Once the impression material has set, the tray is removed, and the mouth is examined for residual material.

The molding plate can then be fabricated on a dental stone model poured from the impression. In general, the appliance is fabricated from a clear methyl methacrylate. The borders are trimmed to accommodate areas that are likely to cause ulceration such as the labial frenum area. The appliance should be highly polished at delivery and at each subsequent adjustment for patient comfort.

Retention buttons are attached to the plate at approximately a 30–40% angle at the time of delivery to aid in retention. The molding plate is then secured extra orally to the cheek bilaterally using steri-strips and an orthodontic elastic at one end. The elastic is stretched to twice its original length to achieve the proper activation force of 2 ounces [11]. The direction of elastic pull is individual to each patient; however, in general it is in a superior and posterior vector. Base tapes such as DuoDERM can be applied to the cheek underneath the steri-strip to aid in retention and help temper hyperreaction irritation of the skin to steri-strip tape adhesive. If necessary zinc-free denture adhesive can be utilized inside the molding plate to aide in retention [12].

Before the molding plate is delivered, final adjustments should be made to ensure proper fit and retention. The child should be observed feeding comfortably with no signs of gagging or distress. Instructions are given to the parents that the plate is to remain in place full time and should be removed briefly once daily for cleaning.

Weekly follow-up appointments should be arranged. At these appointments the molding plate will be modified with selective removal of acrylic, and selective application of soft denture material is used to guide the alveolar segments into a more normal position [11]. The molding plate should be adjusted if any ulcerations are present. If gingivoperiosteoplasty is planned as part of the surgical repair, the adjustments must continue until the alveolar segments are touching [13, 14].

The nasal molding is initiated when the reduction is such that the cleft gap is 5 mm or less. A nasal stent is formed using stainless steel wire in the shape of a "swan neck" with a small loop on one end attached to the existing molding plate [15]. The small loop is used to retain an intranasal bilobed kidney-shaped hard acrylic component. A layer of soft denture liner is added to the acrylic for patient comfort and to prevent ulceration to the nasal mucosa. The upper lobe of the bilobed nasal stent is inserted 3–4 mm inside the nose

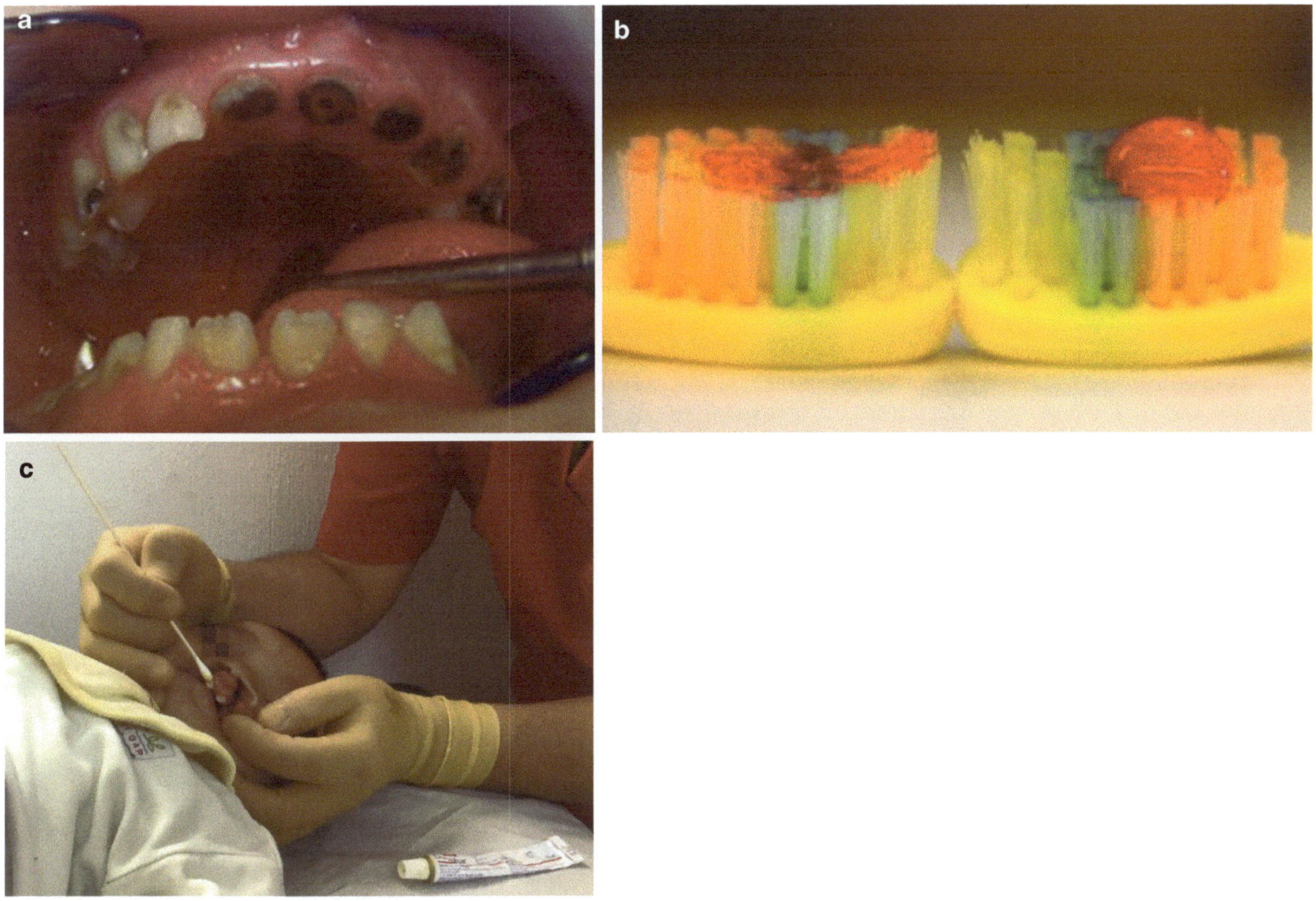

Fig. 26.7 (**a**) *Multiple dental caries*. (**b**) *Toothpaste caption*: the recommendations are to use no more than a smear or rice-sized amount of fluoridated toothpaste should be used for children under age 3; no more than a pea-sized amount should be used for children ages 3–6. (**c**) *Therapies with fluoride varnish*

and gently lifted forward of the dome until a slight bit of tissue blanching is noted. The lower lobe of the stent lifts the nostril apex and defines the top of the columella (Fig. 26.9a).

One nasal stent will be required for the unilateral cleft patient. Two nasal stents will be necessary for the bilateral cleft patient (Fig. 26.9b). The appropriate location of attachment of the nasal stent to the molding plate can be determined by pulling the cleft lip segments together while centering the columella and philtrum [13]· Minor adjustments to the nasal stent location and projection can be accomplished using orthodontic pliers.

The shapes of the medial and lateral crus, the cartilaginous septum, and the alar cartilage tip are carefully molded to resemble a normal shape with weekly modifications to the nasal stent [18].

In the bilateral cleft patient, lengthening of the columella is often necessary. A columella band is fabricated with soft denture liner material that joins the left and right lower lobes of the nasal stents, spanning the columella. The band will sit at the nasolabial junction and helps to define and control the vectors of force as the nasal tip continues to be projected forward. Additional lip taping of the premaxillary segment pulling downward and engaged into the retention buttons with elastics is utilized. The opposing forces of the upward pressure of the two nasal stents and downward pull of the tape on the premaxillary lip tissues will allow for the columellar tissues to stretch (Fig. 26.9b).

The one-stage primary cheilorhinoplasty is typically performed at 4–6 months of age, generally at the older end of this range for bilateral clefts. Some surgeons feel a gingivoperiosteoplasty is beneficial to perform at the time of lip and nose repair [15]. Figure 26.1 details the stages of NAM. See box: Guidelines for Nasal Device.

**NAM Guidelines: Nasal Device**

- Nasal molding is initiated when the cleft gap is 5 mm or less.
- Form a nasal stent using stainless steel wire in the shape of a "swan neck" with an intranasal bilobed kidney-shaped hard acrylic component.
- A layer of soft denture liner is added to the bilobed acrylic kidney-shaped acrylic component.
- Be careful to maintain the bilobular shape.
- Attach it to the existing molding plate.
- Adjustments to the nasal stent location and projection can be accomplished using orthodontic pliers.
- Explain to parents how to place the NAM (plate and the nasal device) and secured extra orally.
- Explain to parents how to remove the NAM and how to clean it twice a day.
- Weekly follow-up appointments should be arranged.
- At weekly follow-up appointments the nasal stent will be modified with selective application of soft denture material.
- Add lip taping and explain to parents how to place and remove it.
- Appointments continue until the objectives are completed.

Timeline of NAM for unilateral and bilateral cases (Fig. 26.10).

## Functional Maxillary Orthopedics (FMO)

FMO is a dentistry specialty that utilizes intraoral devices, which are not fixed to any tooth or oral structure, to prevent and correct oral system dysfunctions [19]. FMO seeks to guide craniofacial development, acknowledging the multiple factors and feedback systems implicated in growth, of which oral musculature is thought to be central [20–22, 23]. FMO seeks to stimulate strengthening of the oral and perioral muscles, with the goal that the muscles will then act to guide improved bony growth [19, 24, 23].

For patients with cleft lip and palate, FMO aims to perform an adequate pre-surgical preparation in the shape and alignment of the maxillary segments, as well as to rehabilitate the altered functions of breathing, suction, and swallowing in the cleft baby [7, 17, 24]. Pre-surgical orthopedic treatment in infants aims to set the course for the functional patterns in later life [17] (Fig. 26.11a, b).

Goals in unilateral cases include (Fig. 26.11c):

- Approximation, alignment, and leveling of the maxillary segments

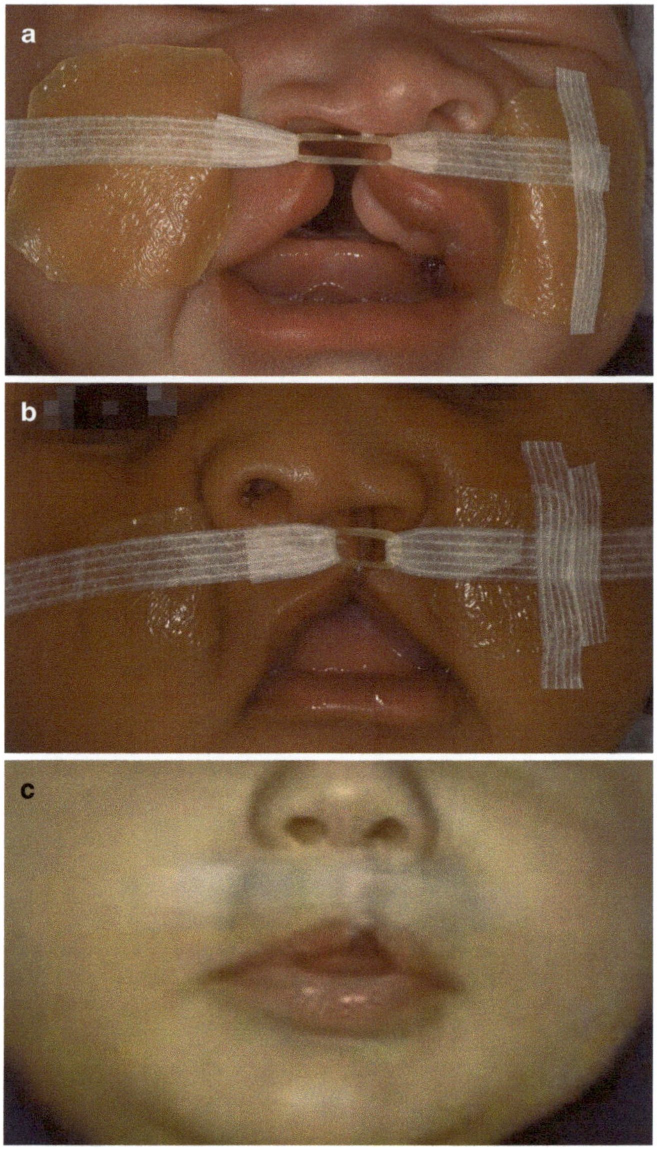


**Fig. 26.8** (**a**) Steri-strips or plastic medical adhesive tape is used for lip taping of patient with wide complete cleft lip. (**b**) DuoDERM gel pads can be applied to prevent inflammation on the cheeks from the adhesive. Lip taping of patient with medium complete cleft lip. (**c**) Lip taping of patient with an incomplete cleft lip

- Progressive closure of the alveolar and palatal gap before lip surgery
- Promotes symmetrical facial growth
- Fosters more or less physiological growth [17]
- Rehabilitates the altered functions of breathing, suction, and swallowing

In addition to the above, in bilateral cases they also include (Fig. 26.11d):

- Progressive correction of premaxilla position with de-rotation and de-tilt

- Reduce nasal septal deformity to improve postoperative nasal function

## Technique

Intraoral plates made of self-curing acrylic are fabricated and placed intraorally as soon as possible after birth (Fig. 26.12).

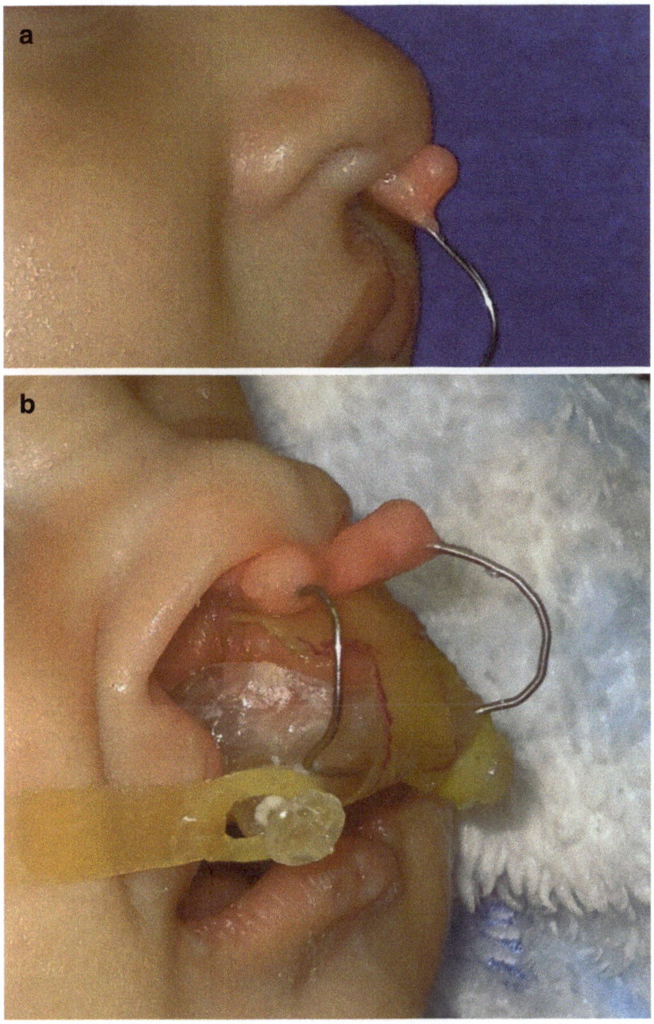


**Fig. 26.9** (**a**) The upper lobe of the bilobed nasal stent is inserted 3–4 mm inside the nose and gently lifted forward of the dome. (**b**) Two nasal stents will be necessary for the bilateral cleft patient. The opposing forces of the upward pressure of the two nasal stents and downward pull of the tape on the premaxillary lip tissues will allow for the columellar tissues to stretch

Due to the constant and rapid growth of the baby in his first year of life, the plate is stimulated [17], with this motion directing maxillary segment relation and facial musculature which is observed to reduce the cleft dimensions [7, 24]. The cleft segments are not compressed, but rather their growth is directed toward alignment of the maxillary arch [17, 24].

Maxillary intraoral impression is made and a cast model created, with wax added on the cast model in order to program the collision areas (Fig. 26.13). FMO plates are made from the model of self-curing acrylic. On the oral surface of the FMO plate and on the side of the minor segment, transverse scratches are made to give the plate a different texture to stimulate the continuous touch of the tongue through proprioception (Pannaci's modification) [7, 24] (Fig. 26.14a) (Video 26.1).

Functional rehabilitation is best aided by ensuring the FMO device is contoured to closely match the palatal contour of the baby and modified if necessary. The plate blocks the passage of liquid to the nasal cavity, acting as an obturator to facilitate nasal breathing while sucking milk from a bottle. It has been observed to expedite feeding [33] and potentially enable breastfeeding.

Treatment course should start as soon as possible after birth and continue to lip repair. New devices are fashioned every 4 weeks, and devices are worn 24 hours per day. It can be continued after lip repair (see next section.) At the first appointment, suction, swallowing, and breathing are evaluated as well as symmetry of tongue movements. Parents are shown how to place and remove the FOP and how to clean with soap and water twice daily.

Mazaheri's Protocol Analysis is applied to all cases in order to ensure that the treatment is proceeding toward objectives [25]. This protocol utilizes a coordinated system that allows the quantitative analysis in millimeters of cleft cases. It facilitates the evaluation and control of the treatment of two-dimensional changes (transversal and longitudinal) that progresses in maxillary segment relation to the cleft; it does not consider the axial axis (Fig. 26.14b) (Video 26.2). Observed clinical outcomes of pre-surgical orthopedic treatment include reduction of cleft width by guiding growth and functional rehabilitation [7, 16, 24, 26].

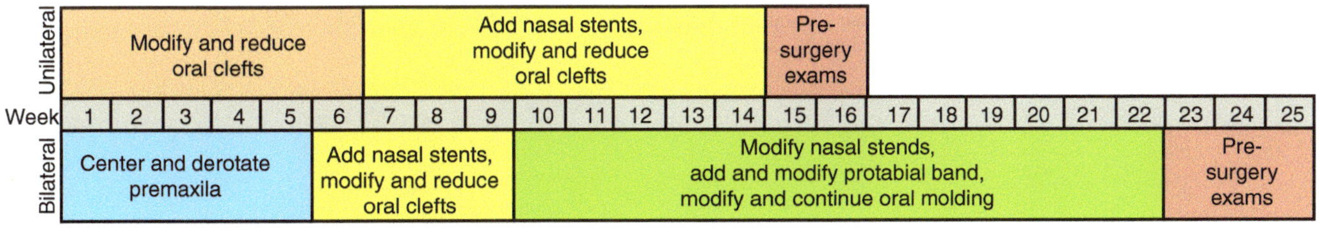


**Fig. 26.10** Timeline of NAM for unilateral and bilateral cases

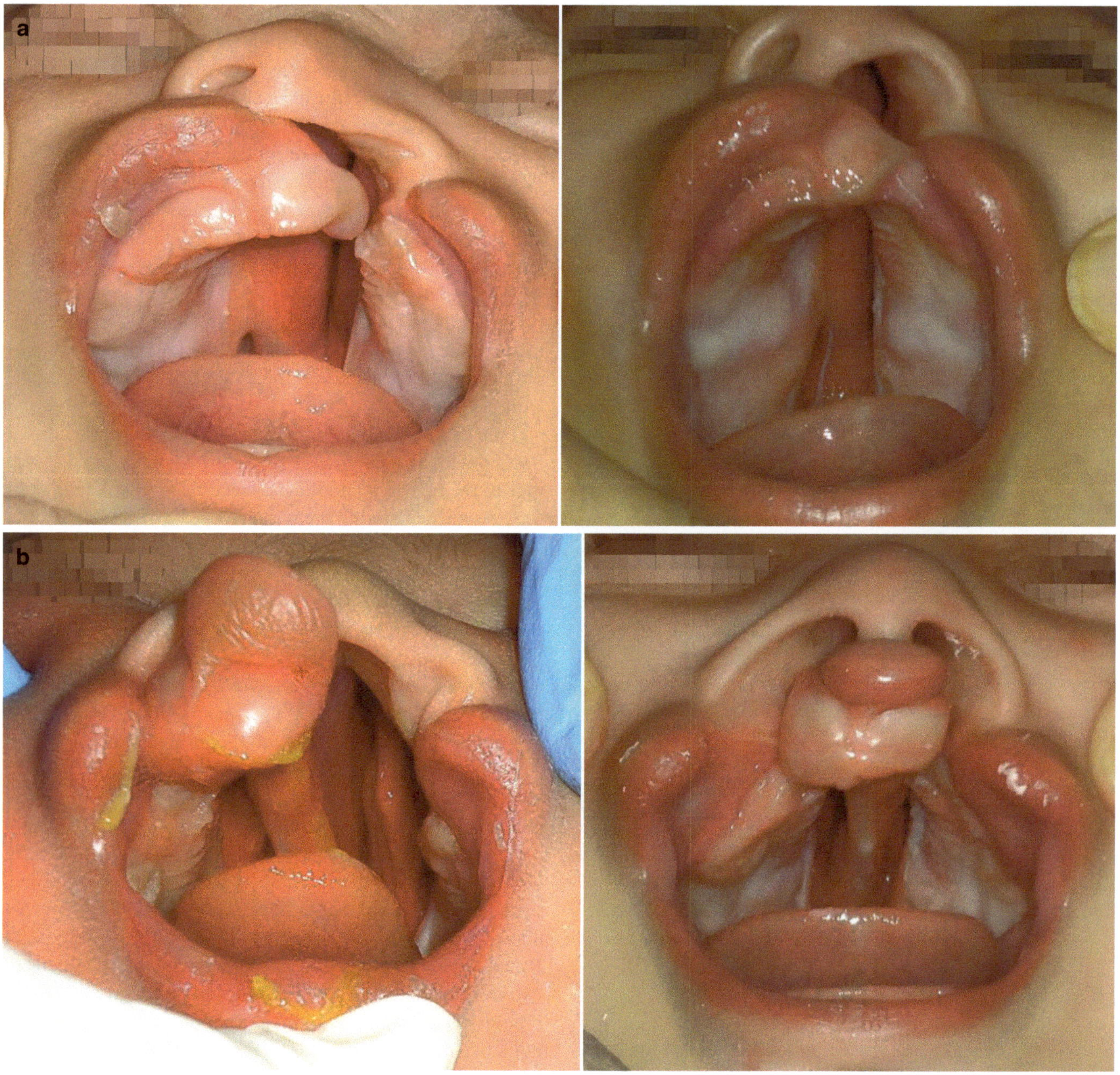


**Fig. 26.11** (**a**) *FMO unilateral sequence treatment*: unilateral cleft lip and palate patient case, 5 months FMO treatment sequence – maxillary arch conformations, increased volume of the maxillary segments; increase of the transversal and sagittal dimensions of the maxilla and decrease of the alveolar and palatal gap, plus molding alar cartilage, increase the nasal symmetry and nonsurgical elongation of the columella. (**b**) *FMO bilateral sequence treatment*: bilateral cleft lip and palate patient case, 6 months FMO treatment sequence – maxillary arch conformation, de-rotation, and de-tilt of the premaxilla, as well as increased volume of the maxillary segments and decrease of the alveolar and palatal gap, plus molding alar cartilage, increase the nasal symmetry and nonsurgical elongation of the columella. (**c**) Approximation, alignment, and leveling of the maxillary segments and the progressive closure of the alveolar and palatal gap before lip surgery are one of FMO's goal in order to improve the conditions for a less aggressive surgery. (**d**) In bilateral cases one of the goals is correct septal deviation as well as correct the rotation and tilt of the premaxilla

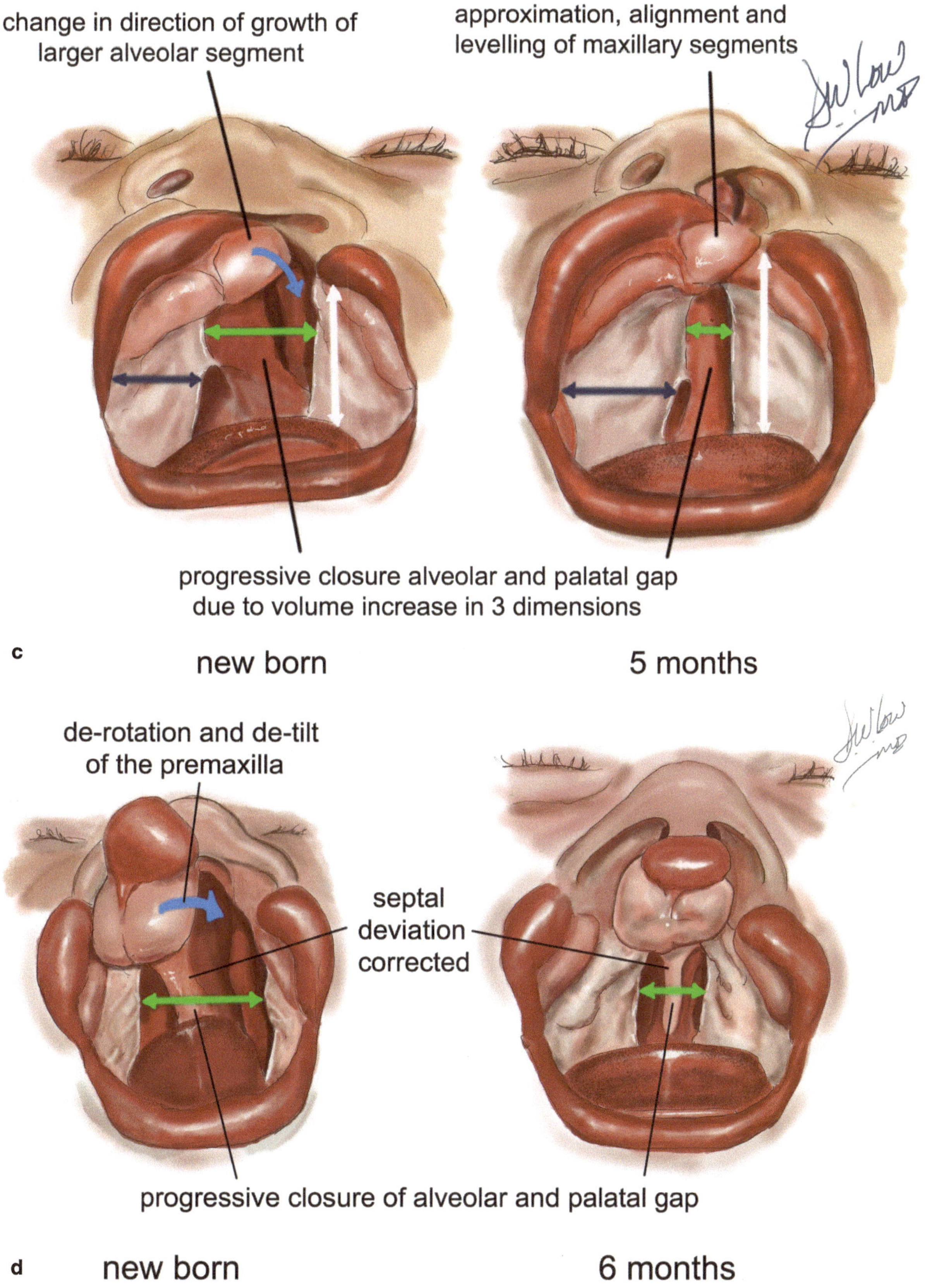


**Fig. 26.11** (continued)

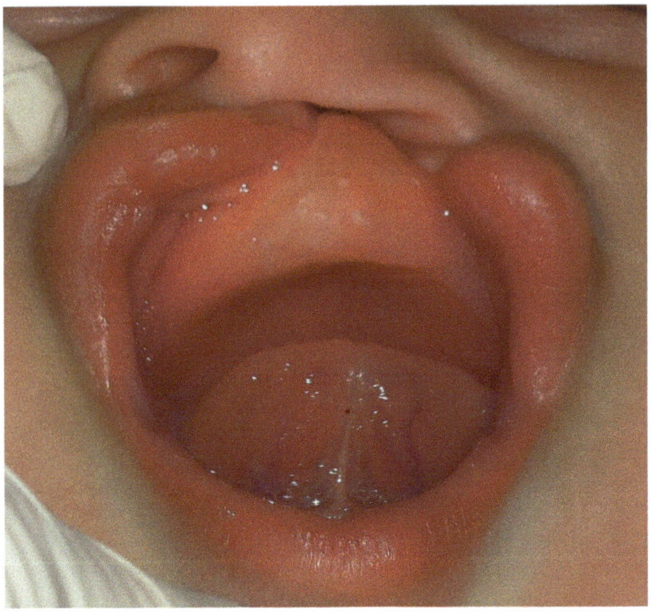

Fig. 26.12 *FMO plate placed intraorally*. The tongue will look to collide the area's plate in the where the scratch marks are located; note the scratches at the palate on the cleft side

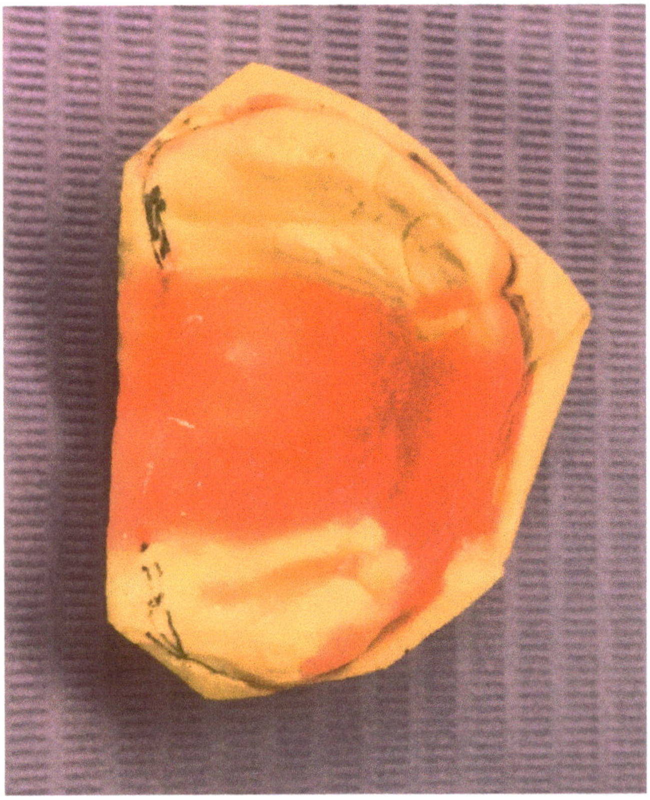

Fig. 26.13 *Wax-up step on the cast model*. The self-curing acrylic FMO plate will be made on it

## Comparing Pre-surgical Orthopedic Techniques

Nasoavolar molding (NAM) and functional maxillary orthopedics (FMO) have similarities and differences, discussed in Table 26.2. Furthermore, we discuss common problems and potential solutions for pre-surgical orthopedic devices (Table 26.3).

**Tips and Tricks**

*Pre-surgical Orthopedics in Low-Resource Settings*

- In a busy center with many patients in pre-surgical orthopedics, it often works well to schedule all appointments on the same day each month (seeing up to 15–25 patients per day). There is a lot of investment in time for the manufacture of the plates, retention buttons, and nasal devices but also economies of scale if the team takes an "all hands on deck" approach. This enables device delivery the same day, an important consideration when patients travel from a distance.
- One reason that FMO has been utilized in some low-resource settings with success is that it is less staff-intensive to create devices without retention buttons, and plate retention seems to be facilitated by using adhesive dental gels for dental prostheses.
- When conditions are met and the alveolar cleft gap is 5 mm or less, the nasal stent is formed by Dr. Grayson's protocol [8] and adapted to the acrylic plate. One nasal device is used for complete treatment even with the FMO device, and at monthly follow-up appointments, the nasal stent is removed from the FOP and placed in the new plate (Figs. 26.11a, b and 26.16a, b).

Most reports agree on the importance of performing an adequate pre-surgical treatment before lip surgery. In clinical practice in low-resource countries, we can mention that preoperative techniques applied to maxillary orthopedics and nasal molding have been effective and that they are also reproducible techniques at very low cost. In settings where surgeon techniques are less consistent than in high-resource settings, the potential benefit of pre-surgical orthopedics may be even larger. In this sense it is important to highlight the role of the dentist who provides these treatments and who must be committed to updating their knowledge. Taking into account the importance of functional benefits, we suggest that

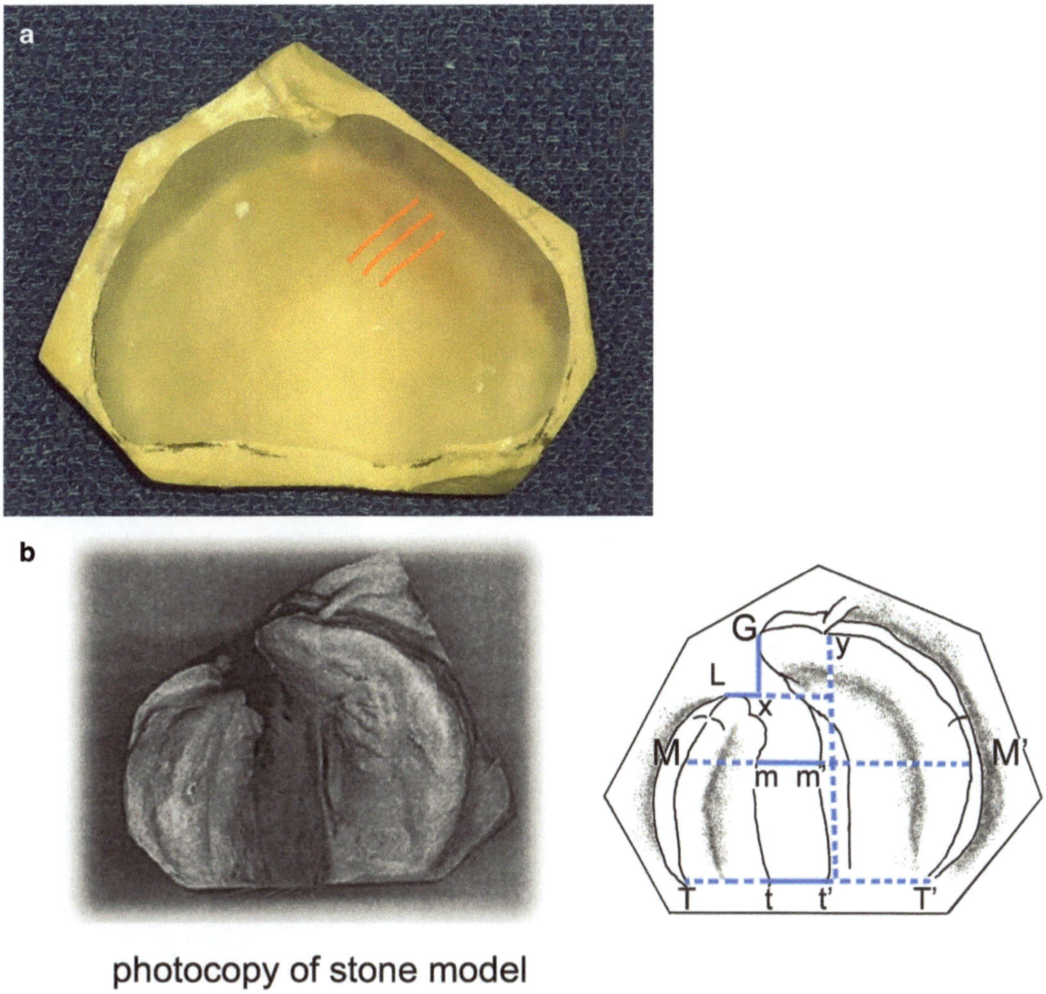


**Fig. 26.14** (**a**) *Self-curing acrylic plate finished.* Note the scratch marks on the surface of the plate and on the cleft side. (**b**) Stone xero-copie is made to place landmarks and obtain measures in millimeters in order to facilitate the evaluation and control of the treatment

**Table 26.2** Similarities and differences between NAM and FMO techniques

| | |
|---|---|
| Similarities | |
| Acrylic intraoral device<br>Device is not tightly affixed to mucosal surfaces<br>Treatment initiated as early after birth as possible<br>Impressions can be taken in dental room / clinic setting | |
| Differences | |
| NAM plate | FMO plate |
| Plate mechanism<br>Plate is held against maxilla with tape to retention button<br>Plate position maintained with retention buttons | Plate is allowed to float freely<br>Denture gel is used to help keep the plate in place |
| Plate fabrication<br>Single plate for course of treatment<br>First plate delivered at second appointment | New impression taken and new plate fabricated monthly<br>First plate delivered at first appointment |
| Plate modification<br>Palatal surface of plate modified at each appointment<br>Follow-up appointments with selective removal of acrylic and application of soft denture material, to guide the alveolar segments into a more normal position<br>Plate and nasal stent adjustment is customized based on clinical assessment of alveolar segments and nose | Wax-up on the stone model to program the collision areas and relief areas<br>Follow-up applying Mazaheri's Protocol Analysis to every new stone model and programming the collision areas and relief areas to guide the alveolar segments into a normal position and closing the palatal gap<br>The programming for the new plate is done on the positive palatal mold on the surface of the stone model.<br>Programming is done on the stone model and the millimetrical control is made with Mazaheri's Protocol (in an objective way) |
| Patient protocol<br>Visits every 1–2 weeks recommended | Visits once monthly recommended |

**Table 26.3** Common complications and solutions of pre-orthopedic therapy (Fig. 26.15a, b)

| Complications | Solutions |
|---|---|
| Soft tissue breakdown may occur in areas of modification of the plate if not properly polished or by excessive activation | Hard acrylic on internal palatal surface should not extend into the nasal cavity (BCLP)<br>Smoothing rough surfaces and relieving over contour areas<br>Lubrication of the mucosal interphase |
| Erythema of the buccal mucosa<br>Nasal septum irritation | Caregivers/parents most recognize this early by regularly monitoring the mucosal surface – immediately alert the clinician<br>The professional must be very careful and methodical<br>Appliance fabrication<br>Appliance insertion<br>Monitor soft tissue at every appointment |
| Full time wear and oral candida infection | Proper hygiene instructions<br>Clean the plate regularly<br>nystatine or amphotericin ointment<br>NAM therapy should continue |
| Occasionally the labial surface of the central incisor may erupt prematurely | Avoid excessive material on top of alveolar ridge |
| Epidermal tissue irritation<br>Rash like lesion<br>Constant removal of the facial tape<br>Tighten the tape too much<br>Allergy to the tape | Base tape DuoDERM, affixed to the chicks 4–5 days<br>Hydration cream<br>Varied the position of the tape |
| Too much adhesive arrests bone growth and cleft closure | Make sure parents and caregivers understand directions on adhesive use, cleaning, and care |

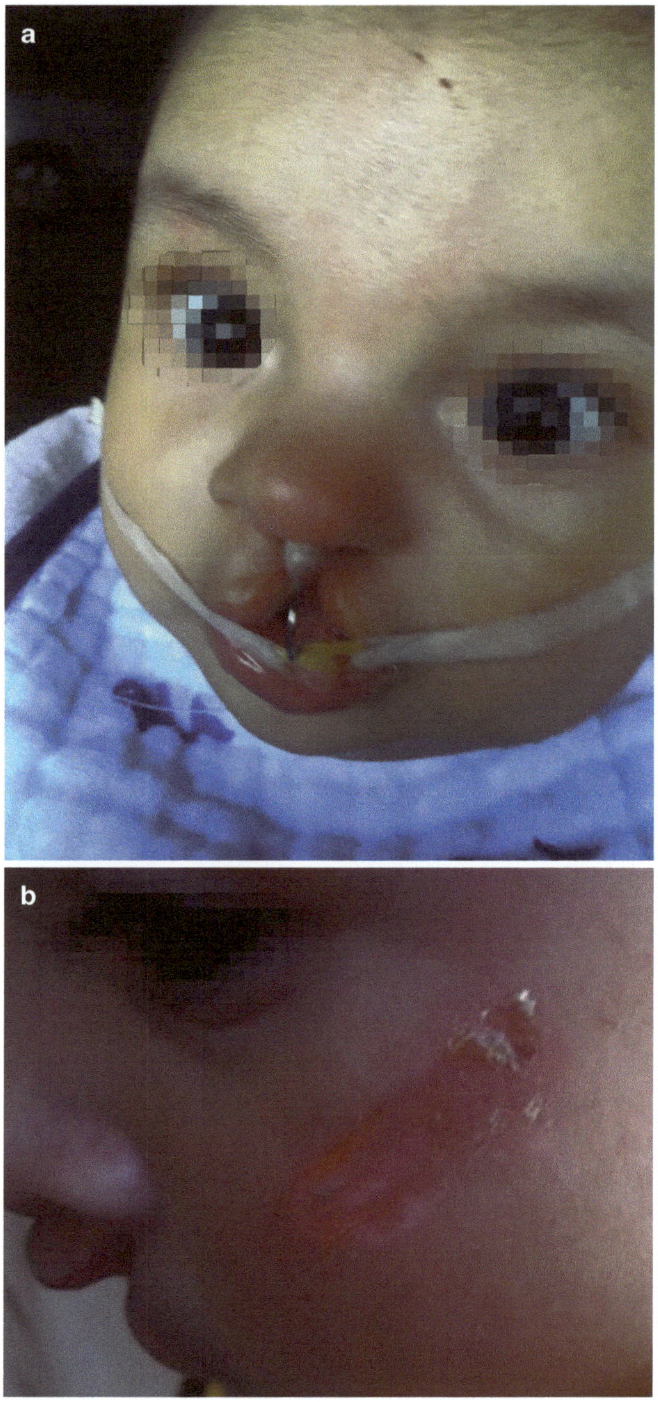


**Fig. 26.15** (**a**) *Soft tissue breakdown*. For excessive activation of NAM. (**b**) *Epidermal tissue irritation*. For allergy to the tape

when planning a treatment, observe not only the morphological effects but also the physiological and functional ones. Healing is synonymous with the restoration of functions, which is why it is important to consider it when preparing the diagnosis and controlling the evolution of the treatment.

## Myofunctional Therapy and Functional Maxillary Orthopedics After Cleft Lip Repair

Although less studied in North American centers, in which orthodontic adjuncts are generally not employed until the age of mixed dentition (6–7 years,) in other regions alternative treatments to promote muscular strengthening are being pursued. The premise of myofunctional therapy, like FMO, is to enable optimal maxillary growth and alignment.

## Functional Maxillary Orthopedics: 6–24 Months of Age

Premised on the functional matrix theory of force-generated osteosynthesis, it is thought that bone growth can be stimulated to favor stock for erupting deciduous teeth [7, 17, 19, 20, 21, 23, 24]. Thus FMO, as described above, can be continued beginning 1 month after lip repair and prior to palate repair, with the goal of improving palatal bone formation, decreased transverse width of alveolar and palatal gap, and improved sagittal growth of maxillary segments. Because infant growth decelerates after 1 year of age, if palatoplasty is performed later, FMO plate change can be decreased to every 6–8 weeks [7, 24]. During this period of treatment, the technique involves helping to place deciduous teeth in correct place on the maxillary arch in order to promote an adequate occlusion and therefore a correct masticatory function (Fig. 26.16c, d). In bilateral clefts, this also helps properly position the premaxilla with reduced risk of lesser segment collapse (Fig. 26.17).

## Soft Palatal Musculature

Inadequate velar mechanism is not restored until after palatoplasty, when velar muscles are repositioned from their sagittal malposition into a transverse sling. However, some practitioners advocate for stimulation of palatal muscles in the interim. This can potentially prevent muscular atrophy, aid in swallowing, and help facilitate middle ear drainage. Without the correct repair of those muscles, the patient lacks an adequate phonological-articulatory development and an adequate ventilation of the middle ear, increasing the risk of hearing loss [27]. Trujillo advocates for muscle stimulation using a cotton-tipped wooden applicator to stimulate the soft palate, alternating the left and right hemi uvula until the nauseous reflex response is obtained [27].

## Cleft Myofunctional Therapy

Patients with facial clefts have anatomical differences in facial and velopharyngeal muscles as well as in the bone tissue of the middle third of the face (described at length in Chap. 6). Their magnitude depends on size and location of the cleft, whether unilateral or bilateral and complete or incomplete, and type and time of surgery done [28, 29, 30]. Growth deficiencies may be due to intrinsic growth, functional distortions, or consequences of surgical intervention.

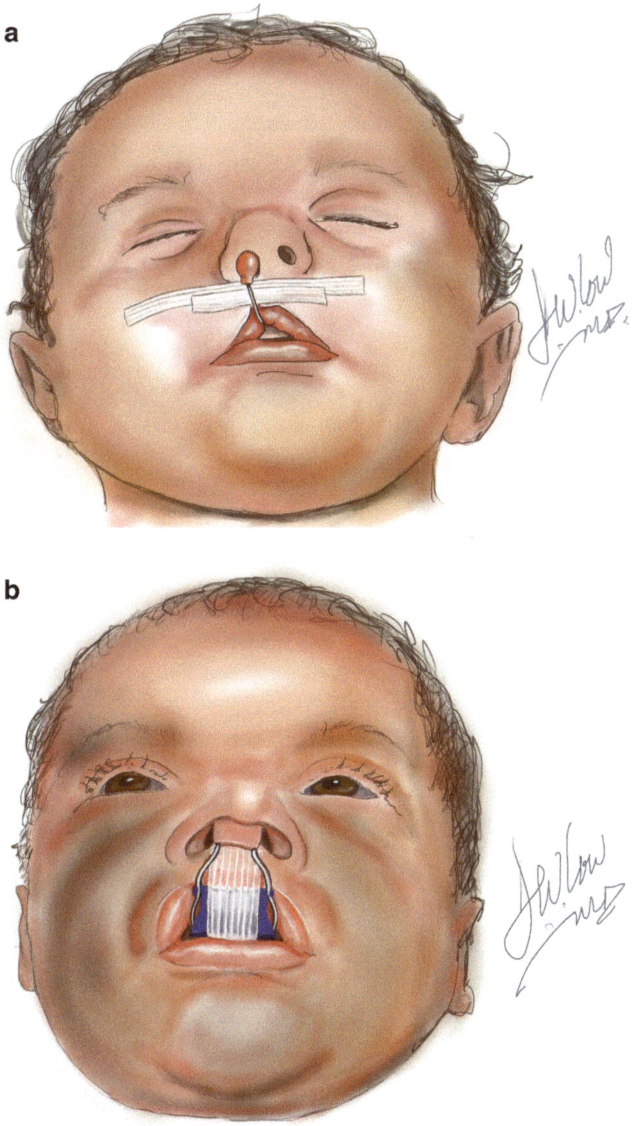


**Fig. 26.16** (**a**) Unilateral NAM device placed on FMO plate with horizontal lip taping. (**b**) Bilateral NAM device placed on FMO plate with vertical lip taping. (**c**) *Cast models XerosCopy sequence*. 20-month sequence unilateral cleft lip and palate case treated with FMO (Pannaci technique); cast models' xero-copie: Birth – 6–20 months. (**d**) *Cast model sequence*. 18-month sequence unilateral cleft lip and palate case treated with FMO (Pannaci technique); 6–20–24 months. FMO plate is made leaving space for erupted teeth. The scratches plate surface on the cleft side are to stimulate the continues touch and collide of the tongue

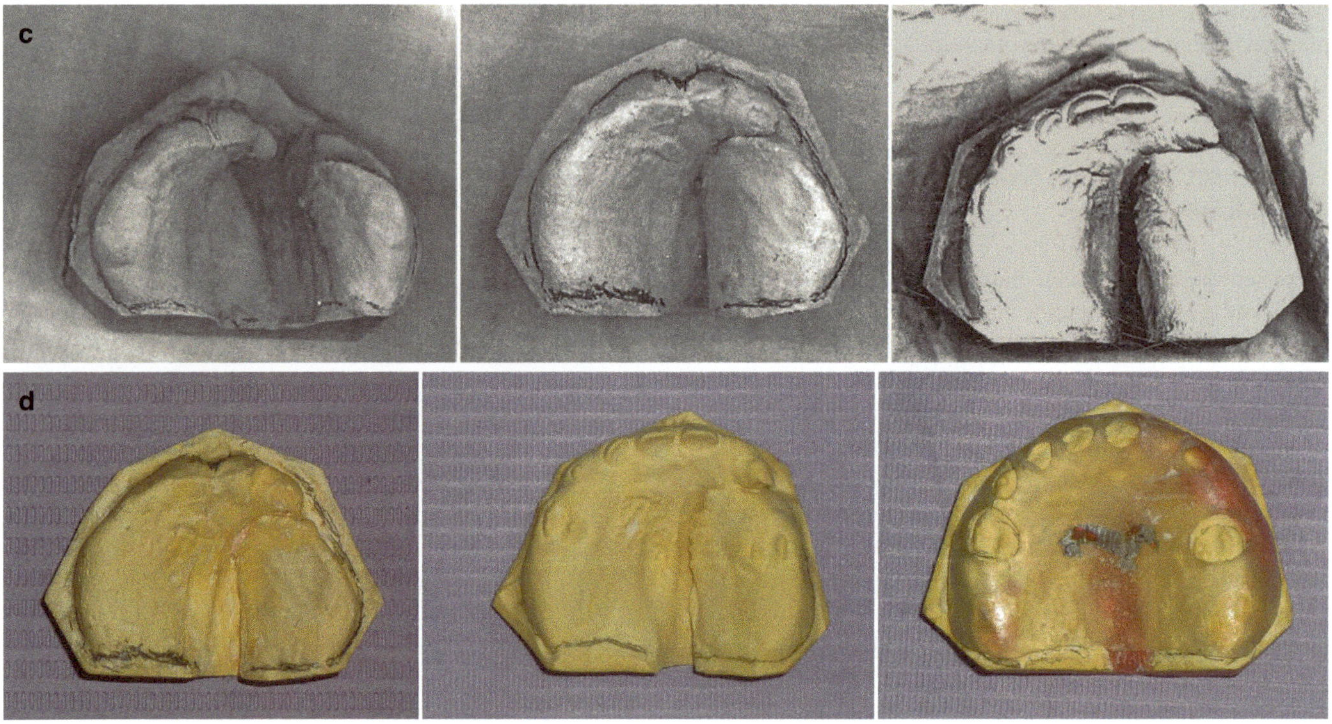


Fig. 26.16 (continued)

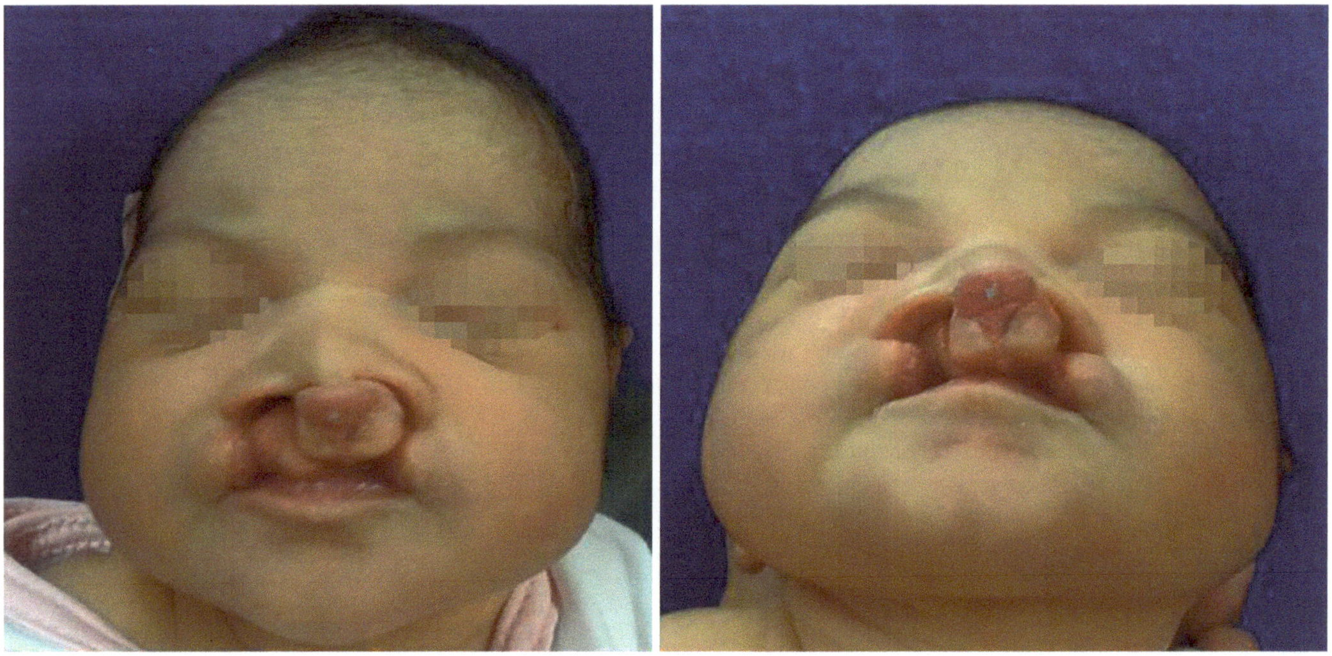

Fig. 26.17 In bilateral clefts, FMO also helps properly position and rotation the premaxilla. This 6-month sequence shows de-tilt and de-rotation of the premaxilla

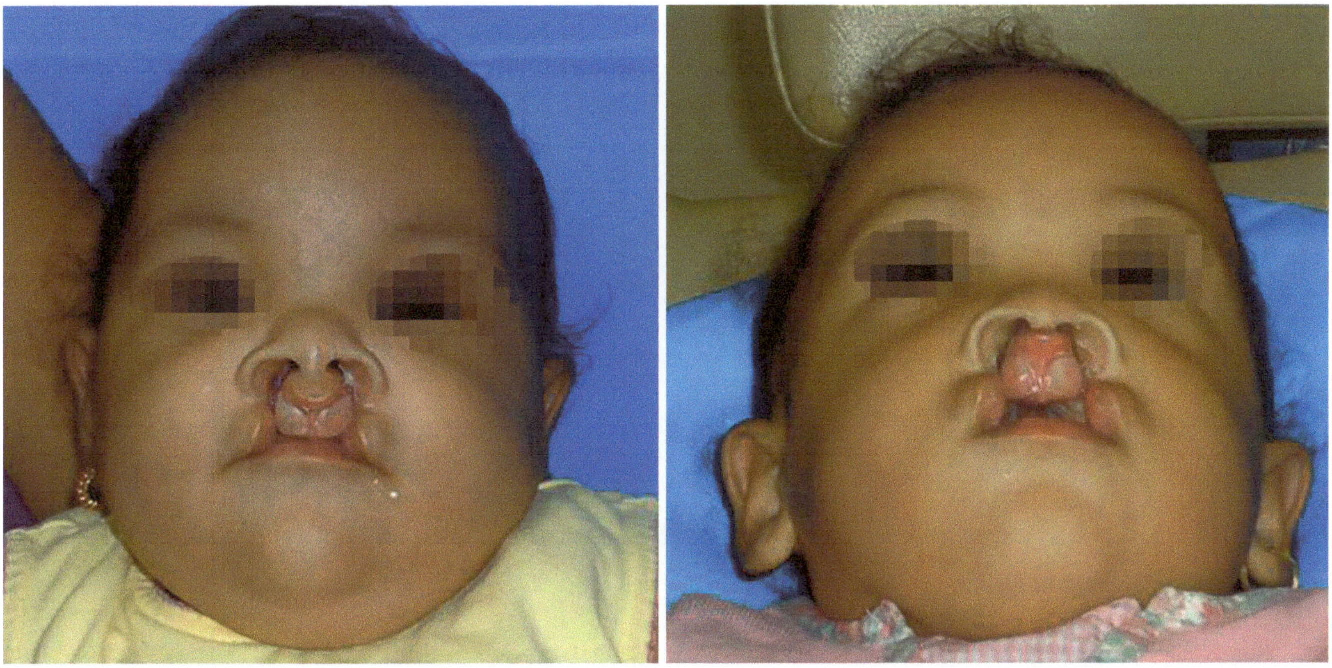

Fig. 26.17 (continued)

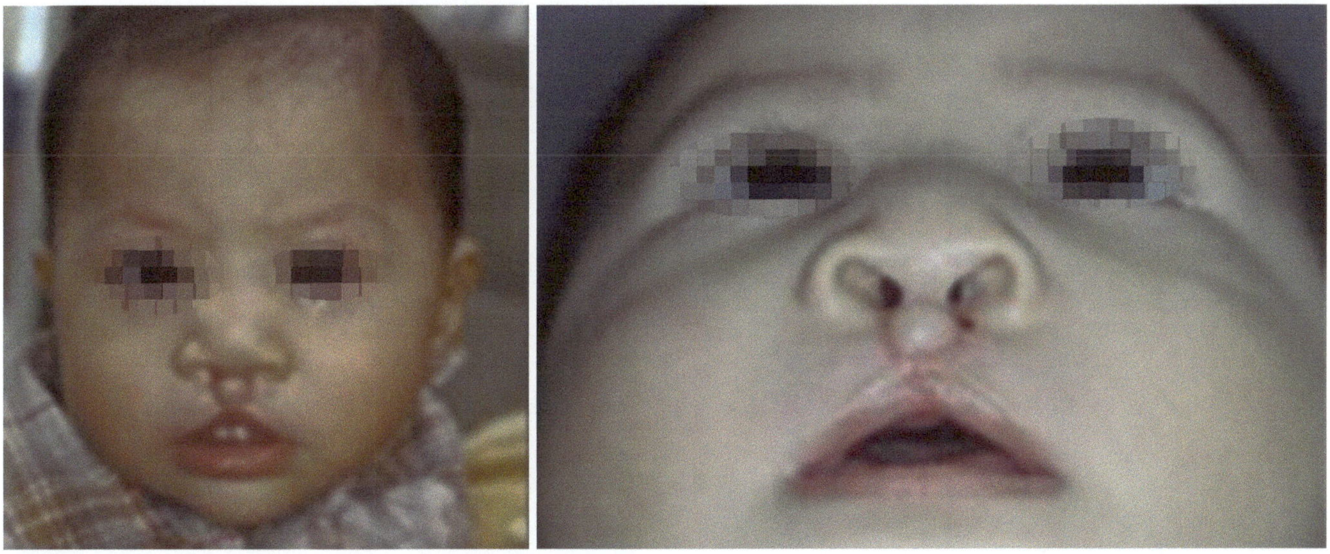

Fig. 26.18 BCLP patient, after lip repair, notice fibrous scar, short upper lip, and lip incompetence

Fibrosis and the increase of tension in many of the scars result in hypotonic and short lips with the consequence of poor facial development (Fig. 26.18). Tongue position after palatoplasty can be depressed and deglutition atypical (Fig. 26.19). In addition, adenoid and tonsillar hyperplasia may be present that diminish airway volumes. Functional rehabilitation of the occlusal plane is an important goal in maxillary orthopedic treatments to achieve a correct masticatory function [19, 21, 23]. Myofunctional therapy is focused on whether stimulating and optimizing orofacial muscle function, particularly at ages 2–6, can promote growth.

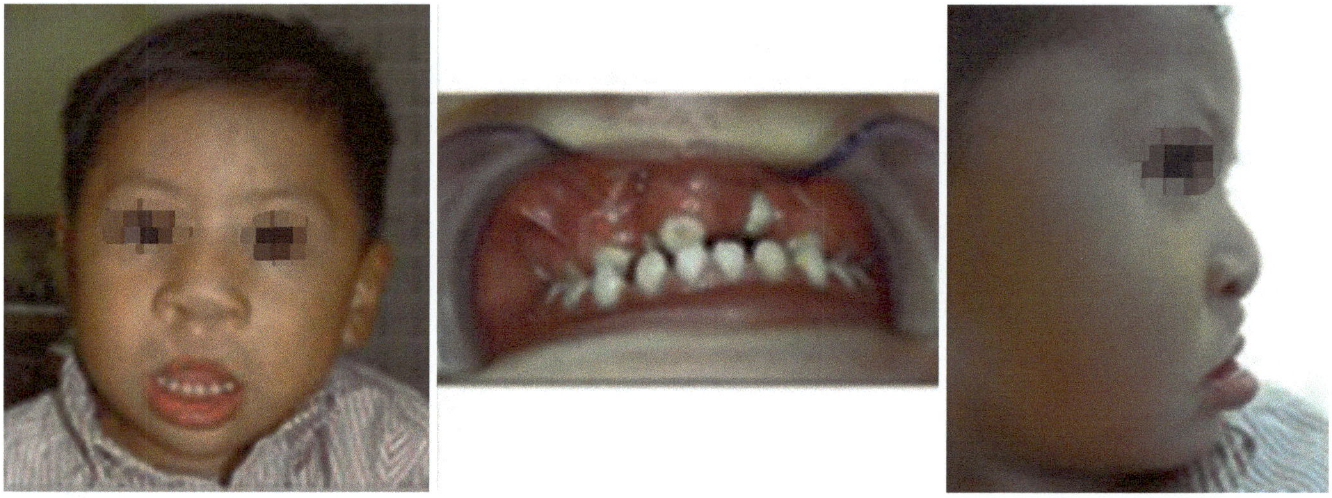

**Fig. 26.19** BCLP intercepted and treated at an early age (2 years) with a facial development protocol immediately after palatal repair. Notice signs of mouth breathing

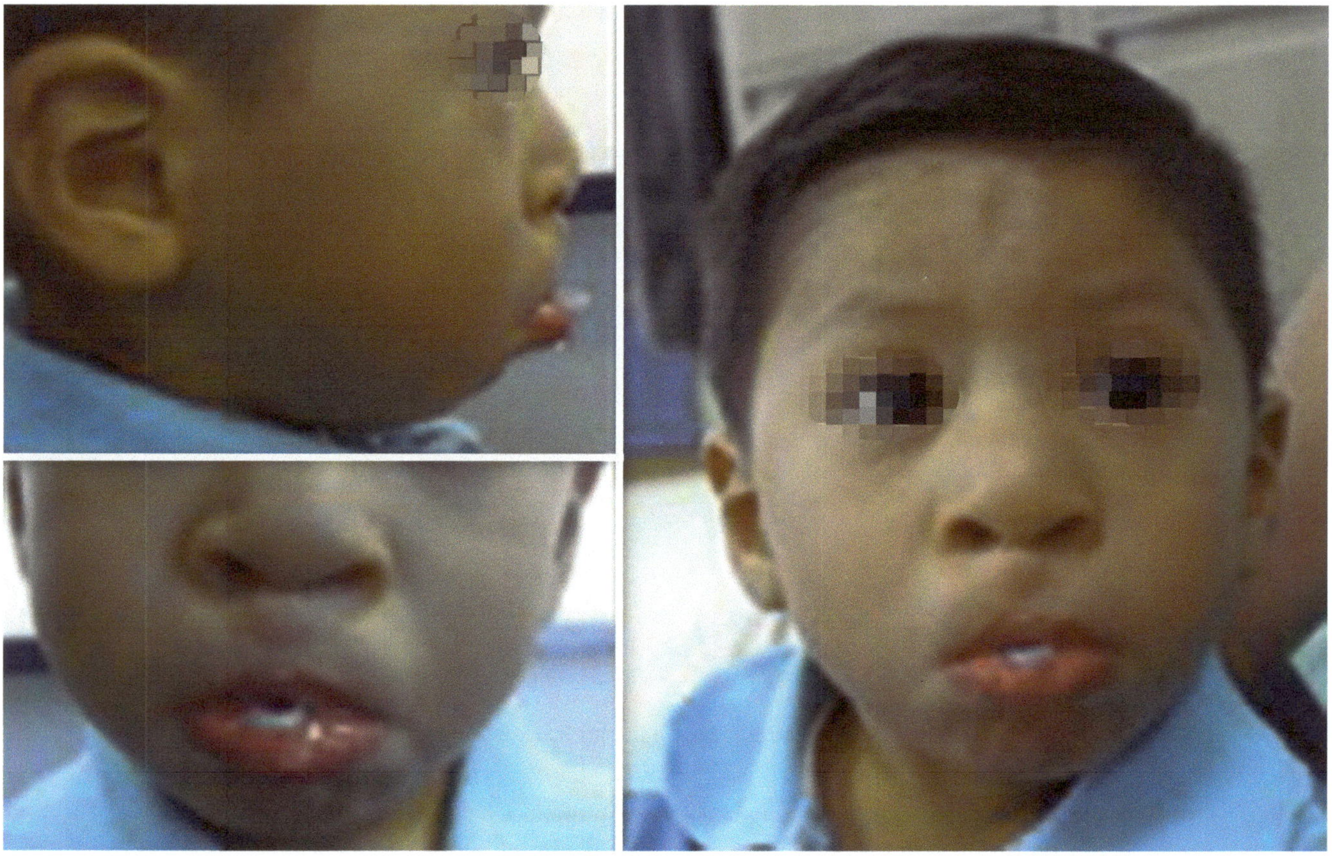

**Fig. 26.20** Use of PMA: 10 min during the day and at night. Breath and lip exercise

Myofunctional devices transmit forces generated by the stretching of the orofacial muscles to the maxilla and mandible to stimulate bone remodeling [31, 32] (Figs. 26.20, 26.21, 26.22, 26.23, 26.24, and 26.25). Instructions are given to start using the PMA for 10 min during the day and to sleep at night. Morning use increases with time until 1 hour of intermittent or constant use (Fig. 26.24a, b). In addition, myofunctional exercises are prescribed for facial muscles and tongue under the speech therapist guide (Video 26.3). This therapy is initiated at a time thought critical for facial

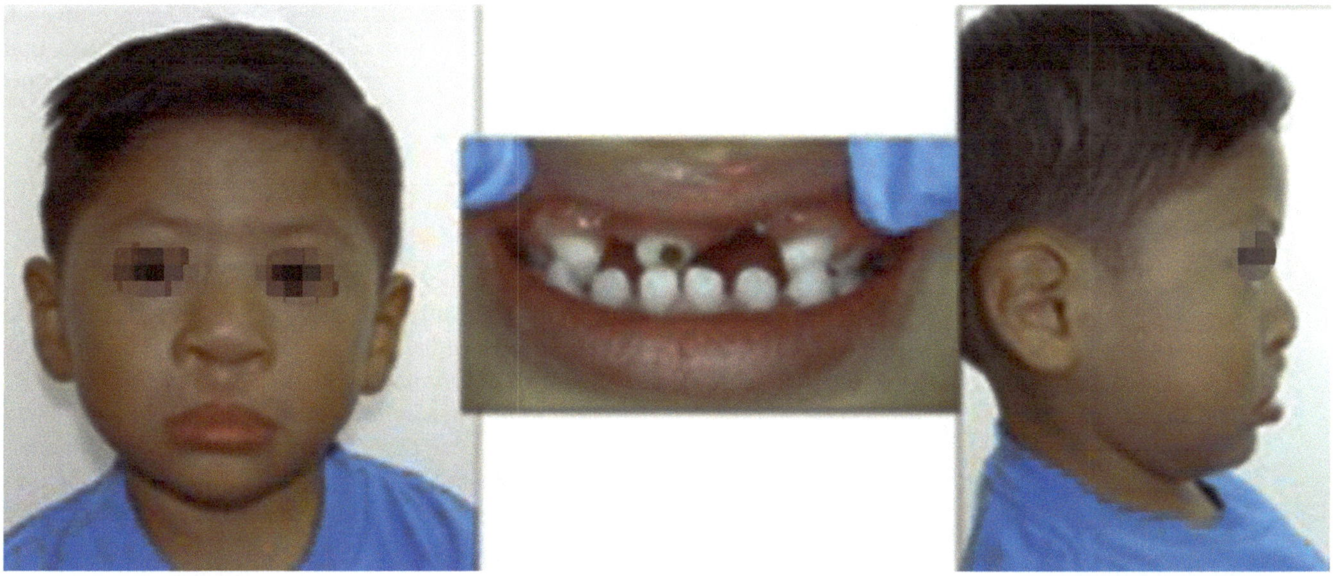

Fig. 26.21 The lip competence was successfully intercepted in a very short period of time (3 months) to improve and promote normal facial development and muscle function

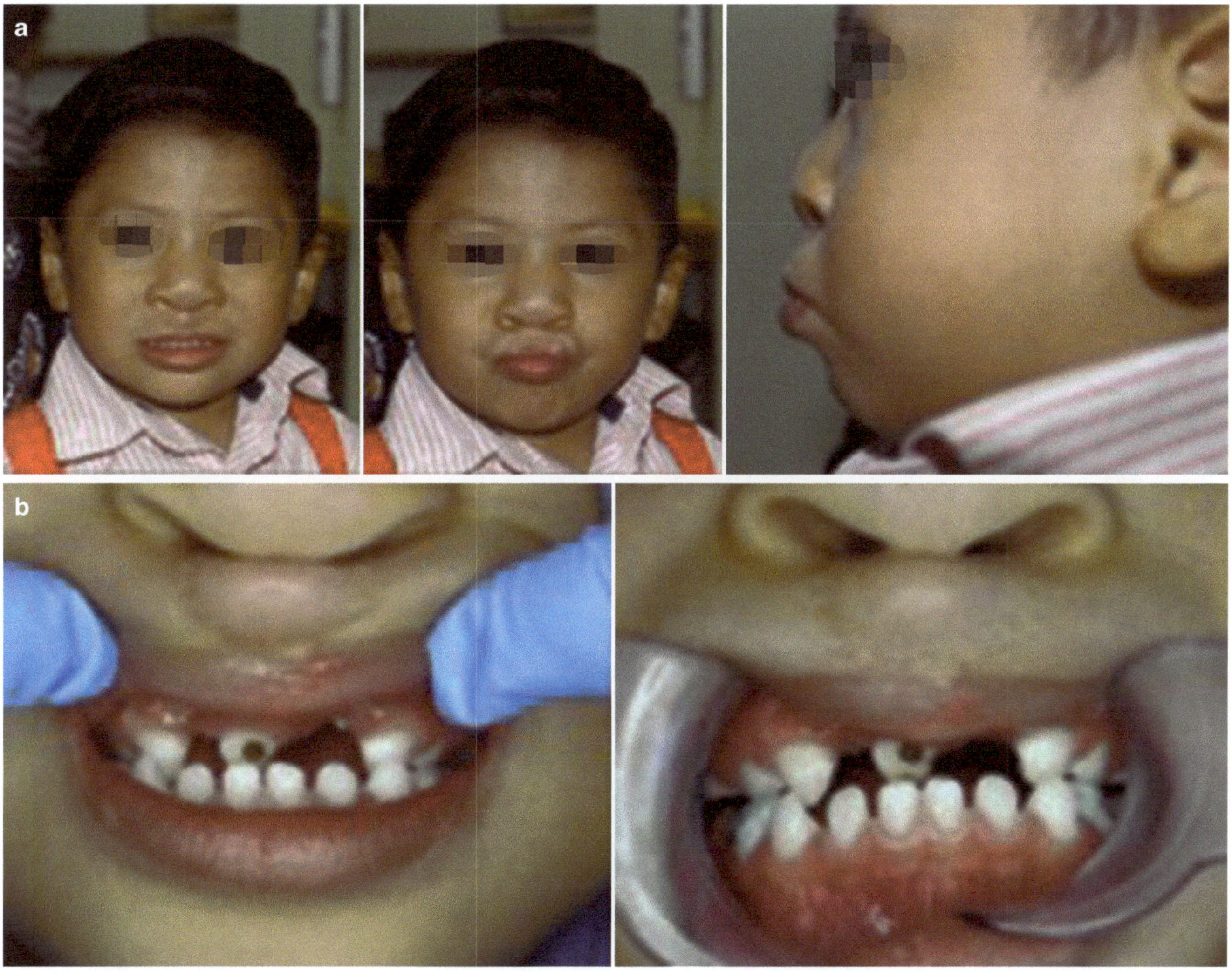

Fig. 26.22 As a result of this facial development protocol through myofunctional orthopedic treatment, the patient gained upper lip length and flexibility and nasal breathing

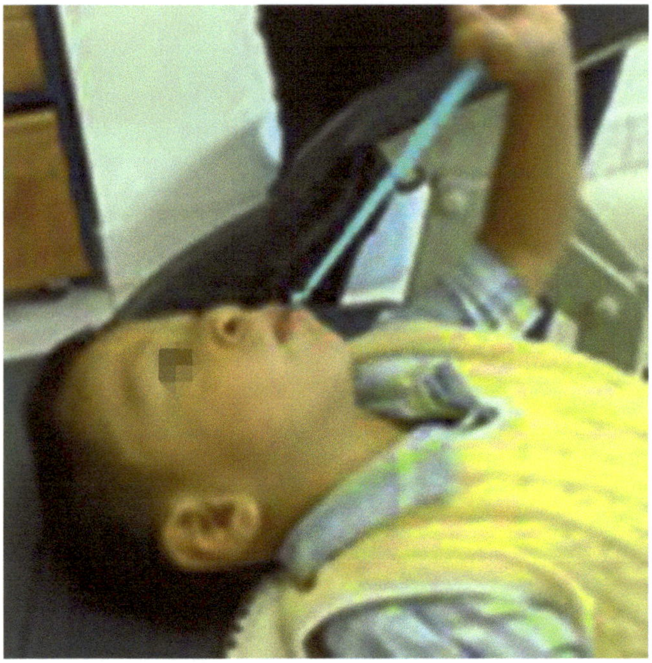

Fig. 26.23 Patient is very cooperative as well as his mother, that helped to start with Planas Direct Tracks (PDT) to further stimulate maxillary growth in three planes of space with the intent on guiding the craniofacial growth and development. Patient and family developed self-confidence which is very important in emotional health and social immersion of the patient while growing. To date there is a notorious improvement on oral functions, swallowing, and lip seal, and he keeps working on the tongue posture at rest with the aid of speech therapist. Thus, all tissues involved can continue expressing their highest growing potential over the following stages

growth, when peers are beginning to note differences in each other; it is thought that normalizing appearance and oral function improves play and reduces relegation during this period.

## Conclusion

Dental care is critical in patients with cleft lip and palate deformities, and initiating good hygiene early is crucial to facilitate oral health. Pre-surgical orthopedics reduce the width of cleft deformities at the time of surgery. Both NAM and FMO utilize an acrylic plate with regular modification to encourage alignment of maxillary segments; nasal remodeling is pursued as an adjunct. Although the utility of pre-surgical orthopedics is questioned in cost-prohibitive environments, we argue that given the surgeon and contextual variability affecting lip repair outcomes, this may be a particularly valuable adjunct in these settings. Finally, while less is well understood about the role for stimulating orofacial muscle development, the orofacial function is likely to be intrinsically related to facial and specifically maxillary growth in patients with clefts. Thus focusing on morphological and functional correction of the stomatognathic system for greater stability in long-term results is an area of excitement with need for future research.

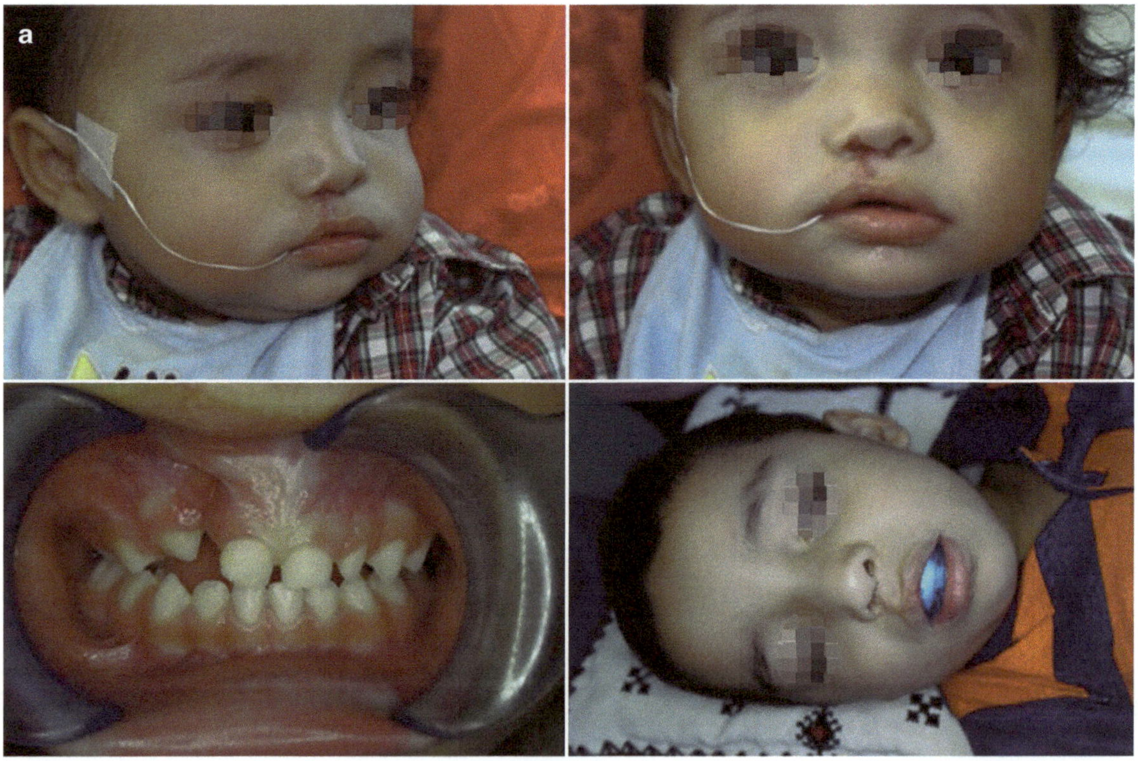

Fig. 26.24 (a, b) Improvements in facial development in a UCLP patient under myofunctional therapy. Improvements in facial development of a BCLP patient under myofunctional therapy

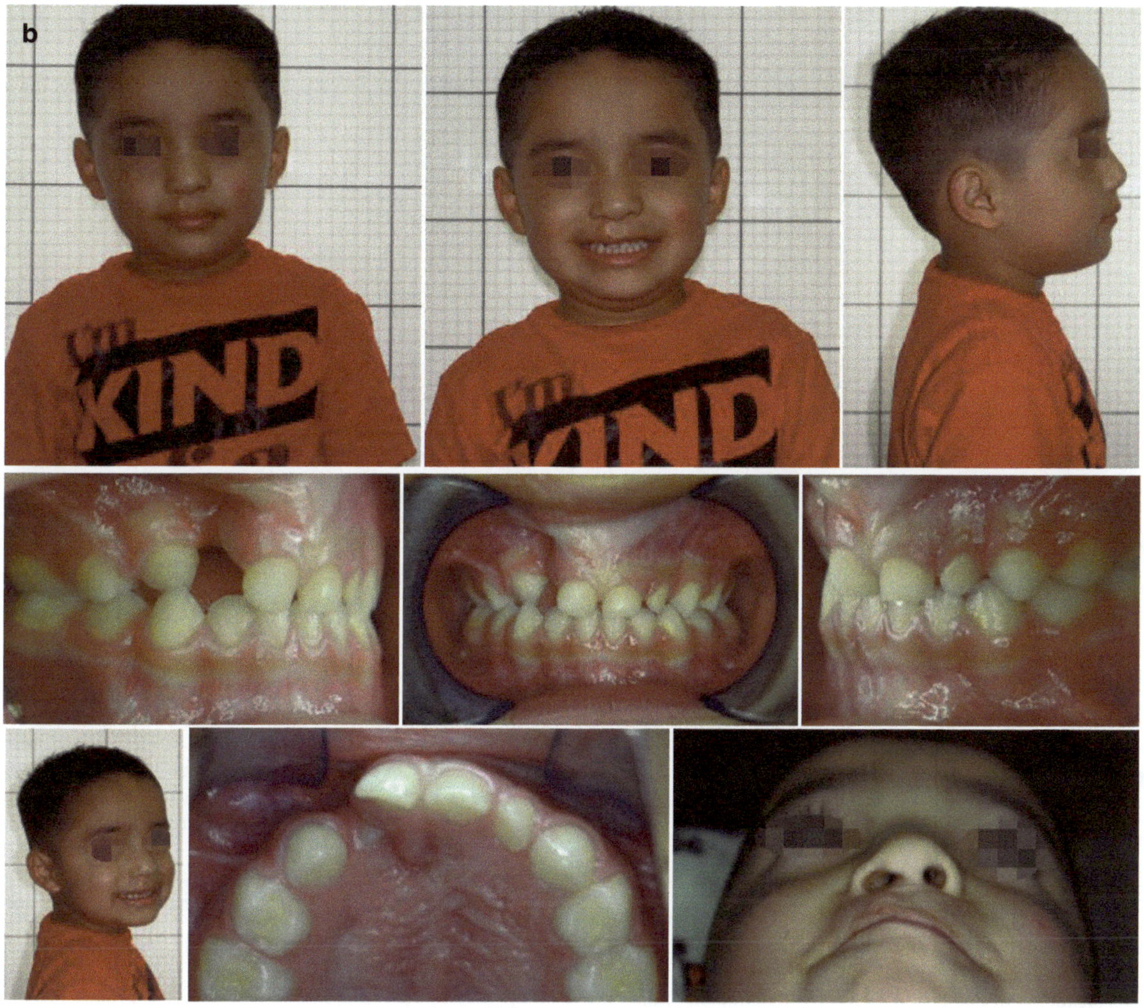


Fig. 26.24 (continued)

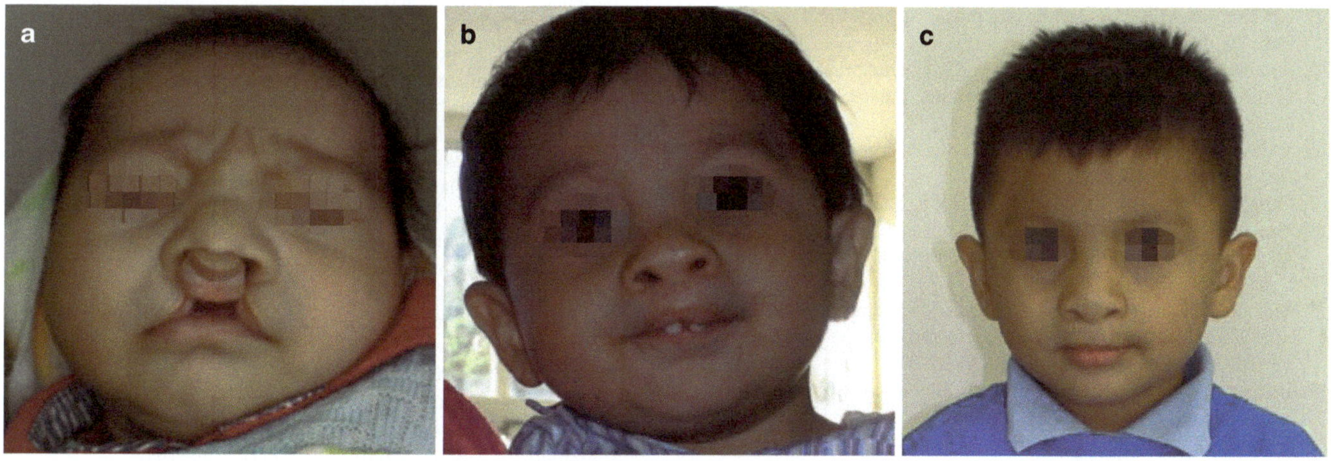


Fig. 26.25 Treatment of a boy with bilateral complete CLP utilizing prefabricated myofunctional appliances (PMA) and myofunctional exercises through age 3

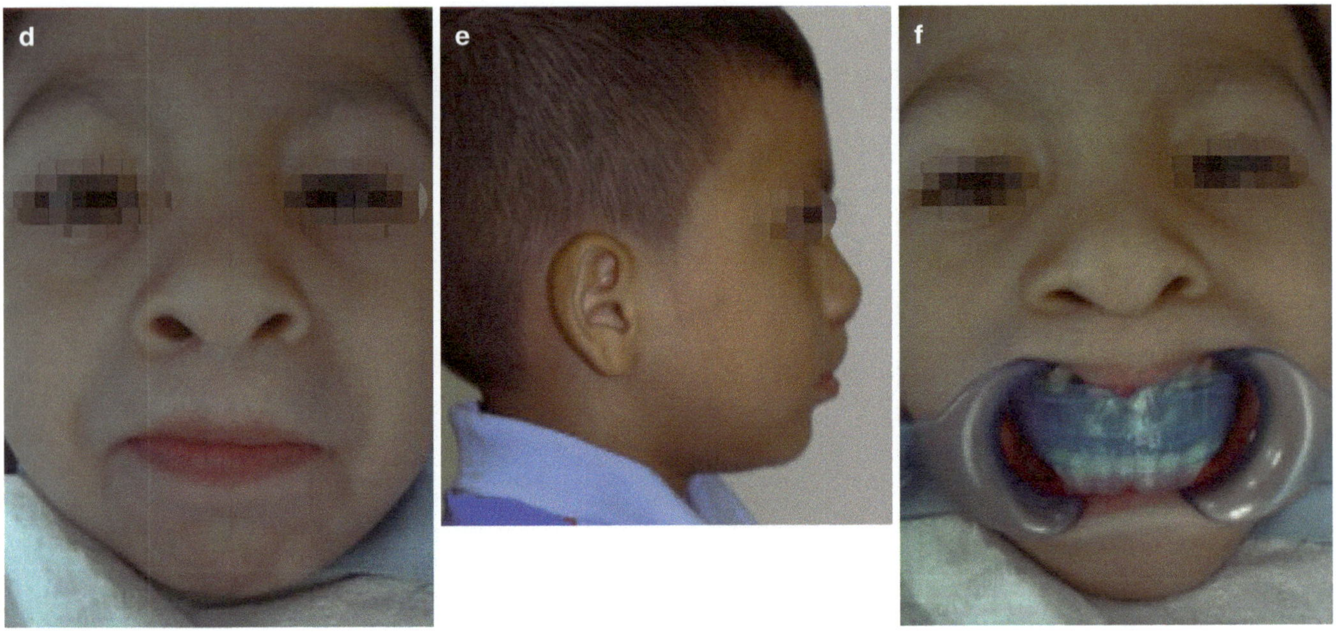


Fig. 26.25 (continued)

## References


1. Sischo L, Clouston S, Phillips C, Broder H. Caregiver responses to early cleft palate care: a mixed method approach. Health Psychol. 2016;35:474–82.
2. Sischo L, Broder H, Phillips C. Coping with cleft: a conceptual framework of caregiver responses to Nasoalveolar molding. Cleft Palate Craniofac J. 2015;52:640–50.
3. American Academy of Pediatric Dentistry. Guideline on infant oral health care: reference manual. Pediatr Den. 2016;37(6):146–50.
4. Grayson BH, Ahmed MM, Kassam SN. The role of pediatric dentists and orthodontists in the presurgical treatment of infants born with cleft lip and palate. In: Rogers D, Hartnick C, Hamdan U, editors. Video atlas of cleft lip and palate surgery. San Diego: Plural Pub; 2014. p. 41–50.
5. Antonarakis G, Palaska P, Herzog G. Caries prevalence in non-syndromic patients with cleft lip and/or palate: a meta-analysis. Caries Res. 2013;47:406–13.
6. Wells M. Oral health status of children with craniofacial anomalies. Pediatr Dent. 2013;35:E79–86.
7. Pannaci T. Pediatric surgery. 1st ed; 2003. p. 255–62, Chap. 14.
8. Grayson B, Santiago P, Brecht L, Cutting C. Presurgical nasoalveolar molding in infants with cleft lip and palate. Cleft Palate Craniofac J. 1999;36:486–98.
9. Matsuo K, Hirose T, Otagiri T, Norose N. Repair of cleft lip with nonsurgical correction of nasal deformity in the early neonatal period. Plast Reconstr Surg. 1989;83:25–31.
10. Brecht LE, Grayson BH, Cutting CB. Nasoalveolar molding in early management of the cleft lip and palate. In: Taylor TD, editor. Clinical maxillofacial prosthetics. Chicago: Quintessence; 2000. p. 63–84.
11. Grayson BH, Mauli D. Nasoalveolar molding for infants born with clefts of the lip, alveolus, and palate. Clin Plast Surg. 2004;31:148.
12. Ezzat CF, Chavarria C, Teichgraeber JF, et al. Presurgical nasoalveolar molding therapy for the treatment of the unilateral cleft lip and palate: a preliminary study. Cleft Palate Craniofac J. 2007;44:8.
13. Smith KS. Presurgical orthopedic management of the cleft patient. In: Turvey TA, editor. Oral and maxillofacial surgery. 2nd ed. p. 783–90, Chap. 38.
14. Smith K, Henry B, Scott M. Presurgical dentofacial orthopedic management of the cleft patient. Oral Maxillofac Surg Clin North Am. 2016;28:169–76.
15. Millard DR, Latham RA. Improved primary surgical and dental treatment of clefts. Plast Reconstr Surg. 1990;86:856.
16. Restrepo N, Carvallo J. Pre-surgical orthopedics in newborn patients with cleft lip and palate. Revista Mexicana de Ortodoncia. 2016;4:e42–7.
17. Grabowski R, Kopp H, Stahl F, Gundlach K. Presurgical orthopaedic treatment of newborns with clefts – functional treatment with long-term effects. J Cranio-Maxillofac Surg. 2006;34:34–44.
18. Liao Y, Wang Y, Chen I, Pai C, Ko W, Wang Y. Comparative outcomes of two nasoalveolar molding techniques for bilateral cleft nose deformity. Plast Reconstr Surg. 2014;133:103–10.
19. Simões W. Functional maxillary orthopedics, through neuro-occlusal rehabilitation. 2nd ed. Mexico: Medical Arts; 2004.
20. Enlow D, Hans M. Essentials of facial growth. Albuquerque: Distributed by TMData Resources; 2008.
21. Petrovic A, Stutzmann J, Lavergne J, Shayne R. Is it possible to modulate the growth of the human mandible with a functional appliance? Int J Orthod. 1991;29:3–8.
22. Falck F, Zimmermann K. Untersuchung zur Kategorisierung des mandibulären Wachstumspotentials von Petrovic, Lavergne und Stutzmann. Fortschr Kieferorthop. 1991;52:98–101.
23. Planas P. Rehabilitación neuro-oclusal (RNO). Madrid: Ripano; 2013.

24. Pannaci T. "Pannaci modification" applied to patients with cleft lip and cleft palate who have lingual dysfunction. San Juan de Dios. 1997;18:43–8.
25. Mazaheri M, Harding R, Cooper J, Meier J, Jones T. Changes in arch form and dimensions of cleft patients. Am J Orthod. 1971;60:19–32.
26. Grayson B, Maull D. Nasoalveolar molding for infants born with clefts of the lip, alveolus, and palate. Semin Plast Surg. 2005;19:294–301.
27. Trujillo L. Prevention of conductive hearing loss in cleft palate patients. Folia Phoniatr Logop. 1994;46:123–6.
28. Losee J, Kirschner R. Comprehensive cleft care. 2nd ed. New York: Thieme; 2015.
29. Sasaki A, Takeshita S, Publico A, Moss M, Tanaka E, Ishino Y, Watanabe M, Tanne K. Finite element growth analysis for the craniofacial skeleton in patients with cleft lip and palate. Med Eng Phys. 2004;26:109–18.
30. Aras I, Olmez S, Dogan S. Comparative evaluation of nasopharyngeal airways of unilateral cleft lip and palate patients using three-dimensional and two-dimensional methods. Cleft Palate Craniofac J. 2012;49:75–81.
31. Quesada Quiros O. The secrets of the trainer and Myobrace appliances and the biofunctional system. 1st ed. Medellín: Amolca; 2016.
32. Ramirez-Yañez G, Farrel C. Guiding craniofacial growth and development with the Myobrace System. 1st ed; 2017.
33. Poplett E. Global engagement: exchange for smiles. University of North Carolina at Chapel Hill. Sept, 2018. https://www.unc.edu/discover/exchange-for-smiles/. Accessed 1 Dec 2019.

# Cleft Orthodontic Care

# 27

Vilma L. Arteaga and Adriana Agell

**Key Points**

- The goals of orthodontic preparation for alveolar bone graft (ABG) are:
  1. Alignment and de-rotation of maxillary incisor at the cleft site
  2. Correction of crossbite of anterior teeth (UCLP)
  3. Expansion of the posterior maxillary segments (BCLP)
  4. The establishing of a U-shape maxillary arch
  5. To restore physiologic continuity of dental arch to enable dental health
  6. Maxillary occlusal plane alignment
  7. To create a convenient path with space to close the palatal floor
- Interceptive orthodontic treatment is indicated before the eruption of permanent lateral incisor or permanent canine in cleft site, during late primary dentition or early mixed dentition.
- The oral health status of patients must be optimized and maintained prior, during, and after the orthodontic/orthognathic procedure.
- Even in low-resource settings, a series of diagnostic records is needed to study the optimal presurgical orthodontic treatment in preparation for orthognathic surgery (OGS)
- Alveolar maxillary segmental distraction is a good option for maxillary protraction in CLP patients and avoids speech problems post-surgery.
- Collaboration and communication between surgeon and orthodontist are extremely important before, during, and after all surgical interventions.

## Introduction

Patients with cleft lip and palate develop skeletal and dental abnormalities due to their intrinsic deformity and imbalance in facial muscular forces. Consequently, dental function for chewing and speaking, oral health, and facial appearance can be adversely affected. As a result of this facial dysmorphism, CLP patients may develop emotional alterations such as body dysmorphic disorder (BDD) [1]. The orthodontist plays a critical role in the multidisciplinary cleft team to assess and treat dental and facial development during the main growth stages.

There are two main phases in the cleft orthodontic care: (1) interceptive orthodontics ("Phase 1") as preparation for alveolar bone graft (ABG) and (2) comprehensive orthodontics, with or without orthognathic surgery (OGS), with possible prosthetic and restorative dental treatment. (See Table 27.1.)

**Electronic Supplementary Material** The online version of this chapter (https://doi.org/10.1007/978-3-030-59105-2_27) contains supplementary material, which is available to authorized users.

V. L. Arteaga (✉)
Maxillofacial Orthodontics and Orthopedics Ortodent, Guatemala City, Guatemala

Juan Pablo II Children Hospital, Operation Smile Guatemala, Guatemala City, Guatemala

A. Agell
Orthodontics and Maxillary Orthopedics, Pediatric Maxillofacial Surgery Unit of Vall D'Hebrón Hospital, Barcelona, Spain

Operation Smile Morocco, Casablanca, Morocco

Gramadent Dental Clinic, Barcelona, Spain

© Springer Nature Switzerland AG 2021

J. W. Swanson, D. W. Low (eds.), *Global Cleft Care in Low-Resource Settings*, https://doi.org/10.1007/978-3-030-59105-2_27

**Table 27.1** Dental stages and orthodontic phases

| Age range | Dental stage | Orthodontic phase |
|---|---|---|
| 0–3 years | Neonatal<br>Primary dentition erupts, teething | Functional maxillary orthopedics (FMO)<br>Nasoalveolar molding (NAM) |
| 3–6 years | Primary dentition<br>Routine dental care begins<br>Crossbite, overjet can be assessed | Myofunctional orthopedics<br>Orthodontic evaluation for palatal expansion need<br>Consideration of face mask |
| 6–12 years | Mixed dentition<br>Begins with permanent mandibular incisor eruption, ends with maxillary canine eruption | Phase 1 Orthodontics<br>Preparation for alveolar bone grafting (ABG)<br>Limited incisor alignment around alveolar cleft<br>Posterior palatal expansion<br>Dental alignment following ABG |
| 12–18 years | Permanent dentition<br>Wisdom teeth (third molar) eruption | Monitoring of jaw growth<br>Phase 2 (comprehensive) orthodontics<br>With or without jaw (orthognathic) surgery<br>Preparation of spaces for future replacement of missing teeth<br>Definitive restoration of missing teeth with implant/prosthesis |

## Anatomical Characteristics

### Maxillary Arch Form and Dimensions

Facial growth in patients with CLP is characterized by a reduced maxilla in three planes of space (anterior projection, vertical height, and transverse width). Contributing factors may include intrinsic growth abnormality related to the cleft deformity, effects of surgical procedures, and contributions from facial muscular function (tongue thrust, oral breathing, and/or atypical swallowing).

In *unilateral cleft lip and palate patients* (UCLP), crossbite is an early common malocclusion, especially in complete clefts. The maxillary minor segment usually grows toward the midline and is shorter on the vertical and sagittal planes. Class III malocclusion is prevalent, and this may be more common in the absence of presurgical orthopedic treatment [2].

In *bilateral cleft lip and palate patients* (BCLP), angle Class II malocclusion is more common. Posterior crossbite is more prevalent than anterior crossbite. The premaxilla may be too protruded or have excessive vertical growth which causes two different occlusal planes when compare to posterior segments. An inclined premaxilla with asymmetric clefts is a major challenge for the orthodontist and surgeon (Fig. 27.1a, b).

Crossbites in CLP patients are associated with speech problems, deviating masticatory muscle function, and the inability to clean teeth, especially those on the cleft site, thus increasing caries risk.

## Phase I Orthodontics at Mixed Dentition

### Presurgical Orthodontic and Orthopedic Management for ABG

#### Objectives of Interceptive Orthodontics and Orthopedics Treatment

1. Alignment and de-rotation of maxillary incisor at the cleft site
2. Correction of crossbite of anterior teeth (UCLP)
3. Expansion of the posterior maxillary segments (BCLP)
4. Establishment of a U-shaped maxillary arch
5. Restoration of dental arch continuity to enable dental health
6. Maxillary occlusal plane alignment
7. Preparation for ABG

## Patient Selection and Clinical Planning

### Timing of Interceptive Orthodontic Treatment

The best time to start orthodontic preparation for ABG is controversial. The evaluation of a panoramic radiograph (OPG) or cone-beam computer tomography (CB-CT) when available is more important than the patient's age.

Historically there are four different age periods [3]:

I. Primary alveolar repair, at the time of palatoplasty, such as gingivoperiosteoplasty (1 year of age).
II. Early alveolar bone graft (EABG), before the eruption of lateral incisor (4–7 years of age) (Fig. 27.2a–e).
III. Conventional alveolar bone graft (LABG), traditionally performed at most centers, before the eruption of permanent canine (7–9 years of age) (Fig. 27.3).

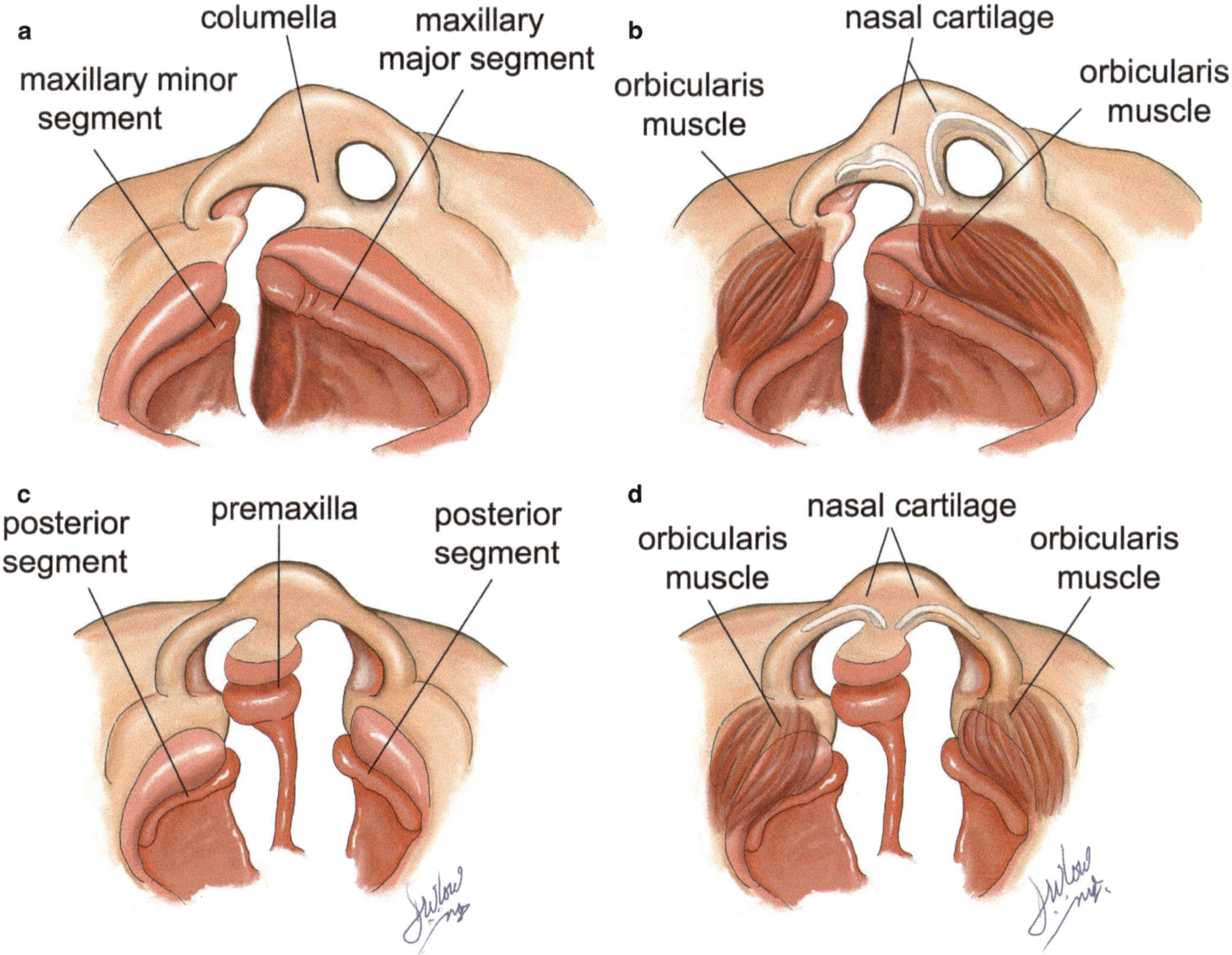


**Fig. 27.1** In a unilateral CLP, the maxillary minor segment grows toward the midline (**a**), and is shorter in the sagittal and vertical plane, due to (**b**) abberant cartilage position and muscle insertion. Similarly, in bilateral CLP, the premaxilla is protruded and tilted (**c**), the vomer driving forward growth unrestrained by the orbicularis muscles (**d**)

IV. Late alveolar bone grafting (TABG), during permanent dentition on orthognathic surgery stage. There is higher risk of wound infection and dehiscence. *This is not recommended.*

Grafted bone site needs stimulation to succeed. It is best to start at time of mixed dentition when the lateral or canine permanent tooth is about to erupt [4]. In EABG protocol, Chinchilla-Asencio approach, the orthodontic preparation starts at time of primary dentition, when the root of primary cleft canine is intact; orthodontic movements of it into the graft site promote bone graft stimulation and regeneration, leaving enough space for permanent teeth eruption [5] (Fig. 27.2a–e).

## Diagnostic Records

When there is no panoramic radiograph (OPG) nor a CB-CT available, clinical assessment may be useful to recognize the anatomical disturbances to be corrected.

Occlusal, periapical films, and OPG will be useful to evaluate the width of clefted area; rotation, presence, or absence of permanent teeth buds; supernumerary teeth in cleft site; as well as the eruption stage and root development of the permanent canine and lateral incisor [6].

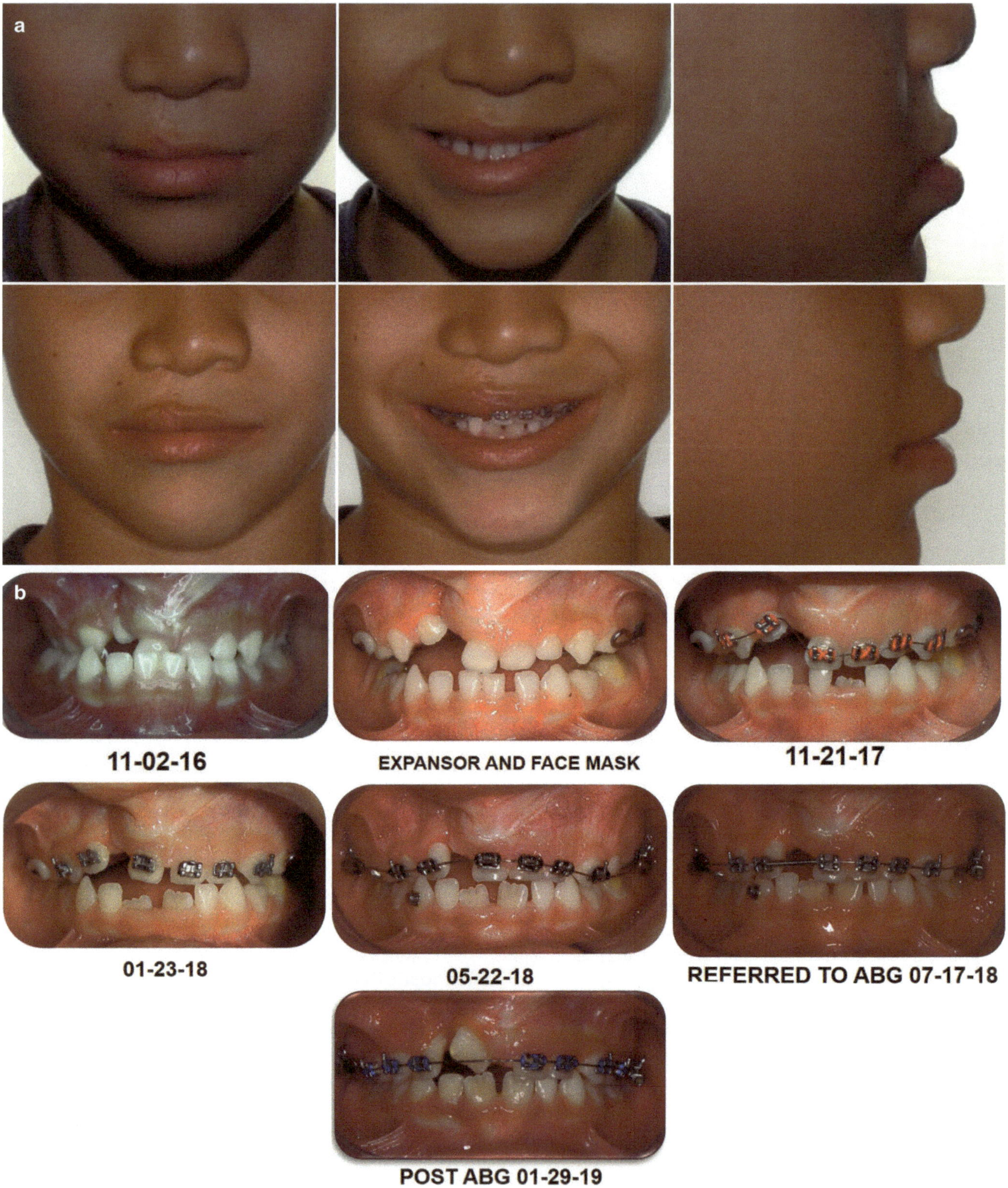


**Fig. 27.2** Early alveolar bone graft EABG. (Case courtesy of Dr. V. Jofre). UCLP 6 years of age. (**a**) Facial view. Face mask protraction. (**b**) Treatment sequence EABG. (**c**) Occlusal view. (**d**) Lateral view; notice vertical growth of minor segment. (**e**) X-rays pre and post EOBG

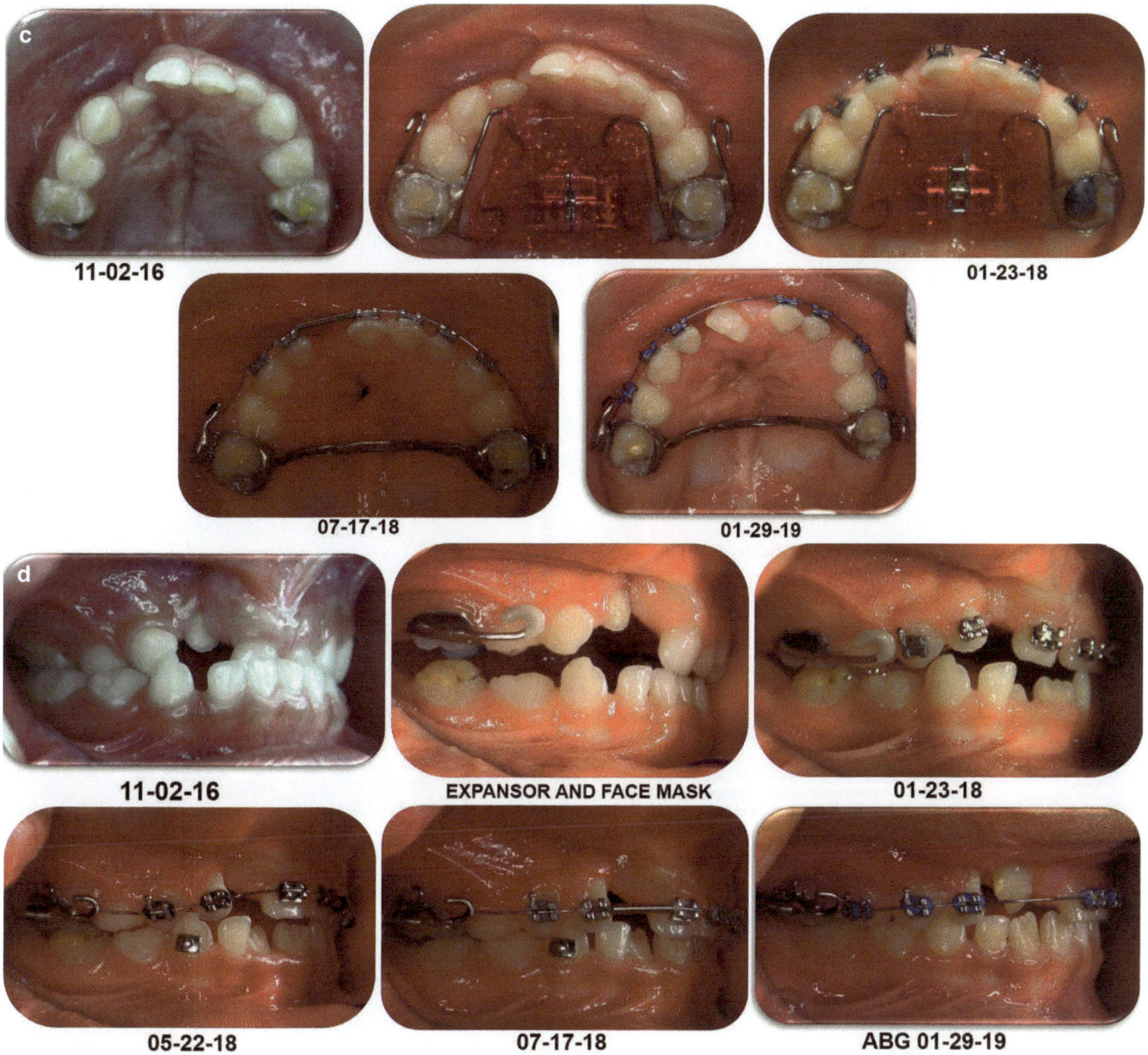


**Fig. 27.2** (continued)

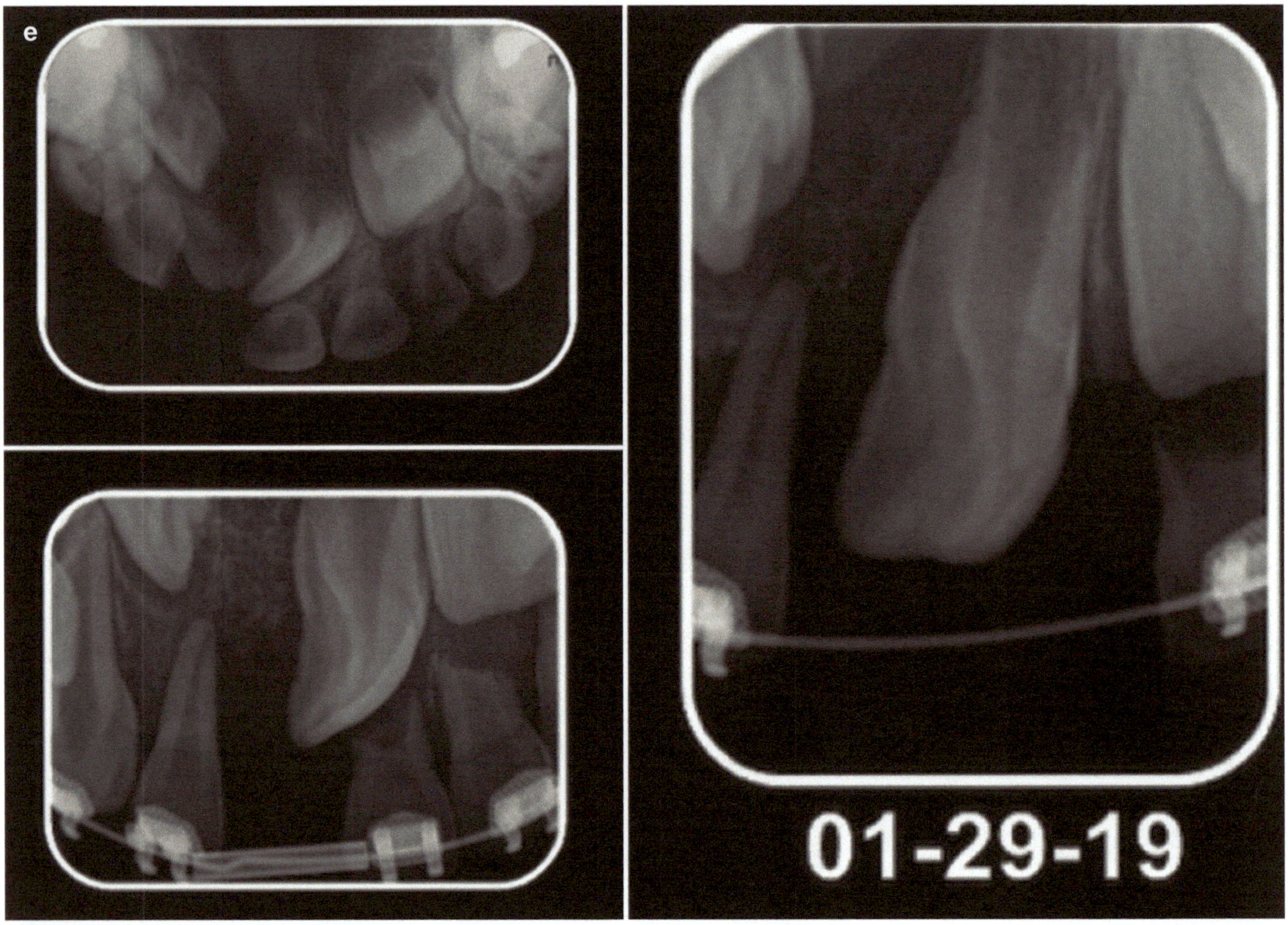


Fig. 27.2 (continued)

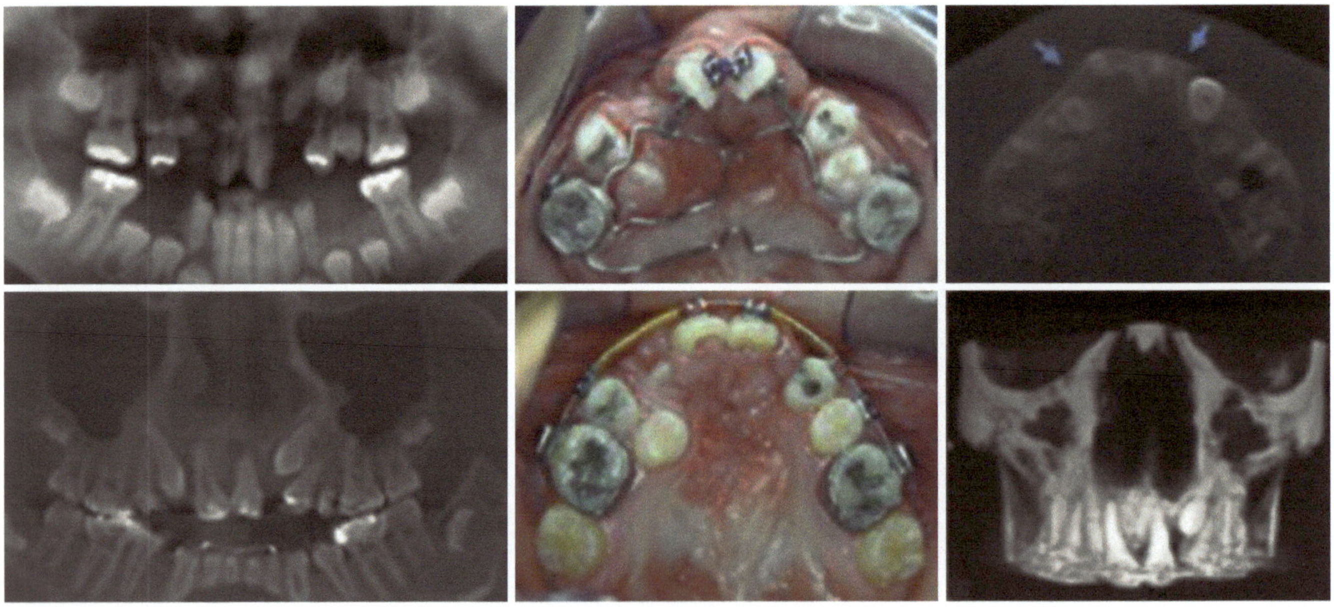

Fig. 27.3 Conventional alveolar bone graft (LABG) before eruption of primary canine

## Procedural Technique

### Maxillary Expansion

In mixed dentition it is often necessary to correct the transverse discrepancies of the maxilla for these reasons:

- To reposition laterally collapsed maxillary segments, allowing the surgeon enough space for alveolar bone grafting
- To create spaces that allow the eruption or alignment of permanent teeth in the frontal area
- To eliminate cross bites to improve facial growth
- To improve nasal breathing
- To improve the position and function of the tongue muscles

### Expansion Methods

1. Removable appliances:

   These are made with screws placed in acrylic that perform different types of expansions depending upon the position of the screw: anterior, central, or triple (anterior and bilateral). This type is not always recommended because of the thickness of the acrylic plate that covers the palate. It may complicate language therapy and requires collaboration of the patient and their parents in its use (Fig. 27.4a).
2. Fixed appliances:
   (a) *Hyrax*: This is the simple method when a parallel expansion is needed, although by modifying the placement of the screw we can achieve more expansion at the minor segment level in patients with UCLP. When positioning the screw anteriorly in the collapsed minor segment and more posteriorly in the major segment, there is greater expansion of the minor segment with minimal expansion of the major segment (Figs. 27.2c, 27.4b, and 27.15) (Video 27.1 Hyrax Laboratory Procedure).
   (b) *Quad helix*: This is an easy and economically manufactured expander. It can be produced directly by the orthodontist in consultation without the need of a laboratory technician. It is made in chrome-cobalt wire of 0.036 inches or 1 mm and welded to bands in the first permanent molars (Fig. 27.5a–c). Its design is personalized for each case, allowing the creation of longer arms if protrusion and expansion of anterior teeth is needed. Activation can be controlled for more anterior than posterior expansion, as well as de-rotation of molars and torque (Fig. 27.6a–c). There is an inverted model welded to bands on maxillary deciduous canines, first primary molars or first premolar; expansion effect is focused in the anterior maxillary region [6, 7] (Fig. 27.7a, b) (Video 27.2 Quad-Helix activation).

### Protraction of the Maxilla

*Midfacial retrusion* is often seen in unilateral cleft patients with an underdeveloped maxilla, which results in skeletal and/or dentoalveolar discrepancies, often showing anterior and/or posterior crossbites with a concave soft tissue profile, triggering functional, esthetic, and psychological problems.

One of the most traditional methods of treatment is the use of an external device for maxillary protraction.

Protraction changes:

- More anterior position of the upper jaw
- More posterior position of the chin point (soft Pogonion – Pg) due to mandibular clockwise rotation

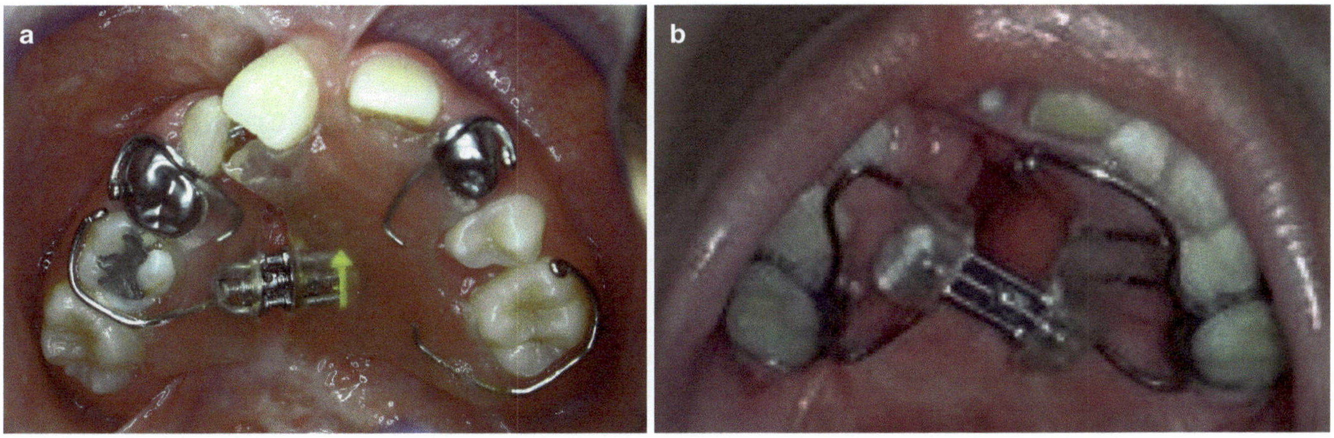


Fig. 27.4 (**a**) Removable expander. Compliance of patient and parents is required. (**b**) Modified Hass expander. Notice inclination of screw; major maxillary segment is used as anchorage

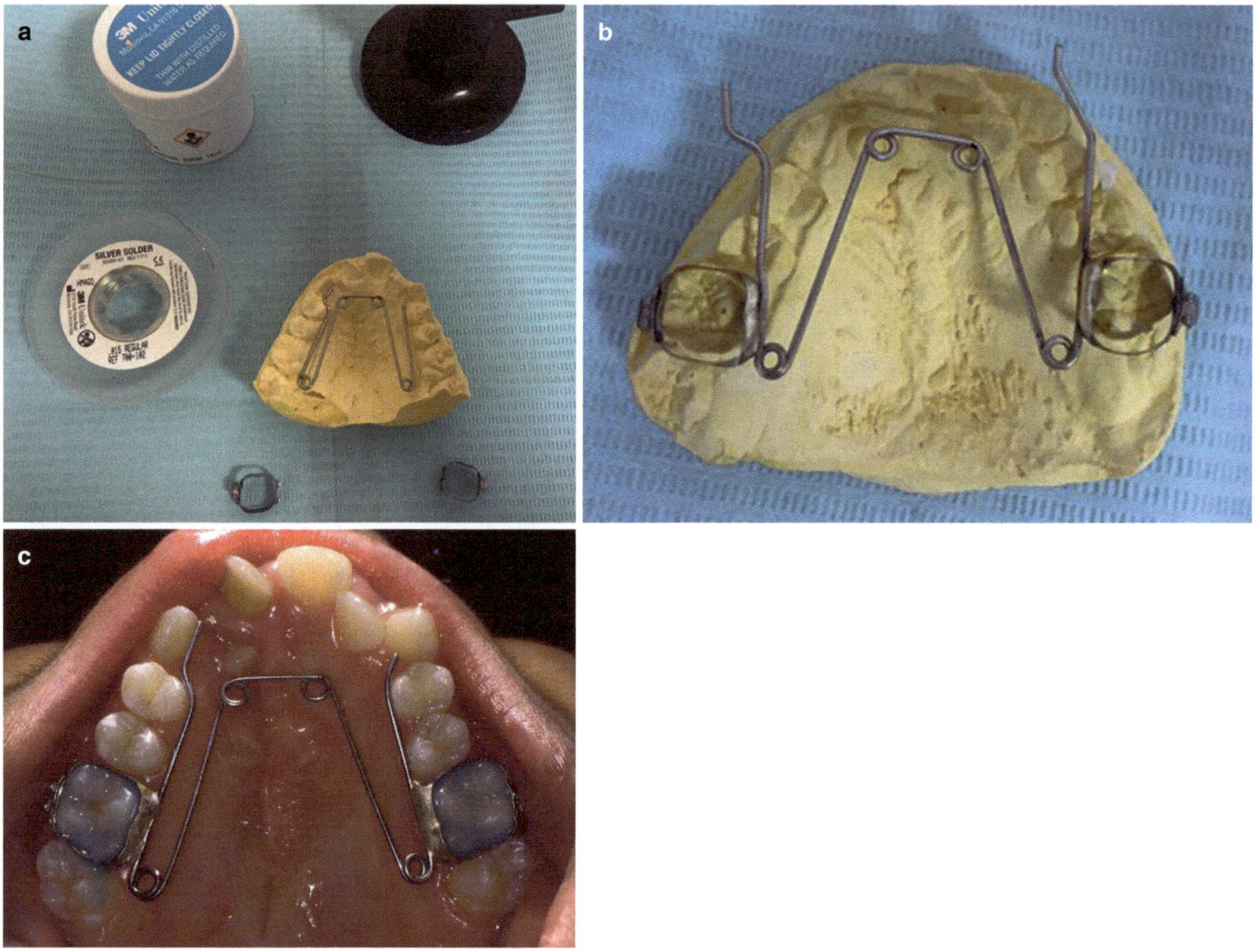


**Fig. 27.5** (**a**) Confection of quad helix. Material needed: Chrome-cobalt wire of 0.036 inches or 1 mm, solder paste, torch, and orthodontic bands. (**b**) Quad helix activated. (**c**) Quad helix clinical view

Components of the treatment [8]:

1. *Expander*: A Hyrax appliance attached to the upper first molars and premolars/deciduous molars with hooks for traction at canine level. If maxillary expansion is needed, activate once a day for 8–10 days, to produce disarticulation of the sutural system, if it is not necessary, can be activated (open) and returned (closed), only to produce sutural disarticulation.

   A Hass-expander with acrylic bite blocks can also be used. Or bite block can be placed in the lower arch to eliminate incisor interference if it is necessary (Fig. 27.8a).
2. Use of the *facemask* for at least 12 hours/day (Fig. 27.8b).
3. *Elastic force* (450–500 g per side) from the canine region oriented downward and forward to the occlusal plane 45°. First 2 weeks 3/8″ 8 oz, increase to 1/2″ 14 oz and finally 5/16″ 14 oz.

Discontinue facemask therapy after a positive anterior overjet (2–5 mm) is obtained and posterior occlusal stability achieved.

## Occlusal Plane Alignment

### Use of Planas Direct Tracks (PDT) on Primary Dentition

As in patients without clefts, crossbites can be treated in unilateral and bilateral cleft patients using PDT in primary upper and lower molars. As described by Planas [9] and Simoes [10], PDT are used as an aid of a quad helix. The PDT tracks are designed such that the distal incline of the upper PDT occludes with the mesial inclined PDT of the lower jaw on correction of anterior crossbites. For posterior segment crossbites, palatal inclined upper PDT occlude with the buccal inclined lower PDT [11] (Fig. 27.7a, c).

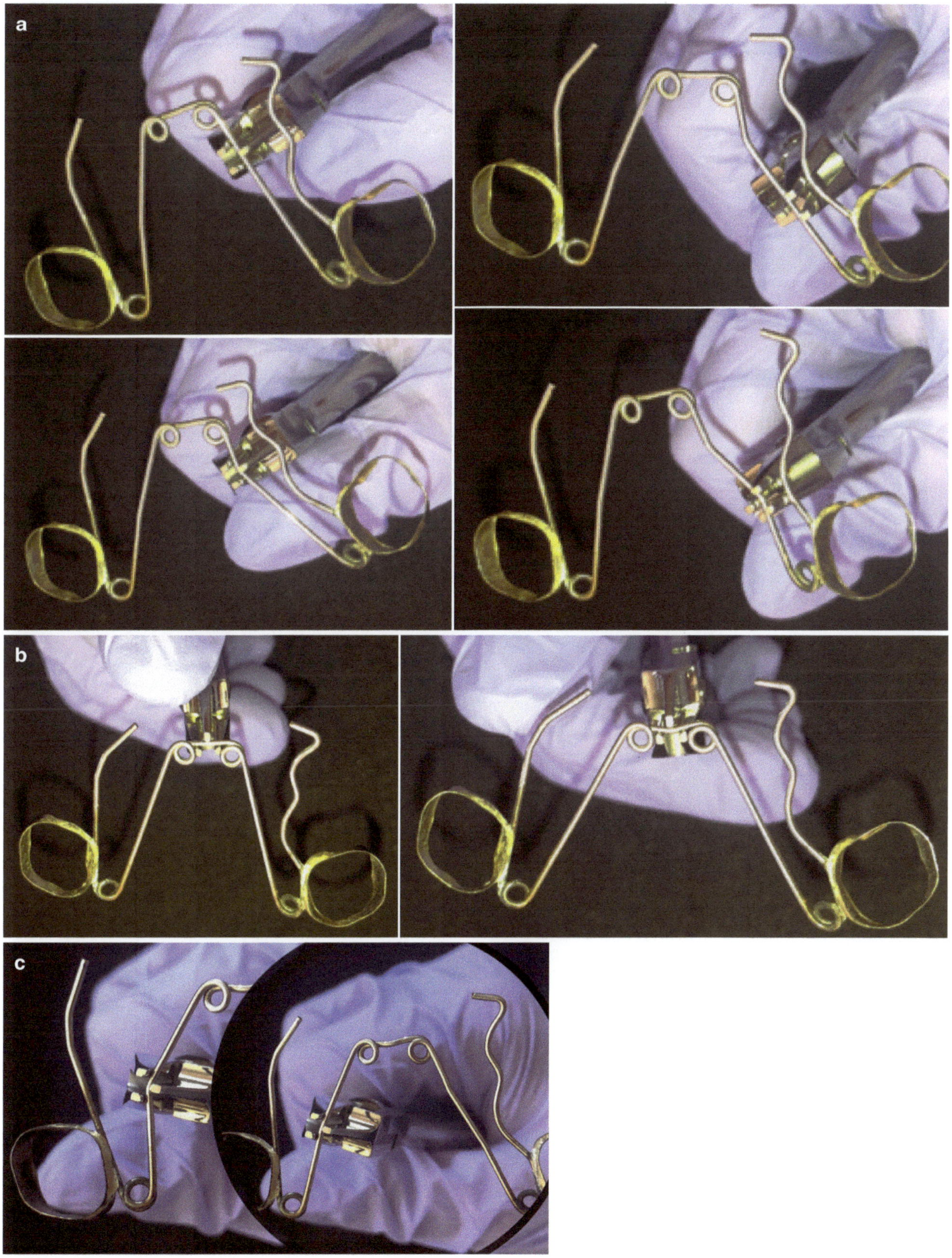


**Fig. 27.6** Quad helix activation (see Video 27.2). (**a**) Anterior and posterior activation in posterior bridge. (**b**) Anterior bridge activation, posterior expansion. (**c**) Posterior bridge activation. Anterior expansion

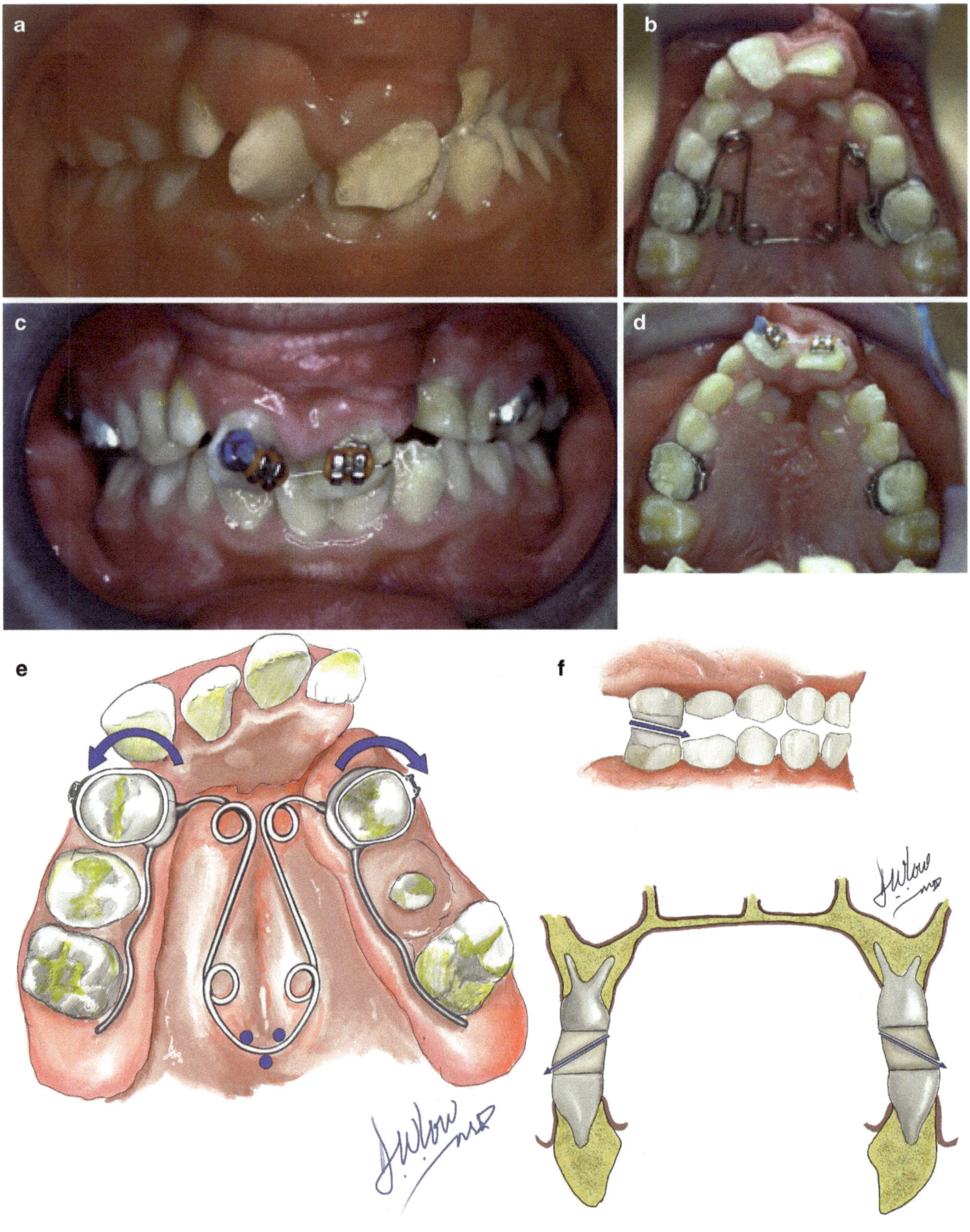


**Fig. 27.7** Reverse Quad Helix expansion in BCLP
(**a**) Initial Frontal view
(**b**) Reverse quad helix modified with lingual boxes soldered to primary molars, easy to remove and comfortable for the patient. Anterior helixes are hold still to primary canines with resin to assure anterior expansion
(**c**) Frontal view. 4 months of interceptive orthopedic and myofunctional therapy. Improvement on over bite
(**d**) Occlusal view. Notice expansion on primary canine distance
(**e**) Reverse quad helix welded to bands in primary canines or permanent first premolars to hold the expansion effects focused in the anterior maxillary region (By Dr. Low)
(**f**) The bonded resin Planas Direct Tracks (PDT) are placed on deciduos molars and used to stimulate maxillary transverse development (By Dr. Low)

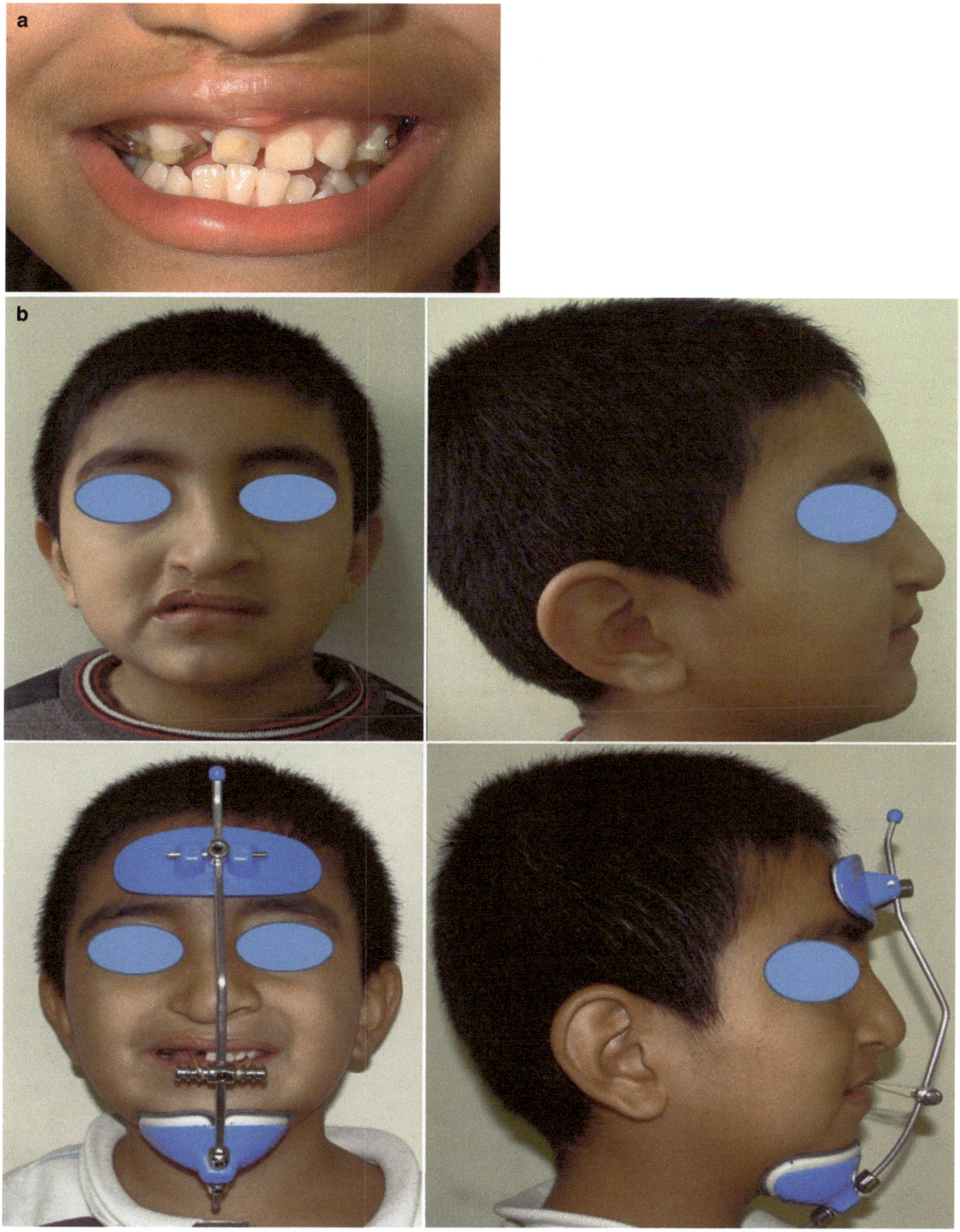


**Fig. 27.8** (**a**) Hass expander with acrylic bite blocks and wire hooks. (**b**) Maxillary protraction with facemask and elastic forces

PDT will remain on primary molars until their exfoliation. Permanent first molars erupt at the same level of premaxilla in BCLP patients if treated with myofunctional appliances as well.

In bilateral cleft, the premaxilla can be extremely malpositioned (>7–8 mm of vertical excess) and most optimal treatment may be orthopedic, orthodontic, or surgical (Table 27.2).

**Table 27.2** Protocol for the treatment of the vertical exceeds of the premaxilla in BCLP base on the dental age of patients, the severity of the vertical excess, and the type of surgical treatment performed

| | |
|---|---|
| Deciduous dentition (also after GAP) or mixed dentition (without bone graft or GAP) | Orthopedic intrusion |
| Mixed dentition (after bone graft or GAP) with vertical excess <7–8 mm | Orthodontic intrusion |
| Mixed dentition (after bone graft or GAP) or permanent dentition with vertical excess >7–8 mm | Surgical intrusion |

Reprinted from Meazzini [4]

## Alignment and De-rotation of Maxillary Permanent Incisors

Maxillary permanent incisors next to cleft site almost always erupt rotated and deviated toward the non-cleft side. Alignment and de-rotation of central incisor is a goal before ABG as well as protrude premaxilla with vertical excess <7–8 mm. Niti arch 0.12 on slot 22 or Utility arch 4 × 2 or 2 × 2 (Rickets) is used; care must be taken to not move the root inside the cleft [12]. De-rotation of central incisor next to cleft area may prevent dehiscence of post-op repaired lip (Figs. 27.9 and 27.10).

## Follow-Up and Management of Complications

Patients are evaluated 8–15 days after ABG. If available, radiographs are obtained of the site 3- and 6-months post-surgery. Liquid diet is prescribed for 7 days and soft diet on the next 6 weeks, given special importance not to chew on

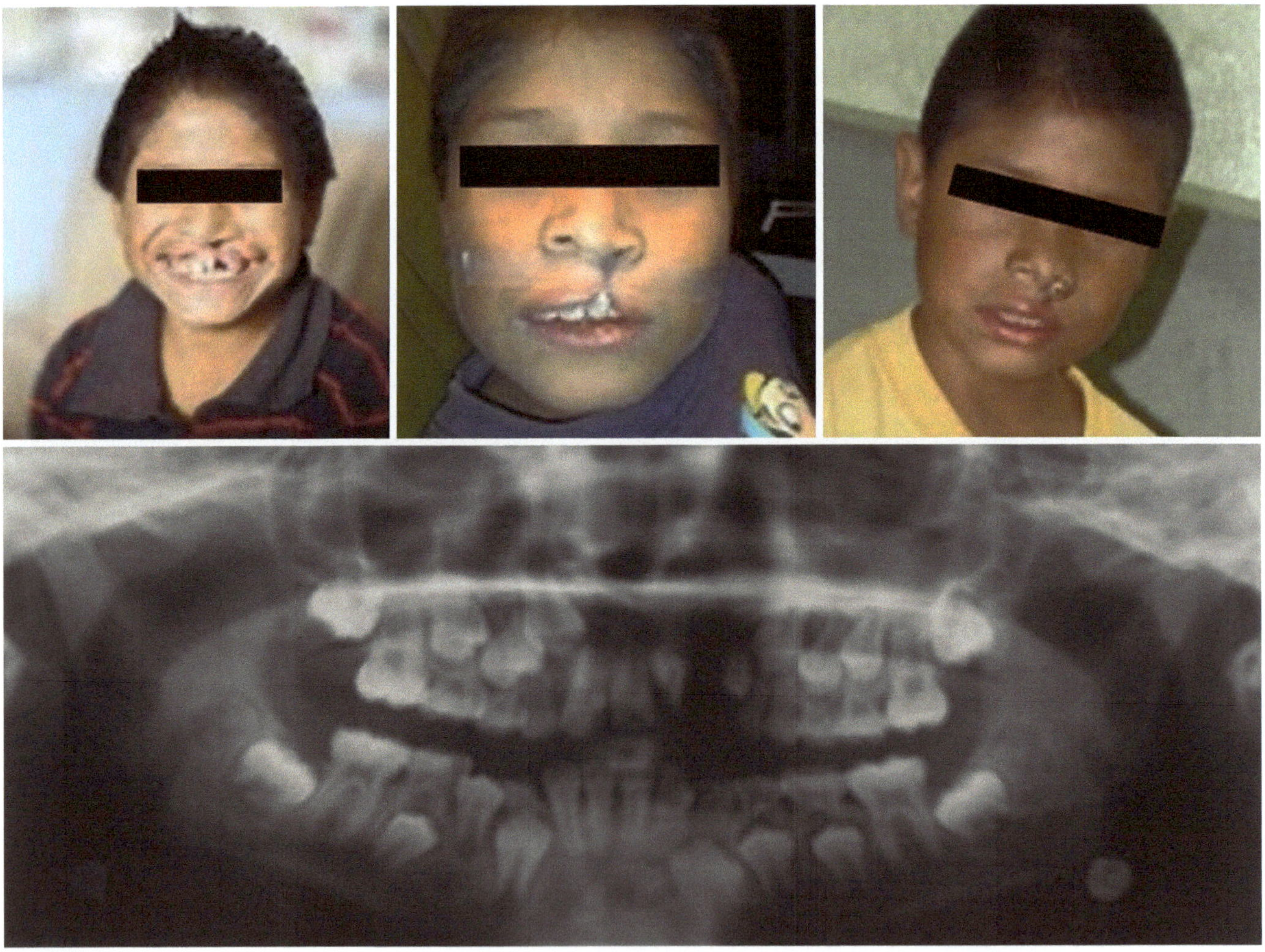

**Fig. 27.9** 10-year-old patient with left UCLP. Left permanent incisor is rotated 90° mesially, it may cause a rupture of the clefted lip once repaired. There is enough space to de-rotate it before surgery. After 4 months of orthodontic preparation, the lip was repaired

hard food. In cases of EABG, after 6–12 weeks, the primary cleft canine is moved toward the site back and forth, with light orthodontic forces to maintain the grafted bone in place. Post graft orthodontic treatment may take 6–8 months [3]. Most cases are maintained with brackets and archwires and others with a fixed palatal arch and wire mesial extensions on the lingual aspect of the posterior teeth on both sides as retainer until all permanent teeth had erupted. A removable maxillary acrylic splint is used at some centers to stabilize maxillary segments and give some mechanical protection to the gingival flaps over the graft; however removable retainers are not generally used, and any splints/retainers pose a hygiene risk if not kept clean.

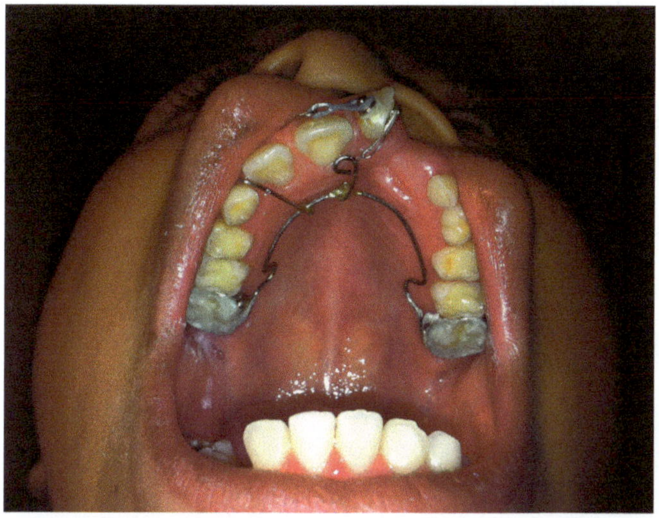

Fig. 27.10 A palatal arch with wire extensions was cemented to the first permanent molars; buttons were placed buccal and lingual and couple forces use to de-rotate 2.1

Education of caregivers and patients on oral hygiene and good care of their orthodontic appliance is crucial to avoid complications. Main complications are graft resorption, infection, and wound dehiscence (Fig. 27.11). The patient or caregiver main concern is a fetid odor coming from the nose or mouth. It can be present on the 8 days post-op appointment. Close cooperation between the surgeon and orthodontist is crucial.

## Phase 2 Orthodontics at Permanent Dentition

With the arrival of permanent dentition and as patients approach skeletal maturity, patients experience the optimal window for orthodontic treatment. They must be carefully assessed for need of orthognathic surgery, if available, because compensation will generally be performed to address occlusal irregularities if no orthognathic surgery is to be undertaken, whereas decompensation would be performed (and exacerbate irregularities) prior to OGS.

In patients with dental posterior crossbites, the expanders described above can be used.

In CLP patients, dental anomalies such as variations in tooth number, shape, and/or position are often found. The

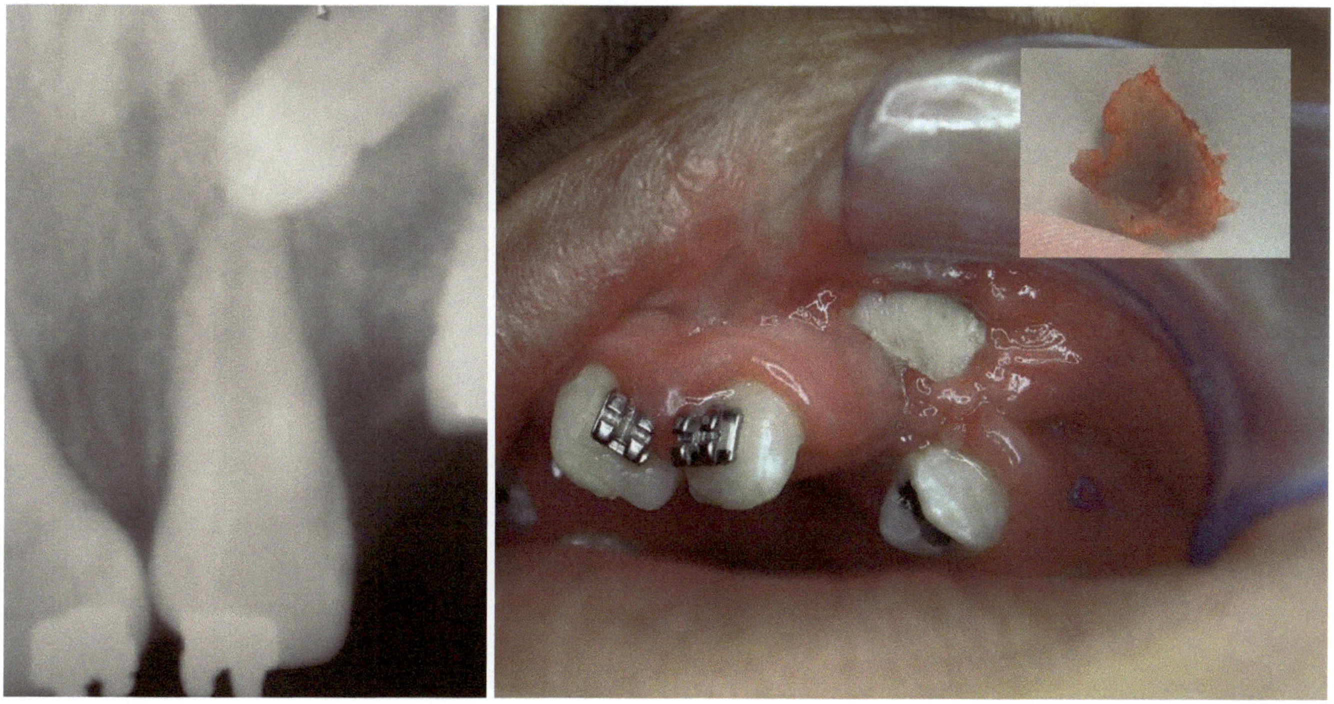

Fig. 27.11 ABG complication on left side of patient on Fig. 27.3. Fifteen days post-surgery, necrotic bone was taken out, ABG site was cleaned and closed, followed by 10 days local and systemic antibiotic

permanent lateral incisor is often affected. The most frequent anomaly is the absence of lateral incisors in the cleft area [13].

## Management of Missing Lateral Incisors

Treatment alternatives for unilateral or bilateral missing lateral incisors are:

A. Orthodontic Space Closure

Parameters in the process of decision-making:

- *Anatomical factors*
  - Position of the molars on the affected side, close space if molar relationship improves without closure of maxillary perimeter.
  - Presence of dental crowding in the unaffected area that would include extractions in the treatment plan without shortening maxillary perimeter.
- *Aesthetic factors*. Take always into account patient's decision.
- *Economic factors*.
- *Space Closure*: (Fig. 27.12a, b)

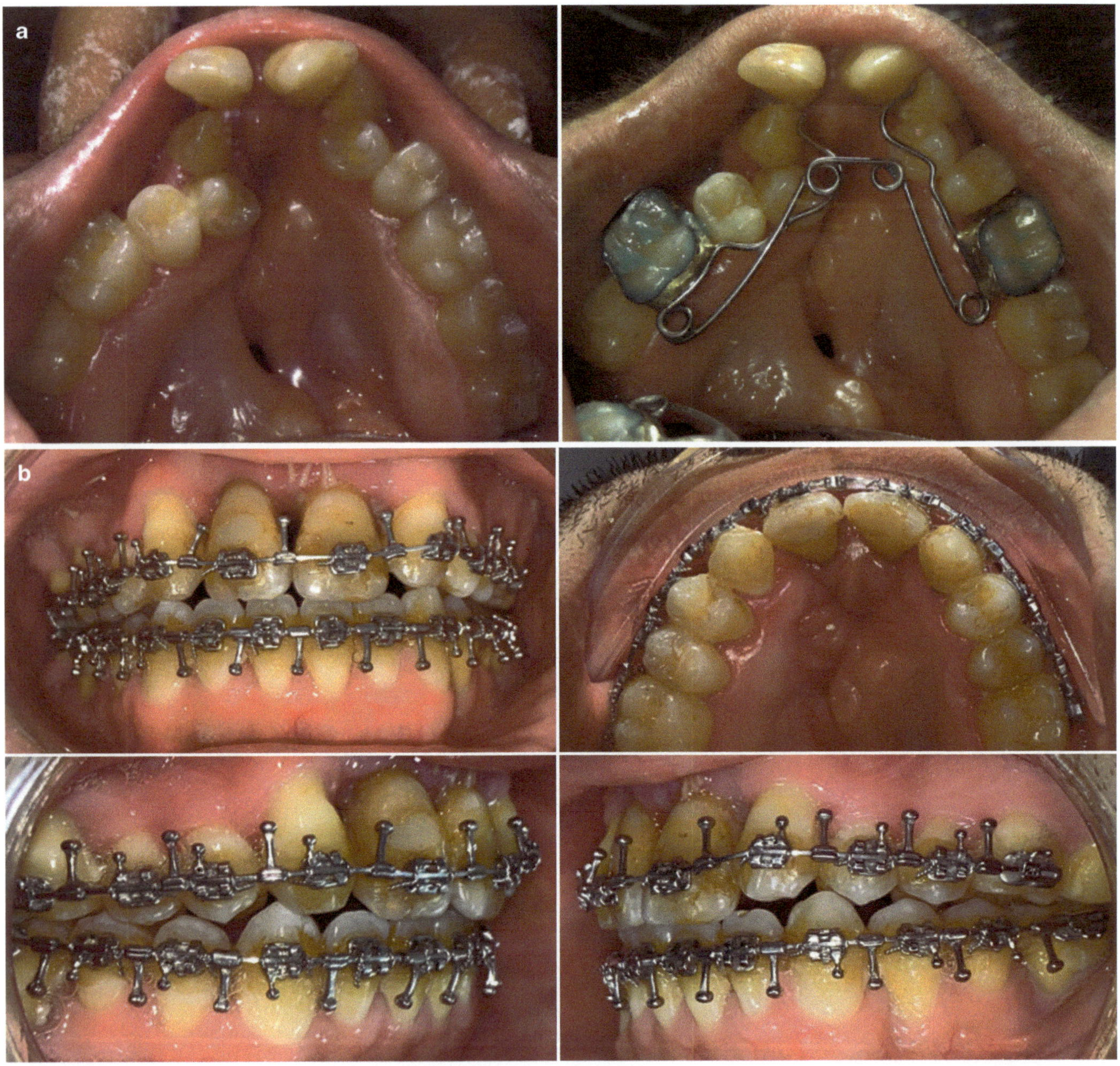


**Fig. 27.12** BCLP OGS patient prepared with space closure through placement of 1.3 and 2.3 in the position of 1.2 and 1.3 in both sides. (**a**) Initial expansion. (**b**) 1 month after OGS

The placement of the canine in the position of the lateral is indicated when:

(a) The canine has naturally deviated through the grafted bone in the lateral position.
(b) The morphology of the canine crown is similar to the lateral.
(c) The *periodontal and hygienic conditions* in the region of the cleft are optimal.
(d) If skeletal discrepancy will be managed with combined orthodontic and surgical approach.

B. Opening Spaces for Prosthetic Replacement
   Parameters in the process of decision-making:
   - *Anatomical factors*
     - In cases without ABG with stable posterior occlusion, restore with fixed bridge or removable prosthesis.
     - Prepare for ABG if planning implant restoration.
     - If managing the discrepancy with orthodontic camouflage.
   - *Aesthetic factors*
   - *Economic factors*

Do not extract or close space if maxillary segments are collapsed unless extraction on mandible is needed due to crowding.

It is important to remember that patients with UCLP have shown reduced bone support at teeth neighboring the cleft. This may cause instability during orthodontic treatment [14].

- *Preparation for Prosthetic restoration or Implant:*

When a prosthetic replacement is possible, it can be done with fixed prostheses. The most common mode is resin-bonded bridges or a removable prosthesis that in some cases are used as obturators and retainers as well. If implant placement is programed, implant surgery is usually carried out after 18 years of age. Additional bone grafting pre-implant may be needed.

## Presurgical Orthodontics in Preparation for Orthognathic Surgery (OGS)

### Patient Selection and Treatment Planning

Of all patients born with CLP, some 25–60% require maxillary advancement to correct maxillary hypoplasia [15, 16] (Figs. 27.13, 27.14, 27.15, 27.16, 27.17, 27.18, 27.19, and 27.20). In cases of skeletal open bite and marked mandibular deficiency and/or asymmetry, a two-jaw approach must be undertaken [5]. The *oral health status* of patients must be optimized and maintained prior, during, and after the orthodontic/orthognathic procedure. Third molar and supernumerary teeth extractions should be performed 6 months before orthognathic surgery to allow adequate healing and ossification of the extraction site, although recent reports by experienced teams show that extractions may be able to performed at time of surgery without additional complication (Fig. 27.19a, b).

Treatment planning is different for each case; even in low-resource settings, it requires a series of diagnostic records, photographs, properly occluded dental study models, orthopantogram and cephalometric radiographs, and ideally CBCT or CT to study the presurgical gnathic and facial relationships.

Collaboration and communication between surgeon and orthodontist are extremely important before, during, and after all surgical interventions. The craniofacial orthodontist interacts with the patient and their family in regular basis. The patient and caregivers should be educated on proper oral hygiene techniques. The overall oral-health status of the patient should be optimized and maintained prior, during, and after the orthodontic/orthognathic procedure.

The psychological impact of facial differences associated with clefts can be overwhelming for patients. Body dysmorphic disorder (BDD), also known as dysmorphophobia, occurs when a person is preoccupied by perceived differences in their appearance to the extent that causes shame, anxiety, or avoidance of social situations. To qualify for a diagnosis of BDD, the perception must cause clinically significant distress in psychosocial functioning. BDD usually onsets in early adolescence [1]. Although a patient's concerns may not reach the extent of a disorder, they may still suffer psychologically. In our experience inadequate attention is often given to mental health, including of cleft patients, in many low-resource settings. It is important for discussion of orthognathic surgery for two reasons: (1) it may create risk factors, such as depression, that need to be addressed when planning OGS, and (2) it may be able to be improved through OGS. A screening interview during the initial consultation can be an effective way of identifying this condition in a CLP patient. Involvement of the cleft team psychologist is very important in preparation for OGS. Psychosocial issues are further discussed in Chap. 31.

### Type of Orthodontic Appliances: Bracket Slot Size

The type of braces and archwires, and also the type of surgical splint, should be specifically discussed by the orthodontic-surgical team, prior to start the orthodontic preparation. Self-ligating type of braces and Niti arches could be useful

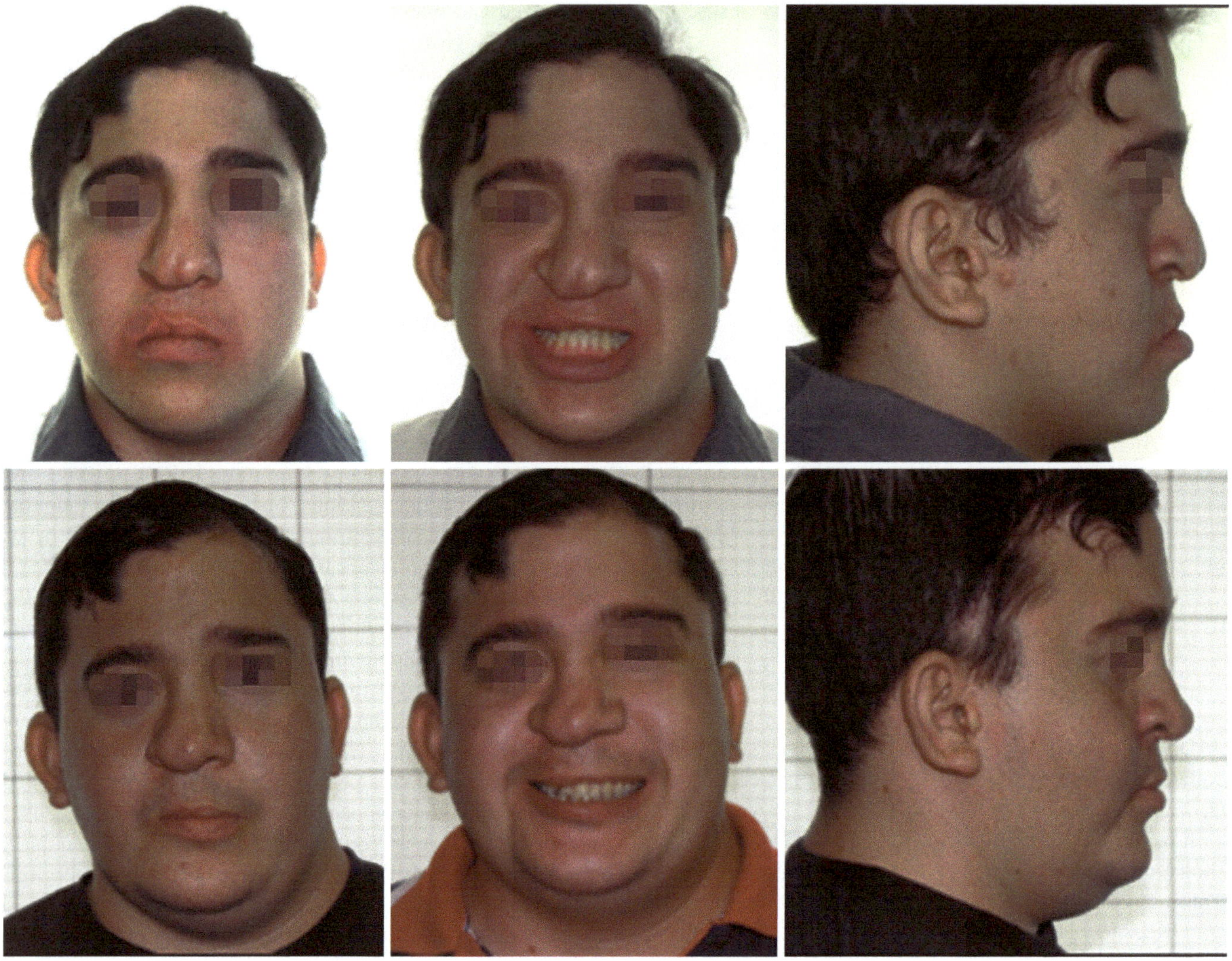

Fig. 27.13 UCLP 19-year-old male patient with severe maxillary hypoplasia, presenting social and emotional difficulties. Patient consultation motive and main concern was the nose. (OGS was done by Dr. Henrique Velez, Dr. Alex Villela and Dr. Hector Cordon)

for arch expansion and alveolar bone reshaping in mild collapsed maxillary cases (Fig. 27.21).

The patient should stay with a rigid (stainless steel) arch for at least 4–6 weeks before surgery. T pins or K hooks should be built onto the orthodontic arches 1 week before surgery to assist intraop stabilization (Fig. 27.17)

### Anterior Maxillary Segmental Distraction (AMSD)

AMSD consist of slow regeneration of bone following corticotomy or osteotomy with the use of an intraoral tooth-borne distractor [15]. AMSD may be especially useful in patients suffering from velopharyngeal insufficiency (VPI) previously treated with pharyngeal flap surgery and who could develop speech problems after orthognathic surgery.

**AMSD Objectives**

1. Create space for impacted teeth and their alignment (Fig. 27.22a–k)
2. Increase the arch length while maintaining the class I molar relationship.
3. Improve crossbites and concave profile

**AMSD Advantages**

1. Less morbidity at surgery
2. Shorter procedure than orthognathic surgery
3. Velopharyngeal sphincter is not affected
4. Stable results with less relapse

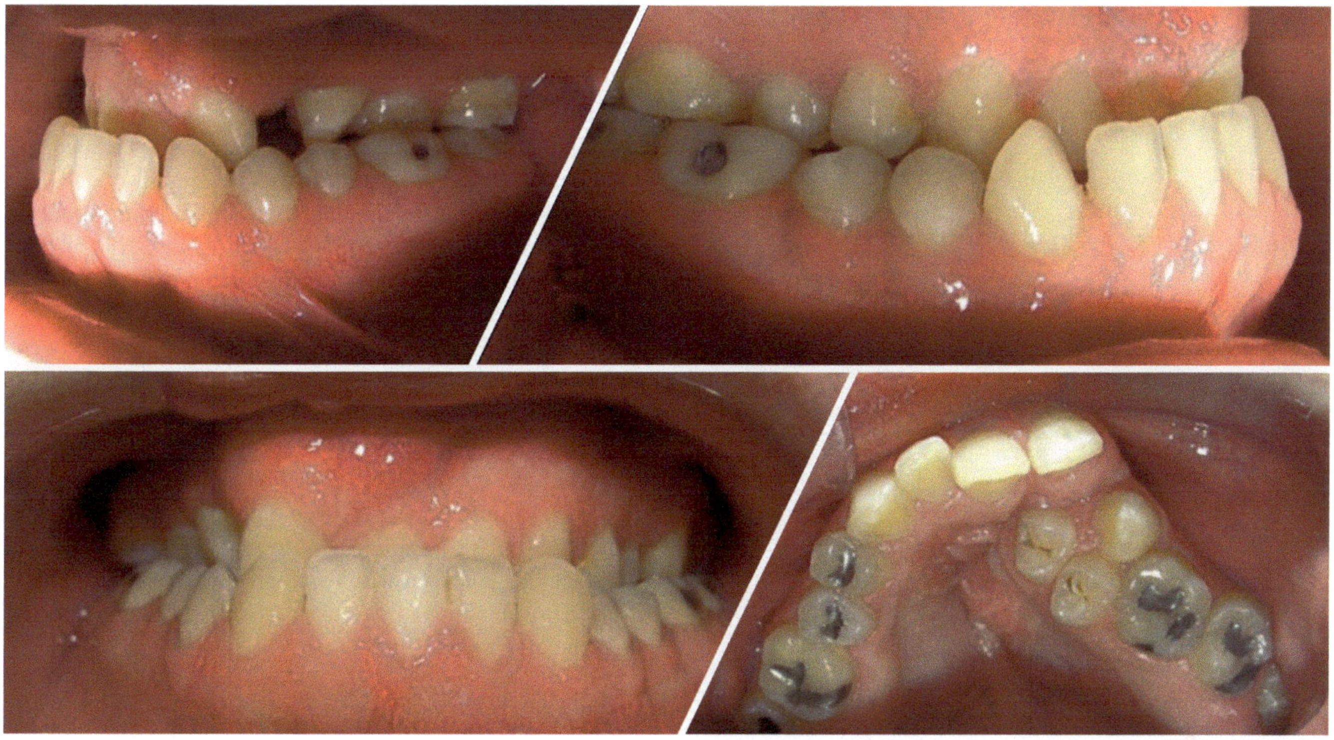

**Fig. 27.14** Intraoral pre-treatment images
Right occlusion
Left occlusion
Frontal, notice complete crossbite
Upper arch occlusal view

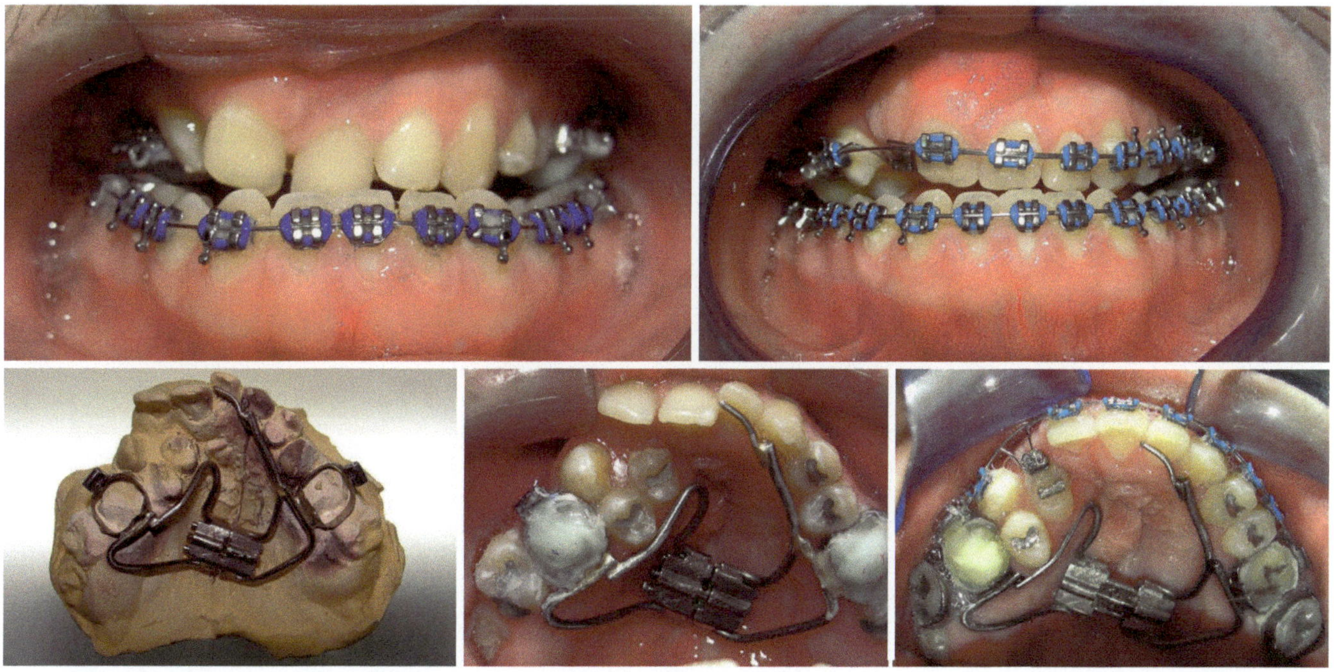

**Fig. 27.15** Maxillary expansion with hyrax type expander. Notice the inclination of the screw. No Surgical Assisted Rapid Expansion (SARPE) needed

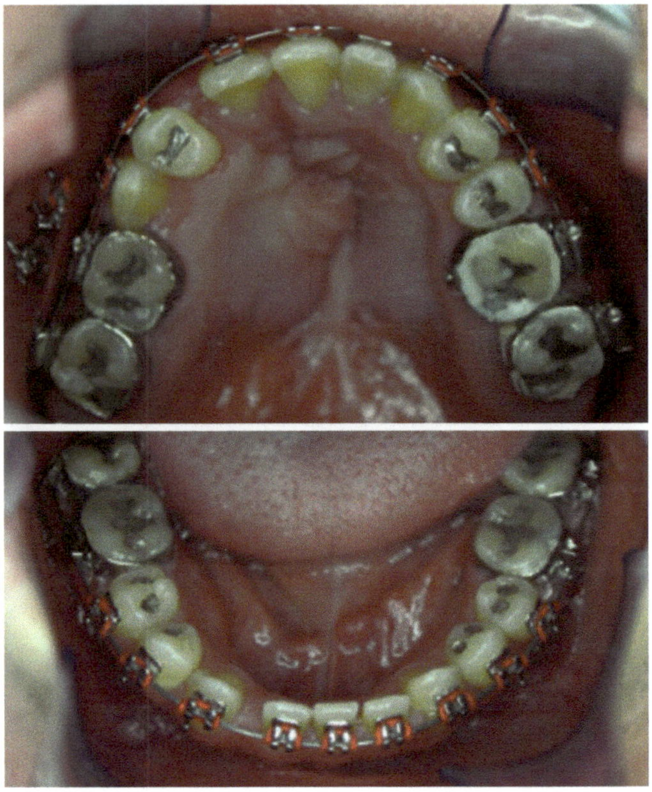

Fig. 27.16 Leveling and alignment of both arches individually

5. Easy fabrication of intraoral distractor, minimal expense, and good patient tolerance

**AMSD Protocol**

1. Initiate non-surgical transverse expansion to correct posterior crossbites, especially in premolar area.
2. Orthodontic preparation, leveling, and aligning tooth on both maxillary segments.
3. A tooth-borne sagittal hyrax distractor is cemented the day before surgery.
4. AMSD is carried out under general anesthesia between the premolars or premolar and molar alveolar bone as decided in the treatment plan in agreement with the maxillofacial surgeon.
5. Distraction commences several days postoperatively at a rate of 1 mm/day with a twice daily rhythm. It continues until device fully expanded (12 mm).
6. A face mask is used with an antero-inferior traction (1/4″ elastics) all time, to avoid counterclockwise rotation of the palatal plane.
7. Liquid diet prescribed for 7 days and then soft diet for 6 weeks.
8. Orthopantography after 4–6 weeks of activation.

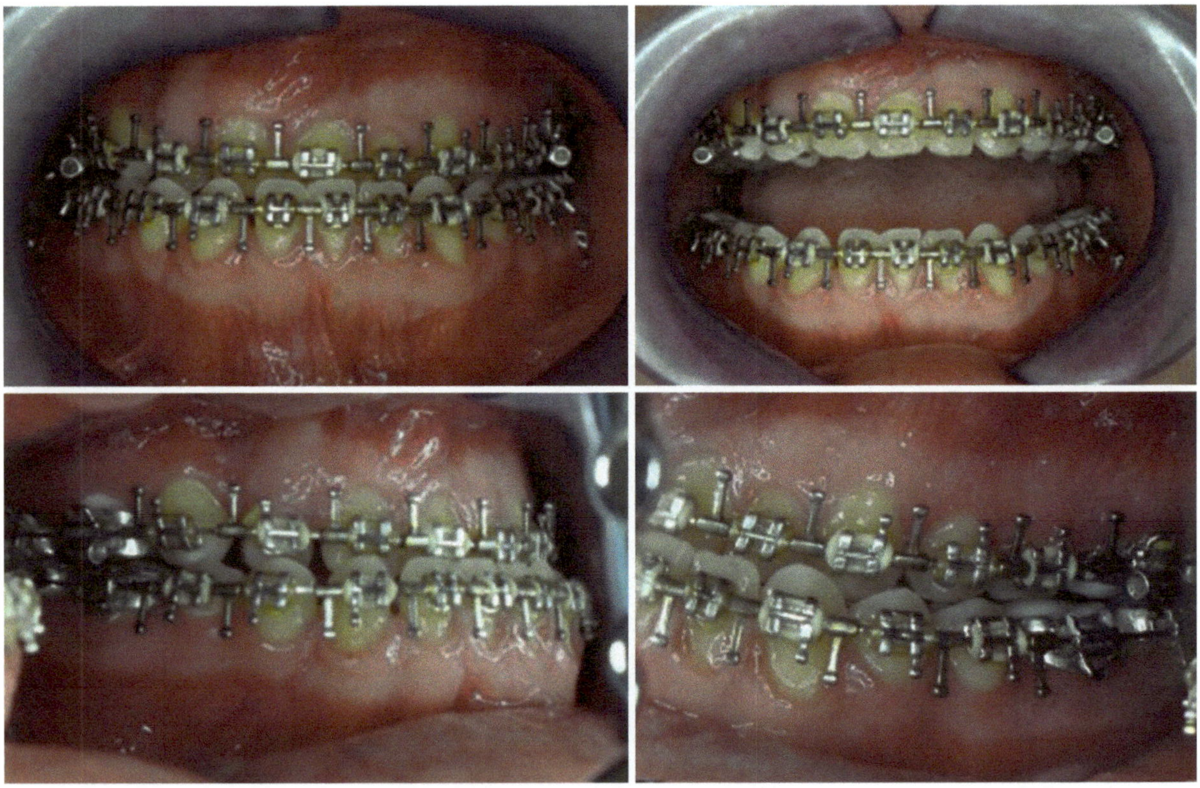

Fig. 27.17 Placement of the rigid 0.17 × 0.25 SS arches 5 months before surgery. SS ligatures were placed the day before surgery. Notice the periodontal health and excellent oral hygiene, imperative for healing after OGS. No surgical splint was needed

**Case Report: Anterior Maxillary Segmental Distraction**

In low-resource settings without orthognathic surgery capabilities, AMSD can improve the anterior dental position in cases of maxillary retrusion. In 23-year-old male BCLP patient with good speech, wide anterior palatal fistula, and severe collapse maxilla, an AMSD was the surgery of choice (Fig. 27.23a, b). The patient had not previously undergone ABG. Preparation was done with transverse palatal expansion, brackets, pre-surgical oral prophylaxis, and restoration of dental caries.

A tooth-borne sagittally oriented hyrax distractor was cemented 1 day before surgery (Fig. 27.23c–e). Under general surgery, an osteotomy was performed between maxillary premolars, a 2-hour surgery. Distractor activation began several days after surgery and was carried out on a rate of 1 mm/day with a twice daily rhythm. When the screw was completely open, an expansion of 12 mm, the device was locked into position for consolidation. A face mask was used with an antero-inferior traction (1/4″ elastics) throughout distraction, to avoid counterclockwise rotation of the palatal plane (Fig. 27.23f). Postoperatively the patient was kept under antibiotics, analgesic, and steroids and maintained a liquid diet for 7 days and then soft diet for 6 weeks. Lateral cephalometric x-rays were taken before and 4 weeks after AMSD (Fig. 27.23g).

## Post-surgical Orthodontic Treatment

Finishing the case after OGS takes from 6 to 10 months. Main objective are to provide the patient with close to ideal occlusal relationship and markedly improved function and aesthetics (Fig. 27.18). Nonextraction UCLP cases will end in Class II molar on the cleft side and molar and canine Class I in the non-cleft side. The cleft team should make every effort to follow patients long-term [5] until growth and facial development is completed.

## Retention

Extensive lip and transpalatal scar tissue have limited stretch capability. Maxillary arch can collapse with relapse on anterior or posterior crossbite even after ABG; permanent retention of maxillary arch form is then necessary. This may be done by a removable palatal prosthesis (Fig. 27.23h and

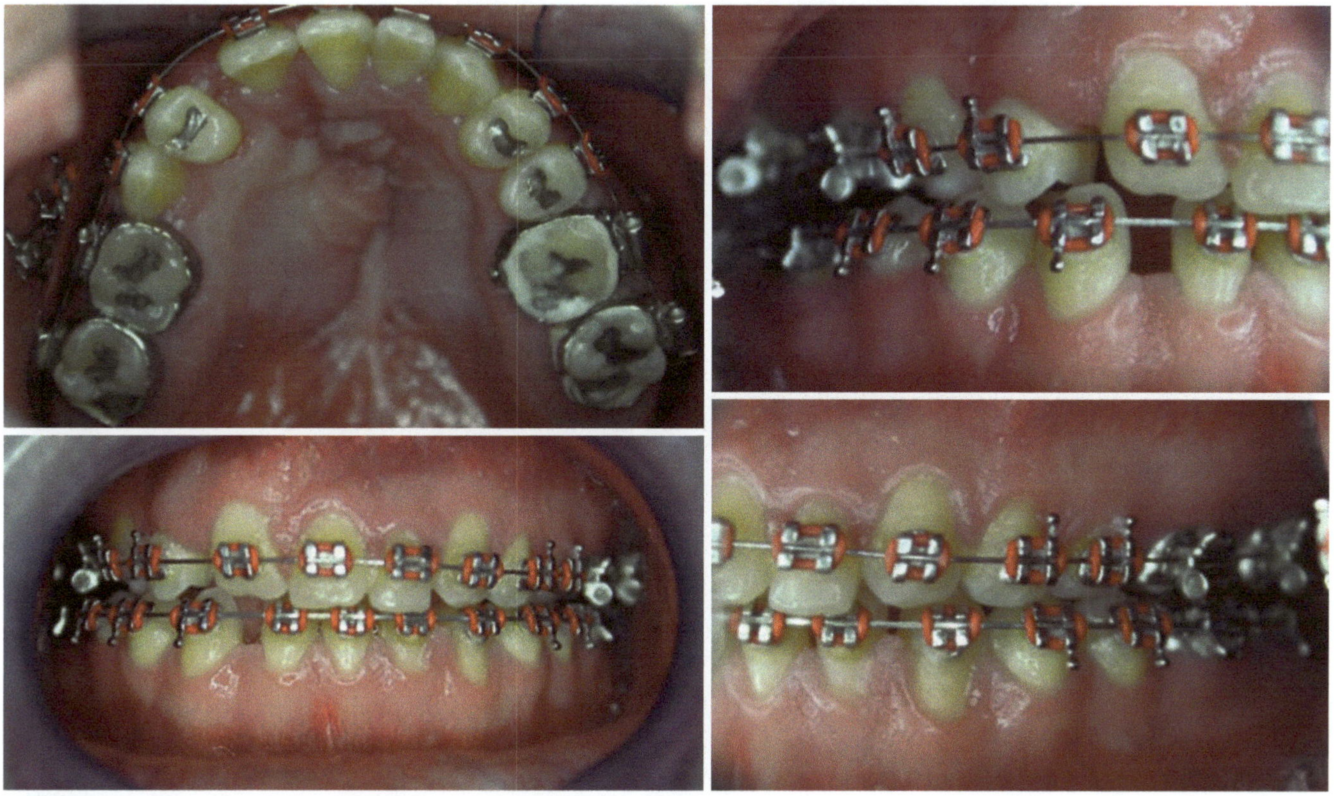

**Fig. 27.18** Intraoral post-surgery images. Patient used intramaxillary elastics (1/4″) in box shaped with Class III vector for 3 months
Upper arch occlusal view
Frontal
Right occlusion
Left occlusion

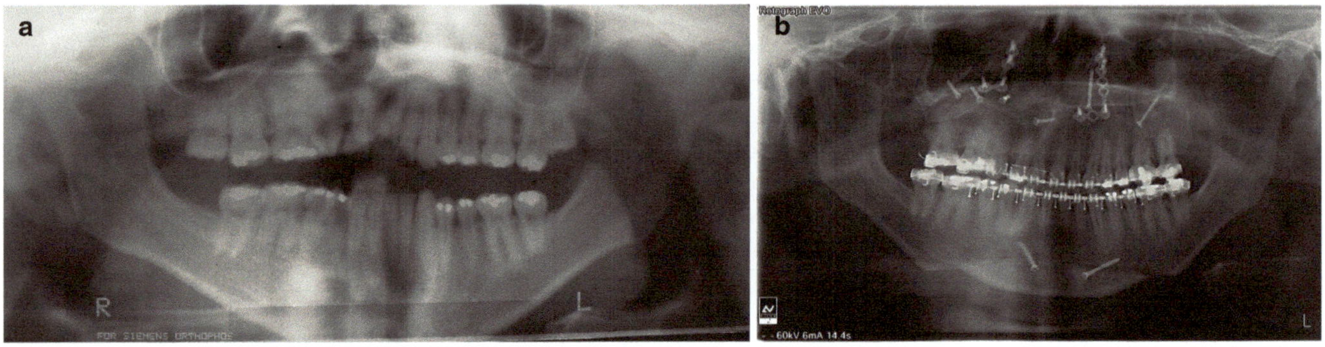


**Fig. 27.19** (**a**) Initial OPG. (**b**) OPG 8 days after OGS

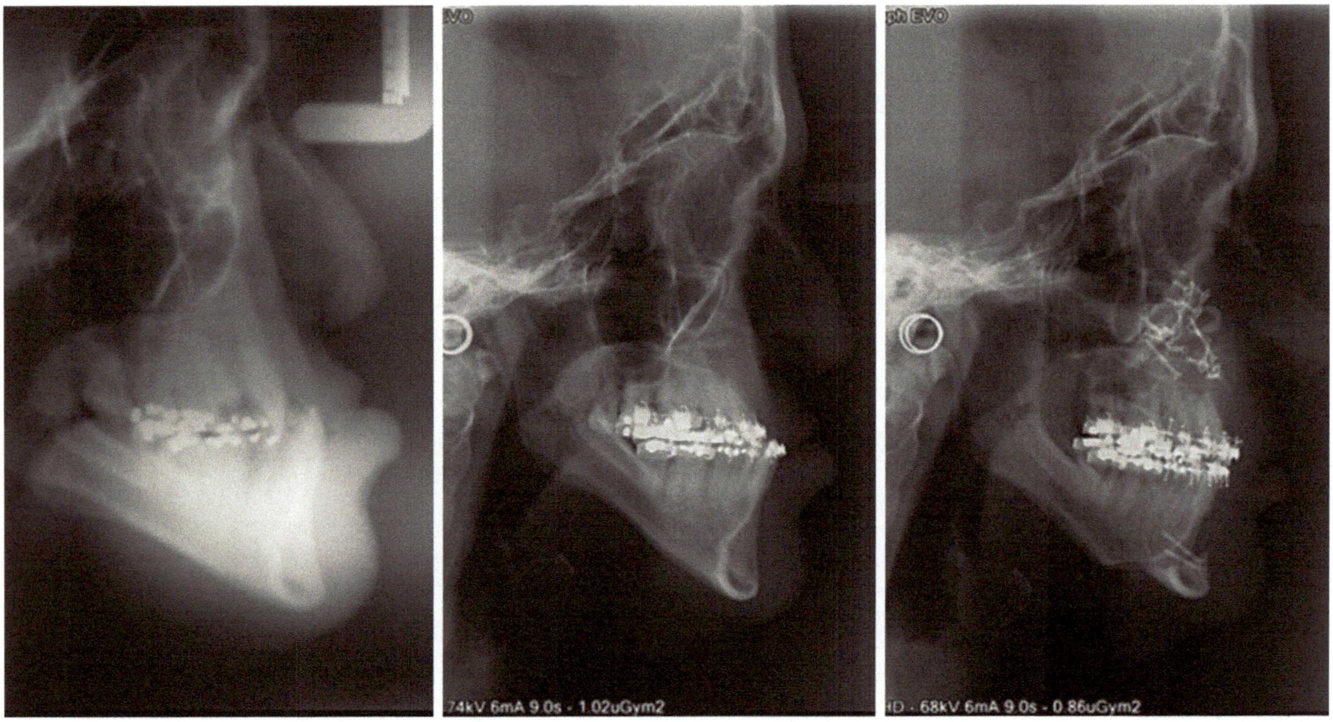


**Fig. 27.20** Initial cephalometric X-ray. Intermediate cephalometric X-ray. Eight days post OGS Cephalometric X-ray

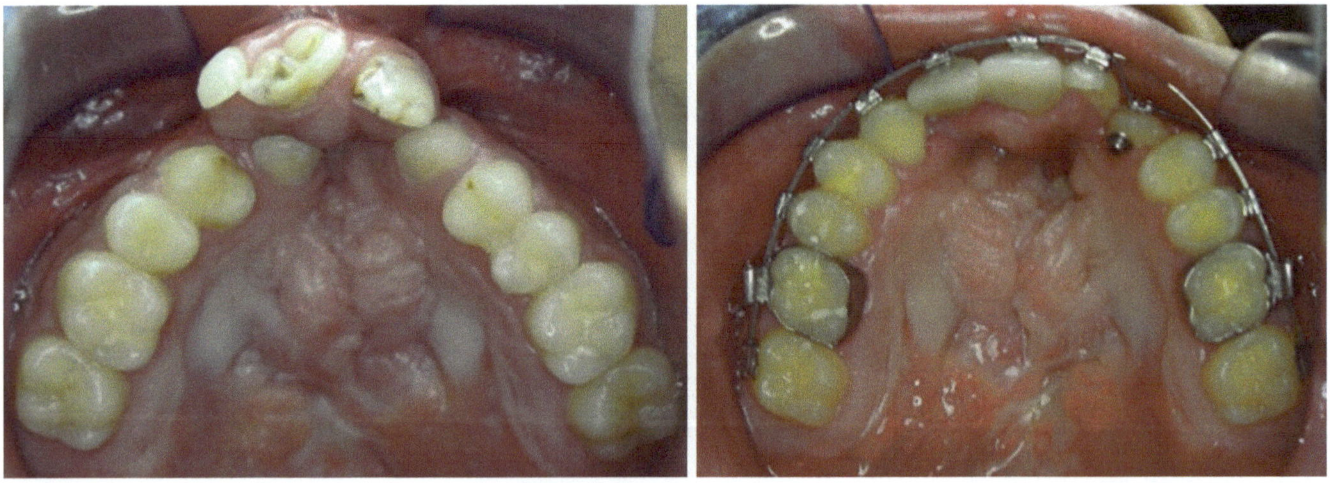

**Fig. 27.21** BCLP patient, maxillary expansion was gained with self-ligating (SL) brackets and Niti arches before ABG

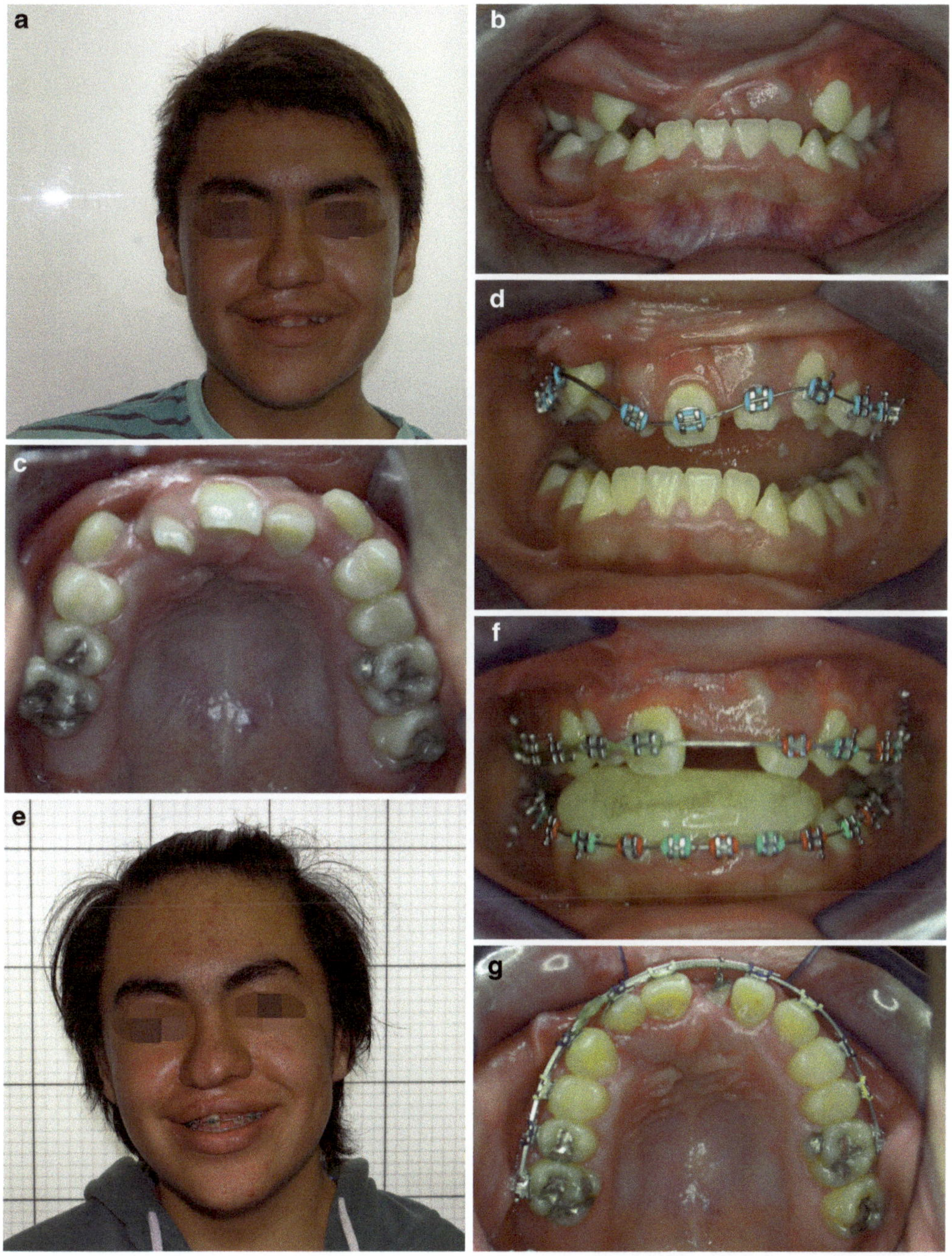

Fig. 27.22 A 15-year-old UCL and cleft alveolus patient with severe anterior crossbite and impacted left maxillary central incisor. (**a**) Initial smile. (**b**) Initial frontal occlusion. (**c**) Occlusal maxillary view. (**d**) Occlusal plane leveling. (**e**) Smile post ASD with space gained for impacted left central incisor. (**f**) Post ASD frontal view. (**g**) Post ASD occlusal view. Distraction was done with elastic chains and open springs in a SS 0.17 × 0.25 archwire. (**h**) 2.1 in place after space was gained. (**i**) OPG, 3 months before ASD. (**j**) OPG after ASD. (**k**) Periapical X-ray of site of osteotomy (mesial to right central incisor). Enough space to traction impacted left central incisor (2.1)

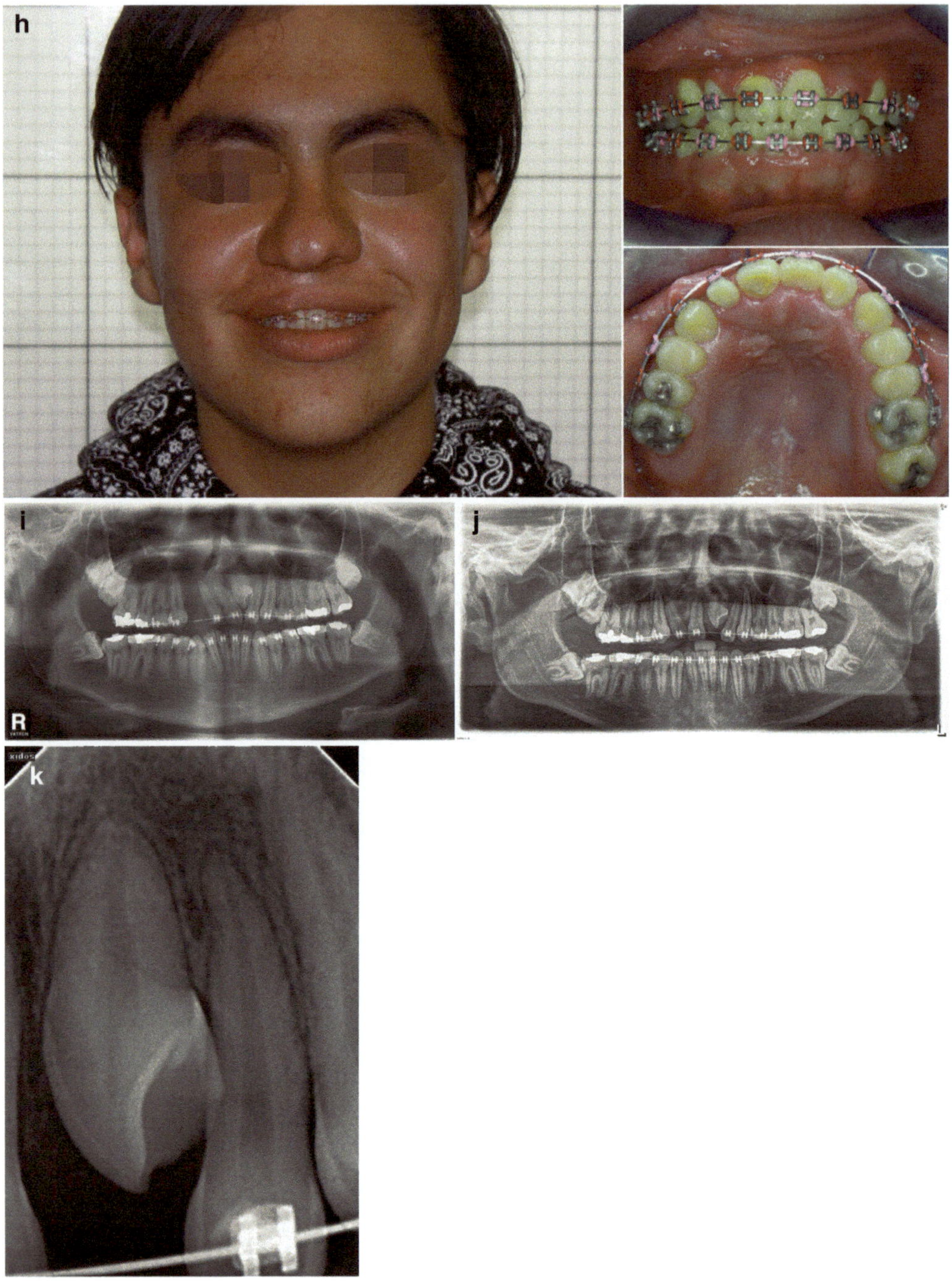


Fig. 27.22 (continued)

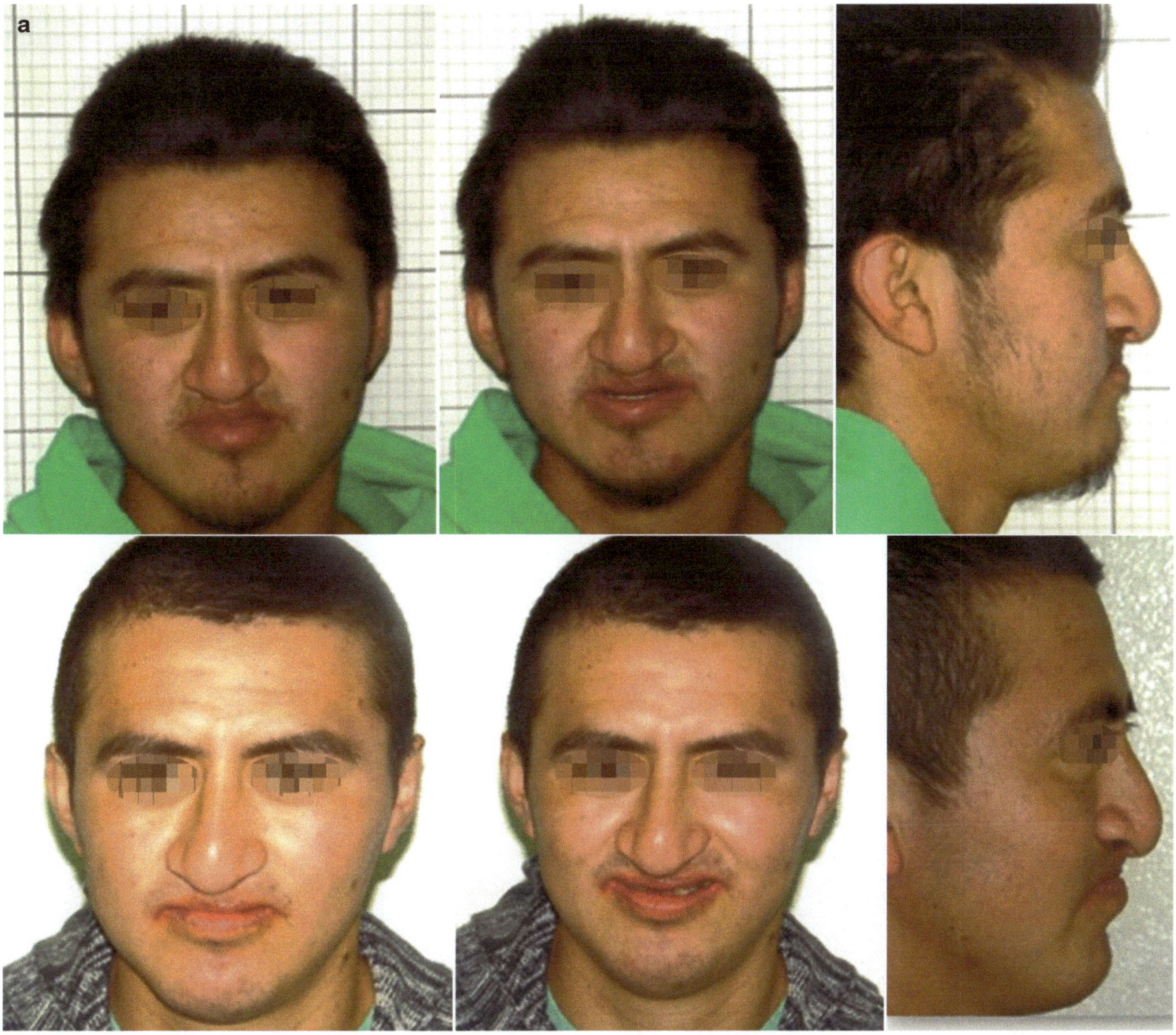


**Fig. 27.23** BCLP patient, 24 years old with no previous ABG. (See text case report) Orthodontic preparation Dr. Rita Morales and Dr. Vilma Arteaga, Surgery done by Dr. Henrique Velez assisted by Dr. Alex Villella, Dr. Hector Cordon. (**a**) Pre and post AMSD facial images. (**b**) Initial intraoral images. (**c**) Maxillary expansion with a V shape expander. (**d**) Orthodontic preparation. (**e**) Intraoral images post AMSD. (**f**) Face mask, anterior and inferior traction used 24 hours/day for 40 days. (**g**) Pre and post AMSD cephalometric X-rays. (**h**) Intraoral occlusion post AMSD

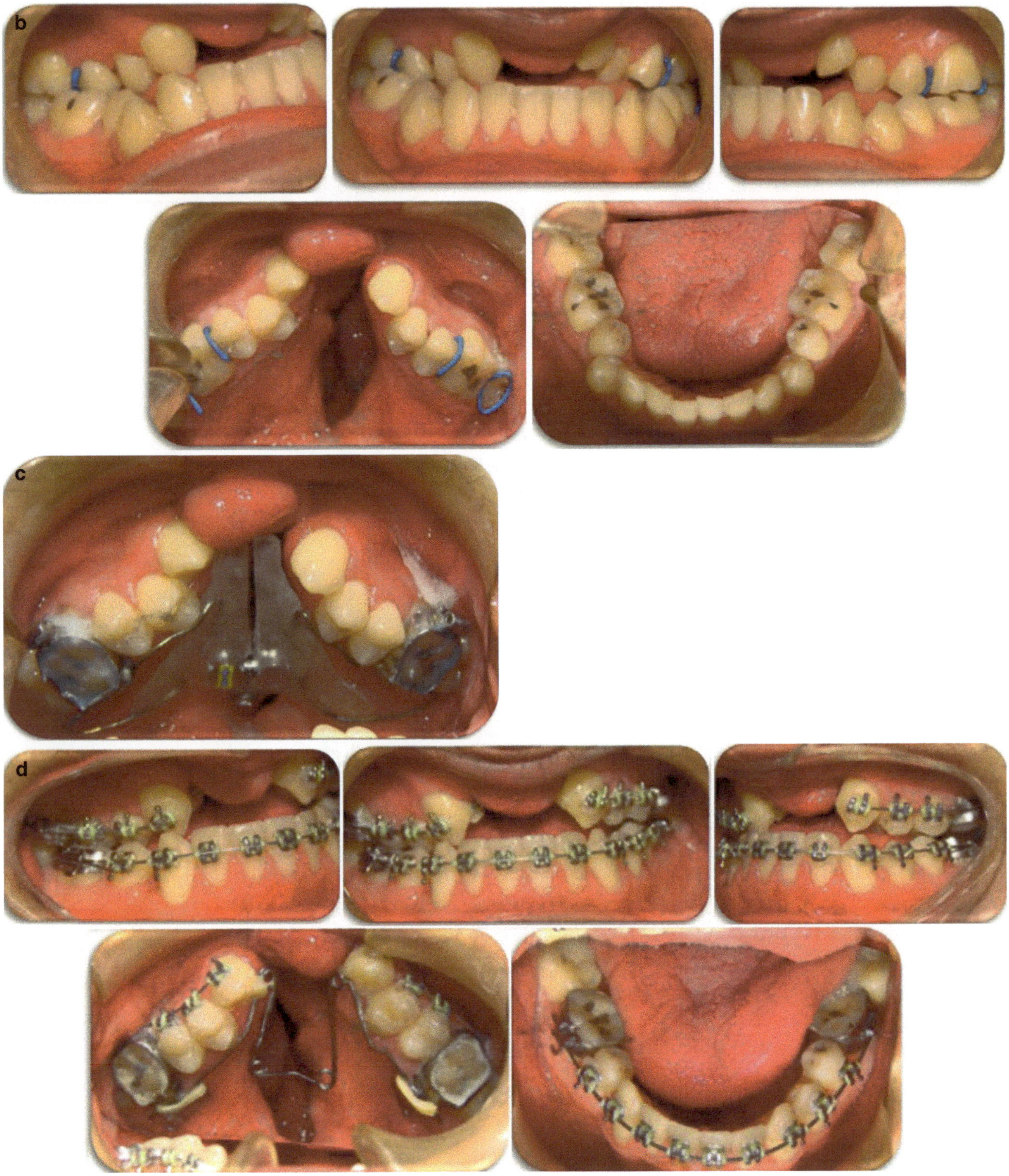

Fig. 27.23 (continued)

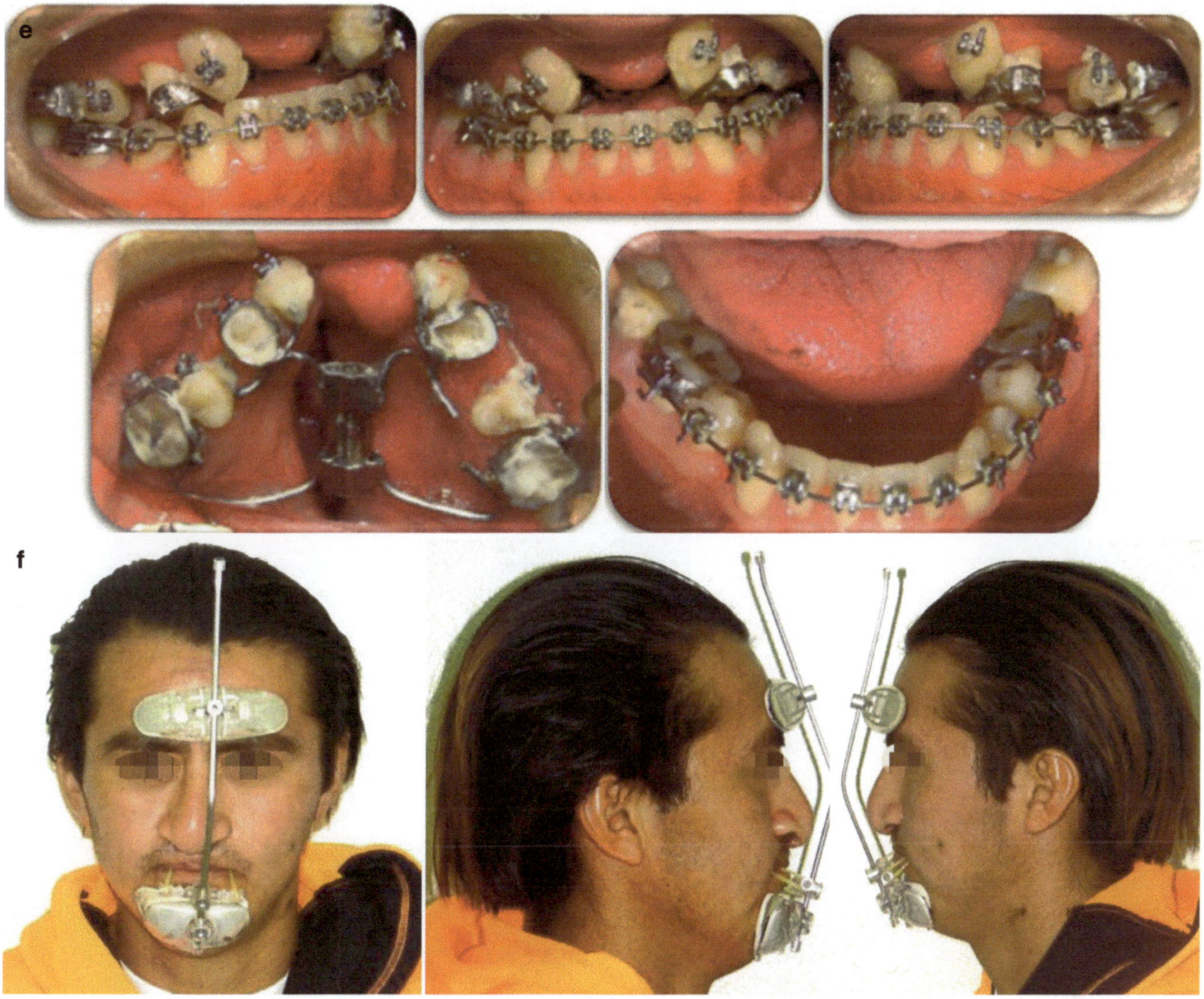


Fig. 27.23 (continued)

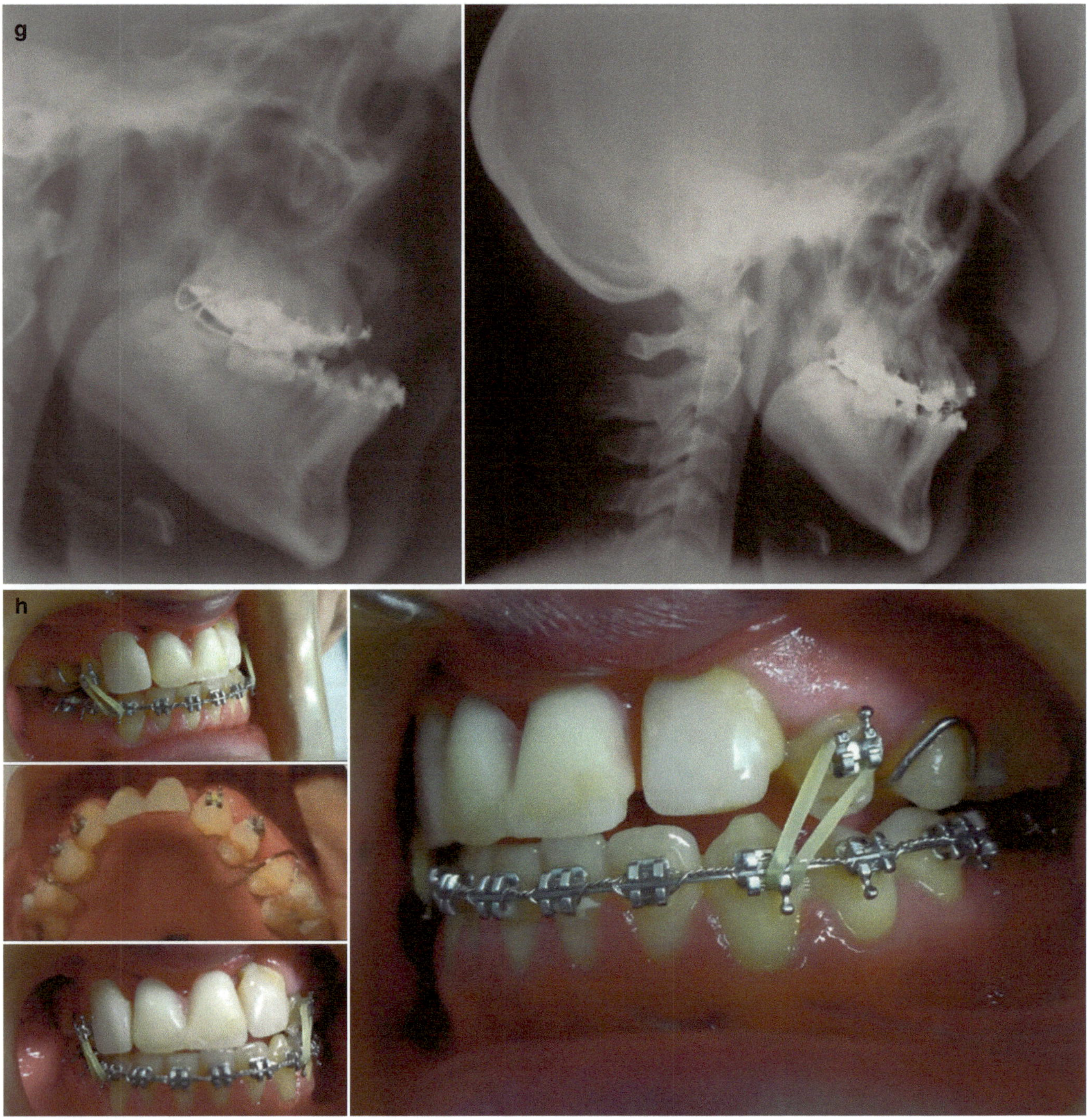


Fig. 27.23 (continued)

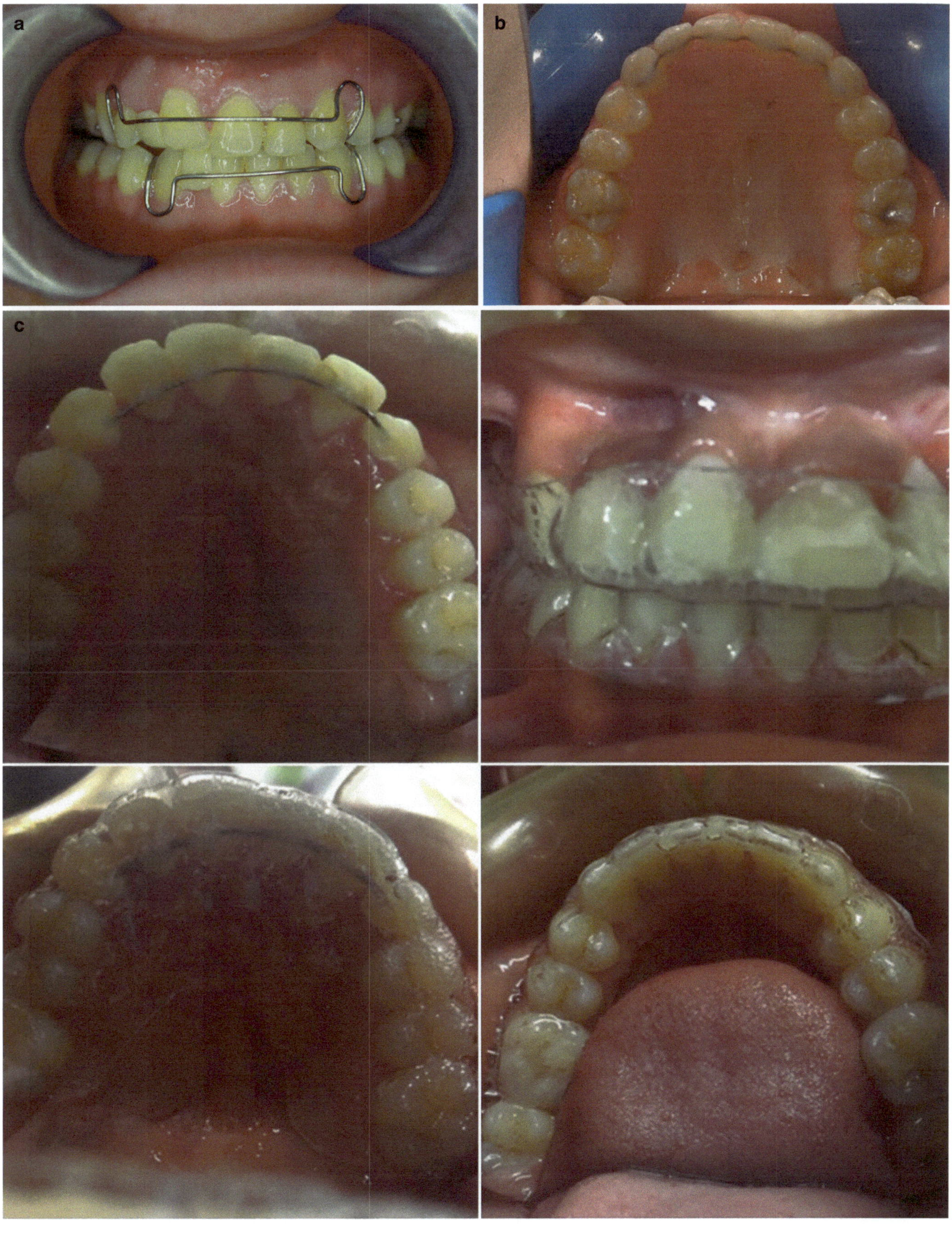


**Fig. 27.24** (**a**) Hawley removable retainers of patient in Fig. 27.13. (**b**) Bonded lingual retention in a UCLP patient. (Courtesy of Dr. Hisham Atwan). (**c**) Essix and lingual fixed retention. (Courtesy of Dr. R. Morales). (**d**) Fixed bridge spanning the cleft. (Courtesy of Dr. Hisham Atwan)

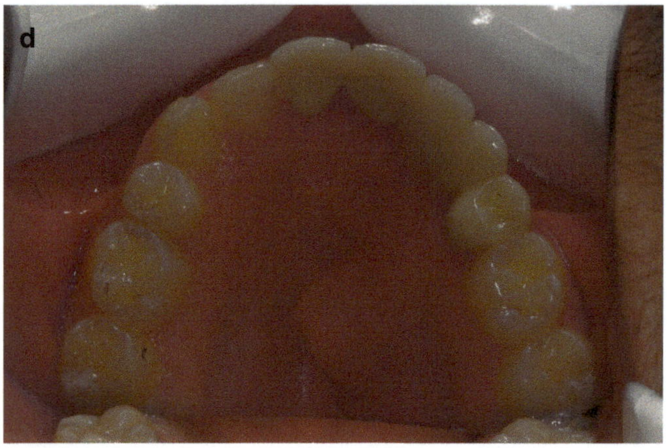


Fig. 27.24 (continued)

27.24a) or bonded retainers (Fig. 27.24b) and in some cases an additional Essix retainer (Fig. 27.24c) or a fixed bridge spanning the cleft (Fig. 27.24d). A transpalatal arch with lateral arms welded to support posterior alveolus may be useful [17].

## Conclusion

Anatomical characteristics of clefts, timing, and sequencing of orthodontic cleft care and clinical planning and protocols have been described. Orthodontic care has been divided in two phases: (1) orthodontic at mixed dentition and (2) orthodontic at permanent dentition. Attention has been given to the importance of proper diagnostic records to study every case and decide for a suitable treatment plan, on orthodontic ABG preparation, maxillary expansion methods, AMSD as an alternative to OGS, and OGS preparation. Continuous education and adequate training are essential to achieve the results that CLP patients require. The role of the orthodontist as a member of a multidisciplinary team is to help cleft lip and palate (CLP) patients reach their full rehabilitation and obtain the best aesthetic and functional outcomes beginning at an early age, as well as develop good self-esteem.

## References

1. Naini F, Gill D. Orthognathic surgery. 1st ed. Oxford: Wiley; 2017. p. 235–42, Chap. 9.
2. Grabowski R, Kopp H, Stahl F, Gundlach K. Presurgical orthopaedic treatment of newborns with clefts – functional treatment with long-term effects. J Cranio-Maxillofac Surg. 2006;34:34–44.
3. Fahradyan A, Tsuha M, Wolfswinkel E, Mitchell K, Hammoudeh J, Magee W. Optimal timing of secondary alveolar bone grafting: a literature review. J Oral Maxillofac Surg. 2018;77:843. https://doi.org/10.1016/j.joms.2018.11.019.
4. Meazzini M, Lematti L, Mazzoleni F, Rabbiosi D, Bozzetti A, Brusati R. Vertical excess of the premaxilla in bilateral cleft lip and palate patients. J Craniofac Surg. 2010;21:499–502.
5. Rodriguez E, Losee J, Neligan P, Liu D. Plastic surgery: craniofacial, head and neck surgery and pediatric plastic surgery. 4th ed. New York: Elsevier; 2017. p. 593–617.
6. Ricketts R. Bioprogressive therapie. Rocky Mountain/Orthodontics: Denver; 1984. p. 245–9.
7. Aizenbud D, Ciceu C, Rachmiel A, Hazan-Molina H. Reverse quad helix appliance: differential anterior maxillary expansion of the cleft area before bone grafting. J Craniofac Surg. 2012;23:e440–3.
8. McNamara J, Brudon W. Orthodontic and orthopedic treatment in the mixed dentition. Ann Arbor: Needham Press; 1995.
9. Planas P. Rehabilitaci6n neuro-oclusal (RNO). Madrid: Ripano; 2013.
10. Simões W. Ortopedia funcional dos maxilares. São Paulo: Editora Artes Médicas; 2003.
11. Ramirez 0Yañez G. Planas direct tracks for early crossbite correction. J Clin Orthod. 2003;37:294–8.
12. Kazemi A, Stearns J, Fonseca R. Secondary grafting in the alveolar cleft patient. Oral Maxillofac Surg Clin North Am. 2002;14:477–90.
13. Meazzini M. Craniofacial anomalies: surgical-orthodontic management. Bologna: Edizioni Matina; 2011. p. 43–67.
14. Oosterkamp B, Dijkstra P, Remmelink H, Van Oort R, Sandham A. Orthodontic space closure versus prosthetic replacement of missing upper lateral incisors in patients with bilateral cleft lip and palate. Cleft Palate Craniofac J. 2010;47:591–6.
15. Rao S, Kotrashetti S, Lingaraj J, Pinto P, Keluskar K, Jain S, Sone P, Rao S. Anterior segmental distraction osteogenesis in the hypoplastic cleft maxilla: report of five cases = إفتراق التكون العظمي للفاصل الأمامي في مرضى نقص تنسج فلج الفك العلوي : عرض لخمس حالات. Sultan Qaboos Univ Med J. 2013;13:447–52.
16. Baker SB, Menon N. Cleft orthognathic surgery. In: Losee JE, Kirschner RE, editors. Comprehensive cleft care. 2nd ed. New York: McGraw Hill; 2016. p. 1171–299.
17. Berkowitz S. Cleft lip and palate. Berlin: Springer; 2006.

# Speech and Resonance Disorders Secondary to Cleft Lip/Palate (CLP)

28

Ann W. Kummer

**Key Points**

- Dental malocclusion secondary to cleft of the primary palate or micrognathia affects the relationship between the tongue tip and the alveolar ridge. This can cause obligatory distortions or compensatory errors during speech sound production.
- Velopharyngeal insufficiency (VPI) occurs in approximately 30% of children with cleft palate, despite the palate repair. This can cause hypernasality and/or nasal emission during speech production.
- Physical management (surgery or a prosthetic device, if surgery is not an option) is the only way to correct VPI.
- Speech therapy cannot correct abnormal structure. Speech therapy is appropriate to correct abnormal function (e.g., abnormal articulation placement) that develops as a compensation for abnormal structure.
- Speech therapy is most effective after surgical normalization of the abnormal structure which caused the disorder.

## Introduction

Children born with cleft lip and/or palate are at risk for disorders of speech sound production (articulation) and disorders of resonance (hypernasality, hyponasality, cul-de-sac resonance, or mixed resonance). There are several potential causes of these disorders, including dental and/or occlusal abnormalities, upper airway obstruction, and most significantly—velopharyngeal insufficiency (VPI).

The purpose of this chapter is to describe how structural anomalies associated with cleft lip and palate can affect both speech and resonance. Information will be given on effective procedures for conducting a perceptual evaluation. There will be a special focus on evaluation techniques that are simple and low-tech yet very effective. Tips will be given on how to perform an intraoral examination.

Common instrumental procedures for evaluation will be described, and the relative advantage of each procedure will be listed. Finally, there will be a review of treatment options, which will include a discussion on when speech therapy is appropriate and when it is not.

## Causes of Speech and Resonance Disorders in Children with Cleft Lip/Palate

### Dental and/or Occlusal Abnormalities

Dental abnormalities, such as supernumerary teeth or ectopic teeth, often occur in children with a cleft of the primary palate, particularly if the cleft extended into the alveolar ridge. Abnormally placed teeth can interfere with bilabial closure or tongue tip movement during speech production. Misplaced teeth can also divert the airstream for certain sounds, causing a lateral distortion.

In addition to dental abnormalities, children with cleft lip and palate often have a retrusive maxilla, and children with Robin sequence have micrognathia. Both of these conditions result in malocclusion of the jaws. Malocclusion can affect the ability to achieve bilabial closure for bilabial sounds (p, b, m). Even more significantly, malocclusion can affect the tongue tip to alveolar ridge relationship, which is necessary for production of all lingual-alveolar sounds (t, d, n, l, s, z, sh, zh, ch, j) (Fig. 28.1).

**Electronic Supplementary Material** The online version of this chapter (https://doi.org/10.1007/978-3-030-59105-2_28) contains supplementary material, which is available to authorized users.

A. W. Kummer (✉)
Division of Speech-Language Pathology, Cincinnati Children's Hospital Medical Center and University of Cincinnati College of Medicine, Cincinnati, OH, USA

© Springer Nature Switzerland AG 2021

J. W. Swanson, D. W. Low (eds.), *Global Cleft Care in Low-Resource Settings*, https://doi.org/10.1007/978-3-030-59105-2_28

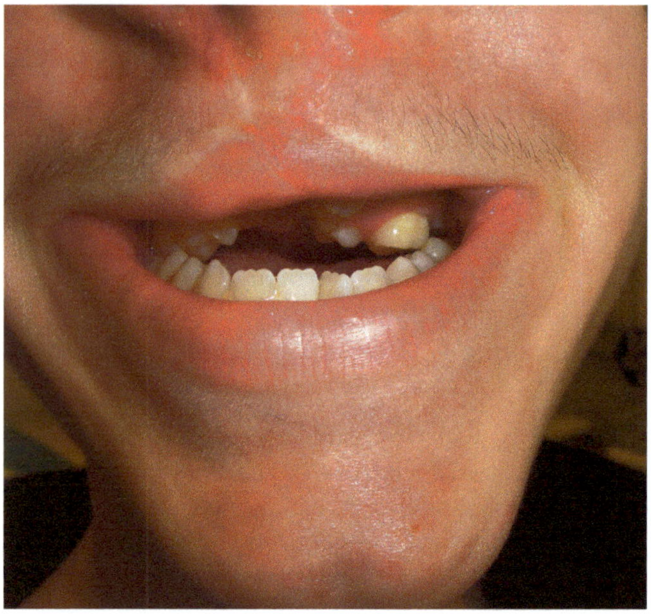

**Fig. 28.1** Class III malocclusion with anterior crossbite and missing teeth. Malocclusion can distort the tongue tip to alveolar ridge relationship, thus affecting speech. (Reproduced with permission from Kummer [1])

Structural anomalies, including those of dentition or occlusion, may cause speech to be characterized by obligatory distortions and/or compensatory errors. *Obligatory distortions* occur when the articulation placement is correct, but an abnormality of the structure results in a distortion of speech [2–4]. Common obligatory distortions due to dental/occlusal anomalies include lateral distortion of sibilant sounds (s, z, sh, zh, ch, j). In contrast, *compensatory errors* are the result of incorrect articulatory placement in response to abnormal structure [2, 3]. An example of a compensatory error is the substitution of a palatal-dorsal placement for a lingual-alveolar sound when dental malocclusion affects the tongue tip placement.

When there are dental abnormalities and/or malocclusion, it is very important to make a differential diagnosis between obligatory distortions, compensatory errors, and functional placement errors. This is because the treatment for each is different. Obligatory distortions require physical management only, whereas compensatory productions require speech therapy — preferably after physical correction of the structure. Functional placement errors (which are not related to abnormal structure) require speech therapy only.

## Upper Airway Obstruction

Obstruction in the upper airway is a common concern in children with clefts and related craniofacial syndromes. It can be caused by glossoptosis secondary to Robin sequence, maxillary retrusion which results in a shallow pharynx, hypertrophic tonsils or adenoids, a deviated septum, or stenotic nares. Upper airway obstruction is sometimes an unwanted consequence of surgery for velopharyngeal insufficiency.

Regardless of the cause, obstruction in the upper airway can cause abnormal resonance, including hyponasality, cul-de-sac resonance, or mixed resonance [4–6]. When this type of resonance is identified by a speech-language pathologist, the child should be referred to an otolaryngologist for physical management.

## Velopharyngeal Insufficiency (VPI)

### Normal Velopharyngeal Function

During nasal breathing, the velum rests against the base of the tongue (Fig. 28.2a). This results in a patent airway for normal nasal breathing. With the production of oral speech sounds, the velum elevates and moves upward and backward to close against the posterior pharyngeal wall. At the same time, the lateral pharyngeal walls move medially to close against (or in rare cases, behind) the velum. The coordinated movement of these structures results in complete closure of the velopharyngeal valve (Fig. 28.2b).

During speech production, there is generation of airflow (from the lungs) and sound (from the vocal folds). This airflow and sound travel in a superior direction through the pharynx. For the production of nasal sounds (m, n, and ng), the velopharyngeal valve is open, and as a result, the airflow and sound are released through the nasal cavity. During the production of oral sounds, however, the valve closes completely. As a result, the airflow and sound are redirected into the oral cavity [7].

### Velopharyngeal Insufficiency (VPI)

Velopharyngeal insufficiency (VPI) is a type of velopharyngeal dysfunction that is caused by abnormal velopharyngeal structure (Fig. 28.3) [3, 8]. A history of cleft palate is the most common cause of velopharyngeal insufficiency. In fact, it has been estimated that approximately 20–30% of children with cleft palate will demonstrate some degree of velopharyngeal insufficiency, despite the palatoplasty [9]. In these cases, the velum is typically not of sufficient length, particularly in midline, to close firmly against the posterior pharyn-

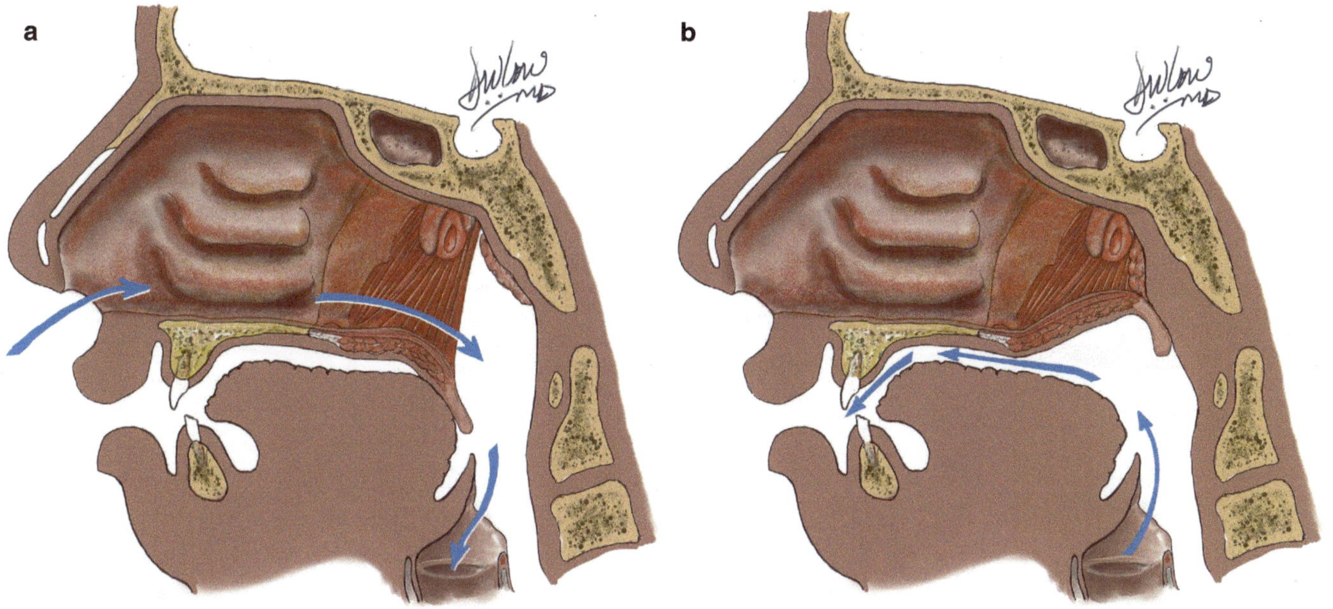


Fig. 28.2 (**a**) Position of the velum during normal nasal breathing. (**b**) Position of the velum during production of oral speech sounds

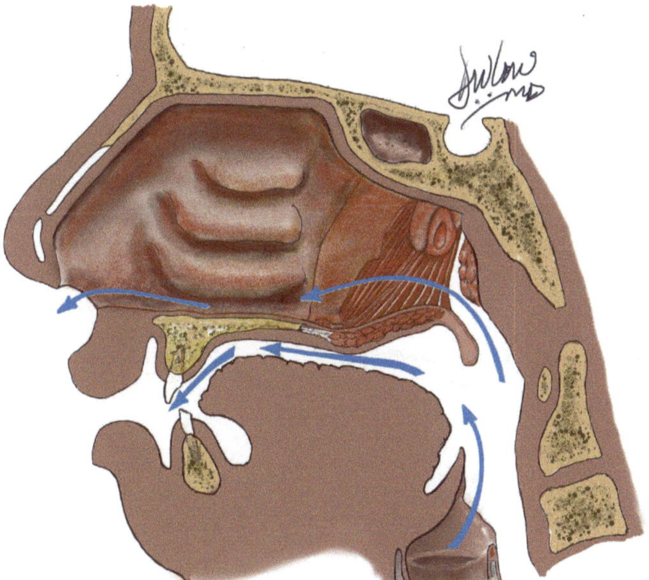

Fig. 28.3 Velopharyngeal insufficiency (VPI) characterized by a short velum

geal wall during oral speech production. This causes a leak of sound and/or airflow into the nasal cavity during speech.

### Effects of Velopharyngeal Insufficiency (VPI) on Speech and Resonance

Velopharyngeal insufficiency can cause hypernasality (a leak of sound) and/or nasal emission (a leak of airflow) during speech. A large velopharyngeal opening will cause hypernasality and also low volume because sound is absorbed by the tissues of the pharynx and nasal cavity. Nasal emission will be inaudible, partly because the hypernasality masks the noise. However, the leak of the airflow will cause the consonants to be very weak in intensity and pressure or omitted. This leak will also cause the child to take more frequent breaths to replace the loss of airflow. Finally, the child may develop compensatory articulation productions, where sounds are produced in the pharynx, rather than the oral cavity, because that is where there is airflow [3, 10, 11]. Compensatory productions include the following: glottal stop (Fig. 28.4a), pharyngeal plosive (Fig. 28.4b), glottal fricative (/h/sound), pharyngeal fricative (Fig. 28.4c), and posterior nasal fricative (Fig. 28.4d). In contrast to a large opening, a very small velopharyngeal opening will result in normal resonance but very audible nasal emission (nasal turbulence/rustle). Overall, because of the physics of sound and airflow, the relative size of the velopharyngeal opening can be predicted based on the specific characteristics of speech (Table 28.1).

## Assessment of Speech and Resonance Disorders

### Perceptual Assessment

The evaluation of speech and resonance involves a perceptual assessment, preferably by a speech-language pathologist who has experience with this population. The initial assess-

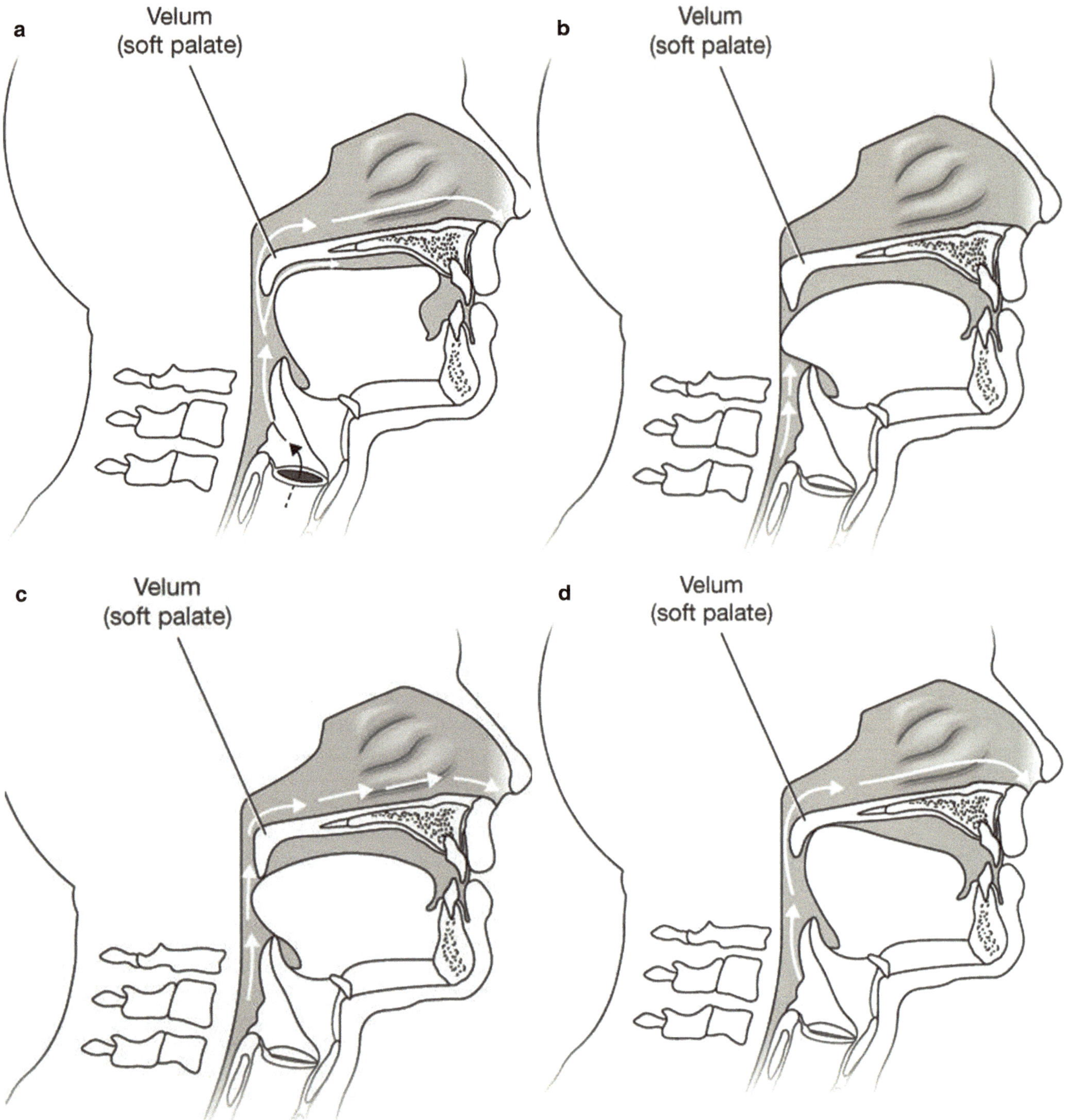


Fig. 28.4 (**a–d**) Compensatory productions for VPI. Compensatory productions occur as substitutions for oral sounds when there is inadequate oral airflow for normal production of the sounds. They are produced in the pharynx (from the glottis to the nasopharynx) where there is airflow, despite VPI. Compensatory productions are developed to improve intelligibility. (**a**) Glottal stop. (**b**) Pharyngeal plosive. (**c**) Pharyngeal fricative. (**d**) Posterior nasal fricative. (Reproduced with permission from Kummer [1])

**Table 28.1** Prediction of the relative size of the velopharyngeal (VP) opening based on the speech characteristics

| Speech characteristics | Relative size of the VP opening |
|---|---|
| Hypernasality, *inaudible* nasal emission, weak or omitted consonants, short utterance length, low volume, compensatory errors | 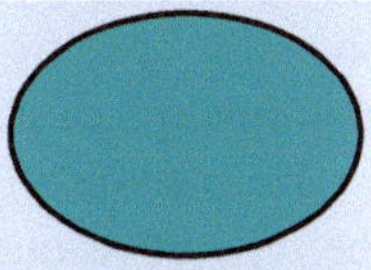 |
| Hypernasality, *audible* nasal emission, weak consonants, may have compensatory errors | 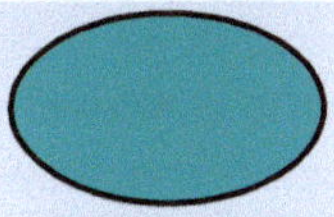 |
| Audible nasal emission and possibly mild hypernasality | 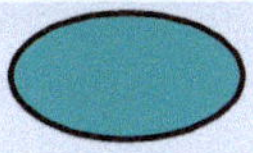 |
| Normal resonance but inconsistent nasal rustle (AKA nasal turbulence) | 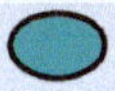 |

ment should be done between ages 3 and 4 years. At this age, the child is communicating with connected speech, is able to cooperate for the perceptual assessment and instrumental testing if needed, and, most importantly, usually has an adequate airway for VPI surgery, if that is diagnosed. (Prior to age 3, the focus of communication development should be on receptive and expressive language development) [12].

## Speech Samples

When assessing speech sound production (articulation), resonance, and velopharyngeal function, it is necessary to obtain a comprehensive speech sample in order to obtain adequate information for a definitive diagnosis [12–17]. Although single-word articulation tests are commonly used by speech-language pathologists, they reveal the child's best speech production, rather than the child's typical production in everyday speech [13]. In the same way, children with VPI achieve better velopharyngeal closure when producing single words than when producing connected speech. Overall, formal single-word tests provide inadequate information for a diagnosis, yet they are expensive and time-consuming to administer.

Instead of using single-word articulation tests, it is better to assess speech production and velopharyngeal function using a connected speech sample. This is because connected speech requires faster and more complex movements and also requires coordination and timing of the speech articulators (including the velopharyngeal valve) [12, 13].

A structured comprehensive speech sample can be obtained by asking the child to repeat consonant-vowel syllables and/or repeat sentences which are loaded with speech sounds with the same placement. In addition, having the child count can be used as a quick screening test. More information about these tests is as follows:

- *Syllable Repetition*: A syllable repetition test allows the examiner to assess only one consonant and one vowel at a time, yet it requires the child to execute more motor movements than with a single word. This test is particularly appropriate for children who do not have the language ability to imitate sentences and also for children who speak a language that is not spoken by the examiner. The syllable repetition test is administered by asking the child to imitate consonant-vowel syllables repetitively (i.e., /pɑ, pɑ, pɑ, pɑ, pɑ, pɑ, pɑ/ (/ɑ/ as in "father") and /pi, pi, pi, pi, pi, pi, pi/ (/i/ as in "pea") [12, 13]. Each consonant in the language can be tested in this manner. Using both the /ɑ/ and /i/ vowels is recommended to rule out phoneme-specific hypernasality, which sometimes occurs on the high vowel /i/. Because this speech sample includes only one consonant and one vowel at a time, it easy to determine if there is an articulation placement error on the consonant, consistent or phoneme-specific nasal emission on the consonant, and/or hypernasality on the vowel. Apraxia of speech should be suspected if prosody is abnormal during the repetition or if the voiceless consonants become voiced or nasal after a few repetitions.
- *Sentence Repetition*: Asking the child to repeat a battery of sentences is a fast, free, and effective way to test speech sound production and velopharyngeal function. Each sentence should contain multiple productions of sounds with the same placement (i.e., bilabial, labiodental, lingual-alveolar, etc.). To separate out the confounding effects of nasal emission or compensatory errors on the listener's ability to judge resonance, the examiner should use a sample of sentences with a large number of low-pressure consonants (i.e., "How are you?" "Why are you here?"). To test for hyponasality, the examiner should use sentences with a high frequency of nasal phonemes (i.e., "My mama made lemonade for me") [12, 13]. (See Table 28.2 for example sentences.)
- *Counting*: Asking the child count from 1 to 20 or 60 to 70 can serve as a quick screening test in any language. A series of repetitions of the word "sixty" (in English) provides a particularly good speech sample for assessment of VPI. This is because this word contains an /s/ in a triple consonant blend in the medial position, which is a difficult combination for achievement and maintenance of velopharyngeal closure. If there are concerns regarding hyponasality or cul-de-sac resonance, counting from 90 to 99 is a good speech sample because it contains the nasal /n/ in connected speech [12, 13].

**Table 28.2** Sample sentences for evaluation of speech and resonance through repetition

| Have the child repeat the following sentences: | |
|---|---|
| p | Popeye plays in the pool. |
| b | Buy baby a bib. |
| m | My mommy made lemonade. |
| w | Wade in the water. |
| j (y) | You have a yellow yo-yo. |
| h | He has a big horse. |
| t | Take Teddy to town. |
| d | Do it for Daddy. |
| n | Nancy is not here. |
| k | I eat cake and cookies. |
| g | Go get the wagon. |
| ŋ (ng) | Put the ring on her finger. |
| f | Fred has five fish. |
| v | Drive a van. |
| l | I like yellow lollipops. |
| s | I see the sun in the sky. |
| z | Zip up your zipper. |
| ʃ (sh) | She went shopping. |
| ʧ (ch) | I ride a choo-choo train. |
| ʤ (j) | John told a joke to Jim. |
| r | Randy has a red fire truck. |
| ɚ (er) | The teacher and doctor are here. |
| θ (th) | Thank you for the toothbrush. |
| Blends | Splash, sprinkle, street. |

**Tips and Tricks: Perceptual Evaluation**

- Children under the age of 5 are often reticent and will not talk to strangers. To get a young child to talk, start out by asking the child either/or questions (i.e., "What do you like best? Puppy dogs or kitty cats? Baseball or soccer? Dancing or singing?"). Once the child starts answering the questions, he or she is more likely to cooperate with repetition tasks. If he still will not repeat the speech samples, then the entire test can be done by having the child answer these questions [12].

## What to Assess

Using the above speech samples, it is important to determine if the child's speech is characterized by obligatory distortions (which are due to structure only) and if there are articulation placement errors. For the placement errors, it is important to determine which are developmental in nature (due to the child's age), compensatory (due to abnormal structure), or functional (due to mislearning).

In addition of assessing articulation placement, the examiner should determine if there is nasal emission on consonants. The focus should be on voiceless sounds, particularly voiceless sounds (e.g., p, t, k, f, s, sh, ch), because there is more airflow on these sounds than on their voiced cognates. If nasal emission is detected, it is important to determine whether it occurs on all pressure-sensitive sounds, including plosives, which suggests a structural etiology, or whether it is phoneme-specific on certain sibilant sounds, which suggests abnormal placement as a cause.

An assessment of resonance should be done to determine the type of resonance (e.g., normal, hypernasal, hyponasal, or cul-de-sac). Some clinicians like to assign a severity rating to abnormal resonance. However, the degree of severity (unless it is very mild) doesn't change the recommendations for the surgical procedure for correction. Therefore, ratings are not essential in clinical situations [12, 13].

**Tips and Tricks: Perceptual Evaluation**

- For confirmation of the presence of hypernasality or nasal emission, put the end of a stethoscope (Fig. 28.5a), straw (Fig. 28.5b), or even a tube in the child's nostril and the other end near your ear. Have the child produce repetitive syllables beginning with oral pressure sounds (i.e., p, t, k, f, s, sh, ch). If you hear sound through the straw, that confirms hypernasality. If you hear airflow through the straw, that confirms nasal emission [12, 13]. (This works a LOT better than using a dental mirror under the nose.)
- To determine if a fistula is symptomatic, use a straw (or tube) as above and have the child produce the /k/ sound and then the /s/ sound in repetitive syllables. Because production of the /k/ sound is almost always behind a fistula, the airflow from the /k/ will go across the fistula and not up into it. In contrast, as the child raises the tongue for an /s/, some of the airflow will be pushed into the fistula. Therefore:
  - If you hear no airflow or sound through the straw on /k/, but you do hear it on the /s/, then the cause is the fistula.
  - If you hear airflow on /k/, then there is VPI.
  - If you hear airflow on both, then you can plug the fistula with chewing gum or edible paper to determine the relative effect of each.

Finally, an assessment of phonation should be done because vocal nodules are common in children with VPI, presumably due to the overall strain in the vocal tract that results from trying to achieve adequate velopharyngeal closure [18]. To assess phonation, the child should be asked to prolong various vowels in isolation at various pitches. The examiner should note the presence of breathiness, hoarseness, pitch breaks, and/or glottal fry

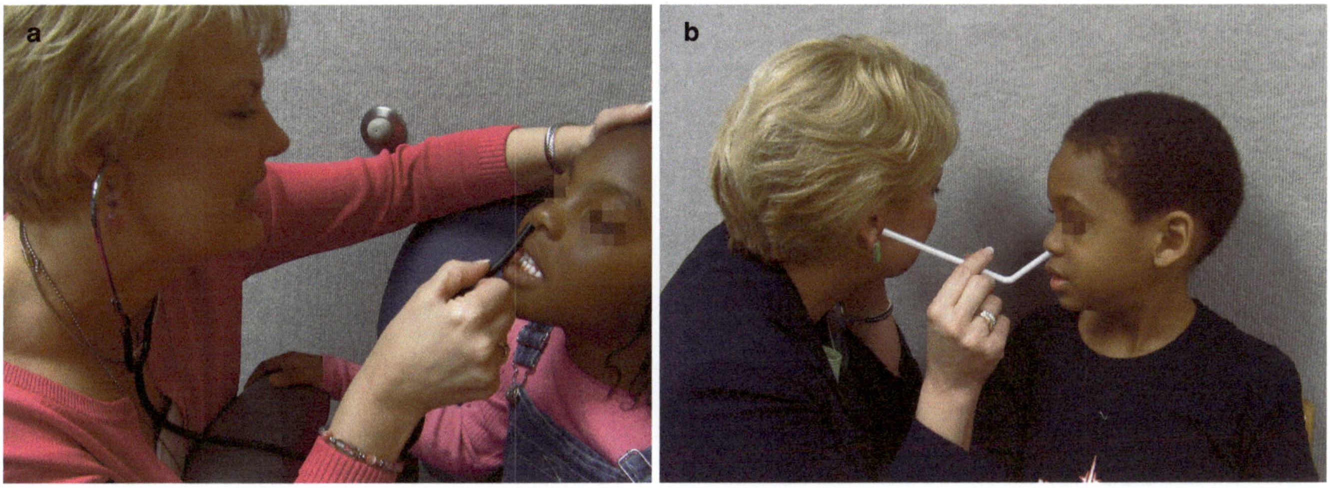


Fig. 28.5 (**a**) Use of a stethoscope to test for hypernasality, nasal emission, and even hyponasality. (**b**) Use of a straw to test for hypernasality, nasal emission, and even hyponasality. (Reproduced with permission from Kummer [1])

## Intraoral Evaluation

An intraoral examination is necessary for all children with a history of cleft and a speech disorder. The examiner should determine whether the tongue tip rests normally under the alveolar ridge. This relationship is essential for normal speech production. In addition, the examiner should look for abnormalities that can affect speech, such as bilabial incompetence, dental/occlusal anomalies (e.g., displaced teeth that interfere with tongue tip movement during speech, anterior crossbite, underbite, Class II or Class III malocclusion, etc.), oronasal fistulae, enlarged tonsils, or dehiscence of the velum. Although velar length and elevation is important for velopharyngeal function, it is hard to estimate because closure occurs above the oral level and depends on the inclination of the pharyngeal wall at that level.

**Tips and Tricks: Intraoral Evaluation**

- When conducting an intraoral evaluation, ask the patient to say /æ/ (as in "fat") rather than /ɑ/ (as in "father") (Fig. 28.6) [19]. With the /æ/ vowel, the back of the tongue goes down on its own so that in most cases, a tongue blade is not necessary. To further open the posterior oral cavity by bringing the tongue forward, the examiner can tell the child to try to touch his tongue to his chin while prolonging this vowel.
- When trying to view the palate to rule out a fistula, put a dental mirror under the palate. Then shine a flashlight on the mirror, which will cause the light to reflect upward to the palate [19].

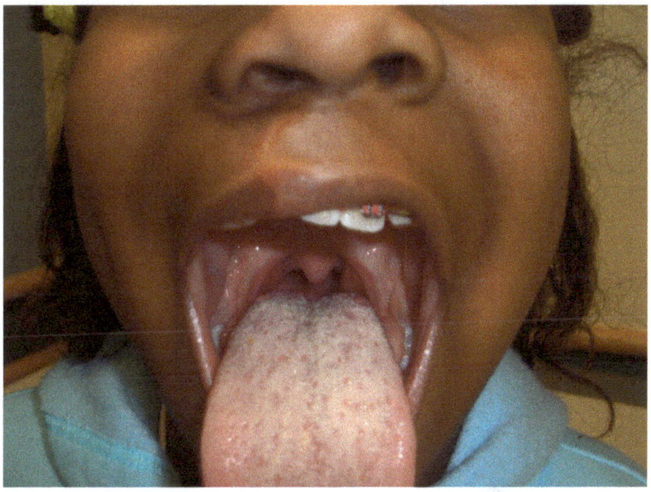

Fig. 28.6 Child phonating with the /æ/ vowel (as in "fat"). With the /æ/ vowel, the back of the tongue goes down on its own so that in most cases, a tongue blade is not necessary. (Reproduced with permission from Kummer [1])

## Instrumental Assessment

The use of instrumentation is not necessary to determine if there is VPI because this can be done through a perceptual evaluation alone. However, instrumentation can augment the perceptual evaluation by providing additional information about velopharyngeal function [20–22]. The relative advantages of each of these instrumental procedures are shown in Table 28.3 [23].

### Nasometry

The Nasometer II (PENTAX Medical, Montvale, NJ) is a computer-based instrument for measuring the acoustic correlates of resonance and audible nasal emission secondary to VPI [24].

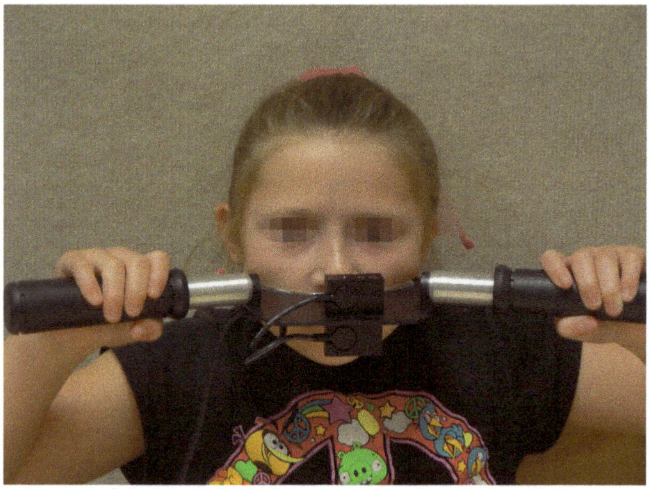

Fig. 28.7 Nasometry. This shows the Nasometer II sound separator in place for data collection. There is a microphone on the top of the plate for sound from the nasal cavity and one on the bottom of the plate for sound from the oral cavity. (Reproduced with permission from Kummer [1])

Table 28.3 Primary advantages of each instrumental procedure over others

| |
|---|
| *Advantages of nasometry* |
| Can obtain objective data regarding the function of the velopharyngeal valve |
| Can clearly delineate normal velopharyngeal function from VPI |
| Can be used for preoperative and postoperative comparisons |
| Can be used to compare outcomes among various surgeons, centers, or surgical procedures by comparing the percentage of patients who achieve normal VPI function following surgery |
| *Advantages of videofluoroscopy* |
| Can see tongue movement during speech |
| Can see the entire length of the posterior pharyngeal wall during speech |
| Can see when there is anterior positioning of the levator muscles |
| Can see the point of velar contact on the posterior pharyngeal wall[a] |
| *Advantages of nasopharyngoscopy* |
| Shows the best resolution of the velopharyngeal valve during speech |
| Can determine the location, size, shape, and cause of the opening, even if it is very small |
| Can see morphology of the nasal surface of the velum to identify an occult submucous cleft |
| Can see the entire adenoid, including irregularities in the surface that can affect the velopharyngeal seal |
| Can see tonsils that intrude into the pharynx, which can affect resonance and VP function |
| Can see pulsations of medially displaced carotid arteries in patients with velocardiofacial syndrome |
| Can view the vocal folds and determine the presence of vocal nodules |
| Can determine the effectiveness of VPI surgery because the ports after a pharyngeal flap or sphincter pharyngoplasty can be viewed directly |
| Is done without radiation or injection of barium in the nasopharynx |
| Allows the parent to hold the child in his/her lap during the procedure |

[a]Some surgeons find this information valuable in order to determine where to place a pharyngeal flap. Others argue that this is not needed because it is important to place the flap as high as possible

The nasometer includes a handheld sound separator plate that fits against the patient's upper lip (Fig. 28.7). There is a microphone on either side of a sound separator plate—one for the oral cavity and one for the nasal cavity. During production of the speech passage, the Nasometer II captures acoustic data from both the nasal cavity and the oral cavity. It then calculates the average ratio of nasal over total (nasal plus oral) acoustic energy for the passage and converts this to a percentage value, called the *nasalance score*. High scores in comparison with normative data suggest hypernasality, whereas low scores in comparison with normative data suggest hyponasality. Standardized passages are available with normative data (Kummer [25]). However, a nasalance score under about 22% is normal for any oral passage, regardless of language.

## Videofluoroscopy

Videofluoroscopy is a radiological procedure that provides visualization of the velopharyngeal valve during speech, along with a simultaneous audio recording [26]. Because videofluoroscopy involves two-dimensional imaging of a three-dimensional structure, a videofluoroscopic speech study requires several views to see all aspects of the velopharyngeal port. The most commonly used views are the lateral, anterior-posterior (AP), and base views. The lateral view shows the velum and velar movement toward the pharyngeal wall (Fig. 28.8a). The AP view shows the lateral walls and their medial movement toward the velum (Fig. 28.8b). The base view shows the lateral and posterior pharyngeal walls and their sphincteric movement (Fig. 28.8c). For both the AP and base views, it is necessary to inject barium into the nasopharynx using a catheter in order to coat the pharyngeal walls for visualization [27].

## Nasopharyngoscopy

Nasopharyngoscopy is a minimally invasive endoscopic procedure that allows direct visualization of the velopharyngeal mechanism during speech [28]. Nasopharyngoscopy allows the examiner to determine the cause and location of the velopharyngeal gap, which is often important for surgical planning. The required equipment includes at least a flexible fiberoptic nasopharyngoscope and a light source. For best practice, a video monitor and a video recording system are included. It is preferable to numb the nasal cavity prior to the procedure, particularly for children. At Cincinnati Children's Hospital Medical Center, we use a premixed, single-patient nasal spray with a one-to-one mixture of oxymetazoline (0.025%) to open the nasal passages and tetracaine (1%) for numbing. The nasopharyngoscope is passed through the middle meatus and then directed back to the pharynx (Fig. 28.9a). Once in the pharynx, the examiner turns the tip of the scope with a lever so that the scope turns down to provide a view of the nasopharyngeal structures from above (Fig. 28.9b). With preparation and patience, children as

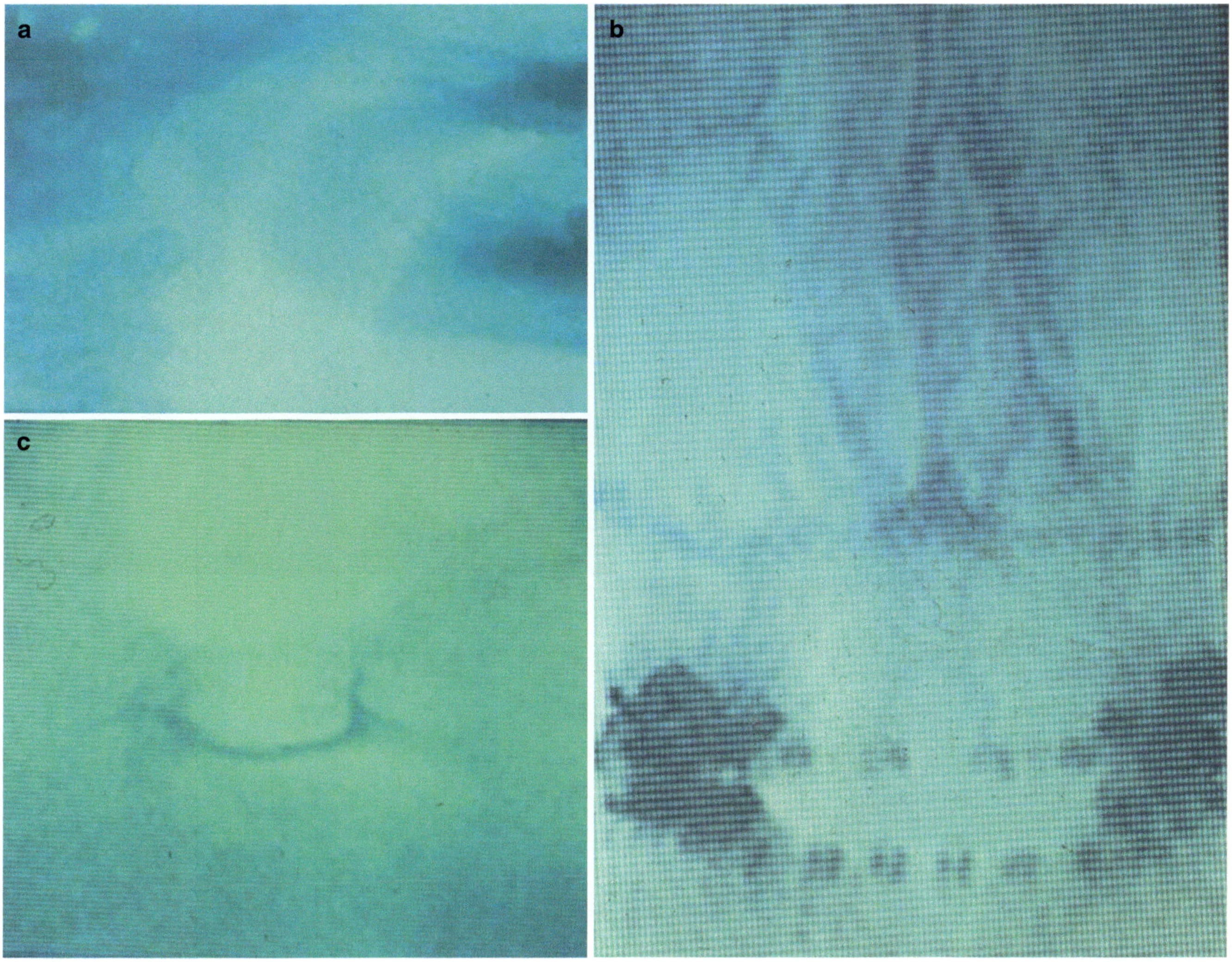


Fig. 28.8 (a–c) Videofluoroscopy. These views show a velopharyngeal opening during speech. (a) This is a lateral view that shows the velum and posterior pharyngeal wall during speech. In this case, the velum is short, causing velopharyngeal insufficiency. (b) This is the anterior-posterior (AP) view which shows the lateral pharyngeal walls wide apart during speech. (c) This is the base view which shows the pharyngeal walls and, again, a large velopharyngeal opening. (Reproduced with permission from Kummer [1])

young as 3 years will tolerate the procedure for this examination.

## Treatment of Speech and Resonance Disorders Secondary to Cleft Lip/Palate

The treatment of speech and/or resonance disorders secondary to cleft lip and palate can include physical management (e.g., surgery, orthodontics, or prosthetics), speech therapy, or a combination of these modalities. Because coordination and appropriate sequencing of interventions is important, these patients are best served by an interdisciplinary cleft or craniofacial team.

For patients with cleft lip/palate who are under the age of 3, the primary goal of communication management is to ensure the development of age-appropriate language skills. As such, parents are counseled on language stimulation at home, and formal intervention is implemented, if needed. At this stage, parents are told to focus on the "quantity" of communication (e.g., the number of words understood, the number of words said, and the number of words put together in a sentence).

After the age of 3, the focus of communication management shifts to the "quality" of communication (e.g., speech sound production, voice, and resonance). At this time, the child is old enough to be cooperative for both a perceptual and instrumental assessment of velopharyngeal function, and the airway is usually big enough for VPI surgery, if needed.

The appropriate type of speech intervention for the child can be determined through the perceptual evaluation, based

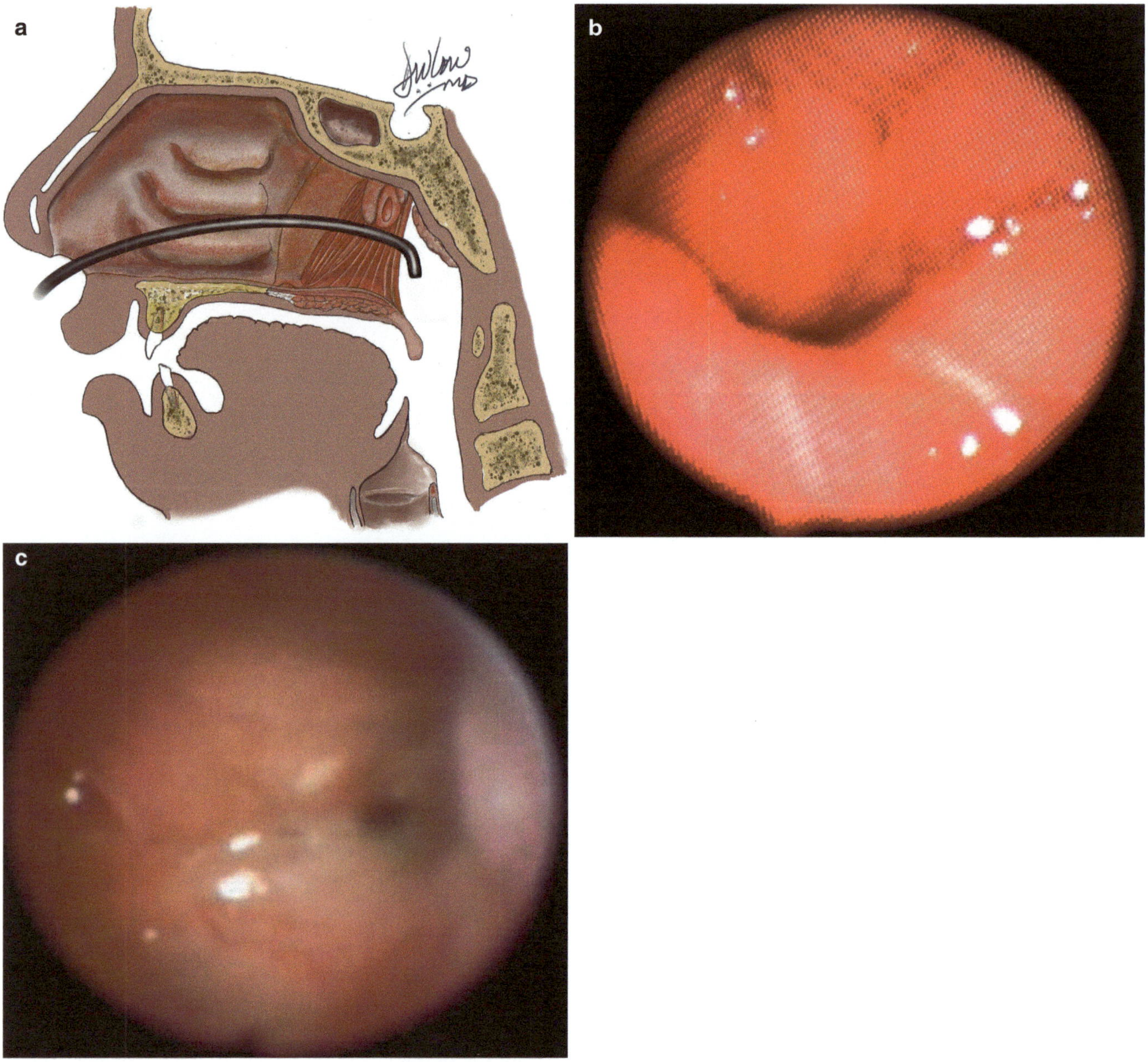

**Fig. 28.9** (**a–c**) Nasopharyngoscopy. (**a**) The nasopharyngoscope is inserted into the middle meatus, and then the tip is turned down to view the velopharyngeal valve from above. (**b**) This shows a submucous cleft on the nasal surface of the velum characterized by a flat velar eminence due to dysplasia of the musculus uvulae muscles. There is a midline velopharyngeal opening as a result. (**c**) This shows a very small yet symptomatic velopharyngeal opening on the (patient's) left. This is important to know for surgical planning. (Figures **b** and **c** reproduced with permission from Kummer [1])

on the speech characteristics. If it is determined that a structural anomaly is causing obligatory distortions (i.e., malocclusion is causing obligatory distortions of sibilants or VPI is causing hypernasality and/or nasal), then physical management is recommended for correction. If certain speech sounds are produced in the pharynx due to the development of compensatory productions, correcting placement and thus, eliminating the associated nasal emission can be done through speech therapy, as long as the structure has been corrected first.

## Surgical Intervention for VPI

Although some centers do not consider VPI surgery until the age of 6 or 7, it is important to recognize that this delay has a negative effect on the ultimate outcomes for speech. Because there is a critical period of time where the brain is "preprogrammed" for speech learning, generally under the age of 5, early surgical intervention for VPI is important for best outcomes. In addition, the longer a child continues

**Table 28.4** Suggested surgical procedures for VPI based on the size and location of the opening

| Size/location of thc opening | Best procedure |
|---|---|
| Midline or large | Pharyngeal flap or buccal flap |
| Narrow coronal opening | Furlow Z-plasty |
| Lateral gap(s) | Unilateral or bilateral sphincter pharyngoplasty |
| Small, localized gap(s) | Pharyngeal augmentation |

to use compensatory productions, the stronger the habit will be and the harder it will be to correct these abnormal patterns. Therefore, VPI surgery should be considered between the ages of 3 and 4, as long as there are no airway issues.

For the best surgical result for each patient, the surgical procedure for VPI should be determined based on the location of the opening and its relative size (Table 28.4).

## Prosthetic Devices

When surgical correction of VPI or a symptomatic fistula is not an option, prosthetic management can be a good alternative. There are three types of removable speech appliances that can be used to assist with speech production: a palatal obturator, a palatal lift, and a speech bulb obturator.

A palatal obturator is a device that can be used to occlude a palatal (oronasal) fistula that is large enough to affect speech or cause problems with nasal regurgitation of food and/or liquids (Fig. 28.10a). A palatal obturator can be used permanently if necessary. It can also be used on a temporary basis when surgical closure is delayed so that it can be done as part of another surgery, such as the bone graft.

A palatal lift is a device that is typically used for velopharyngeal incompetence, where the velum is of normal length, but has inadequate velar elevation and movement due to a neurophysiological cause (Fig. 28.10b). A palatal lift can also be used in some cases of velopharyngeal insufficiency (due to abnormal structure) if there is sufficient length of the velum beyond the natural level of velar elevation. The palatal lift has an oral base section that clasps on to the teeth and a posterior tail that elevates the velum to hold it in place against the posterior pharyngeal wall for speech.

Finally, a speech bulb obturator, also known as a speech aid appliance, can be used for velopharyngeal insufficiency when there is a large velopharyngeal gap (Fig. 28.10c). It also includes an oral base section, but there is a bulb of acrylic on the end of the tail. When in place, the bulb is positioned up and behind the velum in the pharynx. As such, it serves to occlude the velopharyngeal opening during speech.

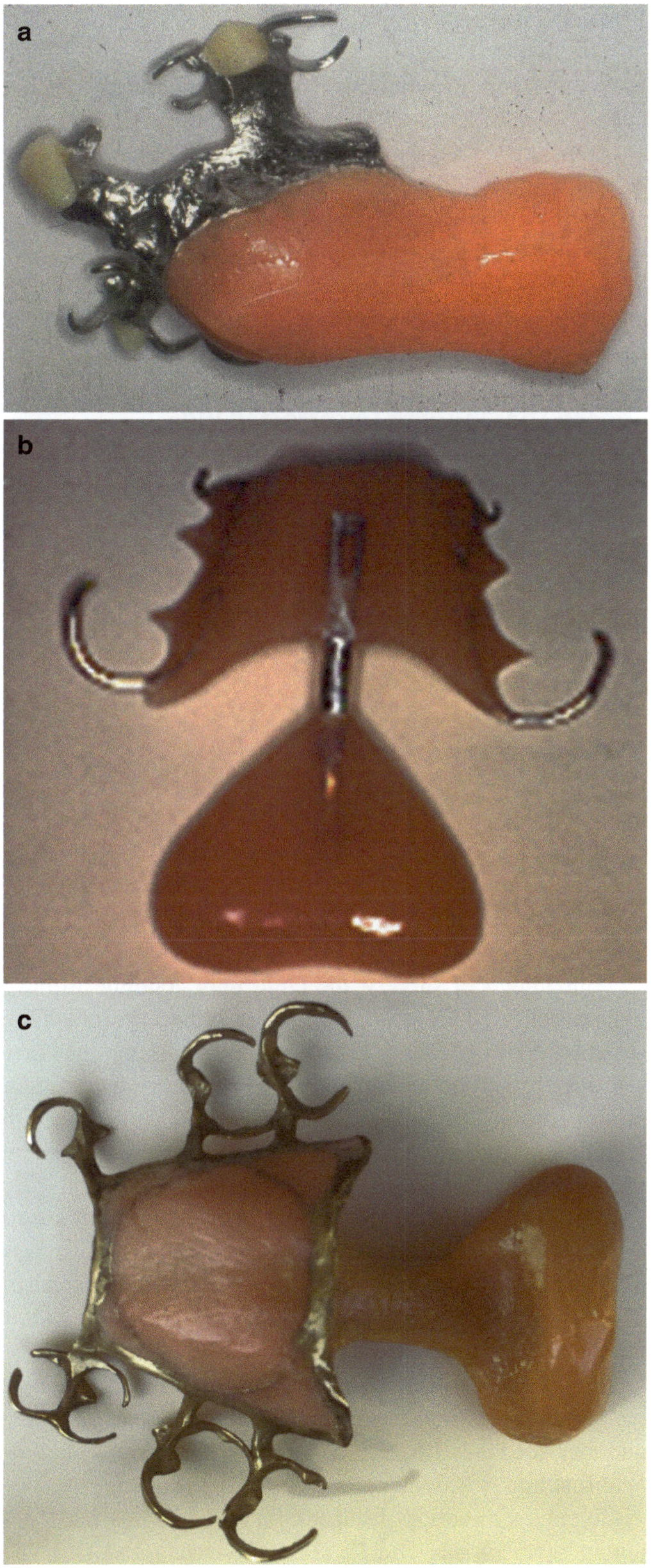


**Fig. 28.10** (**a–c**) Prosthetic devices. (**a**) Palatal obturator used to close a fistula. (**b**) Palatal lift used to raise the velum. This can be used for velopharyngeal incompetence (poor movement of the velum) but can also be used for velopharyngeal insufficiency (a short velum) by extending the tail beyond the point of interdigitation of the levator muscles. (**c**) Speech bulb obturator used to fill in the nasopharyngeal opening that occurs with a short velum. (Reproduced with permission from Kummer [1])

## Speech Therapy

It is important to emphasize that speech therapy cannot change abnormal structure and, therefore, cannot correct hypernasality or nasal emission due to VPI—even if there is only a small gap! Speech therapy can only correct placement errors, including compensatory productions in the pharynx, which cause nasal emission to persist after correction of VPI [29]. Speech therapy is always best done after correction of the abnormal structure that caused the development of these compensatory errors in the first place.

### Speech Therapy with Uncorrected VPI

It is almost impossible to work on oral speech sound production with an open velopharyngeal valve. If the child is 3 years or older and has VPI, yet surgical correction is being delayed due to airway concerns, work can still be done on articulation placement, however, with the use of a swimmer's nose plug. It is also recommended that the nose plug is used at home during practice and even during play as much as possible.

### Speech Therapy After Surgery

Speech therapy is effective in correcting abnormal placement of speech sounds that occurs in order to compensate for abnormal structure (including malocclusion and VPI). Speech therapy is most effective after physical correction of the abnormal structure (which was the cause of the disorder).

Following VPI surgery, the child may continue to have hypernasality or nasal emission. This is because changing structure does not change function. Nasal emission may persist due to the continued use of compensatory articulation productions in the pharynx. These can be corrected with articulation therapy focused on normal oral articulation placement.

When there is a very large velopharyngeal opening due to a short velum, lateral pharyngeal wall movement often does not develop because the velum is not there to close against. Therefore, following a pharyngeal flap, hypernasality and/or nasal emission may persist because of the lack of adequate lateral wall movement. To correct this, the speech-language pathologist uses auditory stimulation, imitation, and then auditory feedback because this is how normal velopharyngeal function is learned in the first 4 months of life.

To enhance auditory feedback for the child, a straw, "listening tube," or the Oral & Nasal Listener (ONL) can be helpful as they amplify the nasal sound during speech [29]. In both cases, the child puts one end of the tube at the entrance of a nostril and the other end (or both ends with the ONL) near or in his ear. When nasality occurs during oral sound production, it is heard loudly through the tube. The child is then instructed to try to eliminate that sound through experimentation.

In the past, some speech-language pathologists used oral-motor "exercises," such as blowing, sucking, whistling, cheek puffing, and even playing wind instruments, in hopes of strengthening the muscles of the velopharyngeal valve for improved function with speech. However, these exercises have been found to be totally ineffective, perhaps because the problem usually is not due to weak muscles [30–32]. Therefore, oral-motor exercises, including the use of blowing and sucking exercises, are never indicated to improve velopharyngeal function. When speech therapy is appropriate, the techniques involve methods to change articulation placement using standard articulation therapy principles [29].

**Tips and Tricks: Speech Therapy Technique**

The following is a technique for eliminating the compensatory production of a pharyngeal (or posterior nasal) fricative for the /s/ sound.

1. Make sure the child produces the /t/ sound with correct placement. If he does not, work on the /t/ sound first.
2. Have the child try to produce the /s/ sound with the nostrils occluded and then open to get the feel for oral versus nasal airflow.
3. Place a straw at the front of the child's closed central incisors during production of the /s/ and note the lack of audible airstream through the straw (Fig. 28.11).
4. Have the child produce a /t/ sound while feeling the tongue tip movement.
5. Put a straw just in front of the child's incisors again. Have the child produce a /t/ while pushing the airstream into the straw.
6. Then, have the child produce the /t/ with the teeth closed, which results in /ts/.
7. Have the child increase the duration of the production until it becomes /tssss/.
8. Have the child produce a /tssss/ sound while consciously trying to push air into the straw. At the same time, have the child feel the airstream flowing over his tongue tip during production.
9. Put one end of a straw or tube (such as a snake whistle) in the child's nostril and the other end in the child's ear for auditory feedback (Fig. 28.12).
10. Have the child produce the /tssss/ with his teeth closed. Tell the child to be sure he doesn't hear anything coming through the tube.

See Videos 28.1, 28.2, and 28.3.

From the Speech Therapy "Cookbook" in Ref. [29], pp. 539-548

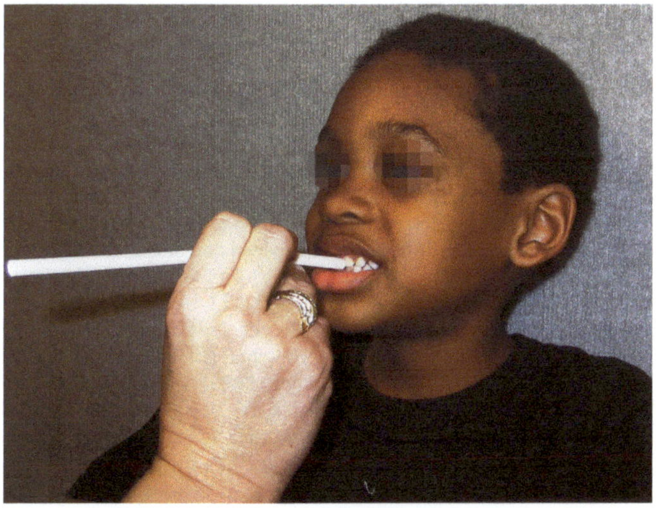

Fig. 28.11 Straw to provide feedback regarding oral airflow. (Reproduced with permission from Kummer [1])

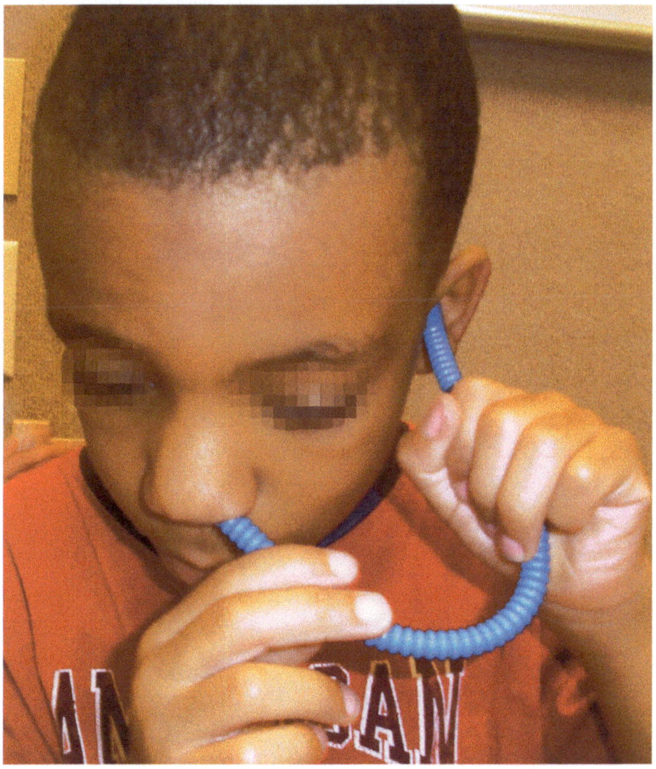

Fig. 28.12 A tube (snake whistle) to provide feedback regarding hypernasality or nasal emission. (Reproduced with permission from Kummer [1])

The success of therapy is not only dependent on the skills of the speech-language pathologist—it is also greatly dependent on involvement of the family in the treatment process. Changing a speech pattern begins with motor learning [33]. During this phase, the speech-language pathologist provides instructions, the child goes through a period of trial and error, and the speech pathologist provides feedback. Once the child is able to achieve the correct placement, the next step is the development of motor memory. This is achieved with frequent (preferably daily) practice at home. Motor memory is required to develop the automaticity of the speech so that the patient uses the sound automatically, without effort or conscious thought [33].

## Summary

The ultimate goal of the speech assessment and then speech management for patients with cleft lip/palate should always be *normal* speech and resonance, not merely "acceptable," "intelligible," or "improved" speech. Considering the advances that have occurred in the last few decades in surgical and therapeutic techniques, this goal is achievable for most affected children, particularly when treated by professionals who specialize in this area.

## References


1. Kummer AW. Cleft palate and craniofacial conditions: a comprehensive guide to clinical management. 4th ed. Burlington: Jones & Bartlett Learning; 2020.
2. Kummer AW. Dental anomalies. In: Cleft palate and craniofacial conditions: a comprehensive guide to clinical management. 4th ed. Burlington: Jones & Bartlett Learning; 2020. p. 149–89.
3. Kummer AW. Resonance disorders and velopharyngeal dysfunction (VPD). In: Cleft palate and craniofacial conditions: a comprehensive guide to clinical management. 4th ed. Burlington: Jones & Bartlett Learning; 2020. p. 259–93.
4. Friel MT, et al. Airway obstruction and the unilateral cleft lip and palate deformity: contributions by the Bony Septum. Ann Plast Surg. 2013;75:37.
5. Mani M, et al. Editor's choice: Objective assessment of the nasal airway in unilateral cleft lip and palate--a long-term study. Cleft Palate Craniofac J. 2010;47(3):217–24.
6. Oosterkamp BC, et al. Craniofacial, craniocervical, and pharyngeal morphology in bilateral cleft lip and palate and obstructive sleep apnea patients. Cleft Palate Craniofac J. 2007;44(1):1–7.
7. Kummer AW. Anatomy and physiology. In: Cleft palate and craniofacial conditions: a comprehensive guide to clinical management. 4th ed. Burlington: Jones & Bartlett Learning; 2020. p. 3–34.
8. Trost-Cardamone JE. Coming to terms with VPI: a response to Loney and Bloem. Cleft Palate J. 1989;26(1):629–70.
9. Witt PD, D'Antonio LL. Velopharyngeal insufficiency and secondary palatal management. A new look at an old problem. Clin Plast Surg. 1993;20(4):707–21.
10. Kummer AW, Briggs M, Lee L. The relationship between the characteristics of speech and velopharyngeal gap size. Cleft Palate Craniofac J. 2003;40(6):590–6.
11. Kummer AW, et al. Comparison of velopharyngeal gap size in patients with hypernasality, hypernasality and nasal emission, or nasal turbulence (rustle) as the primary speech characteristic. Cleft Palate Craniofac J. 1992;29(2):152–6.
12. Kummer AW. Speech and resonance assessment. In: Cleft palate and craniofacial conditions: a comprehensive guide to clinical management. 4th ed. Burlington: Jones & Bartlett Learning; 2020. p. 297–324.

13. Kummer AW. Perceptual assessment of resonance and velopharyngeal dysfunction. Semin Speech Lang. 2011;32(2):159–67.
14. Kuehn DP, Henne LJ. Speech evaluation and treatment for patients with cleft palate. Am J Speech Lang Pathol. 2003;12(1):103–9.
15. Hirschberg J, Van Demark DR. A proposal for standardization of speech and hearing evaluations to assess velopharyngeal function. Folia Phoniatr Logop. 1997;49(3–4):1529–167.
16. Paal S, et al. Evaluation of speech disorders in children with cleft lip and palate. J Orofac Orthop. 2005;66(4):270–8.
17. Smith BE, Kuehn DP. Speech evaluation of velopharyngeal dysfunction. J Craniofac Surg. 2007;18(2):251–61.
18. D'Antonio LL, et al. Laryngeal/voice findings in patients with velopharyngeal dysfunction. Laryngoscope. 1988;98(4):432–8.
19. Kummer AW. Orofacial examination. In: Cleft palate and craniofacial conditions: a comprehensive guide to clinical management. 4th ed. Jones & Bartlett Learning: Burlington; 2020. p. 325–52.
20. Hinton VA. Instrumental measures of velopharyngeal function. In: Lossee JE, Kirschner RE, editors. Comprehensive cleft care. New York: McGraw-Hill; 2009. p. 607–17.
21. Karnell MP. Instrumental assessment of velopharyngeal closure for speech. Semin Speech Lang. 2011;32(2):1629–178.
22. Kummer AW. Overview of instrumental procedures. In: Cleft palate and craniofacial conditions: a comprehensive guide to clinical management. 4th ed. Burlington: Jones & Bartlett Learning; 2020. p. 353–65.
23. Lam DJ, et al. A comparison of nasendoscopy and multiview videofluoroscopy in assessing velopharyngeal insufficiency. Otolaryngol Head Neck Surg. 2006;134(3):394–402.
24. Kummer AW. Nasometry. In: Cleft palate and craniofacial conditions: a comprehensive guide to clinical management. 4th ed. Burlington: Jones & Bartlett Learning; 2020. p. 367–98.
25. Kummer AW. The MacKay-Kummer simplified nasometric assessment procedures-revised (SNAP-R). 2005. Retrieved from https://www.researchgate.net/publication/273060845_The_MacKay-Kummer_SNAP_Test-R_Simplified_Nasometric_Assessment_Procedures_Revised_2005.
26. Kummer AW. Videofluoroscopy. In: Cleft palate and craniofacial conditions: a comprehensive guide to clinical management. 4th ed. Burlington: Jones & Bartlett Learning; 2020. p. 399–416.
27. Kummer AW, Clark S, Redle E, Thomsen L, Billmire DA. Current practice in assessing and reporting speech outcomes of cleft palate and velopharyngeal surgery: a survey of cleft palate/craniofacial professionals. Cleft Palate Craniofac J. 2012;49(2):146–52.
28. Kummer AW. Nasopharyngoscopy. In: Cleft palate and craniofacial conditions: a comprehensive guide to clinical management. 4th ed. Burlington: Jones & Bartlett Learning; 2020. p. 417–50.
29. Kummer AW. Speech therapy. In: Cleft palate and craniofacial conditions: a comprehensive guide to clinical management. 4th ed. Burlington: Jones & Bartlett Learning; 2020. p. 515–48.
30. Lof GL. Science-based practice and the speech-language pathologist. Int J Speech Lang Pathol. 2011;13(3):189–96.
31. McCauley RJ, et al. Evidence-based systematic review: effects of nonspeech oral motor exercises on speech. Am J Speech Lang Pathol. 2009;18(4):343–60.
32. Ruscello DM. Nonspeech oral motor treatment issues related to children with developmental speech sound disorders. Lang Speech Hear Serv Sch. 2008;39(3):380–91.
33. Watson MM, Lof GL. Epilogue: what we know about nonspeech oral motor exercises. Semin Speech Lang. 2008;29(4):339–44.

# 29 Audiology, Otology, and Airway

Aurora G. Vincent, Derek J. Rogers, and Luv Javia

**Key Points**

- Children with a cleft palate are at increased risk of eustachian tube dysfunction, persistent middle ear effusion, and chronic hearing loss.
- Over many years after cleft palate repair, eustachian tube dysfunction improves, but often not before speech and language development has been stunted.
- An otoscopic exam by an otolaryngologist combined with acoustic immittance testing can reliably and feasibly diagnose middle ear dysfunction in children and guide surgical interventions.
- Myringotomy with tympanostomy tube placement is the accepted treatment for eustachian tube dysfunction in children, as it has been demonstrated to relieve middle ear effusion and improve hearing loss.
- Finally, certain syndromes associated with cleft palate predispose patients to a difficult airway, and understanding interventional strategies to manage these airway concerns can prevent morbidity and mortality.

## Introduction

Appropriate treatment of children with palatal and facial clefts is multifactorial. Evaluation and treatment of these patients should include an evaluation of hearing with possible subsequent management of hearing loss. This chapter reviews the relevant ear and eustachian tube anatomy in cleft patients. It examines audiologic testing requirements in low-resource areas and suggests when to place tympanostomy tubes. It describes and illustrates the procedure of bilateral myringotomy with tympanostomy tube placement (BMT). Finally, it describes associated airway concerns for this population of patients and management strategies.

## Anatomy

**Pearls and Pitfalls**

- Abnormal insertion of palatal muscles in a child with a cleft palate worsens eustachian tube dysfunction and retention of middle ear fluid.
- Patients with Pierre Robin sequence and Stickler syndrome not only can have cleft palates but also micrognathia and glossoptosis which can lead to dangerous obstructive breathing.

The anatomy of the ear and eustachian tube in children with a cleft palate can be variable, some appearing relatively normal and others with severe deformity, but clinicians should expect some patterns in the anatomy. Children, in general, are more prone to middle ear dysfunction than adults; otitis media with effusion (OME) is estimated to have a cumulative prevalence of 80–90% by 4 years of age [1, 2]. The eustachian tube in children, in general, courses more horizontally from the nasopharynx to the middle ear space (Fig. 29.1). This is in contrast to an adult eustachian tube, which courses more vertically and allows easier drainage of the middle ear space. Infants with a cleft palate are at a greater disadvantage due to the abnormal insertion of the levator veli palatini (LVP) and tensor veli palatini (TVP) muscles (Fig. 29.2) [3, 4]. Contraction of the palatini muscles normally dilates the eustachian tube. In cleft patients, because of the abnormal insertion of these muscles,

A. G. Vincent
Otolaryngology, Head and Neck Surgery, Madigan Army Medical Center, Tacoma, WA, USA
e-mail: aurora.g.vincent.mil@mail.mil

D. J. Rogers
Pediatric Otolaryngology, Madigan Army Medical Center, Tacoma, WA, USA
e-mail: derek.j.rogers.mil@mail.mil

L. Javia (✉)
Children's Hospital of Philadelphia, University of Pennsylvania Perelman School of Medicine, Philadelphia, PA, USA
e-mail: javia@email.chop.edu

© Springer Nature Switzerland AG 2021

J. W. Swanson, D. W. Low (eds.), *Global Cleft Care in Low-Resource Settings*, https://doi.org/10.1007/978-3-030-59105-2_29

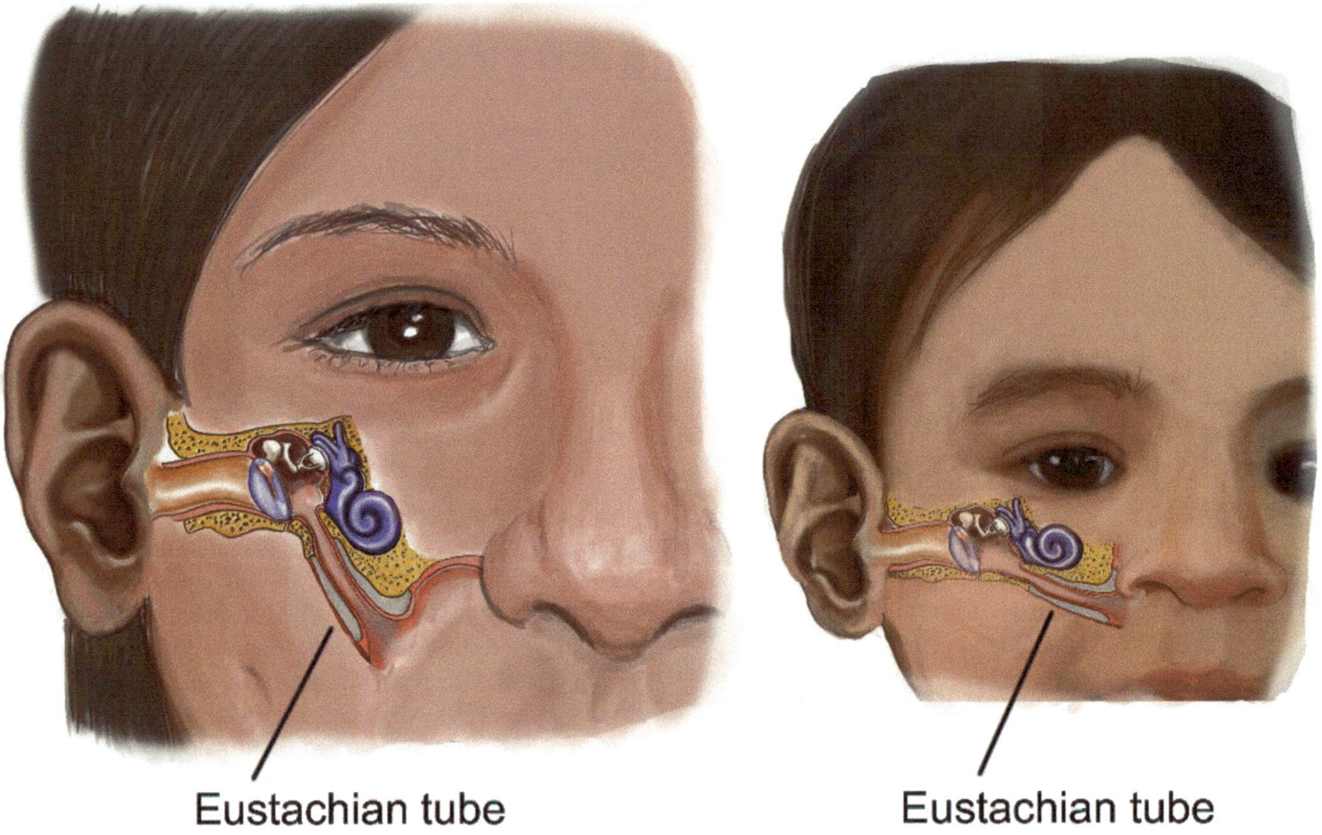


**Fig. 29.1** Comparison of normal eustachian tube anatomy in an adult and in an infant. The eustachian tube courses more vertically in an adult, allowing gravity to aid the drainage of fluid from the middle ear

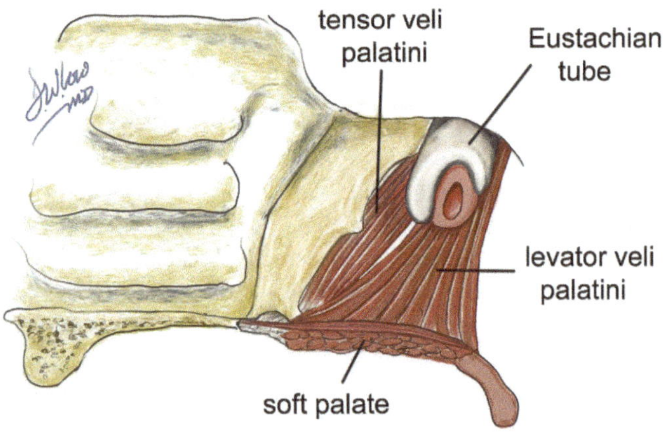


**Fig. 29.2** Normal relationship of the tensor veli palatini, levator veli palatini, and the eustachian tube. In a cleft palate, the abnormal insertions of the palatini muscles diminish their ability to open the eustachian tube and aid drainage of fluid from the middle ear space

their ability to dilate the eustachian tube is reduced, thus further blocking drainage of mucus from the middle ear space.

The cleft and palatini muscles may not be the only abnormally formed structures in this population. Cleft palate often occurs in isolation, but it can be associated with other malformations and syndromes [5]. Most commonly, an isolated cleft palate occurs in velocardiofacial syndrome (now called chromosome 22q11.2 deletion syndrome) due to a microdeletion on chromosome 22q11.2 [6]. Children with del22q11.2 syndrome have been described as having laryngeal abnormalities in up to 14% of patients: 3% with subglottic stenosis, 9% with glottic web, 9% with laryngeal paralysis, and 3% with laryngomalacia. These laryngeal findings can affect the patient's voice and respiratory status or make intubation challenging [7]. Cleft palate is also commonly observed in Pierre Robin sequence (PRS) and Stickler syndrome. In Pierre Robin sequence, there is hypoplasia of the mandible which results in a posterior and superior displacement of the tongue, preventing palatal shelf fusion. However, the small mandible and glossoptosis can result in respiratory distress in the immediate perinatal period if severe in degree. Glossoptosis causes obstruction of the airway at the oropharyngeal level and can result in cyclical breathing. Cyclical breathing is where the neonate is pink and has adequate oxygenation with crying, but then as soon as the baby stops crying, the tongue falls back against the posterior oropharyngeal wall and obstructs the airway. This results in the baby becoming cyanotic. The baby then grunts and cries, temporarily relieving the obstruction and restoring some ventilation, turning the baby pink again. This can continue in a cyclical fashion and, if it is not managed, can result in the neonate tiring and losing their airway.

Others that can develop a cleft include but are not limited to fetal alcohol syndrome, otopalatodigital syndrome, achondroplasia, Larsen syndrome, and Noonan syndrome. Larsen syndrome can be associated with tracheal stenosis or tracheobronchomalacia. Noonan syndrome can be associated with micrognathia. Achondroplasia and Larsen syndrome can have associated sensorineural hearing loss in addition to conductive losses from middle ear disease [5].

## Audiologic Testing

**Pearls and Pitfalls**

- Children with a cleft palate are at increased risk of hearing loss due to fluid buildup in the middle ear space.
- A middle ear effusion can reliably and feasibly be diagnosed with a portable otoscopic exam and acoustic immittance testing.
- When available, a portable audiometer can diagnose the degree of hearing loss.

Audiologic testing is necessary to determine the status of the middle ear and overall hearing capability in children with clefts. Eustachian tube dysfunction is the main cause of middle ear disease and subsequent hearing loss in children with a cleft palate [8]. Children with cleft palate have been shown to be more prone to middle ear dysfunction than children without a cleft [5, 9], and a middle ear effusion is typically associated with a conductive hearing loss of 25–30 dB [1]. Importantly, if untreated, a prolonged middle ear effusion with hearing loss can subsequently lead to poor speech and language development. Longitudinal studies have shown that patients with a cleft palate who have hearing loss will eventually gain normal hearing, but it may not occur until age 10–15 years [5, 10]. An estimated 40–45% of children with a repaired, isolated cleft palate will have middle ear dysfunction at age 7 years, while only 3% of these children will have persistent middle ear dysfunction by age 16 years [5].

Children with a cleft in the setting of other malformations or a syndrome have been shown to have poorer hearing than children with an isolated cleft palate, even when cleft repair has been completed in early childhood and even after accounting for sensorineural hearing loss that can accompany specific syndromes [5]. While only 3% of children with a repaired, isolated cleft palate will have persistent middle ear disease in their late teenage years, an estimated 25–30% of syndromic children will have persistent dysfunction [5].

Definitive testing for infants, such as otoacoustic emissions (OAE) measurement and auditory brainstem response (ABR) testing, is not always available or feasible. A cleft team should, at a minimum, always have an otoscope and a tympanometer (a device for acoustic immittance testing). A middle ear effusion can be evaluated directly with a portable otoscope (Figs. 29.3 and 29.4) and indirectly with a tympanometer (Fig. 29.5). An otoscopic exam should be attempted in every patient. An otoscope can confirm a patent ear canal and, often, an intact tympanic membrane (TM). Further, it can visualize otorrhea from a draining effusion and diagnose an acute middle or external ear infection. Even if one does not have a tympanometer, a pneumatic bulb otoscope can be used to evaluate if there is fluid in the middle ear or not. The speculum of the otoscope is secured in the ear canal (forming an airtight seal), and a bulb attached to the otoscope can be gently squeezed, thus pushing air into the external auditory canal. If the tympanic membrane moves, fluid is unlikely. If the tympanic membrane does not move with insufflation, fluid is likely; however, note that if the otoscope is not seated well/sealed into the ear canal, the tympanic membrane may not move either as air escapes around the poorly seated speculum. Sometimes the tympanic membrane moves with insufflation but not as much as one would expect; this can be indicative of negative pressure and eustachian tube dysfunction.

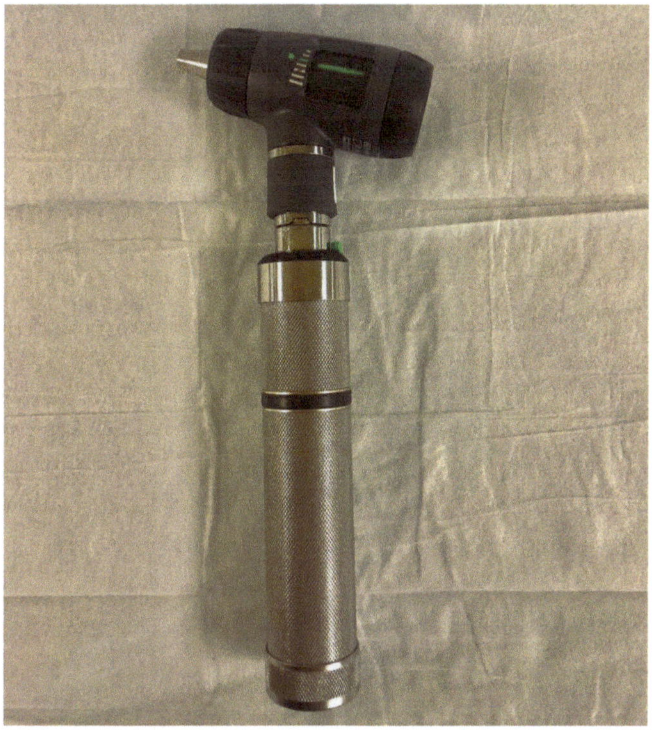

Fig. 29.3 Example portable otoscope. Multiple sizes of disposable tips can be used to examine ear canals of children and adults

The otoscopic exam is not perfect, however. Infants often move during examination and have small caliber ear canals, even in the setting of normal anatomy. This makes clear visualization of the TM difficult. Further, a simple effusion without acute infection can have relatively clear fluid that can be difficult to discern behind the TM. Thus, an otoscopic exam, while useful, cannot always definitively diagnose the presence or absence of fluid in the middle ear space. These issues can be mitigated in many instances: if simple distraction strategies do not work with the child, the patient can be held in the parents lap facing outward with the parent giving the child a secure hug to

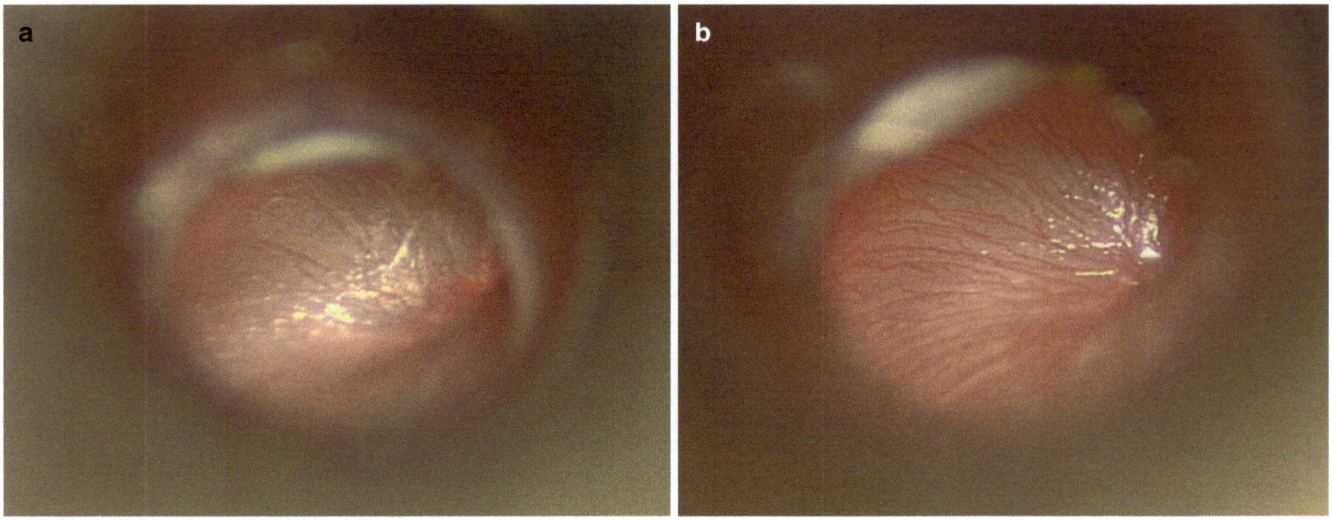


**Fig. 29.4** Normal TM with clear middle ear (**a**). Serous otitis media – fluid in the middle ear (**b**)

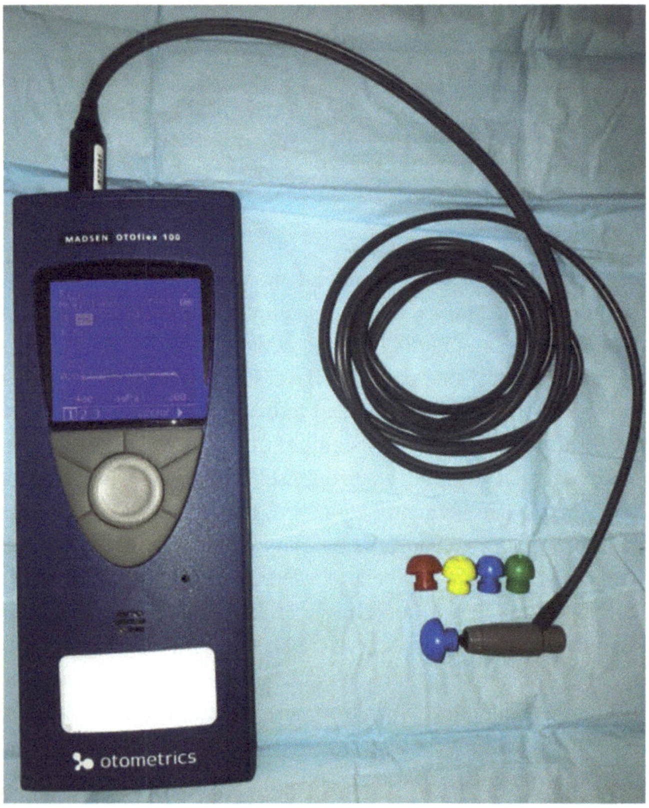


**Fig. 29.5** Example tympanometer with multiple ear bud sizes. The tympanometer is displaying a type B tympanogram result

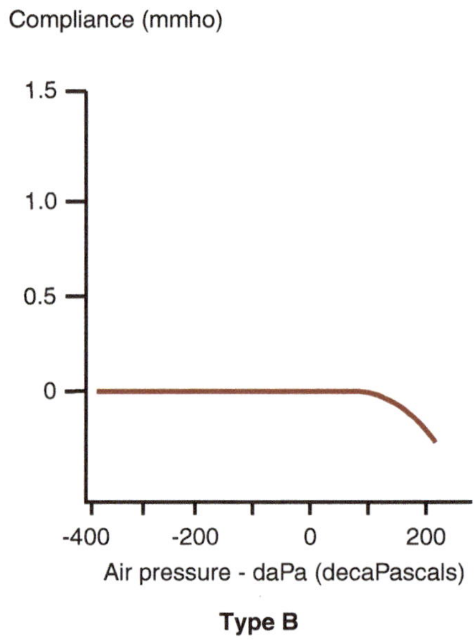


**Fig. 29.6** Example type B tympanogram with no pressure peak indicative of either (1) fluid in the middle ear space or (2) a tympanic membrane (TM) perforation. If there is fluid in the middle ear space and an intact TM, then the ear canal volume will be low (as in this example). If there is a TM perforation, then the ear canal volume will be large

restrain their upper body and hands while another helper such as a nurse or healthcare worker holds the child's head securely on the parent's shoulder/arm. This strategy can greatly facilitate an exam. In patients with very narrow ear canals, a microscope may need to be used to examine the ears, if available.

After normal or near-normal external ear anatomy has been confirmed, a tympanometer can be used to perform acoustic immittance testing and better evaluate the fluid status of the middle ear. An appropriately sized ear bud is selected such that a tight seal is created between the device and the external ear canal. Leakage of air around the earbud will give poor test results. After snugly positioned in the ear canal, the device can assess the mobility of the TM. Further, it can measure the volume of the ear canal and, indirectly, evaluate the presence or absence of a TM perforation. Fluid present in the middle ear space will prevent normal movement of the TM, thus resulting in a "flat line" or type B tympanogram result (Fig. 29.6). A type B tympanogram is also

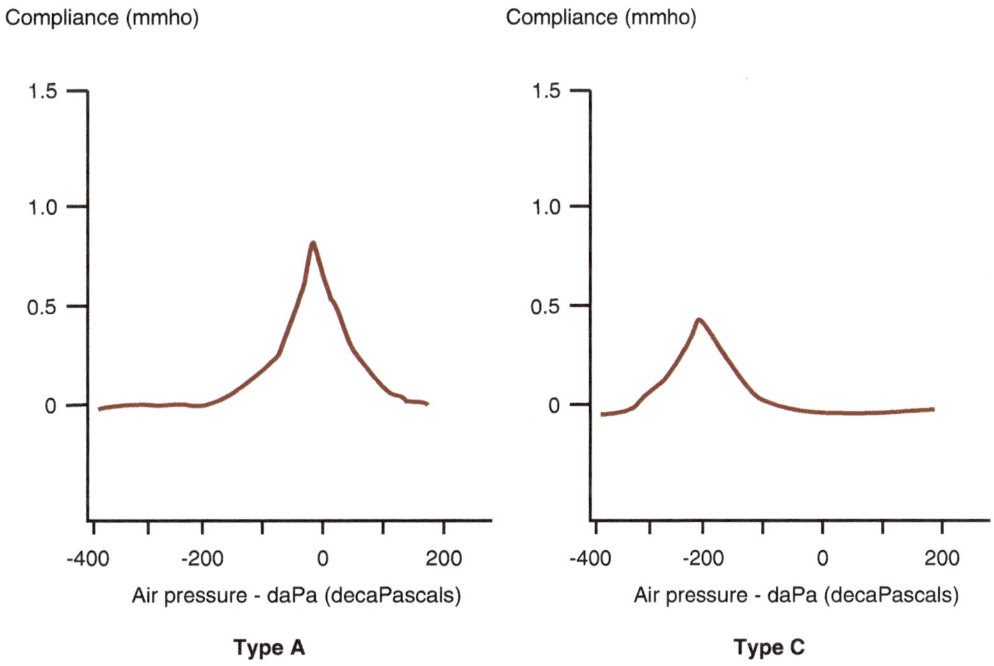


**Fig. 29.7** Example result of types A and C tympanograms. Type A has a pressure peak near 0 daPa, while type C peaks at a negative daPa suggesting negative middle ear pressure

present when there is a TM perforation, as air passes easily between the middle and external ear spaces without the TM moving. The otoscopic exam combined with the estimated ear canal volume (also measured by a tympanometer) can help the clinician decide whether or not there is fluid in the middle ear. In the absence of a middle ear effusion or TM perforation, a tympanogram will have a type A or C result (Fig. 29.7). Some middle ear effusions may result in a type C tympanogram if the TM is severely retracted.

When an audiologist is available, an economical portable audiometer can be used for more formal hearing testing to determine a patient's overall hearing status. Visual response assessment (VRA) and play audiometry are different methods of testing hearing in young children who are not old enough to cooperate with ear-specific testing via headphones or insert earbuds. This type of testing can, nonetheless, determine if a child has hearing loss and can guide clinical decision making. In VRA, the child is conditioned to look at the sound source: the child is rewarded through visual reinforcement (such as a clapping toy monkey) with a correct response. This can be used in children between 6 months and 2 years of age but does require good neck control/strength. Conditioned play audiometry involves having the child perform a task, such as putting a block in a basket, when they hear a sound. Play audiometry is typically employed in children between 2 and 5 years of age but does rely on the child's cooperation. Soundfield testing is usually attempted first, where the sound is presented to both ears at the same time through a speaker. This tests the best hearing ear; thus some cases of unilateral hearing loss may be missed, but bilateral losses should be caught. Headphones can be used during testing to test each ear for better delineation of hearing levels specific for each ear. Figure 29.8 demonstrates an example audiogram after play audiometry in a toddler with normal hearing thresholds, while Fig. 29.9 demonstrates hearing thresholds in a child with hearing loss. Having access to trained audiologists can be an unsurmountable obstacle in resource poor areas when trying to get an audiologic assessment. Recently, there have been reports of using portable, automated audiologic assessment devices and mobile health programs on smartphones to assess hearing [11, 12]. These can be deployed with some basic training of local health officials. If even this is not feasible, then the World Health Organization (WHO) has published manuals on ear and hearing health that describe using a very basic voice test to roughly assess hearing in individuals; even still, this can be challenging to apply in children (Table 29.1) [13]. Additionally, the mother or caregiver should be questioned about whether they feel their baby can hear appropriately; concern from the caregiver or mother should trigger a more extensive and detailed audiologic evaluation. If further evaluation is not available, the WHO manual suggests a noisemaker should be used behind the baby at a level of about a whispered

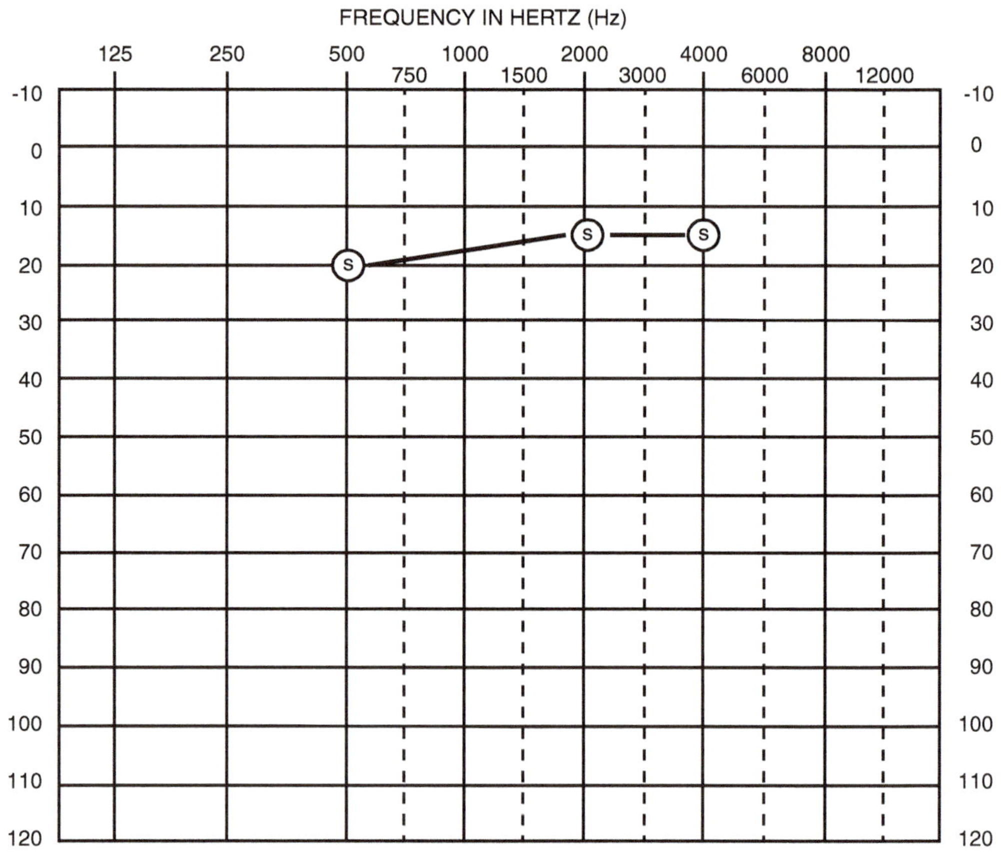


**Fig. 29.8** Audiogram output after soundfield testing of a child's hearing. The "s" depicted on the chart indicates that testing was performed as soundfield and is not ear-specific. The results represent the status of the better hearing ear. All tested frequencies were perceived at a decibel lower than 25. Thus, this child has normal hearing

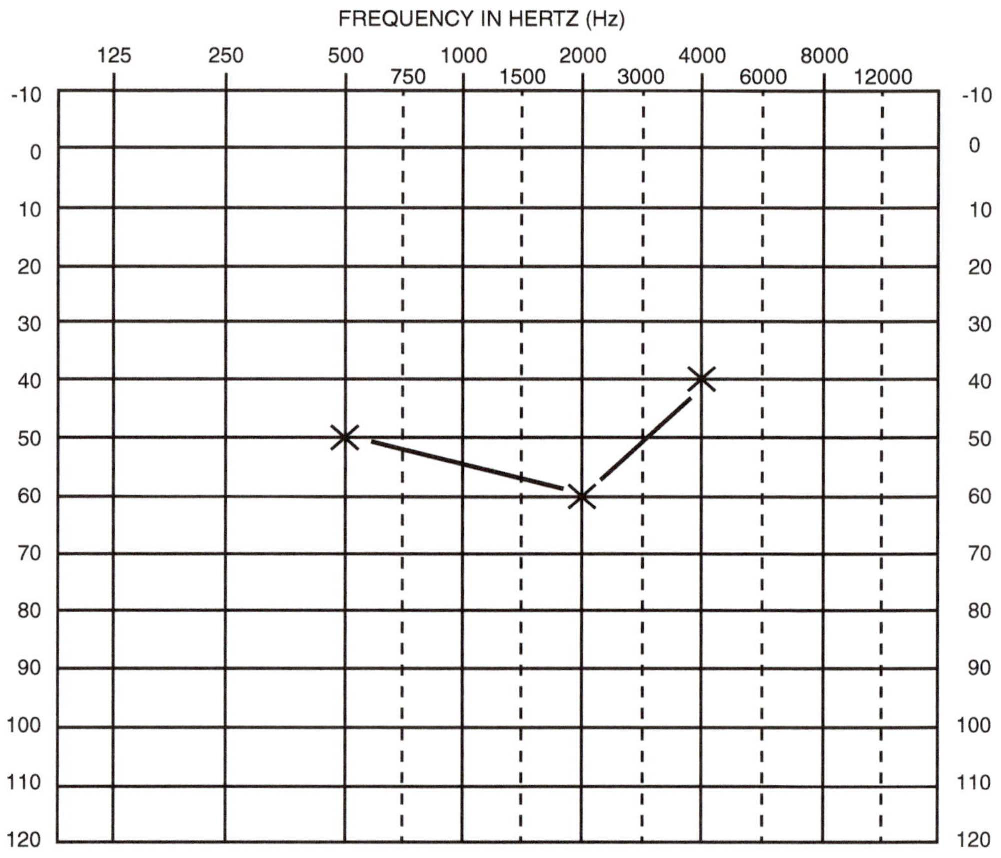


**Fig. 29.9** Example audiogram output demonstrating hearing loss. All tested frequencies were perceived at a decibel higher than 25

**Table 29.1** Voice test as described in [13]

| Grade of impairment | Level tested with audiometer | Level tested with voice test |
|---|---|---|
| Normal hearing | 25 dB or better | Able to hear whispers |
| Slight impairment | 26–40 dB | Able to hear and repeat words spoken in conversational voice at 1 m |
| Moderate impairment | 41–60 dB | Able to hear and repeat words using loud voice at 1 m |
| Severe impairment | 61–80 dB | Able to hear some words when shouted into the ear |
| Profound impairment (deafness) | 81 dB or greater | Unable to hear and understand even a shouted voice |

voice or fingers can be rubbed behind the babies ears; the baby should turn their head in the direction of the sound.

## Management of Hearing Loss

**Pearls and Pitfalls**

- Tympanostomy tubes can be placed to relieve OME and improve hearing.
- Tympanostomy tubes should be placed cautiously when 6–12 month follow-up cannot reliably be expected.

Surgical insertion of grommets (ventilation tubes or tympanostomy tubes) has been demonstrated to relieve fluid buildup in the middle ear space and improve associated hearing loss within the first year after insertion [1, 14]. While 80–90% of children will develop OME, only an estimated 26% of cases will persist beyond 3 months [2, 15]. Thus, in otherwise normal children, tubes are often inserted after effusion and hearing loss have persisted for 3 months or more, thereby demonstrating they are unlikely to spontaneously improve. Children with a cleft palate, however, are known to be more susceptible to persistent middle ear effusions and subsequent hearing loss [2, 6], so tympanostomy tube placement is sometimes undertaken sooner or even prophylactically. When considering tympanostomy tube placement for children living in low-resource areas, however, the clinician should evaluate the child's ability to reasonably have 6-month or annual follow-up with an otolaryngologist. Tube placement carries the risk of tube otorrhea requiring tube removal or exchange. Without follow-up, a child with tympanostomy tubes could develop chronic drainage and canal irritation. Further, if the tubes become obstructed, then the child is prone to effusions and ear infections which cannot appropriately be treated with ear drops. Also, tube placement carries a risk of tympanosclerosis [1]. Thus, in low-resource areas, tube placement should be performed cautiously and, perhaps, only for severe cases of hearing impairment when follow-up is unlikely.

After tube placement, children should have an otoscopic exam every 6–12 months to establish the presence/absence and functionality of the tubes. Ideally, children would also undergo a hearing test after tube placement to determine if their preoperative hearing loss has resolved. Tubes should not be inserted when there is absence of a middle ear effusion or when the child has normal hearing. Also, congenital sensorineural hearing loss or conductive hearing loss due to bony malformations of the middle ear or ear canal amenable to cochlear implantation, ossicular reconstruction, or atresia reconstruction may not be supported in low-income and low-resource areas. For these children, hearing aids may be an option to improve hearing and development.

## Myringotomy With or Without Ear Tube Placement

**Pearls and Pitfalls**

- BMT can be safely, efficiently, and effectively performed in the operating room with a microscope and small instrument set.
- Cerumen removal should be limited to wax directly obstructing a view of the TM, as excessive removal can cause troublesome bleeding.
- Myringotomy should be made in the anterior-inferior quadrant of the TM to avoid damage to middle ear structures.

Myringotomy with placement of tympanostomy tubes for children is typically undertaken in the operating room (OR) under sedation or general anesthesia. Preferably, an operating microscope is used. When not available, however, tube insertion can be attempted with magnifying loupes, provided the child is older and the canal large enough and straight enough to allow TM visualization. Also, there exist semiautomatic tube inserter devices to aid placement in an awake or asleep child without a microscope, but these devices are less precise and riskier than standard microscopic insertion by an otolaryngologist.

Figure 29.10 demonstrates an example setup in the OR for BMT. A common myringotomy instrument set is shown in Fig. 29.11, though the minimum necessary instruments are shown in Fig. 29.12. Multiple sizes of different instru-

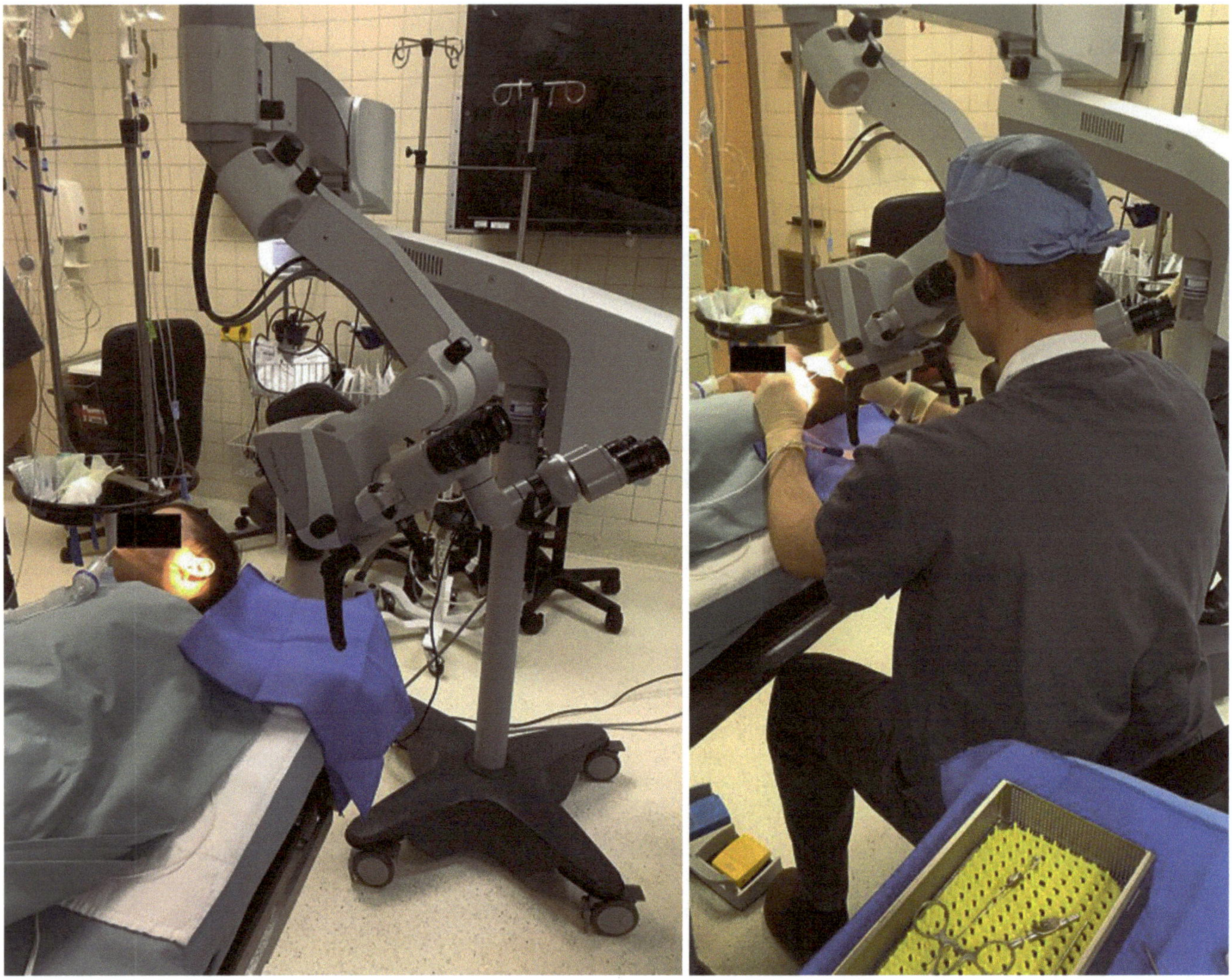

**Fig. 29.10** Example operating room (OR) setup for bilateral myringotomy with tympanostomy tube placement (BMT). The microscope base is positioned at the head of the bed or alongside the bed near the patient's feet to allow visualization of each ear. The surgeon sits for the operation and wears gloves, though sterile gloves are not necessary. The patient may be intubated if other procedures will occur in conjunction with BMT (as in this case), or the patient may be sedated with a mask to avoid intubation if only BMT is to be performed. Sterile draping is not necessary for BMT

ments, if available, make the operation smoother for different ages of children with different sizes of ear canals, but a speculum of any size that allows visualization of the TM and passage of an ear tube through its distal end is sufficient. Similarly, ototopical drops are often applied over the tube lumen after insertion, but sterile water or saline can be used when drops are not available, or this step can be omitted. Ototopical drops include oxymetazoline, a topical vasoconstrictor used for hemostasis and preventing tubes from becoming blocked due to a blood clot. There are multiple different sizes and shapes of tympanostomy tubes (Fig. 29.13). Generally, Tytans are reserved for atretic ear canals that will not permit placement of larger tube. Also, T-tubes are more likely to remain in place for a longer time than Pope or Sheehy tubes, which can be beneficial for patients expected to have a prolonged need for tubes but risky in patients expected to outgrow their eustachian tube dysfunction in a year or two. T-tubes should be used with caution as they can have a 10% perforation rate. Finally, there are multiple sizes of myringotomy blades

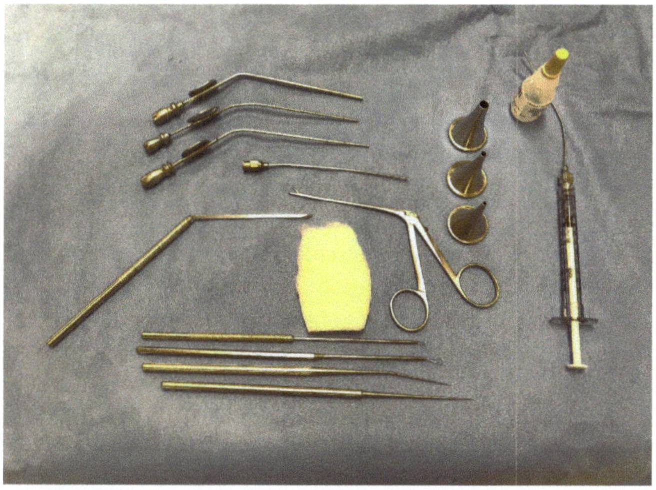

Fig. 29.11 Typical BMT set. Instruments include multiple sizes of suction, multiple cerumen curettes, multiple picks, multiple sizes of specula, a myringotomy blade, an alligator forceps, ototopical drops, a syringe and applicator, and a cotton ball

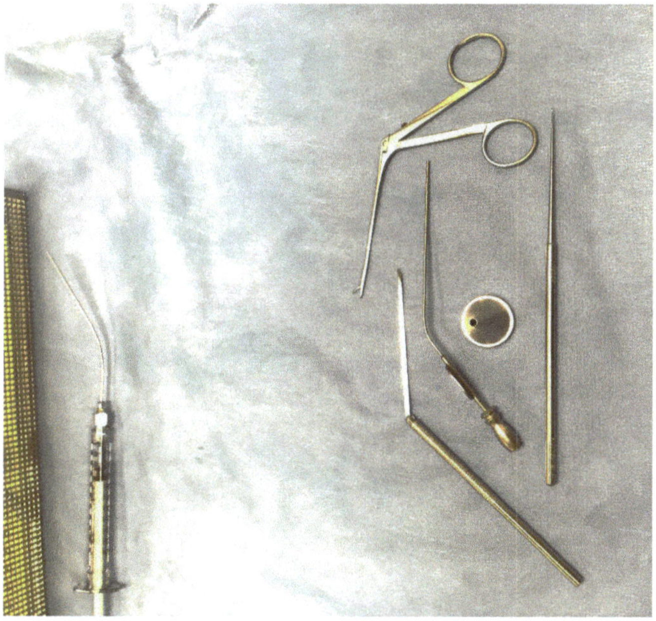

Fig. 29.12 Minimum necessary instruments to complete tympanostomy tube placement. Instruments include a myringotomy blade, suction, speculum, alligator forceps, and Rosen pick

(Fig. 29.14). The size of blade does not matter so long as it can pass through the ear canal without damaging ear canal skin and successfully perforate the TM.

After a child is sedated and positioned, a speculum is inserted into the ear canal (Fig. 29.15). Cerumen is judiciously removed from the ear canal; aggressive wax removal can cause bleeding of the canal skin, which can make subsequent TM visualization and tube placement difficult. Thus, only cerumen blocking direct visualization of the TM is removed, either with a curette, suction, or alligator forceps. Next, the TM is examined, and the anterior-inferior quadrant is identified (Fig. 29.16). The anterior-inferior quadrant is the ideal location for myringotomy to avoid damage to structures of the middle ear space. A myringotomy is made, ideally in a radial orientation, just large enough to fit the tympanostomy tube (Fig. 29.17). If the myringotomy is too small, placement of the tube can cause imprecise tearing of the TM. If the myringotomy is too large, then the tube may not sit stably in the TM. The surgeon should be wary of the ear canal when making a myringotomy to avoid causing troublesome bleeding from the canal skin. Care should particularly be given to avoiding the often prominent anterior ear canal wall as trauma in this region can lead to bleeding onto the freshly placed ear tube in the anterior inferior quadrant of the TM and thus a non-functional ear tube.

After myringotomy, fluid of the middle ear space is suctioned out. Occasionally, if fluid is thick and difficult to remove, saline can gently be flushed through the myringotomy into the middle ear space to help remove the effusion. Next, the tube is placed with an alligator forceps such that one flange is in the middle ear space and one flange is in the ear canal (Fig. 29.18). Ototopical drops (such as oxymetazoline) or saline is applied over the tube lumen, and, if desired, a cotton ball is temporarily placed in the conchal bowl to prevent drainage.

Postoperatively, patients receive antibiotic drops (such as ciprofloxacin or ofloxacin) to the ears: five drops to each ear twice a day for 5 days. If the middle ears were noted to have copious fluid during surgery, it is not rare for there to be drainage for 3–5 days after surgery; but this should dry up shortly thereafter. Subsequently, if the child gets an upper respiratory infection, cough, or cold, mucous or

Fig. 29.13 Different types of tympanostomy tubes. From left to right, the tubes are a titanium Tytan, a Pope beveled grommet, a Sheehy collar button, a Goode T-tube, and a Goode T-grommet

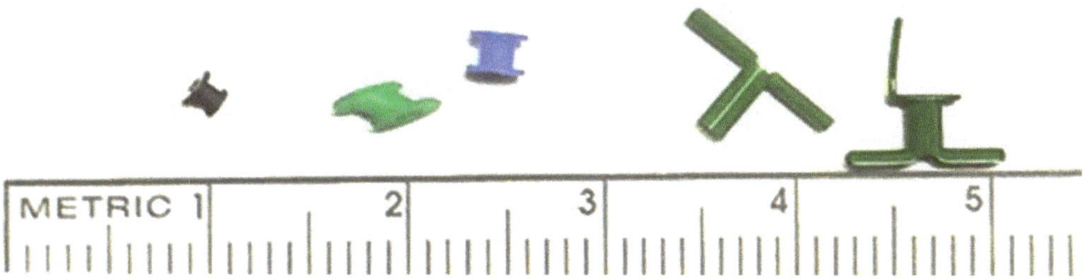

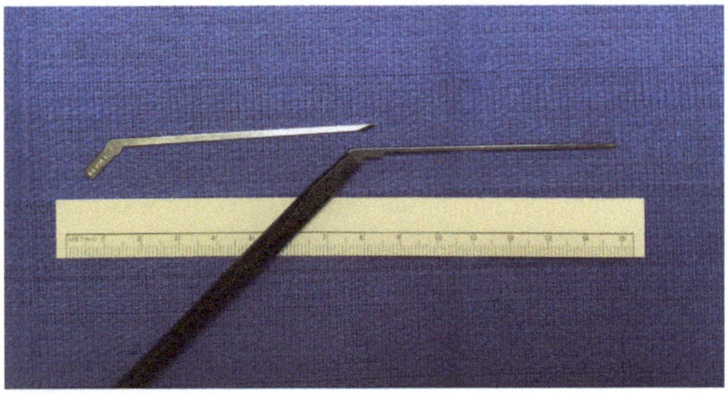

Fig. 29.14 A standard (left) myringotomy blade and a micro (right) myringotomy blade

serous discharge can be seen from the ears in a patient with ear tubes. This is the ear tube doing its job by relieving the fluid from the ear. Sometimes the ears can get infected, and pus can be seen draining from the ear. Whether the ear has serous/mucoid discharge or purulent discharge, we suggest five drops of antibiotic drops (such as ciprofloxacin/dexamethasone or ofloxacin) to each ear twice a day for 7 days. If topical drops are not available, consider a course of oral antibiotics if the drainage does not resolve in a few days. Ear tubes should not cause pain. If there is ear pain, the ear should be evaluated for the possibility of an ear infection. If a patient with ear tubes has bloody otorrhea, the ear should be evaluated for granulation tissue. With an otoscope, one

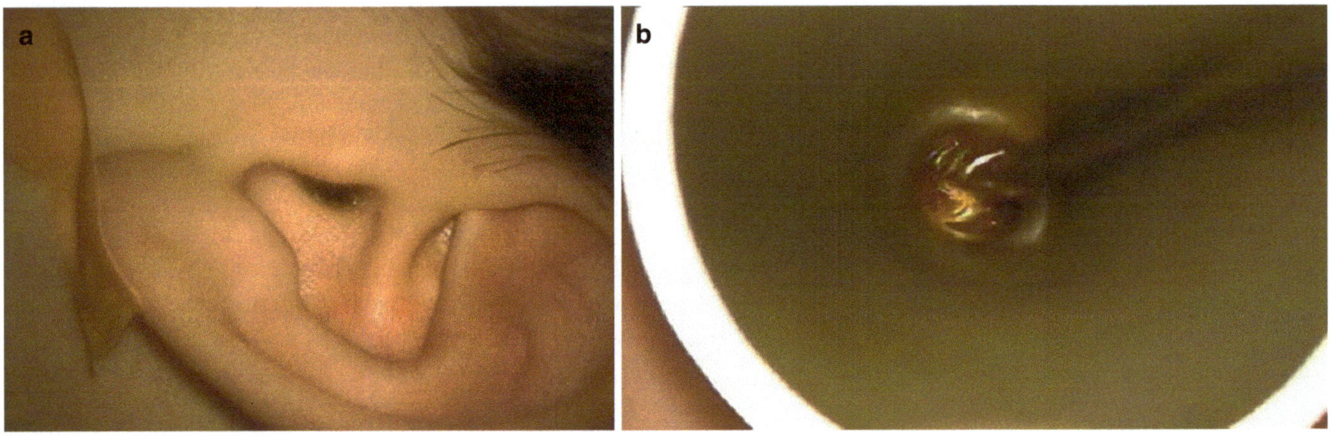


Fig. 29.15 View of the left ear through the operating microscope. Part (**a**) shows the ear before speculum placement. Part (**b**) shows the ear canal on a higher magnification after placement of the speculum. A cerumen curette is used to remove cerumen obstructing TM visualization from the canal

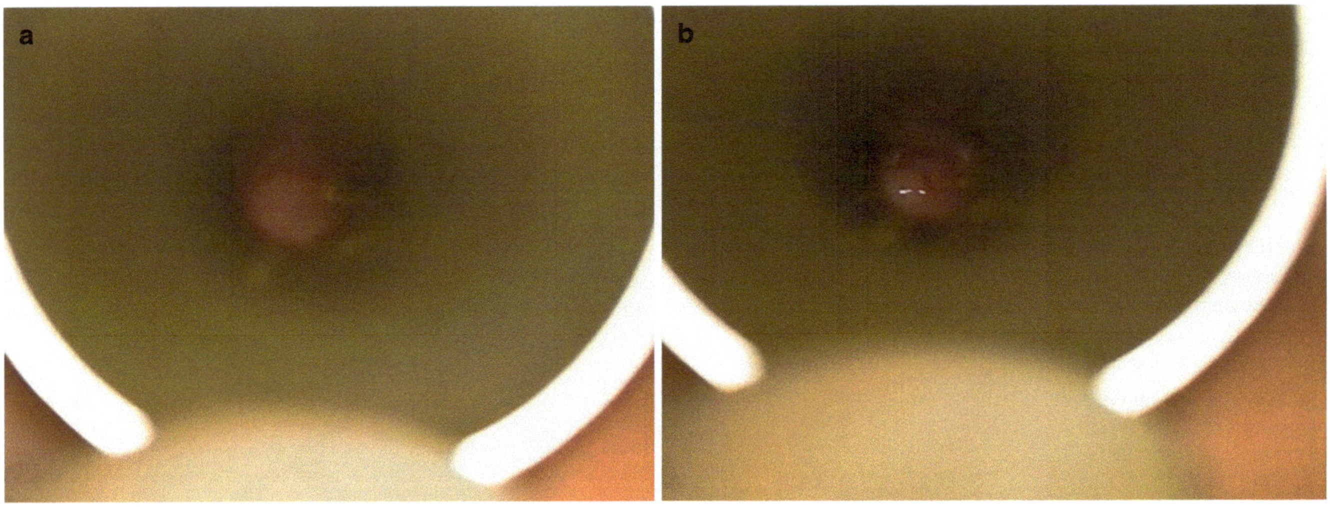


Fig. 29.16 After cerumen removal, the left TM is visualized in its entirety, and the anterior-inferior quadrant is identified (**a**). After myringotomy is made, an effusion can be seen emanating through the hole from the middle ear space into the ear canal (**b**)

should look for fleshy, pink tissue adjacent to or obstructing the tube; this is suggestive of granulation tissue which is benign but can be treated with a 7–10-day course of a steroid containing drop, such as ciprofloxacin/dexamethasone.

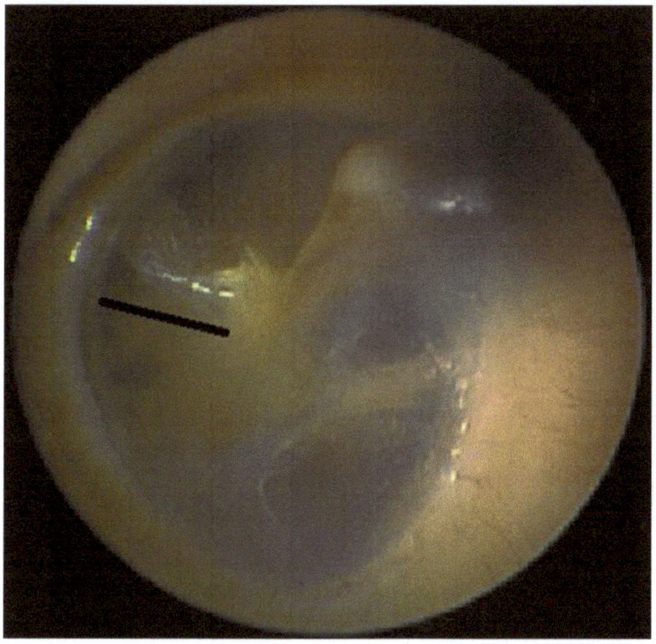

Fig. 29.17 Left-side tympanic membrane. This view was achieved with an endoscope; the entire TM is not commonly visualized all at once, as in this photo, in young children with an operating microscope. The black line illustrates the ideal placement of a myringotomy in a radial fashion in the anterior-inferior quadrant

## Common Airway Issues

### Pearls and Pitfalls

- Children with cleft palate may be at risk of obstructive sleep apnea and airway stenosis.
- During adenotonsillectomy, a cuff of inferior adenoid tissue should be left to mitigate the risk of VPI.
- Patients with Pierre Robin sequence or isolated micrognathia may have an increased risk of difficult intubation and postoperative obstructive breathing due to severe glossoptosis.

The surgeon should be aware of commonly associated airway issues when treating patients with a cleft palate. PRS, for example, is a common cause of cleft palate, as mentioned above, and the syndrome most commonly associated with PRS is Stickler syndrome [6, 16, 17]. Developmentally, PRS is not caused by a specific genetic deletion or mutation. It starts with microgenia/micrognathia, which leads to glossoptosis and displacement of the tongue. This structural shift in tongue position then prevents the midline fusing of the palate, thus resulting in a secondary cleft palate. Glossoptosis in these patients can cause obstructive sleep apnea and, in some cases, acute airway compromise, which may necessitate tracheostomy [18]. Surgeons should be aware of and prepared for an acute airway emergency in patients with PRS or similar disorders when inducing anesthesia. Some cleft surgeons may choose not to operate on children with PRS or craniofacial syndromes due to these increased risks (see Chap. 27).

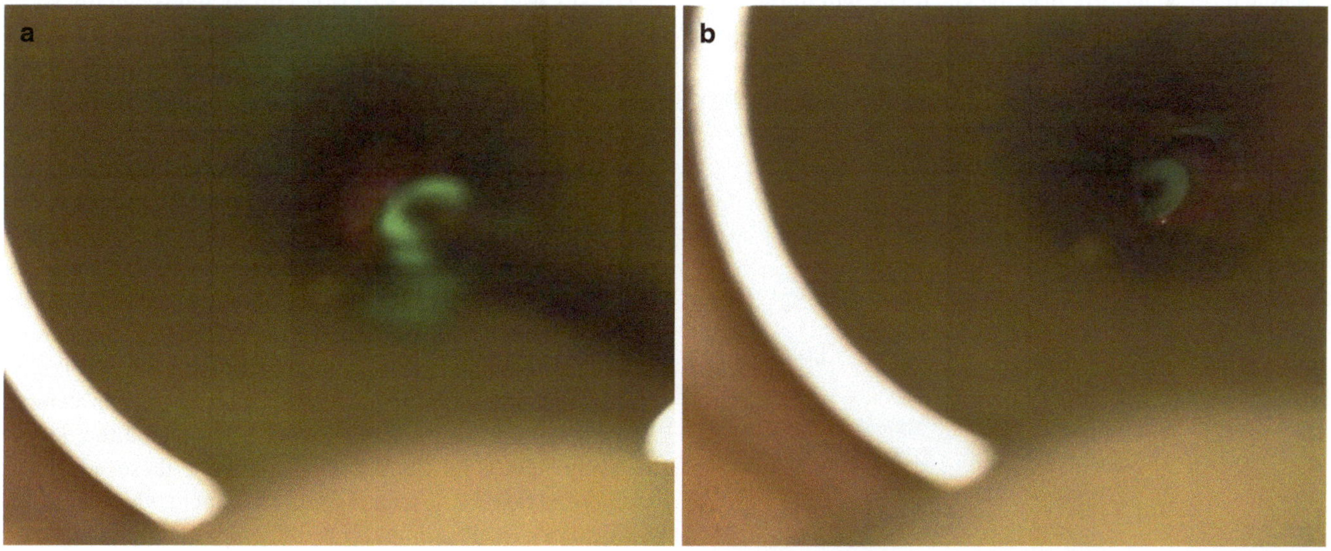


Fig. 29.18 Placement of a Pope tympanostomy tube into a myringotomy. The pope is introduced with an alligator forceps (**a**). If needed, it can then be finely positioned with a Rosen pick. After placement, it can be seen appropriately positioned in the myringotomy with one flange in the middle ear space and one flange in the ear canal (**b**)

With advances in prenatal care, sometimes micrognathia can even be predicted prior to delivery of the child. Ultrasound findings suggestive of micrognathia include a prominent upper lip with a receding chin in a midsagittal view. If polyhydramnios is present, this is more ominous and suggests the presence of not only micrognathia but also glossoptosis. If ultrasound findings suggest micrognathia and glossoptosis, then having an airway specialist such as an anesthesiologist or otolaryngologist at the delivery can be life-saving.

Children with micrognathia and glossoptosis can have a very challenging airway to access. This is relevant not only if such a child is in distress and needs to be intubated but also if they present for routine surgery. In fact, a child with PRS may be asymptomatic at baseline, but once induced during anesthesia, they may become a difficult or critical airway. It is important to anticipate such difficulties by examining the patient's face in profile in the preoperative setting.

Several strategies can be employed to help manage children with micrognathia safely; the management strategy ultimately used by a practitioner will be dependent upon the practitioner's experience and availability of resources. Simple maneuvers such as moderate neck extension and a jaw thrust with bag-mask ventilation can be easy to apply but very effective at stabilizing a child in distress. An oral airway used during bag-mask ventilation and jaw thrust further pulls the tongue anteriorly and creates a protected channel for ventilation. Similarly, a nasopharyngeal airway, also known as a nasal trumpet, can be inserted through the nasal cavity and into the nasopharynx to provide a channel for ventilation. Direct laryngoscopy and bronchoscopy (Fig. 29.19) may not be possible if there is significant micrognathia, as the larynx remains more anteriorly than the small jaw will allow for in terms of exposure. A supraglottic airway device, also known as a laryngeal mask airway (LMA), can be life-saving in situations where intubation is difficult with direct laryngoscopy (Fig. 29.20). An LMA can be inserted through the oral cavity and down into the hypopharynx blindly and quickly. The LMA sits over the larynx (it is not inserted through the vocal cords as is done with a traditional endotracheal tube) and can be used to ventilate the patient. More advanced techniques involve doing a fiberoptic intubation with the endotracheal tube loaded onto a fiberoptic scope (Fig. 29.21a). With the endotracheal tube loaded onto the fiberoptic scope, the scope is advanced either through the nasal cavity and down through the vocal folds and into the trachea or through an LMA which has been placed, through the vocal folds and into the trachea (Fig. 29.21b). Then the endotracheal tube is advanced down the scope and into the trachea; the in-dwelling scope can help visualize final placement of the tube in the trachea. Finally, video laryngoscopes are increasingly being used in centers and can help to see the airway when traditional direct laryngoscopy fails (Fig. 29.22). Unfortunately, these advanced techniques do require training and equipment which may not be available in all settings. If a child with micrognathia does not have a stable airway, it may become necessary to perform a tracheostomy.

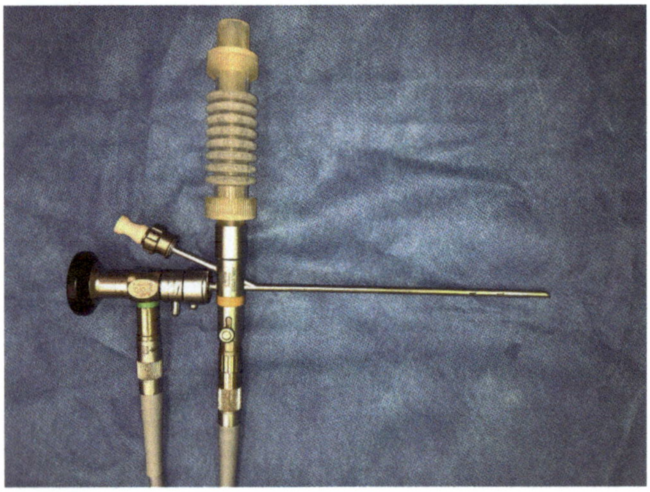

**Fig. 29.19** A ventilating bronchoscope may not be able to visual the airway in patients with severe micrognathia (Karl Storz; Tuttlingen, Germany)

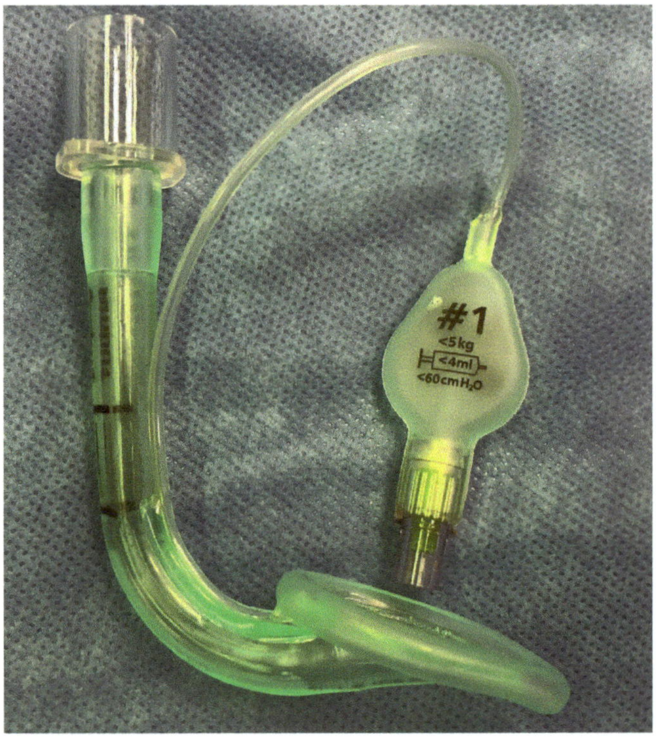


**Fig. 29.20** A supraglottic airway device/laryngeal mask airway can be inserted into the airway quickly and is often useful in patients with poor airway exposure via laryngoscopy due to micrognathia (Ambu; Copenhagen, Denmark)

Standard initial surgical treatment for children with obstructive sleep apnea (OSA) includes adenotonsillec-

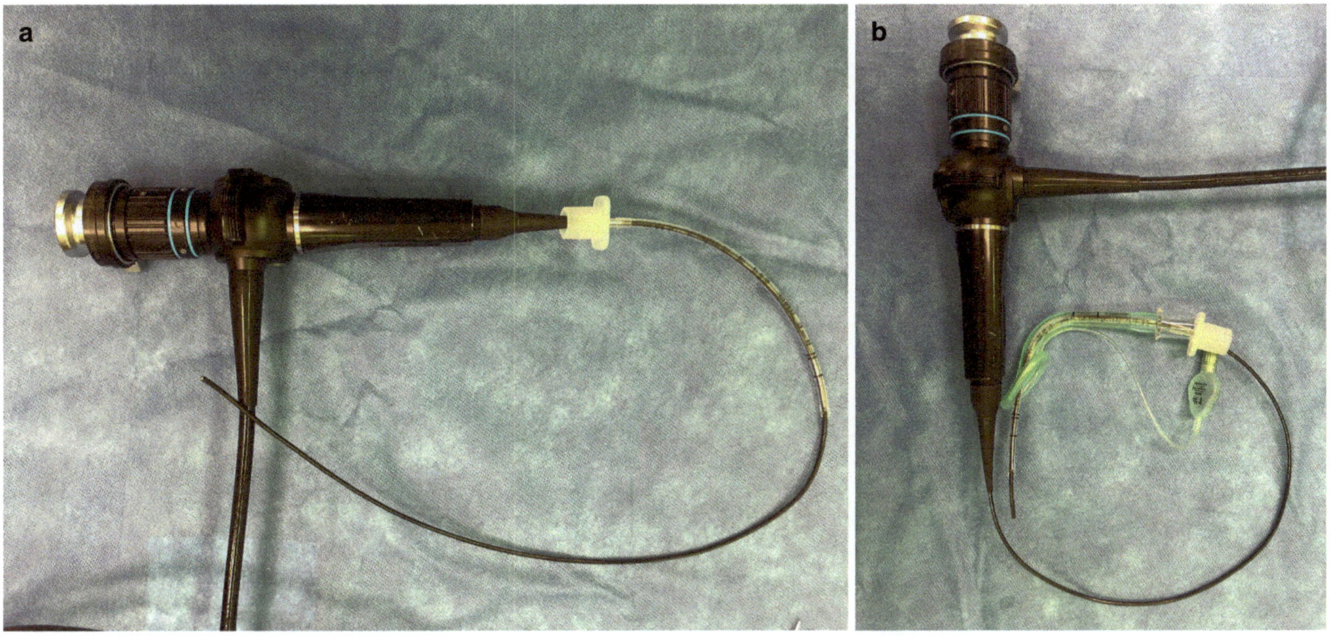

Fig. 29.21 An endotracheal tube can be loaded onto a flexible laryngoscope for intubation (**a**). After placement of a supraglottic airway device into the airway, an orotracheal intubation is possible employing a flexible bronchoscope loaded with an endotracheal tube (**b**)

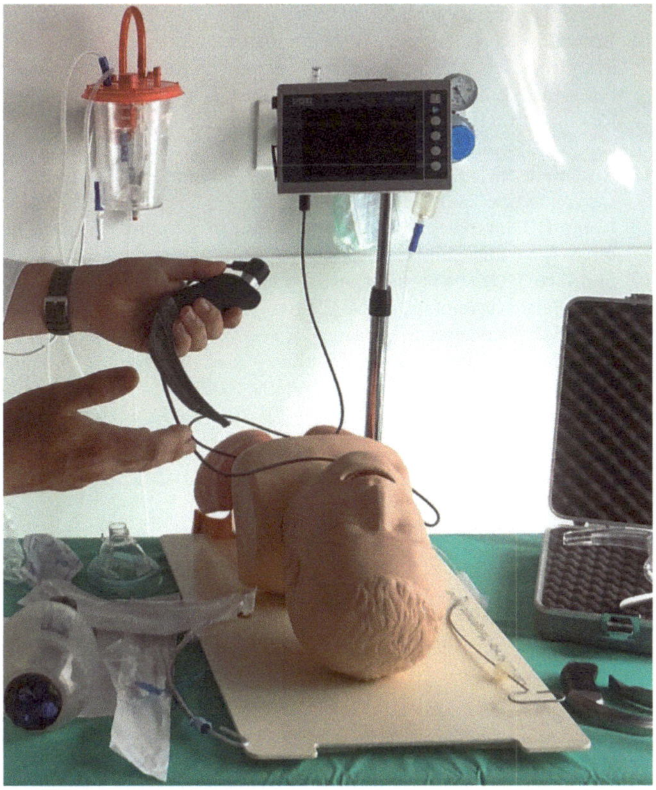

Fig. 29.22 Video laryngoscopes can help to improve visualization during difficult intubations (Karl Storz; Tuttlingen, Germany)

tomy, but there are special considerations for children with a cleft palate. First, while the adenoid pad can be reduced to improve OSA and eustachian tube dysfunction, aggressive removal of the adenoid pad can exacerbate velopharyngeal insufficiency (VPI), a problem this population is already at higher risk of developing. To avoid excessive VPI, a cuff of adenoid tissue can be left inferiorly to allow contact with the soft palate when it elevates. Next, the decision to proceed with adenotonsillectomy should be undertaken carefully and conservatively in underserved areas where patients will not reliably and reasonably have access to emergency services after surgery. Surgical removal of the tonsils carries a 2–5% risk of postoperative hemorrhage that, in some cases, can be life-threatening if not controlled in the operating room. Thus, when acute follow-up cannot be guaranteed, adenotonsillectomy should be avoided.

Last, children with cleft palate can also have subglottic stenosis (Fig. 29.23), and, especially in underserved low-income areas, children can present with malnourishment. In these cases, airway size and tracheal diameter are often smaller than expected, and the surgeon and anesthesia team should be prepared to intubate with a tube a half size smaller than generally expected. Ideally, a cleft team should include a pediatric otolaryngologist or, if not available, an anesthesiologist as one of its members to help optimally manage a difficult airway in cleft patients.

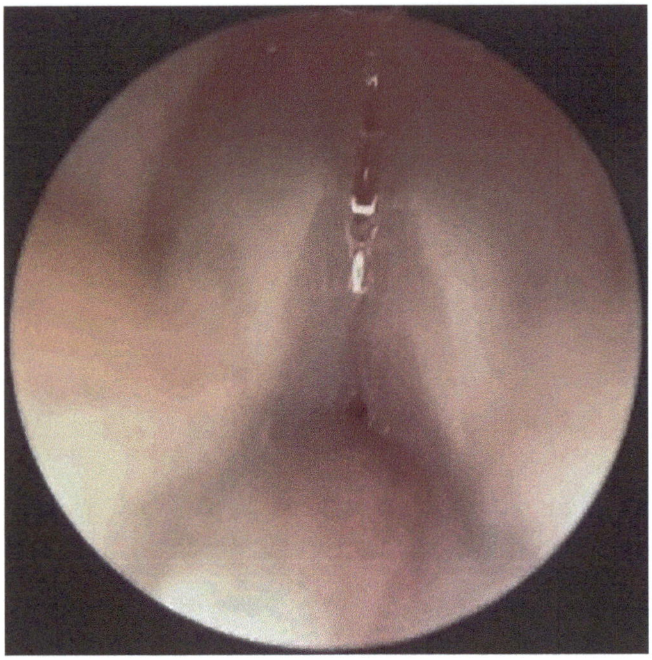

Fig. 29.23 Direct laryngoscopy of the larynx: high-grade subglottic stenosis with only a pinpoint airway

## References


1. Lous J, Burton MJ, Felding J, Ovesen T, Rovers M, Williamson I. Grommets (ventilation tubes) for hearing loss associated with otitis media with effusion in children. Cochrane Database Syst Rev. 2005;(1):CD001801. https://doi.org/10.1002/14651858.CD001801.pub2.
2. Shaffer AD, Ford MD, Choi SS, Jabbour N. The impact of tympanostomy tubes on speech and language development in children with cleft palate. Otolaryngol Head Neck Surg. 2017;157(3):504–14.
3. Sharma RK, Nanda V. Problems of middle ear and hearing in cleft children. Indian J Plast Surg. 2009;42(Suppl):S144–8.
4. Garcia-Vaquero C, Mir C, Graterol D, Ortiz N, Rochera-Villach MI, Lleonart ME, Lorente J. Otologic, audiometric and speech findings in patients undergoing surgery for cleft palate. BMC Pediatr. 2018;18:350.
5. Flynn T, Persson C, Moller C, Lohmander A, Magnusson L. A longitudinal study of hearing and middle ear status of individuals with cleft palate with and without additional malformations / syndromes. Cleft Palate Craniofac J. 2014;51(5):e94–e101.
6. Wang TD, Milczuk HA. Cleft lip and palate. In: Cummings otolaryngology. 6th ed. Philadelphia: Elsevier, Inc; 2015. p. 2915–32.
7. Leopold C, De Barros A, Cellier C, et al. Laryngeal abnormalities are frequent in the 22q11 deletion syndrome. Int J Pediatr Otorhinolaryngol. 2012;76:36–40.
8. Timmermans K, Vander Poorten V, Desloovere C, Debruyne F. The middle ear of cleft palate patients in their early teens: a literature study and preliminary file study. B-ENT. 2006;2(Suppl. 4):95–101.
9. Sheahan P, Miller I, Sheahan JN, Earley MJ, Blayney AW. Incidence and outcome of middle ear disease in cleft lip and/or cleft palate. Int J Pediatr Otorhinolaryngol. 2003;67:785–93.
10. Handzic-Cuk J, Cuk V, Risavi R, Katusic D, Stajner-Katusic S. Hearing levels and age in cleft palate patients. Int J Pediatr Otorhinolaryngol. 1996;37:227–42.
11. Hussein SY, Swanepoel DW, Mahomed F, et al. Community-based hearing screening for young children using an mHealth service-delivery model. Glob Health Action. 2018;11:1–7.
12. Yancey KL, Cheromei LJ, Muhando J, et al. Pediatric hearing screening in low-resource settings: incorporation of video-otoscopy and an electronic medical record. Int J Pediatr Otorhinolaryngol. 2019;126:1–6.
13. World Health Organization. Primary ear and hearing care training resource: Trainer's manual, intermediate level. Geneva: World Health Organization; 2006. p. 96.
14. Browning GG, Rovers MM, Williamson I, Lous J, Burton MJ. Grommets (ventilation tubes) for hearing loss associated with otitis media with effusion in children. Cochrane Database Syst Rev. 2010;(10):CD001801. https://doi.org/10.1002/14651858.CD001801.pub3.
15. Rosenfeld RM, Kay D. Natural history of untreated otitis media. Laryngoscope. 2003;113:1645–57.
16. Robin P. Glossoptosis due to atresia and hypotrophy of the mandible. Am J Dis Child. 1934;48:541.
17. Shprintzen RJ. The implications of the diagnosis of Robin sequence. Cleft Palate Craniofac J. 1992;29:205–9.
18. Cruz MJ, Kerschner JE, Beste DJ, et al. Pierre robin sequences: secondary respiratory difficulties and intrinsic feeding abnormalities. Laryngoscope. 1999;109:1632–6.

# Psychosocial, Educational, and Cultural Aspects of Cleft Care

# 30

Leanne Magee and Caleb J. Figge

**Key Points**

1. On broad measures of psychosocial functioning, children and adults with clefts are not at risk for greater difficulties compared to unaffected peers.
2. Individuals' subjective perceptions of their appearance and their beliefs about how visible their differences are to others, rather than their objective outward differences, are the best predictors of psychological adjustment to appearance differences.
3. Rates of learning disabilities are two to three times greater in patients with CL/P than the general population, with 30–40% estimated to have a learning disability.
4. 74% of children reported teasing about facial appearance, most typically between the ages of 8–11 years. One effective approach for many patients with appearance differences dealing with teasing is to (1) acknowledge the appearance difference, (2) provide a brief but honest explanation, and (3) guide the conversation onto other topics.
5. Studies of adaptive functioning in low- and middle-income countries (LMIC) identify overlapping functioning expectations with high-income countries but also culturally distinct domains and priorities, indicating measures developed in high-income countries may miss relevant information or require adaptation.

## Introduction

This chapter broadly reviews relevant psychosocial issues for patients and families coping with cleft lip and/or palate (CL/P), including issues related to quality of life, mental health, and social and educational functioning. Recommendations are made for assessing psychosocial risk and providing psychosocial support for children and families coping with cleft as it relates to treatment decision-making, coping with medical and surgical interventions, optimizing social, developmental and educational functioning, and enhancing quality of life during all stages of development.

The research exploring psychosocial outcomes among patients with cleft indicates that on broad measures of psychosocial functioning, children and adults with clefts are not at risk for greater difficulties compared to unaffected peers [1]. However, many studies have identified specific areas of risk for patients with CL/P. Individuals with visible differences such as CL/P commonly experience negative perceptions of the self and difficulties with social interaction, which can, in turn, contribute to negative feelings, thoughts, and changes in behavior [2]. Patients and families affected by CL/P may experience challenges adjusting to diagnosis, coping with treatment, difficulties in school functioning, social challenges, and appearance concerns, described below, which contribute to psychosocial functioning, quality of life, and medical outcomes.

It is critical to note the objective type, extent, and severity of a visible difference do not predict the level of psychological distress [2]. Rather, individuals' subjective perceptions of their appearance and their beliefs about how visible their differences are to others are the best predictors of psychological adjustment to appearance differences [2]. However, highly

L. Magee (✉)
Division of Plastic and Reconstructive Surgery, Department of Child and Adolescent Psychiatry and Behavioral Sciences, Children's Hospital of Philadelphia and University of Pennsylvania, Philadelphia, PA, USA
e-mail: mageel@email.chop.edu

C. J. Figge
Department of Mental Health, Johns Hopkins Bloomberg School of Public Health, Baltimore, MD, USA

© Springer Nature Switzerland AG 2021

J. W. Swanson, D. W. Low (eds.), *Global Cleft Care in Low-Resource Settings*, https://doi.org/10.1007/978-3-030-59105-2_30

visible appearance differences, such as CL/P, are likely to have a greater influence on social interactions and consequently, body image, and self-esteem.

## Family Adjustment to Diagnosis

Receiving news that a baby is diagnosed with CL/P can be a shock for many parents, often contributing to feelings of anxiety, grief, and guilt [3]. Families exhibit variable experiences of stress and resilience throughout the child's course of care, which can be affected by factors unique to the parent's coping style, broader sociocultural or religious beliefs about cleft, and the experiences with their medical providers. Timing of diagnosis can impact family coping; those who receive a cleft diagnosis prenatally have been found to have more time to process emotions and seek education about cleft and its treatment [4], whereas families who receive a diagnosis after birth must adjust and learn about care while navigating their infants' early days and challenges.

Treatment teams are encouraged to assess the family's understanding of diagnosis information and be open to answering all questions asked so parents feel included and valued as a part of their child's care team. Many parents of children with cleft emphasize the benefits of hearing from their treating providers that their child's diagnosis is not their fault, and they greatly value communication from their providers that conveys empathy, confidence, and willingness to provide support [5]. Often, families benefit from being connected to family support organizations where available.

## School Functioning

Children with CL/P face elevated risks for school difficulties. Though overall rates of intelligence are in the average range for children with CL/P, affected children may exhibit increased risk for deficits in cognitive and behavioral functioning, which are, in turn, associated with lower school achievement and increased need for academic supports [6]. For some, cleft palate is associated with neurocognitive differences, including verbal memory deficits, problems with visuospatial and executive functioning, developmental delays, speech and language delays, and reading and language-based learning disabilities [7]. Rates of learning disabilities are two to three times greater in patients with CL/P than the general population, with 30–40% estimated to have a learning disability [6, 7].

To optimize the educational experience, team members should ask parents and children about strengths and challenges in school, whether the child is performing at grade level, and the type, amount, and satisfaction with educational supports if available. School services may include learning supports as well as accommodations that allow the child to access the classroom or otherwise function in the school setting, such as special education instruction, resource room support, reduced or altered workload, speech therapy, hearing support, vision, physical therapy, occupational therapy, testing accommodations, nursing support, personal care assistant, or behavioral support.

Testing is often needed to determine if additional school supports are warranted (see Fig. 30.1). Psychoeducational testing assesses achievement and skills in essential academic areas and may identify learning disabilities or other needs for accommodations to facilitate classroom performance. For children with more complex neurological or neuroanatomical differences, neuropsychological evaluation assesses brain/behavior relationships, including memory, language, visual perceptual skills, fine motor skills, attention, and executive function. For children whose school performance is being affected by emotional or behavioral functioning, psychological testing by a clinical psychologist may be indicated. Assessments should consider cognitive, behavioral, and academic outcomes in the context of the child's broader medical and developmental status. The best educational plans will consider the child's unique needs, the general risks for learning difficulties associated with cleft, and the resources available to patients in their school setting.

## Social Functioning

Children with cleft experience challenges navigating social relationships, including coping with visible differences in facial appearance, changes in appearance over time, speech difficulties, and absence from activities due to surgical and medical treatments. Many children experience teasing, which can include verbal, relational, and physical bullying. Children with chronic health conditions are reported to be teased five times more often than unaffected peers [8], with one study among EuroCleft centers reporting that 74% of children reported teasing about facial appearance, most typically between the ages of 8 and 11 years [9].

Clinicians are in a unique role to help families navigate social issues related to appearance and identity through the lifespan, including inquiring whether they are receiving any unwanted questions, comments, or behaviors related to their appearance or speech. Psychosocial team members can help children with CL/P cope with teasing and bullying by working to develop a script for responding to commonly asked questions or comments about cleft, so parents and children are prepared to manage challenges with confidence. Acknowledging the appearance difference, providing a brief but honest explanation, and guiding the conversation onto other topics are effective approaches for

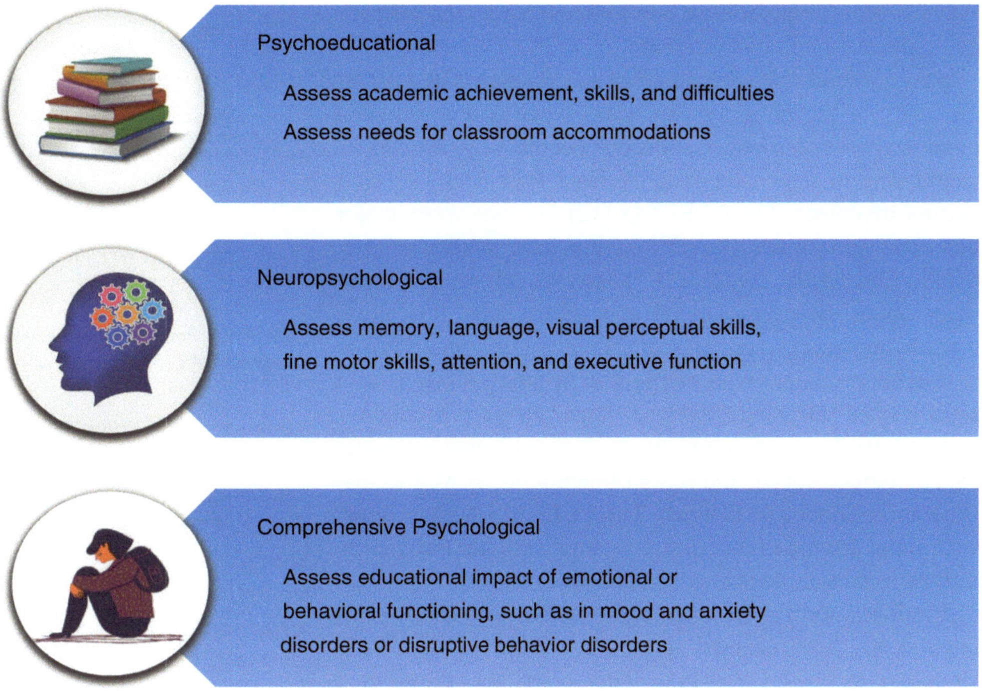


**Fig. 30.1** Types of assessment for educational, cognitive and psychological concerns

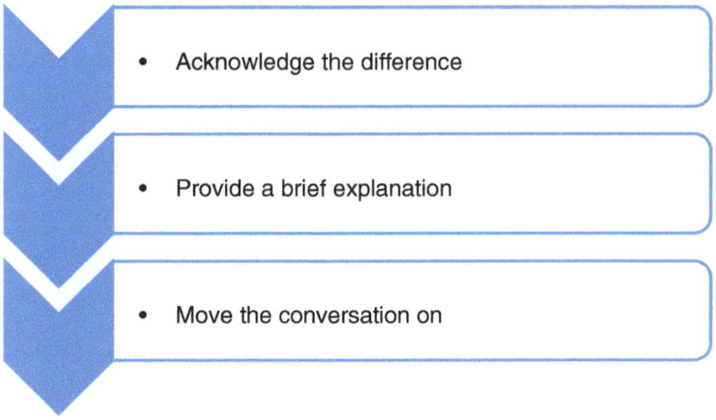


**Fig. 30.2** Responding to questions and comments about appearance difference

many patients with appearance differences ([10]; see Fig. 30.2). Children experiencing more significant difficulties navigating social relationships will benefit from the provision of supportive psychotherapy with an emphasis on social skills. Skills include prosocial responses, including active ignoring of teasing, leaving the situation, seeking support of a nearby friend or adult, using direct communication to request the bully stop, or using humor to deflect negative attention [10].

Providers can promote positive self-image in patients by using neutral, descriptive language when discussing the condition and its treatment. The American Cleft Palate-Craniofacial Association recommends using person first language, e.g., instead of "cleft patient" use "patient with a cleft." This simple change at all levels of care will help to place the whole person and not just their condition at the center of their treatment. Providers should also employ neutral terms that preserve the precision of their descriptions to avoid using negative or stigmatizing language. Terms like "defect," "malformation," and "deformity" could be switched to "difference," or "diagnosis." Lastly, clinicians may help patients and parents better accept and integrate information about their care by providing accessible explanations of typical interventions. For instance, surgeons are encouraged to say "surgery" in lieu of "repair" or "fix" to help avoid implications of brokenness, which can affect self-esteem.

## Psychosocial Screening

### Models and Tools for Measuring Psychosocial Functioning

Given these risk factors, ongoing psychosocial screening of patients and families affected by cleft is recommended through all stages of development to assess quality of life. Health-related quality of life (HRQOL) focuses on perceived physical and mental health over time [11], including physical, emotional, social, and cognitive factors as well as aspects of medical conditions and treatment, financial impact of health conditions, and community resources, policies, and practices that affect health and healthcare. It is important to assess HRQOL, as well as psychosocial functioning more broadly, on an ongoing basis to best understand the changing impact of medical conditions and their treatment on the individual's broader experience and to demonstrate the efficacy and clinical benefit of treatments.

Psychosocial risk screening can be completed by various members of the patient's care team when using validated parent-report measures. Condition-specific measures are a useful way to screen for issues related specifically to cleft and its treatment. The CLEFT-Q [12] assesses three major domains: appearance, facial function, and quality of life. Within appearance, the CLEFT-Q assesses self-reported concerns about the overall facial appearance, lips, jaw, nose, nostrils, teeth, and cleft lip scar. There is also a checklist to assess for problems with eating and drinking, as well as a speech scale assessing functional impairments in communication. Lastly, there is a quality of life module that measures psychological, social, and school functioning as well as distress about speech difficulties. The CLEFT-Q was designed with input from patients in 6 countries and validated in an international sample across 12 countries.

Similarly, the Psychosocial Assessment Tool (PAT; [13]) has recently been adapted into a craniofacial version, PAT-Craniofacial (PAT-CV; [14]). This brief, parent-reported screener of psychosocial risk includes subscales assessing family structure and resources, family problems, social support, stress reactions, child problems, sibling problems, family functioning, and belief systems as well as stressors related specifically to the craniofacial condition and its treatment. Scores indicate a family's current risk status (*Universal*, *Targeted*, or *Clinical*) and appropriate intervention recommendations. The PAT has been adapted to a wide range of pediatric health populations, including those with specific diseases like craniofacial conditions, and translated into multiple languages. Though the PAT and other screeners can be administered by most clinical staff, collaboration between surgeons and specially trained psychosocial providers allows for the most effective and efficient evaluation and intervention over time.

Once screening is completed, it is important to consider the level of psychosocial need and associated interventions. The Pediatric Psychosocial Preventative Health Model (PPHM) outlines three levels of risk with associated interventions ([15]; see Fig. 30.3). Families at the *Universal* level experience expected levels of concern and distress about the child's condition, but demonstrate resilience and effective adjustment. Universal families benefit from general resources to support coping and compliance, including psychoeducation about treatment, case management services, collaboration with schools, general supportive counseling, brief medical play, or referral to condition-specific support networks. Families at the *Targeted* level experience continued or worsened vulnerability in conjunction with the stressors of medical treatment. Targeted families benefit from psychosocial interventions and ongoing monitoring to address specific symptoms and determine continued or increasing

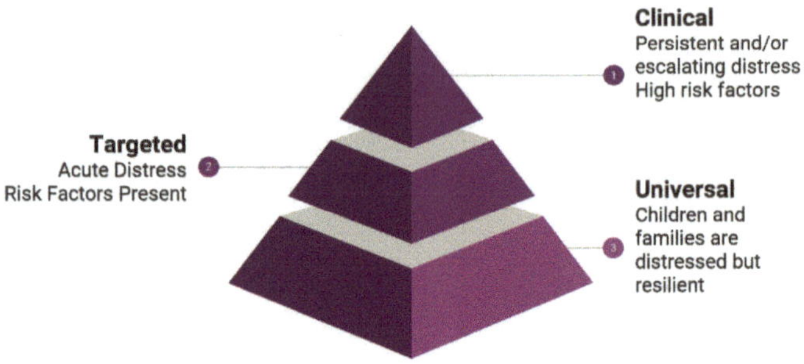
Clinical
Persistent and/or escalating distress
High risk factors
Targeted
Acute Distress
Risk Factors Present
Universal
Children and families are distressed but resilient

**Fig. 30.3** Pediatric psychosocial preventative health model (PPHM) levels of risk

support needs, such as a course of therapy for help with adjustment to diagnosis and treatment, compliance with medical care, or reducing procedural anxiety. Families at the *Clinical* level require the highest level of support and monitoring, as they exhibit multiple pre-existing, chronic, and complex difficulties requiring intensive intervention with a behavioral health specialist such as a psychologist or psychiatrist. Clinical families may require crisis intervention, legal supports, or consultation with child welfare agencies, psychiatric medication, or interventions designed to assure the safety of the patient and family. Ongoing assessment of a family's risk level allows for the tailoring of preventive, evidence-based, and cost-effective psychosocial care designed to enhance patient outcomes and quality of life.

## Mental Health Screening Across Global Contexts

There are many challenges to adequate and accurate mental health screening in LMIC contexts. Geographical distances from healthcare settings and difficulties affording healthcare can contribute to infrequent visits to providers and limited or no follow-up care. Services may be available inconsistently due to provider availability (e.g., transitory mission groups) or limited training in mental healthcare. Low or no literacy and language barriers can contribute to difficulty communicating concerns and recommendations between patients and providers, and there may be a lack of culturally validated mental health instruments available in the patients' native languages. These challenges directly affect the patient and family's mental health status by adding or exacerbating stressors surrounding the patient's healthcare provision and indirectly affect them through worsening medical outcomes associated with limited access (e.g., non-adherence to treatment recommendations). The unique challenges highlight the importance of providing feasible strategies for families to self-monitor functioning, utilizing innovative technologies to increase access (e.g., telemedicine, MHealth), and disseminating culturally validated mental health screeners that are freely available and can be reliably administered by non-mental health professionals or lay providers.

Mental health symptoms and associated problems lack universal, synonymous terms across cultural contexts. In screening for symptoms associated with cleft, it is important to consider ethnocultural conceptualizations of mental health problems that are rooted in local concepts of health and illness. Patients may report linguistically marked, culturally salient symptomatology that expresses distress in locally intelligible terms, or "idioms of distress" [16]. The *Diagnostic and Statistical Manual* – 5th Edition defines cultural idioms of distress as "ways of expressing distress that may not involve specific symptoms or syndromes, but that provide collective, shared ways of experiencing and talking about personal or social concerns." Common examples of idioms of distress include "thinking too much" across a wide range of populations [17], "ataque de nervios" in Latinx populations, and "shenjing shuairuo," or neurasthenia, which is currently the most widely used psychiatric diagnosis in China.

Incorporating open-ended questions of symptoms and problems may be a useful addition to existing screening assessments to capture idioms and other culturally relevant expressions of problems associated with cleft. Several screening assessments exist that are validated across multiple cultural contexts. The World Health Organization (WHO) has published a toolkit for mental health screening in global contexts, which includes several freely accessible measures in multiple languages (https://www.who.int/mental_health/resources/toolkit_mh_emergencies/en/).

For contexts with no formally trained mental health professionals, there are several freely available broad psychosocial functioning instruments that can be reliably administered and scored by lay providers. For example, the Strengths and Difficulties Questionnaire (SDQ; [18]), which provides scores across a range of domains, is available in over 85 languages. Additionally, parents and families are encouraged to self-monitor the degree of *functional impairment* for the person with CL/P as a screener for pursuing additional services. For example, clinical staff can assess whether the person's thoughts or behaviors are making it difficult for them to be successful in meeting individual, family, and community expectations (self-care, social relationships, school, religious, occupational, etc.) and provide additional support as needed. See Fig. 30.5 for additional screening recommendations.

## Adaptive Functioning

An important consideration among mental health providers is whether and to what degree an individual's cleft and associated mental health symptoms interfere with their adaptive functioning, or ability to meet individual, family, and community expectations (see Fig. 30.4). Poor or worsening functioning in daily activities is often an indicator of deteriorated health or mental health status, suggesting the child may benefit from additional supports or psychosocial interventions. Further, functional impairment domains often align more strongly with subjective family perceptions of salient problems than mental health symptoms. For example, a child may more likely be flagged for intervention if excessively truant from school than if exhibiting signs of low mood. Thus, screening for functional impairment can help determine service needs and identify specific targets for treatment.

A child's roles and expectations are contextually specific, shaped by a range of social-ecological factors pertinent to

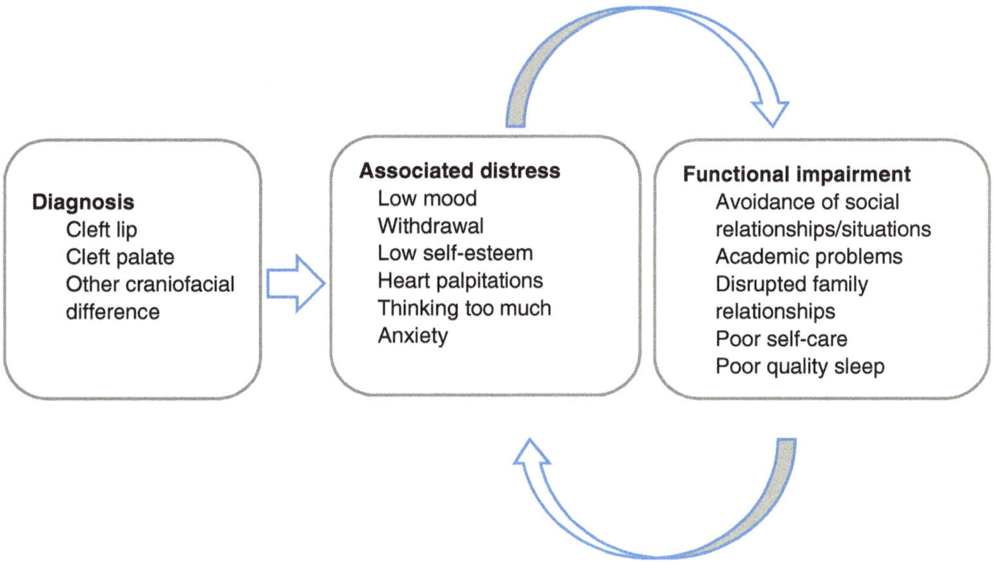


**Fig. 30.4** Signs of psychosocial distress in patients affected by cleft and related conditions

their ethnocultural experiences. Assessing for culturally relevant adaptive functioning domains can elucidate treatment targets salient to the population and activate culturally appropriate and accessible services. Studies of adaptive functioning in low- and middle-income countries identify overlapping functioning expectations with high-income countries but also culturally distinct domains and priorities, indicating measures developed in high-income countries may miss relevant information or require adaptation. Accordingly, a 10-year review of global and disorder-specific functional impairment measures [19] revealed most scales do not adequately address cultural context. Incorporating adaptive functioning and related impairment questions into screening procedures can assess for the impact of health and mental health conditions on child functioning and identify contextually salient and appropriate treatment targets and services.

## Psychosocial Support

It is natural for children and families to experience fears, worries, and anxieties about diagnosis, surgery and other medical procedures related to CL/P. These concerns can be eased by encouraging patients and families to develop effective coping skills by working with specially trained psychosocial clinicians where available.

A *pediatric psychologist* specializes in providing assessment, intervention, and consultation services to children who need support adjusting to a medical diagnosis, adhering to treatment recommendations, or making decisions about medical and surgical interventions. Pediatric psychologists can also provide support related to the trauma of an illness or procedure and help treat patients who are experiencing mental health issues such as anxiety and depression, social skills difficulties, or issues in family or school functioning associated with their medical condition and its treatment.

A *social worker*'s role is to offer support, information, and education to patients and families so they are appropriately connected to needed hospital and community resources. Social workers can answer questions about insurance, school access, employment and legal rights, and child advocacy and protection.

A certified *child life specialist* can prepare children and their families for medical experiences by explaining what will happen, and why, in terms a child can understand. Child life specialists can provide age-appropriate recreational, developmentally supportive, and therapeutic play activities to help children develop coping skills, facilitate expression of feelings, and support them through all stages of their healthcare experience. They can orient children to the hospital before an admission, use toys to demonstrate common medical interventions, and provide play experiences to help distract and support patients and their families during their medical care.

In medical settings without dedicated psychosocial support staff, physicians, nurses, and other clinical staff can work to provide valuable psychosocial support. Clinicians can meet with families to ensure they understand the nature of their child's condition and recommendations for treatment, as well as the risks and benefits of surgery and the alternatives to surgery when available. Clinicians can also help families to identify questions or concerns they may want to share with the medical team and discuss ways that the family can best prepare their child for surgery and recovery. Lastly, clinical staff can address any comorbid mental health concerns that may be affecting the patient or family's functioning at home and school or with their medical team and provide community-based referrals when available. (See Fig. 30.5.)

Among patients and families who are considering elective surgical procedures, the decision-making process can be complex. As children get older, and functioning is maximized, they may be eligible for surgical procedures that normalize or enhance their appearance. When possible, decisions about elective procedures should be made collaboratively, with input from the surgeon, parents, and child. Though

**Solutions from the Field: Patient and Family Support**

In treatment settings where staff are reliably available, the integration of social and support groups may be an important aspect of mental healthcare for patients and families. Providers may wish to consider adding formal programming, in which a clinician such as a nurse or physician leads group-based educational sessions about common treatments and provides an opportunity for families at the same stages of care to connect with each other. Alternatively, clinic staff can work to connect patients and families earlier in their care journey with families who have already been through similar procedures, so that the experienced families can share their experiences and give tips for coping. It is best when these ambassador families can receive some screening and instruction about the types of information to share to ensure it is safe and appropriate to the treatment plan. Lastly, providing informal opportunities for families to connect and socialize during their clinic visits can go a long way in decreasing feelings of stress and isolation. Shared meals, group play, and simple introductions between families may help create supportive connections that last beyond their clinical visit.

| School performance | Mental health symptoms | Adaptive functioning | Functional impairment |
|---|---|---|---|
| What is your child's school and classroom setting?<br><br>Is your child performing below, at, or above grade level?<br><br>Does your child have any formal learning supports?<br>What supports are included?<br>Are supports sufficient in supporting learning needs? | What problems has your child faced related to their cleft?<br><br>Any concerns for your child with...<br>• Sadness<br>• Anger<br>• Attention or focus<br>• Anxiety or worry<br>• Fearfulness<br>• Stomach /headaches | What does your child do to take care of him/herself?<br><br>What activities is your child involved in?<br><br>Does your child participate in religious ceremonies (attending services, praying)?<br><br>What does your child do to help the family?<br><br>What does your child do to help the community? | In the past month, has your child had any difficulties with:<br>• Taking care of their body<br>• Friends<br>• Doing well in school<br>• Sleeping<br>• Praying<br>• Helping the family<br>• Helping the community |

**Fig. 30.5** Psychosocial screening questions

many older children and adolescents want to be involved in the decision-making process, it is common for patients who have undergone many surgeries to feel "burnout" and to decline beneficial surgeries. Adolescents in particular are likely to make decisions based on the short-term without carefully considering long-term benefits. Psychosocial clinicians can work with patients and their treatment team to facilitate communication about the current and future benefits of a surgical operation, addressing the patient's fears and concerns, and helping patients weigh the risks and benefits of pursuing elective procedures.

Childhood and adolescence can be challenging for all children, and having a cleft condition requiring multiple medical and surgical procedures adds a unique stressor to an already difficult time. Ensuring the medical team is attending to the patient's and family's shifting psychosocial needs throughout the course of treatment will contribute to optimizing treatment outcomes and ultimately serve to enhance the patient's quality of life.

## Conclusions

Child and adolescent social, emotional, behavioral, and academic development in the context of CL/P is complex and is best supported by a multidisciplinary team of specialists and clinicians. Psychosocial support staff serve as critical team members trained in screening and treatment planning to improve quality of life, psychosocial and educational outcomes, and engagement with care for patients with CL/P. As such, careful consideration and integration of culturally sensitive psychosocial assessment and treatment recommendations work to make a child's cleft care as comprehensive, effective, and supportive as possible.

## References


1. Stock NM, Feragen KB. Psychological adjustment to cleft lip and/or palate: a narrative review of the literature. Psychol Health. 2016;31:777.
2. Rumsey N, Harcourt D. Body image and disfigurement: issues and interventions. Body Image. 2004;1:83.
3. Pope AW, Tillman K, Snyder HT. Parenting stress in infancy and psychosocial adjustment in toddlerhood: a longitudinal study of children with craniofacial anomalies. Cleft Palate Craniofac J. 2005;42:556.
4. Speltz ML, Endriga MC, Fisher PA, Mason CA. Early predictors of attachment in infants with cleft lip and/or palate. Child Dev. 1997;68:12.
5. Byrnes AL, Berk NW, Cooper ME, Marazita ML. Parental evaluation of informing interviews for cleft lip and/or palate. Pediatrics. 2003;112:308.
6. Richman LC, McCoy TE, Conrad AL, Nopoulos PC. Neuropsychological, behavioral, and academic sequelae of cleft: early developmental, school age, and adolescent/young adult outcomes. Cleft Palate Craniofac J. 2012;49:387.
7. Conrad AL, Richman L, Nopoulos P, Dailey S. Neuropsychological functioning in children with non-syndromic cleft of the lip and/or palate. Child Neuropsychol. 2009;15:471.
8. Pinquart M. Systematic review: bullying involvement of children with and without chronic physical illness and/or physical/sensory disability-a meta-analytic comparison with healthy/nondisabled peers. J Pediatr Psychol. 2017;42:245.
9. Semb G, Brattström V, Mølsted K, Prahl-Andersen B, Zuurbier P, Rumsey N, et al. The Eurocleft study: Intercenter study of treatment outcome in patients with complete cleft lip and palate. Part 4: relationship among treatment outcome, patient/parent satisfaction, and the burden of care. Cleft Palate Craniofac J. 2005;42:83.

10. Clarke A, Thompson A, Jenkinson E, Rumsey N, Newell R. A stepped-care approach to psychosocial intervention. In: CBT for appearance anxiety. Malden: Wiley; 2013.
11. Centers for Disease Control and Prevention. Concept|HRQOL|CDC: CDC; 2016. https://www.cdc.gov/hrqol/index.htm
12. Klassen AF, Riff KWYW, Longmire NM, Albert A, Allen GC, Aydin MA, et al. Psychometric findings and normative values for the CLEFT-Q based on 2434 children and young adult patients with cleft lip and/or palate from 12 countries. CMAJ. 2018;190:E455.
13. Kazak AE, Prusak A, McSherry M, Simms S, Beele D, Rourke M, et al. The psychosocial assessment tool (PAT)©: pilot data on a brief screening instrument for identifying high risk families in pediatric oncology. Fam Syst Health. 2001;19:303.
14. Crerand CE, Kapa HM, Litteral J, Pearson GD, Eastman K, Kirschner RE. Identifying psychosocial risk factors among families of children with craniofacial conditions: validation of the psychosocial assessment tool–craniofacial version. Cleft Palate Craniofac J. 2018;55:536.
15. Kazak AE. Pediatric psychosocial preventative health model (PPPHM): research, practice, and collaboration in pediatric family systems medicine. Fam Syst Health. 2006;24:381.
16. Hinton DE, Lewis-Fernández R. Idioms of distress among trauma survivors: subtypes and clinical utility. Cult Med Psychiatry. 2010;34:209.
17. Kaiser BN, Haroz EE, Kohrt BA, Bolton PA, Bass JK, Hinton DE. "Thinking too much": a systematic review of a common idiom of distress. Soc Sci Med. 2015;147:170.
18. Goodman R. The strengths and difficulties questionnaire: a research note. J Child Psychol Psychiatry. 1997;38(5):581–6.
19. Winters NC, Collett BR, Myers KM. Ten-year review of rating scales, VII: scales assessing functional impairment. J Am Acad Child Adolesc Psychiatry. 2005;44:309.

# Optimizing Postoperative Pediatric and Nursing Care

# 31

Florence C. Kuyt and Emmanuella Amoako

**Key Points**

- Vigilant postoperative care is essential to patient safety and impacts outcomes of surgical treatment.
- Team dynamics should aim to facilitate good communication among physicians and nurses, local hospital staff, and visiting medical providers.
- The ward should be equipped, and staff prepared, for postoperative conditions common after cleft surgery: bleeding, airway difficulties, pain management, and feeding promotion.
- Discharge planning is most effective when it is tailored to specific patient needs (distance to travel, specific risk factors), maximizes chance of a good surgical outcome, and promotes follow-up, and the family understands and agrees with the plan.

## Introduction

Postoperative care of patients and their compliance with instructions after cleft surgeries are important contributors to the outcomes of the procedures.

Setting up a ward that facilitates an acceptable standard of care in countries with low resources can be challenging. Yet, with well-defined goals, organization, common sense, a bit of creativity, and flexibility, the team can provide excellent care and meet safety standards.

Patient safety is the ultimate goal and should never be compromised.

Challenges are severalfold:

1. *Location and facilities*: While some sites might be able to offer well-appointed hospitals, often the ward space provided is crowded and noisy and lacking necessary supplies. Laboratory tests, imaging studies, intensive care, and running water are often unavailable, and electricity can be sporadic.
2. *Staff*: Not every care provider has advanced training or has been encouraged to question and take initiative. With good guidance, teaching, integration of everybody's skills and expertise, and understanding of the local culture, postoperative staffs can form a cohesive team and provide excellent care.
3. *Patients*: Many patients and their families have had limited exposure to modern medical care, sometimes not even to plumbing and hygiene. Entrusting the care of a family member to strangers, sometimes from a different culture or faith, can be stressful.

**COVID-19 Pandemic Special Considerations**

Although patients and staff should have been prescreened, possibility of infection or exposure during hospitalization remain

- Check current recommendations for safe elective surgeries using sources such as for example WHO, CDC, and Johns Hopkins [1–3]
- Know your in-country Health Ministry and local recommendations, and incidence and prevalence of COVID-19
- Confirm availability of COVID-19 testing and treatment centers

**Electronic Supplementary Material** The online version of this chapter (https://doi.org/10.1007/978-3-030-59105-2_31) contains supplementary material, which is available to authorized users.

F. C. Kuyt (✉)
Neonatologist, Children's Hospital Oakland Pediatric, California, USA

Clinical Specialty Advisor, Operation Smile's Medical Council, Virginia Beach, VA, USA

E. Amoako
Pediatrician, Cape Coast Teaching Hospital, Cape Coast, Ghana

Part-time lecturer, School of Medical Sciences, University of Cape Coast, Cape Coast, Ghana

© Springer Nature Switzerland AG 2021

J. W. Swanson, D. W. Low (eds.), *Global Cleft Care in Low-Resource Settings*, https://doi.org/10.1007/978-3-030-59105-2_31

- Implement strict adherence to distancing, hand washing and masks, and keep areas well aerated
- Implement strict protocol for evaluation, isolation and treatment referral
- Have a designated isolation room, PPE, surgical and N95 masks
- Avoid aerosol-producing procedures, but if necessary, follow safety protocols
- Avoid aerosolizing procedures, use MDI bronchodilators rather than nebulizers
- Practice Distancing, Good Hygiene, and wear a Mask

This chapter is a guide to:

1. Evaluate the ward and equip it with the essentials for a safe outcome.
2. Provide guidelines for care of patients.
3. Evaluate and manage common postoperative complications.
4. Educate patients in discharge instructions.

## Ward Assessment and Setup

Evaluating the conditions on the ward systematically is imperative. Conditions vary from modern, well-designed units with all amenities to bare-bone spaces. A walk-through with an eye to logical placement of a nursing station, medication and supply storage, an emergency area, and access to bathrooms will help determine the needs and the most practical layout (Fig. 31.1).

Never assume good function; test everything:

- Each light and plug should be checked carefully and power failures anticipated.
- Each piece of equipment should be tested for proper function.
- Wall oxygen outlets do not mean supply.
- Faucets and sinks do not mean water supply or drainage.
- Beds and bedding might be inadequate.
- Clear signage is helpful.

Safety and hygiene should never be compromised. Hand sanitizer and gloves must be available, as blood-borne diseases like HIV and hepatitis are common. PPE (Personal Protective Equipment) needs to be available to deal with the additional risks of transmission for organisms like COVID-19.

**Field Solutions**
- Headlamps and flashlights
- Solar power and solar lights
- Multi-plug extension cords

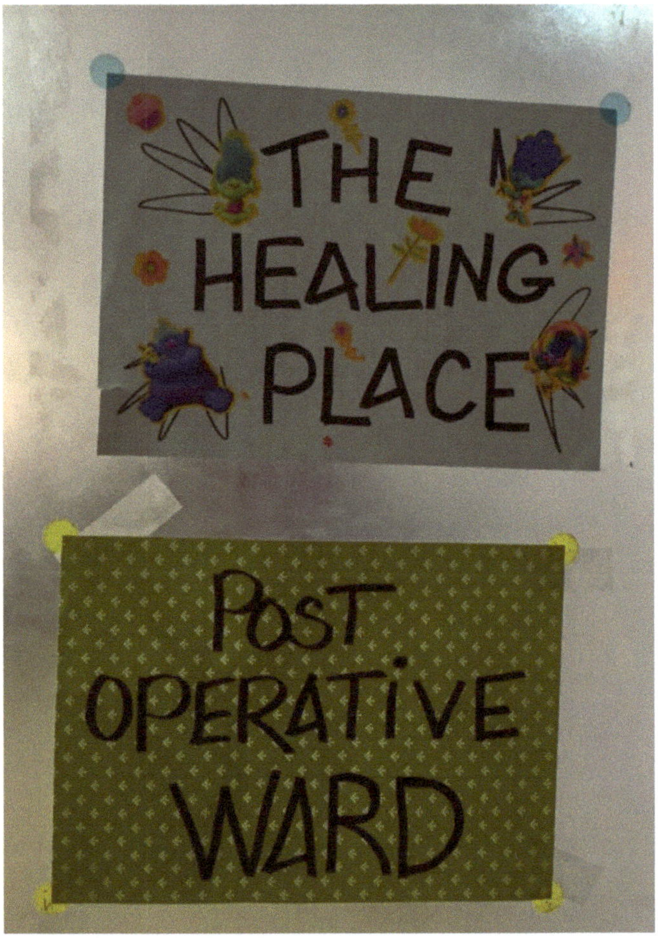


Fig. 31.1 Welcome! (Photo courtesy of J Kesselman RN)

- Oxygen tank and regulator
- Extra-large pails to store and dispose of water
- Water stations with purified water for hand washing and drinking
- Co-bedding of patients or mats on the floor to increase patient capacity, if culturally acceptable and infectious situation permits
- Empty water bottles for needle disposal
- Large labeled garbage bags for contaminated material
- Small bags taped to cart or bed for garbage
- Improvised barriers to shield patients from drafts or excessive heat

Making the setting welcoming and friendly also plays an important role. Decorations, bubbles, art supplies, and child life activities can do marvels to decrease stress in the pediatric population.

Translators must always be present (Table 31.1, Figs. 31.2, 31.3, and 31.4).

**Table 31.1** Suggested supplies to set up ward

| |
|---|
| Crash box with meds and supplies (PALS/ALS guidelines) and difficult airway box |
| Biomedical supplies |
| Adapters and extension cords |
| Monitor, leads, and probe for $O_2$ saturation (skin electrode pads) |
| Dinamap/blood pressure cuff |
| Suction machine |
| Defibrillator |
| Fans/heater |
| Medications (see Table 31.4) and medicine cups |
| $O_2$ tank and regulators (check if the tank is full) |
| Bag-valve-mask |
| Masks of all sizes, nasal trumpets, and oral airways |
| $O_2$ tubing, $O_2$ masks, and nebulizer masks |
| Suction catheters and Yankauer and suction tubing |
| Difficult airway supplies |
| Gloves, sanitizer, alcohol swabs, surgical and N95 masks, PPE |
| Tongue blades |
| Gauze 2x2 and 4x4, Q-tips |
| Tape |
| IV boards and No-No's to limit flexion and touching surgical site |
| IV catheters, IV tubing with microdrip or volume chamber, IV poles |
| Tourniquet |
| Needles, syringes 3 cc or 5 cc for flush, syringes 10 cc or 20 cc for feeding |
| NS flushes (or NS bag) |
| LR and NS bags, D5 1/2NS if available |
| Scissors |
| Garbage bags |
| Needle disposal container |
| Thermometers, stethoscope, pulse ox |
| Ice packs |
| Wire cutters |
| Hand soap, toilet paper, paper towels |
| Water and juice (or powdered sugar drink, non-acidic, not red or purple) |
| Bottles/containers for juices for patients, cups |
| Beds (or mats), bed sheets/blankets |
| Mirror |
| Mosquito nets |
| Chairs |
| Patient gowns and name bracelets |
| Diapers |
| Charts, markers, labels |
| Flashlights, headlamps |

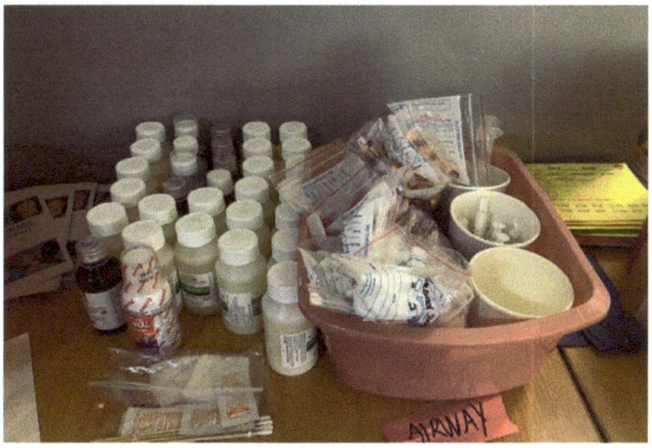


**Fig. 31.2** Supplies. (Photo courtesy of J Kesselman RN)

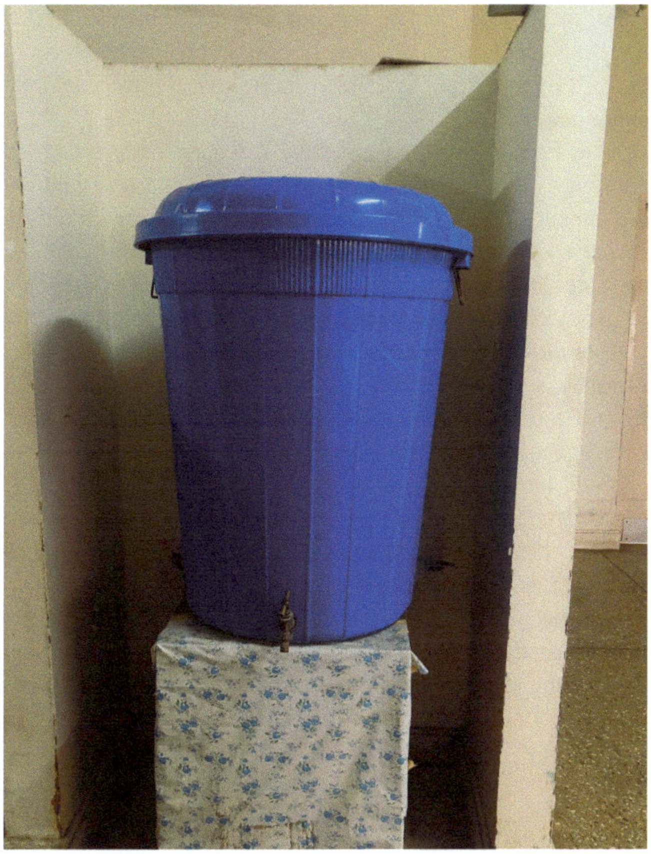

**Fig. 31.3** Water pail

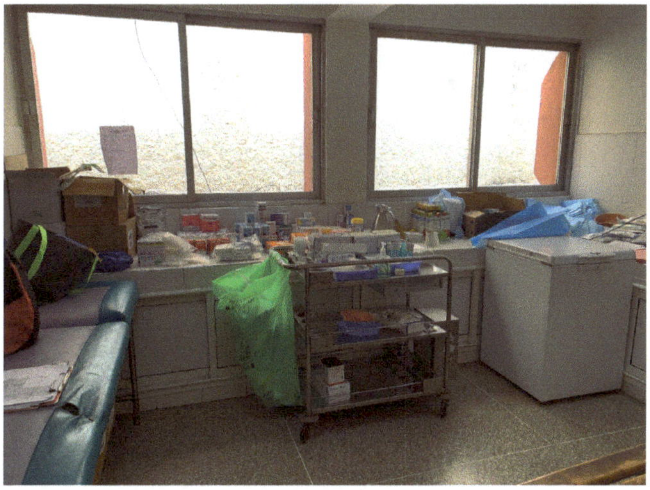

**Fig. 31.4** Supply room setup

## Emergency Preparation

Patient safety from admission until discharge is imperative.

Organization saves lives. A separate and well-maintained emergency area with organized and labeled supplies should be set up, where all possible anticipated complications can be addressed. Supplies should be laid out and ready to use. The emergency box should be stocked with recommended PALS and ALS medications and supplies. Additional isolation room and PPE must be available during dangerous epidemic situations.

The team members must have a leader, have access to emergency supplies, and know how to operate resuscitation equipment. A safety session with the entire team should be rehearsed prior to admitting the first patient, to familiarize the staff with the location and use of the resuscitation equipment.

A rapid communication system with the operating room staff or on-call team needs to be well delineated, especially if distance, stairs, or separate buildings are involved. The location of a more acute level of care should be known, and a contingency plan for transfer should be in place, whether to hospital intensive care or to another facility. The identity of the charge person and the responsibilities for each team member should be clear, and each member should feel comfortable raising concerns and asking questions. A call system should be instituted to identify a core team, including surgeon, anesthesiologist, and nurse, in the event a surgical emergency occurs when the full team is not on site (Table 31.2, Figs. 31.5, 31.6, and 31.7).

**Table 31.2** Emergency supplies

| |
|---|
| Crash box with PALS/ALS medications and supplies |
| Difficult airway box |
| Bed with sufficient lighting and electrical access |
| Oxygen source with regulator, humidifier, tubing. Secure the tank! |
| Bag-valve-mask, all size masks, nebulizer mask |
| Bronchodilators and racemic epinephrine or epinephrine |
| Airways (oral and nasal) |
| Pressure applicator: gauze, black tea bag, Afrin (oxymetazoline), Tongue blade |
| Gloves |
| IV (intravenous) supplies, IV catheters, intra-osseous needle |
| PPE, surgical and N95 masks |

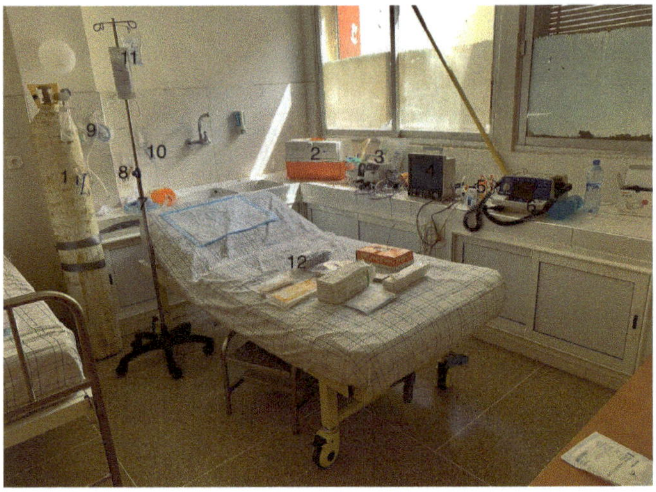


**Fig. 31.5** ER setup with numbered items (1). $O_2$ tank and regulator with oxygen tubing and mask, secured to wall (2). Emergency crash box (3). Suction machine with catheters (4). Monitor with pulse oximeter (5). Nebulizer with bronchodilator (6). Defibrillator (7). Bag-valve-mask all sizes (8). Compression pack and Afrin (9). Face masks all sizes (10). Respiratory meds: albuterol, racemic epinephrine (11). IV pole and IV start supplies (12). Miscellaneous supplies: gauze, gloves, alcohol swabs, sanitizer

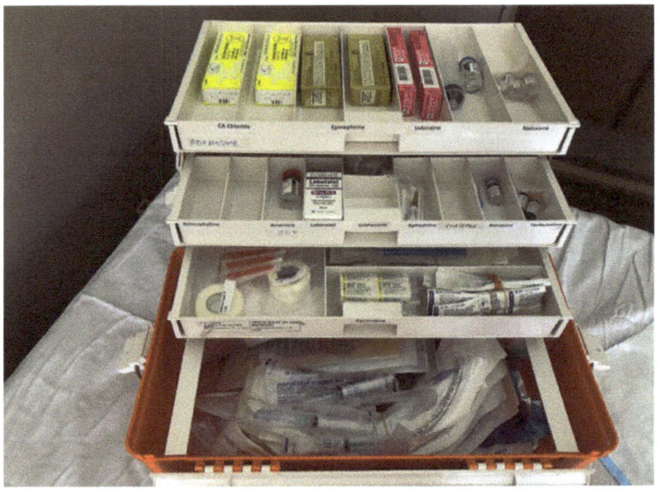

**Fig. 31.6** Emergency medication box. (Photo courtesy of J Kesselman RN)

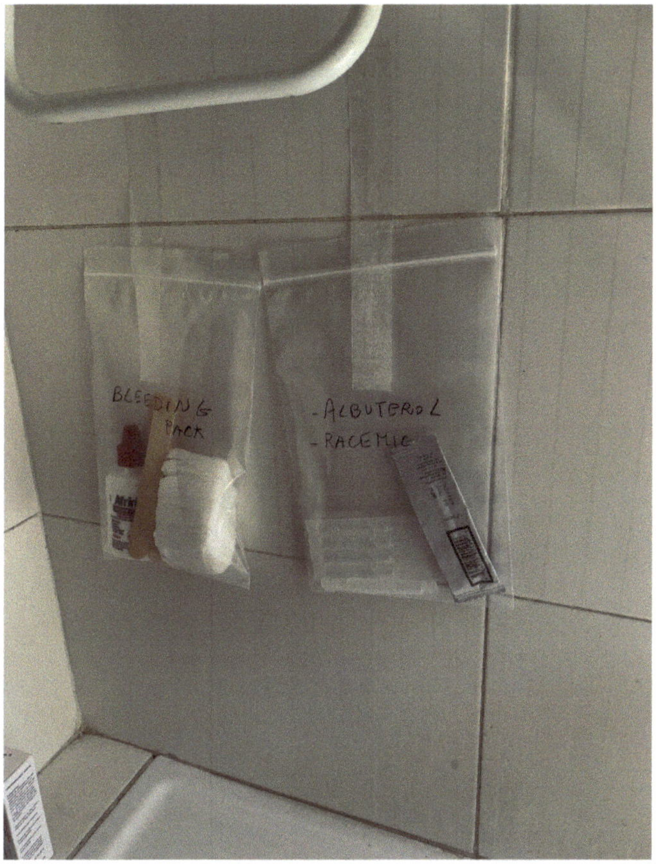


**Fig. 31.7** Bleeding and breathing kits. *Bleeding kit with tongue blades, gauze, and Afrin (oxymetazoline). Respiratory kit with unit doses of racemic epinephrine and albuterol*

**Tips and Tricks**

- Local SIM cards or walkie-talkies can help communication.
- A Gurney or wheelchair must be available on ward for rapid transport to emergency room setup or operating room.
- Access to the emergency room (ER) setup must be immediate: there is no time to look for a key!
- Prepare easily accessible bleeding kits in advance, with tongue blades, gauze, tea bags, and oxymetazoline.
- Prepare easily accessible breathing kits with bronchodilators, racemic epinephrine, mask, or spacer.

**Table 31.3** Assessment on admission to ward

| | |
|---|---|
| Level of consciousness | Alertness level, orientation, agitation |
| Respiratory status | Respiratory rate, ease of breathing, color, obstruction, stridor, or abnormal respiration<br>Pulse oximetry |
| Hemodynamic status | Skin turgor, mucous membranes wetness, capillary refill time, heart rate, blood pressure |
| Surgery site | Nose: patency, stents, or packing<br>Mouth: lip, tongue stitch, packing, teeth extraction, palate, graft site, orthodontics, wires<br>Mandible, donor graft sites, wound (dry, swollen, bruised, sutures, surgical glue, steristrips) |
| Intravenous line | Patency, security, necessity |
| Positioning | Decubitus, head elevation to avoid pooling of blood or secretions in back of throat or swallowing<br>Head of bed elevation at 45 degrees for ABG and orthognathics<br>In parent's arms<br>Prone position might be best for micrognathic patients |
| Limb restriction | Restriction of limbs in infants and toddlers to avoid touching the face and mouth |
| Pain level | Evaluate all patients "3 years and over" using 0–10 scale or the FACES pictogram<br>Elevated heart rate and/or blood pressure can indicate pain<br>Irritability (can also be caused by hot or cold weather, hunger or thirst, emergence of anesthesia) Fig. 31.8 |

## Patient Assessment on Admission

### Evaluation and Examination

Systematic assessment is paramount to safe recovery, in the recovery room and on the ward. The anesthesiologist should summarize the intraoperative course and specific issues detected.

Unless the ward is well staffed and equipped, keeping the patients in the recovery area until stable and on room air is advisable. Oxygen is rarely available for transport. Always know the backups available for more intensive care needs. Surgical notes and anesthesia records should be carefully reviewed for essential information about the procedure, intraoperative medications, types of blocks and anesthesia, and cardiorespiratory stability and complications (Table 31.3, Fig. 31.9).

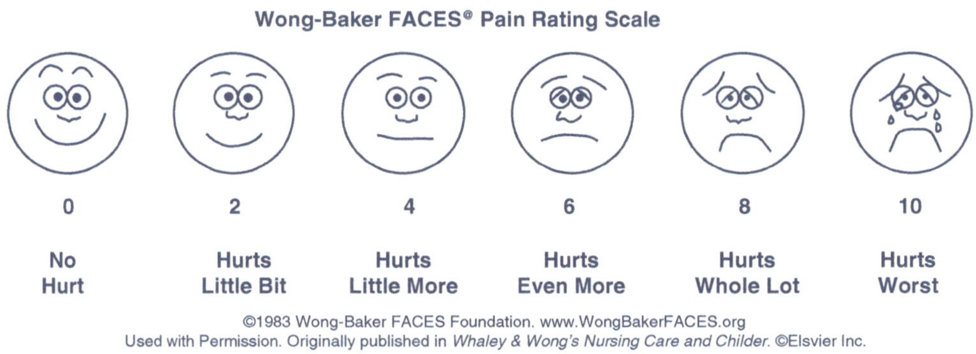


**Fig. 31.8** FACES scale

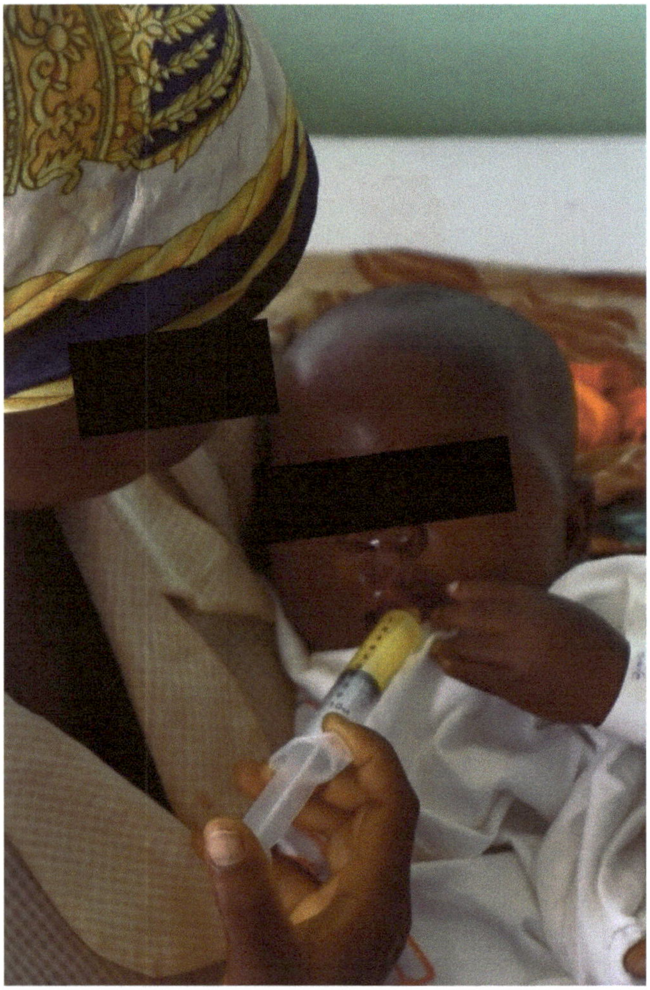

**Fig. 31.9** Cleft lip patient in mother's arms, syringe feeding. *Well-positioned bilateral cleft lip surgery patient syringe feeding in mother's arms*

**Tips and Tricks**

- Place sicker patients closest to the emergency area.
- Place patients with same surgeries in the same area to facilitate rounds and teaching.
- Post a master schedule with location of each patient's room, and/or mark each room door with the patients' names or numbers.

## Fluids

**Tips for the Field: Evaluating Mucous Membranes**

Oral mucous membranes might appear to have a whitish coating. Differential diagnosis would be:

- Desquamation or sloughing secondary to the vasoconstriction of the local anesthetics (most likely diagnosis).
- Milk coating, which would easily scrape off with a tongue blade.
- Thrush (oral candidiasis): usually more widespread and can involve the tongue. It requires treatment with topical antifungals.

The majority of the patients can be encouraged to advance to oral fluids rapidly, in accordance with the guidelines for their procedure. Clear liquids via a syringe or cup or breastfeeding can be started in recovery. Monitoring of intake and evaluation of mucosa, tearing, turgor, and urine output need to be part of every assessment.

Many considerations are important when assessing the need for maintaining an intravenous line:

1. Ability of the patient to handle oral hydration
2. Risk of bleeding requiring immediate IV access
3. Insensible losses: climate, temperature of the patient
4. Safety of the IV (intravenous) setup:
   - Is there a volutrol chamber or microdrip to protect accidental fluid overload of small infants?
   - Is the staff able to provide safe IV line management, sterile technique, and IV medication dilution and administration?
   - Is the bottle shatterproof?
5. Possibility of saline-locking if IV might be needed later
6. Intravenous solutions: For long-term maintenance hydration, are glucose-containing fluids like D5 1/2NS available?

Field Solutions

If only normal saline (NS) is available and prolonged IV fluid infusion is needed, consider infusing simultaneously NS and D10W or D5 water at the same rate to make D5 1/2NS or D2.5 1/2NS to provide some glucose and decrease sodium intake.

Cold, diluted non-acidic juices are liked best.

Pediatric IV rate maintenance 4-2-1 rule:

- 4 ml/kg/h for first 10 kg
- +2 ml/kg/h for 10–20 kg
- +1 ml/kg/h for >20 kg
- Bolus = 20 ml/kg LR or NS
- In the absence of IV pumps, consider ordering the amount to be infused over 6 or 12 hours.

Drip infusion:

- The drop factor is printed on the IV tubing, and represents the number of drops that = 1ml
- How to calculate the number of drops per minute needed to deliver the amount ordered:

Desired Volume x Drop Factor/60
= # drops/min to infuse

## Medications and Blocks

Be aware of patient's past allergies. Review medication complications and side effects (Fig. 31.10, Table 31.4).

1. *Pain*

Before treating for pain, assess whether the patient's agitation and confusion might be from anesthesia emergence rather than pain. Involving a parent can provide a reassuring environment.

(a) *Blocks*: Ideally, all patients will have received local infiltrations and long-lasting nerve blocks. Bupivacaine can confer 12–24 hours of relief. Infraorbital blocks provide good numbing to lips and anterior mouth; suprazygomatic blocks are effective for the posterior palate [4]. Blocks can leave visible puncture marks and bruising, but placement should be confirmed by anesthetic and surgical records.

(b) *Acetaminophen and NSAIDs*. Acetaminophen (paracetamol) and ibuprofen are the safest to manage pain on the wards. Paracetamol remains the medication of choice in palate surgery mostly because of concern that impaired platelet aggregation can result from nonsteroidal anti-inflammatories (NSAIDs) [5]. Keeping patients on medication around the clock for the first 24 hours helps avoid breakthrough pain. NSAIDs can be added in stable patients with uncontrolled pain. If needed, those two medications can be used in alternation every 3 hours to maximize pain control. Paracetamol and ketorolac can be given intravenously.

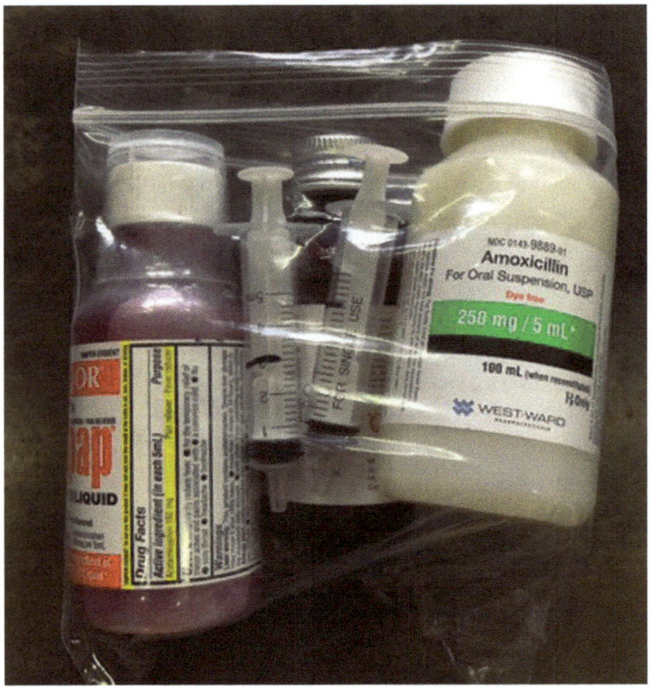


**Fig. 31.10** Discharge medication packet. (Photo courtesy of J Kesselman RN). Meds with labeled syringes for dosing. In addition, these should be labeled with patient's name, dose, and timing

**Table 31.4** Medications frequently used on the ward

| |
|---|
| Amoxicillin or amoxicillin-clavulanate |
| Acetaminophen liquid and pills |
| Ibuprofen liquid and pills |
| Albuterol/salbutamol: unit doses, solution, or inhaler |
| Racemic epinephrine or epinephrine 1:1000 |
| Afrin nasal spray (oxymetazoline) |
| Ondansetron (the IV solution can be given orally) |
| Dexamethasone (the IV solution can be given orally) |
| Antibiotic ointment |
| Oral rehydration packets |
| Cefazolin |

(c) *Ice*: After orthognathic surgery and alveolar bone grafts, ice packs 20 minutes on/20 minutes off for the first 24–48 hours reduce swelling and can reduce pain.

(d) *Opiates*, especially codeine and tramadol, have variable metabolism in children and should be avoided in a ward setting, because of possible respiratory depression [6, 7]. Well-trained staff can administer intravenous pain medication or sedatives in a PACU/recovery room. Nalbuphine is a mixed agonist/antagonist opioid stimulator, which has fewer side effects than morphine at same levels of pain relief [8]. Reversal medications should always be available.

**Tips and Tricks for Comfort**

- Parental/family involvement
- Normalizing environment with own clothes/ blanket
- Distraction
- Drink/food
- Medication
- Fans

**Doses**

*Acetaminophen/paracetamol*

Kids:

- Oral: 10–15 mg/kg/dose PO every 4–6 hours orally for up to 30 kg and max 5 doses max 75mg/kg/day.
- Suppositories: 25 mg/kg/dose but should be avoided because of erratic absorption. They melt in hot weather unless refrigeration is available. Avoid in older children and adults.
- IV: 12.5 mg/kg/dose over 10–15 minutes, max 75 mg/kg/day; use if >2 years old.

Adults:

- Oral: 500–1000 mg q4–6 hours, max 4 g/day
- IV: 625 mg q4 hours, max 3.75 g/day

*Ibuprofen*:

- Kids: 10 mg/kg orally every 6–8 hours, max 40 mg/kg/day
- Adults: 400–600 mg q6–8 hours

*Ketorolac*:

- Kids: 0.5 mg/kg/dose, max 15 mg IV q6

Adults: 30 mg IV q6

2. *Antibiotics*

All patients receive one prophylactic intravenous dose of antibiotic in the operating room. Conflict remains as to length of treatment, but the World Health Organization (WHO) recommends no further antibiotics beyond the first 24 hours after surgery, with the exception of orthognathics and alveolar bone grafts where a 7–10 days course might be standard [9]. The postoperative treatment remains the prerogative of the surgeons. Simple cleft lip patients do not require additional antibiotics. Surgeons mostly agree to 1–3 days of prophylactic coverage for cleft palates (amoxicillin 25 mg/kg/dose given BID). Conflicting studies exist on whether oral antibiotics decrease the incidence of oronasal fistula (ONF) [10–12]. Some studies suggest that placement of an antibiotic pack on the hard palate for 5 days decreases the incidence of ONF [13]. The most widely used antibiotics are amoxicillin or amoxicillin-clavulanate and clindamycin in cases of penicillin allergy. Purulent or perforated otitis, dental abscess, pneumonia, or cellulitis should be treated with their normal course.

**Field Questions**

- Is the treatment necessary? (Overuse of antibiotics contributes to increased resistance and superbugs.)
- Is refrigeration available for reconstituted suspension? Studies suggest amoxicillin/clavulanate degrades rapidly when stored at room temperature [14].
- Will the patient take the medication or possibly sell it?
- If asking the patient to buy the medication: Can they afford it? Is it readily available in pharmacies?

3. *Tranexamic Acid (TXA)*
   The antifibrinolytic TXA might be used when there is increased concern with bleeding. It is usually given intravenously for the first 12–24 hours [15]. Its topical use is also advocated.
4. *Oxymetazoline*
   Oxymetazoline is a selective α-adrenergic receptor agonist used as a topical decongestant. Its vasoconstriction reduces bleeding [16].
5. *Other Common Medications*
   High-caloric supplements, vitamins, iron, and folic acid are often needed but difficult to procure because of poor funding.
6. *Antiretrovirals*: Most patients diagnosed with HIV receive antiretrovirals through in-country public health programs. Being HIV positive is NOT a contraindication to surgery.
7. *Permethrin or Benzyl Benzoate*: Scabies and lice are common and cause major housekeeping and laundry issues for families that have no access to extra clothing, bedding, or laundry. They are never a contraindication to surgery. Patients should be treated prior to surgery and isolated to decrease risk of contamination to other patients and to staff.
8. *Medications for chronic conditions* need to be continued without interruption.

**Tips and Tricks**

- Use rounds to teach patients' families how to draw up medications appropriately. Doses and timing should be clearly labeled.
- Consider decreasing medication cost by drawing doses from one bottle for all patients, especially for patients who will be discharged without medications or who are expected to fill their own prescription.
- Consider giving anticipated discharge medicines to patients on admission with labeled doses and instructions, and use rounds to teach how to administer them.

## Nutrition

Proper nutrition is undeniably linked to better healing, improved immunity, and decreased infection rates [17, 18]. Many patients come with various degrees of malnutrition, vitamin deficiencies, and anemia but will benefit from surgical repair. Delivering good nutrition can be a challenge, both because of poverty and access issues and feeding difficulties from the maxillofacial anomalies and the special diets required after surgery. Maintenance of breastfeeding is extremely important. Breast milk provides the best, safest, and cheapest nutrition. Teaching families how to prepare nutritious liquid and soft diets with staple ingredients (with and without blenders) helps compliance. Multivitamins, iron, folic acid, RUTF (ready-to-use therapeutic food), and zinc, if obtainable, are beneficial.

**Tips and Tricks**

- Know the local staples and which protein-rich foods and dairy products are available.
- Teach how to make nutritious soups and pureed food.

## Charting and Rounds

Every healthcare center has its own medical record rules. Paper charts will likely be the norm. Preformatted forms facilitate the recording process. Unless the patient is unstable, checking vital signs every 4 hours is adequate. Anomalies must be assessed and intervention and outcomes recorded.

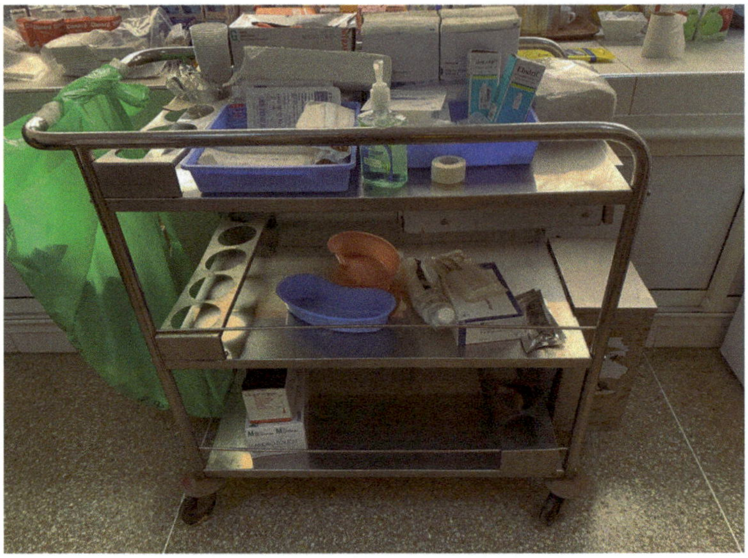

**Fig. 31.11** Cart for rounds

**Table 31.5** Example of bedside information card

| | | | | | | |
|---|---|---|---|---|---|---|
| NAME ______ MR# ______ | | | | | | |
| SURGEON: | | | | | | |
| Age: | M/F | Wt: | Allergies: | | | |
| CL | CP | Fistula | Others: | | | |
| Surgical glue | Y/N | Discharge teaching ☐ | | | | |
| Antibiotic – POD 1: (dose/time:________) | ☐ | ☐ | ☐ | ☐ | | |
| POD 2: | ☐ | ☐ | ☐ | ☐ | | |
| Acetaminophen – POD 1: (dose/time:________) | ☐ | ☐ | ☐ | ☐ | ☐ | ☐ |
| POD 2: | ☐ | ☐ | ☐ | ☐ | ☐ | ☐ |
| Ibuprofen – POD 1: (dose/time:________) | ☐ | ☐ | ☐ | ☐ | | |
| POD 2: | ☐ | ☐ | ☐ | ☐ | | |
| VS/q4 hours – POD 1: | 12 PM | 4 PM | 8 PM | 12 AM | 4 AM | 8 AM |
| POD 2: | 12 PM | 4 PM | 8 PM | 12 AM | 4 AM | 8 AM |
| Pain scores: Q4hrs: 0–10 | | | | | | |
| Consider tracking in and out | | | | | | |
| Mark specific issue (e.g., stridor, bleeding) | | | | | | |

**Tips and Tricks** (Table 31.5)
A bedside card permits assessment at a glance of:

- When last vital signs were taken
- When medications were last given
- What specific concern needs to be monitored closely

**Field Solutions**
- A cart on wheels stocked with the equipment for care and medications makes rounds very efficient (Fig. 31.11).
- Timing patients on the same medication on same schedule makes rounds more efficient.
- Patient care rounds are a golden opportunity for involving the family, starting to model care, giving instructions, and teaching medication administration.

## Common Complications and Troubleshooting

### Bleeding

Postoperative bleeding is one of the most dreaded complications, but many cases can be handled without return to the OR.

**Examination**
- Localize the site of bleeding by dabbing gently or by rinsing and suctioning gently from the side, and assess whether dealing with oozing or brisk and continuous bleeding.
- Pink saliva, nose bleed, oozing from the lip, and bleeding from tooth extraction site are all common and normal.
- Note whether the blood is bright red or dark or clotted and if there is evidence of dehiscence.
- Emesis of old, dark, swallowed blood is quite common.

**Management**
- Apply pressure with gauze attached to a tongue blade or directly by a gloved hand for 10 minutes before re-examining (Fig. 31.12).
- Keep the patient calm.
- In case of intraoral rapid bright red blood loss, call surgeon immediately while applying pressure, placing an IV, and transferring the patient to the OR (Fig. 31.14).

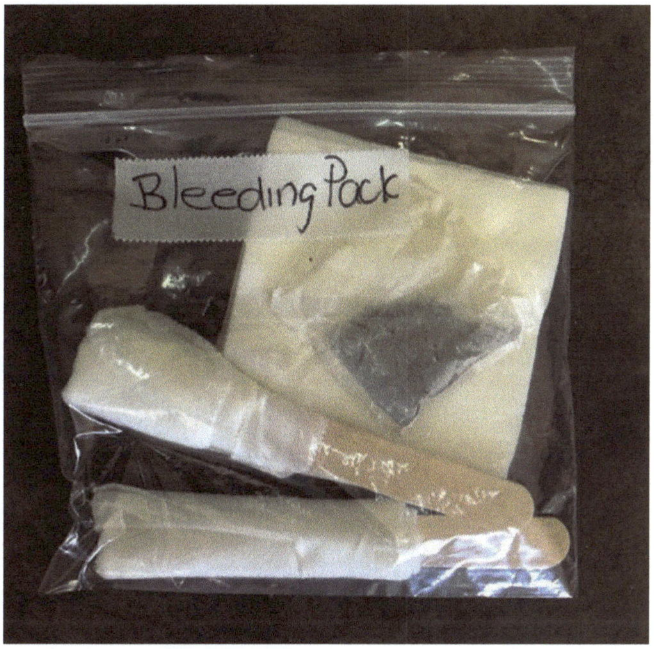


**Fig. 31.12** Kit for bleeding management. *Gauze around tongue blade, gauze, tea bag, Afrin (oxymetazoline) not shown.* (Photo courtesy of J Kesselman RN)

**Field Solutions**
- Moistened black tea bags in lieu of gauze have been reported to help with vasoconstriction [19].
- Oxymetazoline spray (Afrin) can be sprayed directly on the site or applied copiously to the gauze used for pressure. The vasoconstriction effect can last up to 12 hours and permits hemostasis for slow bleeding [16].
- It is important to prevent aspiration and swallowing large amounts of blood, which could lead to emesis by keeping the patient in a supine position.

**Algorithm 31.1: Bleeding Management**

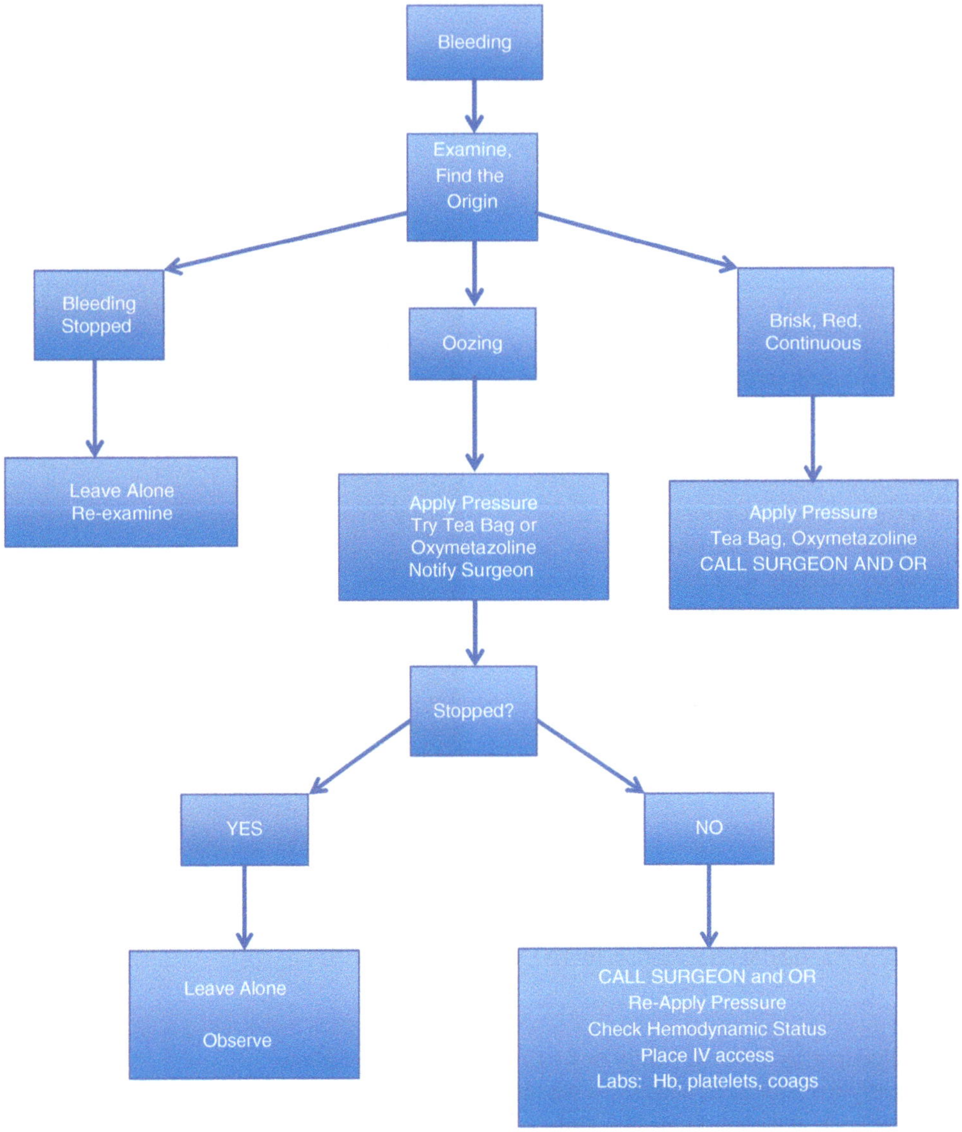


> **Tips and Tricks**
> - In case of persistent bleeding without obvious cause, consider underlying bleeding disorder.

## Respiration

(Fig. 31.13)

(a) *Obstruction*

Obstructive breathing caused by the tongue or a floppy airway is common and is often resolved by repositioning (small neck roll, mandibular lift, decubitus or prone position) or by a nasal airway.

Nasal packing or congestion requires a patent oral airway.

Children with Pierre Robin sequence or micrognathia, or those who underwent a complete palate closure including soft palate, might require nasal airway and/or prone positioning.

Dexamethasone can be helpful to minimize tissue swelling.

Palatal flap dehiscence, detaching surgical packing, or forgotten throat pack also can cause distress. The surgeons should evaluate those immediately, as they will understand the postoperative anatomy best.

(b) *Stridor*

Stridor can be caused by airway edema from intubation and surgery. The harsh inspiratory sound and use of accessory muscles are diagnostic and not alleviated by repositioning alone. If the patient can maintain good saturation and air movement, then time, humidified air, and keeping calm might be sufficient. Nebulized racemic epinephrine and dexamethasone are helpful. Epinephrine can cause a rebound after 20 to 30 minutes. Continuous close monitoring is essential.

(c) *Wheezing and Reactive Airway*

Many patients are at risk of reactive airway disease:

- Young infants less than a year of age
- Patients recovering from an upper respiratory infection
- Patients with a past history of reactive airway or asthma
- Environmental factors such as open pit fires, pollution, and cigarettes

Inhaled anesthetics, like sevoflurane, and endotracheal intubation can be bronchial irritants. Nebulized bronchodilators are the treatment of choice. Steroids should be considered in severe cases. Increased wheezing after treatment might represent improved air movement (Figs. 31.14, and 31.15).

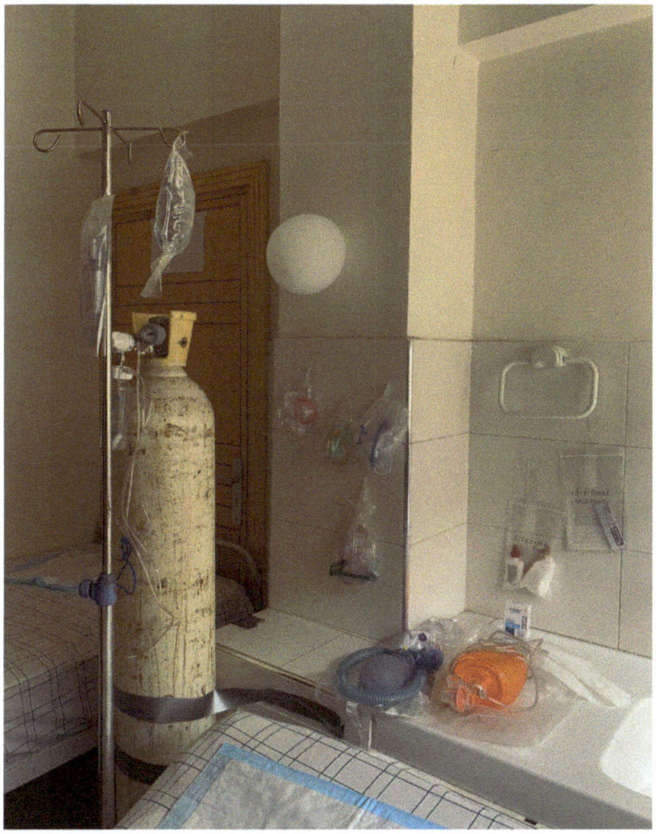

**Fig. 31.13** Respiratory management setup

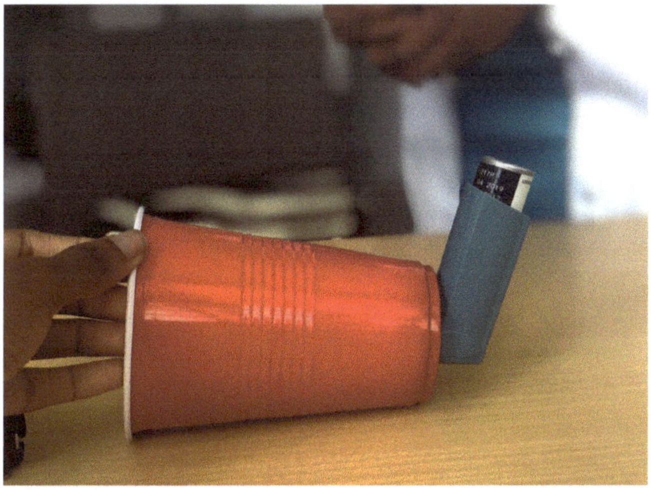

**Fig. 31.14** Spacer

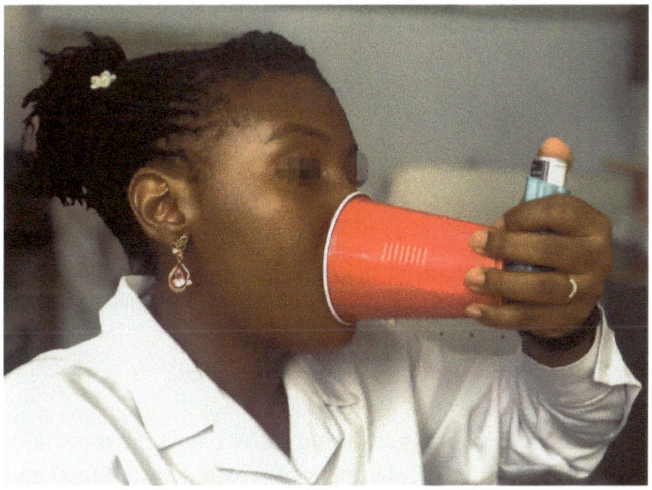

**Fig. 31.15** Spacer user (1). Make a hole at bottom of the cup to insert the mouth piece of the metered dose inhaler (2). Apply to face making tight seal if possible (3). Activate one puff and then breathe in very deeply and hold as long as possible (holding breath might be difficult for young children) (4). Repeat after 1 minute up to the number of puffs desired

**Field Solutions**

- When nebulized bronchodilators are not available, four to eight sequential puffs from a metered dose inhaler with spacer can provide good relief.
- When spacers are not available, one can be made easily with a cup or an empty plastic bottle.
- Critically assess whether dealing with wheezing or stridor or both.

## Dehydration and Vomiting

High ambient temperatures, fever, loss of IV access, or pain can contribute to fluid losses. Most patients do well taking small amounts of fluids frequently. Evaluating mucosa, tearing, perfusion, turgor, and urine output is essential.

Postoperative vomiting triggered by anesthetic drugs or blood in the stomach is common. Ruling out gastroenteritis is important.

Oral rehydration with electrolyte solution is an option, but in more severe cases, 10–20 ml/kg of lactate of Ringer (LR) or normal saline (NS) bolus should be administered and repeated as necessary.

**Tips for the Field**

- Ondansetron IV or orally (PO) for severe nausea or vomiting.
- Compazine suppositories and metoclopramide are less effective alternatives.
- Dexamethasone (often given intraoperatively) is also a good anti-emetic.

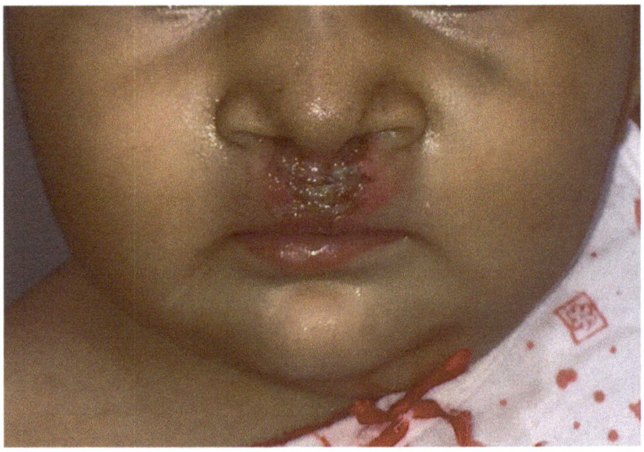

**Fig. 31.16** Cleft lip repair infection leading to dehiscence. (Photo courtesy of Dr. Swanson. Notice the cellulitis, mild swelling, and crusty exudates)

## Fever and Infection

Fever within the first 24 hours occurs commonly, is usually benign, but remains a diagnosis of exclusion requiring evaluation (Figs. 31.16 and 31.17) [20].

- *COVID-19*
  Needs to be considered during active pandemic especially if fever, dry cough, shortness of breath, loss of smell and taste, diarrhea, nausea and vomiting, unusual rashes, muscles soreness, new confusion, exposure to COVID-19 positive person.
- Wound infections
  Redness and possible cellulitis, drainage of cloudy fluid, abscess formation, or wound dehiscence can signify infection.
- Infections endemic to the area
  Clinicians should have a high degree of suspicion for diseases endemic to the area. Malaria has a high morbidity and mortality rate in children less than 5 years of age and should be diagnosed immediately. Primary malaria or relapse sec- ondary to the stress of surgery can occur in previously well patients and may present with fever, chills, rigor, headache, and malaise or vomiting. Always be aware of the local pathogens, like dengue fever, chikungunya, or encephalitis.
- Common community-acquired infections Infectious disease outbreaks can spread rapidly, including those linked to lack of vaccines, gastroenteritis, and other viral illnesses.

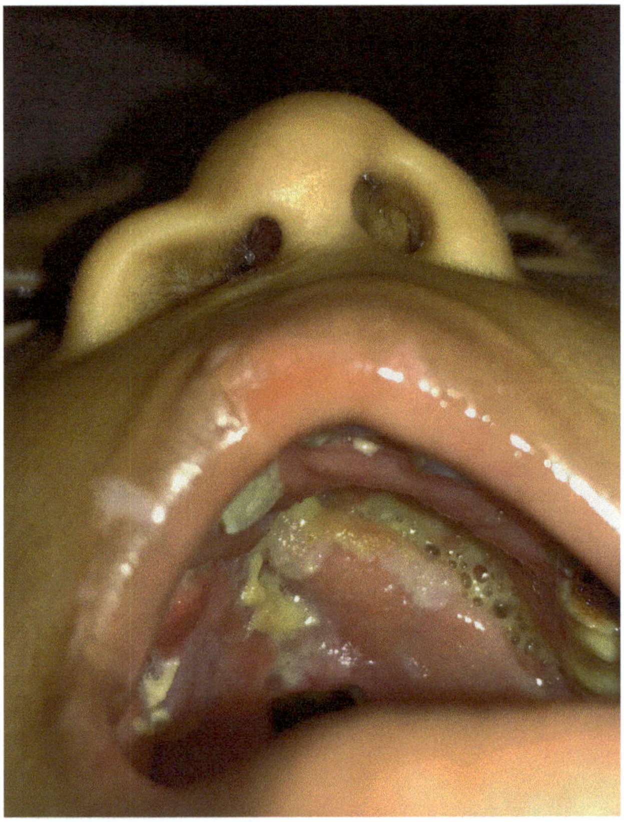

**Fig. 31.17** Postoperative palatal infection with risk of dehiscence. (Photo courtesy of Dr. Swanson)

- Otitis is common in patients with maxillofacial anomalies [21].
- Osteomyelitis can occur after orthognathic surgery.
- *Non-infectious fevers*: Overdressing, high environmental temperature, as well as dehydration can cause temperature elevation. Surgery can trigger inflammation and release of cytokines and cause fever.

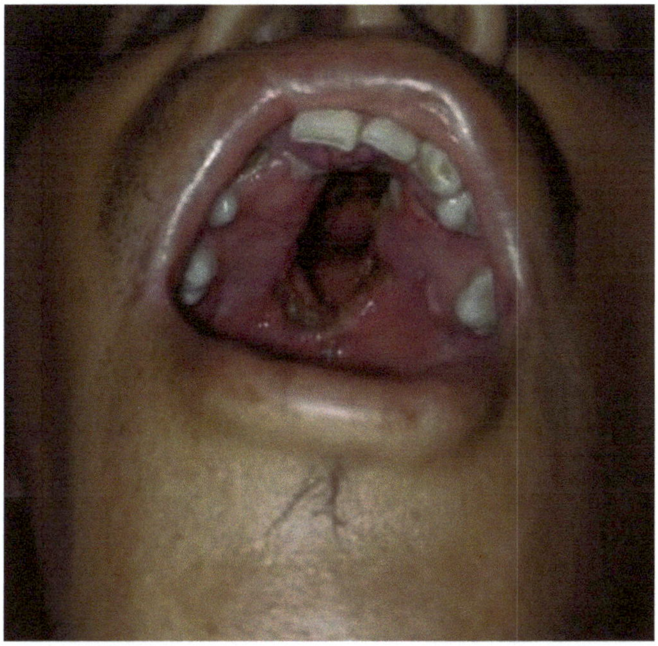

**Fig. 31.18** Acute dehiscence of soft and hard palate 5 days after surgery. (Photo courtesy of Dr. Edwar Alvarez)

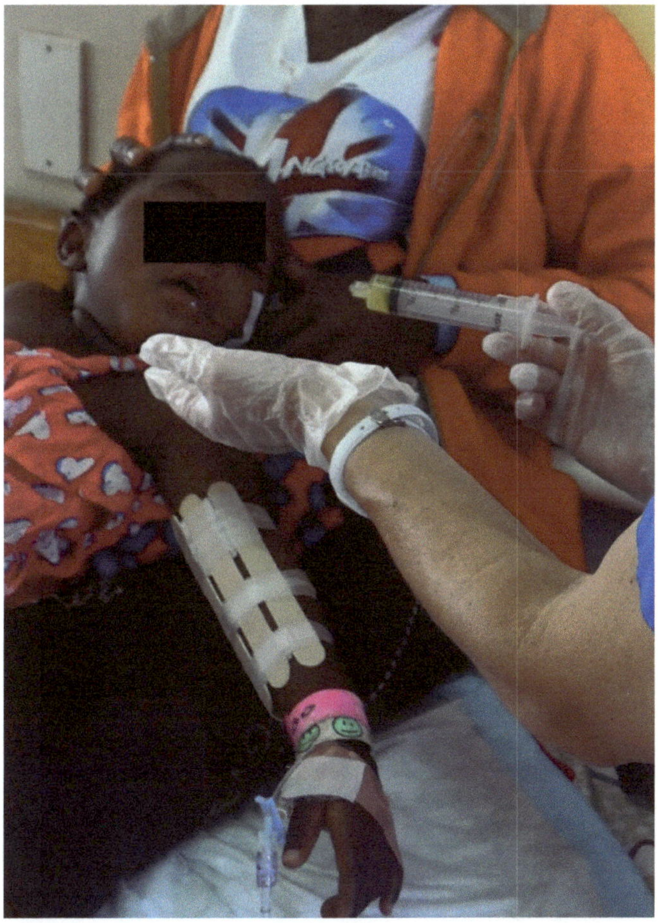

**Fig. 31.19** Arm restraints and "No-No's" after cleft palate surgery. *Notice arm restraints made out of tongue blades and tape*

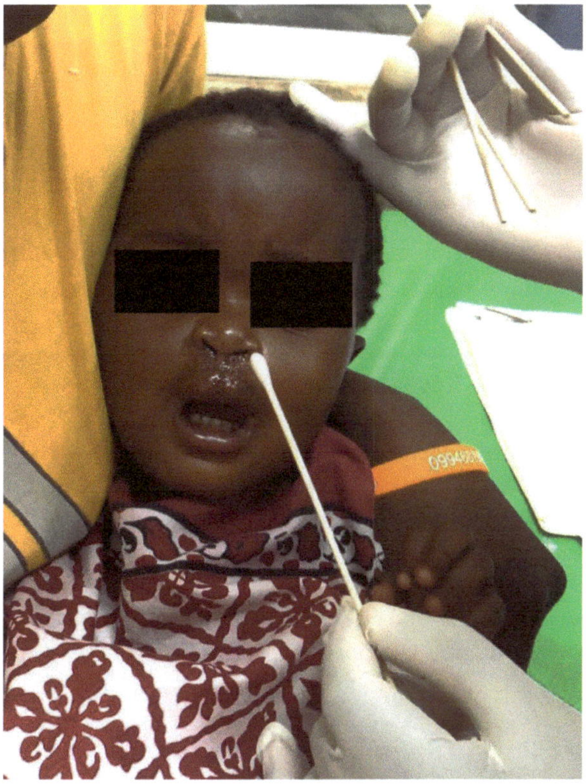

**Fig. 31.20** Lip care technique. (Photo courtesy of J Kesselman RN). *(1) Wash hands. (2) Use cotton swab and boiled/soapy water. (3) Start at the nasal end of the incision. (4) Use gentle circular motions starting away from the incision. (5) Do not rub on the incision itself. (6) Dry. (7) Apply ointment if prescribed*

**Tips and Tricks: Malaria**

- Rapid diagnostic test kits for malaria are inexpensive and should be available.
- Alternatively, thick and thin blood smears can be requested from a laboratory.
- Drug protocols are mostly available locally, and treatment is usually short.

**Field Solutions**

Isolate and group patients with contagious illnesses in a separate space: viral illness, gastroenteritis, scabies, or lice. Implement specific COVID-19 guidelines if suspected.

## Dehiscence

Dehiscence of the wound occurs more frequently in bilateral cleft lip repairs and occasionally in palate repair [22, 23]. The surgeon should promptly evaluate the possibility of immediate re-repair, but delayed wound breakdown might require later secondary revision (Fig. 31.18).

## Oronasal Fistula (ONF)

ONF is a common long-term complication occurring in 5–35% of patients after CP surgery. ONF presents with food regurgitation through the nose and nasal voice. The efficacy of preventing fistulas with antibiotics is still being studied [11]. The consensus remains that embryology of the defect, tension in the repair, technique, and surgical skill all play important roles [23].

## Procedure-Specific Care and Instructions

The patients' understanding of postoperative care is essential for a good outcome but can be complicated by unfamiliarity with medicine, poor hygiene habits, language barriers, and cultural differences. Most patients with maxillofacial anomalies will benefit from long-term care by orthodontists and speech therapists and referral to audiology and possibly myringotomy (Figs. 31.19 and 31.20) [21].

### Cleft Lip and Rhinoplasty Procedures

The majority of cleft lip and rhinoplasty patients can start eating after recovering from anesthesia and can be discharged within 24 hours. The consensus is to allow breastfeeding immediately. Patients can progress to a normal diet as tolerated. They should rinse with clear water after every feeding and resume normal oral hygiene.

Much care needs to be taken in protecting the lip and nose from any trauma. In young children, this might require immobilizing arms against flexion, feeding cautiously with spoon or cup rather than brisk bottle feeding, and avoiding all activities that might cause a fall.

Antibiotics are usually not prescribed except in cases of complex rhinoplasty or bilateral lip repair. Wound care will depend on the surgeon's practice.

Cleaning of the wound should be done with clean gauze or Q-tip, with soapy sterile or cooled boiled water, making sure not to rub or apply too much pressure. Use of hydrogen peroxide on the wound itself is discouraged, as it disrupts the healing process [24]. Most surgeons use self-absorbing sutures. Some surgeons cover the wound with steristrips or surgical glue. Ointments should be applied only if no surgical glue was used, as they might dissolve this layer of protection. Nasal packing or stents will be removed at the surgeon's discretion.

Surgeons will direct patients to massage the scar of the lip repair several times a day after the first several weeks [25] (Figs. 31.21, 31.22, and 31.23, Table 31.6).

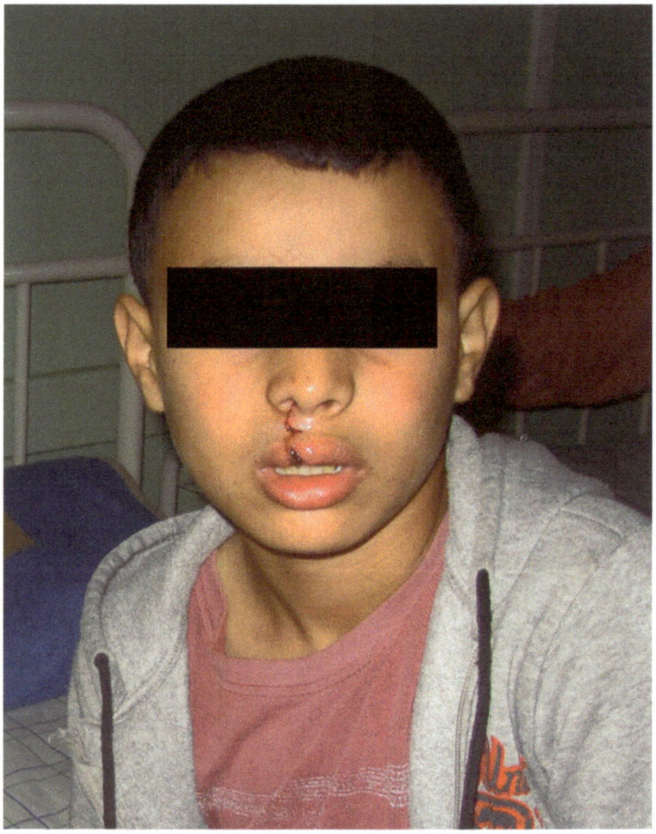

**Fig. 31.21** Lip repair with Dermabond (surgical glue). *Notice the typical slightly shiny coating of the surgical glue over the incision*

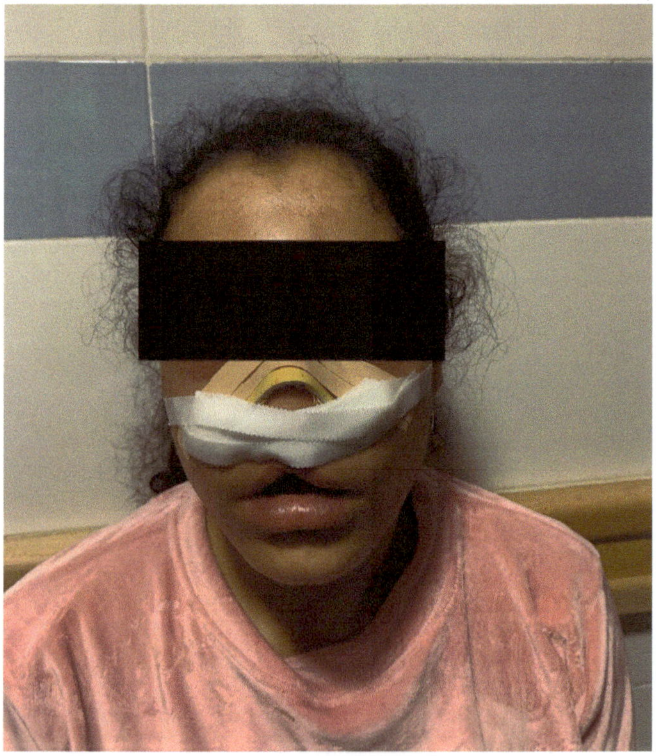

**Fig. 31.22** Mustache dressing or "drip guard". *Rolled-up gauze is gently taped under the nose to collect secretions or bleeding*

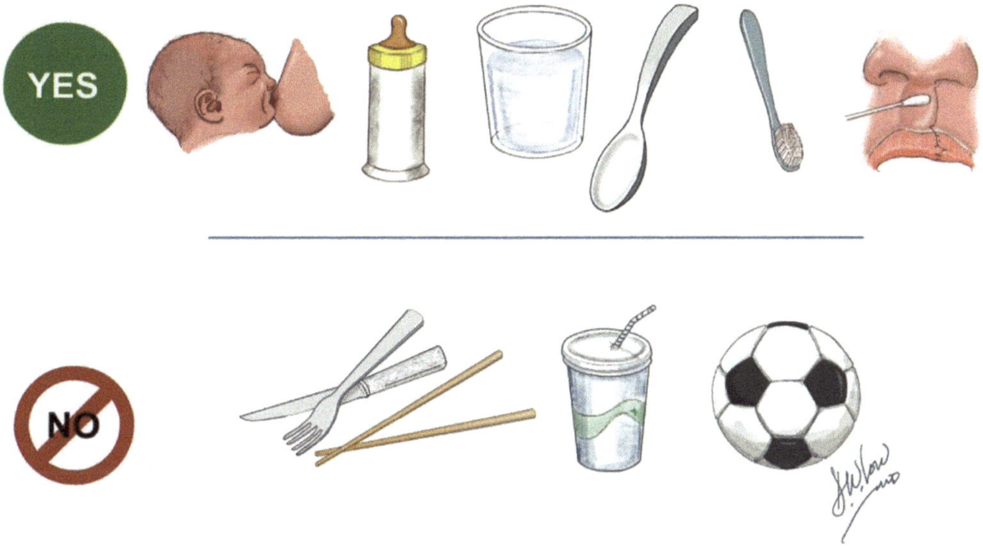


Fig. 31.23 Postoperative lip care pictorials to instruct families of what is ok and what to avoid

Table 31.6 Discharge instructions for cleft lip and rhinoplasty surgery

| |
|---|
| Diet: Breastfeeding, syringe or cup or spoon feeding, and progress to regular food as tolerated |
| Care: Rinse mouth with clean water after every meal. Brush teeth carefully |
| Site care: Keep dry, clean gently with boiled (soapy) water twice a day, apply ointment if no surgical glue, steristrips will fall off, and sutures will dissolve spontaneously |
| Caution: Immobilize elbows, protect the face, and keep fingers out of the mouth. Avoid running, trauma to face, and playing with balls, until healed |
| Rhinoplasty sutures to be removed on ________________ at ____________________ |
| Medication as prescribed |
| Return to health center immediately if high fever, lethargy, redness, swelling, or pussy drainage |
| Start massaging scar gently in circular motion three times/day after 1 month |
| Follow-up appointment on ________________ at __________ ____________________ |

**Tips and Tricks**

- Hand the patient a mirror to look at the new smile!
- Prepare the patient for the increase swelling and bruising over the first 24–48 hours.
- Emphasize the importance of compliance: Revision surgery does not allow for optimal cosmetic and functional results.

## Cleft Palate Repair

The majority of acute complications are likely to occur during the first 24 hours. Most patients will have a tongue stitch taped to the cheek, to pull the tongue forward in case of obstruction, and to help examination. This stitch is usually removed after the first postoperative night. A thorough oral exam on admission is important.

Optimal positioning is on the side, or supine with head elevation at 45 degrees, or in a parent's arms.

Patients can start drinking clear liquids when recovered from anesthesia, but advancing to full liquids should be delayed in case there is a need to return to the OR. Breastfeeding can resume immediately. It is safer to keep the IV in place until good oral intake and stability are established. The importance of good adherence to the modified diet and oral care needs to be stressed. Diet progresses slowly to nutritious liquid diet over the first week (staple soups mashed or blended smoothly, milk, thinned porridge) and advanced to soft mechanical diet for 3 weeks. Acidic, spicy, carbonated, and hot drinks are not permitted. Iced drinks can help with pain. Patients should use a spoon, a cup, or a syringe. Pacifiers and straws are forbidden. If surgeon permits use of a bottle, it should have a soft free-flowing silicone nipple. Patients are instructed to rinse with clean water after every meal and to use a soft toothbrush with caution. Orthodontists will explain care if an obturator was made.

Most patients attain good pain control with nerve and local blocks and paracetamol and ibuprofen.

The majority of the patients can be discharged after 1–2 days if taking appropriate nourishment and comfortably following instructions and do not need antibiotics beyond 24 hours [9] (Figs. 31.24, 31.25, 31.26, 31.27, and 31.28, Video 31.1, Table 31.7).

## Alveolar Bone Grafts and Orthognathic Procedures

Patients are typically in a lot more pain and develop substantial swelling. The head of their bed should be elevated to 45 degrees. Ice packs should be applied 20 min on/20 minutes off for the first 24–48 hours to both the surgical and donor sites. Care should be taken not to be inflicting frostbites.

Anti-emetics should be given prophylactically to prevent vomiting.

Wire cutters should be at the bedside of wired orthognathic patients for emergencies.

A 7- to 10-day course of antibiotics is customary.

Strict adherence to instructions is essential, including rinsing mouth with lukewarm water after every meal, and with an oral disinfectant three times a day, making sure not to rinse forcefully or spit, but rather let the water drip out by gravity. Diet progresses over a week from liquid to mechanical soft for 4–6 weeks. Teeth should be brushed as described by orthodontist. Vaseline should be applied to the lips and nostrils to prevent cracking.

Temporary numbness in trigeminal nerve area can occur (Table 31.8).

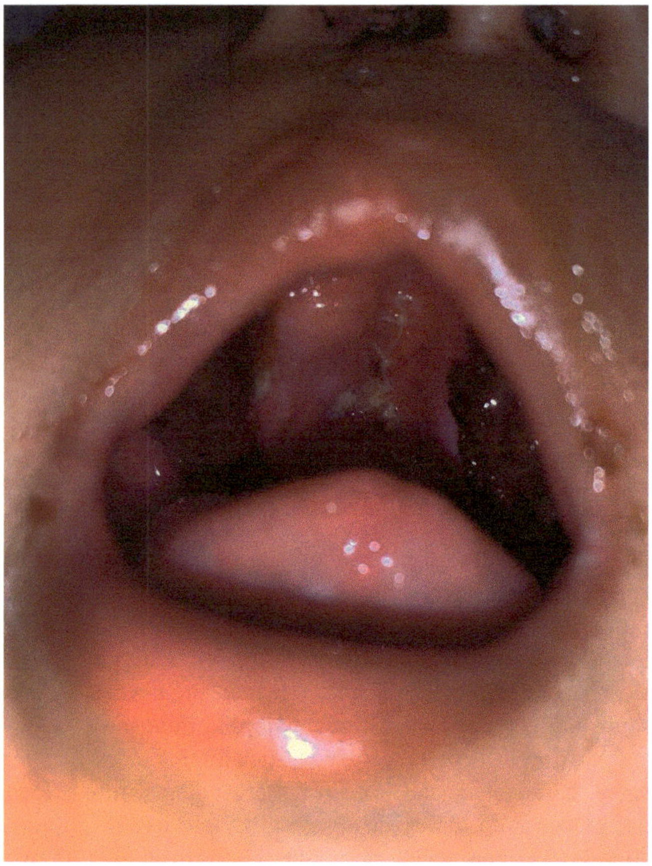

**Fig. 31.24** Palate repair with Surgicel. *Note Surgicel bilaterally (darker). It usually disintegrates spontaneously within 5 days. It can be swallowed, or spit out, but occasionally can dangle in throat and cause discomfort. The empty space it covers will granulate over with fresh tissue and close the gaps in the palate*

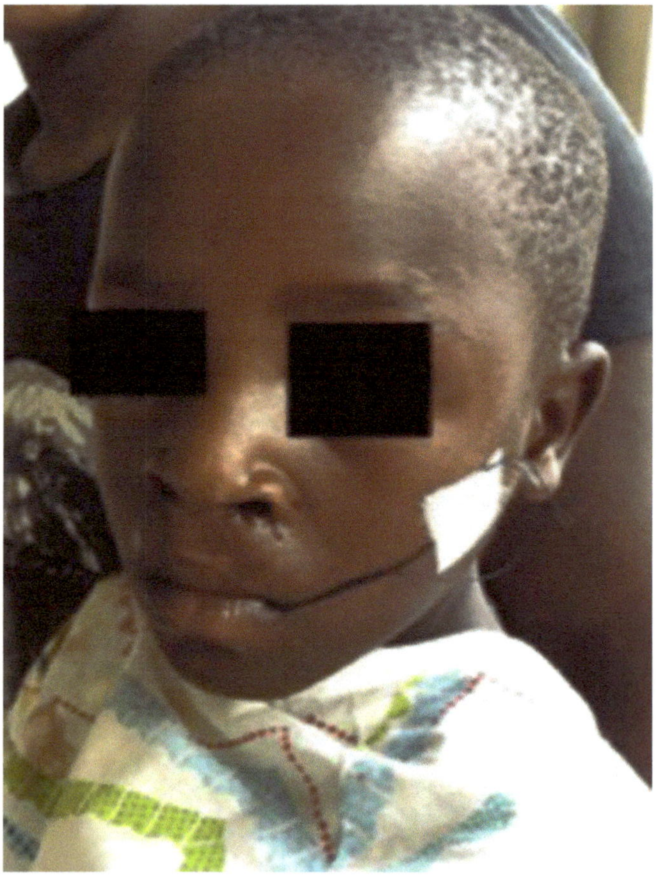

**Fig. 31.25** Tongue stitch taped to the cheek. (Photo courtesy of J Kesselman RN)

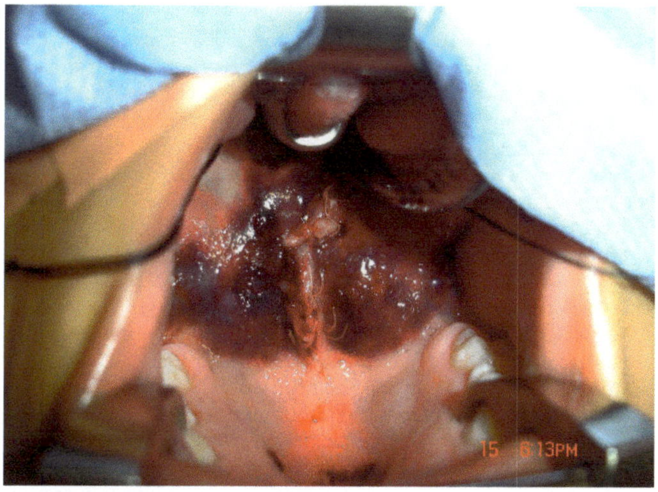

**Fig. 31.26** Hematoma of the soft palate identified 1 day after surgery. (Photo courtesy of Dr. Edwar Alvarez)

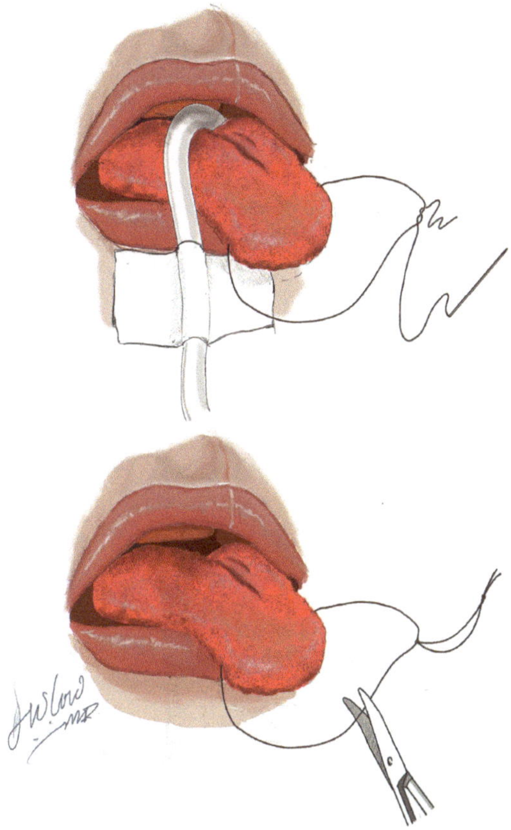

**Fig. 31.27** Tongue stitch removal pictorial. (*1*) *Reassure the patient that the procedure is pain-free. (2) Loosen the tape on the cheek. (3) Carefully place scissors inside the large suture loop outside of the mouth. (4) Cut and pull. Done!*

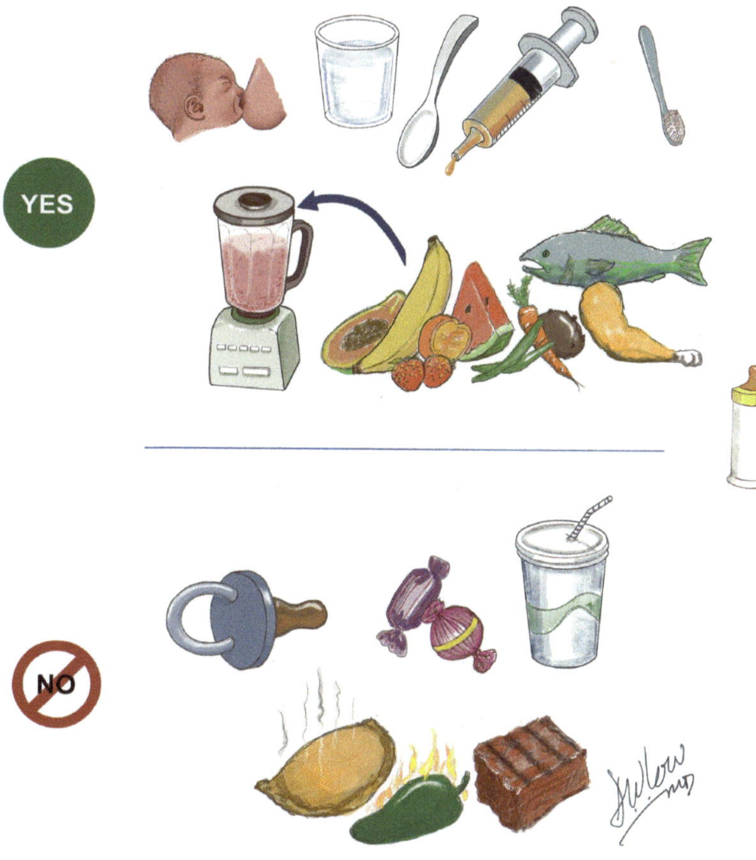


**Fig. 31.28** Postoperative palate care pictorial. Surgeons decide if feeding from bottle with soft free-flowing nipple is allowed or not

**Table 31.7** Discharge instructions for cleft palates and fistula repair

| |
|---|
| Diet: Use only cup, syringe, and spoon. Breastfeeding is acceptable. Liquid/soft food for 1 week, mechanical soft food for 2–4 weeks. NO hard pieces, only smooth food. NO spicy or acidic food, NO hot food, NO carbonated drinks |
| Caution: NO bottle feeding except if surgeon agrees to use a *soft free-flowing* silicone nipple, NO straws, NO pacifiers, NO candy, NO chewing. NO fingers or objects in mouth. Immobilize arms if needed |
| Care: Rinse mouth with clean water after every meal. Brush teeth carefully |
| Normal activity but no contact sports for 1 month |
| Medications as prescribed |
| Return to health center immediately for high fever, lethargy, poor intake, respiratory distress |
| Follow-up appointment on ________________ at __________ ____________________ |

**Table 31.8** Discharge instructions for ABG and orthognathics

| |
|---|
| Diet: Liquid diet for a week and then progress to mechanical soft for 6 weeks. NO chewing, NO straws, NO high temperatures, NO spicy food, NO added fat, NO carbonated drinks |
| Mouth care: After every meal – rinse gently with water, moving head side to side, letting it drip out. Rinse with disinfectant three times a day for 2 weeks. Brush teeth per protocol (do not brush alveolar graft area, do brush around wires) |
| Site care: Keep dry or apply antibiotic ointment twice a day if no surgical glue |
| Lip and nose: Apply ointment to prevent cracks |
| Antibiotics: 7- to 10-day coverage |
| Pain medication: Acetaminophen and NSAID and ice as needed |
| Elastic bands: Need to be worn 24/7 at ALL times. Change daily using diagram provided by orthodontist |
| Wires: Wire cutters with patient at all times in case of emergency only |
| Resume cautious normal activity but no contact sport |
| Return to health center/call orthodontist immediately for recurrent swelling, bleeding or pain, bad odor from mouth or nose, food coming up through nose, feeling of space or hole at suture area, and white tooth-like protrusion = graft dehiscence |
| Follow-up appointment on ________________ at __________ ____________________ |

## Conclusion

With good organization and communication, and a cohesive team, excellent postoperative care of cleft surgery patients can be achieved in low-resource settings, and underserved patients' lives can be dramatically improved.

## References


1. www.who.int/emergencies/diseases/novel-coronavirus-2019/technical-guidance
2. www.cdc.gov
3. www.hopkinsmedicine.org/coronavirus/
4. Reena, Kasturi HB, Abhijit P. Postoperative analgesia for cleft lip and palate repair in children. J Anaesthesiol Clin Pharmacol. 2016;32(1):5–11.
5. Zhao-Fleming H, Hand A, Zhang K, et al. Effect of non-steroidal anti-inflammatory drugs on post-surgical complications against the backdrop of the opioid crisis. Burns Trauma. 2018;6:25.
6. Tobias JD, Green TP, Coté CJ. Codeine: time to say "no". Section on Anesthesiology and Pain Medicine, Committee on Drugs. Pediatrics. 2016;138(4):e20162396.
7. FDA Statement from Douglas Throckmorton, MD, deputy center director for regulatory programs, Center for Drug Evaluation and Research, on new warnings about the use of Codeine and Tramadol in children and nursing mothers. April 20, 2017.
8. Zeng Z, Lu J, Yin P, et al. A comparison of nalbuphine with morphine for analgesic effects and safety: meta-analysis of randomized controlled trials. Nature Sci Rep. 2015;5:1092.
9. Allegranzi B, et al. New WHO recommendations on intraoperative and postoperative measures for surgical site infection prevention: an evidence-based global perspective. Lancet Infect Dis. 2016;16(12):288–303.
10. Aznar ML, Schonmeyr B, Echaniz G, Nebeker G, Wendby L, Campbell A. Role of postoperative antimicrobials in cleft palate surgery: prospective, double-blind, randomized, placebo-controlled clinical study in India. Plast Reconstr Surg. 2015;136(910):59–66.
11. Rottgers SA, Camison L, Shakir S, Grunwaldt L, Nowalk AJ, Natali M, Losee JE. Antibiotic use in primary palatoplasty: a survey of practice patterns, assessment of efficacy, and proposed guidelines for use. Plast Reconstr Surg. 2016;137(2):574–82.
12. Hollier LH. Discussion: antibiotic use in primary palatoplasty: a survey of practice patterns, assessment of efficacy, and proposed guidelines for use. Plast Reconstr Surg. 2016;137(2):583–4.
13. Reddy RR, Reddy SG, Banala B, Bronkhorst EM, Kummer AW, Kuijpers-Jagtman AM, Bergé SJ. Placement of an antibiotic oral pack on the hard palate after primary cleft palatoplasty: a randomized controlled trial into the effect on fistula rates. Clin Oral Invest. 2018;22(5):1953–8.
14. Stanley CN, Igala SE. Effect of different storage conditions on the stability and efficacy of some reconstituted oral antibiotic suspensions sold in Port Harcourt. J Pharma Res Int. 2017;20:3): 1–10.
15. Durga P, Raavula P, Gurajala I, Gunnam P, Veerabathula P, Reddy M, Upputuri O, Ramachandran G. Evaluation of the efficacy of tranexamic acid on the surgical field in primary cleft palate surgery on children- a prospective, randomized clinical study. Cleft Palate Craniofac J. 2015;52(5):e183–7.
16. Krempl GA, Noorily AD. Use of oxymetazoline in the management of epistaxis. Ann Otol Rhinol Laryngol. 1995;104(9):704–6.
17. Quain AM, Khardori NM. Nutrition in wound care management: a comprehensive overview. Wounds. 2015;27(12):327–35.
18. Global Guidelines for the Prevention of Surgical Site Infection, WHO 2016, 4.10, p. 102–6.
19. Soltani R, Haghighat A, Fanaei M, Asghari G. Evaluation of the effect of green tea extract on the prevention of gingival bleeding after posterior mandibular teeth extraction: a randomized controlled trial. Evid Based Complement Alternat Med. 2014;2014:857651, 4 pages.
20. Liang HH, Zhang MX, Wen YM, Xu XL, Mao Z, She YJ, Liu PZ. The incidence of and risk factors for postoperative fever after cleft repair surgery in children. J Pediatr Nursing. 2019;45:89–94.
21. Kuo CL, Tsao YH, Cheng HM, Lien CF, Hsu CH, Huang CY, Shiao AS. Grommets for otitis media with effusion in children with cleft palate: a systematic review. Pediatrics. 2014;134(5):983–94.

22. Schonmeyr B, Wendby L, Campbell A. Early surgical complications after primary cleft lip repair: a report of 3108 consecutive cases. Cleft Pal-Craniofacial J. 2018;52(6):706–10.
23. Sadhu P. Oronasal fistula in cleft palate surgery. Oronasal fistula in cleft palate surgery. Indian J Plast Surg. 2009;42(Suppl):S123–8.
24. Loo Eng Kiat A, Wong YT, Ho R, Wasser M, Du T, Ng WT, Halliwell B. Effects of hydrogen peroxide on wound healing in mice in relation to oxidative damage. PLoS One. 2012;7(11):e49215.
25. McKay E. Assessing the effectiveness of massage therapy for bilateral cleft lip reconstruction scars. Int J Ther Massage Bodywork. 2014;7(2):3–9.

# Operating Room Function and Biomedical Equipment

# 32

David Aldrete Flores, Gisela H. Sánchez Sosa, Yader Arce, and Keith L. Ballance

**Key Points**

- Ensuring safe surgery in low-resource settings (LRSs) requires essential biomedical equipment and instrumentation, with appropriate planning to ensure that it is functional given that backups are not often available.
- Operating room (OR) equipment needs to be complete for any possible anesthetic or surgical eventuality, and a "common back table" concept can reduce autoclave throughput when multiple tables are in use or multiple are to be done in a day.
- Equipment improvisations, such as fashioning a needle-point cautery tip, can tailor instrumentation to cleft care beyond what is typically available in these settings.
- Infrastructure inspection assures sufficient oxygen, water, electricity, and the design of backup plans.
- Preventive maintenance improves the function and prolongs the life of instruments and essential equipment.

## Introduction

Functioning biomedical equipment – anesthesia monitors, suction, electrocautery, and lighting – keeps a patient safe through surgery and must be ready at moment's notice should an emergency arise. In low-resource settings (LRSs), the challenges of biomedical readiness are numerous: often dated equipment in varied state of function, scarce trained biomedical personnel, unreliable infrastructure, and difficulty in acquiring spare parts. Clinical technology continues to rapidly advance, improving safety and effectiveness in all domains, but increasing complexity and cost exacerbate the challenges in LRSs. The field of biomedical engineering seeks to integrate technology to provide solutions for the technical challenges in clinical practice and to ensure patient and medical staff safety [1].

Many cleft organizations have historically brought external supplies and equipment to assure consistency on a temporary basis for the cleft surgery they perform. However, there has been increasing attention to how surgical systems in LRS hospitals can be strengthened broadly through investment in equipment, team training, and protocols that transcend cleft surgery. Thus, this chapter addresses how to implement biomedical standards for cleft surgery but takes the perspective of trying to enhance the hospital's systems for delivering surgical care more broadly in so doing.

First, the chapter discusses operating room equipment and setup, acknowledging that creating an effective OR environment requires creativity, patient-centered thinking, and familiarity with essential medical equipment. Complying with local and international safety standards is the goal, even if the hospital's infrastructure is not prepared for it. Second, intraoperative equipment use and patient care protocols are addressed. Third, the core steps and methodologies of preoperative infrastructure assessment are detailed, with a goal to reduce the risks that could reach the patient. Finally, equipment maintenance and elements of developing local biomedical talent are discussed. Clinical engineering is important to

D. A. Flores
Division of Biomedical Engineering, Operation Smile, Guadalajara, Jalisco, Mexico
e-mail: daldrete@medmec.com

G. H. Sánchez Sosa
Division of Biomedical Engineering, Tecnológico de Monterrey, Guadalajara, Jalisco, Mexico

Y. Arce
Operacion Sonrisa Nicaragua, Managua, Nicaragua

K. L. Ballance (✉)
Surgical Instruments Maintenance Department, Operation Smile, Virginia Beach, VA, USA

© Springer Nature Switzerland AG 2021
J. W. Swanson, D. W. Low (eds.), *Global Cleft Care in Low-Resource Settings*, https://doi.org/10.1007/978-3-030-59105-2_32

ensuring the safe operation, calibration, and cost-effective maintenance of equipment [2].

## Operating Room Equipment and Setup

An ideal room setup enables efficient staff flow around the patient and minimizes contamination of surgical sites. In developing countries, cleft operations are commonly performed in spaces of all shapes and sizes, including multiple operating tables placed in a standard operating theater. For cleft surgical procedures, operating on multiple surgical tables in a single room does not seem to cause higher rates of infection [12]. Although working in such spaces requires creativity, it can actually lead to better flow than in larger more complex operating theaters because the amount of essential equipment is quite minimal. Thoughtfully positioning the surgical table and equipment is key to creating an efficient workflow and flow of people and supplies and maintaining an aseptic environment [6].

### The "Common Back Table" Concept

Contrary to typical instrument preparation, in which all instruments are opened onto the surgical field and must be cleaned/sterilized following the procedure, many cleft teams employ a "common back table" concept when multiple cleft procedures are performed sequentially. Sterile instrument sets and supplies (gauze, marking pens, syringes, etc.) are opened onto a large back table, which is kept sterile throughout the day (Fig. 32.1, far left). Instruments and supplies are then passed onto a small trolley or table (typically, a mayo stand) corresponding to the specific patient case, when their use is anticipated. When two operating tables are used in the same room, the small table of each is served from the common back table. This approach has several advantages: a smaller set of instruments is used for each case from the entire set, which results in shorter instrument cleaning (and case turnover) time and enables smaller autoclaves to be used between cases.

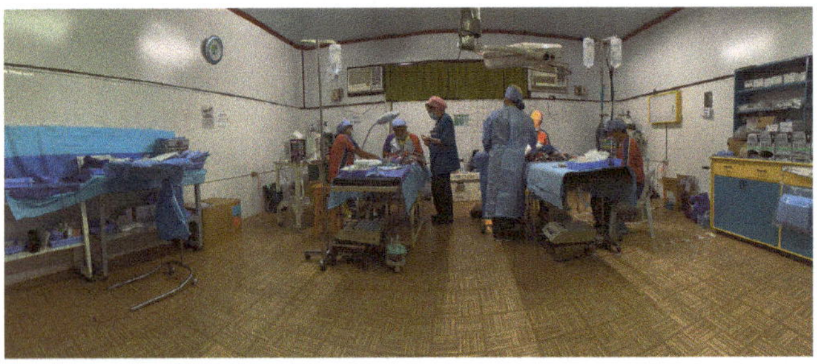

**Fig. 32.1** Functional installation of simultaneous procedures

### Traffic Flow in the Operating Room

The collisions of the personnel when moving inside the OR is something that occurs relatively frequently and increases when the space of the room is small [6, 7]. For this reason, the staff flow should be considered. When only one surgical table is used in the room, personnel circulating on the opposite side of the anesthesia machine is preferable, as sutures, surgical instruments, medications, etc., are delivered (Fig. 32.2). If more than one surgical table is installed in the same OR, central traffic flow between both surgical tables is generally preferred, so that both surgical tables can be easily accessed through the same path (Fig. 32.2).

### Essential Surgical Equipment

Table 32.4 describes essential surgical equipment appropriate for most cleft procedures. In addition, anesthesiologists utilize stethoscopes, laryngoscopes, and various airway devices and often prepare several emergency medicines which are immediately available (in plastic bag or tapes to wall). Surgeons often utilize operating loupes (glasses which magnify tissue view by 2.5–4×) and headlights to better visualize the palate (and act as a backup to overhead light failure).

### Equipment Arrangement

Each cleft surgical case requires staff, equipment, and furniture which are outlined in Table 32.2.

#### Surgical Table

The surgical table is the center of the movement in the room. Staff move around it to operate, monitor the patient, supply anesthesia, and deliver instruments and supplies, while trying at all times to preserve the asepsis of the environment. To position the surgical table, two fundamental things are taken into account: (a) the incidence of light in the surgical area and (b) the ease of entry of the transfer table to it.

Ideally, the head of the stretcher should be positioned under the direct incidence of light coming from the surgical lamp and the other end pointing to the door to facilitate the entrance of the stretcher inside the room (see Fig. 32.3), always preferring to leave the path of the stretcher as close to the door as possible. If a second surgical table is used in the

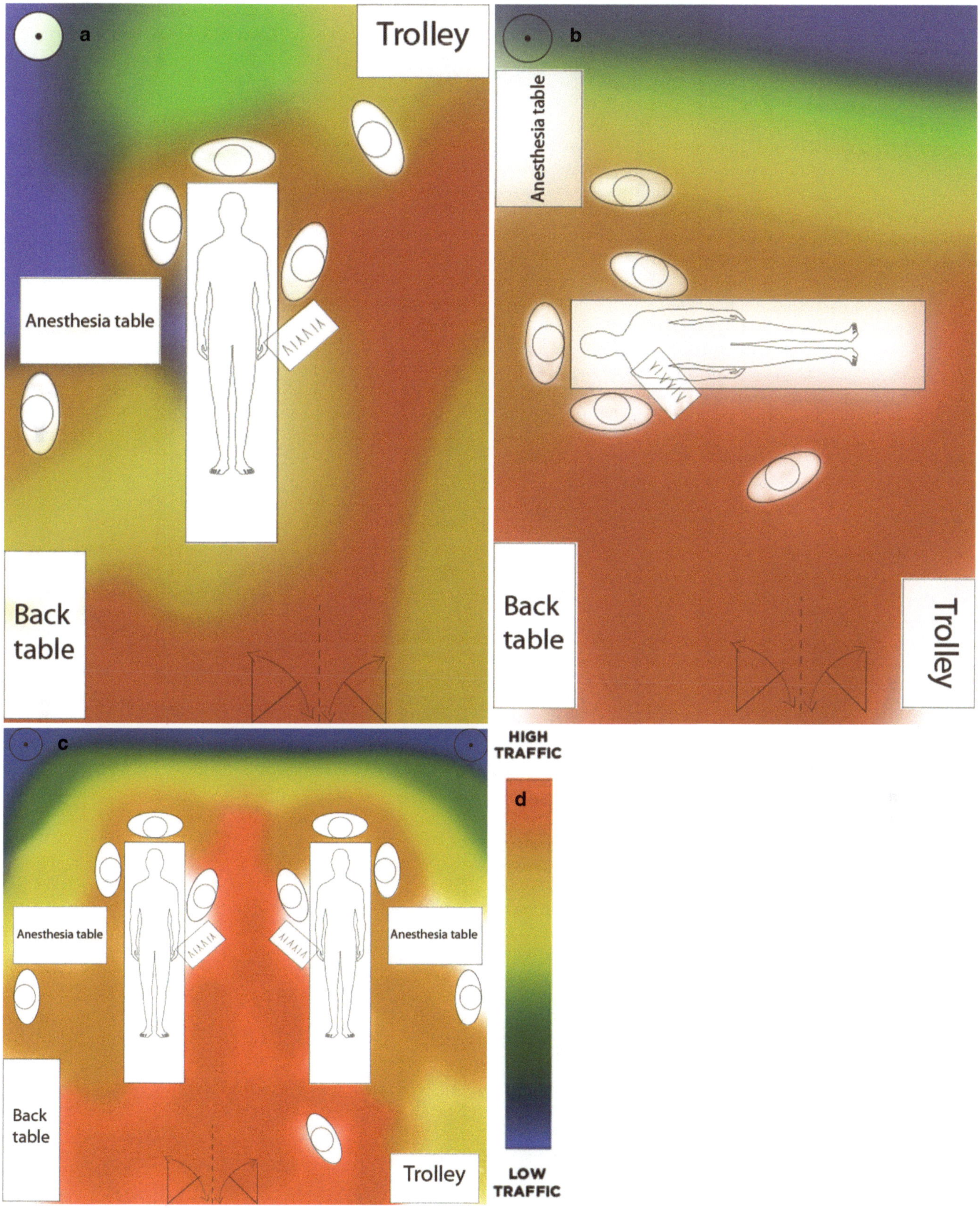


Fig. 32.2 (**a**) Traffic flow of personnel within an OR in an isolated procedure in an adequate position of the surgical table, (**b**) traffic flow of personnel within an OR in an isolated procedure in an unfavorable surgical table position, (**c**) traffic flow in simultaneous procedures and Color scale (**d**) reflects high traffic (red) to low traffic (blue)

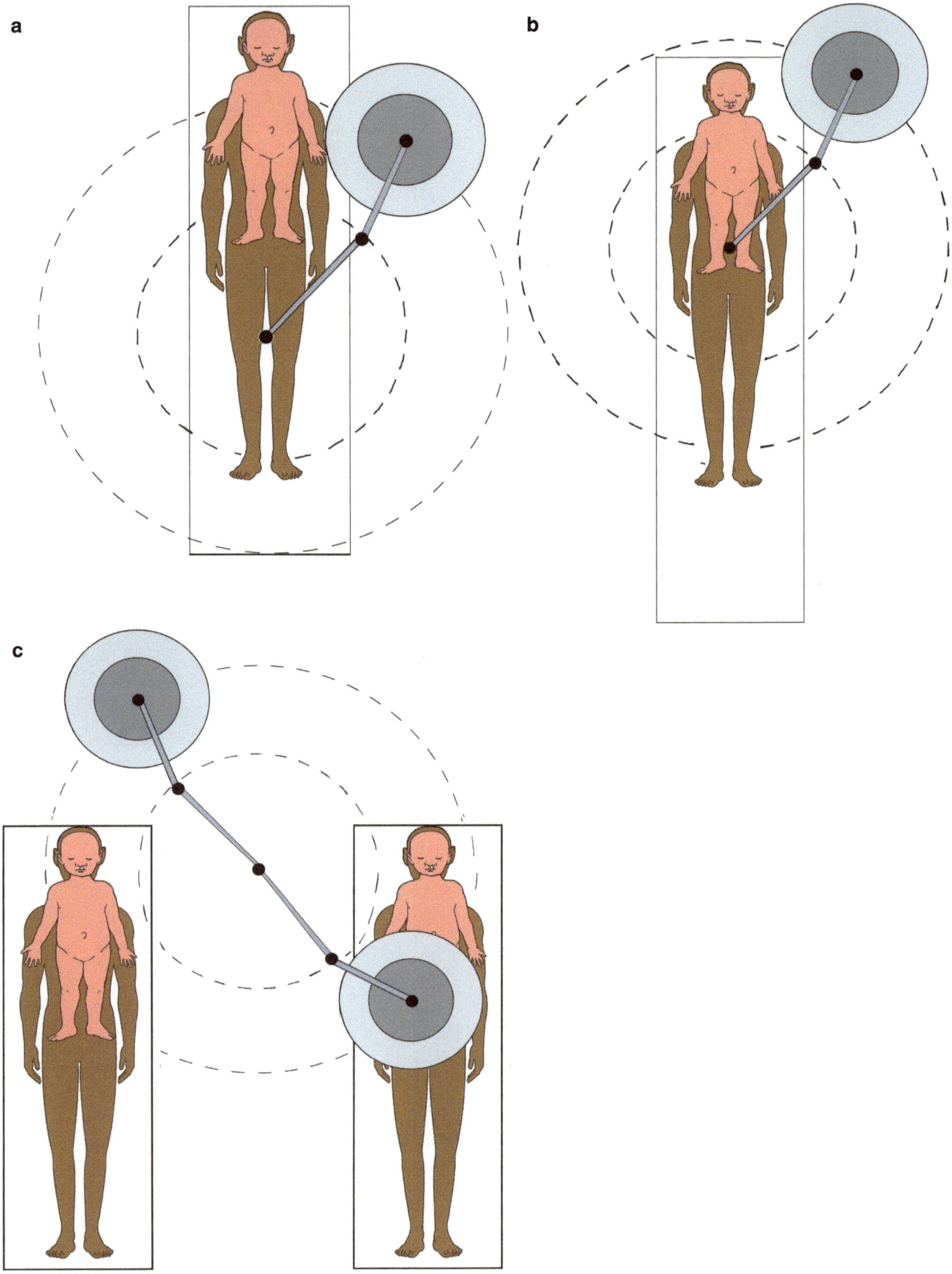


**Fig. 32.3** Position of the surgical table as a function of the incidence of light in the surgical site: (**a**) isolated procedure with incidence of light in the abdominal area, (**b**) isolated procedure with incidence of light in the head, and (**c**) simultaneous procedures with incidence of light in both heads

same OR for simultaneous procedures and the surgical lamp has two satellite, table placement should support illuminating both surgical areas.

### Anesthesia Machinery

The anesthesia equipment (vital sign monitor, anesthesia machine, and vaporizer) is ideally placed where it does not impede surgeon flow around the head of the table and enables entry of the stretcher. Good options include alongside the OR table opposite where the stretcher will enter (Fig. 32.4) or, in a narrow space, off the top or side of the head of the table.

### Other Equipment

Once the position of the surgical table, the path of the stretcher, and anesthesia machinery are determined, the position of the back table and trolley (small table, mayo stand) can be determined (Fig. 32.5).

In order to maximize the space within the OR, it is possible to place the electrosurgical unit (ESU) and the suction machine under the feet side of the surgical table, where they'll be on a small bench. In this way, the flow of medical personnel within the work space is improved, and the path of the cables and hoses that would otherwise traverse workspace can be eliminated (Fig. 32.6).

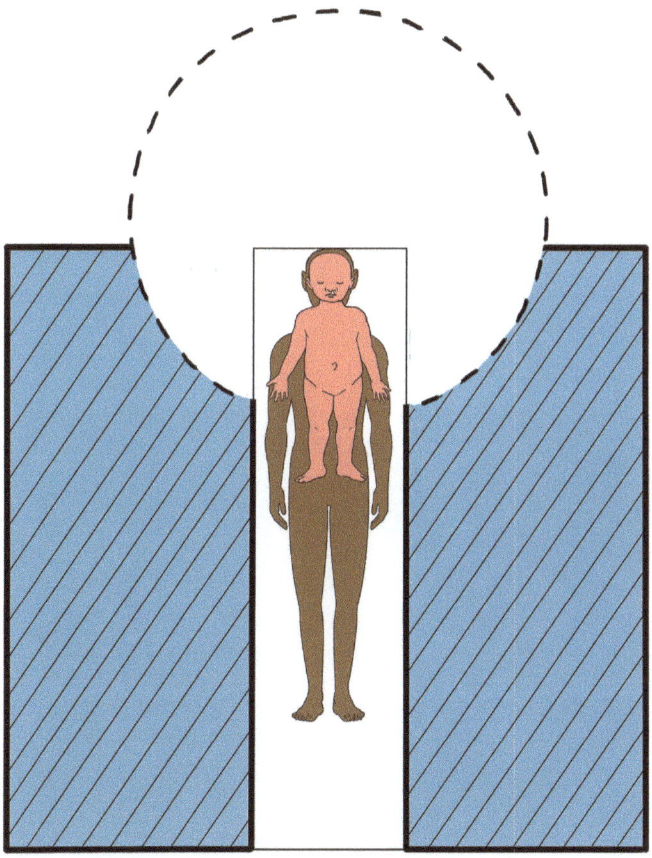

Fig. 32.4 The shaded part indicates the ideal place where an anesthesia machine can be placed without obstructing a cleft care procedure; the circle indicates the area that should not be obstructed

### Support Systems

Once everything is in place, the next step is to plan the electrical supply for medical equipment under the surgical table, oxygen supply for the anesthesia machine, and the scavenging for the waste anesthetic gas disposal (WAGD) following these guidelines:

1. Do not put cables or hoses in any area where the surgeon moves.
2. Do not put cables or hoses in any area where the stretcher moves.
3. Do not pass cables or hoses through main traffic flow areas.
4. All cable or hose must be taped to the floor or wall.
5. No cable or hose must pass through any area where it can be punctured by any door or window.
6. If possible, pass a single electric cable to connect the equipment under the surgical table
7. Patient monitoring cables (pulse oximetry, blood pressure, electrocardiogram leads, capnography) can be wrapped together in a hose.

This approach minimizes cable damage and tripping hazards and improves stretcher mobility.

### Space Required in the Operating Room

The space necessary in a cleft care surgery is calculated based on the personnel, furniture, and medical equipment that need to be inside the OR for the procedure (Table 32.2).

Minimum suggested space for an effective working space is estimated as follows:

(a) At the head part of the table, where the surgeons will work, at least 1 m of space is needed.
(b) On the anesthesia machine side of the table, 1 m is needed.
(c) On the opposite side of the anesthesia machine, the scrub nurse is positioned and occasionally the stretcher and the staff to move the patient, a meter and a half is required.

Since a normal surgical table measures 2 m × 0.5 m, we can estimate an optimal minimal space of 4 m × 3 m (12 $m^2$) per surgical table (Fig. 32.5).

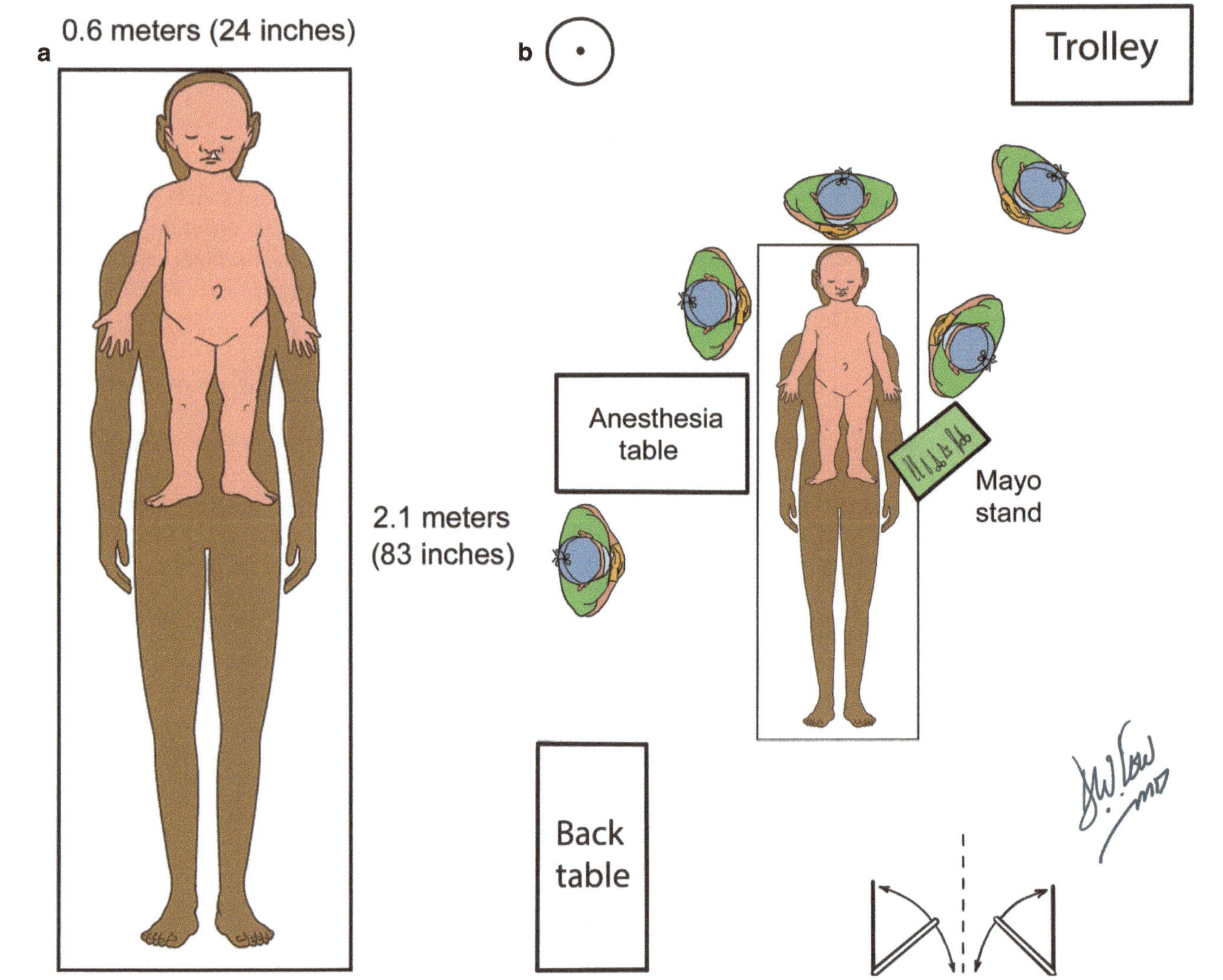


**Fig. 32.5** (**a**) Normal dimensions of a surgical table and (**b**) relation of furniture and medical equipment with respect to the surgical table in a cleft care procedure

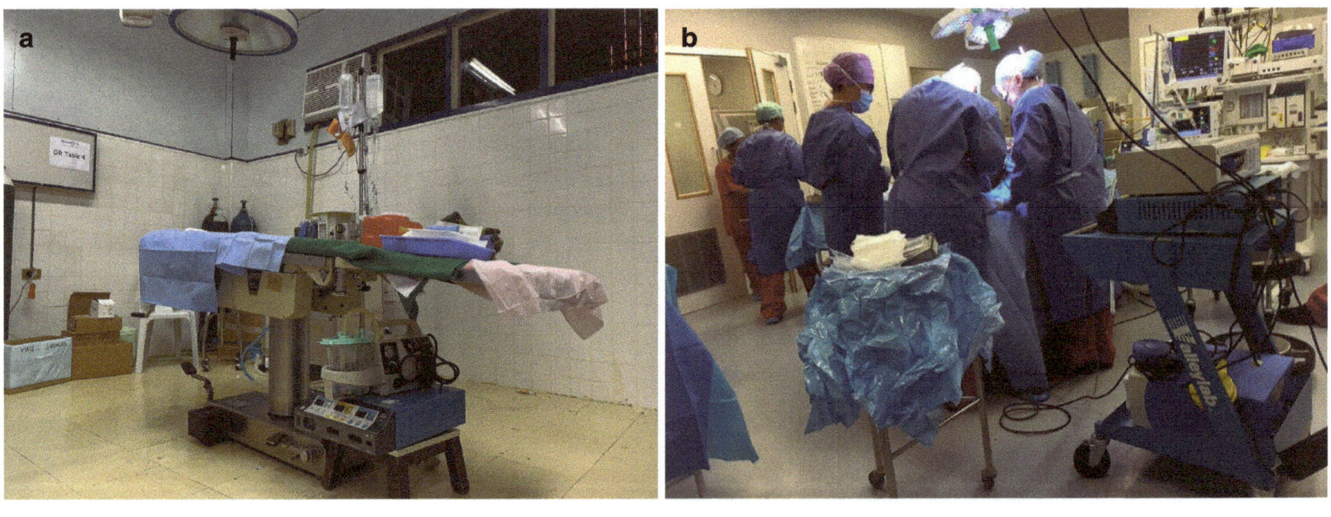


**Fig. 32.6** (**a**) ESU and suction machine under the surgical table. (**b**) Normal position of the electrosurgery unit, where the cables of the ESU can be observed toward the patient, being able to cause tripping

## Outside the Operating Room

An adequate space to sterilize instruments, equipped with a reliable water supply and packet wrapping supplies, is essential (Fig. 32.7). This may be a standard hospital sterilization area, an area in the OR suite dedicated to sterilization during cleft surgery, and/or small autoclaves outside of each operating room.

### Postanesthesia Care Unit (PACU)

This space must have the capacity of beds to meet the demand generated by surgeries in the OR. In addition to this, it must have a vital sign monitor, a suction machine, and the ability to supply oxygen to patients (Fig. 32.8).

### Intensive Care Unit (ICU)

The hospital must have a space to treat the most severe patients, which must have at least a vital sign monitor, a suction machine, oxygen supply, and a mechanical ventilator. As a contingency, an emergency plan must be designated to transfer the patient to the nearest appropriate unit using a transfer ventilator.

Defibrillator, crash box, and difficult airway box are located in the OR suite/PACU area, as described in Table 32.4.

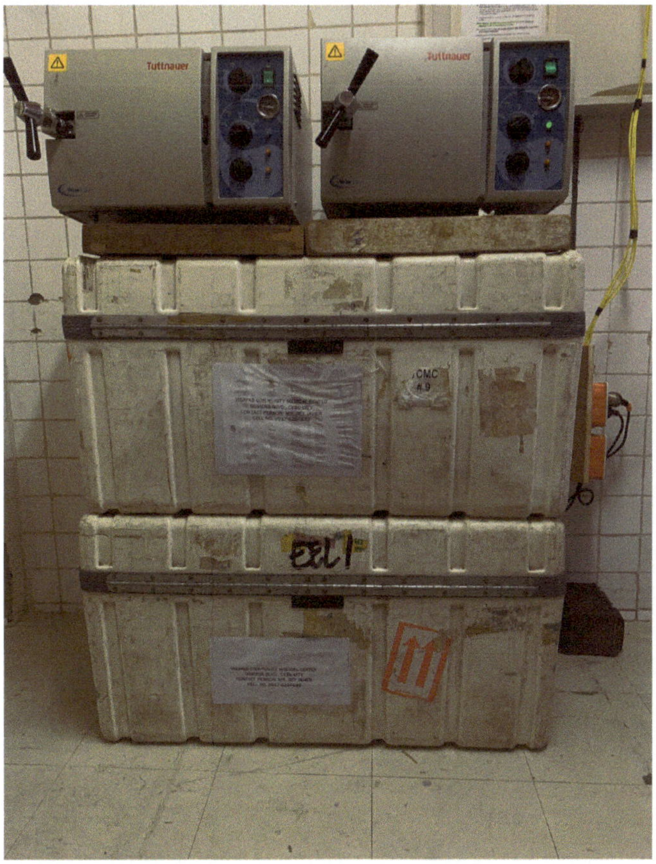


**Fig. 32.7** Sterilization area installed in a hospital with no reliable autoclave in site

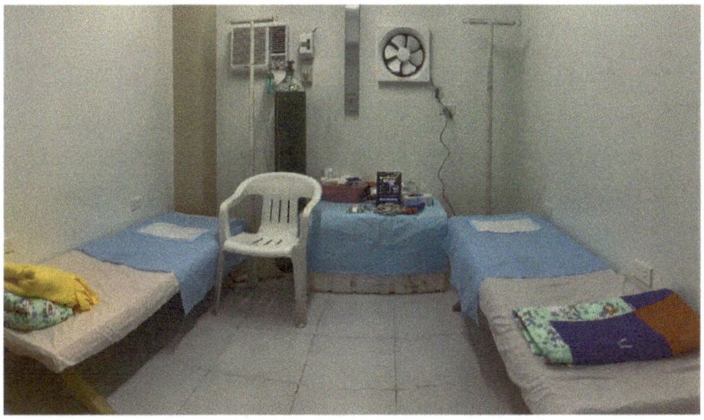

**Fig. 32.8** PACU installed in the Philippines

## Intraoperative Patient Care and Equipment Use

Performing a "time-out" or "surgical pause" before the start of every case enables the surgeon, anesthesiologist, and circulating nurse to confirm the patient, planned procedure, and operative site and side. It also facilitates discussion of any unusual anesthesia, nursing, or surgical issues relevant to the case and helps to set a pattern of proactive team communication.

A throat pack, if used during surgery, should be announced and a sign on the wall or OR table, or sticker, used to identify its presence. A suture or fabric leash on the throat pack that is left outside the mouth provides an additional visual reminder to all team members to prevent a retained foreign body that could cause airway obstruction during extubation.

Several innovative solutions have been developed to replicate instrumentation that may not be available in low- to middle-income country (LMIC) settings. For instance, in the absence of a fine-tipped surgical marking pen or quill-tip stylus, a wooden cotton-tipped applicator can be shaved down to a point and dipped in methylene blue to make fine marks on the lip.

**Solutions from the Field: Needle-Point, Protected Electrocautery Tip**

Needle-point cautery enables fine tissue cauterization with less collateral thermal injury. Insulation along the metal shaft reduces risk of burns to tissue (lips, nose, cheeks) that the cautery shaft may touch when the tip is directed at deeper intended tissue. Cauterization tips with these enhancements are often not available in LMICs.

A 1.5 cm section can be cut from an 8-French soft nasopharyngeal suction tube, or similar silicone or soft plastic tubing, and slid over the shaft of the cautery, leaving a 3 mm exposed tip. Additionally, a 22 gauge needle can be slid inside this insulation tube (Fig. 32.9) to create a needle-tipped cautery device (literally). We find that smaller gauge needles (and smaller) are more likely to warp or melt when bipolar current is delivered and are avoided. A current setting of 8–10 is often sufficient given the concentrated energy. The tip assembly should be inspected before each use to ensure there is no migration of parts or exposed metal at the top of the insulation sleeve, which could result in a burn.

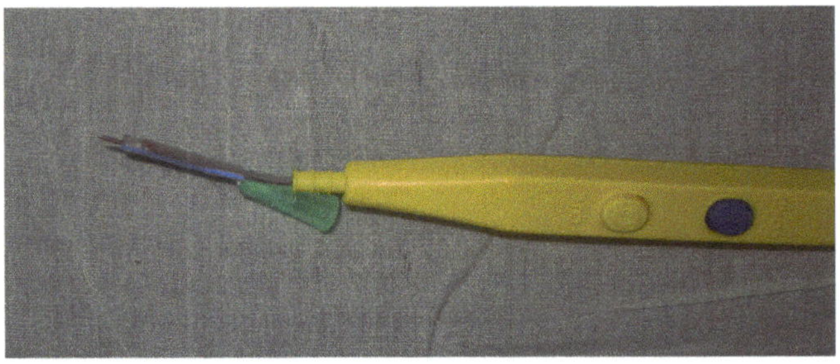

**Fig. 32.9** An improvised needle-point, insulated cauterization tip. (Photo courtesy Yader Arce)

**Solutions from the Field: Light-Handle Covers**
Reusable, sterilizable surgical light-handle covers are often absent in LMIC ORs. If sterile gloves are readily available, a sterile light-handle cover can be improvised by knotting the fingers, turning it inside out, and sliding it over the light hand. It can be held in place by cutting an elastic band from the wrist area that can be wrapped around the glove several times (Fig. 32.10).

## Infrastructure Inspection

The clinical engineer should perform an inspection to evaluate the medical devices and hospital's infrastructure before surgical procedures begin. The most critical points for this inspection are electricity and oxygen.

## Electrical Power Supply

A reliable electrical power supply is critical to the function of essential medical devices. Examples of electrically supplied equipment in even small LMIC hospitals are the refrig-

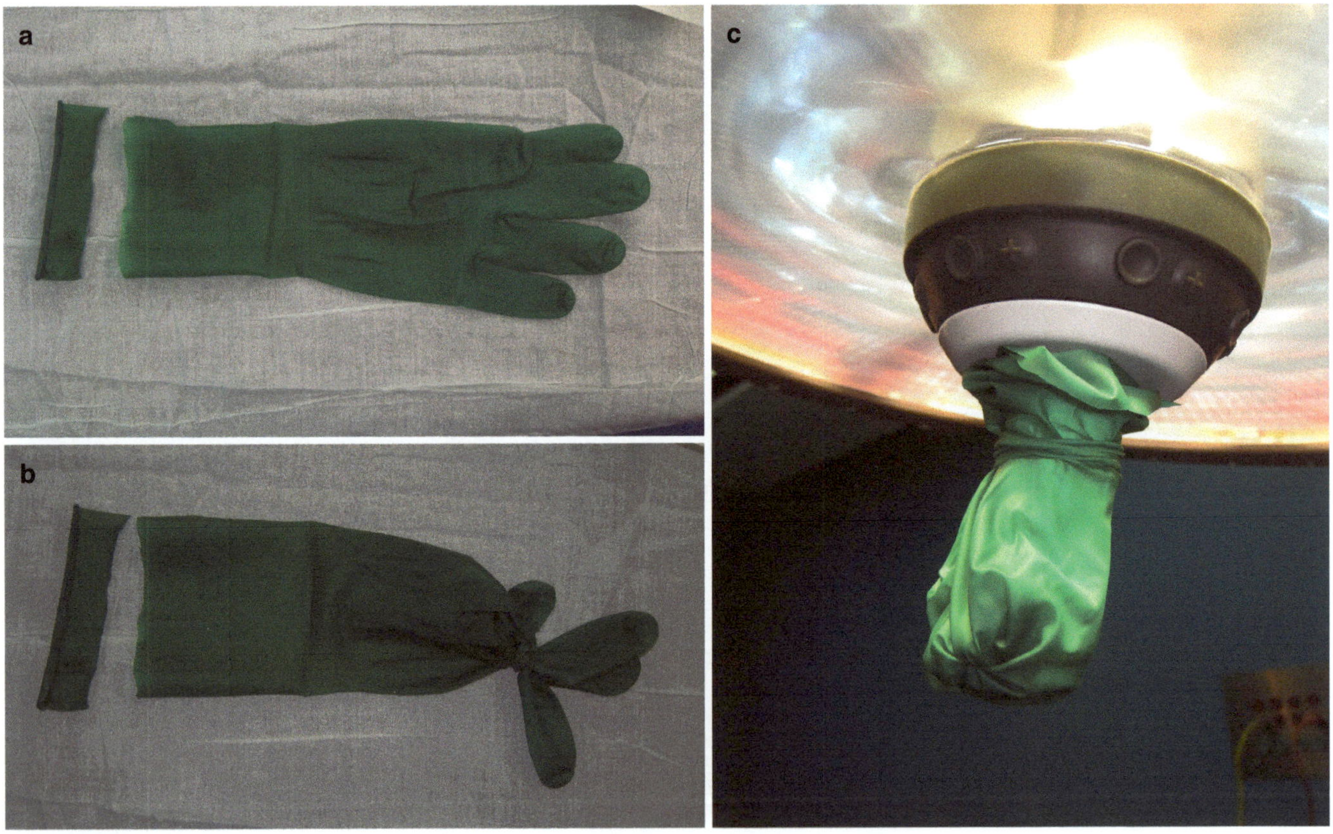

**Fig. 32.10** (**a–c**) An improvised sterile light-handle cover from a surgical glove. (Photos courtesy Yader Arce)

erators used to store vaccines and incubators used to treat newborns. One of the most common faults during surgical procedures is inadequate electrical infrastructure in the OR, so inspection and verification of electrical installation are two of the first tasks that must be performed when readying a space for surgical procedures.

## Electrical Load

Circuit breakers for OR electricity should be inspected. On an ideal electrical installation, each circuit breaker should be clearly identified with its related load capacity (Fig. 32.11). For example, in ORs equipped to perform cleft care surgery, at least the equipment listed on Table 32.1 is required; this means electrical installation must be able to support a load of at least 40 amperes. For this reason, it is important to verify which circuit breaker provides power to each electrical outlet in the OR and the kind of cable used [3], so quick action can be taken to prevent an accident in case of a power failure on any of the medical devices used during the surgical procedure.

## Voltage Supply

Currently, most medical devices that require electrical power supply can operate with voltages of 110–240 volts; however, in emerging countries, ORs usually have many donated medical devices from different parts of the world, which have different power supply requirements, and not all of them may work with the hospital voltage supply. For this reason, it is vital to inspect all the electrical outlets in the OR and verify the label specifications of each medical device to avoid electrical damage of medical devices [4].

## Electrical Ground

The physical ground or earth in hospitals helps to prevent electrical discharges in patients and medical staff and fire hazards caused by sparks of electrostatic discharges (ESD). Electric discharges can be originated by energized medical devices, faults in the electrical installation, ESD, and atmospheric discharges among other reasons. To prevent electrical discharges, electrical receptacles on medical devices should have a direct electrical path to ground, which, in

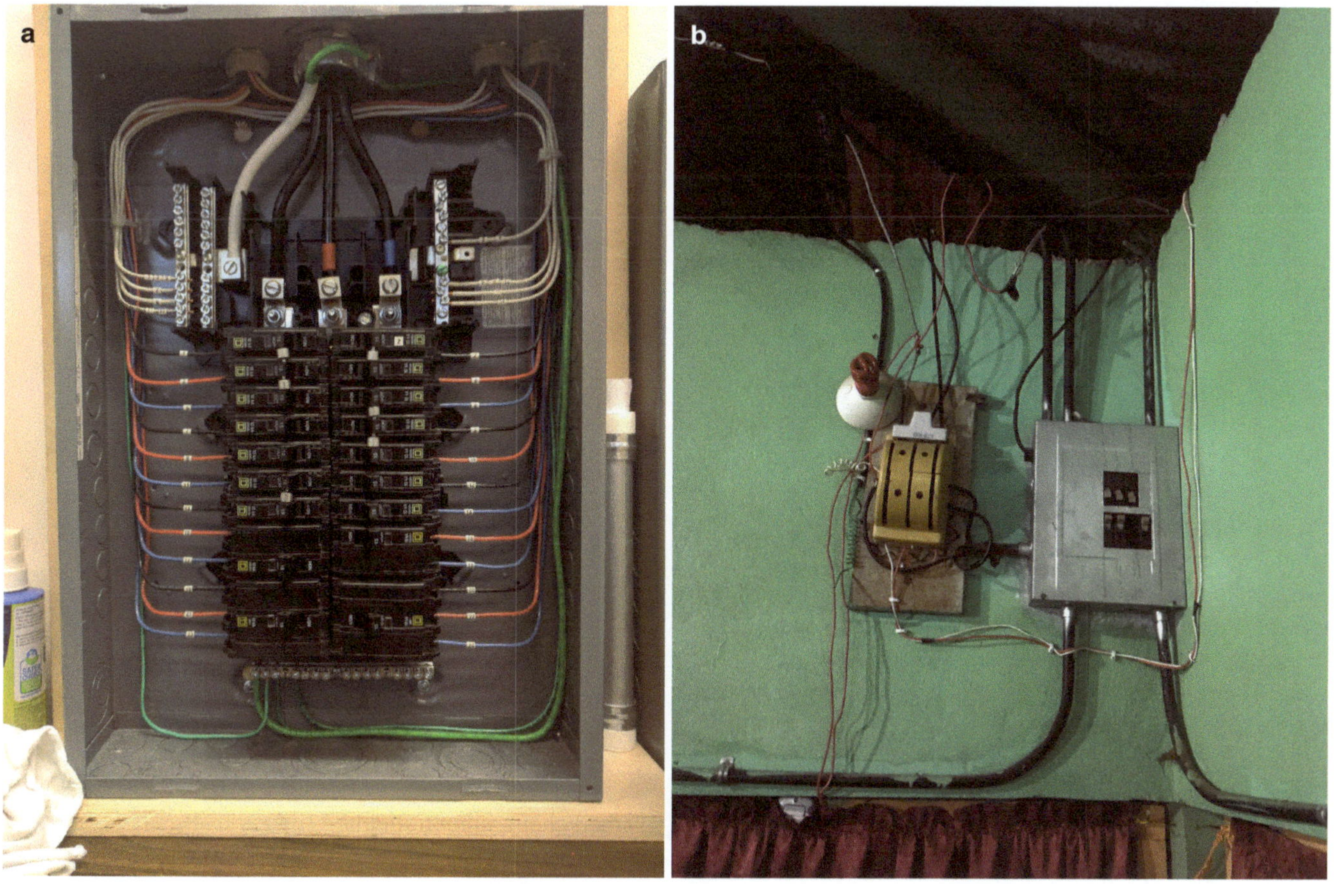


**Fig. 32.11** (**a**) Ideal installation of the circuit breaker panel, with identified, divided circuits and with cables according to the required amperage. (**b**) Installation commonly found in low-resource setting hospitals, with wiring not suitable for the required amperage

**Table 32.1** Electrical medical equipment and its approximate current consumption

| Electrical equipment | Power consumption |
|---|---|
| Ceiling lamp | ≈ 6A |
| Surgical table | ≈ 8A |
| Electrosurgical unit | ≈ 8A |
| Suction machine | ≈ 1A |
| Surgical headlight | ≈ 1A |
| Anesthesia machine | ≈ 5A |
| Vital sign monitor | ≈ 1A |
| General lighting | ≈ 3A |
| Negatoscope | ≈ 1A |
| Air conditioner | ≈ 8A |

**Table 32.2** (a) Essential medical staff for a cleft care procedure, (b) essential medical furniture for a cleft care procedure, and (c) essential medical equipment for a cleft care procedure

| | |
|---|---|
| **(a) Staff inside OR** | |
| Surgeon | Circulating nurse |
| Surgeon's assistant | Biomedical engineer[a] |
| Anesthesiologist | Hospital porter[a] |
| Scrub nurse | |
| **(b) Medical furniture (for 2 OR tables)** | |
| Surgical table | Sterile back table |
| IV pole | Surgical tray trolley |
| Two anesthesiologist chairs | Two hospital trolley |
| Two surgeon chairs, if needed | Two kick buckets |
| **(c) Medical equipment** | |
| Ceiling lamp | Electrosurgical unit |
| Surgical table | Suction machine |
| Anesthesia machine | Oxygen tank |
| Vaporizer | Stretcher[a] |
| Vital sign monitor | |

[a]Non-permanent staff/equipment

emerging countries, is not always available. This is not easy to solve; many times the metal structure of the hospital (beams) could act as an alternative for electrical ground.

## Power Generators

An electrical generator powered by diesel is commonly used in hospitals as a fallback measure in case of a power outage. Power generators can be connected to the electrical installation to supply power to critical areas of the hospital. Critical areas on hospitals usually considered are the OR, intensive care units (ICU), and emergency rooms (ER), among others. This should be inspected and function verified if possible.

## Oxygen Supply

In a hospital environment, oxygen is the most important gas as it is used in most areas (anesthesia machines in the OR, mechanical ventilators in the ICU).

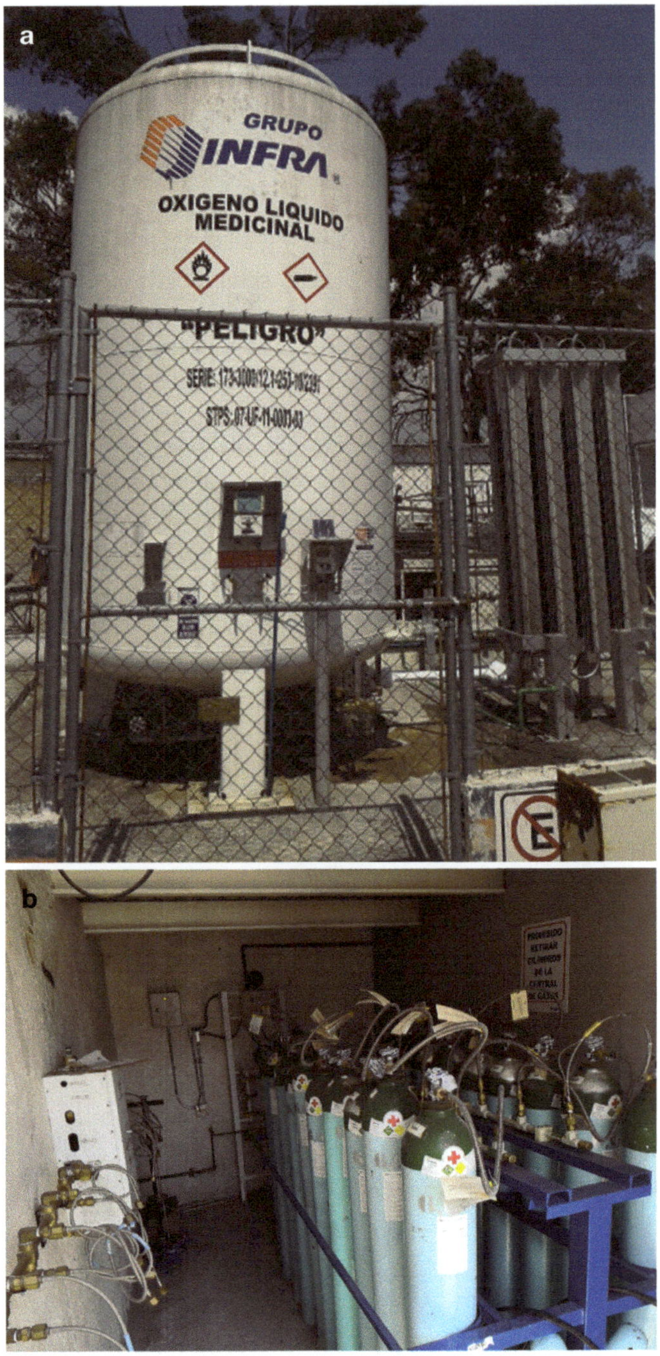


**Fig. 32.12** (**a**) Cryogenic oxygen tank and (**b**) manifold gas supply system

## Oxygen Wall Outlets

There is not a unique standard for gas wall outlets and connectors, so it is possible to find different connector types in the same OR. Wall gas outlets are usually connected to a central gas supply, which can be a cryogenic tank or a tank manifold (Fig. 32.12). Typically, the status of the gas supply at the wall outlet is not known, so additional measures should be taken to evaluate gas supply by using a pressure gauge or

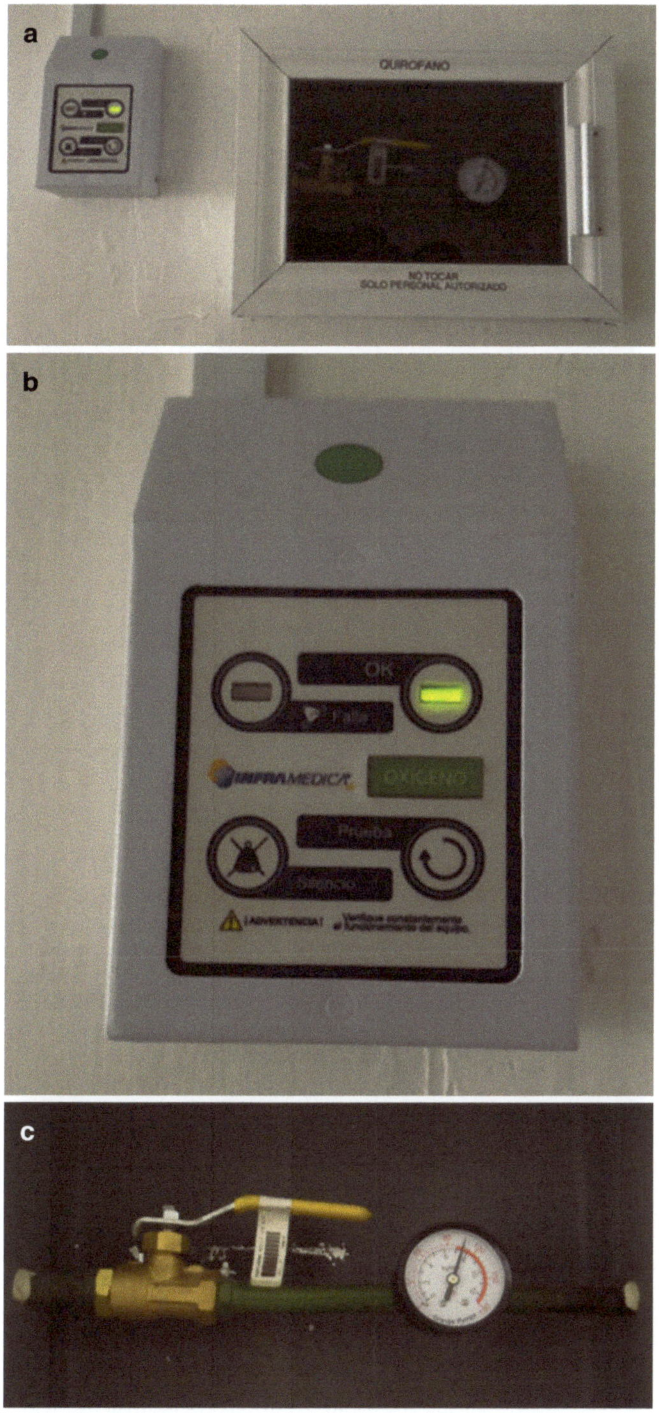


**Fig. 32.13** (**a**) Photo of low/high oxygen pressure alarm and pressure gauge on the wall, (**b**) detail of the alarm, and (**c**) detail of the manometer

an alarm system and be able to determine if a problem exists as soon as possible (Fig. 32.13).

## Central Cryogenic Tank and Manifold

When a central gas supply through a cryogenic tank is used, usually a permanent contract exists between the hospital and an external medical gas supplier, which can remotely monitor the amount of oxygen remaining in the tank, ensuring a continuous gas supply for the hospital. However, not all hospitals have this type of resource, either because of the cost of installation or the remote location of the hospital. In these cases, other types of gas supply are used.

When the hospital does not have a constant or automatic monitoring system for central gas supply, they rely on personnel and protocols implemented in the hospital to monitor gas supply manually. Usually, the gas tank manifold is checked many times per day to avoid running out of gas. Delivery delays should be taken into account when directing restock.

## Gas Tanks

When the hospital does not have wall outlets for gas supply, single oxygen tanks are used for each area where oxygen is required. To connect a tank to a medical device, usually a pressure regulator is required (Fig. 32.14) to reduce the oxygen tank pressure to the working pressure of the medical device (around 50–55 psi) [5].

> **Safety Tip**
> When using an anesthesia machine with direct supply from an oxygen tank, it is recommended to replace the oxygen tank with a new one when the pressure gauge on the regulator indicates 500 psi or less.

Using oxygen tanks inside the OR is the riskiest option for gas supply, because ORs usually are not prepared to secure tanks safely in a fixed location. The pressure inside an oxygen tank can easily reach 2000 psi, and in case the tank falls, it can cause an explosion or turn into a projectile. It is essential to place the tank in the location of least transit inside the OR and secure it with a chain if possible. A table or chair can also be used to secure the tank in place in case no other means are available.

Oxygen sources also pose a fire risk in operating rooms, given the flammability of oxygen gas. Ignition sources, such as electrocautery, when combined with a flammable substance (oxygen or chlorhexidine prep solution that has pooled or not dried), create a fire or explosion. For this reason, fire risk needs to continually be assessed and mitigated. Particular risks include cauterization near an "open" oxygen course such as nasal cannula or proximity of hoses conveying concentrated oxygen, particularly if a leak may be present.

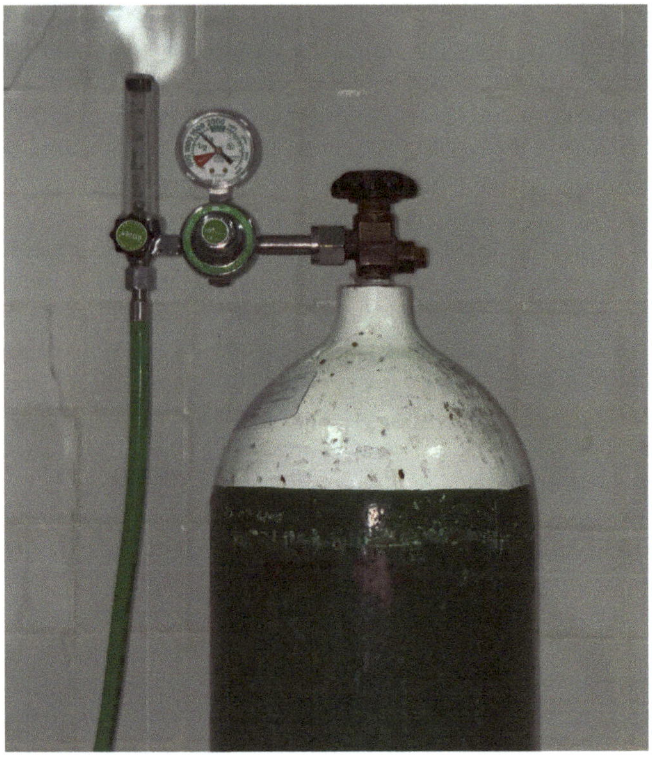

**Fig. 32.14** Oxygen pressure regulator

## Equipment Maintenance

The maintenance of medical equipment can be classified into three broad categories:

(a) Predictive, which anticipates failures based on previous experience or duration of use of certain components
(b) Preventive, which is a periodic evaluation to guarantee that the equipment is working properly, increasing the security that patient care is utilizing functional devices
(c) Corrective, which involves restoring the integrity and operation of the equipment after a fault has occurred, is the most expensive of the three, and is used when the equipment no longer works, causing downtime that constrains or interrupts patient care (and potentially clinical revenue) [8]

Hospitals with low-resource settings commonly run without a proper maintenance department or even an equipment inventory [9]. Consequently, extensive time (and scarce money) is often directed to external help only after an item is causing severe problems. Applying these maintenance types is described in Table 32.5.

## Implementation of a Local Biomed Program

The vast majority of problems that can occur in medical equipment in developing countries is really basic such as loose parts, wear of mechanical parts, and broken cables, among others, which can be easily identified and repaired with the tools shown in Table 32.3 [10, 11].

**Table 32.3** Indispensable tools set to repair medical equipment: (a) electric tools, (b) manual tools, and (c) consumables

| **Tool required** | |
|---|---|
| **(a) Electric** | |
| Multimeter | Flashlight |
| Soldering iron | |
| **(b) Manual** | |
| Tweezers | Jewel screwdrivers |
| Wire cutters | Crescent wrench |
| Wire strippers | Hex wrench set (Allen; metrics and standard) |
| Needle nose pliers | Torx wrench set |
| Phillips screwdrivers | Knife |
| Flathead screwdrivers | Solder sucker |
| Scissors | Tape measure |
| **(c) Consumables** | |
| Electric tape | Roll of solder |
| Duct tape | Fasteners |
| Cyanoacrylate (super glue) | Fuses |
| Epoxy glue | Batteries (AAA, AA y 9 V) |
| Sandpaper | Latex gloves |
| Desoldering wick | |

**Table 32.4** Essential medical equipment

| | |
|---|---|
| Vital signs monitor | Real-time monitoring of patient: *oxygen saturation* [$sPO_2$] (from a digit probe), noninvasive *blood pressure* [NIBP] (from a cuff on arm or leg), electrocardiogram [ECG] (from leads on stickers to chest), and *capnography* [$CO_2$] (the carbon dioxide exhaled with each breath, from a probe connected to the endotracheal tube), among others. Monitor is typically placed on the anesthesia machine or table in the OR. Vital sign monitors are also essential for each patient in the postanesthesia care unit (PACU) |
| Anesthesia vaporizer | Mixes volatile anesthesia agent with fresh gas flow (mixture of medical gases: air, oxygen, and nitrous oxide) to deliver general anesthesia. Requires the patient to be breathing spontaneously (not chemically paralyzed) or anesthesiologist delivering breaths by squeezing a rubber bladder. Generally feasible for most cleft procedures, except for orthognathic surgery |
| Anesthesia machine | Able to deliver anesthesia agents, as well as mechanically deliver breaths to a patient who is chemically paralyzed. If vaporizers are in use, one anesthesia machine should be available in the OR suite in case a patient requires prolonged paralysis or mechanical assistance |
| Ventilator | A ventilator is best suited to a patient requiring long-term ventilation, such as in intensive care. A ventilator should be available in the ICU in case of need for prolonged sedation or respiratory failure postoperatively |
| Electrosurgical unit (ESU) | Used to cut or coagulate tissue, its benefits include the ability to make precise cuts with limited blood loss through electric current. Particularly essential for control of bleeding in the palate or pharynx |

**Table 32.4** (continued)

| | |
|---|---|
| Suction machine | An electrical motor generates suction, essential to clearing the airway for anesthesia and surgery. Utilized as a backup to hospital-integrated wall-suction systems, where available |
| Defibrillator | Used to shock a heart with aberrant electrical activity not delivering regular pulses of blood flow, as part of an advanced cardiac life support (ACLS) intervention. Best located in the OR surgical suite when surgery is underway |
| Autoclave | Use elevated temperature and pressure in a sealed chamber to sterilize surgical instruments and reusable gauze or linens. A test strip should always be used to assure proper temperature attained. Small portable autoclaves facilitate rapid turnover between cleft procedures, in addition to or instead of a larger central hospital autoclave |
| Difficult airway box | Contains airway adjuncts (such as nasopharyngeal tubes, bougie stylette, video laryngoscope, fiber-optic laryngoscope, or naso-endoscope) to be used in a difficult airway or when an airway is suddenly lost. Best located in the OR surgical suite when surgery is underway |
| Crash cart (or box) | Contains medications to be used for an ACLS intervention, as well as dantrolene for malignant hyperthermia. Best located in the OR surgical suite when surgery is underway |

**Table 32.5** Implementing the three maintenance types in LMIC hospitals

| | |
|---|---|
| Predictive maintenance | To apply this quickly and appropriately, a checklist should be developed based on the needs, equipment, and inventory of the hospital in order to evaluate performance and identify any abnormalities |
| Preventive maintenance | Preventive maintenance aims to take into account failures early in medical equipment helping to increase the useful life of the equipment<br>This procedure is based on inspecting the equipment periodically in accordance with the manufacturer's recommendations and solving any damage detected by the engineer in an early manner |
| Corrective maintenance | If a problem occurs during the use of the equipment, the root cause of it should be evaluated in order to restore its functionality and performance<br>The maintenance department should run strenuous tests on all parameters before returning it to use |

Because many of the electrical problems found in low-resource setting hospitals are caused by electrical spikes, it is useful to have several fuses of different value to quickly solve those problems.

Implementing a local biomedical workshop is something that almost every hospital can afford in comparison of the cost of repairing equipment by an external company. This requires only a small space with good lighting, some tools, and personnel.

**Solutions from the Field: Implementing a Local Biomed Program in Rural Nicaragua**

In an order to field test the concept of an embedded full-time biomedical technician, in two rural Nicaraguan hospitals, biomedical technicians were trained through a partnership model (Fig. 32.15). At 1 year, there was an 85% reduction of equipment failures effecting or delaying patient care. In addition, the investment costs of running the program were below 10% of the projected savings and direct and indirect costs of nonfunctional equipment.

## Surgical Instrumentation

Surgical instrumentation in a low-resource setting may be challenging on several fronts. The following discussion will concern handheld stainless steel surgical instrumentation only. When a surgical instrument is labeled as "reusable," manufacturers of these devices must provide complete written instructions for the handling, cleaning, packaging, and sterilization of the products to support the label claim. The manufacturer's instructions should be strictly complied with. However, in a low-resource setting, this information is not known or simply not complied with. Education and training will increase the quality of care as a result of some classroom instruction.

Availability of quality instrumentation is the primary obstacle to successful outcomes. Normally due to budget restrictions, decisions are made to purchase low-quality, low-price instrumentation. Secondly, lack of knowledge for maintenance techniques, cleaning and inspection methods, and proper handling procedures adds to the cost of sustaining a viable inventory. Normally there is no one in the house to repair, sharpen, and educate the staff on these subjects.

As a result of these factors, surgical instruments become basically disposable to some extent. The shortened life of instruments becomes a costly burden to any hospital or medical arena that is providing surgeries. Improper inventory control is another area that presents challenges in a low-resource setting as well. The worst time to find out an instrument is missing or defective is in the OR. This discussion will be promoting the benefits of preventive maintenance.

## Preventive Maintenance

On-site maintenance of surgical instruments is normally managed by scrub nurses and/or the sterile processing

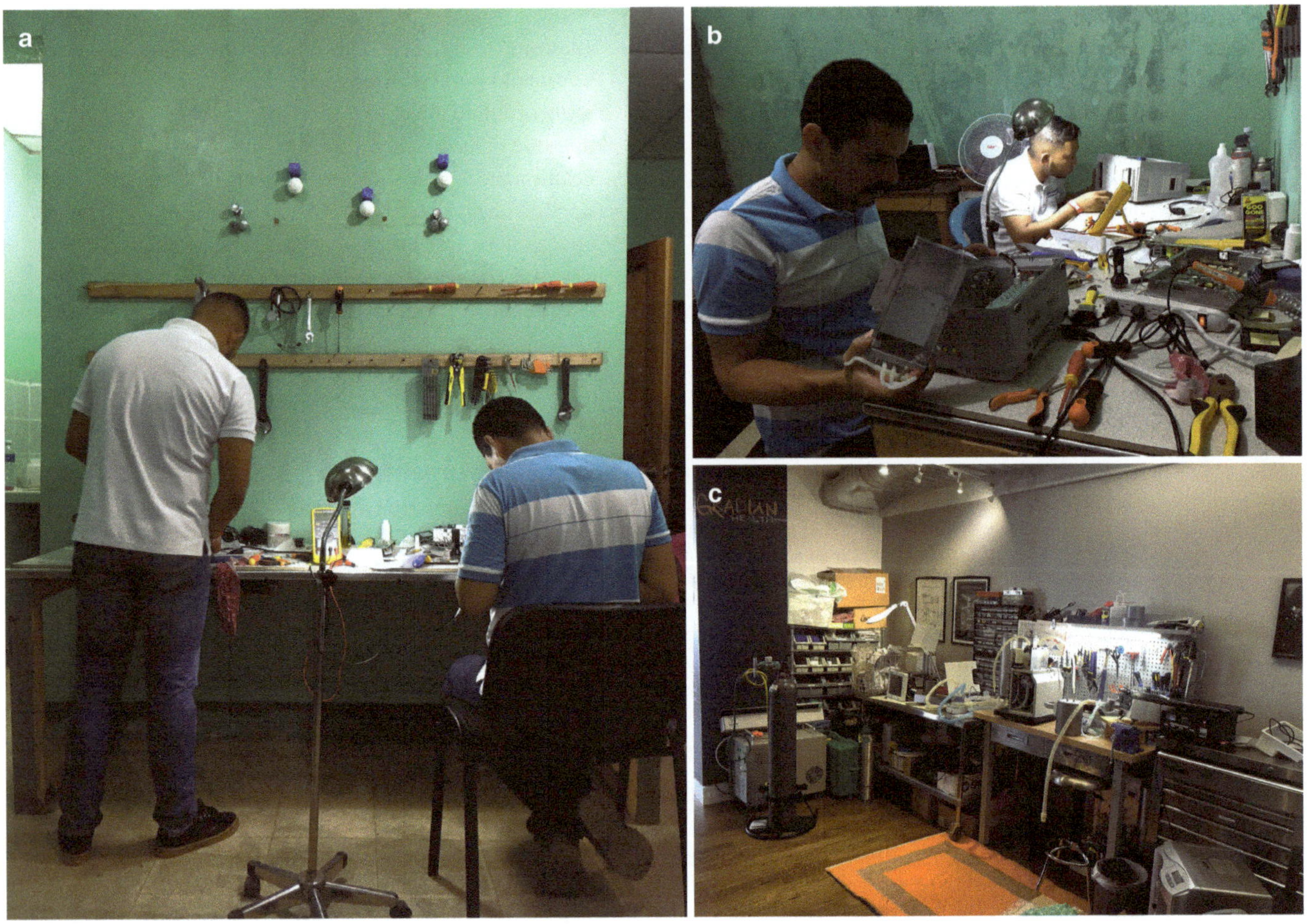


**Fig. 32.15** (**a**, **b**) Biomedical technicians working with just the minimum tools required to do maintenance in a workshop developed in Nicaragua. (**c**) Maintenance workshop in the USA

department. Proper care can prevent instrument damage and prolong the lifespan of most instruments. Involved simple steps like cleaning, inspection, drying, and storage will help keep the instruments from unnecessary damage. Optimally maintained surgical instrumentation requires significant time and resources; the cost pales in comparison to expensive repairs or replacements, as well as potential for patient harm.

## Cleaning

Cleaning an instrument is a critical step in reprocessing it after patient use. The goal of cleaning is to render devices safe for handling and to prep them for reuse. This begins at the point of use and prepares them for the subsequent steps of processing.

Cleaning which is ineffective in removing foreign material from the inside and outside of an instrument will interfere with the efficacy of the subsequent sterilization process. After surgery, instruments should immediately be rinsed in warm [not hot or cold] running water. In low-resource settings, it is common to manually clean all the instruments under the faucet, with untreated water. Dirty water used during cleaning can and will create bio buildup and corrosion issues during the sterilization process.

Moistening and removing gross debris at the point of use can help prevent debris from drying on instruments. Treating instruments with an approved cleaner reduces rusting, corrosion, and debris buildup and inhibits biofilm formation. Improper cleaning of blood and tissue will result in the same issues.

Tissue and debris can become lodged in crevices, box locks, and other areas. Mechanical cleaning is preferred over manual because it is reproducible (e.g., ultrasonic washer, washer dryer). Manual cleaning is subject to variation. All instruments should be visually inspected for cleanliness, correct alignment, corrosion, pitting, kinks, burrs, cracks, wear, chipping of inserts, missing parts, and sharpness of cutting edges.

Efficacy of cleaning has traditionally been evaluated visually. Items that are not clean or do not function allow for the opportunity to remove the instrument from service until cleaned or repaired. The visual inspection phase is most effective if it is done in a well-lit space and with a magnifying lamp by a trained person. Included are some visual guidelines to follow.

### Drying

Residuals like water, surgical debris, and moisture will contain chloride ions that leave brown or dark spots on the surgical instruments. Only a clean and dry instrument should be sterilized. For example, if blood remains on an instrument for more than 20 minutes, it will stain or mark. One of the most damaging procedures is to autoclave an instrument with dried blood. The acidity of blood activated by the temperatures of the autoclave will become a baked-on stain that is extremely difficult to remove. All instruments should be properly dried before being sterilized and stored. If not, corrosion and residual buildup will occur and shorten the life of the instrumentation. This involves hand wiping away all moisture on surface of instruments with a dry soft absorbent cloth. Pay special attention to all hinged instruments, including cutting edges and tips.

### Storage

Instrumentation needs to be stored in a climate-controlled room without threats of insect and rodent infestation. These spaces should have easy access to the operating theater and, if possible, some type of air filtration systems to insure infection control. Instrument storage, the sterilization department, and operating theater should never be on the ground floor. Proper storage of instruments should be done in a metal sterilization container or covered in a sterilization wrap. All sterilization procedures should follow the manufacturer's instructions.

### Lubrication

One of the most effective and the easiest methods of keeping instruments in optimum condition is to lubricate them after every cycle of cleaning. Instruments with moving parts like box locks, hinges, screw joints, and articulation joints should be lubricated regularly. Correct lubrication will keep the moving parts from scraping and rubbing, which prevents straining of the articulation zones and dulling from shearing. All instruments with moving parts should be lubricated with a water-based surgical lubricant (steam penetrable) before autoclaving.

## Conclusion

There are several common problems that can be addressed in a low-resource setting that will greatly improve and eliminate normal issues that are detrimental to the efficacy and life of the instrumentation. Proper care begins with thorough inspection and proper cleaning techniques followed by a scheduled preventive maintenance program. The enemies of instrumentation are water or moisture of any variety. Improper drying is problematic at any level. Cleaning with inappropriate solutions is common issue globally, such as using dirty water, cold or hot water, bleach, improper detergents, and any solution containing chloride or iodine. The addition of ultrasonic cleaning will be a great investment that will eliminate the most common problems and will greatly extend the life of the surgical instrument inventory. Lastly, the purchase of high-quality instruments should be considered a long-term investment and cost-cutting decision. Purchasing the cheapest priced instrumentation will ultimately cost more and lower the quality of the surgeries and directly affect patient outcomes.

## References

1. Bronzino J. The biomedical engineering handbook, volume II. 2nd ed. Boca Raton: CRC Press; 2000. p. 170.1–2.
2. Hossain A, Rashid MA, Islam R, Ahmad M. Current status of skilled clinical engineer in developing countries. Procedia Soc Behav Sci. 2015;195:1688–93.
3. National Fire Protection Association. NFPA 70: National Electrical Code, 2017 Edition, Quincy; 2016. p. 43–5.
4. World Health Organization. Medical device donations: considerations for solicitation and provision. Geneva: World Health Organization; 2011.
5. National Fire Protection Association. NFPA 99: Health Care Facilities Code. 2018 Edition. Boston; 2018. p. 28–68.
6. Taaffe K, Lee B, Ferrand Y, Fredendall L, San D, Salgado C, et al. The influence of traffic, area location, and other factors on operating room microbial load. Infection Control & Hospital Epidemiology Cambridge University Press. 2018;39(4):391–7.
7. Birgand G, Azevedo C, Toupet G, et al. Attitudes, risk of infection and behaviours in the operating room (the ARIBO project): a prospective, cross- sectional study. BMJ Open. 2014;4:e004274. https://doi.org/10.1136/bmjopen-2013-004274.
8. World Health Organization. Medical equipment maintenance program overview. Geneva: World Health Organization; 2011.
9. World Health Organization. Introduction to medical equipment inventory management. Geneva: World Health Organization; 2011.
10. Malkin R. Medical instrumentation in the developing world. 1st ed. Memphis: Engineering World Health; 2006. p. 105–14.
11. Kaewgun T, Yantapan K, Anupongongarch P. Multi-function electrical safety tester for medical equipment application. In: 2016 International Conference on Biomedical Engineering (BME-HUST), Hanoi; 2016. p. 57–60.
12. Schönmeyr B, Wendby L, Campbell A. Early surgical complications after primary cleft lip repair: a report of 3108 consecutive cases. Cleft Palate Craniofac J. 2015;52(6):706–10.

# Part V

# Cleft Education, Innovation, and Surgical Outcomes

# Cleft Lip and Palate Simulators in Surgical Training

33

Dale J. Podolsky, David M. Fisher, Karen W. Y. Wong Riff, James M. Drake, and Christopher R. Forrest

## Introduction

Cleft lip and palate surgery is challenging. Good outcomes rely on experience, tactile knowledge of soft tissue, anatomic awareness, delicate tissue handling, as well as precise dissections. Technical errors can result in aesthetic and functional consequences that may be difficult or impossible to correct. Specifically for cleft palate surgery, the small confines of the infant oral cavity make it difficult to supervise a trainee [1]. This in addition to limited instrument manipulation within the oral cavity and the delicate anatomy of the velum makes cleft palate surgery uniquely difficult to learn. There is also evidence that adverse outcomes such as palatal fistula and poor speech correlate with surgeon experience [2, 3]. For cleft lip repair, mastery of the pre-incision markings, understanding of the geometric relationships of the lip elements, and addressing the nasal deformity require a three-dimensional (3D) appreciation of the deformity and methods of correction that can be difficult to understand. For these reasons, a platform to practice cleft surgery outside of the operating room to gain experience without compromising patient outcomes is advantageous.

Cadavers provide a realistic environment to learn anatomy and surgical procedures and are widely used [4] for surgical training outside of the operating room. However, they can be costly and difficult to access [5]. Animal models have also been utilized [6], and a cleft palate goat model has been developed [7]. However, there is always the ethical discussion of practicing on animals, and such a model is difficult to implement widely. For the reasons described above, the use of simulation is finding an increasing role in cleft surgical education [1, 8–16].

## Surgical Simulation

Surgical simulators have been shown to improve operating room performance [17, 18]. Generally, surgical simulators are either physical models or virtual environments [11, 19]. Physical simulators provide a synthetic workspace and are developed using material to mimic human tissue. In cleft palate surgery, a physical representation of the infant oral cavity allows practicing instrument manipulation within the small confines of the workspace. However, disadvantages of physical simulators are the inability to reuse them after each use. Virtual simulators, on the other hand, allow unconstrained repeat practice [20], but they can lack realism and tactile feedback. Efforts in implementing haptic feedback where a virtual environment can be translated to a physical one are promising, but more work is necessary to reach higher levels of fidelity [21].

Simulators can also be classified as either task trainers or complete end-to-end simulations of complex procedures. Task trainers simulate a portion of a procedure or allow performance of a particular task (e.g., insertion of an IV, insertion of a Foley catheter). End-to-end simulators allow performance of an entire procedure. Task trainers or full simulators can also be either physical or virtual environments.

D. J. Podolsky (✉)
Division of Plastic & Reconstructive Surgery, University of Toronto, Toronto, ON, Canada
e-mail: dale.podolsky@mail.utoronto.ca

D. M. Fisher · C. R. Forrest
Division of Plastic & Reconstructive Surgery, University of Toronto, Toronto, ON, Canada

The Cleft Lip and Palate Program, Division of Plastic & Reconstructive Surgery, The Hospital for Sick Children, Toronto, ON, Canada
e-mail: christopher.forrest@sickkids.ca

K. W. Y. Wong Riff
Division of Plastic and Reconstructive Surgery, Hospital for Sick Children, Toronto, ON, Canada
e-mail: karenw.wong@sickkids.ca

J. M. Drake
Division of Neurosurgery, The Hospital for Sick Children, Toronto, ON, Canada
e-mail: james.drake@sickkids.ca

© Springer Nature Switzerland AG 2021
J. W. Swanson, D. W. Low (eds.), *Global Cleft Care in Low-Resource Settings*, https://doi.org/10.1007/978-3-030-59105-2_33

## Cleft Simulators

Many physical [14, 16, 22–25] and virtual [19, 26, 27] simulators for cleft surgery have previously been described. The majority of the physical simulators would be considered task trainers where only a portion of the procedure can be performed. An exception to this are the cleft lip (Fig. 33.1) [13] and palate simulator (Fig. 33.2) [11] developed at the Hospital for Sick Children in Toronto, Canada, and now commercially available (Simulare Medical Corp., Toronto, Canada) [25]. These high-fidelity simulators allow performance of the entire procedure from start to finish. They are complete representations of cleft anatomy allowing detailed dissections, incisions, and performance assessment of particular surgical steps using real surgical instruments. These higher-fidelity simulators are developed using 3D printing, polymer, and adhesive techniques to emulate realistic tissue feel and dissection planes. The primary disadvantage of these higher-fidelity simulators relates to increased cost associated with their production. The Simulare cleft simulators cost between US$200 and US$300 per simulator. The Simulare cleft lip and palate simulators can be found at http://www.simularemedical.com.

These high-fidelity cleft simulators allow the trainee surgeon the opportunity to perform all critical steps of the procedure. The high-fidelity cleft palate simulator comprises a cleft of the secondary palate [11]. Von Langenbeck, Bardach, and Furlow repairs have been performed on the simulator. The simulator incorporates detailed anatomy with distinct velar musculature. This allows precise dissection and the ability to visualize the anatomy of the palate, which can be difficult to understand and appreciate.

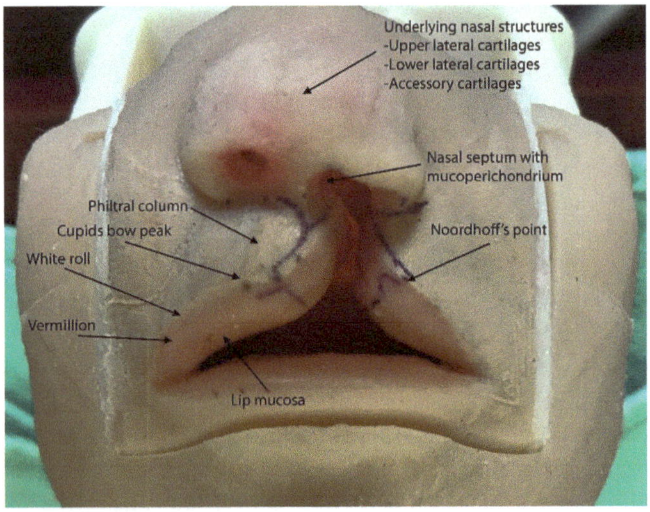


Fig. 33.1 High-fidelity cleft lip simulator demonstrating markings for a rotation advancement-type repair

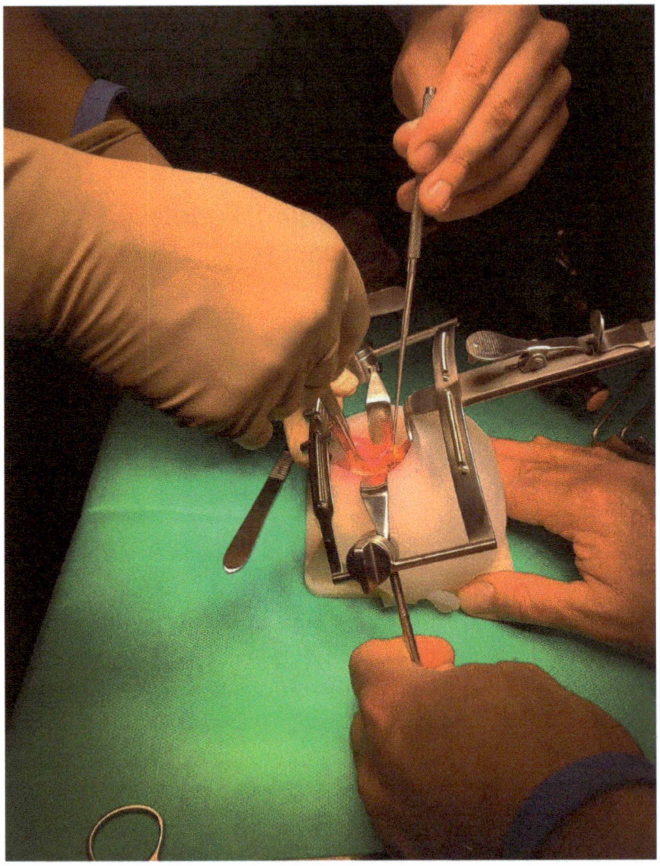

Fig. 33.2 Utilization of a high-fidelity cleft palate simulator during a cleft palate simulator training workshop

The cleft lip simulator also allows performance of critical steps of a repair (Fig. 33.1) [13]. The simulator includes accurate surface features, multilayered tissues, and complete nasal anatomy. Steps of the procedure that can be performed include performing the markings, removal of lip marginal tissue, repositioning of the septum, primary rhinoplasty, and closure. Both rotation advancement and anatomical subunit approximation techniques have been performed successfully on the simulator.

The platform utilized by Smile Train [27] walks the user through a 3D virtual cleft lip or palate procedure. These simulators provide a valuable exercise in understanding fundamental concepts of the procedure, anatomy, and procedural steps. The Smile Train cleft simulator can be found at https://www.smiletrain.org/medical/training/virtual-surgery-simulator. More recently, a free app for smart phones has been developed demonstrating step-by-step demonstrations of procedures for cleft and craniofacial reconstructions. This is available for download at https://www.myface.org/civa.

## Simulators from the Field

High-fidelity cleft simulators can be expensive and cost prohibitive for widespread adoption. As a result, several groups have developed more economical alternatives that use commonly available material and provide instructions for do-it-yourself assembly. The "Shazmak" simulator is such an example, developed by cleft surgeons Dr. Mohamed El-Shazley and Dr. Mohamed Makmoul in Egypt. This simple simulator utilizes a foam sheet to simulate mucosa covering a plastic sheet representing the hard palate, with red tubing to create the greater palatine neurovascular pedicle and red elastic material for the levator veli muscles. The model is placed within a transparent cup to simulate the confines of the infant oral cavity (Fig. 33.3) and can be built by students from an instruction sheet (Shazmak simulator assembly instructions are available by contacting Dr. Mohamad El-Shazley at elshazly@aun.edu.eg.). Similarly, a simulator developed by Pang et al. describes using a pig's tongue and surgical gloves to simulate the soft palate and oral cavity [28]. Although these low-cost models may not incorporate complete anatomy, they allow trainees to practice fundamental skills in cleft palate repair such as cutting and suturing within small confined areas and to emphasize key procedural steps such as release and repositioning of the levator veli musculature. They represent an effective starting point with respect to practicing technique before progressing to more complex surgical steps. Lower-cost production of higher-fidelity simulators is also being pursued [29] but is not yet available.

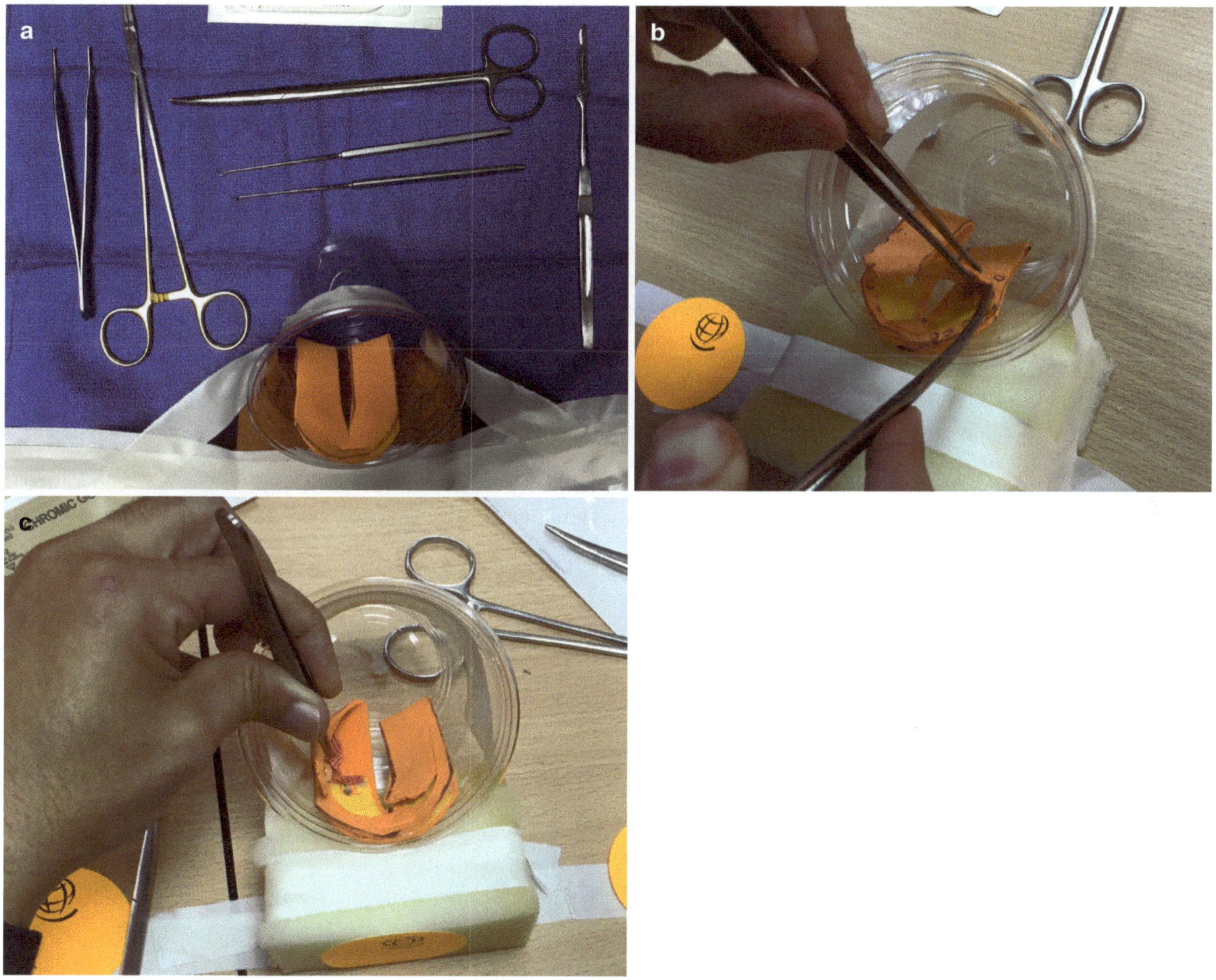


**Fig. 33.3** Shazmak simulator; with basic instrumentation (**a**), being dissected in the submucosal layer (**b**) to expose the greater palatine neurovascular pedicle (**c**). (Courtesy of Drs. Mohamed El-Shazley and Mohamed Makmoul.)

## Cleft Simulator Validation

The types of validation utilized for simulators have typically included face, content, and construct validity. These specific descriptions are being replaced by the unitary framework proposed by Messick [30]. In this framework, a simulator or educational tool is never thought of as valid or invalid but whether it has evidence to support its effectiveness and use. In this framework, five domains of building evidence are described and are (1) content, (2) process response, (3) internal structure, (4) relations to other variables, and (5) consequences. *Content* refers to the expertise of the simulator's development team, *process response* refers to quality control during the evaluation stage of the simulator, *internal structure* refers to the reliability of the process, *relationship to other variables* is most commonly used to describe performance in relation to experience level, and *consequences* are used to describe the process of using the simulator to provide feedback for performance improvement.

There is a large variability in the level of validation for the cleft simulators that have been developed. Almost all have only demonstrated "content validity [30]," more commonly known as "face validity [31]" in the older system of educational assessment. The gold standard measure of a simulator's effectiveness is whether its use leads to fewer negative patient outcomes. None of the cleft simulators developed to date have proven this. This is in part due to the reluctance of supervising surgeons to allow trainees to practice independently and the long time frames in assessing outcomes in cleft surgery. The simulator with the largest body of evidence is the cleft palate simulator developed at The Hospital for Sick Children in Toronto, Canada [11]. The simulator has been shown to improve performance after repeated use in a simulated environment [12], confidence, as well as knowledge [8, 11]. The simulator has also been shown to distinguish between skill levels [9, 12] ("relationship to other variables [29]" formerly known as "construct validity [32]"), a hallmark of a valid simulator.

## Assessing Performance in Cleft Surgery

The most frequently utilized tools to assess technical performance are checklists that comprise both a procedure-specific and global rating scale [33]. Procedure-specific scales allow assessment of specific components of the procedure. Global rating scales provide a more generalized assessment of technical skill and are thought by some to be more reliable than procedure-specific scales [34]. A validated cleft-specific technical assessment tool [12] entitled CLOSATS (cleft palate objective structured assessment of technical skill) has been developed by our group and assessed in trainees [32]. In this study, the CLOSATS and a previously developed global rating scale [33] determined that repeat use of the cleft palate simulator leads to improved performance over time. In addition, using standard setting techniques, a minimum number of 6.3 simulation sessions were required to reach competence. Standard setting methods were utilized to determine the minimum acceptable score [35]. This number represents a framework for supervising surgeons to develop a longitudinal training program and to determine whether trainees meet minimum acceptable scores.

## International Implementation of Cleft Simulators

These cleft simulators have been implemented in a variety of settings around the world. A study utilizing the cleft palate simulator in Santiago, Chile (Fundación Gantz), demonstrated that the simulator can be successfully implemented within an international setting using video recording for the purpose of technical assessment (Fig. 33.4). Intraoral video recording of cleft palate repair is necessary for technical assessment. This required the development of a novel, low-cost video recording setup using a USB-connected endoscope in conjunction with a Dingman retractor attachment (Fig. 33.5). In this study, 16 surgeons from South America used the simulator during a 2-day workshop. The workshop proved that implementation of the simulator is easily done and a low-cost endoscope provided sufficient resolution to perform the assessments. The assessments demonstrated adequate reliability. Using previously determined minimum acceptable scores, the assessment data demonstrated that surgeons with high levels of experience may fail to meet minimum scores. One conclusion of the study is that experi-

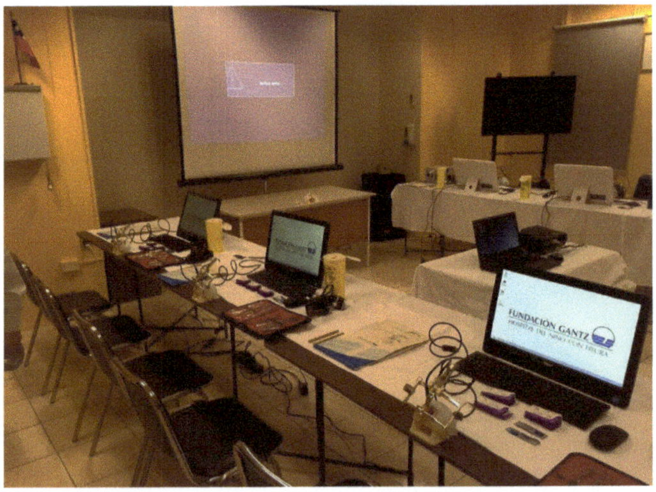

Fig. 33.4 Comprehensive cleft palate training workshop at Fundación Gantz in Santiago, Chile

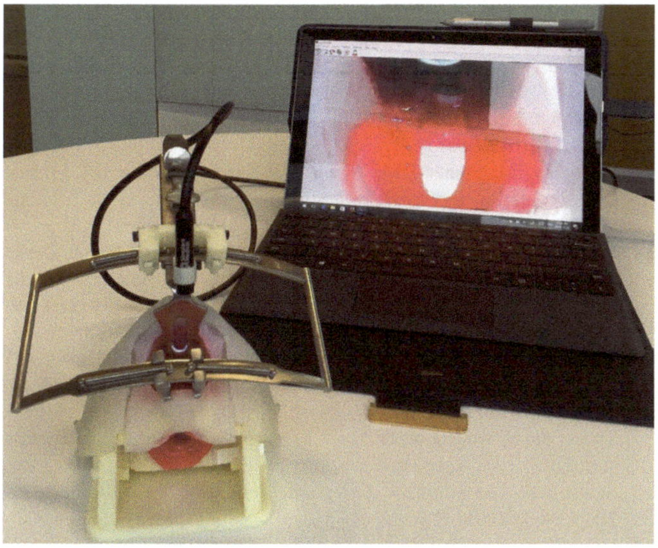

**Fig. 33.5** Cleft palate simulator with USB-connected endoscope coupled to a novel Dingman attachment piece

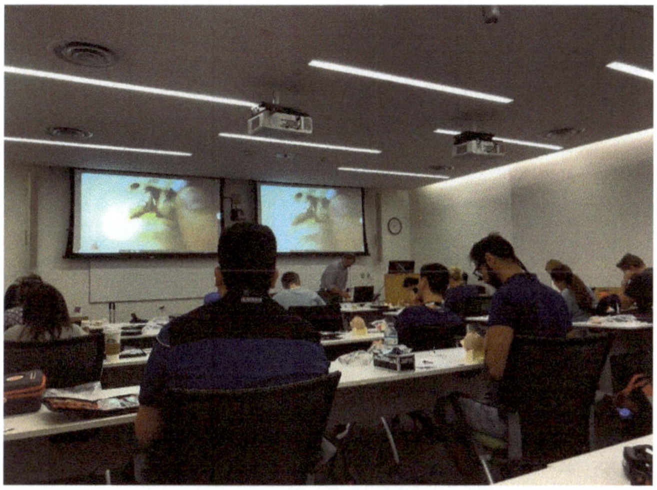

**Fig. 33.6** Comprehensive cleft lip simulation training workshop

ence alone may not be enough to determine competence in cleft palate repair.

Similar types of workshops have been implemented for cleft lip repair. Figure 33.6 demonstrates a cleft lip training workshop at The Hospital for Sick Children in Toronto, Canada. During this workshop, an expert cleft surgeon performed a simulated lip repair that was projected on a large screen. The trainees, each with their own simulator, emulated each procedural step in real time following the expert surgeon.

Nongovernmental organizations (NGOs) involved in delivering cleft surgeries in low- and middle-income countries may desire more objective and accurate methods to assess whether surgeons are competent to perform cleft surgeries independently. NGOs are under increasing scrutiny by governments to perform safe surgeries in other countries [36]. A simulator provides a platform to perform an objective assessment of skill level. The work by Ericsson [37, 38] highlights why experience as measured by the number of years in practice or case number may not be adequate to assess competence. He describes the concept of deliberate practice, where feedback and conscious effort to improve are required to reach skill mastery. A surgeon's level of experience alone does not take into account the level of deliberate practice. Therefore, an objective measure of skill is required, and a simulator in conjunction with assessment tools provides this within a safe environment.

## The Future of Cleft Simulation

The implementation of new technology to cleft simulation will play an important role in the future. Augmented and virtual reality are becoming increasingly more realistic. However, the integration of more realistic haptic-enabled instruments where a user can sense surgical workspaces is necessary to provide more meaningful simulated virtual training experiences. Three-dimensional printing has enabled development of complex medical models and anatomical structures that are not possible to develop using standard manufacturing techniques. In addition, 3D printing is continually becoming more cost-effective and more reliable providing the prospects of cheaper models that can be developed quicker, while maintaining the same level of detail and accuracy.

The integration of new technology within the realm of cleft simulation will play an important role in the future. It is not only the development of more sophisticated and realistic simulators that is required but also the optimum method of implementation. Cleft surgical training requires meeting specific needs within the international cleft community. The large burden of cleft [39] within low- and middle-income countries requires creative approaches that are cost-sensitive and can be implemented within lower-resource environments. Furthermore, access to expertise in these environments is often lacking.

An interesting concept is the utilization of remote teaching platforms to teach surgery and to assess performance. The cleft lip and palate simulators in conjunction with low-cost video recording equipment are the fundamental building blocks required to implement a remote teaching environment. A simulator with recording equipment can be sent to a remote center anywhere in the world. The simulator with video recording of the simulated procedure can be sent back to a center of expertise to assess performance and to provide feedback. Access to the Internet in low-resource environments is improving [40]. Internet access provides the ability to perform live teaching sessions and real-time feedback.

This may play a significant role in training future cleft surgeons in geographical areas that lack expertise. This concept has been successfully implemented in other surgical specialties [41–43].

## Conclusions

Simulation has an important role to play in surgical training. Cleft simulators allow trainees and surgeons to practice cleft surgery to gain experience outside of the operating room. There is growing interest in cleft simulator development, and the latest simulators have the fidelity necessary to practice a cleft palate and cleft lip repair from start to finish in highly realistic physical environments. Utilization of these simulators in conjunction with assessment tools provides the framework to assess technical performance to integrate training strategies that rely on objective measures of assessment. These tools can be implemented in international settings and will play a growing role in cleft surgical training paradigms in both developed and developing countries.

**Conflict of Interest** Drs Dale Podolsky, David Fisher, Karen Wong Riff, James Drake, and Christopher Forrest are shareholders of Simulare Medical Corp, which produces and sells the Simulare cleft lip and palate simulators.

## References


1. Podolsky DJ, Fisher DM, Wong Riff KW, Looi T, Drake JM, Forrest CR. Infant robotic cleft palate surgery: a feasibility assessment using a realistic cleft palate simulator. Plast Reconstr Surg. 2017;139(2):455e–65e.
2. Rintala AH, Haapanen ML. The correlation between training and skill of the surgeon and reoperation rate for persistent cleft palate speech. Br J Oral Maxillofac Surg. 1995;33:295–8.
3. Witt PD, Wahlen JC, Marsh JL, Grames LM, Pilgram TK. The effect of surgeon experience on velopharyngeal functional outcome following palatoplasty: is there a learning curve? Plast Reconstr Surg. 1998;102(5):1375–84.
4. Kshettry VR, Mullin JP, Schlenk R, Recinos PF, Benzel EC. The role of laboratory dissection training in neurosurgical residency: results of a national survey. World Neurosurg. 2014;82(5):554–9.
5. Lloyd GM, Maxwell-Armstrong C, Acheson AG. Fresh frozen cadavers: an under-utilized resource in laparoscopic colorectal training in the United Kingdom. Color Dis. 2011;13(9):e303–4.
6. La Torre M, Caruso C. The animal model in advanced laparoscopy resident training. Surg Laparosc Endosc Percutan Tech. 2013;23(3):271–5.
7. Weinzweig J, Panter KE, Patel J, Smith DM, Spangenberger A, Freeman MB. The fetal cleft palate: v. elucidation of the mechanism of palatal clefting in the congenital caprine model. Plast Reconstr Surg. 2008;121(4):1328–34.
8. Cheng H, Podolsky DJ, Fisher DM, Wong KW, Lorenz HP, Khosla RK, et al. Teaching palatoplasty using a high-fidelity cleft palate simulator. Plast Reconstr Surg. 2018;141(1):91e–8e.
9. Ghanem A, Podolsky DJ, Fisher DM, Wong Riff KW, Myers S, Drake JM, et al. Economy of hand motion during cleft palate surgery using a high-fidelity cleft palate simulator. Cleft Palate Craniofac J. 2018:1055665618793768.
10. Podolsky DJ, Cheng H, Fisher DM, Wong Riff KW, Drake JM, Forrest CR. Reply: evaluation and implementation of a high-fidelity cleft palate simulator. Plast Reconstr Surg. 2018;142(6):980e–1e.
11. Podolsky DJ, Fisher DM, Wong KW, Looi T, Drake JM, Forrest CR. Evaluation and implementation of a high-fidelity cleft palate simulator. Plast Reconstr Surg. 2017;139(1):85e–96e.
12. Podolsky DJ, Fisher DM, Wong Riff KW, Szasz P, Looi T, Drake JM, et al. Assessing technical performance and determining the learning curve in cleft palate surgery using a high-fidelity cleft palate simulator. Plast Reconstr Surg. 2018;141(6):1485–500.
13. Podolsky DJ, Wong Riff KW, Drake JM, Forrest CR, Fisher DM. A high fidelity cleft lip simulator. Plast Reconstr Surg Glob Open. 2018;6(9):e1871.
14. Vadodaria S, Watkin N, Thiessen F, Ponniah A. The first cleft palate simulator. Plast Reconstr Surg. 2007;120(1):259–61.
15. Senturk S. The simplest cleft palate simulator. J Craniofac Surg. 2013;24(3):1056.
16. Devinck F, Riot S, Qassemyar A, Belkhou A, Wolber A, Martinot Duquennoy V, et al. Suture simulator - Cleft palate surgery. Ann Chir Plast Esthet. 2017;62(2):167–70.
17. Kazan R, Cyr S, Hemmerling TM, Lin SJ, Gilardino MS. The evolution of surgical simulation: the current state and future avenues for plastic surgery education. Plast Reconstr Surg. 2017;139(2):533e–43e.
18. Cosman P, Hemli JM, Ellis AM, Hugh TJ. Learning the surgical craft: a review of skills training options. ANZ J Surg. 2007;77(10):838–45.
19. Schendel S, Montgomery K, Sorokin A, Lionetti G. A surgical simulator for planning and performing repair of cleft lips. J Craniomaxillofac Surg. 2005;33(4):223–8.
20. Pfandler M, Lazarovici M, Stefan P, Wucherer P, Weigl M. Virtual reality-based simulators for spine surgery: a systematic review. Spine J. 2017;17(9):1352–63.
21. Escobar-Castillejos D, Noguez J, Neri L, Magana A, Benes B. A review of simulators with haptic devices for medical training. J Med Syst. 2016;40(4):104.
22. Matthews MS. A teaching device for Furlow palatoplasty. Cleft Palate Craniofac J. 1999;36(1):64–6.
23. Zheng Y, Lu B, Zhang J, Wu G. CAD/CAM silicone simulator for teaching cheiloplasty: description of the technique. Br J Oral Maxillofac Surg. 2015;53(2):194–6.
24. Cote V, Schwartz M, Arbouin Vargas JF, Canfarotta M, Kavanagh KR, Hamdan U, et al. 3-Dimensional printed haptic simulation model to teach incomplete cleft palate surgery in an international setting. Int J Pediatr Otorhinolaryngol. 2018;113:292–7.
25. Rogers-Vizena CR, Saldanha FYL, Hosmer AL, Weinstock PH. A new paradigm in cleft lip procedural excellence: creation and preliminary digital validation of a lifelike simulator. Plast Reconstr Surg. 2018;142(5):1300–4.
26. Kobayashi M, Nakajima T, Mori A, Tanaka D, Fujino T, Chiyokura H. Three-dimensional computer graphics for surgical procedure learning: web three-dimensional application for cleft lip repair. Cleft Palate Craniofac J. 2006;43(3):266–71.
27. Kantar RS, Plana NM, Cutting CB, Diaz-Siso JR, Flores RL. Internet-based digital simulation for cleft surgery education: a 5-year assessment of demographics, usage, and global effect. J Surg Educ. 2018;75(4):1120–6.
28. Pang X, Yang C, Shi B, Li CH. Teaching palatoplasty using a high-fidelity cleft palate simulator. Plast Reconstr Surg. 2018;142(6):978e–80e.
29. Reighard CL, Green K, Rooney DM, Zopf DA. Development of a novel, low-cost, high-fidelity cleft lip repair surgical simulator using computer-aided design and 3-dimensional printing. JAMA Facial Plast Surg. 2019;21(1):77–9.

30. Ghaderi I, Manji F, Park YS, Juul D, Ott M, Harris I, et al. Technical skills assessment toolbox: a review using the unitary framework of validity. Ann Surg. 2015;261(2):251–62.
31. van der Wiel SE, Koch AD, Bruno MJ. Face and construct validity of a novel mechanical ERCP simulator. Endosc Int Open. 2018;6(6):E758–E65.
32. Kenney PA, Wszolek MF, Gould JJ, Libertino JA, Moinzadeh A. Face, content, and construct validity of dV-trainer, a novel virtual reality simulator for robotic surgery. Urology. 2009;73(6):1288–92.
33. Reznick R, Regehr G, MacRae H, Martin J, McCulloch W. Testing technical skill via an innovative "bench station" examination. Am J Surg. 1997;173(3):226–30.
34. Laeeq K, Waseem R, Weatherly RA, Reh DD, Lin SY, Lane AP, et al. In-training assessment and predictors of competency in endoscopic sinus surgery. Laryngoscope. 2010;120(12):2540–5.
35. Szasz P, Bonrath EM, Louridas M, Fecso AB, Howe B, Fehr A, et al. Setting performance standards for technical and nontechnical competence in general surgery. Ann Surg. 2017;266(1):1–7.
36. Welling DR, Ryan JM, Burris DG, Rich NM. Seven sins of humanitarian medicine. World J Surg. 2010;34(3):466–70.
37. Ericsson KA. Acquisition and maintenance of medical expertise: a perspective from the expert-performance approach with deliberate practice. Acad Med. 2015;90(11):1471–86.
38. Ericsson KA. Deliberate practice and acquisition of expert performance: a general overview. Acad Emerg Med. 2008;15(11):988–94.
39. Poenaru D. Getting the job done: analysis of the impact and effectiveness of the Smile Train program in alleviating the global burden of cleft disease. World J Surg. 2013;37(7):1562–70.
40. Nations U. World's most vulnerable countries on track to achieve universal internet access by 2020 - UN report: United Nations; 2018. Available from: https://www.un.org/sustainabledevelopment/blog/2018/01/worlds-vulnerable-countries-track-achieve-universal-internet-access-2020-un-report/.
41. Okrainec A, Vassiliou M, Kapoor A, Pitzul K, Henao O, Kaneva P, et al. Feasibility of remote administration of the Fundamentals of Laparoscopic Surgery (FLS) skills test. Surg Endosc. 2013;27(11):4033–7.
42. Okrainec A, Vassiliou M, Jimenez MC, Henao O, Kaneva P, Matt Ritter E. Remote FLS testing in the real world: ready for "prime time". Surg Endosc. 2016;30(7):2697–702.
43. Choy I, Fecso A, Kwong J, Jackson T, Okrainec A. Remote evaluation of laparoscopic performance using the global operative assessment of laparoscopic skills. Surg Endosc. 2013;27(2):378–83.

# Cleft Surgeon Training Models

# 34

Meghan McCullough and Alex Campbell

## Introduction

Skilled providers are the backbone of healthcare delivery systems, and effective training programs are central to any strategy for markedly increasing surgical services in low- and middle-income countries (LMICs). For the advanced surgical training required for cleft surgery, a traditional model had been for surgeons in LMICs to travel to visit institutions in high-income countries (HICs). While these are potentially valuable opportunities, they are limited in number, the environment is often dissimilar to the home institutions from which trainees visit, and increased regulatory barriers often prevent trainees from hands-on training through patient care. These limitations constrain the ability of HIC visitation to scale up the global surgical workforce. The Lancet Global Surgery 2030 report states that "NGOs should have a training component hardwired into their programs to ensure the durability of their effect" [1]. Humanitarian organizations, academic institutions, and hospitals are working to develop better strategies to train, distribute, and support surgical specialists in order to improve equity of access across all populations. The complexity of providing safe, quality surgery combined with the sheer scale of need necessitates creativity, innovation, and lasting dedication. Success requires a disruption in the classical approach to surgical education and strategies to shift the majority of training opportunities to the LMICs where expertise is ultimately required [2].

M. McCullough (✉)
Keck School of Medicine, University of Southern California, Los Angeles, CA, USA
e-mail: Meghan.McCullough@med.usc.edu

A. Campbell
Division of Plastic Surgery, Penn State Hershey College of Medicine, Hershey, PA, USA

Operation Smile Inc, Virginia Beach, VA, USA

Mobile Surgery International, Mexico City, Mexico

Premium Care Plastic Surgery, Cartagena, Colombia

This chapter covers a range of models for international collaboration in the training of cleft surgery, and various organizations are discussed as illustrative examples. Many other organizations are conducting valuable programs to advance the education of in-country trainees, and further documentation and coordination within the global surgery field should help unify training efforts and share best practices [3].

## Mission Trips

International collaborations have most commonly taken place through short-term service trips, often referred to as "missions." Primarily focused on delivering surgical care and comprehensive services to otherwise untreated patients, they have been critiqued for placing less emphasis on sustainability. Many organizations engaged in missions have responded by investing in education to provide surgical training experiences to local surgeons. Rotoplast, Global Smile Foundation, ReSurge International, Operation Smile, and Transforming Faces all cite inclusion of local providers on missions as an important element of their engagement [4–9].

Surgical mission trips have the ability to bring together visiting and local surgeons for rigorous periods of hands-on training taking advantage of volume and repetition inherent to the mission setting. Evaluation and treatment of large numbers of patients in an intimate local setting provide a platform for exchange of ideas and intensive instruction both in the clinical setting and in the operating room [10] (Fig. 34.1). Weaknesses of mission-based training include shortcomings of "on the spot" intraoperative instruction by the visiting surgeons and the tension between throughput of operative volume and a slower pace for teaching and learning. Although considered to be valuable experiences by mentors and trainees, a common sentiment is that the learning accompanying surgical missions does adequately transfer knowledge and skills to enable trainees to operate independently when mission teams are away.

© Springer Nature Switzerland AG 2021

J. W. Swanson, D. W. Low (eds.), *Global Cleft Care in Low-Resource Settings*, https://doi.org/10.1007/978-3-030-59105-2_34

In response to the need for more clear training objectives, better continuity of instruction, and more specific evaluation mechanisms, several organizations have developed formalized curriculum to monitor the progression of individual trainees over time:

- ReSurge International developed the ReSurge Global Training Program (RGTP). The program is modeled after the US surgical residency training paradigm with core competencies in medical knowledge, patient care, communication, and professionalism. Local surgical trainees participating in the program are directly observed by visiting educators and evaluated on their understanding of surgical indications during preoperative patient evaluations, their technical abilities in the operating room, and their postoperative management of patients following surgery. A recent review of the RGTP details the structure and delivery of the program during its first 3 years and shows promising impact developing competent reconstructive surgeons in partner countries [11].
- Operation Smile similarly developed a cleft surgery training program to utilize its extensive platform of missions to train cleft surgeons from partner countries [12]. The program pairs local trainees with senior visiting surgeons over the course of four to five missions in a 1- to 2-year period. Through these trainings, participants complete a "cleft fellowship" and gain competency and independence in cleft surgery. The mentors and candidates participate in a formalized educational curriculum, mentored surgical training, and a competency-based evaluation system to ensure that their training is progressing in an intentional and evidence-based fashion. The evaluation form rates both technical and nontechnical skills and grades trainees on a 1 through 5 scale based on their degree of autonomy in performing essential steps of individual cleft procedures. Figure 34.2 shows average improvement in lip- and palate-specific competencies observed among a cohort of trainees over a single mission-based training experience. Data from the pilot program demonstrates a statistically significant increase in both technical and nontechnical skills over

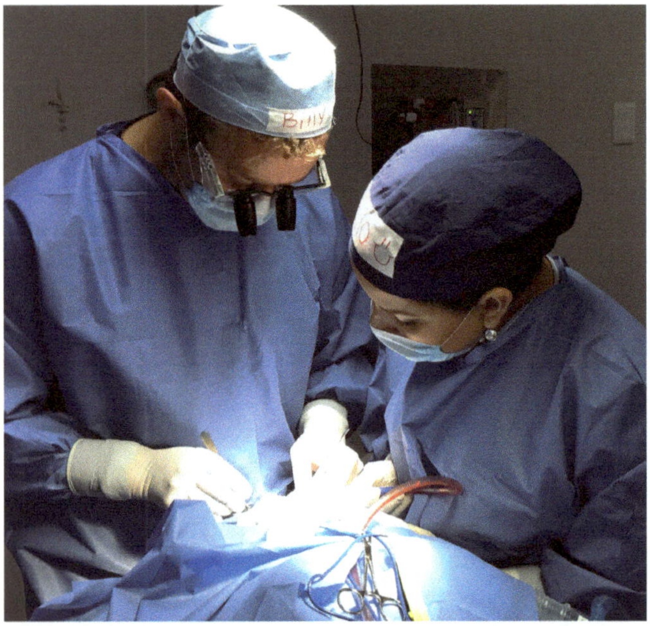

**Fig. 34.1** Surgical mission trips bring together visiting and local surgeons for intensive hands-on training taking advantage of patient volume and procedure repetition

**Fig. 34.2** Average percentage improvement in lip- and palate-specific competencies observed among a cohort of trainees over a single mission-based training experience through a formal cleft surgeon training program. (Reproduced from McCullough et al. [12] through a Creative Commons license)

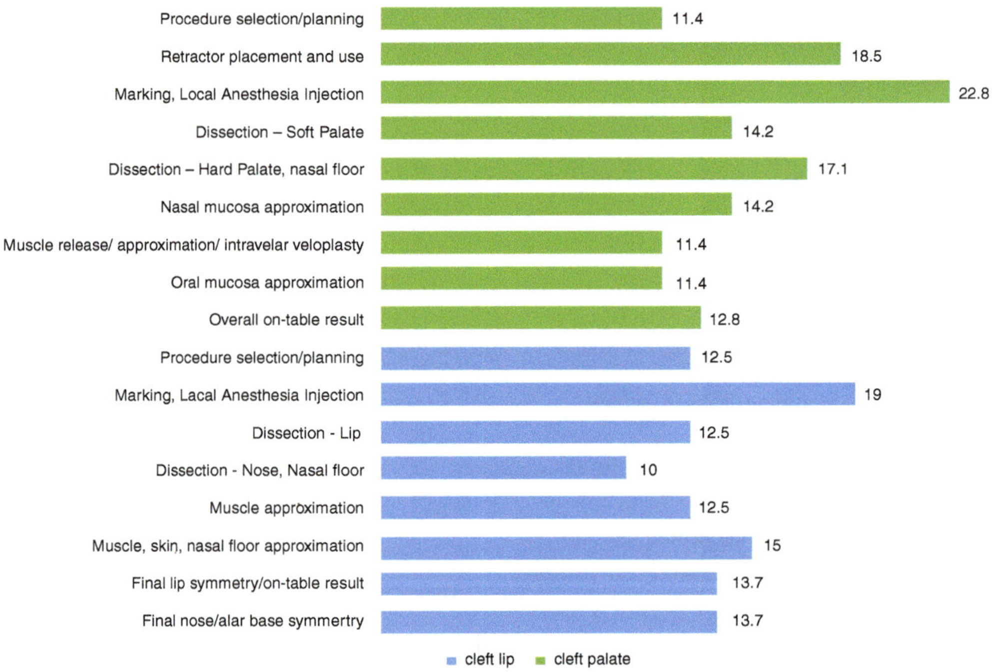

the course of the training as well as high levels of subjective satisfaction with the program [12].

**Side Bar: Educational Surgical Missions Focused on Specific Needs**

A short-term mission trip may be particularly conducive to education when it is focused on bringing expertise to a specific problem. For instance, an organization in one South American country identified a high rate of nasolabial and palatal fistulas, the treatment of which was avoided by local surgeons who were unfamiliar with how to treat them. In response, a weeklong educational mission was convened with the first 2 days focused on lectures, workshops, and live cast surgeries, with the subsequent 4 days focused on treating approximately 80 patients with pairs of more and less experienced surgeons operating together. At the conclusion of the week, all participants reported an improved understanding of both the treatment and prevention of fistulas.

## Advantages

- Short-time commitment enables mentor surgeons from HICs to use vacation time to attend trips and still meet the demands of full-time work commitments at home.
- The model integrates education into existing service delivery platforms.
- High volume and multiple experienced mentors facilitate effective transfer of skills.
- Structured training pathways with multiple experiences over time allow for progressive acquisition of ability and autonomy.

## Disadvantages

- Ensuring continuity can be challenging, and without formalized curriculums and structured tracking of trainees, efforts can become fragmented.
- Total time to train surgeons is relatively long as training opportunities are intensive but spaced over several educational experiences.

## Long-Term Collaborations Through Partner Hospitals

In response to concerns of fragmentation, duplication of efforts, and limited follow-up inherent to short-term trips, many organizations have sought to establish long-term partnerships to ensure continuity of care across sustained visits to a single site. The emphasis of these partnerships is primarily educational, with operative care by the visiting teams either a secondary goal or reserved for challenging cases. These long-term partnerships can provide more consistent educational inputs, as well as support for infrastructure development. Examples of such collaborations range from interactions between individual surgeons to multi-institutional consortiums.

Universities have long been involved in supporting humanitarian efforts at partner hospitals, individually and through multi-institutional collaborations:

- The University of Pennsylvania has a 30-year partnership with the University Children's Hospital in Krakow, Poland, in which a professor of craniofacial surgery made 68 trips to perform direct patient care in conjunction with local surgeons [13].
- The University of Wisconsin Division of Plastic Surgery and the Universidad Nacional Autonoma de Nicaragua, UNAN-Leon, have partnered in a plastic surgery training initiative for 24 years. The US institution supports its counterpart with textbooks, journals, and computer-based learning technology as well as twice yearly faculty and resident exchanges [14].
- The University of Washington created the Partners in African Cleft Training (PACT), a training program to improve and expand access to cleft lip and palate care in sub-Saharan Africa. Since its founding in 2007, the program has trained more than 90 African healthcare providers from nations including Côte d'Ivoire, Ethiopia, Ghana, Liberia, Nigeria, Senegal, South Africa, and Tanzania. PACT is now working to develop three specialized training centers in Ghana, Nigeria, and Ethiopia that will serve as models of interdisciplinary cleft care [15]. Innovations such as using an inexpensive endoscope to video and broadcast a palatoplasty for participants to better see, as well as a simpler and easier way to repair palatal mouth gag, have arisen from the partnership.

Large humanitarian organizations may also partner with the same hospitals over the course of many years to develop human talent and local capacity:

- The Smile Train embraces a sustainable model of empowering local medical professionals by providing free training and equipment as well as financial support to local partners to allow them to provide comprehensive cleft care in their communities. The Smile Train has partnered with more than 2100 medical professionals in 1100 partner hospitals and has supported attendance at more than 1500 medical conferences and trainings. Many Smile

Train partner surgeons perform hundreds of cleft surgeries a year and are there on the ground to provide continued follow-up care and comprehensive services [16].

- ReSurge identifies promising reconstructive plastic surgeons in the countries served through its mission trips, partnering with these local medical professionals to develop ongoing year-round programs. ReSurge provides financial support, training, and ongoing mentorship with access to a global network of clinical experts, with the goal of building surgical capacity. In Nepal, ReSurge partnered with Dr. Shankar Man Rai to develop the country's first surgical outreach center, which later enabled him to form the first plastic surgery residency program in Nepal's history [17]. In Zambia, ReSurge supports its only plastic surgeon, Dr. Goran Jovic. In addition to performing surgeries in Lusaka, Dr. Jovic, a pilot, flies to remote areas of Zambia to treat underserved patients, while helping doctors and surgeons in rural areas advance their medical skills and services [18].
- Operation Smile has likewise supported capacity building by establishing longer-term collaborations at specific sites in which local volunteer surgeons provide most care, with or without the support of international missions. As their presence in these regions has matured, the organization has focused on capacity building and sustainability through the creation of locally governed foundations. These foundations help drive the education and training of local medical professionals, investment into equipment and infrastructure, and funding for clinical activities. Initially the organization used only international teams to provide care, but by 2012, this had shifted to 33% of patients being treated by international teams, with the other 67% of patients receiving treatment from local providers [19]. Numerous countries are now fully self-sufficient, providing care year-round without the need for visiting international teams.
- The Noordhooff Craniofacial Foundation (NCF) partners with the Chang Gung Memorial Hospital (CGMH) in Taiwan to deliver cleft programs to developing nations still in need of adequate cleft care. The lessons learnt through the development of the Chang Gung Cleft and Craniofacial Center from humble beginnings to its current international standing have enabled key insights into devising strategies for training surgeons in LMICs. Identification of "seed" physicians and key personnel, and their subsequent training and support at a major cleft center, is central to the Chang Gung Cleft and Craniofacial Center's efforts to empower LMIC providers' autonomy in delivering the highest standard of care to patients with cleft in their own countries [20, 21].

**Side Bar: Special Considerations in Long-Term Relationships – Balancing HIC Trainee and LMIC Trainee Needs**

It is not uncommon for surgery residents from HICs to complete an international rotation in LMICs. Research shows that these experiences enhance the training of the visiting surgical residents, but it is less clear that host institutions benefit equally [22–25]. As institutional partnerships between academic centers in HICs and LMICs become increasingly common, the surgical community must look beyond the needs of visiting trainees to the needs of students, residents, faculty and staff in host institutions, and communities.

### Advantages

- Continuity in educational efforts is improved with longitudinal relationships over repeated exposures.
- The model fosters sustainability by empowering local medical professionals to provide quality cleft care to those in need in their own communities.
- Ongoing partnerships promote long-term inputs in the form of education, equipment, and funding in order to provide continuous care for patients locally with decreased reliance on international providers.

### Disadvantages

- Approach requires significant commitments in time and travel on numerous occasions on the part of HIC surgical educators.
- Total time to train surgeons is relatively long as training opportunities are intensive but spaced out over many educational experiences.
- Balancing the educational needs of both HIC and LMIC trainees takes careful planning.

## Self-Contained Hospitals

The gold standard for cleft care in developing regions are comprehensive cleft centers (CCCs), which are causing a paradigm shift in how clefts are treated in LMICs (Fig. 34.3). These centers function as permanent hospitals, utilizing local staff and offering a broad range of services year-round. This enables the treatment of each patient comprehensively and longitudinally, from early nutrition and orthodontics to surgery and speech therapy. The continuity of care in conjunc-

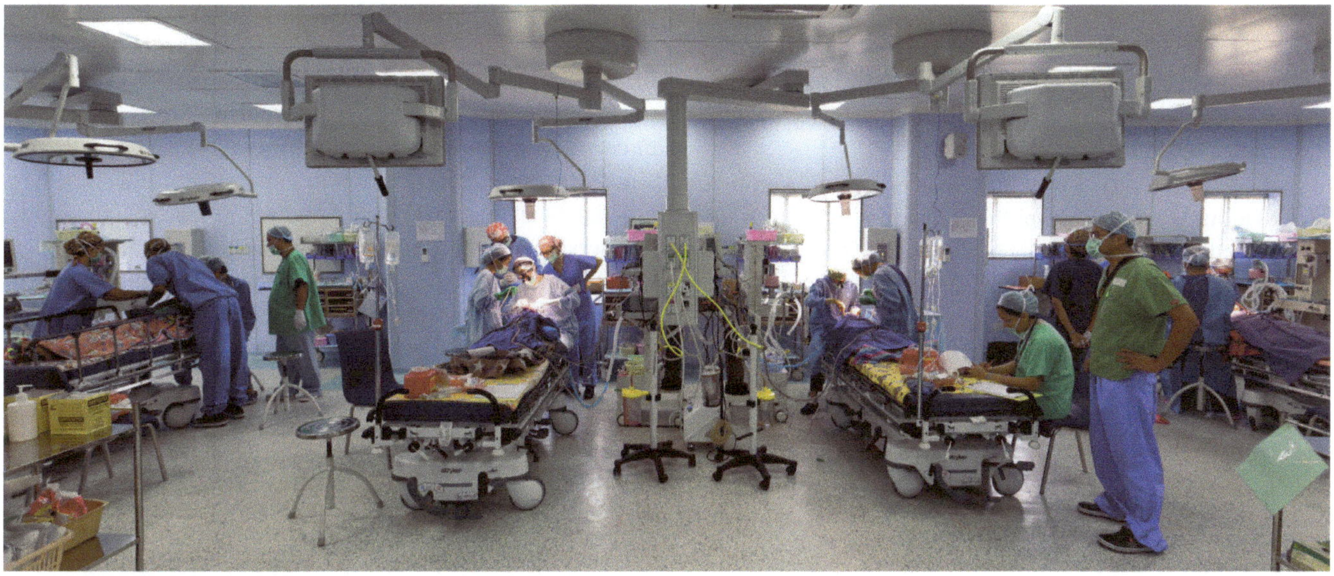

**Fig. 34.3** The gold standard for cleft care in developing regions is comprehensive cleft centers (CCCS), centers function as permanent hospitals utilizing local staff, and offering a broad range of services year-round

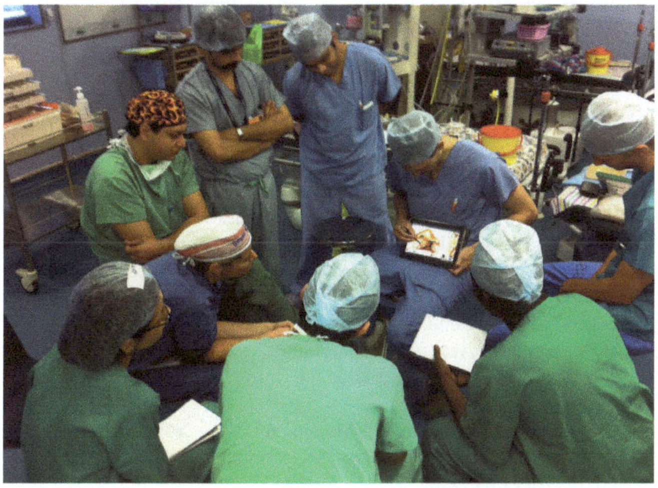

**Fig. 34.4** CCCs are able to capitalize on a focused scope of practice, high patient volumes, and multidisciplinary approach to support unique training programs capable of training surgeons effectively and relatively rapidly

tion with the consistent postoperative follow-up produces surgical outcomes on par with academic university centers in HICs [26]. CCCs are able to capitalize on a focused scope of practice, high patient volumes, and multidisciplinary approach to support unique training programs targeted to the needs of the local patients (Fig. 34.4). Trainees can be trained effectively and relatively rapidly to provide cleft care in this type of high-volume subspecialized center. There is also ample opportunity for research and academic contributions that further advance best practices in LMICs [27].

- The GSR Institute of Craniofacial Surgery (Hyderabad, India) was formed in 2000 and now performs 1500(+) surgeries per year. This center hosts robust rotations and fellowships for national and international fellows from all over the world and has trained more than 100 surgeons from different areas of India and abroad in cleft surgery [28, 29].
- The Sri Ramachandra Cleft and Craniofacial Center (Chennai, India) was established in 2000 and now provides approximately 800 cleft surgeries per year. The center hosts formal fellowships in cleft surgery and has trained dozens of providers to date [30].
- The Inga Health Foundation (Bangalore, India) was established in 2006 and runs three state-of-the-art pan-India treatment centers, performing 8000 surgeries to date. Inga Health intends to set up multiple dedicated multidisciplinary centers across India and offers fellowships to train surgeons and allied professionals [31].
- The Guwahati Comprehensive Cleft Care Center (Guwahati, India) was established in 2011 and by 2013 was performing more than 2500 cleft surgeries per year. Education and training were prioritized from the beginning, and 12 fellows completed full training in cleft surgery between March 2011 and March 2014 [32]. The center provided unprecedented operative exposure and fellows averaged over 40 cases per month in which they were the primary surgeon, with an average of 15 primary cleft lip repairs per month and 9 cleft primary palate repairs per month.

## Advantages

- High volume and immediate repetition provide for intensive learning experience under consistent and experienced mentorship.
- Exposure is focused over the course of several months providing relatively rapid acquisition of skills and knowledge.

## Disadvantages

- Centers may operate parallel to, instead of integrated within, local care and educational systems.

## Future Directions

A challenge of all international work, educational efforts included, is a lack of coordination to limit duplication. Increased communication across institutions, organizations, and collaborations is important to better coordinate efforts and make opportunities available to the individuals they are meant to serve. Several governing bodies have attempted such organization including Global Partners in Anesthesia and Surgery (GPAS) and the College of Surgeons of East, Central, and Southern Africa (COSECSA), posting summary boards of relevant opportunities or training activities based on area [32–35]. The Mexican Association of Cleft Lip, Cleft Palate, and Craniofacial Anomalies (MACLCPCA) is currently engaging all cleft surgery charities operating in Mexico to coordinate efforts with those provided by local professionals as part of a national cleft coverage plan [36].

Another limitation to current education programs is a lack of rigorous monitoring and evaluation. While many collaborations cite descriptive benefits to trainees, very few undertake objective measurement of improvements in trainee knowledge and skill. A recent program has attempted to adapt competency-based training goals and assessments, modeled on trends in North American training norms, to cleft training in LMICs [12]. However, particularly with the variability of surgical experience and proficiency, it can be difficult to evaluate and compare competencies. Nonetheless, efforts should be made to measure and document the specific impact of educational collaborations in order to better understand efficacy, respond to changing needs, and inform decisions to scale.

## Conclusion

In recent years, multiple collaborations have been undertaken to augment local training systems, and a wide variety of educational initiatives have been implemented. But surgical education is challenging, and these challenges only become amplified in the global arena where resources are limited and patient demand is high. Analysis of current initiatives is important to critically evaluate efforts in order to understand their impact on both providers and health systems. Moreover, coordination to unify efforts and share best practices is essential to building effective strategies. Partnerships are becoming more widespread, but research on effectiveness is sparing. Understanding the unmet needs of communities is important, and an emphasis should be placed on sharing best practices and outcomes.

## References


1. Meara JG, Greenberg SL. The Lancet Commission on Global Surgery Global surgery 2030: evidence and solutions for achieving health, welfare and economic development. Lancet. 2015;386(9993):569–624.
2. Campbell A. Disruptive innovation in surgical education. J Am Soc Maxillofac Surg. 2016;1(1):6e–7e.
3. Shrime MG, Sleemi A, Ravilla TD. Charitable platforms in global surgery: a systematic review of their effectiveness, cost-effectiveness, sustainability, and role training. World J Surg. 2015;39:10–20.
4. Smile Train. Grants and programs. Available at: https://www.smiletrain.org/medical/grants-and-programs. Accessed 28 Feb 2019.
5. Magee WP Jr. Evolution of a sustainable surgical delivery model. J Craniofac Surg. 2010;21(5):1321–6.
6. Corlew S, Fan VY. A model for building capacity in international plastic surgery: ReSurge international. Ann Plast Surg. 2011;67(6):568–70.
7. Rotaplast. Available at: https://rotaplast.org/. Accessed 28 Feb 2019.
8. Global Smile Foundation. Education. Available at: https://gsmile.org/education/. Accessed 28 Feb 2019.
9. Transforming Faces. Available at: https://transformingfaces.org/. Accessed 28 Feb 2019.
10. Campbell A, Sherman R, Magee WP. The role of humanitarian missions in modern surgical training. Plast Reconstr Surg. 2010;126(1):295–302.
11. Sue G, Covington W, Chang J. The ReSurge global training program: a model for surgical training and capacity building in global reconstructive surgery. Ann Plast Surg. 2018;81(3):250–6.
12. McCullough M, Campbell A, Siu A, et al. Competency-based education in low-resource settings. World J Surg. 2018;42(3):646–51.
13. Swanson JW, Skirpan J, Stanek B, et al. 30-year international pediatric craniofacial surgery partnership: evolution from the "third world" forward. Plast Reconstr Surg Glob Open. 2016;4(4):e671.
14. Nayar HS, Bentz ML, Baus GH, et al. The imperative of academia in the globalization of plastic surgery. J Craniofac Surg. 2015;26(4):1102–5.
15. Partners in African Cleft Training (PACT). Available at: https://www.seattlechildrens.org/clinics/craniofacial/partners-african-cleft-training/. Accessed on 5 Jan 2019.
16. Smile Train Annual Report FY 2017. Available at: https://www.smiletrain.org/sites/default/files/smile-train-annual-report-fy17.pdf. Accessed 28 Feb 2019.
17. ReSurge International. Dr. Shankar Man Rai Bio. Available at: https://www.resurge.org/story/dr-shankar-man-rai-bio/. Accessed on 5 Jan 2019.
18. ReSurge International. Zambia. Available at: https://www.resurge.org/zambia/. Accessed 28 Feb 2019.

19. Magee WP, Raimondi HM, Beers M, Koech MC. Effectiveness of international surgical program model to build local sustainability. Plast Surg Int. 2012;2012:185725.
20. Noordhoff MS. Establishing a craniofacial center in a developing country. J Craniofac Surg. 2009;20 Suppl 2:1655–6.
21. Goh RC, Wang R, Chen PK, Lo LJ, Chen YR. Strategies for achieving long-term effective outcome in cleft missions: the Noordhoff Craniofacial Foundation and Chang Gung Memorial Hospital. J Craniofac Surg. 2009;20 Suppl 2:1657–60.
22. Campbell A, Sullivan M, Sherman R, Magee WP. The medical mission and modern cultural competency training. J Am Coll Surg. 2011;212(1):124–9.
23. Aziz SR, Ziccardi VB, Chuang SK. Survey of residents who have participated in humanitarian medical missions. J Oral Maxillofac Surg. 2012;70(2):e147–57.
24. Yao C, Swanson J, McCullough M, Taro TB, Gutierrez R, Bradshaw A, Campbell A, Magee WP, Magee WP III. The medical mission and modern core competency training: a 10-year follow-up of resident experiences in global plastic surgery. Plast Reconstr Surg. 2016;138(3):531e–538.
25. Riviello R, Lipnick MS, Ozgediz D. Medical missions, surgical education, and capacity building. J Am Coll Surg. 2011;213(4):572–4.
26. Persing S, Patel A, Clune JE, Steinbacher DM, Persing JA. The repair of international clefts in the current surgical landscape. J Craniofac Surg. 2015;26(4):1126–8.
27. Campbell A, Restrepo C, Mackay D, Sherman R, Varma A, Ayala R, Sarma H, Deshpande G, Magee B. Scalable, sustainable cost effective surgical care: a model for safety and quality in the developing world. Part III: impact and sustainability. J Craniofac Surg. 2014;25:1685–9.
28. Hyderabad Cleft Society. Available at: http://www.craniofacialinstitute.org/. Accessed on 28 Feb 2019.
29. Hyderabad Cleft Society Annual Report 2018. Available at: https://www.baoms.org.uk/_userfiles/pages/files/members/ssig%20cleft/cleft_annual_report_2018.pdf. Accessed on 28 Feb 2019.
30. Cleft and Craniofacial Center. Sri Ramachandra University. Available at: http://www.cleftcare.in/index.html. Accessed 28 Feb 2019.
31. Inga Health Foundation. Available at: http://ingahealth.org/who-we-are/. Accessed 28 Feb 2019.
32. Nagengast E, Campbell A, Restrepo C, et al. Reverse innovation in surgical education: value in training surgeons in developing regions. Ahead of Publication.
33. Global Partners in Anesthesia and Surgery. Available at: http://www.globalsurgery.org/. Accessed 28 Feb 2019.
34. Ibrahim A. Sub-specialization in plastic surgery in sub-saharan Africa: capacities, gaps and opportunities. Pan Afr Med J. 2014;19:13.
35. Butler M, Ozgediz D, Poenaru D, et al. The global paediatric surgery network: a model of subspecialty collaboration within global surgery. World J Surg. 2015;39(2):335–42.
36. Mexican Association of Lip, Cleft Palate and Craniofacial Anomalies. Available at: https://www.amlph.com.mx/. Accessed 28 Feb 2019.

# 35 Educator Workshops: Visiting Educators, Curricula, and Digital Education

Anna Luan and James Chang

## The Need for Global Cleft Surgery Education

Orofacial clefts occur in approximately 1 in 700 births, or more than 160,000 births globally each year [1, 2], and can present a significant psychological and socioeconomic burden on both the patient and their family. In areas lacking qualified surgeons to perform cleft operations, many of these patients are left untreated and suffer from considerable social stigma. In addition to the psychosocial impact, cleft repair addresses both form and function, allowing treated patients to rejoin society and contribute to the local economy [3]. Recent studies of data from ReSurge International, a non-profit organization which provides plastic and reconstructive surgery care, have shown orofacial cleft repair to be very cost-effective, with a cost per disability-adjusted life year (DALY)-averted of $31 [4]. Unfortunately, despite increasing awareness regarding the global burden of surgical disease, surgical capacity in low- and middle-income countries (LMICs) for treating cleft lip and palate remains inadequate.

Traditionally, involvement in global surgery has taken the form of the international mission trip model, in which surgical personnel travel abroad for a designated period of time to perform surgeries before returning to their home country. However, concerns exist regarding the cost and sustainability of such an approach, as well as the potential consequences on the local medical infrastructure. Thus, more recently, focus is now turning towards the building of surgical capacity in LMICs [5]. Increasingly, visiting plastic surgeons to LMICs have recognized that they serve a valuable role not only in providing direct surgical care but also as educators to train local healthcare professionals [6, 7]. By training local providers and building surgical capacity at the host institution, the impact of a visiting surgeon is more sustainable and cost-effective. Through visiting educator trips, local healthcare personnel are trained to provide care in the intervening months between short-term trips and, over time, can ultimately learn to perform complex procedures independently.

A. Luan · J. Chang (✉)
Division of Plastic and Reconstructive Surgery, Stanford Medical Center, Stanford, CA, USA
e-mail: aluan@stanford.edu; jameschang@stanford.edu

## Visiting Educator Curriculum Development and Implementation

While varying curriculum models exist, ReSurge has adopted a competency-based training structure modeled after surgical residency training programs in the United States. Competency-based training models are based not on number of years or completion of a set number of cases but instead use specific knowledge, skills, or attitudes as a benchmark of competency for practice [8]. ReSurge has developed competency-based milestone ratings of trainee surgeons modified from US plastic surgery residency curriculums to focus on pertinent topics in low-resource settings [9]. In competency-based curriculum models, important principles and/or procedures are identified and broken down into stepwise benchmarks of progress [10]. An example of milestones for cleft lip surgery is shown in Fig. 35.1. We have utilized these milestone ratings on 1-week duration visiting educator trips in LMICs including in Asia, Africa, and South America. Repeat assessments on subsequent trips allow for longitudinal tracking of trainee progress over time. Other organizations such as Operation Smile [11] have also developed and piloted similar competency-based evaluation instruments utilizing essential steps in preoperative, intraoperative, and postoperative cleft care.

A critical step in the process of setting up visiting educator trips is the identification of appropriate host institutions. During this initial vetting process, hospitals must be evaluated for several criteria. First, there must be a demonstrated clinical and educational need. Next, there must exist host surgeons who are invested in establishing a long-term col-

© Springer Nature Switzerland AG 2021

J. W. Swanson, D. W. Low (eds.), *Global Cleft Care in Low-Resource Settings*, https://doi.org/10.1007/978-3-030-59105-2_35

Fig. 35.1 Example of milestone ratings for cleft lip surgery

**Score 1 :** Able to evaluate patients for the need for cleft lip surgery; able to advise family on feeding and other future treatment
**Score 2:** Able to assist in unilateral and bilateral cleft lip surgery; understands the concepts of staged interdisciplinary treatment in the care of the cleft lip patient
**Score 3:** Able to independently perform unilateral and bilateral cleft lip surger; manages complications related to unilateral and bilateral cleft lip surgery
**Score 4:** Able to independently perform secondary lip surgery and cleft rhinoplasty; understand the anatomy and surgical priciples of secondary cleft lip and nasal deformities
**Score 5:** Able to perform complex maxillofacial surgery related to cleft lip and palate, including alveolar bone grafting and LeFort osteotomy; manages a multidisciplinary cranio facial team

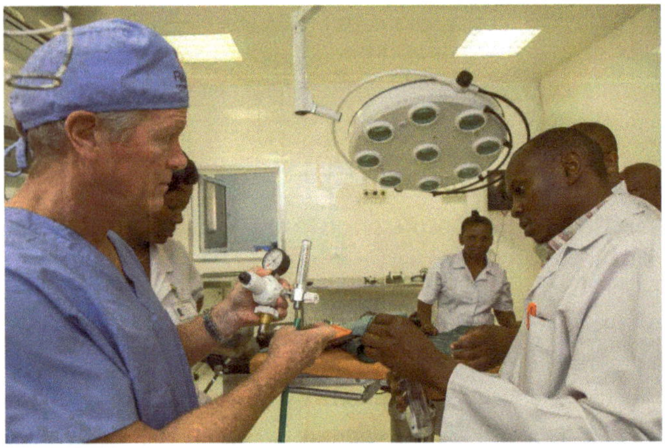

Fig. 35.2 Direct teaching during visiting educator trip

laboration. Finally, to ensure a longitudinal relationship between the visiting educators and host institution, it must be logistically feasible to provide surgical care in the host country on a long-term basis [12].

Once a host hospital and surgeons are coordinated, appropriate local patients should be identified for the visiting educator trip. Suitable patients should have a surgical condition that is sufficient in complexity for host surgeons to gain educational value but should also be comfortably within the specialized skillset of the visiting educator and the projected capabilities of the host surgeons.

The selection of personnel for visiting educator trips should be comprehensive in all aspects of the patient's care. A typical cleft visiting educator group from ReSurge includes one or two reconstructive surgeons, one anesthesiologist, one pediatrician, and one nurse and/or therapist. Each team member is responsible for directed teaching with their local counterpart (Fig. 35.2). Hospital space is typically arranged by the host institution. Medical equipment may be provided by either the host institution or the visiting educators.

SAMPLE RESURGE INTERNATIONAL VE TRIP SCHEDULE

SUNDAY
Team arrives

MONDAY
PREOP Clinic Evaluation (9AM - 4PM)

TUESDAY
OR (8AM - 6PM)

WEDNESDAY
OR (8AM - 8PM)

THURSDAY
OR (8AM - 8PM)

FRIDAY
Lecture (8AM -12PM)

- Cleft palate repair
- Facial Paralysis
- Hypertelorism
- Lefort Osteotomies and Distraction
- Nasal Reconstruction

SATURDAY
Team leaves

Fig. 35.3 Sample visiting educator (VE) trip schedule. OR, operating room

Sample schedules for a visiting educator trip are outlined in Fig. 35.3. Generally, each visiting educator trip is comprised of lectures, demonstrative surgical cases, observation and assessment of surgical trainees, and real-time feedback. Visiting educators participate in evaluation of patients in the preoperative clinic setting, typically scheduled for the first day of the visiting educator trip. Lectures are tailored toward the visiting educators' area of expertise and the surgical cases selected, and can be either distributed across the duration of the trip or concentrated in one or a few sessions. Resources such as lecture slides and videos are made to be available free of charge and on an open-source basis.

We recommend establishing an "operating rhythm" of regularly scheduled trips, generally approximately four times each year for each host institution. This schedule allows for longitudinal collaboration with the host institution and surgeons. Recently, we have also designated one of these trips each year as a trip in which we focus on issues regarding patient safety (anesthesia, operating room safety, identification of perioperative complications).

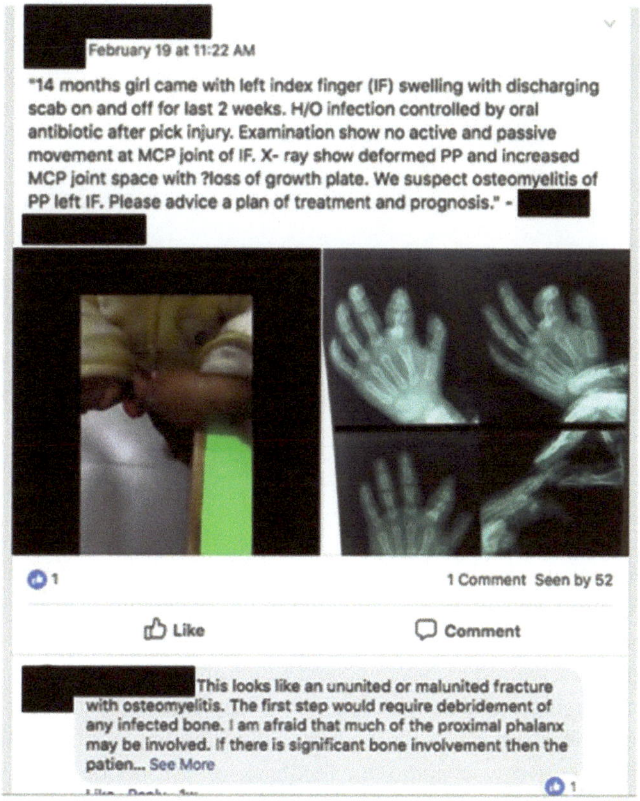


**Fig. 35.4** Sample case-based community discussion in ReSurge Grand Rounds online group

## Tele-mentoring and the Utilization of Digital Technology in Education

Tele-mentoring is the use of information technology to provide guidance from an expert remotely to a trainee. The time and resources required for visiting educator trips limit the frequency of international trips due to visiting surgeons' existing clinical and personal responsibilities at home. The ability to provide education and mentorship remotely ensures continuity of interactions between in-person visiting educator trips and is a useful adjunct to on-site training.

The most simple and easily implementable form of tele-mentoring takes the form of non-procedural tele-mentorship. Various Internet-based portals may be utilized to create an online community for discussion and feedback for trainees or mentees. For example, ReSurge Grand Rounds is an online community that facilitates multidirectional discussion about complex cases. In this setting, multiple experts (mentors) may contribute with their insights and give feedback about cases presented to the group by trainees (Fig. 35.4). Reports from other surgical fields [13, 14] also support the benefits of international tele-mentoring through collaborative case-based discussion communities. In addition to case-based guidance, discussion regarding general topics in surgical care may also be facilitated through online forums. The ReSurge experience has shown that many prefer to interact through existing platforms, such as Facebook, due to familiarity and as it bypasses the need to log in to a separate website or program. In these discussion groups, resources are shared and advice exchanged with the exclusion of any protected health information. This form of tele-mentorship provides not only guidance regarding surgical care but can also aid in professional development and career mentorship.

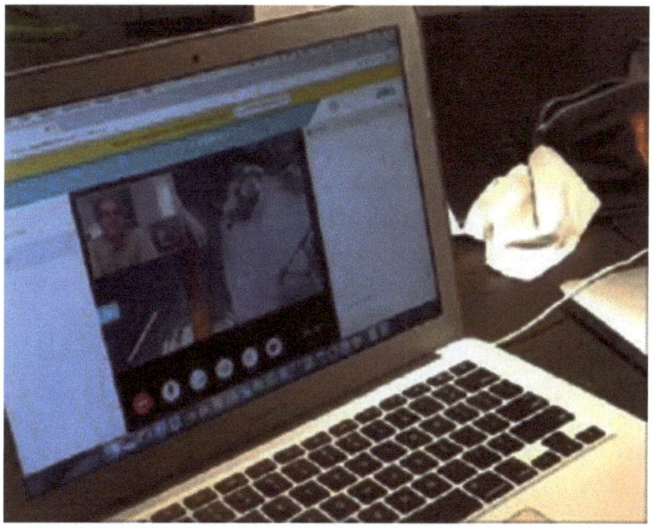

**Fig. 35.5** Sample screen of video and audio feed to tele-mentor surgeon, from McCullough et al. [23]

Over the last few decades, direct surgical tele-mentoring has also emerged as an innovative adjunct in surgical educa-

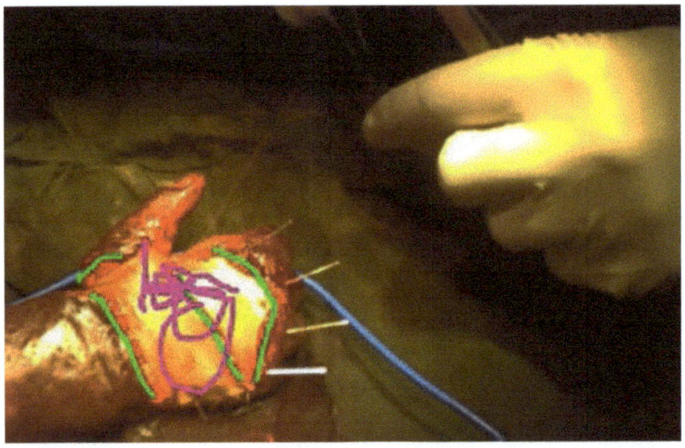

Fig. 35.6 Example of "tele-stration," from McCullough et al. [23]

tion. In this form of tele-mentorship, audio and visual technology is further utilized to provide real-time remote feedback and guidance, including its use in the intraoperative setting (Fig. 35.5). Since its inception, advances in technological capabilities have allowed for dramatic improvements in imaging and data transmission. Many platforms incorporate visualization of the operative field in conjunction with one- or two-way audio for feedback or instruction. Some also permit telestration, which is the drawing of illustrations overlaid onto the video (Fig. 35.6).

Initial efforts in development of tele-mentoring applications in surgery focused on laparoscopic and endoscopic procedures, in which video images visualized by the primary surgeon are simultaneously transmitted to a remote surgeon. In 1996, Moore et al. demonstrated feasibility of tele-mentorship with a surgeon in a control room supervising an inexperienced surgeon in urologic procedures and found no statistical difference in patient outcomes or operative time [15]. Soon after, Lee et al. successfully provided international tele-mentoring from the United States for several cases in Thailand and Austria [16]. Since then, multiple other groups have successfully established remote tele-mentorship programs, including in the fields of endoscopic skull base surgeries and endovascular repairs [17, 18]. Snyderman et al. identified the most common mentoring interventions to include identification of anatomy, extent of exposure, extent of resection, and surgical technique. Recently, potentially due to the anticipated influence of tele-mentoring in surgery, highly specialized robots such as the Karl Storz VisitOR1 robot [19, 20] and the InTouch Health RemotePresence-7 robot have been created for this specific purpose.

While tele-mentoring has quickly gained traction in the laparoendoscopic space, open surgeries such as cleft operations present the additional challenge of providing high-quality imaging not inherently built in to the operation. The development of wearable technologies may provide the ability to project high-fidelity images of the operating surgeon's view to a remote mentor surgeon without obstructing the field of view.

Google Glass (Google, Inc.; Mountain View, California), a wearable device worn like a pair of glasses, has been used by several groups to pilot tele-mentoring in the surgical setting. For example, in inguinal hernia surgery, Datta et al. utilized Google Glass to transmit video from the operating room in real time via a web-based streaming platform, where remote expert surgeons could give feedback which in turn appeared in the Google Glass display field [21]. Using this technology, surgeons were trained remotely in Haiti, Paraguay, Brazil, Ecuador, and the Dominican Republic, and trainees found Internet connectivity, image quality, and transmission rates to be acceptable.

However, despite the potential promise of Google Glass as a wearable technology for tele-mentorship, the quality of video transmitted is a limitation to its safe and reliable use [22, 23]. The device's occasionally inconsistent reproduction of detail, color, brightness, depth, and motion render it potentially inadequate as a platform for tele-mentorship (Fig. 35.7). Finally, there can be a discrepancy between the line of sight of the captured camera video and the operating surgeon's true field of view if the angle of the mounted camera is not adjusted carefully or if the surgeon's loupes compete for the same space [22] (Fig. 35.8). Despite these shortcomings, trainees and proctors who have used Google Glass for remote tele-mentorship consider the technology to be useful as a teaching instrument [23].

HoloLens (Microsoft Corp.; Redmond, Washington), a mixed reality head mount device manufactured by Microsoft, is another option for wearable tele-mentoring technology. Tepper et al. used HoloLens with Skype to broadcast mixed reality scenes in the operating room with bidirectional communication and tele-stration [24]. The benefit of a mixed reality device such as HoloLens is that complex two- and three-dimensional data may be projected on the wearer's visual field, such as holograms of virtual surgical plans. This may be useful for incorporating surgical markings in cleft lip repair or in flap design in cleft palate surgery.

The most notable barriers to the widespread adoption of tele-mentoring are technological limitations as well as the cost of equipment and necessary infrastructure. For successful tele-mentorship, requirements include a reliable network connection and speed of data transmission, high quality of the video feed, and security of patient data. Currently, commercially available wearable technology can cost several thousand dollars per device [24], although these prices may decrease over time as the technology becomes more readily available. Despite this, the cost of equipment for tele-mentoring devices remains lower than the cost of a surgical mission trip. Current wearable technology may require mod-

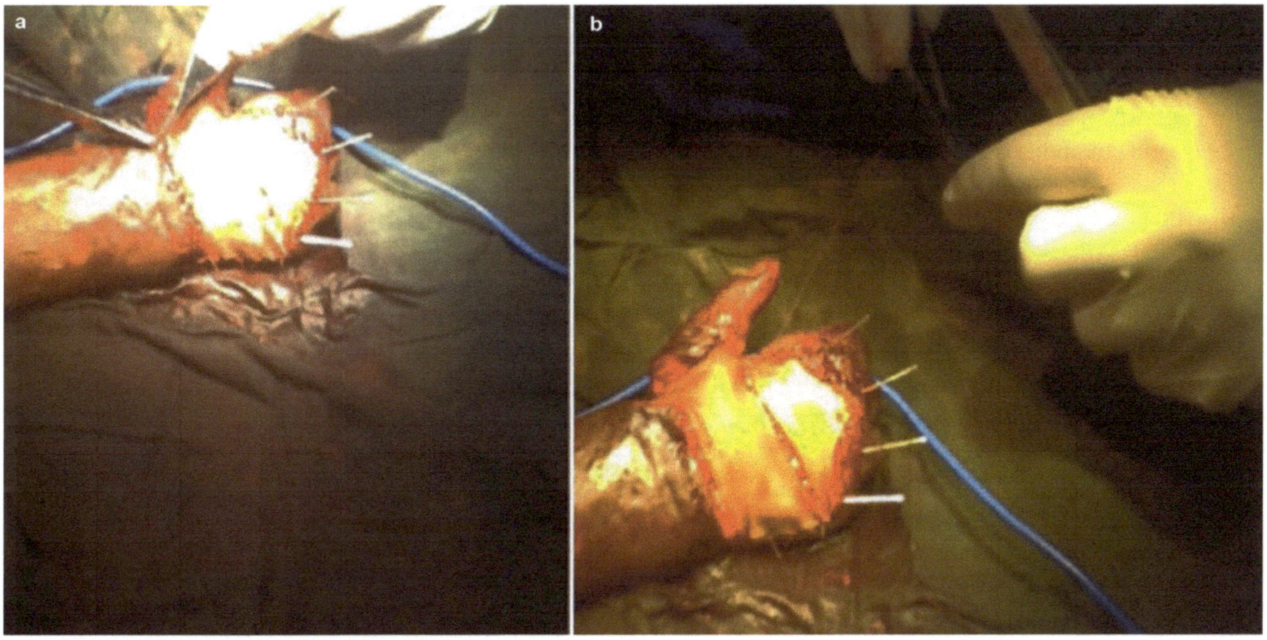


Fig. 35.7 Example of distortion of light with Google Glass video (**a**) and with correction (**b**), from McCullough et al. [23]

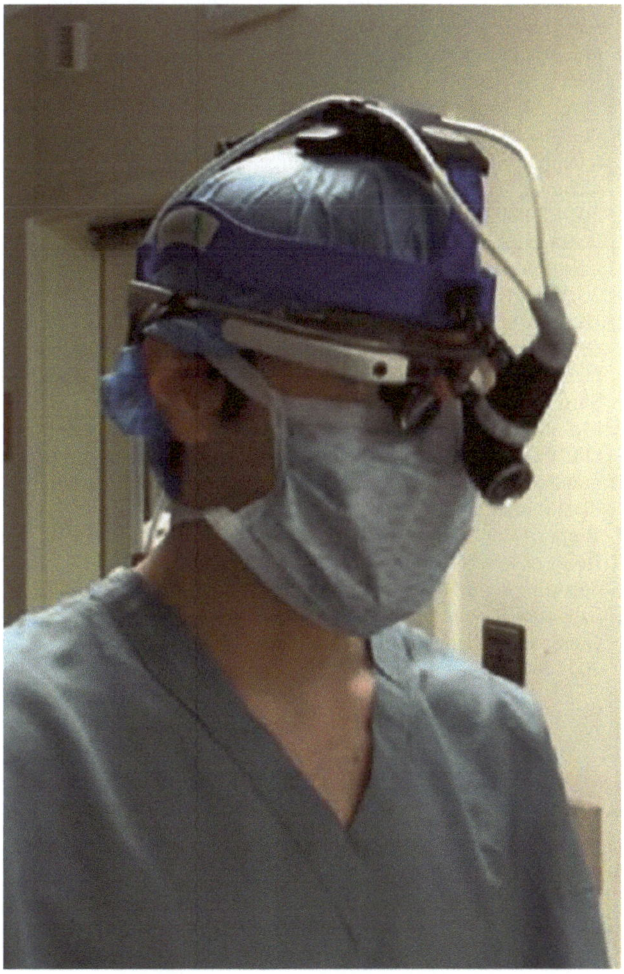

Fig. 35.8 Google Glass worn with surgical loupes, from Sahyouni et al. [25]

ifications or augmentation with additional software to be sufficient for complex cleft operations.

Finally, some aspects of tele-mentoring remain unclear, in particular the legal implications of direct surgical tele-mentorship. We suggest that the primary surgeon must be capable of performing the procedure independently to maintain primary responsibility for the operation, with the mentor surgeon available for advice as needed. In order to maintain this distinction, one must determine a set of credentials or qualifying skillset for the primary surgeon. Thus, direct real-time tele-mentorship may be reserved for particularly complex cases or if unexpected situations arise intraoperatively. As the field surgeon becomes increasingly familiar with an operation and its complications, the use of tele-mentoring for the procedure may be expected to decrease over time.

## Conclusion

Surgical capacity for the repair of orofacial clefts remains insufficient in LMICs. Through visiting educator trips and the development of a longitudinal educational curriculum, local surgeons and healthcare personnel in LMICs can be trained in surgical principles and techniques, thereby building a sustainable expansion of the host country's surgical capacity. Recent developments in technology may also prove to be a useful adjunct to the formal curriculum. Direct and indirect tele-mentorship using Internet-based platforms and wearable devices can provide more readily accessible mentorship and guidance in the intervening months between visiting educator trips.

**Tips and Tricks: Visiting Educator Trips**

- Identify host institutions by the presence of motivated host surgeons and logistical feasibility of long-term collaboration.
- Select patients who are challenging but representative of common presentations, to match visiting educators' skillset and projected capabilities of host surgeons.
- Involve the entire team in teaching their counterpart; typical visiting educator teams include one or two reconstructive surgeons, one anesthesiologist, one pediatrician, and one nurse and/or therapist.
- Make lectures and educational resources open access.
- Establish an "operating rhythm" of regularly scheduled trips to maintain longitudinal education and to assess milestones of trainee surgeons.

## References


1. Mossey PA, Modell B. Epidemiology of oral clefts 2012: an international perspective. Front Oral Biol. 2012;16:1–18.
2. Gorlin RJ, Cohen MM, Hennekam RCM. Syndromes of the head and neck. 4th ed. Oxford England; New York: Oxford University Press; 2001.
3. Poenaru D, Lin D, Corlew S. Economic valuation of the global burden of cleft disease averted by a large cleft charity. World J Surg. 2016;40:1053–9.
4. Nasser JS, Billig JI, Sue GR, Chang J, Gosain AK, Chung KC. Evaluating the economic sustainability of plastic and reconstructive surgical efforts in the developing world. Plast Reconstr Surg Glob Open. 2018;6:194–5.
5. Butler MW. Developing pediatric surgery in low- and middle-income countries: an evaluation of contemporary education and care delivery models. Semin Pediatr Surg. 2016;25:43–50.
6. DeGennaro V Jr, Degennaro VA. Linking surgical missions with training of developing-country surgeons. J Craniofac Surg. 2013;24:699.
7. Plana NM, Diaz-Siso JR, Culnan DM, Cutting CB, Flores RL. The first year of global cleft surgery education through digital simulation: a proof of concept. Cleft Palate Craniofac J. 2018;55:626–9.
8. Nguyen VT, Losee JE. Time- versus competency-based residency training. Plast Reconstr Surg. 2016;138:527–31.
9. Sue GR, Covington WC, Chang J. The ReSurge global training program: a model for surgical training and capacity building in global reconstructive surgery. Ann Plast Surg. 2018;81:250–6.
10. Knox AD, Gilardino MS, Kasten SJ, Warren RJ, Anastakis DJ. Competency-based medical education for plastic surgery: where do we begin? Plast Reconstr Surg. 2014;133:702e–10e.
11. McCullough M, Campbell A, Siu A, et al. Competency-based education in low resource settings: development of a novel surgical training program. World J Surg. 2018;42:646–51.
12. Rockwell WT, Agbenorku P, Olson J, Hoyte-Williams PE, Agarwal JP, Rockwell WB. A model for university-based international plastic surgery collaboration builds local sustainability. Ann Plast Surg. 2015;74:388–91.
13. Jaffer U, Vaughan-Huxley E, Standfield N, John NW. Medical mentoring via the evolving world wide web. J Surg Educ. 2013;70:121–8.
14. Obura T, Brant WE, Miller F, Parboosingh IJ. Participating in a Community of Learners enhances resident perceptions of learning in an e-mentoring program: proof of concept. BMC Med Educ. 2011;11:3.
15. Moore RG, Adams JB, Partin AW, Docimo SG, Kavoussi LR. Telementoring of laparoscopic procedures: initial clinical experience. Surg Endosc. 1996;10:107–10.
16. Lee BR, Bishoff JT, Janetschek G, et al. A novel method of surgical instruction: international telementoring. World J Urol. 1998;16:367–70.
17. Snyderman CH, Gardner PA, Lanisnik B, Ravnik J. Surgical telementoring: a new model for surgical training. Laryngoscope. 2016;126:1334–8.
18. Porretta AP, Alerci M, Wyttenbach R, et al. Long-term outcomes of a telementoring program for distant teaching of endovascular aneurysm repair. J Endovasc Ther. 2017;24:852–8.
19. Ponsky TA, Schwachter M, Parry J, Rothenberg S, Augestad KM. Telementoring: the surgical tool of the future. Eur J Pediatr Surg = Zeitschrift fur Kinderchirurgie. 2014;24:287–94.
20. Ponsky TA, Bobanga ID, Schwachter M, et al. Transcontinental telementoring with pediatric surgeons: proof of concept and technical considerations. J Laparoendosc Adv Surg Tech A. 2014;24:892–6.
21. Datta N, MacQueen IT, Schroeder AD, et al. Wearable technology for global surgical teleproctoring. J Surg Educ. 2015;72:1290–5.
22. Hashimoto DA, Phitayakorn R, Fernandez-del Castillo C, Meireles O. A blinded assessment of video quality in wearable technology for telementoring in open surgery: the Google Glass experience. Surg Endosc. 2016;30:372–8.
23. McCullough MC, Kulber L, Sammons P, Santos P, Kulber DA. Google glass for remote surgical tele-proctoring in low- and middle-income countries: a feasibility study from Mozambique. Plast Reconstr Surg Glob Open. 2018;6:e1999.
24. Tepper OM, Rudy HL, Lefkowitz A, et al. Mixed reality with HoloLens: where virtual reality meets augmented reality in the operating room. Plast Reconstr Surg. 2017;140:1066–70.
25. Sahyouni R, Moshtaghi O, Tran DK, et al. Assessment of Google Glass as an adjunct in neurological surgery. Surg Neurol Int. 2017;8:68.

# Educator Workshops: Skills Training

# 36

Rami S. Kantar, Allyson R. Alfonso, and Usama S. Hamdan

**Key Points**

- Comprehensive, simulation-based, multidisciplinary, cleft care surgical skills workshops are well received in low-resource settings.
- These workshops provide a platform for capacity building in low-resource settings.
- Collaborations between cleft foundations, academic leaders in cleft surgery, and key stakeholders from the biomedical industry sector are essential.

## Introduction

The incidence of cleft lip and/or palate (CLP) in developing countries is estimated to be close to 250,000 per year [1]. Barriers preventing international equitable access to comprehensive cleft care are numerous but can mostly be attributed to lack of appropriate skills and expertise or lack of resources. While international volunteer cleft surgery initiatives may alleviate this backlog, sustainable solutions must rely on empowering local surgeons in order to achieve autonomy in patient care [2].

R. S. Kantar (✉)
New York University Langone Health Hansjörg Wyss, Department of Plastic and Reconstructive Surgery, New York City, NY, USA

The University of Maryland Medical System, Baltimore, MD, USA

A. R. Alfonso
New York University Langone Health Hansjörg Wyss, Department of Plastic and Reconstructive Surgery, New York City, NY, USA
e-mail: allyson.alfonso@nyulangone.org

U. S. Hamdan
Global Smile Foundation, Boston, MA, USA

Tufts University School of Medicine, Boston, MA, USA

Harvard Medical School, Boston, MA, USA

Boston University School of Medicine, Boston, MA, USA

## Traditional Models of Foundation-Based Cleft Surgery Education

### Visiting Trainees

The traditional cleft surgery mission model, by bringing together multiple surgeons to operate on many cleft patients over a 1-week period, provides an incredible learning opportunity for young plastic surgeons, particularly those with an interest in cleft surgery. Historically, residents and fellows have traveled overseas (typically from high-income countries) to participate in these missions. Fellowships offered through cleft care foundations enable trainees to gain significant exposure to surgical and perioperative care, as well as research opportunities [3, 4]. Trainees who partake in these fellowships are more likely to participate in humanitarian outreach in the future [5, 6]. Further, they consistently report growth personally and professionally in developing key proficiencies outlined by the Accreditation Council for Graduate Medical Education (ACGME) [7]. However, potential concerns are raised about visiting trainees operating in these settings: Does their education create excess risk for vulnerable populations? Does devoting time to the pace of their learning reduce the number of local patients who can receive treatment? And does their operative experience come at the cost of a local surgical trainee who would otherwise receive that opportunity?

### Local Trainees

International cleft surgery educational initiatives may inadvertently disregard the needs of local trainees or potentially prioritize surgical quantity over quality, resulting in what is termed "safari surgery" [8, 9]. This can have potentially devastating consequences on the development of local cleft care infrastructure in low-resource settings and might demoralize local surgeons by overstepping on their clinical practices

© Springer Nature Switzerland AG 2021

J. W. Swanson, D. W. Low (eds.), *Global Cleft Care in Low-Resource Settings*, https://doi.org/10.1007/978-3-030-59105-2_36

[10]. In an attempt to address these issues, many cleft care foundations have focused their efforts on educating and training local surgeons. Historically, some programs such as the Operation Smile Physician Training Program involved hosting surgeons from low-resource settings in the USA [7]. Now, most programs are focused on training that occurs in the low-resource setting. Recent studies demonstrate improvement in surgical skills and competency among local cleft surgeons through these programs [4, 11].

## Workshops

Workshops can serve as a nice adjunct to clinical experiences. They can be a supplement to surgical missions, with participants freed from the tight schedule of clinical care, or a stand-alone program. They can take multiple forms, including one-on-one practice sessions, small group workshops, and video-broadcast forums. It is thought that workshops with hands-on skills training and adept instructor feedback are likely to provide the greatest enrichment to practical skills. Simulation-based cleft care workshops are a feasible solution.

## Simulation-Based Comprehensive Cleft Care Surgical Skills Workshops: A New Model for Foundation-Based Cleft Surgery Education

Simulation has emerged as a valuable component of surgical education in developed countries in light of growing work hour limitations, mandatory faculty supervision, as well as a growing trend toward surgical subspecialization [12]. Training in cleft surgery has witnessed similar trends, with the recent rise of a number of digital as well as haptic simulators in developed countries [13–16]. Available data suggest that these simulators are an important adjunct for teaching cleft surgery knowledge and surgical skills and are generally well received by their users [13, 14, 17, 18]. Nevertheless, financial as well as organizational restraints have limited the application and widespread adoption of cleft surgery simulation in low-resource settings.

Collaborative relationships between international cleft surgery foundations, academic leaders in cleft surgery, and key stakeholders from the biomedical sector have the potential to translate successes in cleft surgery simulation from developing countries to low-resource settings through comprehensive educational surgical skills workshops. As an example, Global Smile Foundation has partnered with academic leaders from North America, Europe, and the Middle East to organize two simulation-based comprehensive cleft care surgical skills workshops in the Middle East and in Latin America [19] (Fig. 36.1). The curriculum included didactic lectures supplemented by hands-on cleft surgery simulation sessions using high-fidelity cleft lip and palate simulators (*Simulare Medical*) (Table 36.1).

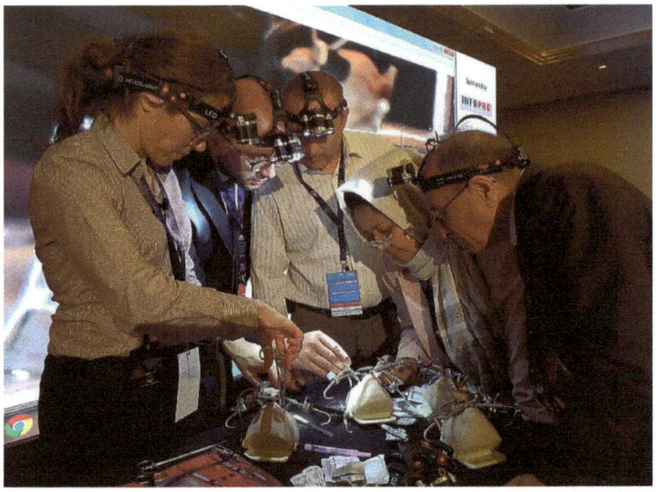

**Fig. 36.1** Real-time expert demonstration of cleft palate repair. (Permissions and copyrights retained by Usama S. Hamdan, MD, FICS)

**Table 36.1** Potential benefits of simulation-based comprehensive cleft care surgical skills workshops

| |
|---|
| *Learning through simulation.* Simulation is evolving into an essential component of contemporary surgical training [20, 21]. For instance, an online cleft surgery visualization simulator has been accessed by surgeons and surgical trainees from more than 130 countries, for a total screen time of nearly 1700 hours [13]. Data also support the effectiveness of cleft surgery simulators in teaching cleft markings and procedural skills, as well as improving procedural knowledge and confidence [14, 15, 17, 18, 22] (Fig. 36.2) |
| *Capacity building and overcoming adversity.* Comprehensive surgical skills workshops provide a unique opportunity for capacity building and empowering surgeons in low-resource settings through high-quality cleft surgery education. This is particularly true in areas that may be suffering from political turmoil resulting in significant strains on healthcare infrastructure and major demographic shifts. This has led us to observe an increasing number of refugees with CLP seeking cleft care at an older age in these regions. While financial strains represent an obstacle to these patients seeking earlier care, lack of cleft expertise in the region remains a significant barrier to care. The first simulation-based comprehensive surgical skills cleft care workshop took place in Beirut, Lebanon, in 2018, attracting participants from 30 countries distributed over five continents (Fig. 36.3) [19]. The second international conference was held in Lima, Peru, in 2019. This 3-day course had 181 registered surgeons, dentists, and speech pathologists from 27 countries. Participants learned from 32 experts in the cleft field and had the opportunity to participate in hands-on surgical simulation sessions for cleft lip and palate, as well as nasoendoscopy for speech therapists |
| *Platform for multidisciplinary learning.* Cleft care is more effective when able to be delivered in a multidisciplinary fashion, with surgeons, speech pathologists, orthodontists, and nurses involved in the longitudinal care of patients with CLP for optimal outcomes. Cleft foundation-driven workshops in low-resource settings provide an ideal platform for participants to appraise multidisciplinary aspects of patient care, as well as network with peers, colleagues, and faculty, and exchange practice experiences across disciplines |

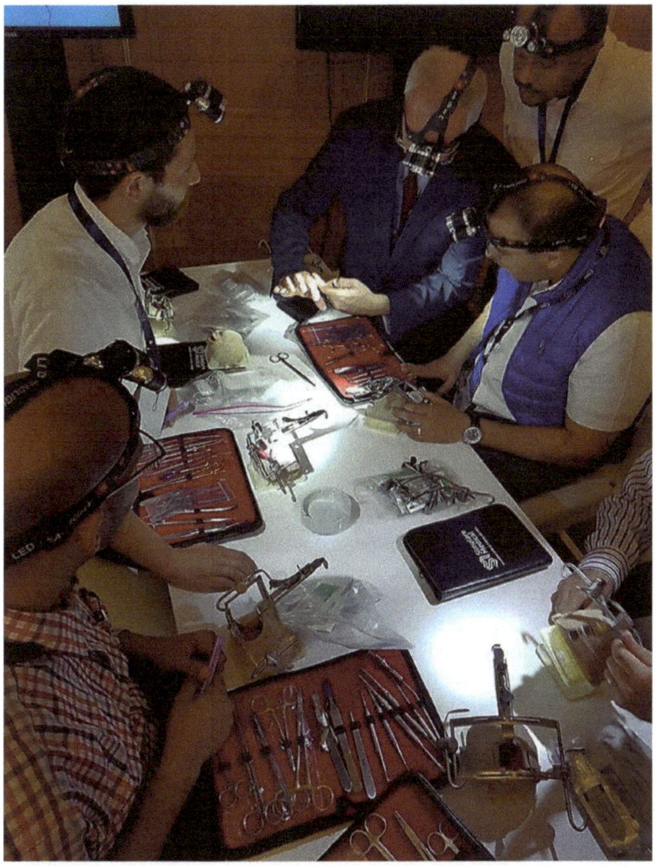

Fig. 36.2 Directed real-time operative feedback from faculty to participants. (Permissions and copyrights retained by Usama S. Hamdan, MD, FICS)

## Pillars of a Successful Comprehensive Cleft Care Workshop

Comprehensive cleft care workshops require meticulous planning, strong partnerships, context-dependent curricular development taught by expert faculty, and a thorough workshop evaluation strategy. International locations must be accessible and convenient with amenities that include large lecture halls and the capacity to provide meals. This reduces barriers to attendance, which maximizes the learning environment and optimizes the use of time during an intensive 3-day workshop. Both learners and faculty must be motivated to attend sessions. Strategies to enhance motivation include curricular content taught by world-renowned leaders in the field, small instructor-to-student ratio during hands-on simulation sessions, and inclusion of topics relevant to the geographic location of the workshop. Educators benefit from the opportunity for open and honest discussion among peers, in addition to demonstrations of variations in surgical technique in a setting that fosters collegial interaction. Currently, survey-based assessments of participants are the main component program evaluation, including satisfaction surveys and measurement of the workshop's perceived impact on practice and procedural confidence. Efforts to follow the long-term influence of these initiatives will be important for program support and sustainability.

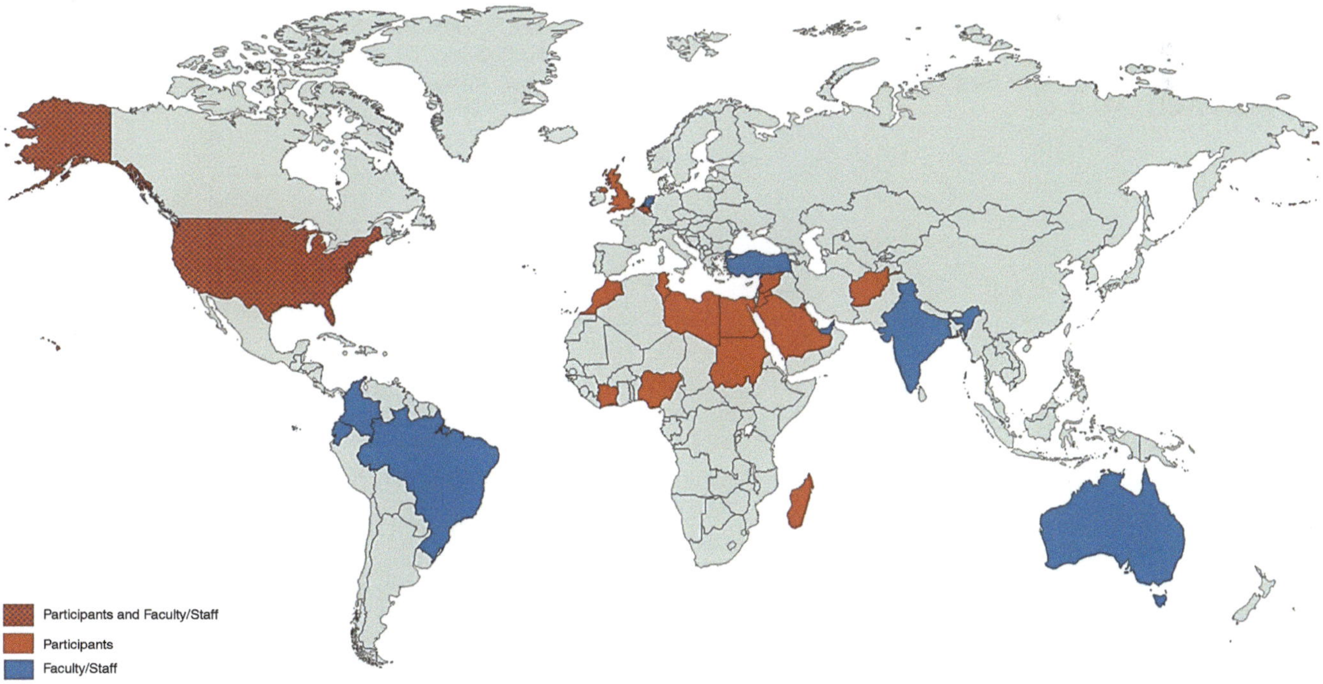


Fig. 36.3 Countries of origin of workshop participants, faculty, and staff. (Permissions and copyrights retained by Usama S. Hamdan, MD, FICS)

## Future Directions and Conclusion

Comprehensive, multidisciplinary, simulation-based cleft care surgical skills workshops provide a unique opportunity for capacity building and a platform for multidisciplinary learning and are made possible through collaborations between cleft foundations, academic leaders in cleft care, regional practitioners, and invested stakeholders from the biomedical industry sector. Educational content should also take into account unique contexts of each region and country, while aiming for the optimal blend of didactic learning and hands-on knowledge and skills acquisition.

## References

1. Michael Mars DS, Habel A. Management of cleft lip and palate in the developing world. England: Wiley Publishing; 2008.
2. Hubli EH, Noordhoff MS. Smile train: changing the world one smile at a time. Ann Plast Surg. 2013;71(1):4–5.
3. Agag RL. Fellowship review: ReSurge International The Jerome P. Webster fellowship. Ann Plast Surg. 2012;69(5):495–9.
4. Taro T, Yao C, Ly S, et al. The global surgery partnership: an innovative partnership for education, research, and service. Acad Med. 2016;91(1):75–8.
5. Jones CM, Campbell CA, Magee WP, Ayala R, Mackay DR. The expanding role of education and research in international healthcare. Ann Plast Surg. 2016;76 Suppl 3:S150–4.
6. Aziz SR, Ziccardi VB, Chuang SK. Survey of residents who have participated in humanitarian medical missions. J Oral Maxillofac Surg. 2012;70(2):e147–57.
7. Campbell A, Sherman R, Magee WP. The role of humanitarian missions in modern surgical training. Plast Reconstr Surg. 2010;126(1):295–302.
8. Dupuis CC. Humanitarian missions in the third world: a polite dissent. Plast Reconstr Surg. 2004;113(1):433–5.
9. Precious DS. Important pillars of charity cleft surgery: the avoidance of "safari surgery". Oral Surg Oral Med Oral Pathol Oral Radiol. 2014;117(4):395–6.
10. Patel PB, Hoyler M, Maine R, Hughes CD, Hagander L, Meara JG. An opportunity for diagonal development in global surgery: cleft lip and palate care in resource-limited settings. Plast Surg Int. 2012;2012:892437.
11. McCullough M, Campbell A, Siu A, et al. Competency-based education in low resource settings: development of a novel surgical training program. World J Surg. 2018;42(3):646–51.
12. Selzer DJ, Dunnington GL. Surgical skills simulation: a shift in the conversation. Ann Surg. 2013;257(4):594–5.
13. Kantar RS, Plana NM, Cutting CB, Diaz-Siso JR, Flores RL. Internet-based digital simulation for cleft surgery education: a 5-year assessment of demographics, usage, and global effect. J Surg Educ. 2018;75(4):1120–6.
14. Podolsky DJ, Fisher DM, Wong KW, Looi T, Drake JM, Forrest CR. Evaluation and implementation of a high-fidelity cleft palate simulator. Plast Reconstr Surg. 2017;139(1):85e–96e.
15. Podolsky DJ, Wong Riff KW, Drake JM, Forrest CR, Fisher DM. A high fidelity cleft lip simulator. Plast Reconstr Surg Glob Open. 2018;6(9):e1871. Latest Articles.
16. Rogers-Vizena CR, Saldanha FYL, Hosmer AL, Weinstock PH. A new paradigm in cleft lip procedural excellence: creation and preliminary digital validation of a lifelike simulator. Plast Reconstr Surg. 2018;142(5):1300–4.
17. Podolsky DJ, Fisher DM, Wong Riff KW, et al. Assessing technical performance and determining the learning curve in cleft palate surgery using a high-fidelity cleft palate simulator. Plast Reconstr Surg. 2018;141(6):1485–500.
18. Plana NM, Rifkin WJ, Kantar RS, et al. A prospective randomized blinded trial comparing digital simulation to textbook for cleft surgery education. Plast Reconstr Surg. 2019;143(1):202–9.
19. Kantar RS, Ramly EP, Almas F, et al. Sustainable cleft care through education: the first simulation-based comprehensive workshop in the Middle East and North Africa region. Cleft Palate Craniofac J. 2019;56(6):735–43. https://doi.org/10.1177/1055665618810574.
20. Waltzman JT, Tadisina KK, Zins JE. The rise of technology in plastic surgery education: is the textbook dead on arrival (DOA)? Aesthet Surg J. 2016;36(2):237–43.
21. Beaubien JM, Baker DP. The use of simulation for training teamwork skills in health care: how low can you go? Qual Saf Health Care. 2004;13 Suppl 1:i51–6.
22. Cheng H, Podolsky DJ, Fisher DM, et al. Teaching palatoplasty using a high-fidelity cleft palate simulator. Plast Reconstr Surg. 2018;141(1):91e–8e.

# Outcome Assessment

# 37

Eugene Park, Carolina Restrepo, Karen W. Y. Wong Riff,
and Alex Campbell

## Introduction

A critical analysis of cleft care around the world reveals large disparities in access to and quality of care [1]. While collaborative research and the adaptation of team-based multidisciplinary care have elevated cleft care in developed nations, cleft surgery in low- and middle-income countries (LMICs) is still often associated with poor outcomes [2]. The number of patients with clefts in these regions often exceeds the capacity of local healthcare systems to treat them, resulting in a global backlog of over 600,000 untreated patients [3]. These patients also face significant geographic and socioeconomic barriers, which contribute to higher rates of complications and lower rates of follow-up [1, 4, 5].

The global scale-up of cleft care over the past several decades has been immense. Charitable organizations have provided more than one million free cleft repair surgeries and trained local surgeons in LMICs to perform these procedures [2]. Historically, the success of these outreach efforts has been measured by the number of patients served, and little emphasis has been placed on the quality of care delivered. Consequently, complication rates following cleft palate repair in these settings often approach 30%, and aesthetic results following lip repair have been difficult to track [6].

In order to bridge this gap in quality, thoughtfully designed improvement measures must be implemented, and outcomes must be tracked in a meaningful way. Until recently, outcomes reporting in cleft care has been limited by a lack of high-quality, validated, cleft-specific assessment instruments. In this chapter, we discuss two very different approaches to assessing outcomes after cleft lip and palate repair. The first focuses on developing a standardized, objective cleft lip assessment tool that can be used by nonmedical personnel, thus increasing its applicability in resource-limited settings. The second utilizes patient-reported outcomes to obtain a more granular picture of how various cleft types affect patient function and quality of life, revealing outcomes that may otherwise be missed by provider assessment.

## Surgical Outcomes Evaluation in Resource-Limited Settings

While complications following cleft lip repairs are widely reported in the literature, aesthetic outcomes are less frequently assessed. Furthermore, aesthetic outcomes after cleft lip repair in LMICs are rarely, if ever, reported. Effective quality improvement initiatives in cleft care must not only reduce complication rates but also help patients achieve the best possible aesthetic results from their surgery. An essential component of achieving such a goal is to develop a method of rigorously analyzing aesthetic outcomes following cleft lip repair in a reproducible way.

The unilateral cleft lip surgical outcomes evaluation (UCL SOE) scale was developed in response to a need for a uniform and simple assessment tool that provides objective evaluations of the results of cleft lip repair. Subjective or qualitative assessments using standardized photographs by a panel of judges have been previously reported by Asher-McDade et al. [7]. The Asher-McDade scale uses a standardized method to evaluate four nasolabial components (nasal

E. Park
Division of Plastic Surgery, Northwestern University Feinberg School of Medicine, Chicago, IL, USA
e-mail: eugene-park@northwestern.edu

C. Restrepo
Operation Smile, Inc, Virginia Beach, VA, USA

K. W. Y. Wong Riff (✉)
Division of Plastic and Reconstructive Surgery, Hospital for Sick Children, Toronto, ON, Canada
e-mail: karenw.wong@sickkids.ca

A. Campbell
Division of Plastic Surgery, Penn State Hershey College of Medicine, Hershey, PA, USA

Operation Smile Inc, Virginia Beach, VA, USA

Mobile Surgery International, Mexico City, Mexico

Premium Care Plastic Surgery, Cartagena, Colombia

© Springer Nature Switzerland AG 2021

J. W. Swanson, D. W. Low (eds.), *Global Cleft Care in Low-Resource Settings*, https://doi.org/10.1007/978-3-030-59105-2_37

form, nose symmetry, nasal profile, and vermilion border) and grades each component on a 5-point scale. While effective in its intended area of use, the scale has limited applicability in global cleft care as it was designed to evaluate patients in late childhood/early adolescence after years of multidisciplinary treatment. In order to practically evaluate patients after cleft lip repair in resource-limited settings, the global cleft charity Operation Smile developed the UCL SOE scale as an instrument to focus on aesthetic results of a single surgical intervention.

The UCL SOE scores symmetry of four individual anthropomorphic components of a cleft lip repair (Cupid's bow, lateral lip, nose, and free vermilion) (Fig. 37.1). Each element is scored on a 3-point scale: 2 (excellent), 1 (mild asymmetry), 0 (unsatisfactory). The scores of the four components are then summed for a total score of 0 (lowest) to 8 (highest). A validation study was performed to evaluate the reliability of the UCL SOE scale when used by both surgeons and laypersons, with the thought that the ability of nonsurgical personnel to use the scale would increase its applicability in resource-limited settings [8]. Twenty-five sets of standardized frontal and basal photographs of on-table immediate postoperative unilateral cleft lip repairs were distributed to 9 experienced cleft surgeons and 12 laypersons. When scores were averaged between three evaluators, inter-rater reliability for surgeons was in the "good" range (intraclass correlation coefficient (ICC) = 0.71) and inter-rater reliability for laypersons was in the "very good" range (ICC = 0.82).

As aesthetic results following cleft lip repair depend heavily on the severity of the initial cleft lip deformity, the unilateral cleft lip severity index (UCL CSI) was developed to be used in conjunction with the UCL SOE scale. The UCL CSI was designed to analyze and categorize unilateral cleft lip deformities according to the amount of lip involved and the degree of nasal asymmetry (Fig. 37.2). The severity index was also validated in a study measuring the inter-rater reliability of the tool when used by both surgeon and laypersons [9]. Twenty-five participants (10 surgeons and 15 laypeople) evaluated 25 sets of presurgical photographs of unilateral

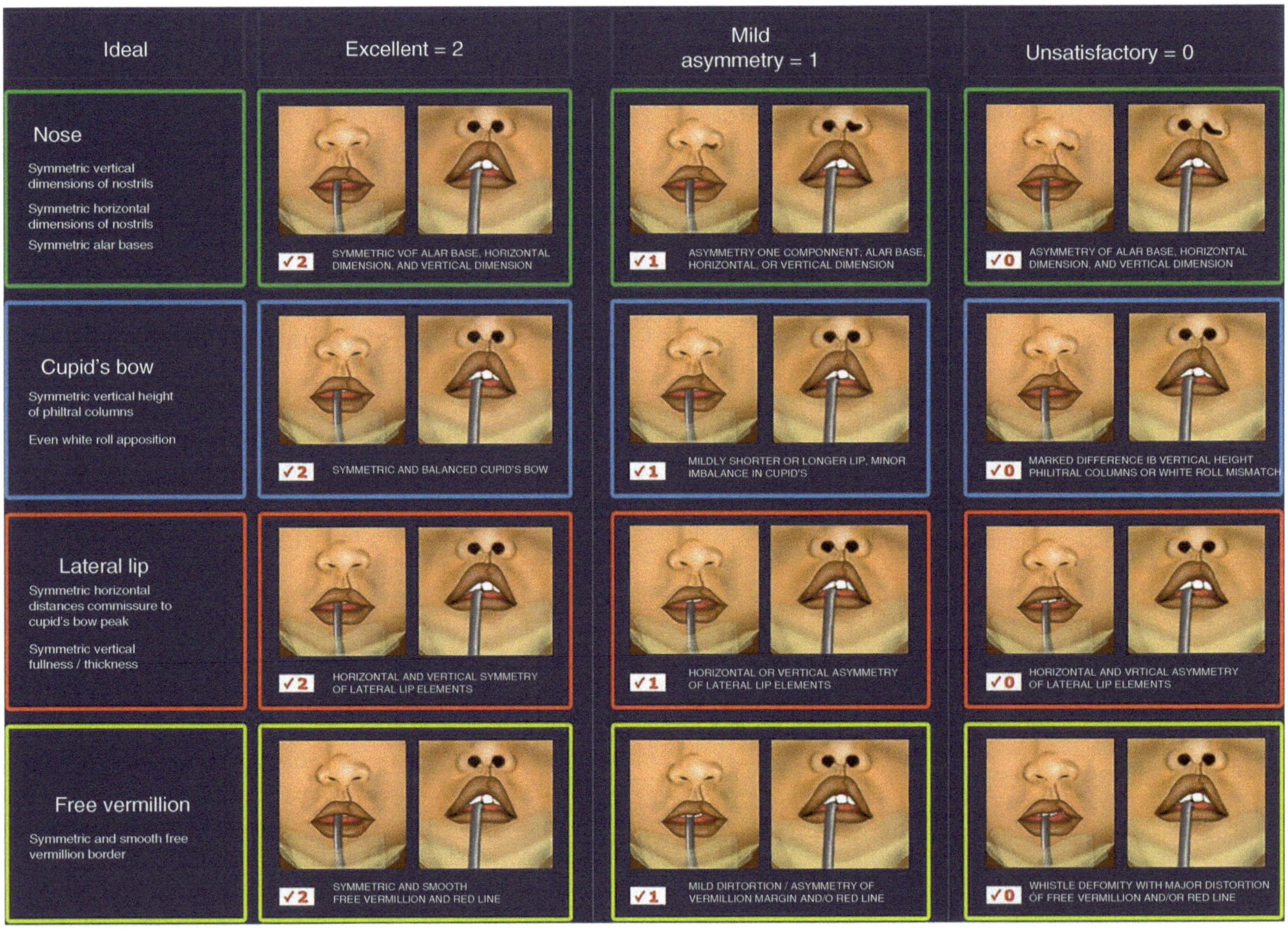


**Fig. 37.1** Unilateral cleft lip surgical outcomes assessment scale. Each element is scored on a 3-point scale: 2 (excellent), 1 (mild asymmetry), and 0 (unsatisfactory). The scores of the four individual components are then summed for a total score of 0 (lowest) to 8 (highest)

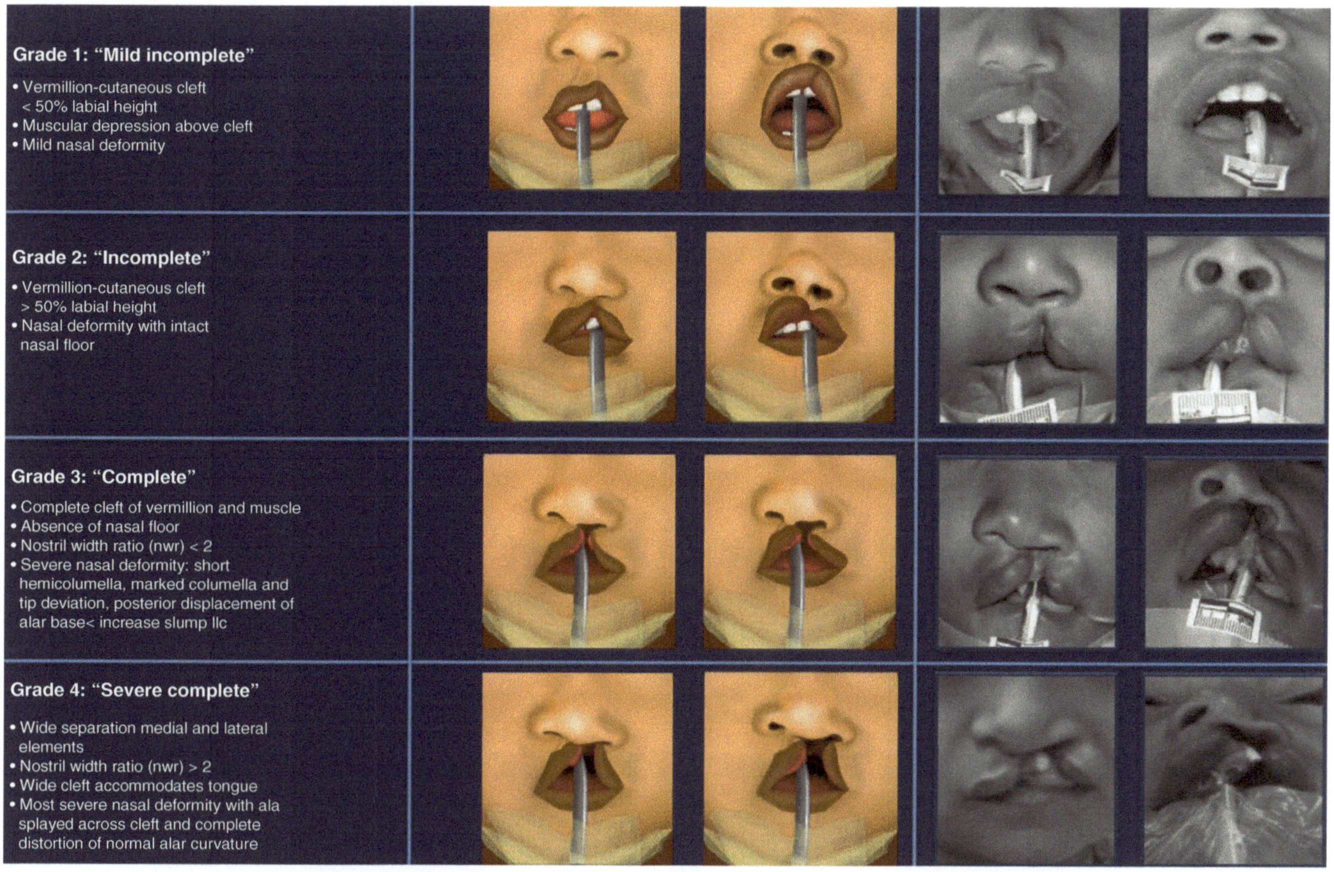


**Fig. 37.2** Criteria and examples demonstrating each of the four grades of the unilateral cleft lip severity index

cleft lip patients. Inter-rater reliabilities for both groups were categorized as very good (ICC > 0.8).

The unilateral cleft lip severity index and surgical outcomes evaluation scale are now utilized globally and provide feedback regarding outcomes to volunteer surgeons as well as OS administrators with a rapid turnaround time. In order to aid in the interpretation of results, a retrospective study was performed applying the severity index and outcomes evaluation scale to 1823 patients who had undergone unilateral cleft lip repair by OS during missions in various countries and at the Guwahati Comprehensive Cleft Care Center (GCCCC) in Assam, India [10]. The results of this study established a normative bell curve of outcomes for each severity of unilateral cleft lip deformity (Fig. 37.3). Based on these normative values, a surgeon can see where his or her results fall in the range of results for a given severity of cleft. Surgeons who fall on the upper end of the spectrum can provide coaching to less experienced surgeons, and results that fall below a standard deviation of the average can be investigated for root cause analyses (Fig. 37.4).

The UCL SOE is, of course, not without limitations. The aesthetic outcomes of a cleft lip repair must be evaluated in a longitudinal manner as scar maturation and the forces of growth can change the appearance of a lip repair over time. One of the main limitations of the UCL SOE is that the outcomes evaluation is performed using a photograph from a single time point, namely, the immediate postoperative period. The distorting effects of local anesthetic injections and surgical swelling can affect the appearance and thus the score given to a repair, and the position of the camera can also influence how the result is viewed by the reviewer. However, the scale does provide an easily accessible tool that can be applied across all missions and work in the developing world and effectively allows the identification of results that are substandard.

The routine use of these tools in OS's work around the world provides a means of quality control and supports the mandate that patients in LMICs receive the same high level of care as patients in the developed world.

## Patient-Reported Outcomes in Cleft Care

Whereas outcomes from some medical conditions can simply be measured in cure or survival rates, outcomes reporting following cleft lip and palate repair must describe a complex panoply of conditions ranging from aesthetic to psychosocial and functional. Numerous studies over the past several

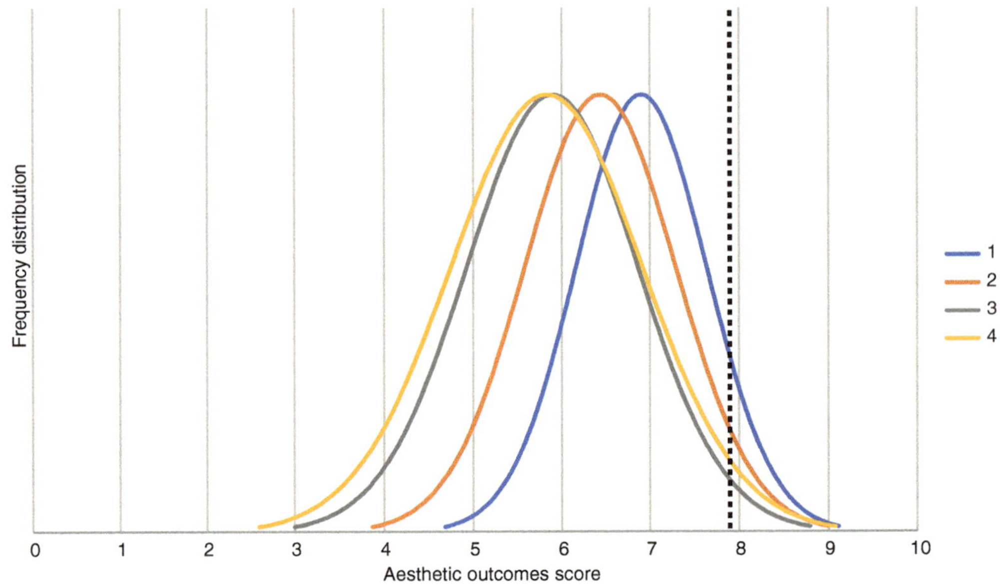


**Fig. 37.3** A large-scale rollout of the unilateral cleft lip severity index and unilateral cleft lip surgical outcomes evaluation scale established normative bell curves for outcomes for each severity of unilateral cleft lip. The dotted line represents the maximum possible score

| Dr. [redacted] | Cases | Nose | Lateral Lip | Vermillion | Cupid's Bow | Total score |
|---|---|---|---|---|---|---|
| Cleft severity 1 | 3 | 1.67 | 2 | 2 | 1.89 | 7.56 |
| Cleft severity 2 | 8 | 1.41 | 1.79 | 1.66 | 1.79 | 6.66 |
| Cleft severity 3 | 3 | 1.22 | 1.66 | 1.89 | 2 | 6.77 |

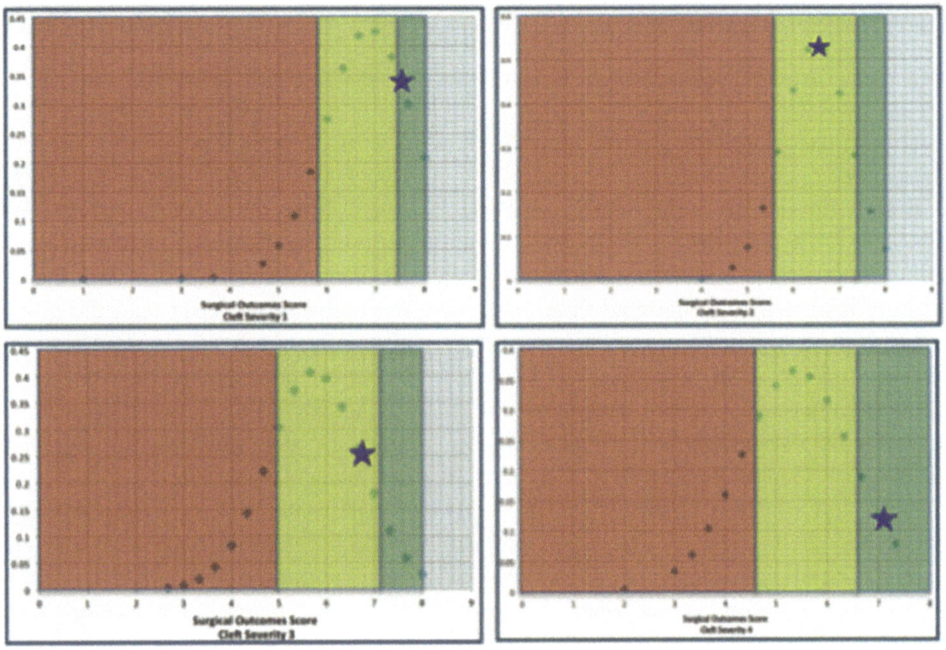

**Fig. 37.4** Sample outcomes report for a surgeon participating in a surgical mission showing where his/her results fall on the histogram curve of outcomes for each severity of cleft

decades have reported on objective measurements of outcome such as complication rates, symmetry, and reoperation rates [11, 12]. These measures, however, do not provide a complete picture of how cleft lip and palate affect patients' lives and their perception of their own well-being. A growing awareness of this discrepancy has led to an increased use of patient-reported outcomes (PROs) in plastic surgery [13].

A major roadblock in the collection of patient-reported outcomes after cleft lip and palate surgery has been the absence of effective, validated, cleft-specific instruments. In

2011, Eckstein et al. performed a literature review to identify questionnaires validated for use in patients with cleft lip and palate. Of the 44 instruments identified, only 9 were relevant to patients with cleft lip and palate, and only 5 of the 9 instruments had undergone a validation process. None of these five validated instruments were created specifically for use in patients with cleft lip and palate, limiting their applicability.

CLEFT-Q is a patient-reported outcomes questionnaire designed to specifically evaluate health-related quality of life (HRQoL) and function in patients with cleft lip and palate. The goal of CLEFT-Q was to improve the treatment provided to patients with cleft lip and palate by measuring physical, psychological, and social health from the patient perspective. An additional goal of CLEFT-Q was to develop a common metric that could be used internationally so that the instrument could be applicable in both high-resource countries and LMICs. In order to design an internationally applicable instrument, CLEFT-Q was developed in a cross-cultural manner through a collaboration between 30 centers in 12 countries [14].

The development of CLEFT-Q followed a rigorous multiphase mixed method approach in accordance with guidelines set forth by the Scientific Advisory Committee, the USA Food and Drug Administration, and the International Society for Pharmacoeconomics and Outcomes Research [14]. Strict adherence to such guidelines ensures a methodologically sound instrument and strengthens the validity of studies performed using the instrument. In the first phase of development, a systematic review of existing instruments was performed in accordance with PRISMA guidelines and confirmed the need for a comprehensive PRO instrument for cleft lip and palate. Next, qualitative studies were performed to expose relevant areas of concern through topics uncovered from the systematic review and through intensive interviews performed on patients with cleft lip and palate in each of the participant countries. This generated a large array of items, which were then carefully filtered through a rigorous process to generate the final list of items to be considered for use in the instrument (Fig. 37.4).

In 2018, a validation study for CLEFT-Q was performed based on item responses from 2434 children and young adults with cleft lip and/or palate using the Rasch model [15]. In Rasch analysis, individuals are placed along a scale based on the probability that they will answer a set of items in a certain manner. The results of this analysis provided evidence of reliability and validity for 12 of 13 scales initially created for CLEFT-Q. Specifically, the analysis showed that lower scores on CLEFT-Q scales were associated with having a speech problem, being unhappy with facial appearance,

**Table 37.1** List of CLEFT-Q scales

| CLEFT-Q scales | | |
|---|---|---|
| *Appearance scales* | *HRQoL[a] scales* | *Facial function scales* |
| Cleft lip scar | Psychological function | Speech |
| Face | School function | |
| Jaws | Social function | |
| Lips | Speech-related distress | |
| Nose | | |
| Nostrils | | |
| Teeth | | |

[a]*HRQoL* health-related quality of life

and needing future cleft-related treatments, providing evidence of construct validity. The 12 scales included in the final iteration of CLEFT-Q are face, nose, nostrils, lips, cleft scar, teeth, jaws, psych, school, social, speech distress, and speech function (Table 37.1). The topics covered span the gamut of issues likely to be encountered by patients with cleft lip and palate and empower CLEFT-Q to become the first validated, internationally applicable PRO tool for use specifically in this population.

In 2019, Wong Riff et al. reported their findings from a large-scale rollout of CLEFT-Q designed to detect differences in the various CLEFT-Q item bank scores among patients with different types of cleft [16]. Patients ranged in age from 8 to 29 years and were enrolled at 30 centers in 12 countries. The results of the group's analysis confirmed clinically apparent differences in appearance, speech, and HRQoL between patients with various cleft types, further confirming the validity of the instrument. Patients with bilateral lip involvement had lower scores for appearance and HRQoL, and patients with more severe cleft palates had lower scores for speech. Additionally, the study introduced the use of radar charts as visual representations of a patient's overall cleft-related well-being as measured by CLEFT-Q. A comprehensive assessment of a patient's outcomes following cleft lip and/or palate repair cannot focus on one metric alone (Fig. 37.5). For example, a patient undergoing Le Fort I advancement for midface hypoplasia may achieve improvement in appearance but may encounter negative effects on speech and resonance. The use of a radar chart allows clinicians to obtain an instant assessment of multiple factors that contribute to a patient's condition and is useful for following changes in these factors over time (Fig. 37.6).

CLEFT-Q holds great potential for elucidating aspects of cleft-related health that are often missed by observer-reported metrics. Future studies will address differences in PROs among various centers and among different countries, which will in turn inspire effective quality improvement measures in the parts of the world that need it the most.

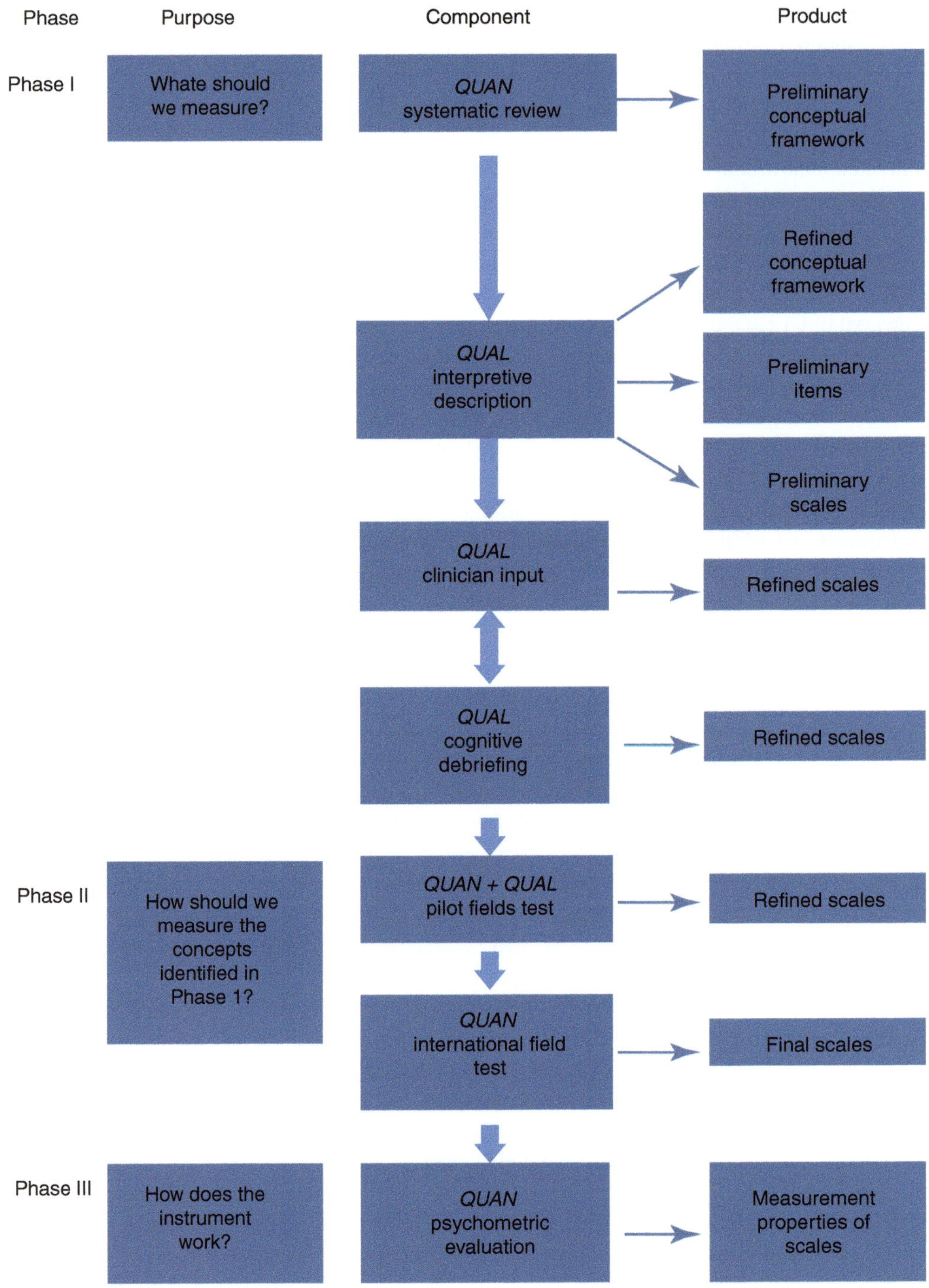


**Fig. 37.5** Flow diagram showing the multiphase mixed method protocol for developing CLEFT-Q

## Improving Patient Follow-Up in Resource-Limited Settings

One of the most challenging barriers to improving cleft outcomes in resource-limited settings is poor patient follow-up. With decreasing costs of mobile technology, cellular phones have become ubiquitous, even in the developing world. Surgeons from Changing Children's Lives Inc. have leveraged this fact to provide long-term follow-up for cleft mission patients in a remote manner using mobile phones [17]. The authors evaluated a group of 56 patients who underwent cleft lip and/or palate repair during a mission to Thailand and found that more than half of these patients' families were reachable by phone 1.5 years after surgery. Foong et al., in 2012, randomized 36 patients undergoing cleft palate repair to receiving or not receiving a phone dedicated to communication with the provider team and found that the group receiving a

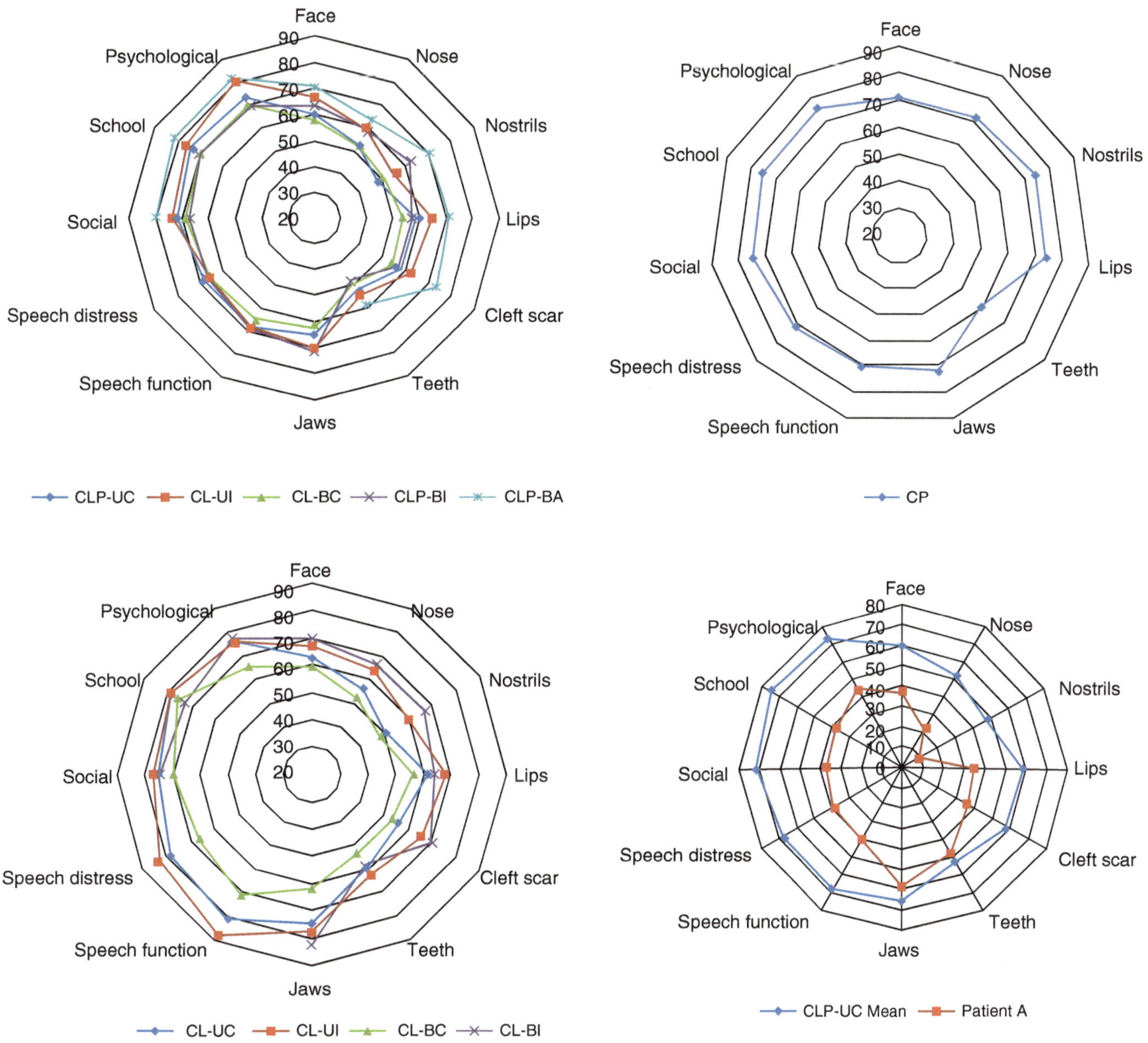


**Fig. 37.6** Radar charts allow simultaneous visualization of all 12 scales measured by CLEFT-Q. This provides an efficient means of following patient outcomes in a longitudinal manner

phone were more likely to return for speech therapy ($p = 0.005$) [18]. Various forms of technology such as teleconferencing software and mobile chat apps have been proposed as means of improving follow-up and providing longitudinal care to cleft patients in a resource-conserving manner.

Providers at the GCCCC launched the District Outreach Follow-Up and Speech Therapy (DOFAST) program with the goal of bringing the follow-up to patients instead of having them travel to the center. Small multidisciplinary teams of providers were sent to outreach camps near patients living more than 200 km away if there were at least 20 patients to be seen. A prospective analysis of results after launching the DOFAST program revealed that postoperative follow-up visits increased from 139 monthly visits (follow-up to surgery ratio of 0.722) to 363 monthly visits (ratio of 1.57) [5]. Additionally, the average cost to the center per patient was lower for local follow-up compared to follow-up at the center (Rs. 303 vs. 1100).

## Conclusions

Outcomes reporting after cleft lip and palate repair often focuses on complication rates, and a large array of factors affecting patient well-being are frequently missed. The cleft lip severity index, cleft lip surgical outcomes evaluation, and CLEFT-Q represent steps forward in a global effort to improve outcomes reporting in cleft care. By providing effective and globally applicable tools for evaluating patients with cleft lip and palate, these tools promise to narrow the gap in the quality of care delivered among different populations and different regions of the world.

## References


1. Yao CA, Swanson J, Chanson D, Taro TB, Gura B, Figueiredo JC, et al. Barriers to reconstructive surgery in low- and middle-income countries: a cross-sectional study of 453 cleft lip and cleft palate patients in Vietnam. Plast Reconstr Surg. 2016;138(5):887e–95e.
2. Kantar RS, Cammarata MJ, Rifkin WJ, Diaz-Siso JR, Hamdan US, Flores RL. Foundation-based cleft care in developing countries. Plast Reconstr Surg. 2019;143(4):1165–78.
3. Carlson LC, Stewart BT, Hatcher KW, Kabetu C, VanderBurg R, Magee WP Jr. A model of the unmet need for cleft lip and palate surgery in low- and middle-income countries. World J Surg. 2016;40(12):2857–67.
4. Schonmeyr B, Restrepo C, Wendby L, Gillenwater J, Campbell A. Lessons learned from two consecutive cleft lip and palate missions and the impact of patient education. J Craniofac Surg. 2014;25(5):1610–3.
5. Jansen LA, Carillo L, Wendby L, Dobie H, Das J, Restrepo C, et al. Improving patient follow-up in developing regions. J Craniofac Surg. 2014;25(5):1640–4.
6. Deshpande GS, Campbell A, Jagtap R, Restrepo C, Dobie H, Keenan HT, et al. Early complications after cleft palate repair: a multivariate statistical analysis of 709 patients. J Craniofac Surg. 2014;25(5):1614–8.
7. Asher-McDade C, Roberts C, Shaw WC, Gallager C. Development of a method for rating nasolabial appearance in patients with clefts of the lip and palate. Cleft Palate Craniofac J. 1991;28(4):385–90; discussion 90–1.
8. Campbell A, Restrepo C, Deshpande G, Tredway C, Bernstein SM, Patzer R, et al. Validation of a unilateral cleft lip surgical outcomes evaluation scale for surgeons and laypersons. Plast Reconstr Surg Glob Open. 2017;5(9):e1472.
9. Campbell A, Restrepo C, Deshpande G, Bernstein SM, Tredway C, Wendby L, et al. Validation of the unilateral cleft lip severity index for surgeons and laypersons. Plast Reconstr Surg Glob Open. 2017;5(9):e1479.
10. Campbell A, Restrepo C, Park E, Navas G, Deshpande G, Swanson J, et al. Influence of severity on aesthetic outcomes of unilateral cleft lip repair in 1,823 patients. Plast Reconstr Surg Glob Open. 2019;7(1):e2083.
11. Park E, Deshpande G, Schonmeyr B, Restrepo C, Campbell A. Improved early cleft lip and palate complications at a surgery specialty center in the developing world. Cleft Palate Craniofac J. 2018;55(8):1145–52.
12. Schonmeyr B, Wendby L, Campbell A. Early surgical complications after primary cleft lip repair: a report of 3108 consecutive cases. Cleft Palate Craniofac J. 2015;52(6):706–10.
13. Chung KC, Pusic AL. Patient-reported outcomes instruments. Outcomes measures in plastic surgery. Clin Plast Surg. 2013;40(2):xi–xii.
14. Wong Riff KW, Tsangaris E, Goodacre T, Forrest CR, Pusic AL, Cano SJ, et al. International multiphase mixed methods study protocol to develop a cross-cultural patient-reported outcome instrument for children and young adults with cleft lip and/or palate (CLEFT-Q). BMJ Open. 2017;7(1):e015467.
15. Klassen AF, Riff KWW, Longmire NM, Albert A, Allen GC, Aydin MA, et al. Psychometric findings and normative values for the CLEFT-Q based on 2434 children and young adult patients with cleft lip and/or palate from 12 countries. CMAJ. 2018;190(15):E455–E62.
16. Wong Riff KWY, Tsangaris E, Forrest CR, Goodacre T, Longmire NM, Allen G, et al. CLEFT-Q: detecting differences in outcomes among 2434 patients with varying cleft types. Plast Reconstr Surg. 2019;144(1):78e–88e.
17. Wes AM, Paul N, Gerety PA, Folsom N, Swanson J, Taylor JA, et al. A sustainable model for patient follow-up following an international cleft mission: a proof of concept. Cleft Palate Craniofac J. 2018;55(7):977–82.
18. Foong DY, Butler DP, Vanna K, Sok Leng T, Gollogly J. A mobile phone initiative to increase return for speech therapy follow-up after cleft palate surgery in the developing world. J Plast Reconstr Aesthet Surg. 2012;65(9):e260–1.

# Part VI

# Optimal Cleft Care Delivery

# Comprehensive Cleft Care Centers: Scalable, Sustainable, and Cost Effective Surgical Care

38

Alex Campbell and Prasetyanugraheni Kreshanti

**Key Points**

- Comprehensive cleft care centers (CCCCs) are capable of providing scalable, sustainable, and cost-effective multidisciplinary surgical care to vulnerable patient populations in resource-limited settings.
- CCCCs function as permanent specialty surgical hospitals staffed by local professionals year-round, offering comprehensive and longitudinal treatment to patients from early nutrition and orthodontics to surgery and speech therapy.
- Establishing a CCCC requires special attention to need identification, site selection, partnerships, financing, facilities, equipment, supplies, leadership, and team building.
- Significant efforts and organization are required to operate on a single individual, including patient recruitment, patient care services, multidisciplinary screening, medical records, surgeons, anesthesia services, 24-hour nursing, blood bank availability, and postoperative care.
- Impact and sustainability are achieved.
- Several economic reviews have shown that care at CCCCs can be "very cost-effective," providing superior care to larger numbers of patients while decreasing costs and increasing investments in the local healthcare system and community.
- The CCCC has the ultimate potential to develop into a regional referral center and center of education and research, providing world-class care to the most needy of patients while contributing to the evolution of global cleft care.

## Introduction

Cleft surgery is the largest and most sustained humanitarian global surgical effort to date, with roots in outreach by humanitarian cleft care organizations to low-resource settings, traveling missionary and military surgeons who have provided care to local patients, and local teams who have developed cleft programs. International cleft mission trips have traditionally proven successful in providing surgical treatment of cleft in areas where treatment was previously unavailable, helping to overcome the misconception that surgery is too difficult and costly in resource-poor regions [1]. Despite these successes, cleft lip and cleft palate remain a stark example of the global burden of surgical disease, with millions of untreated – or inadequately treated – patients worldwide. The need for a new paradigm in global surgery has been increasingly recognized by governments, funding agencies, and professionals in order to exponentially expand care, while emphasizing safety and quality.

Comprehensive cleft care centers (CCCCs) have emerged as the gold standard for cleft care in low- and middle-income countries (LMICs), capable of providing scalable, sustainable, and cost-effective surgical care to vulnerable patient populations in resource-limited settings [2, 3]. CCCCs function as permanent specialty surgical hospitals staffed by local professionals year-round, offering comprehensive and longitudinal treatment to patients from early nutrition and orthodontics to surgery and speech therapy (Table 38.1).

A. Campbell (✉)
Division of Plastic Surgery, Penn State Hershey College of Medicine, Hershey, PA, USA

Operation Smile Inc, Virginia Beach, VA, USA

Mobile Surgery International, Mexico City, Mexico

Premium Care Plastic Surgery, Cartagena, Colombia

P. Kreshanti
Cleft and Craniofacial Center Cipto Mangunkusumo Hospital, Plastic Surgery Division, Department of Surgery, Faculty of Medicine Universitas Indonesia, Jakarta, Indonesia

© Springer Nature Switzerland AG 2021

J. W. Swanson, D. W. Low (eds.), *Global Cleft Care in Low-Resource Settings*, https://doi.org/10.1007/978-3-030-59105-2_38

**Table 38.1** Timeline of surgical treatment for cleft lip and cleft palate

| Surgical treatment of cleft lip and palate by age | | |
|---|---|---|
| Age | Treatment | Cleft team members |
| Prenatal | Prenatal imaging, diagnosis, and counseling | Multidisciplinary |
| Newborn | Feeding assessment, medical assessment, genetic counseling, treatment information | Multidisciplinary |
| 0–3 months | Presurgical orthopedics | Orthodontist, plastic surgeon |
| 3–6 months (or after presurgical orthopedics) | Primary cleft lip repair | Plastic surgeon |
| 12 months (delayed if airway or medical concerns) | Primary cleft palate repair with intravelar veloplasty, myringotomy, and tubes if needed | Plastic surgeon, otolaryngologist |
| 3–4 years diagnosis of velopharyngeal insufficiency (3–4 years) | Secondary palate repair lengthening or pharyngoplasty, speech obturator | Speech pathologist, plastic surgeon otolaryngologist, orthodontist |
| School-age years | Treatment of secondary lip and nasal deformities | Plastic surgeon |
| 7–9 years (mixed dentition) | Secondary alveolar bone graft | Orthodontist, plastic surgeon, oral surgeon |
| 7–9 years (mixed dentition) | Presurgical orthodontics | Orthodontist |
| Skeletal maturity | Le Fort I | Plastic surgeon, oral surgeon |
| Skeletal maturity | Definitive open rhinoplasty | Plastic surgeon |

Centers offer a markedly enhanced portfolio of multidisciplinary services and have demonstrated improved safety and surgical outcomes on par with academic university cleft centers in high-income countries (HICs) [4–8]. Several economic reviews have shown that care at CCCCs can be "very cost-effective," providing superior care to larger numbers of patients while decreasing costs and increasing investments in the local healthcare system and community (Figs. 38.1 and 38.2) [9–11]. This facilitates further development of CCCCs into regional referral centers capable of additional impact through education and training, enhanced patient services, and clinical research.

This chapter discusses key ingredients for establishing and maintaining a successful comprehensive cleft care center and presents several original studies that have emerged from CCCCs.

## Establishing a Comprehensive Cleft Care Center

### Need Identification and Site Selection

CCCCs may arise from multiple potential origins, ranging from a plastic surgery division of a local hospital that seeks to create a multidisciplinary cleft program to an underserved area in a host country in which government, charity organizations, and local businesses see an opportunity to collaborate. In some cases, repeated cleft outreach missions to a site instigate formation of a CCCC. Feasibility studies

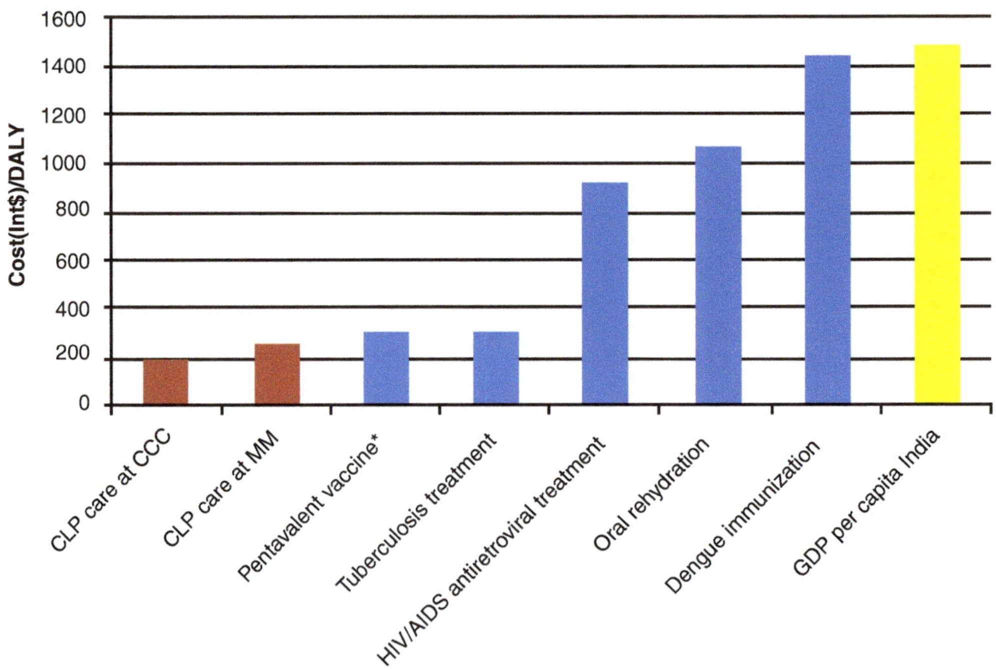


**Fig. 38.1** Cost per DALY of different prevention and treatment strategies for common global health conditions as compared with CLP treatment via a mission or center strategy. (Reproduced with permission from Hackenberg et al. [9])

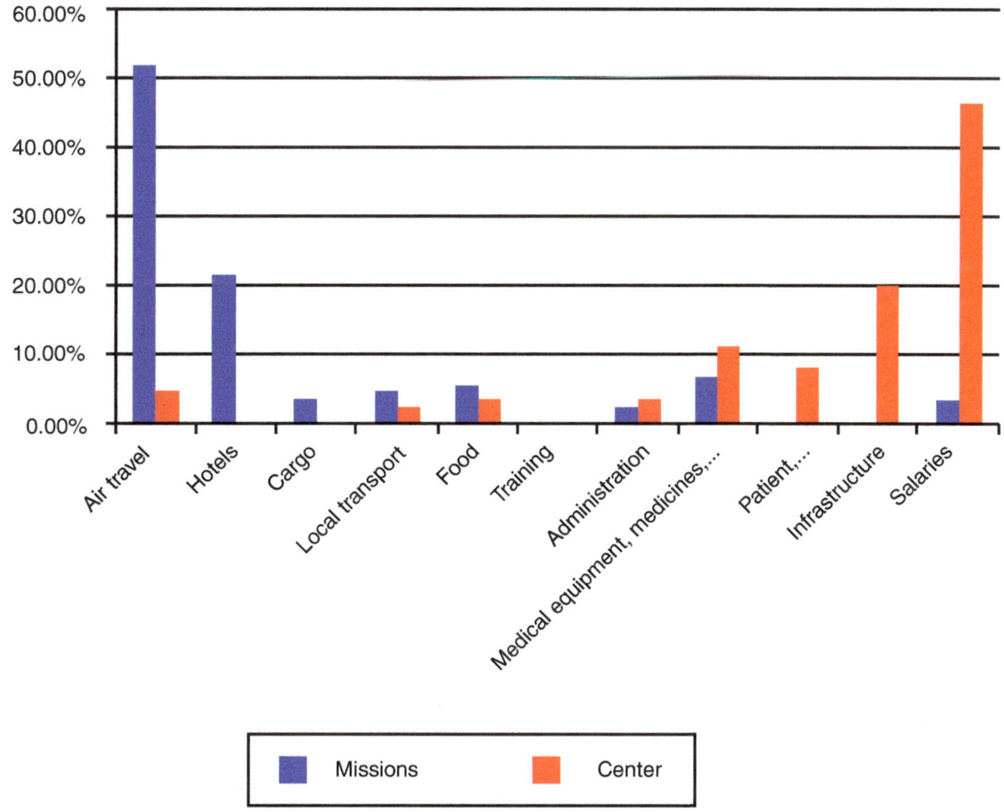


**Fig. 38.2** Comparison of categorical expenditures between missions and full-time center activity in Assam, India. (Reproduced with permission from Nagengast et al. [10])

must be undertaken to determine the need and ability of establishing a CCCC. The political and economic environment as well as the attitude of the local government, hospitals, and medical societies must be aligned for optimal success. The site for a CCCC must be chosen with respect to patient demographics, existing infrastructure, available space, local transportation systems, patient access, and proximity to governing and regulatory bodies. Larger cities where some form of expertise and hospital services already exist tend to be the most productive locations for a CCCC. It is also important to have sufficient volume of patients in order to justify the resources required for a multidisciplinary cleft care team and more importantly because higher-volume centers have been associated with better outcomes [12–15].

## Partnerships

Close collaboration among dedicated partners is essential to creating and sustaining a successful CCCC. Ideal is a public-private partnership involving local government, health authorities, charitable organizations, and donors. This combines expertise in medical care and training, organizational structure and management, local healthcare infrastructure, and finance. These partnerships also facilitate initial access to patients, facilities, transportation, and media and play a critical role in developing local support.

Initial medical missions are often carried out to initiate a presence in the region, evaluate the patient recruitment and turnout, and begin establishment of more advanced treatment capabilities.

## Financing

The foundation of partnerships supporting the CCCC must involve a fundamentally sound mechanism to finance the center indefinitely. Parties typically invest into the project in terms of monies provided, human resources, and infrastructure. This involves funding the upfront capital expenditures required to build a CCCC, as well as ongoing monetary support for running costs required for the center to fulfill its mission long term. Agreements are often successful that involve reimbursement to the center on a fee-per-surgery basis motivating productivity. Meticulous records enable managers and donors to understand resource utilization and performance and make the case for ongoing investment. Successes of the CCCC become successes of all of the stakeholders and typically encourage continuation of funding commitments, while attracting additional corporate, philanthropic, and university sponsors providing additional programmatic support in line with their individual interests and mandates.

## Facilities

Different models exist depending on local capabilities and goals of the project.

- The most common is when the sponsoring organization provides funding for equipment and financial aid to individual local surgeons to provide cleft surgeries and multidisciplinary services utilizing existing personnel and hospital facilities. This allows surgeons to treat patients in their communities that are otherwise neglected by underfunded local healthcare systems, with training of key professionals and strategic investments bridging the gap in care.
- On a larger scale, sponsoring organizations can partner with institutions such as universities, governmental hospitals, and private healthcare systems to establish comprehensive cleft centers at existing facilities. Funding of surgeries and support for patients provide access to care, while training of professionals and support of multidisciplinary services allow institutions to improve quality, expand services, and increase scale. Institutions also bring unique strengths in education, training, and research.
- The most advanced model is to create a stand-alone CCCC, with facilities for all aspects of care including operating rooms, postanesthesia recovery units, and inpatient facilities (Fig. 38.3). The center can then provide all services at a single site including medical evaluations, surgery, speech therapy, nutrition services, child life counseling, dental care, otolaryngology, and orthodontics. These are often adjacent to local hospitals with contracts for radiology, laboratory, blood bank, and intensive care unit services.
- A slightly modified version of the stand-alone is the mobile surgical hospital (MSH). This is essentially a stand-alone subspecialty hospital built onto a mobile platform, complete with operating rooms, full-time team, pre- and postoperative wards, and multidisciplinary services. Double-sided expandable tractor-trailers have been converted into mobile hospitals, able to travel long distances to quickly establish a CCCC where there is significant number of patients awaiting care (Fig. 38.4). The ease of deployment and ability to remain for prolonged periods of time allow the rapid treatment of large numbers of patients.

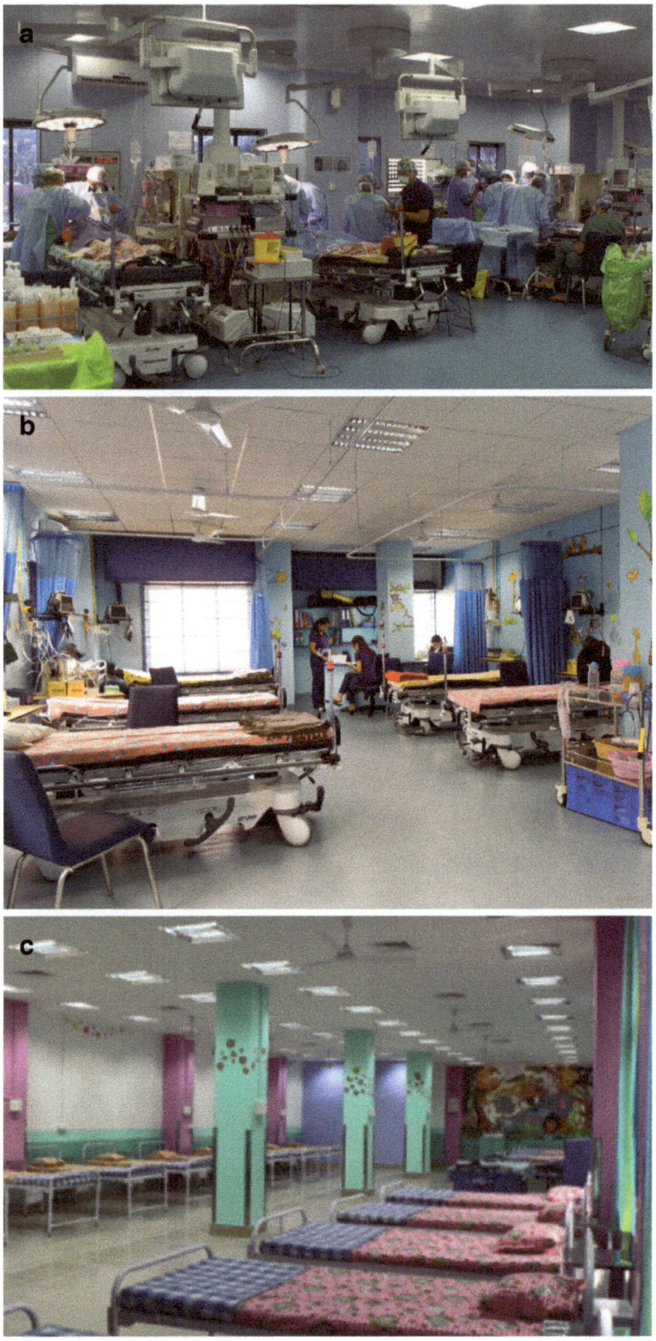

**Fig. 38.3** A state-of-the-art comprehensive cleft care center featuring a modern integrated operating suite with open layout (**a**); recovery room with monitoring, central gases, and emergency equipment (**b**); and inpatient creating a child friendly environment focused on quality pediatric care, education, and rehabilitation (**c**)

## Equipment and Supplies

- Acquisition, preparation, and maintenance of equipment and supplies are central to quality cleft surgery, and equipment and supply needs in an LMIC cleft center are generally equivalent to those in HICs. At a minimum, complete surgical trays, sutures and dressings, reliable and modern anesthesia equipment, resuscitation packs, perioperative monitors, and sterile materials are required for cleft surgery regardless of the setting (Table 38.2)

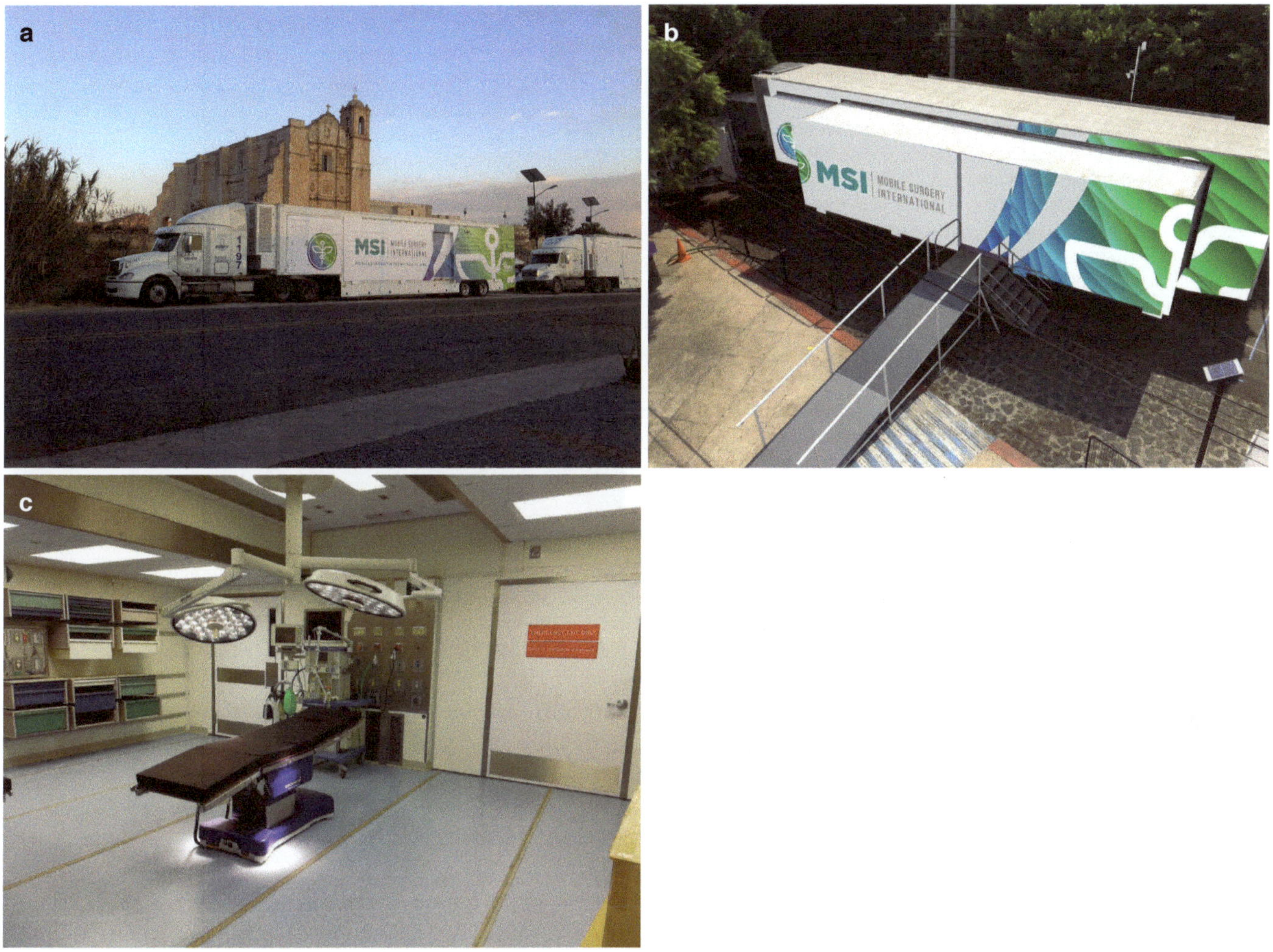


**Fig. 38.4** The mobile surgical hospital (MSH) is a stand-alone subspecialty hospital built onto a mobile platform (**a**), complete with operating room (**b**), postoperative ward (**c**), a full-time team, and multidisciplinary services

## Leadership and Team Building

Comprehensive cleft centers offer fully articulated cleft care teams designed to deliver an entire care package full-time and year-round, providing the highest level of safety and quality.

| | |
|---|---|
| Cleft surgeon(s) | Speech therapist |
| Anesthesiologist(s) | Child life specialist |
| Pediatrician(s) | Medical records specialist |
| Nurse manager | Medical photographer |
| Operating room nurses | Biomedical technician |
| Recovery room nurses | Patient recruitment team |
| Pre-/postoperative nurses | Patient care team |
| Dentist/orthodontist | Clinical coordinator(s) |

The team generally begins the operations with a core nucleus consisting of a cleft surgeon, speech therapist, orthodontist, and nurse coordinator. The center is then developed around these key specialties in order to mature and expand services. Educational exchanges, through twinning programs between an emerging CCCC in an LRS and a mature cleft program in an HIC or through extended visitorships by experienced professionals, can help support initial clinical efforts and to train local counterparts (Fig. 38.5). As volume increases and teams are expanded, emphasis should be placed on achieving optimal outcome for each patient, as opposed to treating the maximum number of patients. Emergency preparedness should be vigorous. Staff at all levels and specialties should train in basic life support (BLS) and pediatric advanced life support (PALS) and advanced cardiac life support (ACLS) or equivalent training provided for anesthesiologists, pediatricians, and recovery room personnel (Fig. 38.6). All team members should participate in continuous education activities including didactic instruction, skills training, and clinical training. Rotation of key team members at a major cleft center can be invaluable in teaching them about best practice advanced treatment modalities.

**Table 38.2** Comprehensive cleft center equipment and supplies

| | |
|---|---|
| Screening and assessment | Vital sign monitors, camera, oto-/ophtalmoscope, lights, tongue blades, and examination equipment, medical records, laboratory facilities, |
| Anesthesia | Anesthesia machine, resuscitation boxes with current, unexpired drugs and pediatric dosage schedules. Airway equipment for pediatric patients including masks, endotracheal tubes, airways, laryngoscopes, positive pressure ventilation systems, noninvasive monitors, and difficult airway management items. Sevoflurane anesthetic agent, and dantrolene. Intravenous fluids and fluid administration sets, blood matching and blood for transfusion, defibrillator, and appropriate emergency equipment |
| Surgery | Appropriately constructed surgical instrument trays for cleft lip, cleft palate, and other cases. Appropriate suture material. Sterilization materials with gowns, gloves, and drapes. Electrocautery and illumination |
| Postanesthesia care | Full resuscitation packs, oxygen and suction equipment at each bedside, vital sign monitors with pulse oximetry, documentation system |
| Postoperative intensive care | Either built-in capability in host hospital or provision made for transport of critical patients |
| Ward nursing units | Vital sign monitoring equipment, intravenous fluids and fluid administration sets, appropriate dressing and cleaning materials, medications for pain, antisepsis, nausea, and other nursing needs |

Adapted from Sherman and Campbell [16]

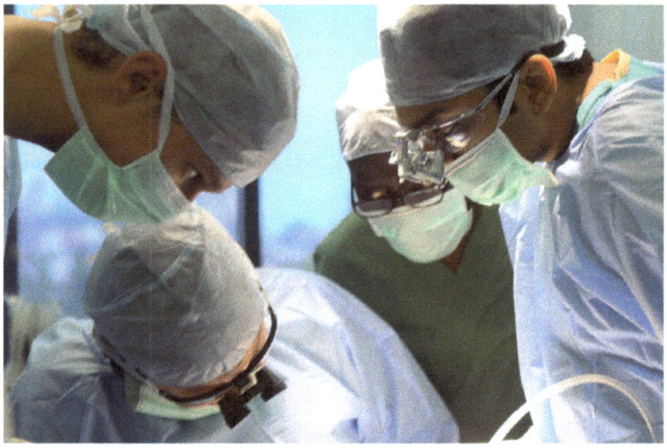

**Fig. 38.5** Often an international team helps to support initial clinical efforts and to train local counterparts and then independently run a cleft center within their own country (Fig. 38.3)

## Quality Care Delivery

Effective cleft care in the LMICs is based on safe anesthesia and quality surgery and depends on a multitude of other contributions in order to provide top care to the patients. Significant efforts and organization are required to operate on a single individual, including patient recruitment, patient care services, multidisciplinary screening, medical records,

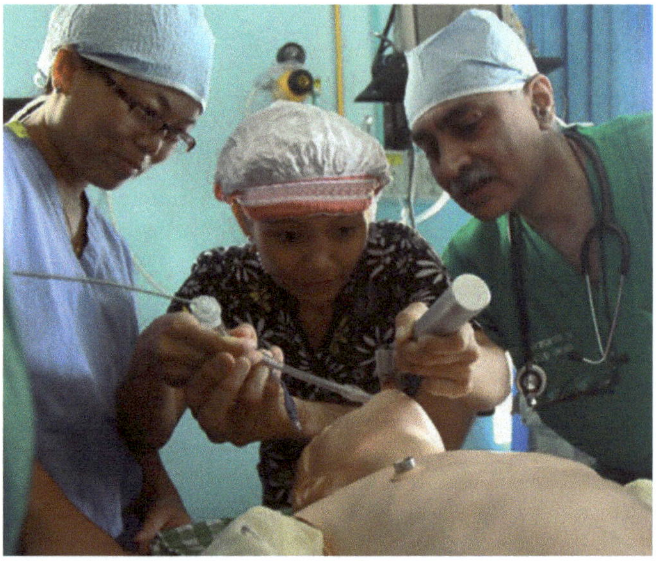

**Fig. 38.6** Staff at all levels and specialties should train in basic life support (BLS) and pediatric advanced life support (PALS) and advanced cardiac life support (ACLS) or equivalent training provided for anesthesiologists, pediatricians, and recovery room personnel

surgeons, anesthesia services, 24-hour nursing, blood bank availability, and postoperative care.

## Patient Mobilization

Patient mobilization is one of the core care challenges in LMICs, and a central step in expansion of care is to make patients aware that opportunities for treatment exist and to facilitate access. This seemingly straightforward notion becomes exponentially more complex with a population that is impoverished, remote, and diverse in religion, ethnicity, and language.

Community health activists throughout the region should be educated on cleft lip and cleft palate, so that they can create awareness in the communities they serve to best identify and treat patients. Local prescreening camps may be organized to locally screen, register, and educate patients and families on their condition and treatments available and to help coordinate transport to the CCCC for medical evaluation and care (Fig. 38.7).

## Patient Care Services

A patient care team is helpful in coordinating clinical services and hospitality to patients coming to the CCCC, often from distant regions. This team assumes responsibility for patients and their families upon arrival to the CCCC, coordinating food, hygiene, and shelter as well logistics needed for all patients to receive multidisciplinary clinical evaluations

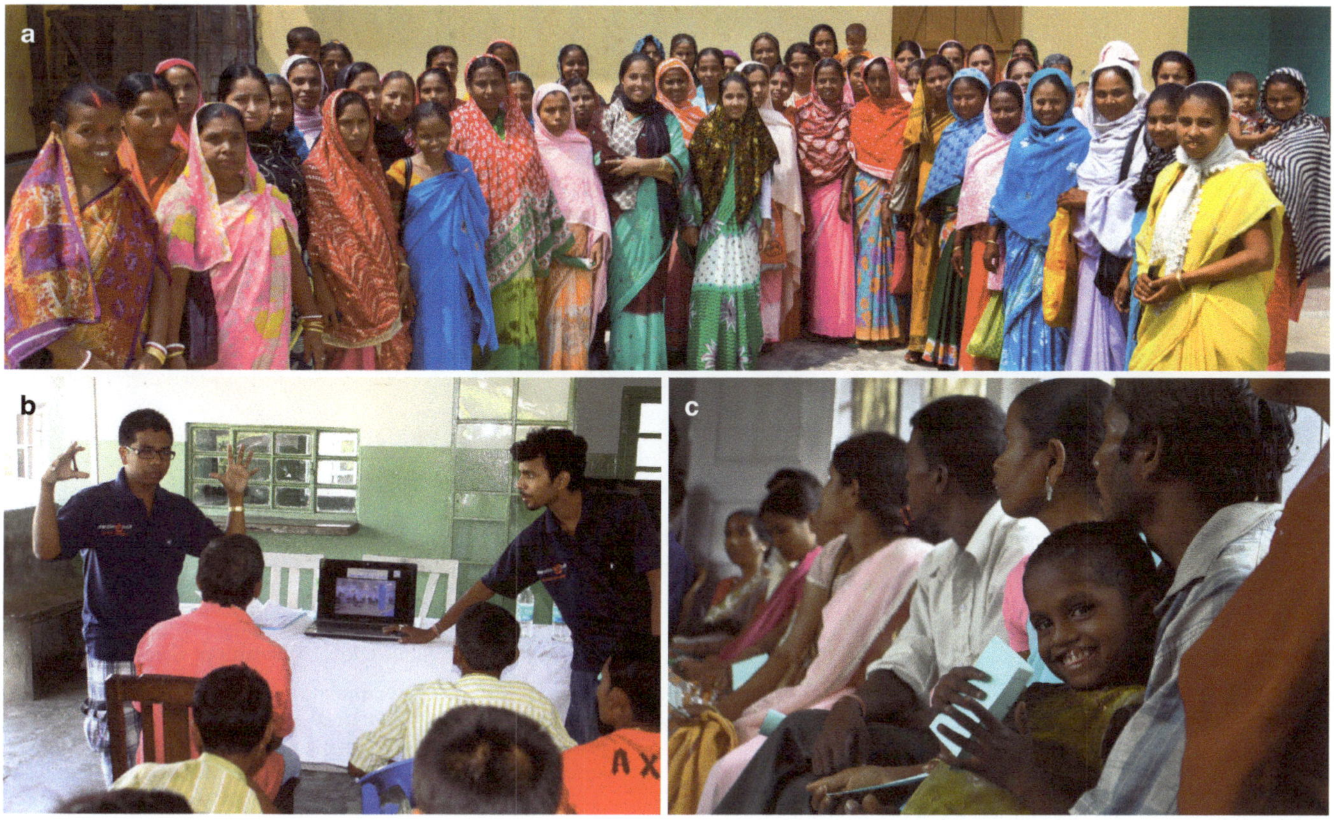

Fig. 38.7 A robust patient mobilization should constantly work to identify patients in need of surgical care and connect them to the CCCC for treatment. Engaging community health activists (**a**) and hosting local prescreening camps (**b**) assist patients to break through the barriers to obtaining care (**c**)

and to synchronize investigations and care plans between professionals. After surgery, the patient care team assists patients with transportation back to their homes and coordinates for postoperative follow-up appointments.

## Patient Assessment

Multidisciplinary preoperative screening and assessment of all patients allows the CCCC to optimally establish plans for provision of medical care of the highest safety, quality, and effectiveness. Individual medical evaluation by surgeons, anesthesiologists, pediatricians, and nurses is designed to detect any risk factors such as congenital anomalies, cardiac or pulmonary pathology, infections disease, illness, and malnutrition. Hemoglobin should be checked on all patients to detect anemia. Age minimums should be adopted and implemented to minimize risk (e.g., 3–6 months minimum for cleft lip and 9–12 months minimum for cleft palate). Preoperative evaluation by multidisciplinary team members (e.g., nutrition, dentistry, orthodontics, speech therapy, and child psychology) is also performed to initiate comprehensive cleft care. Any patients requiring treatment of medical conditions (e.g., anemia, malnutrition, illness) or preoperative preparation (e.g., NAM, speech therapy) are selected out to receive appropriate interventions to optimally prepare them for surgery (Fig. 38.8).

## Informed Consent

Simple and direct communication with patients in their native language is essential for quality surgical care. Consents for families to read and sign should be comprehensive and clear, informing them of the nature of the operation and its risks, use of anesthesia, potential blood transfusion, HIV, and hepatitis testing in the case of needle stick, with permission for taking photographs and permission to utilize data and photographs for research, publication, and social media if applicable. When language differences exist, skilled interpreters are necessary to assure proper informed consent prior to surgery.

## Documentation

Patient care should be documented meticulously throughout evaluation, treatment, and follow-up with records stored in a

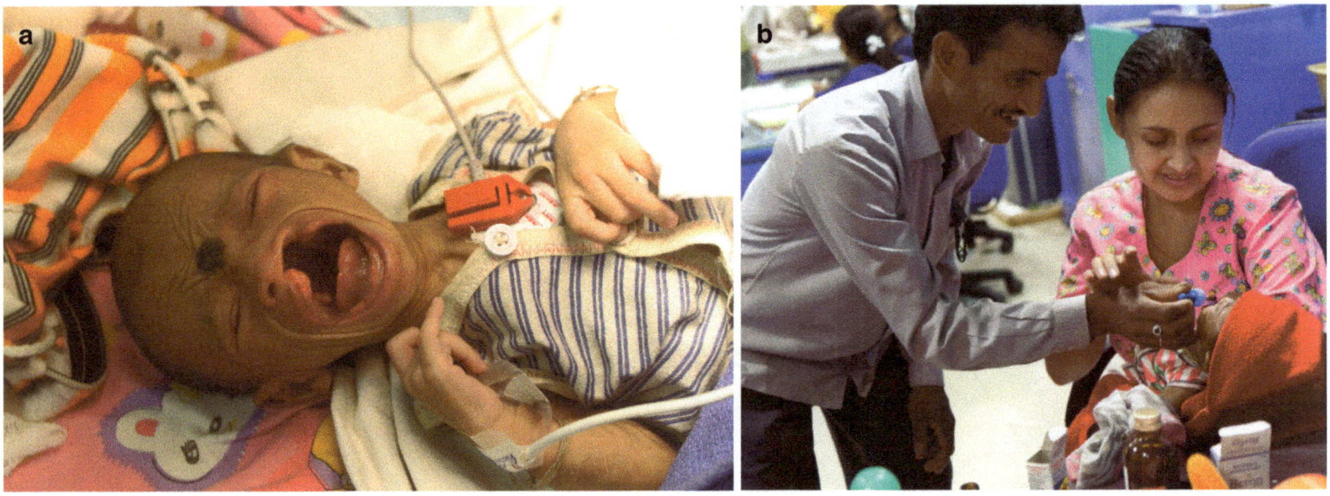

**Fig. 38.8** An intensive screening process identifies patients with medical conditions such as malnutrition (**a**) so that these patients are selected out to receive appropriate interventions and optimally prepare them for surgery (**b**)

secure and accessible location. Medical records should be comprehensive, explicit, and clear to provide details of the patient's history, examination findings, and interventions performed. Pre- and postoperative photographs of patients are a critical part of the medical record, and providers need to be disciplined in taking standardized views throughout the process in order to follow the patient's course and to evaluate outcomes. Electronic health records may be appropriate in some settings, and simple/affordable options may be available. Simple, available medical records tend to be utilized more often than complex records with greater barriers to attain and use.

## Surgical Care

The central focus of the CCCC should be on safe surgery with excellence in outcomes. Policies, procedures, and protocols should be developed to guide all aspects of care. One such example is the Operation Smile Global Standards of Care (Table 38.3) [17]. On the day of surgery, patients should be examined once again by the pediatrician, anesthesiologist, operating surgeon, and nurses as part of a "double-check" system designed to enhance safety and communication. As operations are initiated, it is wise to be conservative with surgical volume and complexity of cases to provide a rigorous standard of care for all patients and to not overextend the limited staff members and create unsafe situations. Operating room procedures should be reviewed periodically to improve safety and efficiency. Surgical techniques and surgical outcomes should undergo continuous evaluation and maturation, so as to create uniform quality and refine best practices. A policies and procedures manual should be developed to establish a long-term guide for center practices.

**Table 38.3** Operation Smile Global Standards of Care

| | | |
|---|---|---|
| 1 | Requirements for preoperative patient screening and assessment | Appropriate equipment, laboratory support, and trained personnel will be available to preform comprehensive and evaluation in order to properly assess our candidates' indications for any possible risks of surgery |
| 2 | Required anesthesia equipment and supplies | Only state-of-the-art, currently calibrated anesthetic delivery and support equipment, supplies, and pharmaceuticals will be used by our medical professionals to provide the safest in reliable anesthesia |
| 3 | Required surgical equipment | Comprehensive, well-maintained surgical instruments, sutures, and supplies will be provided for each patient, customized to the particular operative procedure received by each of our patients |
| 4 | Required for the recovery room – PACU | All our patients will receive specialized recovery care as they awaken from anesthesia, in an environment fully equipped with specialized instrumentation, personnel, and pharmaceuticals |
| 5 | Postoperative intense care | Any of our patients requiring additional postoperative care to support their successful recovery will be managed in a suitable, well-staffed intensive care environment |
| 6 | Patient consent | All of our patients and their families will receive understandable information and education in their native language, allowing them to make informed decision about surgery |
| 7 | Surgical priority | Our patients will receive surgery based on appropriate, well-tested, and proven priority systems, developed to maximize the expected benefit with primary consideration to safety and the allocation of time and resources |
| 8 | Preventing transmission of blood-borne pathogens | Universal precaution protocols will be followed to help minimize infection, transmission of disease, and wrong-site surgery |

**Table 38.3** (continued)

| | | |
|---|---|---|
| 9 | Pain management | Alleviation of pain and anxiety during every phase of our perioperative care is of primary concern. Each patient will receive the safest, most effective analgesic medication under strict monitoring from our doctors and nurses |
| 10 | Operation Smile team | Operation Smile believes a team approach to the care of our patients provides the highest level of care and safety. Team compositions are comprehensive, deep, and broad in their expertise; drilled in fluid teamwork and effective communication; and most importantly unified by the single desire to achieve the very best outcome for each of our patients |
| 11 | Volunteer credentials | Each of our volunteers is extensively interviewed, credentialed, and proctored prior to joining the operative team. Skills required from each of our specialist meet or exceed those of his/her core discipline. Ongoing mentoring, evaluation, performance review, and professional growth are central to maintaining top volunteer cops |
| 12 | Minimum patient follow-up | Effective postoperative care is essential for a good surgical result and effective planning for further treatment. Postoperative care requires good documentation and extensive education of parents and clinicians to be effective. When and wherever possible, our patients will receive short, intermediate, and long-term follow-up and care |
| 13 | Proper translation | Operation Smile missions will have sufficiently qualified translators to ensure proper communication among team members, support personnel, families, and patients. Proper translation is considered to be a matter of safety, quality, and respect of our patients' rights |
| 14 | Documentation | The purpose of documentation is to protect the patients, protect the healthcare personnel, and provide accurate record for the basis of outcome assessment. Each of our patients will be monitored through a well-documented and protected medical record, whether paper or electric |

## Nursing

Nurses are involved with all areas of clinical care, and a talented and well-trained nursing team is essential to the ongoing support and promotion of all medical programs at a CCCC. The nursing department can consist of three tiers to cover the OR, PACU, and inpatient ward with nurses cross-trained across divisions. A nurse manager should oversee all nursing divisions, which are headed by unit heads. Nursing coordinators in clinical care, quality assurance, and education provide additional support.

## Postoperative Care and Patient Education

Postoperative care should be standardized among surgeons and pediatricians and the nurses provided with specific education and training regarding postoperative care protocols. Nurses then lead a targeted education program that includes individual and group teaching to patients and parents. Patients can view instructional videos on the postoperative ward and should receive discharge materials including pictographs written in the local language (Fig. 38.9). These straightforward steps have been shown to improve patient understanding and decrease postoperative complications [18].

## Patient Follow-Up

Social, economic, and geographical challenges in LMICs can create intense challenges to patient travel and follow-up. Helpful strategies for follow-up programs include block scheduling of follow-up appointments, improved discharge teaching, clear patient discharge records, repeated telephone reminders, and assistance with transportation, food, and shelter when needed [19]. Patients returning to follow-up should be evaluated in a multidisciplinary fashion and scheduled for future examinations, therapy, and procedures as indicated. Patients who were "no-shows" should be called repeatedly to schedule a future appointment. When groups of patients are based in remote locations, outreach follow-up camps can also be helpful (Fig. 38.10). The use of smart phone applications like WhatsApp® can be utilized for following the appearance of patients with cleft lip and continuous speech monitoring of the patients following repair of cleft palate.

## Comprehensive Programs

Identification of talented, ambitious, and compassionate professionals is essential to the development of quality multidisciplinary services. Equally important is the support of their professional and clinical development.

**Dentists** Dentists provide oral prophylaxis, restorations, extractions, presurgical orthodontics (nasoalveolar molding and orthodontic corrections), and obturators. Helpful additions are the development of dental care protocols and dental outreach education programs on toothbrushing and tobacco cessation. More sophisticated orthodontia services to appropriate patients should be undertaken with a dedicated cleft orthodontist.

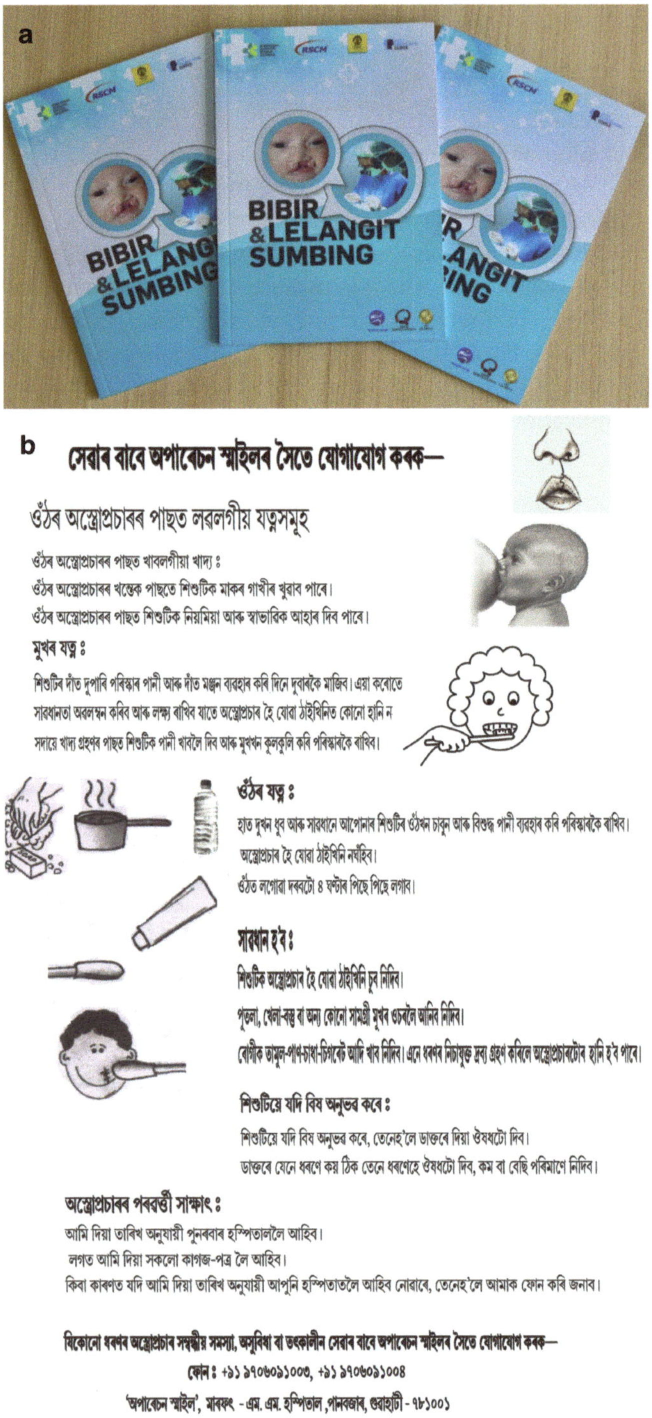


Fig. 38.9 (**a**, **b**) Standardized postoperative protocols and a culturally focused patient education program have been proven to improve patient understanding and compliance, while decreasing complications

**Speech Therapists** Speech therapists provide screening, diagnosis, therapy protocols, teaching, and ongoing treatment. There are severe challenges to providing cleft-specific speech therapy for patients in LMICs, which necessitate the creation of unique strategies and materials. Videos, booklets, and handouts can be developed to facilitate patient and parent teaching at the center, and district outreach speech therapy clinics can be provided in conjunction with local follow-up camps. A significant expansion of speech therapy outreach programs is possible through development of regional centers that can provide ongoing therapy. Speech therapists evaluate patients in their communities and prescribe specific speech therapy sessions to be administered by trained local resource teachers so that patients near a given outreach center can receive regular sessions closer to home. Speech therapists from the center can provide regular oversight, program audits, and periodic site visits for ongoing patient evaluations and treatment planning.

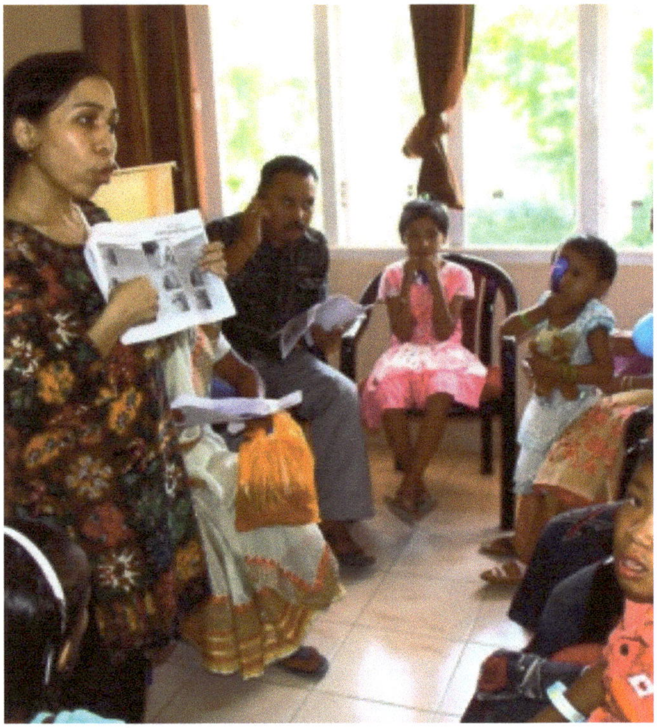

Fig. 38.10 District outreach programs can improve patient follow-up and access to services such as postoperative speech therapy

An **otolaryngologist** ideally should evaluate all cleft patients and provide treatment as appropriate. Because of the typical late median age of patient presentation in LMICs, there are far more chronic problems of the middle ear, with much higher demand for tympanoplasty and mastoid exploration than for myringotomy.

**Child Life Specialists** Child life specialists are very important to provide perioperative services and counseling to all patients and families receiving surgery at the CCCC. They prepare children for surgery while minimizing emotional trauma. This creates a child-focused and child-friendly environment that markedly improves the overall care experience.

## Impact and Sustainability

The CCCC is committed to medical and surgical care to patients afflicted with facial deformities and to assist patients with breaking through the barriers that prohibit them from obtaining services. The CCCC has the ultimate potential to develop into a regional referral center and center of education and research, providing world-class care to the most needy of patients while contributing to the evolution of global cleft care.

## Education and Training

An emphasis on education and training at the CCCC is central to sustainability and expanding impact. CCCCs are able to capitalize on a focused scope of practice, high patient volumes, and multidisciplinary approach to support unique training programs targeted to the needs of the local patients [20]. Educational programs based at the center should be designed and implemented in all specialties including plastic surgery, anesthesiology, nursing, speech therapy, dentistry, and child life. With excellent mentoring and large clinical volume, initial trainees become seasoned and highly experienced providers, going on to become the medical leaders and instructors (Fig. 38.11). This should happen across specialties, expanding the quality of all services within the CCCC and beyond. Numerous centers have gone on to develop excellent fellowship programs, training professionals to staff additional CCCCs [21].

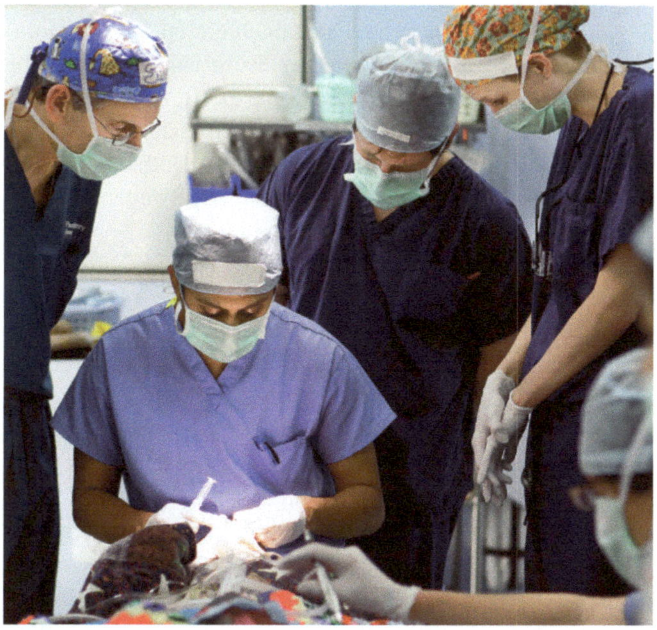

Fig. 38.11 With excellent mentoring and large clinical volume, initial trainees become seasoned and highly experienced providers, going on to become the medical leaders and instructors

## Research and Outcomes

The CCCC has the capacity to develop formalized efforts in research and outcomes to document, analyze, and critique various aspects of clinical care. The goal is to improve the quality of care at the CCCC and ultimately to contribute to the knowledge, standards, and practices of cleft care in LMICs. Data collection should be meticulous and well organized from the start, and an institutional review board should oversee all research projects. University partnerships both locally and internationally facilitate collaboration and combination of complimentary resources to best design and implement objective investigations into topics long debated in the literature. Participation in groups such as the International Confederation of Cleft Lip and Palate and Related Craniofacial Anomalies helps to promote and facilitate cleft care throughout the world.

## Regional Referral and Resource Center

Efforts to improve the quality of surgical care have led many organizations to advocate the use of high-volume hospitals for complex surgical procedures and for those requiring comprehensive multidisciplinary care.

The high volume of patients treated at a CCCC is important to the evolution of care, acting as a catalyst for the development of the structure, processes, and techniques that ultimately lead to better quality and outcomes. Surgical capacity and sustainability increase while complications and costs generally decrease. The CCCC can evolve to become a regional referral cleft center, with patients from adjacent regions traveling to the CCCC for specialized care. Teams from the CCCC can also travel to regional hospitals on outreach missions to provide surgery and multidisciplinary care to more remote populations. Additional regional and global impact is achieved through continued investments into education and training, comprehensive services, and research and outcomes.

Spotlight: Comprehensive Cleft Care Centers

The below represents some known examples of CCCCs of various models that have achieved global recognition as centers of excellence in LMICs. The reader is encouraged to read more deeply into the publications from successful

CCCCs in LMICs, listed in this section and in "References" at the end of the chapter.

- Smile Train supports more than 1100 partner hospitals in 85 partner countries, funding surgeries for patients that otherwise would not receive care. It also provides training and funding for equipment and comprehensive services to empower local doctors to provide free cleft repair surgery and comprehensive cleft care in their own communities. Since 1999, the organization has supported more than 1,000,000 cleft surgeries worldwide through this model [22, 23].
- The Sri Ramachandra University Cleft and Craniofacial Center was established in 2000 through partnership with the Smile Train and Sri Ramachandra Medical College and Research Institute (SRMC) in Chennai, India. Headed by Dr. Jyotsna Murthy, the center provides approximately 800 cleft surgeries per year and has completed more than 12,000 surgeries to date [24, 25].
- The Inga Health Foundation (Bangalore, India) was established in 2007 by Dr. Krishna Shama Rao and runs three state-of-the-art regional treatment centers for cleft and craniofacial surgery in partnership with university and private hospitals in Bangalore, Mumbai, and Srinagar. Inga Health has performed more than 8000 surgeries to date and intends to set up multiple dedicated multidisciplinary centers across India to expand clinical care and training [26].
- Operation Smile Colombia established its multidisciplinary care center in Bogotá, Colombia, in 2007 as an investment into long-term sustainability after nearly 20 years of missions in the country. The center provides a full portfolio of multidisciplinary services and has an operating room where ambulatory surgeries are performed (e.g., cleft lip, cleft lip revision, rhinoplasty). Cases requiring inpatient care (e.g., cleft palate, complex cases) are performed in partnership with local hospitals. The center performs approximately 500 surgeries per year and provides an additional 500 surgeries per year through outreach missions throughout Colombia [27, 28].
- The GSR Institute of Craniofacial Surgery (Hyderabad, India) was formed in 2000 by Dr. Srinivas Gosla Reddy in partnership with Smile Train and now performs more than 1500 surgeries per year, while providing advanced multidisciplinary services and innovative patient care programs. This center hosts robust rotations and fellowships for national and international fellows from all over the world and has trained more than 100 consultants from different areas of India and abroad in cleft surgery [29–31].
- The Guwahati Comprehensive Cleft Care Center (Guwahati, India) was established in 2011 by Operation Smile as part of a public-private partnership to create a high-volume CCCC in a region of intense need. It features a state-of-the-art surgical facility with modern integrated operating suite with an open layout, advanced surgical equipment, and sophisticated anesthesia and monitoring capabilities. By 2013 the center was performing more than 2500 cleft surgeries per year, while hosting advanced fellowship training and producing ample clinical research [32]. The center was transitioned to local leadership and is operated by Mission Smile and has completed 16,000 surgeries to date.
- Mobile Surgery International (Mexico) operates a state-of-the-art MSH that includes a modern integrated operating suite with an open layout, advanced surgical equipment, sophisticated anesthesia and monitoring capabilities, central medical gases, and sterilization facilities. An expandable unit measuring 22′8″ × 53′1″ accommodates a complete perioperative treatment area with two surgical tables, three recovery room beds, and supporting facilities. Two additional expandable units have been customized to serve as patient wards. A resident team of professionals provide quality surgical care, comprehensive services, education and training, research and outcomes, and organizational optimization. The MSH is planned for multiple long-term deployments (6 months to 1 year) throughout Mexico to provide services and establish sustainability [33].
- The Cleft and Craniofacial Center, Cipto Mangunkusumo Hospital-Universitas, Indonesia, is among the few hospital-based cleft centers in the entire country providing multidisciplinary and sustainable cleft and craniofacial care. In 2012 all services were centralized at the current center, where the team has performed more than 1700 cleft and craniofacial surgeries to date. In 2015, the team started a collaboration with the Gothenburg cleft team, Sahlgrenska University Hospital, Sweden, to optimize research protocols and activities.
- The Chang Gung Craniofacial Center (CGCFC) in Taipei, Taiwan, was started in 1978 by a single surgeon, Dr. Samuel Nordhoff, whose vision was to assist children from poor families born with cleft lip and palate to receive the best possible care [34]. Since its inception, the team has been devoted to providing wholistic, patient-oriented medical care in a multidisciplinary approach and is comprised of dedicated craniofacial surgeons, craniofacial dentists, speech and language pathologist and therapists, psychologists, and social workers. CGCFC has treated over 30,000 patients with cleft lip and palate and hosted more than 600 international visiting fellows from more than 50 countries [32]. CGCFC is widely recognized as the gold standard in cleft care by authorities in HICs and LMICs alike.

## References


1. Campbell A, Sherman R. Global cleft care. In: Losee JE, Kirschner RE, editors. Comprehensive cleft care. 2nd ed. New York: McGraw-Hill Medical; 2015.
2. Campbell A, Restrepo C, Mackay D, Sherman R, Varma A, Ayala R, Sarma H, Deshpande G, Magee B. Scalable, sustainable cost effective surgical care: a model for safety and quality in the developing world. Part I: challenge and commitment. J Craniofac Surg. 2014;25:1674–9.
3. Campbell A, Restrepo C, Mackay D, Sherman R, Varma A, Ayala R, Sarma H, Deshpande G, Magee B. Scalable, sustainable cost effective surgical care: a model for safety and quality in the developing world. Part II: program development and quality care. J Craniofac Surg. 2014;25:1680–4.
4. Park E, Restrepo C, Deshpande G, Schonmeyr B, Campbell A. Improved cleft lip outcomes at a surgical specialty hospital in the developing world. Cleft Palate Craniofac J. 2018;55(8):1145–52.
5. Patel A, Clune JE, Steinbacher DM, Pershing J. Comprehensive cleft center: a paradigm shift in cleft care. Plast Reconstr Surg. 2013;131(2):312e–3e.
6. Deshpande G, Campbell A, Restrepo C, Jagtap R, Dobie H, Keanan T, Sarma H. Early complications after cleft palate repair: a multivariate statistical analysis of 709 consecutive patients. J Craniofac Surg. 2014;25:1614–8.
7. Schonmeyr B, Wendby L, Campbell A. Early surgical complications after primary lip repair: a report of 3108 consecutive patients. Cleft Palate Craniofac J. 2015;52(6):706–10.
8. Schonmeyr B, Wendby L, Restrepo C, Campbell A. Surgical complications in 1408 primary cleft palate repairs operated at a single center in Guwahati, Assam, India. Cleft Palate Craniofac J. 2016;53(3):278–82.
9. Hackenberg B, Ramos M, Campbell A, Resch S, Howaldt HP, Caterson EJ. Measuring and comparing the cost-effectiveness of surgical care delivery in low-resource settings: cleft lip and palate as a model. J Craniofac Surg. 2015;26(4):1121–5.
10. Nagengast E, Caterson EJ, Magee W, Hatcher K, Ramos M, Campbell A. Providing more than health care: the dynamics of humanitarian surgery efforts on the micro-economy; comparing a comprehensive cleft care center with Mission model. J Craniofac Surg. 2014;25:1622–5.
11. Alkire B, Vincent J, Meara J. Chapter 21: Benefit-cost analysis of a cleft lip and palate surgical subspecialty hospital in India. In: Debas HT, Donkor P, Gawande A, Jamison DT, Kruk ME, Mock CN, editors. Essential surgery: disease control priorities, vol. 1. 3rd ed. Washington, DC: The International Bank for Reconstruction and Development/The World Bank; 2015.
12. Sandy JR, Williams A, Bearn D, Mildinhall S, Murphy T, Sell D, Murray J, Shaw W. Cleft lip and palate care in the United Kingdom – the Clinical Standards Advisory Group (CSAG) Study. Part 1: background and methodology. Cleft Palate Craniofac J. 2001;38(1):20–3.
13. Williams A, Bearn D, Mildinhall S, Murphy T, Sell D, Shaw W, Murray J, Sandy JR. Cleft lip and palate care in the United Kingdom – the Clinical Standards Advisory Group (CSAG) Study. Part 2: dentofacial outcomes and patient satisfaction. Cleft Palate Craniofac J. 2001;38(1):24–9.
14. Sell D, Grunwell P, Mildinhall S, Murphy T, Cornish TA, Bearn D, Shaw WC, Murray J, Williams A, Sandy JR. Cleft lip and palate care in the United Kingdom – the Clinical Standards Advisory Group (CSAG) Study. Part 3: speech outcomes. Cleft Palate Craniofac J. 2001;38(1):30–7.
15. Bearn D, Mildinhall S, Murphy T, Murray JJ, Sell D, Shaw WC, Williams AC, Sandy JR. Cleft lip and palate care in the United Kingdom – the Clinical Standards Advisory Group (CSAG) Study. Part 4: outcome comparisons, training, and conclusions. Cleft Palate Craniofac J. 2001;38(1):38–43.
16. Sherman R, Campbell A. Global aspects of cleft care. In: Losee JE, Kirschner RE, editors. Comprehensive cleft care. 2nd ed. New York: McGraw-Hill Medical.
17. Operation Smile Global Standards of Care. Available at: https://www.operationsmile.org/sites/default/files/Operation%20Smile%20Global%20Standards%20of%20Care.pdf. Accessed 10 Mar 2019.
18. Schonmeyr B, Restrepo C, Wendby L, Gillenwater J, Campbell A. Lessons learned from two consecutive cleft missions and the impact of patient education. J Craniofac Surg. 2014;25:1610–3.
19. Jensen L, Carrillo L, Wendby L, Dobie H, Das J, Restrepo C, Campbell A. Improving patient follow up in developing regions. J Craniofac Surg. 2014;25:1640–4.
20. Nagengast E, Campbell A, Restrepo C, et al. Reverse innovation in surgical education: value in training surgeons in developing regions. Publication Pending.
21. Campbell A. Disruptive innovation in surgical education. J Am Soc Maxillofac Surg. 2016;1(1):6e–7e.
22. Smile Train. Available at: https://www.smiletrain.org/our-cause/our-work. Accessed 28 Feb 2019.
23. Louis M, Dickey R, Hollier LH. Smile Train: making the grade in global cleft care. Craniomaxillofac Trauma Reconstr. 2018;11(1):1–5. Published online 2017 Dec 11.
24. Cleft and Craniofacial Center. Sri Ramachandra University. Available at: http://www.cleftcare.in/index.html. Accessed 28 Feb 2019.
25. Murthy J. Smile Train in India. Ann Plast Surg. 2012;68(3):236–9.
26. Inga Health Foundation. Available at: http://ingahealth.org/who-we-are/. Accessed 28 Feb 2019.
27. Operación Sonrisa Colombia. Centro de Atención Multidisciplinario (CAM) de Bogotá. Available at: http://colombia.operationsmile.org/programas/centros-de-atencion-multidisciplinarios/cam-bogota/. Accessed 28 Feb 2019.
28. Magee WP, Raimondi HM, Beers M, Koech MC. Effectiveness of international surgical program model to build local sustainability. Plast Surg Int. 2012;2012:185725.
29. Hydrabad Cleft Society. Available at: http://www.craniofacialinstitute.org/. Accessed on 28 Feb 2019.
30. Hydrabad Cleft Society Annual Report 2018. Available at: https://www.baoms.org.uk/_userfiles/pages/files/members/ssig%20cleft/cleft_annual_report_2018.pdf. Accessed on 28 Feb 2019.
31. Reddy SG, Reddy LV, Reddy RR. Developing and standardizing a center to treat cleft and craniofacial anomalies in a developing country like India. J Craniofac Surg. 2009;20 Suppl 2:1664–7.
32. Noordhoff MS. Establishing a craniofacial center in a developing country. J Craniofac Surg. 2009;20 Suppl 2:1655–6.
33. Campbell A, Restrepo C, Mackay D, Sherman R, Varma A, Ayala R, Sarma H, Deshpande G, Magee B. Scalable, sustainable cost effective surgical care: a model for safety and quality in the developing world. Part III: impact and sustainability. J Craniofac Surg. 2014;25:1685–9.
34. Posta. Oaxaca receives the "mobile hospital" to perform free surgeries. 10 March 2019. Available at: https://www.posta.com.mx/oaxaca/oaxaca-recibie-al-hospital-movil-para-realizar-cirugias-gratuitas. Accessed 10 Mar 2019.

# Empowering Local Partners

# 39

Karoon Agrawal, Amanda A. Gosman,
and Shankar Man Rai

Cleft lip and palate are visible congenital deformities which attract attention, so much that they have taken a centre stage for medical missions globally. Orofacial clefts present a considerable medical and psychological burden in every community – be it in either a developed or developing nation. Being a high-incidence congenital anomaly at approximately 1:500 to 1:2500 live births, this creates enormous burden for healthcare facilities, especially in low- and low-middle-income group countries (LMIC). Various local and global organizations have been working tirelessly over the last five decades to address this considerable need and doing so with increasing success. But, in order to best serve the populations most in need, it is imperative that local partners play a major role in this ongoing journey. Local partners come in many forms: experienced or aspiring clinicians, who are often under-resourced, governments and surgical societies and churches and local non-governmental organizations (NGOs) that form a link between visiting clinicians and the remote or vulnerable populations they seek to serve. In this chapter, we explore three examples of collaboration with local partners which have each sought to strengthen cleft care. First, we explore the development of the first cleft care team in Nepal and the practical strategies that have enabled it to grow and serve a remote population as the national cleft referral centre. Second, we look at a surgical team-NGO partnership model, which has focused on empowering local doctors to deliver the highest quality care to children in remote parts of India. And third, we discuss the formalization of collaboration among cleft teams, and its expansion to engage a national cleft society, in order to improve the consistency of care in Mexico.

K. Agrawal (✉)
Smile Train, New Delhi, India

A. A. Gosman (✉)
University of California San Diego, San Diego, CA, USA
e-mail: agosman@health.ucsd.edu

S. M. Rai (✉)
National Academy of Medical Sciences, Kirtipur Hospital, Kathmandu, Nepal

## Creating a Local Team

*Shankar Man Rai*

In the early 1970s, there were very few cleft centres providing comprehensive cleft care in the developing world. Cleft surgeries were primarily performed by infrequently visiting surgeons from developed countries. Interplast, now ReSurge International, a non-profit organization based in California was one of the first organizations to provide organized cleft surgeries in the developing world; since then, many other organizations have followed.

### Origins of Local Cleft Teams

Due to a very small number of surgeons trained adequately in cleft surgical care in the developing world, there was a huge unmet need in cleft care. While providing the much-needed cleft surgical care, these organizations also focused on providing opportunities for local surgeons to learn cleft surgery from the visiting surgeons. The Smile Train and ReSurge International also started empowering local surgical groups to perform cleft surgical services on a regular basis by providing funding, since training alone was not enough to provide an organized comprehensive cleft care in developing countries.

The initial impetus for surgeons as well as for the supporting organizations was to perform cleft surgeries, but it was soon realized mainly by the local teams that surgery alone was not enough. A need for a multidisciplinary comprehensive cleft care became eminent. Unlike in high-income countries where a multidisciplinary cleft team is formed before starting a cleft programme, creation of a

© Springer Nature Switzerland AG 2021
J. W. Swanson, D. W. Low (eds.), *Global Cleft Care in Low-Resource Settings*, https://doi.org/10.1007/978-3-030-59105-2_39

multidisciplinary cleft team in the developing world usually starts only with cleft surgery with slow addition of other disciplines. This is the reason why most of the cleft programmes in the developing world were started by surgeons.

## Teaching and Learning Cleft Surgery

Teaching cleft surgery also has its challenge. When the cleft lip patients are small children, the surgeon cannot spend a lot of time in teaching under anaesthesia safety reasons. Learning cleft palate is another challenge since it is not easy to look inside the patient's oral cavity, while the surgeon is working there unless an operating microscope is being used which is a very rare case. The author, who decided to take up plastic surgery after witnessing by chance a remarkable change in the face of a child after cleft lip surgery performed by a visiting plastic surgeon, always thinks that he would have decided otherwise if the visiting surgeon was doing a cleft palate surgery, in which case he would not have been able to see anything inside the mouth of the patient.

When access to cleft surgery was uncommon, there was a huge back log of cleft cases with many adult individuals with cleft deformities. The large volume of cases as well as adult cleft patients also gave opportunity for surgeons to learn cleft surgery quickly. The author had observed that the average duration to teach a new surgeon to be able to perform most of the cleft surgeries was 3 months in the beginning, while now when most of the patients are small children and the back log of adult cleft cases has been mostly cleared, it takes about 1 year [10].

## Key Team Roles

Initial local cleft team consisted of a surgeon, an anaesthetist, nurses, and a coordinator (Fig. 39.1). Later, when more and more children were being brought for surgery, a paediatrician joined the team since pre-operative evaluation of the child was essential.

In the developing world, the patient and the family usually cannot access the cleft service easily even though it may be provided free of cost. Thus a coordinator or a scout—a special cleft team member, not usually part of cleft teams of the developed world—is needed to seek out and identify individuals with cleft deformities. They can also independently screen the cleft individuals for surgery. Thus they recruit new patients with cleft deformities as well as coordinate the follow-up in the community after surgery.

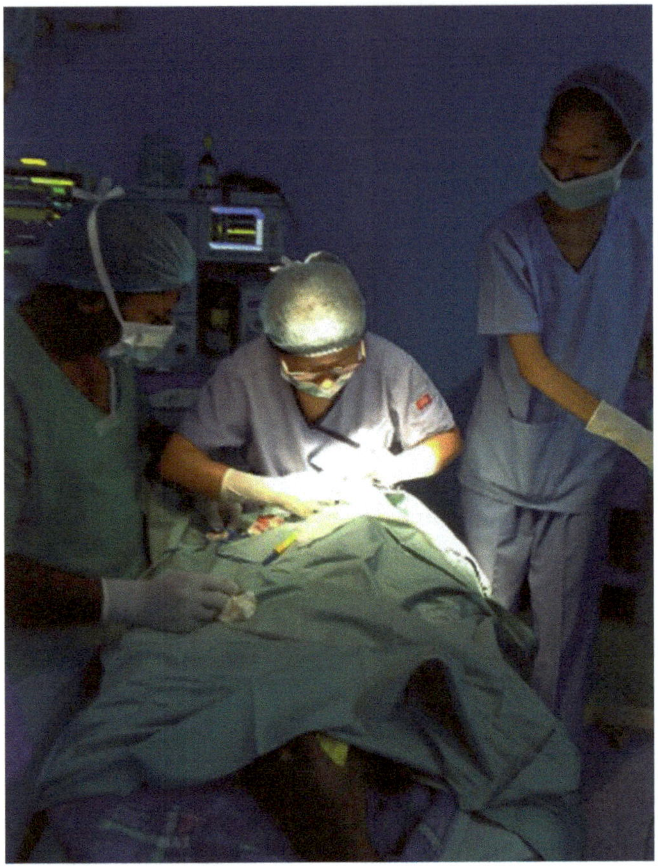

**Fig. 39.1** Surgeon performing cleft lip repair

## Practical Solutions for Comprehensive Cleft Care

Access to speech therapy in the developing world is even more difficult than to surgery merely due to the lack of the experts in this field. Compared to the duration of time spent on cleft surgery, the time spent on speech therapy is much more protracted, thus requiring even more number of professionals in this field. The other complexity with speech therapy is the fact that children needing speech therapy will be from distant places and frequent travel is difficult even if the therapy is provided free of cost (Fig. 39.2). This requires that the speech therapy be provided in many remote areas, rather than hoping that the families will bring their children to the hospitals.

Thus to provide the speech therapy to cleft children, we have found the following to be practical:

(a) Task shifting is the only way to provide this much needed care to a large number of individuals in the developing world. In Nepal, several nurses have been trained in assisting speech pathologists over the years to cater this service in the remote villages. The nurses are multi-tasking since they help in the surgery, pre-operative screening, postoperative care as well as the speech therapy.

(b) Organizing week-long speech therapy camps in remote areas nearer to the homes of the cleft families. Provision of free food and lodging have to be arranged for the child as well as one family member, preferably mother who would spend a lot of time with the child (and continue speech coaching) at home. The rooms for lodging in the night can be used for providing speech therapy in the day time by the speech assistants under the supervision of a speech pathologist. These camps can be repeated in the same or nearby places every 3–6 months.

(c) Involvement of the family member during the whole process of speech therapy so that the family member can continue the therapy in between the sessions with the speech assistant during the camp and at home in between the speech camps.

In most of the developing world, speech pathology and audiology is performed by a single professional unlike in the developed countries where these are two completely different specialties (Fig. 39.3). This has helped the developing world to have the same services with fewer number of professionals to be paid.

Individuals with cleft deformities are known to have dental problems. Oral hygienists have the greatest role to play in preventive and restorative oral/dental health. Having all the different dental specialists (e.g. dental surgeon, endodontists, periodontists, orthodontists) is not usually practical in the remote areas of the developing world. A well-trained dental surgeon and an oral hygienist could provide a large spectrum of dental care to children (Fig. 39.4). An orthodontist is also a must once the cleft programme develops to a higher level.

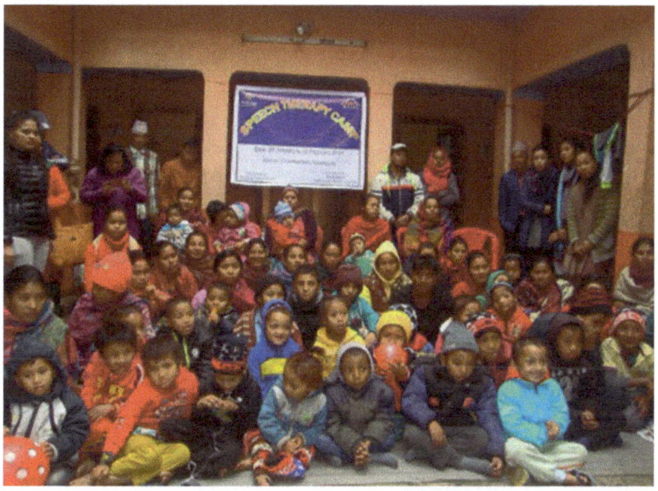


Fig. 39.2 A speech therapy camp in rural Nepal

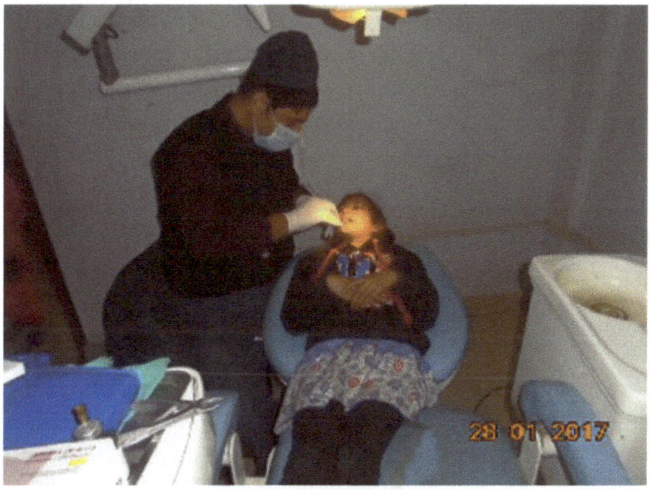


Fig. 39.4 Well-trained oral surgeons and dental hygienists can perform a wide range of dental care to children

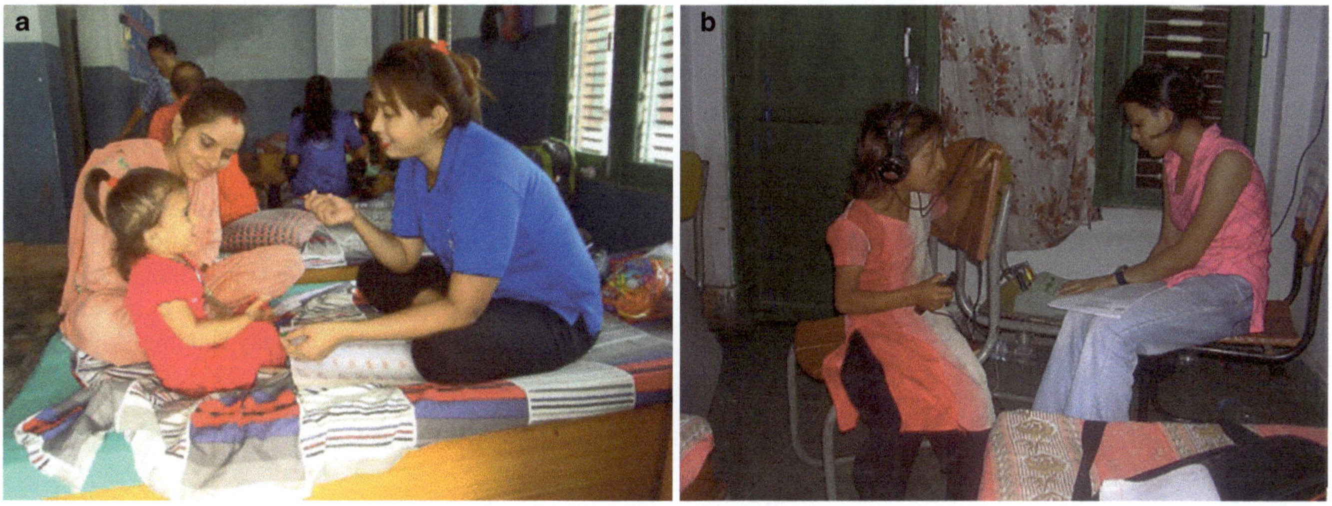


Fig. 39.3 (**a** and **b**) Speech pathology and audiology is performed by the same health professional, an example of task-sharing

Having an orthodontist providing this very specialized care in the periphery for poor people is the ideal level of care.

Dental care and speech therapy can be combined during the delivery of the service in the peripheral sites since the children can also be provided the dental care in between the speech therapy sessions. This maximizes the use of limited funds.

## In the Future

Comprehensive cleft care by a local team ideally has to be incorporated into the regular government healthcare system. This is not seen historically in any of the developing countries where this service has been provided by non-governmental organizations. However, organizations must work closely with the national health system to ensure their integration within it. Ideally, with recognition of the importance of basic cleft services by the government and its provision of these, NGOs can move on to more advanced levels of cleft care and address other challenging problems in its delivery.

# Local Surgeon Partners: The Smile Train Model

*Karoon Agrawal*

Recognizing the global need of healthcare support, many non-governmental organizations have come forward to share the burden. Smile train was established in 1999 with an innovative concept of encouraging and supporting local partner hospitals and surgeons, in performing cleft care following strict safety norms and high-quality standards (Louis 2018). This model has stood the test of time over past two decades.

## Evolution of Charity for Cleft

Cleft surgery is well suited for delivery through medical missions and has a long history of delivery through plastic surgery camps by individuals or groups of surgeons visiting LMICs. Interplast (now ReSurge) and Operation Smile, pioneered by Donald Laub in 1969 and William and Kathy Magee in 1983, respectively, were two of the earliest cleft charities. In 1999, Charles Wang and Brian Mullaney conceived of a different model. Encouraging and training local specialists to deliver care could be potentially more cost–effective and efficient than an approach reliant on transporting North American doctors with their equipment. With the launch of this model, Smile Train (ST) and this innovative concept were born in 1999 [4]. That local surgeons are available year round to take care of both previously operated and unoperated children was revolutionary in many of the sites that ST launched. The concept strengthened the role of surgeons and gave them important recognition and compensation as well.

## Details of the Programme

Since 1999, ST has funded over 1,300,000 surgeries through 1100+ partner hospitals in more than 85 countries. ST funds 2100+ partner surgeons to perform these surgeries, through the principle that "if you teach a man to fish, you feed him for a life". Through these surgeon partnerships, it fosters local health systems and cleft treatment initiatives, thereby creating a lasting resource to provide surgical treatment for cleft lip and palate.

Safe surgery and high standard of postoperative care have always been emphasized; in recent years, ST has also begun to embark on comprehensive care through partner hospitals. This includes providing orthodontic and speech therapy supports to many partners and commencing nutritional support for the children of cleft lip and palate in many countries where there is urgent need. Nursing care training modules have been developed for nutritional support and safe postoperative care (Fig. 39.5). In partnering with hospitals, apart from surgeons, anaesthetists and nurses are also encouraged to become part of the cleft care team. Discussions with anaesthetists facilitate safety, and equipment is provided to fill gaps.

## Why Local Partners

In our experience, the involvement of local surgeons has alleviated typical problems of other cleft outreach models: shortage of surgeons, an overwhelming number of patients awaiting treatment, limited spaces in an operative schedule, poor postoperative care and long-term follow-up, little support from local medical personnel and difficulty in performing multistage surgeries. When local surgeons are involved and financially benefit from participation, the scenario seems different. Involvement in the mission is a great recognition for the local surgeons. The honour and financial compensation they receive stimulates high devotion, availability and willingness to provide follow-up. The quality of work is good, as are efforts to improve. This is the essence of capacity building.

## Partnering with Local Hospitals

Over the years ST has established its network of partner hospitals in more than 85 developing nations. The partner hospitals are identified by the programme directors and assessed

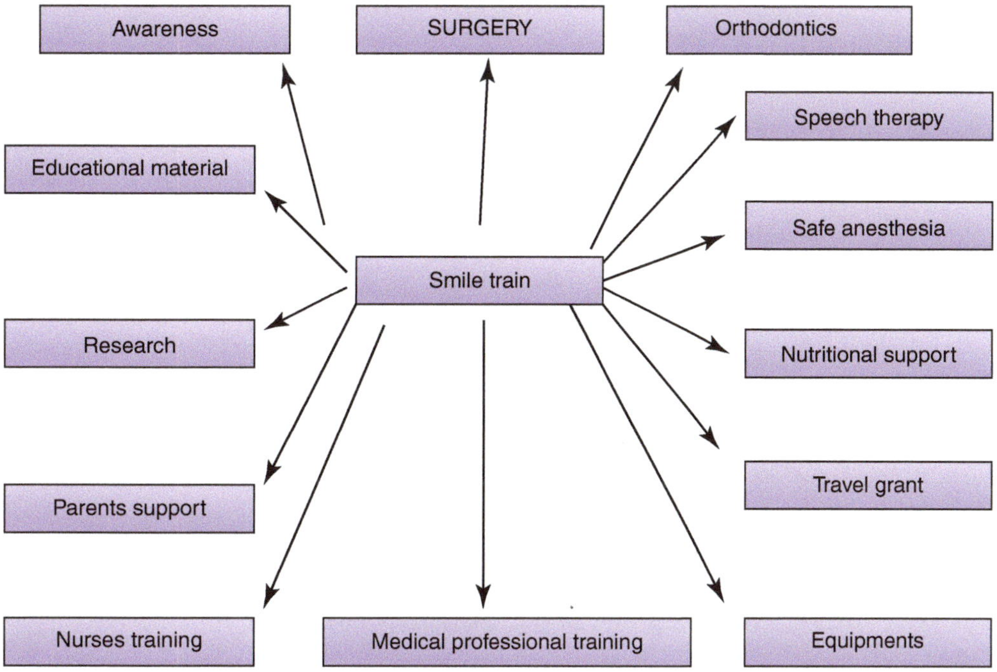


**Fig. 39.5** Smile Train providing services to the children with cleft lip and palate

by the members of medical advisory board. Sometimes, the infrastructure is assessed by the panel of safety protocol auditors. The selection of partner hospital and credentialing of the surgeon are decided collectively. The selected hospital signs the MOU and agrees to follow various guidelines provided by the ST (Fig. 39.6).

These guidelines have been developed over the past two decades by the medical advisory board and are basically directed towards delivery of safe and quality care to every child.

## Safety and Quality Assurance

Along with safety, the top priority of the ST is to ensure the partner surgeons are competent and are able to deliver high-quality cleft care. The surgeons are credentialed based on their surgical results. They are certified by their respective authorities mandatorily.

ST reviews ~5% of cases every year. Failing the quality assessment, the surgeon is advised and motivated to undergo specific training through variety of educational programmes specially designed to suit the requirement of a cleft surgeon. The partner surgeons and anaesthetists are encouraged to attend updates, workshops and CMEs at regular intervals. ST is regularly updating its resources in the field of training and education. Figure 39.7 enlists the training and educational avenues under the umbrella of ST. This figure also enlists the various resources available with ST for training and educational programme. Some of them are specially developed for ST.

## Expansion of Services

Initially, Smile Train was restricted to surgical care. Now the goal is to provide comprehensive care through multidisciplinary management. Orthodontics and speech therapy have become integral part of cleft care under ST. Orthodontics and speech therapy are supported in many centres wherever the specialists and infrastructure are available. In some countries nutritional support is being encouraged and propagated. Speech apps for kids, Habla y Lenguaje (Spanish) and Speech Games and Practice (English), are being developed to potentially empower speech therapists and parents and to facilitate speech therapy at home.

## Economic Impact

Independent researchers studied the economic and global health impacts of ST services over a 10-year period [5]. They found that each cleft surgical procedure averted 2–3 disability-adjusted life years (DALYs), granting economic benefit and gained productivity for each individual of some USD$40,000. For the collective 500,000 patients treated during this time period, this constituted a boost to the global economy of $20 billion. Given the programme cost of approximately $197 million during this time period, this represented a modest cost of $147 per DALY averted, representing a "return on investment" of between 40–105 dollars per dollar spent. These findings reinforce the objectives of ST in supporting welfare creation through local partnerships with communities around the world.

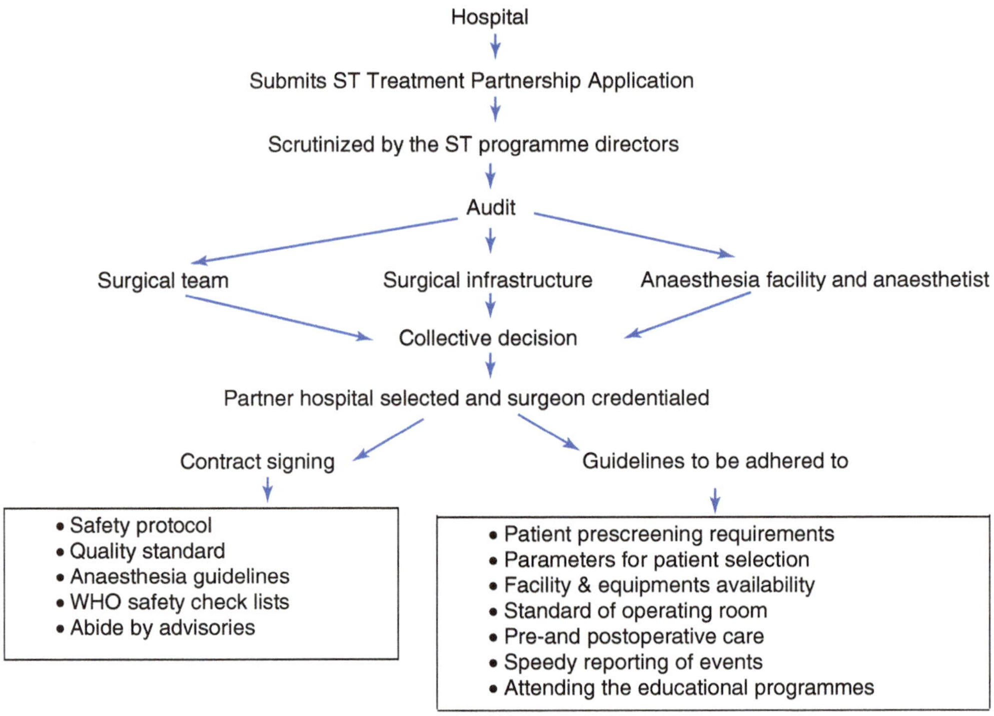


**Fig. 39.6** ST Procedure of partnership with local hospitals

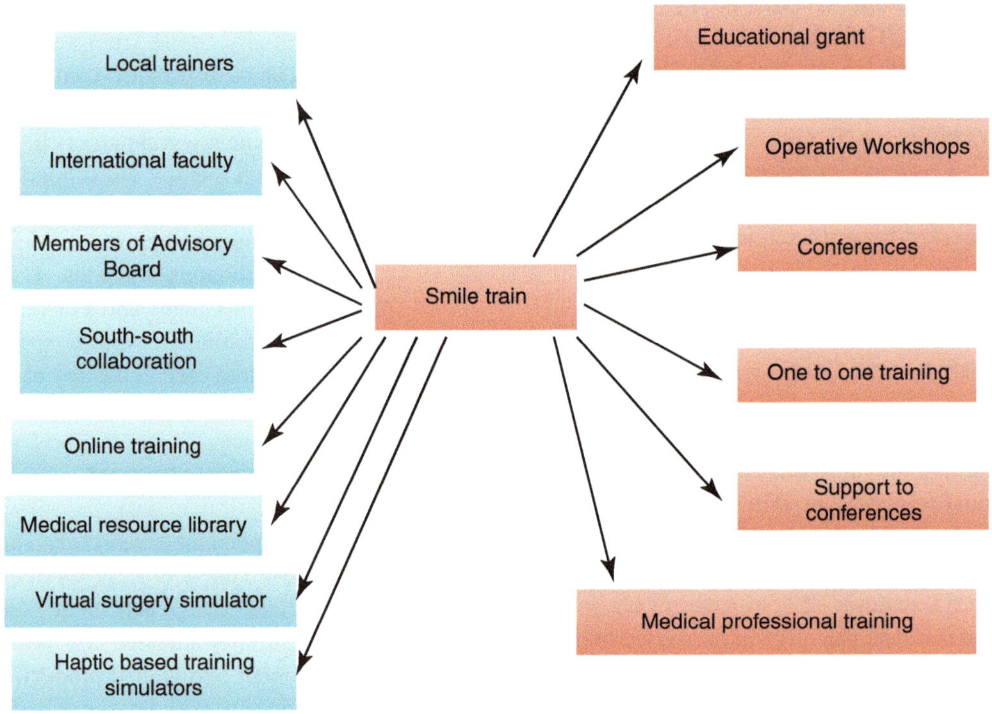


**Fig. 39.7** Training and educational avenues under the umbrella of Smile train

## Sustainability

The growth of ST over the years reflects the success of its model. It is expanding its services as well as extending its presence to more and more LMICs for providing effective and efficient care to the children with CLP, affirming its sustainability. The success of any organization depends upon its good intention, global presence, sustainability and good management. ST's experience suggests that the service and organization becomes viable and popular by empowering and funding the local partners; hence all its activities revolve around establishing and supporting local talent.

## From a Trans-border Partnership to Engaging a National Cleft Society

*Amanda A. Gosman*

### Roots in Local Cooperation

Collaborative partnerships are a critical component of multidisciplinary cleft team care. The development of an international multidisciplinary cleft team across the USA-Mexico border is no exception. The multidisciplinary cleft and craniofacial team in Tijuana, Mexico has been under the leadership of Dra. Alicia Sigler since 2006. For more than a decade, we have collaborated on the development of a cross-border health system between the cleft and craniofacial centres in Tijuana and San Diego, 25 miles apart but separated by an international border.

Initially members of the San Diego team would participate in the biweekly clinics in Tijuana Mexico. As schedules and logistics became more constrained, we deployed telemedicine so that the San Diego-based providers could participate remotely [6]. Through the Tijuana clinic, we identified complex patients in need of a higher level of care than we could offer at the Hospital Infantil, and we worked with their foundation to provide care for complex patients combined with a visiting professor programme. In 2008 we launched our collaborative international health telemedicine conference which has been running as a CME conference out of University of California San Diego (UCSD) School of Medicine four times a year for the past decade. The initial educational collaboration involved a didactic component by visiting professor and Dra Sigler's mentor, Dr. Fernando Ortiz Monasterio, from Mexico City and included a live interactive telemedicine broadcast of a free fibular reconstruction of the mandible in an 8-year-old patient with haemifacial microsomia [7]. This collaborative educational event became a quarterly CME conference and was combined with a full day of surgical care ("jornadas") with international participants that joined in-person and remotely through the telemedicine broadcast to multiple academic centres in several countries.

### Expansion to an Education- and Care-Focused Coalition

In 2010 we founded Connectmed International, a non-profit organization to support the development of an international network of educational initiatives and multidisciplinary care (Fig. 39.8). Over the past decade, we have collaborated with our Mexican colleagues on providing educational opportunities for surgical trainees from several countries, medical students, orthodontists, speech pathologists, nurses, researchers and psychologists. Our model of cross border care focuses on building multidisciplinary capacity and has elevated the level of care provided to patients on both sides of the border. The opportunity to learn for our international colleagues and to work side by side in the provision of care has allowed us to develop a patient-centred delivery system that facilitates the best logistical option with the highest quality for each individual patient. Fresh Start Surgical Gifts has been an essential partner in supporting our ability to perform complex craniofacial cases in San Diego when the resources or funding was not available in Tijuana. Ongoing collaborative initiatives include direct patient care through quarterly surgical journeys at the CER Hospital in Tijuana, annual self-esteem camps for patients with craniofacial differences in Tijuana and San Diego, support of original research in multiple disciplines, biannual visiting professor programme, support of NAM training and programmes in Tijuana and Ensenada and support of ongoing educational conferences.

### Collaboration with the National Cleft Society

One of the most important collaborative initiatives is with the Asociacion Mexicana de Labio, Paladar Hendido y Anomalias Craneofaciales, A.C.(AMLPH) (https://www.amlph.com.mx). AMLPH is a multidisciplinary organization with 32 comprehensive centres for cleft and craniofacial care across Mexico (Fig. 39.9). We have been proud participants and supporters of their annual educational programming and worked closely with their leadership to ensure that all our outreach efforts in Mexico are aligned with their mission. AMLPH has done a tremendous job launching their national evidence-based guidelines for cleft care (https://www.amlph.com.mx/que-es-labio-y-paladar-hendido/guias-de-practica-clinica-de-lph/) [8] as a

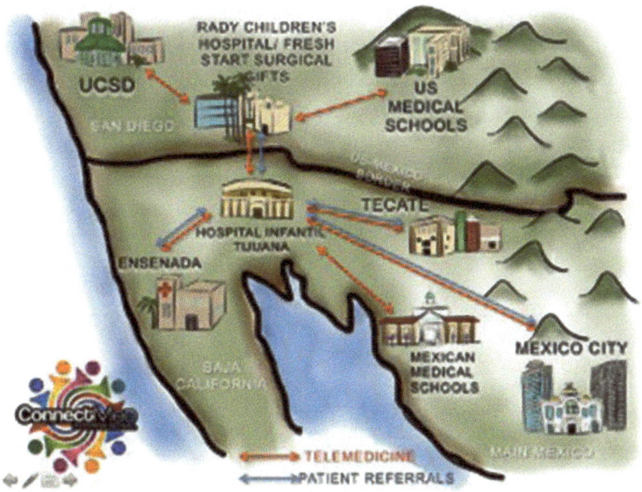


**Fig. 39.8** Schematic of ConnectMed, to utilize telemedicine and a referral network to facilitate educational initiatives and multidisciplinary care among a network of organizations

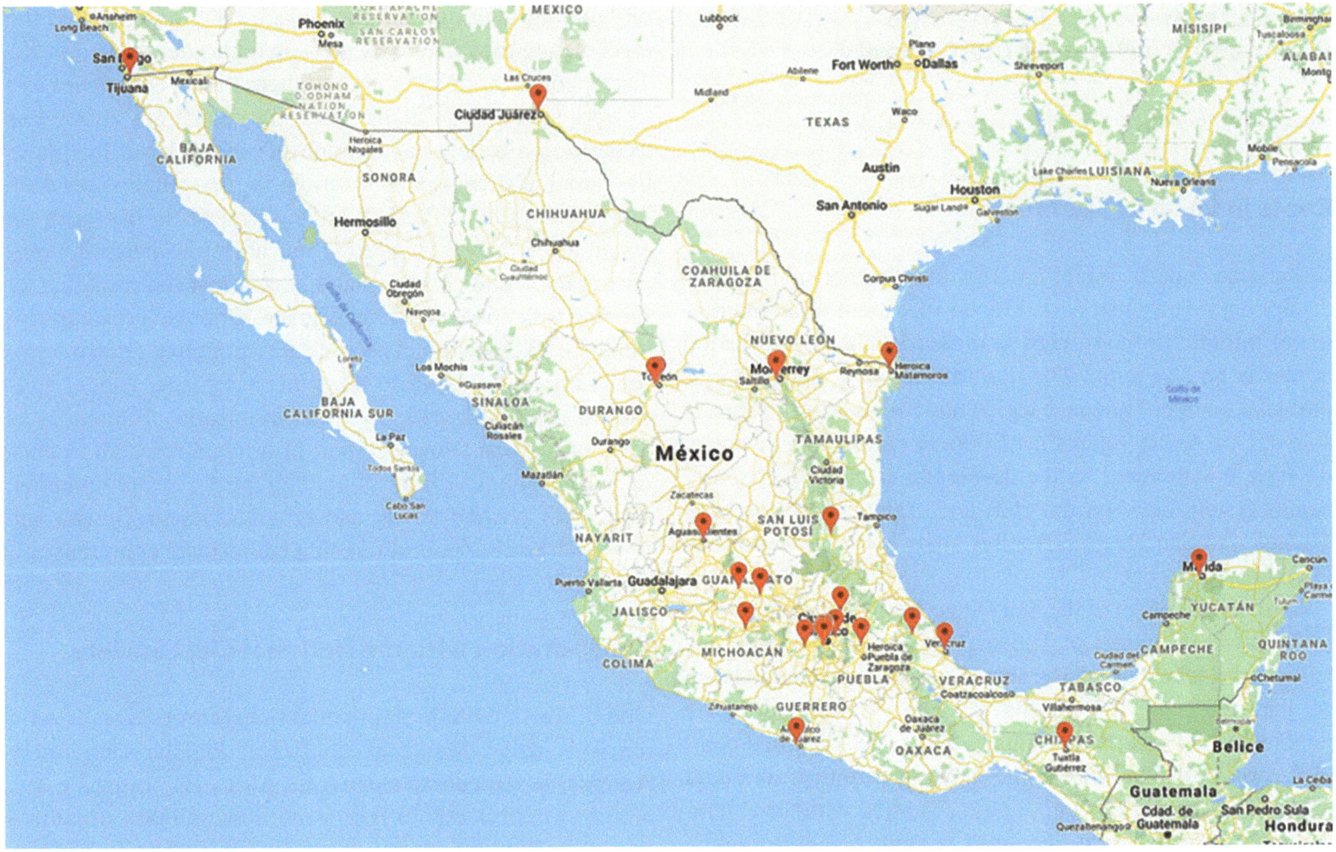


**Fig. 39.9** Cleft care teams belonging to the Mexican Association of Cleft Lip, Palate, and Craniofacial Anomalies (AMLPHAC) are located throughout Mexico

part of their evolving Mexicleft initiative. Dr. Sigler has played a pivotal role in AMLPH as a liaison to international organizations participating in cleft care in order to align these efforts with the national guidelines developed by the organization for best practices. Oversight of international collaboration by the national leaders of multidisciplinary cleft care in Mexico has been a critical initiative to improve the quality of care and can be a model for other countries. We have worked closely with AMLPH to understand the positive and negative aspects of international collaboration in cleft care in Mexico and to develop joint educational programming to strengthen the capacity to provide the best multidisciplinary care on both sides of the border [9].

## References


1. Mossey P. Epidemiology under pinning research in the aetiology of orofacial clefts. Orthod Craniofac Res. 2007;10(03):114–20.
2. Mossey P, Little J, Munger RG, Dixon MJ, Shaw WC. Cleft lip and palate. Lancet. 2009;374(9803):1773–85.
3. Louis M, Dickey RM, Train HLHJS. Making the grade in global cleft care. Craniomaxillofac Trauma Reconstr. 2018;11:1–5.
4. Kalra S. Cleft lips and palates: a societal perspective. J Cleft Lip Palate Craniofac Anom. 2014;1(2):100–3.
5. Corlew DS, Alkire BC, Poenaru D, Meara JG, Shrime MG. Economic valuation of the impact of a large surgical charity using the value of lost welfare approach. BMJ Glob Health. 2017:1–9. https://doi.org/10.1136/bmjgh-2016-000059.
6. Whitehead E, Dorfman V, Tremper G, Kramer A, Sigler A, Gosman A. Telemedicine as a means of effective speech evaluation for patients with cleft palate. Ann Plast Surg. 2012;68(4):415–7.
7. Gosman A, Fischer C, Agha Z, Sigler A, Chao J, Dobke M. Telemedicine and surgical education across Borders: a case report. J Surg Educ. 2009;66(2):102–5.
8. Amlph.com.mx. Guías de Práctica Clínica de LPH – Asociación Mexicana de Labio, *Paladar Hendido y Anomalías Craneofaciales* [online]. 2019. Available at: https://www.amlph.com.mx/que-es-labio-y-paladar-hendido/guias-de-practica-clinica-de-lph/ [Accessed 23 Jun. 2019].
9. Schoenbrunner A, Kelley K, Buckstaff T, McIntyre J, Sigler A, Gosman A. Description of Mexican cleft surgeons' experience with foreign surgical volunteer missions in Mexico. Ann Plast Surg. 2018:1.
10. Rai SM, Nakarmi K, Basnet S, Shakya P, Nagarkoti K, Ghartimagar M, Karki B, Hirachan S. Age of individuals undergoing cleft lip and cleft palate surgeries in Nepal. J Nepal Med Assoc. 2013;52:192.

# Short-Term International Cleft Outreach

40

Melissa Kanack, Charanya Vijayakumar, Usama S. Hamdan, and Raj M. Vyas

**Key Points**

- *Short-term* outreach lasts between 1 day and 8 weeks, often performed by volunteers with limited time to volunteer their services.
- High-quality outreach involves carefully planned and evaluated site establishment, preoperative, perioperative, and postoperative stages.
- Short-term outreach should still aim to increase regional capacity and sustainability of multidisciplinary cleft services.
- Teams should undergo previsit emergency preparedness training and on-site training at the beginning of any outreach trip.
- Technology, including virtual or augmented reality, can aid in building capacity and providing comprehensive cleft services

M. Kanack
Department of Aesthetic & Plastic Surgery, UC Irvine School of Medicine, Irvine, CA, USA

C. Vijayakumar
Department of Plastic & Reconstructive Surgery, Sri Ramachandra Institute of Higher Education and Research (SRIHER, Chennai, Tamil Nadu, India

U. S. Hamdan
Global Smile Foundation, Boston, MA, USA

Tufts University School of Medicine, Boston, MA, USA

Harvard Medical School, Boston, MA, USA

Boston University School of Medicine, Boston, MA, USA

R. M. Vyas (✉)
Department of Aesthetic & Plastic Surgery, UC Irvine School of Medicine, Irvine, CA, USA

Global Smile Foundation, Boston, MA, USA

## Introduction

Cleft lip and palate is a congenital condition that affects facial appearance, carries significant social stigma, and interferes with the functions of speech and feeding. Because it is not life-threatening, despite high morbidity, cleft lip and palate care is often underprioritized by state and local health agencies handicapped by limited resources and access to specialized expertise. Each year, scores of nongovernmental global health organizations mobilize medical volunteers to provide cleft surgery and related care to thousands of affected children worldwide. Many efforts are focused on the short-term needs of endemic and under-resourced regions and motivated by the impressive ability to make an immediate, lasting impact in these populations.

*Short-term* international outreach is defined as lasting between 1 day and 8 weeks, with medical care provided by volunteers who are typically from higher-income countries [1]. This model is often viewed as an attractive option for qualified individuals who are interested in international work but have limited time to volunteer their services. Therefore, in order to optimize impact, it is paramount that short-term outreach be thoughtfully planned and carefully executed with a clear emphasis on quality and safety. Although short term, overseas outreach should always aim to increase the regional capacity and sustainability of comprehensive cleft services.

## Quality

Every short-term cleft outreach organization must draft and follow its own quality assurance and quality improvement protocols. Much like the approach to care for a surgical patient, organizing a successful, high-quality outreach program can be divided into site establishment, preoperative, perioperative, and postoperative stages [2] (Table 40.1).

*Site Establishment:* New outreach programs or expansion into new locations should begin with a site visit by at least a surgeon and anesthesiologist who represent the sponsoring organization and who will participate in the anticipated out-

© Springer Nature Switzerland AG 2021

J. W. Swanson, D. W. Low (eds.), *Global Cleft Care in Low-Resource Settings*, https://doi.org/10.1007/978-3-030-59105-2_40

**Table 40.1** Quality

| |
|---|
| Key quality imperatives by stages |
| Site establishment<br>Initial site visit with surgeon, anesthesiologist, OR/PACU RN<br>Establish need for planned services<br>Coordinate with local organizations<br>Assess local availability of equipment and surgical supplies<br>At least 12 months before first planned trip |
| Preoperative<br>Establish goals with local partners<br>Build the multidisciplinary outreach team<br>Plan for local training, quality improvement, and/or research endeavors |
| Perioperative<br>First operation on an older patient<br>Schedule younger patients earlier in the day<br>All airway cases (cleft palate, VPI) completed 48 hours prior to team's departure<br>One OR prepared each night for emergency prior to team leaving |
| Postoperative<br>Provide detailed postoperative care instructions in native language<br>Maintain accessible medical records and standardized patient photography<br>Track quality improvement data including outcomes and complications |

reach. Many organizations recommend that the visit also involve operating room (OR) and post-anesthesia care unit (PACU) nurses [3]. The Volunteers in Plastic Surgery (VIPS) guidelines state that site visits should establish the need for planned services, coordinate with other organizations providing similar services at that site, and evaluate the facilities, local staff, logistical support, and safety infrastructure [3]. An understanding of local governmental norms with proper medicolegal and ethical attention is necessary for long-term, secure, and trusting partnerships. Site visits should take place at least 6–12 months before the first planned outreach trip; often a second or third site visit is needed to ensure the goals of short-term outreach are achieved. The local availability of equipment and surgical supplies should be assessed. Historically these were brought in by teams as cargo (at great expense), but they are increasingly available in many countries locally.

*Preoperative:* In planning for a surgical mission or outreach program, the goals of the program should be established and shared with local partners. Team composition should reflect sufficient quantity of providers to match the anticipated case volume, as well as clinicians representing as many possible disciplines of team care (Table 40.2). The primary goal is always to provide state-of-the-art surgical care, and this mandates all volunteers have the highest degree of specialty/subspecialty training and routinely care for children with the full spectrum of cleft conditions in their domestic clinical practices. Additional goals may include education and training of local professionals, establishment of a multidisciplinary comprehensive cleft center, and quality improvement or research endeavors.

**Table 40.2** Team roles

| |
|---|
| Surgeons<br>Plastic surgeons (with pediatric/craniofacial training)<br>Pediatric otolaryngologists-head and neck surgeons<br>Oral and maxillofacial surgeons |
| Anesthesiologists<br>Pediatric<br>General<br>Certified nurse anesthetists |
| Other physicians<br>Pediatric intensivist |
| Nurses<br>OR<br>PACU<br>Postop |
| Other surgical team members (may vary)<br>Nutritionist<br>Biomedical engineers<br>Administrative staff<br>Volunteers<br>Speech therapists<br>Students/residents |
| Dental<br>Pediatric dentists<br>General dentists<br>Dental assistants<br>Dental hygenists<br>Dental students |
| In-country team<br>On-site coordinator<br>Local plastic surgeon<br>Healthcare facility staff<br>Lecture coordinator<br>Local host organizations<br>Translators |

In some sites, as local capacity begins to build, lip repair and then palate repair are feasible by local surgeons. However, some cleft palate repairs, fistula repairs, secondary speech surgery, and alveolar bone grafting are often not able to be addressed by local providers. Surgical outreach missions can be particularly helpful when they complement local capabilities. In these situations, focusing care on these more difficult cases and teaching through them optimizes value of the mission. Staffing and equipping team to best treat these cases is important, for instance, with surgeons who are experienced with fistula repair or speech surgery, speech therapists familiar with diagnosis of velopharyngeal insufficiency, and equipment such as nasoendoscopy.

*Perioperative*: Surgical scheduling should prioritize younger patients being scheduled earlier in the day, with the exception of the first operation of the trip being an older patient in case of equipment failure or malfunction. Priority should be given to patients and families traveling from further distances, and these patients might require preoperative admission for logistical and medical considerations. Cases that involve the airway, including cleft palate repair or surgery for velopharyngeal insufficiency, should be scheduled earlier in the day and completed prior to 48 hours before the team's departure in order to allow adequate time for airway monitoring [2]. All equipment should be carefully inspected prior to performing any procedures, and an operating room should be prepared prior to leaving the outreach site each night in case of emergency. Several additional facets of perioperative quality – patient selection, safety, emergency preparedness, and mindful use of resources – are covered in the remainder of this chapter.

*Postoperative:* Detailed postoperative care instructions and education must be provided in the native language of patients and families. In addition to daily rounds in both the morning and evening for evaluation of postoperative patients, outreach teams should have a defined structure for tracking short- and long-term surgical outcomes and complications. Ideally, monitoring outcomes after short-term outreach is facilitated by partnerships with local personnel trained by the visiting team who remain in close communication with the medical supervisors of the outreach organization. Quality improvement data related to perioperative complications and events (e.g., unanticipated ICU admission, return to the operating room, re-intubation) should also be collected and analyzed by the host organization along with the entire visiting team prior to departure [3]. Longer-term outcomes, such as fistula rates and speech hypernasality, should also be followed and addressed on future outreach trips. Maintaining medical records that are accessible at future surgical missions and include standardized patient photography is essential for tracking outcomes, maintaining continuity of care, and initiating quality improvement measures. Electronic medical record (EMRs) can be used increasingly in these settings and should be encrypted, HIPAA compliant, and accessible by domestic and overseas providers.

## Safety and Emergency Preparedness

Short-term outreach trips often bring together a team of volunteers from different areas and backgrounds who have not previously worked together. Limited resources in an unfamiliar setting can augment complications and slow resolution. During an emergency, providers must respond immediately with seamless collaboration and defined roles. All volunteers and trip participants undergo previsit emergency preparedness training including a site-specific virtual hospital tour demonstrating the location of emergency and safety supplies (blood bank, fire extinguishers, etc.). At the first on-site team meeting, specific emergency responsiveness roles are assigned, and emergency simulations are undertaken to reinforce each team member's role and responsibilities (Fig. 40.1). Global Smile Foundation, a nonprofit global outreach foundation, recommends establishing a portable emergency cart with instruments and medications necessary to respond to common (and uncommon) perioperative emergencies: securing an airway, performing cardiopulmonary resuscitation, treating adverse anesthetic reactions, stopping unanticipated bleeding, and more [4] (Fig. 40.2). An on-call schedule and reliable means of telecommunication are also established to ensure a prompt and sufficient response to emergencies – no matter the hour. Safety and emergency preparedness are covered in more detail in the following chapter.

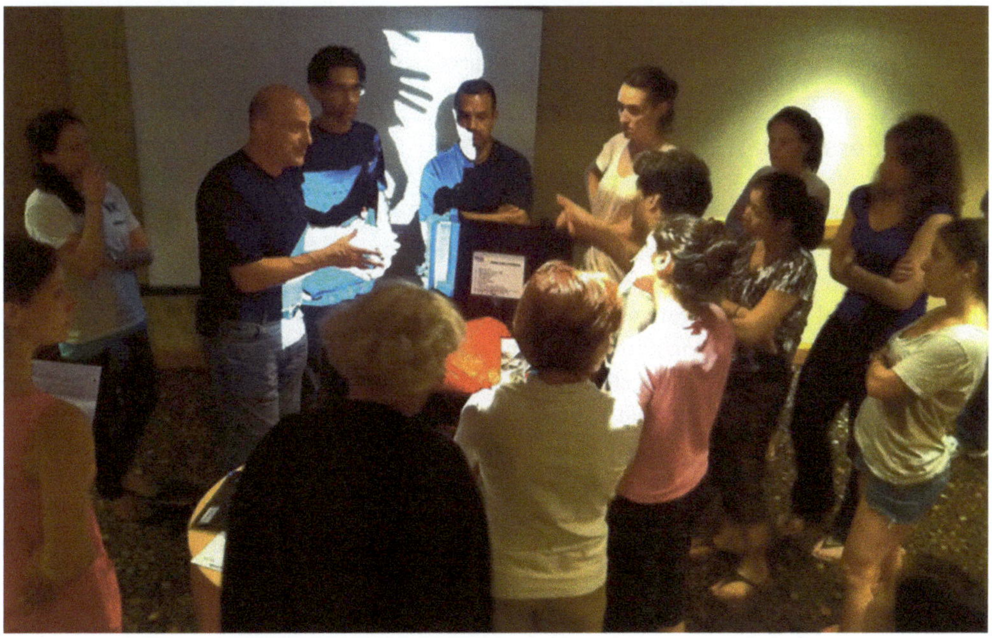

**Fig. 40.1** On-site team safety huddle at the beginning of a short-term outreach program

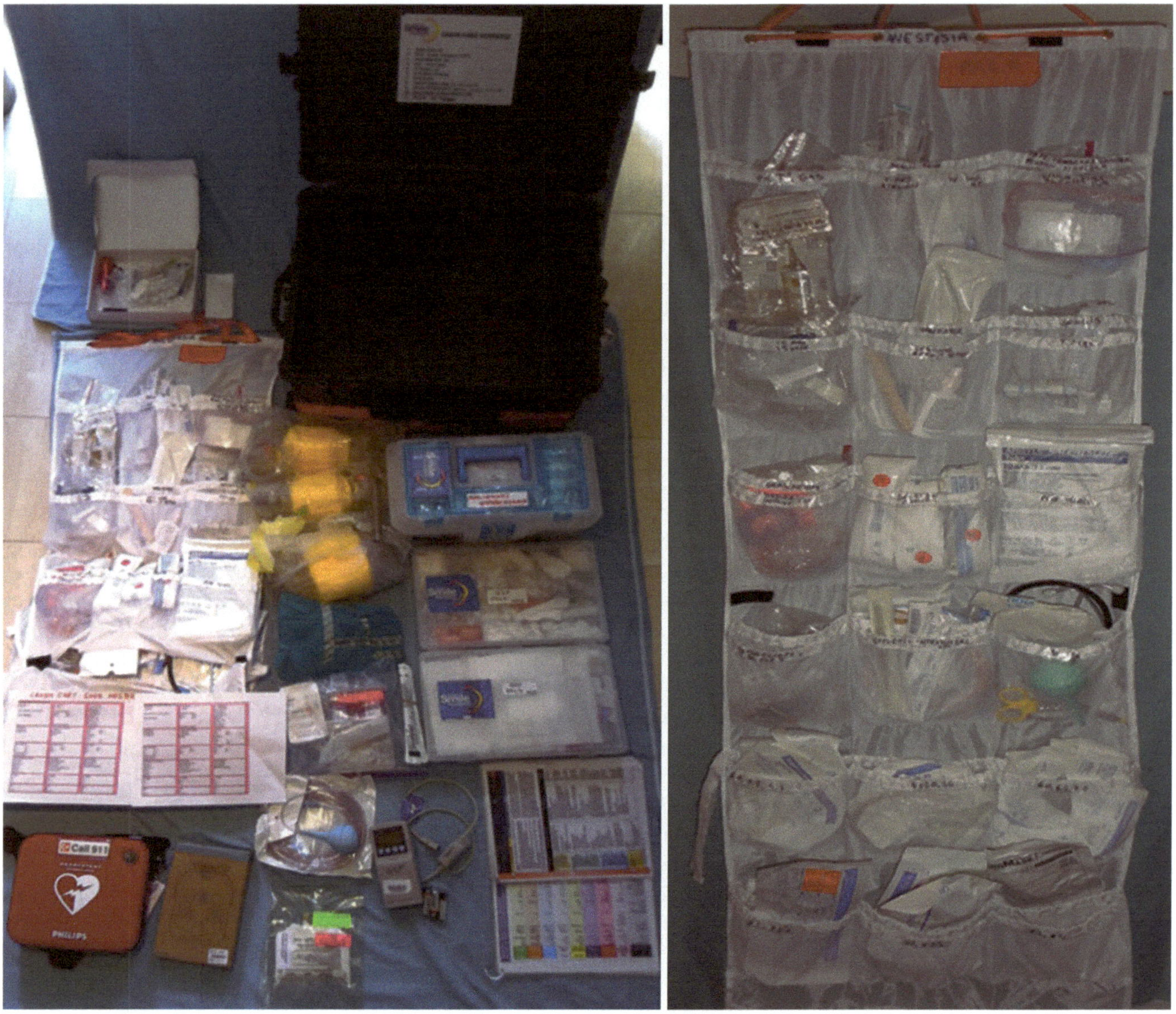

Fig. 40.2 Example of Global Smile Foundation's emergency response cart and supplies

## Mindfulness Toward Resources

A key portion of the initial site visit is identification of available resources. Outreach teams should be prepared to supply both disposable and durable equipment necessary for the planned surgical and perioperative care. Equipment taken for granted in the outreach organization's home country, such as backup power generators and anesthesia machines, may not be available or may not be reliable at overseas partner sites. Photographic documentation of available equipment in the hospital is recommended at the time of the site visit(s). Availability of surgical instruments and sterilization capacity should also be assessed, as the team may need to bring their own instruments and possibly even portable sterilization equipment. Presence of a blood bank and availability of blood for transfusion should also be assessed.

An inventory of surgical sutures, IV medications, and other single-use materials (gowns, gloves, drapes) should be taken as many or most of these materials likely need to be purchased, brought as luggage, or shipped in advance. The standard of care followed in developed nations of not reusing single-use/disposable items should generally be maintained during overseas outreach [3]. In addition, surgical planning must take into account a simplified approach for postoperative follow-up; for example, use of only absorbable sutures for skin closure in a cleft lip repair may be recommended to avoid the need for suture removal [2]. A major limiting resource during short-term surgical outreach is operating room time. Surgeons must be mindful of being expeditious while maintaining quality and safety in order to optimize this precious resource.

When faced with constraints regarding use of general anesthesia in limited resource settings, outreach programs must give serious consideration to the choice of procedures and the age of patients who can be treated. In such scenarios, adolescents and adults may suitably undergo surgery under just local anesthesia. Judicious use of nerve blocks and local anesthetic infiltration can provide adequate anesthesia for more extensive surgeries without use of sedation, including cleft lip repair [5].

## Political and Social Partnerships

Successful international cleft outreach depends on forming partnerships with the local and national government as well as private organizations based in the community. Established organizations may receive invitations from government officials or regional healthcare organizations and providers. Administration at the local hospital hosting the outreach campaign must be engaged and supportive of its goals. These partnerships help ensure that the outreach addresses an identified unmet need in the community and facilitates local perception of the visiting outreach program as positive rather than intrusive (Fig. 40.3).

An important goal of networking within the local community is to identify a local liaison or coordinator. This key team member helps to identify and recruit patients from local healthcare organizations and providers while also assisting in the planning and execution of tasks during the outreach program [6]. It is mandatory to also identify a committed host surgeon who will assist with preoperative patient selection, acquire cleft surgical skills and knowledge during the outreach trip, and provide follow-up care to treated patients [2].

Medicolegal coverage for the visiting outreach team should be planned well in advance and in coordination with domestic and host agencies. Establishing affiliations with regional professional academies and universities both solidifies the educational partnership with host countries and is helpful in identifying local medical volunteers (students, residents, etc.) for aid with administration, translation, and patient support.

## Patient Identification and Mobilization

Ideally, two phases of patient identification occur. The first involves screening by a local/regional surgeon or patient coordinator in the weeks or months prior to the arrival of the outreach team. The second is performed by the outreach team at the start of the trip to confirm that patients are appropriate surgical candidates and make specific surgical plans. Several cleft organizations as well as VIPS have developed guidelines for patient selection. For pediatric patients with cleft lip and/or palate, these include age, weight, ASA class, and hemoglobin requirements as well as lack of significant comorbidities or congenital syndromes [2] (Table 40.3). Utilizing an EMR or cloud-based platform allows for patient screening information and photographs to be shared among outreach teams in advance in order to enhance communication and ensure more accurate preoperative planning by surgeons (Fig. 40.4).

Each patient should be evaluated by several clinicians. The first evaluation is performed by surgeons, who determine if surgery can and should be performed. If the patient is deemed an appropriate surgical candidate, he or she is then evaluated by an anesthesiologist and/or pediatric intensivist

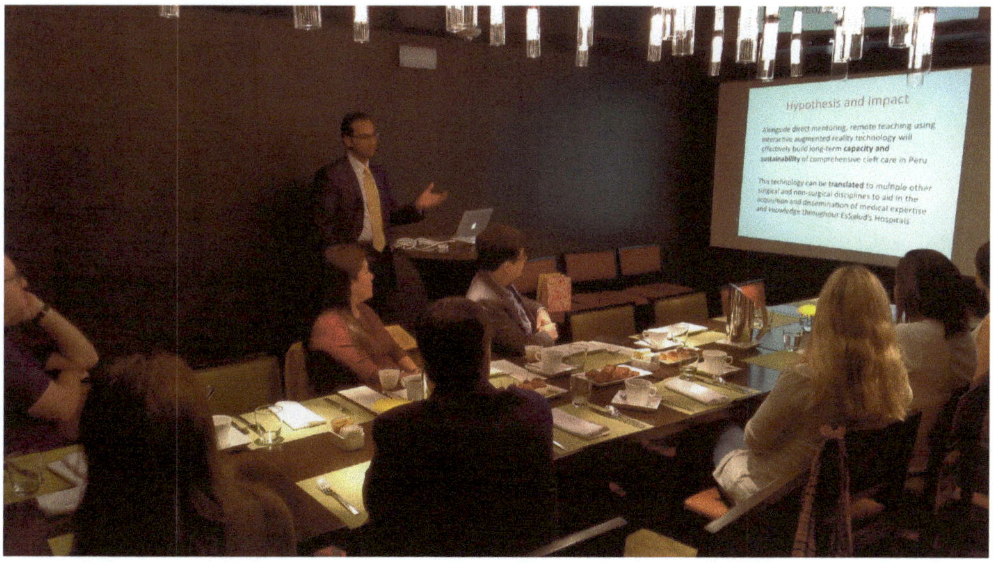


**Fig. 40.3** Members of Global Smile Foundation's team meeting with local community, government, and healthcare leaders in Peru

to determine anesthetic risk stratification and that no health condition precludes surgery; this includes careful cardiac and respiratory evaluation. Nutritional status and presence of respiratory or other concurrent infections are additional important considerations [3]. Speech evaluation of velopharyngeal function is important in older patients for whom palatal revision, fistula repair, or secondary speech surgery is being considered. Finally, dental assessment is important in dentulous patients to evaluate for gingival or dental disease that could complicate surgery.

**Table 40.3** Guidelines for safe patient selection

| Cleft lip patients | Cleft palate patients | Microtia patients |
|---|---|---|
| At least 10 weeks old<br>Weigh at least 10 lbs<br>Hbg at least 10 g/dL | 10–18 months old | 5–8 years old |
| For all patients<br>ASA class I<br>No extensive comorbidities or congenital syndromes associated with increased anesthetic risk<br>No concurrent respiratory tract or febrile illness<br>No contraindications to general anesthesia<br>No obvious evidence of malnutrition (Hgb < 10, growth percentiles well below expected for age) | | |

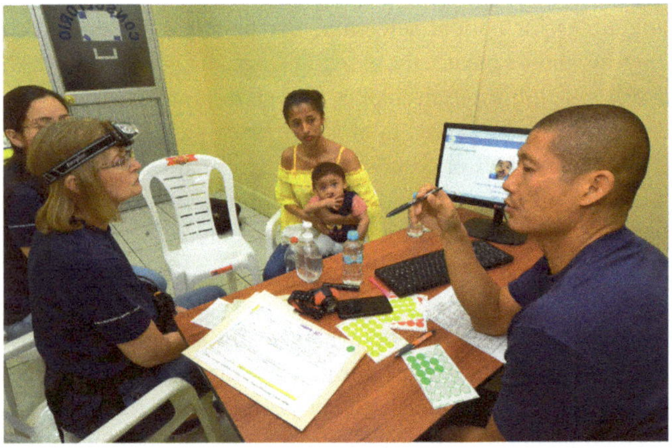

**Fig. 40.4** A patient undergoing preoperative screening during a short-term outreach program

If the patient is considered a surgical candidate following these evaluations, they are then seen by an administrative team to obtain surgical/photographic consent and standardized preoperative photographs [2]. Standardized pre- and postoperative photographs are important for assessing quality and critically analyzing surgical results and should be taken for every patient undergoing surgery and at all follow-up visits. Patients who are not deemed fit for surgery at the time of the trip or patients who are presenting for postoperative reviews can still be further evaluated by dental and speech therapy teams (Fig. 40.5).

Prioritizing patients for surgery due to limited OR time is a major consideration during short-term outreach. Though tempting, surgical outreach trips should not aim to operate on the greatest number of patients possible as this mentality risks sacrifice of quality and increases chances of complications. The International Task Force on Volunteer Cleft Missions recommends that teams "adopt the aim of achieving the maximum benefit for each patient" even if this means that fewer patients receive surgery [5]. Work hour and case volume restrictions also prevent staff fatigue and related errors. Beyond health status and ability to safely tolerate surgery, other considerations for patient selection include age, severity of deformity or facial difference, distance traveled, and the need for additional procedures in the future [2].

## Fund Raising, Publicity, and Social Media

The primary sources of funding for short-term cleft outreach programs include private donations, nongovernmental organizations (NGOs), governmental agencies, and the recipient

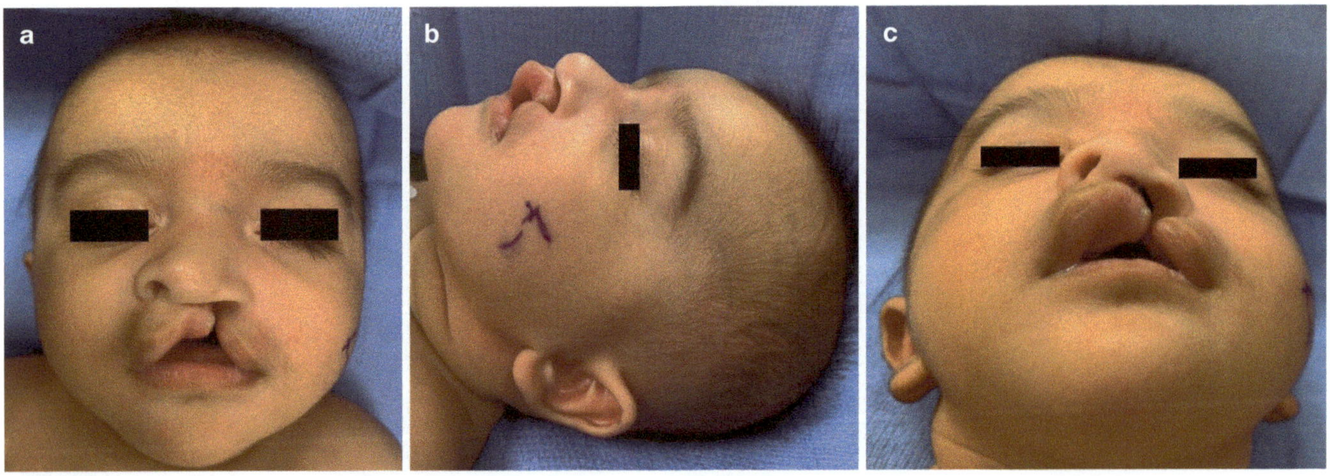


**Fig. 40.5** Standardized preoperative photos of a patient with a cleft lip. Photos should include frontal (**a**), lateral (**b**), and worms-eye (**c**) views

nation itself (typically in the form of hospital facilities and/or lodging for team members) [6]. In order to continue to raise funds and awareness, surgical outreach trips and their sponsoring organizations are often publicized in the members' home countries; this is only increasing with the popularity of social media which is now widely utilized by outreach organizations and team members for both educational and advertising purposes. Although social media posts of children with cleft lip repairs can harness social and financial capital, volunteer agencies must remember the American Society of Plastic Surgeons' code of ethics requires patient consent be obtained prior to publication of photos or other media [12]. Clear discussion regarding the planned use of the media and signed patient/parent consent is mandatory prior to publication of photos on any social media platform or website. This is also true for personal social media accounts and websites, and volunteers are advised to avoid publishing photos of patients without explicit, language-appropriate consent.

## Comprehensive Cleft Care

Surgical care is only one dimension of care for patients with cleft lip and palate. Establishing a comprehensive cleft care team is the ultimate goal of overseas cleft outreach. To this end, programs should incorporate a multidisciplinary team which includes dentists, orthodontists, and speech therapists as visiting staff. These team members can participate in follow-up evaluations for patients who have already had surgery with local professionals and provide training specific to cleft patients. They are critical in knowledge and skill transfer for services such as nasoalveolar molding (NAM) and nasoendoscopy for velopharyngeal insufficiency. Interpreter services are critical for addressing language barriers as well as understanding nuances of speech evaluation and therapy methods in the native language of patients [7]. Advanced technology has recently helped establish telemedicine and internet-based speech therapy sessions for postoperative follow-up of patients treated on cleft outreach trips. Mobile speech therapy addresses travel and financial barriers for patients and families who may live far from the institute or hospital-based speech therapy programs [7, 8].

## Building Capacity and Sustainability

Patel et al. describe a "diagonal" approach to international cleft care, where the immediate benefits of short-term surgical outreach trips are combined with efforts to increase local capacity and independence in caring for cleft patients [9]. Diagonal approaches that build local capacity include a long-term presence of the outreach team at a particular site, with regularly scheduled trips by the outreach group comprised of (mostly) the same team of multidisciplinary volunteers and host professionals. This usually requires the establishment of a self-sustained revenue source, as opposed to relying on external funding, and critical partnerships with host agencies. Newer technologies, such as virtual and augmented reality, have recently been shown to aid in the safe and effective transfer of surgical knowledge and skills [10]. Such platforms allow "hands-on" remote visits by outreach surgeons who can virtually "scrub in" to live cleft surgery, enabling surgical proctoring and teaching that goes beyond progress achieved during regularly scheduled outreach trips (Fig. 40.6). Vyas and colleagues found that outreach visits and augmented reality-based remote visits worked synergistically and significantly to accelerate knowledge and skill

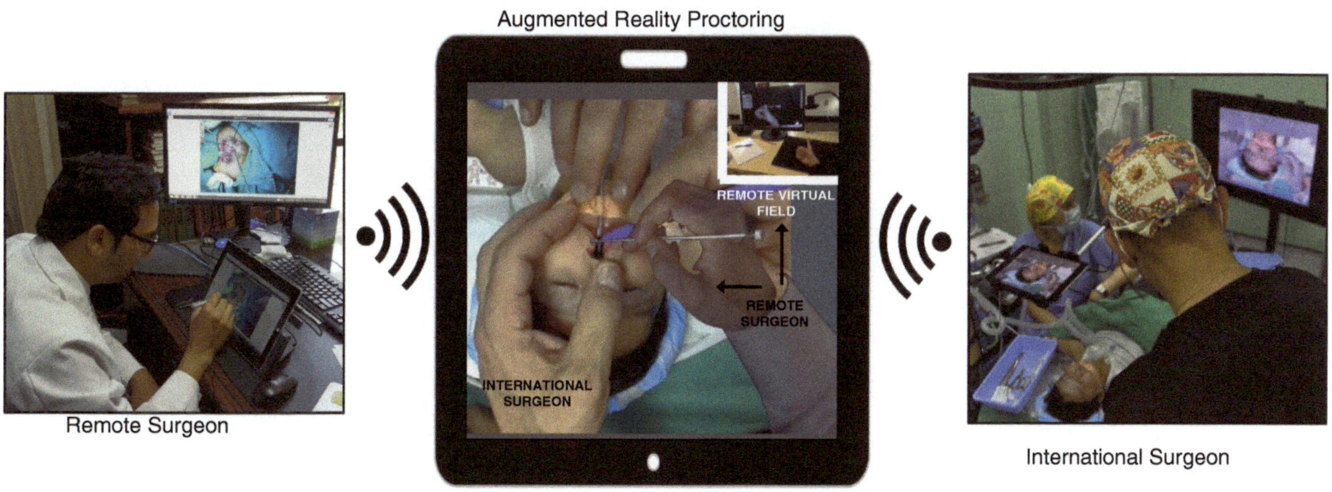


**Fig. 40.6** Augmented reality platform enables remote surgeon to "scrub in" to overseas cleft surgery, providing longer-term "hands-on" guidance

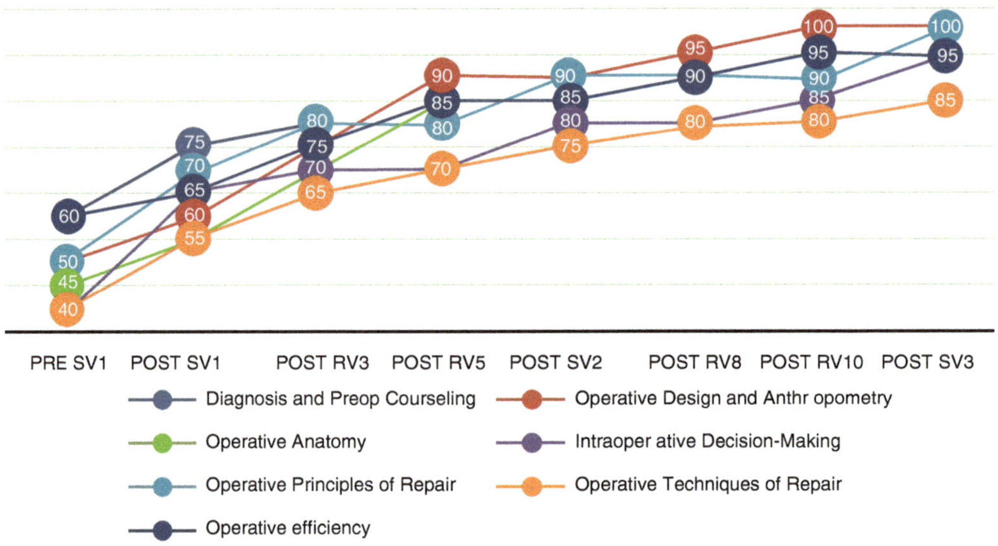


**Fig. 40.7** Increased overseas cleft capacity reported after site visits (SV) and remote (AR-guided) visits (RV)

transfer to new providers of cleft surgery, creating the foundation for sustainable delivery of cleft care [11] (Fig. 40.7). This technology can also be utilized by dentists, orthodontists, and speech pathologists working to establish comprehensive cleft services at overseas outreach sites.

In addition to training local professionals, building local infrastructure and improving durable medical equipment are other important aspects of building international capacity. Outreach groups should consider donation of essential equipment and supplies transported for the trip as well as soliciting donations from regional benefactors throughout the year. This simplifies future outreach campaigns and allows local surgeons to incorporate improved technology and resources into their practice, thereby expanding the regional capacity to treat children with cleft deformities.

## References


1. Skyes KJ. Short-term medical service trips: a systematic review of the evidence. Am J Public Health. 2014;104:e38–48. https://doi.org/10.2105/AJPH.2014.301983.
2. Vyas RM, et al. International surgical outreach initiatives: planning, execution, and safety. In: Rogers DJ, Hartnick CJ, Hamdan US, editors. Video atlas of cleft lip and palate surgery. 1st ed. San Diego: Plural Publishing; 2014.
3. Schneider WJ, et al. Volunteers in plastic surgery guidelines for providing surgical care for children in the less developed world. Plast Recon Surg. 2011;127(6):2477–86.
4. Vyas RM, et al. Implementation of an emergency response protocol for overseas surgical outreach initiatives. Plast Recon Surg. 2013;131(4):631e–6e.
5. Eberlin KR, et al. Adult cleft lip repair under local anesthesia: an effective technique for resource poor settings. Cleft Palate Craniofac J. 2013;50(1):59–63.
6. Yeow VKL, et al. International task force on volunteer cleft missions. J Craniofac Surg. 2002;13(1):18–25.
7. Furr MC, et al. Extending multidisciplinary management of cleft palate to the developing world. J Oral Maxillofac Surg. 2011;69(1):237–41.
8. Glazer CA, et al. Multidisciplinary care of international patients with cleft palate using telemedicine. Arch Facial Plast Surg. 2011;13(6):436–8. https://doi.org/10.1001/archfacial.2011.72.
9. Patel PB, et al. An opportunity for diagonal development in global surgery in cleft lip and palate care in resource-limited settings. Plast Surg Int. 2012; https://doi.org/10.1155/2012/892437.
10. Kim Y, et al. Virtual reality and augmented reality in plastic surgery: a review. Arch Plast Surg. 2017;44(3):179–87.
11. Vyas R, et al. Using virtual augmented reality to remotely proctor overseas surgical outreach: Building long term international capacity and sustainability. Plast Reconstr Surg. 2020;146(5):622–9
12. American Society of Plastic Surgeons. Code of Ethics. https://www.plasticsurgery.org/documents/Governance/asps-code-of-ethics.pdf. Updated September 25, 2017. Accessed March 17, 2019.

# Creating a Culture of Care and Safety

# 41

Elie P. Ramly, Ruben Ayala, and Usama S. Hamdan

**Key Points**

- Great multidisciplinary care can be delivered in low-resource settings, but guiding cleft care standards should be well understood and then thoughtfully adapted.
- Potential sources of adversity encountered by teams in low-resource settings – hierarchy, language barriers, unfamiliar equipment, fatigue – can be broadly addressed in ways that strengthen a team's sense of mission and unity.
- Community partnerships bring in critical stakeholders and help a cleft program endure.
- Quality assurance and emergency response protocols promote the safety of patients and team members alike. Proper implementation of protocols can prevent surgical and other perioperative complications and mitigate their repercussions. Team member participation in developing protocols ensures that they are appropriate to the context and most likely to be followed.
- Looking for opportunities to teach and learn, formally and informally, improves quality of care and strengthens team dynamics.

## Introduction

Comprehensive cleft care is a multidisciplinary team endeavor and is most effective when delivered through a patient-centered culture. Success in cleft outreach is highly dependent on a good grasp of the people, environment, and resources that make care delivery possible. While untreated craniofacial conditions have multiple undue repercussions, surgical care in outreach settings can be fraught with significant perioperative morbidity [1–5]. Excellent clinical care, team organization, and quality assurance protocols are foundational to high-quality care in low-resource settings. Several common barriers – such as hierarchy, language, and unfamiliar equipment – must be addressed and mitigated in order to institute a culture of safety. Beyond immediate care delivery, surgical missions can be effective vehicles for local capacity building and the establishment of sustainable cleft care ecosystems. This chapter describes logistic and operational considerations important for the delivery of safe and effective cleft care in underserved settings.

## Team Components and Dynamics

### Adapting the Multidisciplinary Team Care Concept

A successful cleft team is bigger than the sum of its parts (Fig. 41.1). As the African proverb states: "To go fast, go alone; to go far, go together." Comprehensive cleft care relies on a multidisciplinary team approach. The American Cleft Palate-Craniofacial Association (ACPA) outlines standards for team care, which provide practical guidance for teams worldwide (Table 41.1) [6]. This chapter provides strategies for adapting the ACPA standards to outreach settings to maximize safety and efficacy while laying foundations for sustainable cleft care.

E. P. Ramly
Global Smile Foundation, Norwood, MA, USA

Hansjörg Wyss Department of Plastic Surgery, NYU Langone Health, New York, NY, USA

R. Ayala
Operation Smile, Virginia Beach, VA, USA
e-mail: rayala@operationsmile.org; http://www.operationsmile.org

U. S. Hamdan (✉)
Global Smile Foundation, Boston, MA, USA

Tufts University School of Medicine, Boston, MA, USA

Harvard Medical School, Boston, MA, USA

Boston University School of Medicine, Boston, MA, USA
e-mail: uh@gsmile.org; http://www.gsmile.org

© Springer Nature Switzerland AG 2021

J. W. Swanson, D. W. Low (eds.), *Global Cleft Care in Low-Resource Settings*, https://doi.org/10.1007/978-3-030-59105-2_41

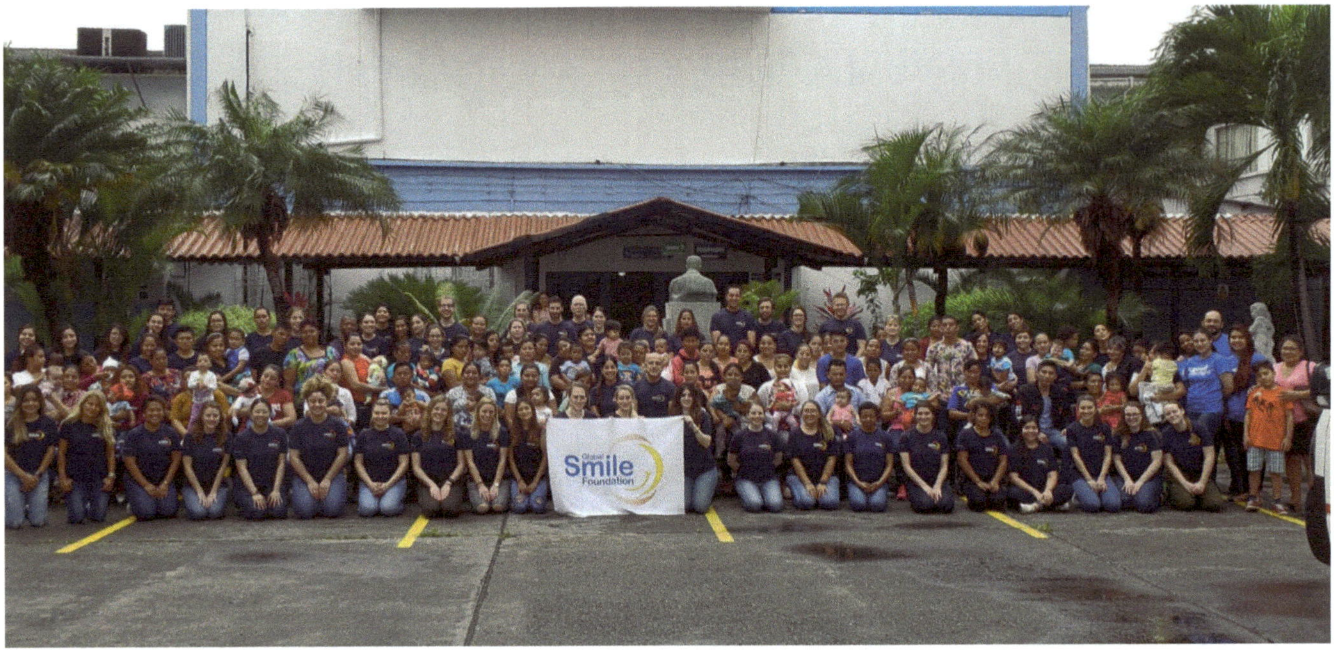


**Fig. 41.1** International and local volunteers, families, and patients at the Global Smile Foundation (GSF)-Fundacion Global Smile-Ecuador Cleft Center in Guayaquil, Ecuador

**Table 41.1** ACPA Standards of Team Care

| |
|---|
| 1. Multidisciplinary *team composition*, which includes a patient care coordinator, cleft surgeon, orthodontist, and speech-language pathologist, with access to psychology, social work, audiology, genetics, dentistry, otolaryngology, and pediatrics/primary care |
| 2. Protocols for *team management*, including collaboration on patient care, referrals to other professionals, and shared records |
| 3. *Patient and family communication* to encourage family/caregiver participation with treatment and help with locating financial assistance |
| 4. *Cultural competence* to treat patients and families with sensitivity to differences and in a non-discriminating manner |
| 5. Mechanisms to assess and treat *psychological and social needs* including cognitive development and refer for further treatment as necessary |
| 6. An *outcomes assessment* process to evaluate patient treatment and satisfaction and make improvements accordingly |

Abbreviated from Standards for Approval of Cleft Palate and Craniofacial Teams, revised 4/19. Available at https://acpa-cpf.org/team-care/standardscat/standards-of-approval-for-team-care/

Optimal cleft care includes the multiple clinical disciplines of surgery, anesthesiology, pediatrics, dentistry, orthodontics, nursing, psychosocial care, and speech-language pathology. The ACPA specifies that some services should be internal to the cleft team, and others can be accessible by referral, but reinforces the principle of assuring the best possible access for patients to this range of services. This philosophy applies well to outreach efforts as well: while accessibility of all services should be prioritized, the form of how the different services are provided may vary. A comprehensive cleft center, or a comprehensive cleft mission, ought to incorporate all of these disciplines; conversely, a small outreach mission focused on primary cleft treatment of infants may focus on surgery, anesthesia, pediatrics, and dentistry. There are also additional critical roles in low-resource settings, such as a biomedical engineer for the evaluation and maintenance of on-site operating room and anesthesia equipment in underserved facilities. In most cleft outreach, there is a physician leader (often called the team leader, or field medical director) who oversees the medical staff and medical decision-making and a coordinator (patient care coordinator, or clinical coordinator) who acts as the central manager of patient flow. Tight coordination and open communication between each of these leaders, and their respective teams, are essential to establish a cooperative dynamic centered on patient safety.

## Anticipating Adversity

Cleft teams often have to deliver care in suboptimal conditions within a short period of time. Treatment facilities may be remote and not fully integrated with other resources within the community. Hospitals may be under-equipped or under-staffed. While technically highly qualified, many visiting team members may not have much experience working outside of their home institution and may be unfamiliar with the site, local culture, or language. Taken together, those factors constitute a fertile environment for the occurrence of adverse events. A number of overarching challenges can perhaps best be addressed systemically, in a way that strengthens team culture:

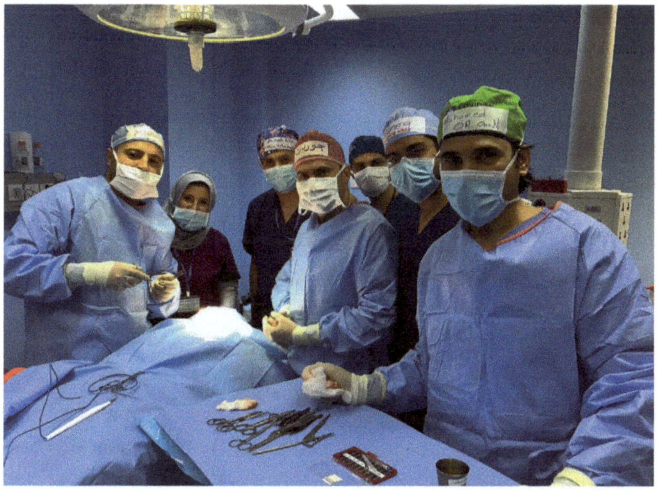

**Fig. 41.2** Open communication is facilitated by visible nametags

- The *hierarchy* of traditional medical structures can often prevent less senior team members from speaking up. Using first names and writing names on caps can make all team members seem more approachable and encourage speaking up! (Fig. 41.2)
- *Language barriers* are common both when international clinicians are collaborating on cleft missions and when local dialects exist. Ensuring team members are proficient in a common language, and the availability of translators, helps overcome these barriers.
- *Unfamiliar medication names and equipment* can cause confusion, particularly in an emergency. Team familiarity with all equipment, especially monitors and defibrillator, prior to the start of surgical cases, is important. Further, a preprinted weight-based dosing sheet for resuscitation medications (with local/generic medication names) can reduce confusion in an emergency.
- *Fatigue* can arise from the stress and duration of workdays. Strict daily end times can be useful to prevent staff exhaustion and the risk of mistakes being made.

Team members often work in a volunteer capacity delivering cleft care in low-resource settings. The esprit de corps that motivates volunteerism must be nurtured and allowed to flourish, and tempering team energy with rule compliance can at times be a tricky balance. Further, because care is often delivered outside of a highly regulated, institutional structure, it often falls to clinicians and organizations to establish norms where they often are not dictated by governing bodies. One way that norms can be developed is through participation among team members. In 2006, Operation Smile began a consensus-based process of establishing and regularly reviewing Global Standards of Care, to establish consistent expectations for its programming across countries. Each standard is structured as a global best practice

**Table 41.2** Operation Smile Global Standards of Care

| Care categories |
|---|
| 1. Preoperative patient screening and assessment |
| 2. Anesthesia equipment and supplies |
| 3. Surgical equipment |
| 4. Post-anesthesia care unit (PACU) |
| 5. Postoperative intensive care |
| 6. Postoperative ward |
| 7. Patient consent |
| 8. Surgical priority |
| 9. Preventing transmission of blood-borne pathogens |
| 10. Pain management |
| 11. Operation Smile team |
| 12. Qualifications for volunteers |
| 13. Patient follow-up |
| 14. Translation |
| 15. Documentation |
| 16. Hospital facility |
| 17. Quality assurance |

Adapted from Operation Smile Global Standards of Care, revised 2/15. Available at https://www.operationsmile.org/content/about-us#medical

(supported by peer-reviewed literature), the Operation Smile context (addressing considerations of missions/centers in low-resource settings), global commitments (which serve as "minimum" requirements and operational specifics in each area), and supporting policies, procedures, and evaluation mechanisms to measure compliance with the standards (Table 41.2). The Global Standards of Care serves as guiding norms for both Operation Smile and other cleft organizations but have perhaps more importantly fostered a culture of shared decision-making and responsibility when it comes to team and patient safety.

## Partnering with the Community

Community involvement is an excellent starting point for building an inclusive culture of cleft care. There are many natural stakeholders of cleft care in a community: pediatricians treating children with clefts and seeking the best possible care on their behalf, and in many cases surgeons performing lip or palate repair, even if occasionally or itinerantly; local healthcare and government authorities responsible for child welfare; parents and families of children with clefts who often form connections; and businesses who may be able to donate funding.

Examples abound of cleft care that grows from mission-based programs to comprehensive cleft care centers in large part due to community involvement. The Guwahati Comprehensive Cleft Care Center (GC4) in the northeast Indian state of Assam is a successful example of such a collaboration. GC4 was established in 2011 in collaboration between Operation Smile, the government of Assam, and private enterprise (Tata Trust). It was found to be more cost-effective than mission-based care, reinvesting resources into creating sustainable infrastructure and employment [7]. Consistent engagement with the local community can help foster a collective feeling of ownership. In Guayaquil, Ecuador, a Cleft Center was established by Global Smile Foundation (GSF) and Fundacion Global Smile-Ecuador at Leon Becerra Hospital in 2012, based on more than three decades of outreach cleft programs in that city. The Cleft Center provides year-long comprehensive speech, dental, and psychosocial services in addition to surgical care coupled with periodic biannual team missions and continuous follow-up (Fig. 41.3a, b). Patients treated in their infancy have since become GSF volunteers as young adults and advocates for comprehensive cleft care. They help to coordinate patient referral and follow-up and disseminate informative cleft awareness at a national level (Fig. 41.4a, b).

Multiple cleft organizations and multiple cleft surgeons operate in the same cities or regions. Seeking shared areas to collaborate, attempting to minimize competitiveness with one another, and creating solutions for those challenges by sharing expertise and resources to maximize patient safety and quality of care should be ideals we all try to uphold.

## Quality Assurance in Outreach Settings

Even when a strong team dynamic is generated, specific protocols applicable to a surgical mission or comprehensive care center can serve as the team's safety net, providing practical tools for preventing complications or mitigating their effects. Recognizing the lack of standardization of safety practices across different humanitarian organizations, a number of quality assurance guidelines, safety checklists, and emer-

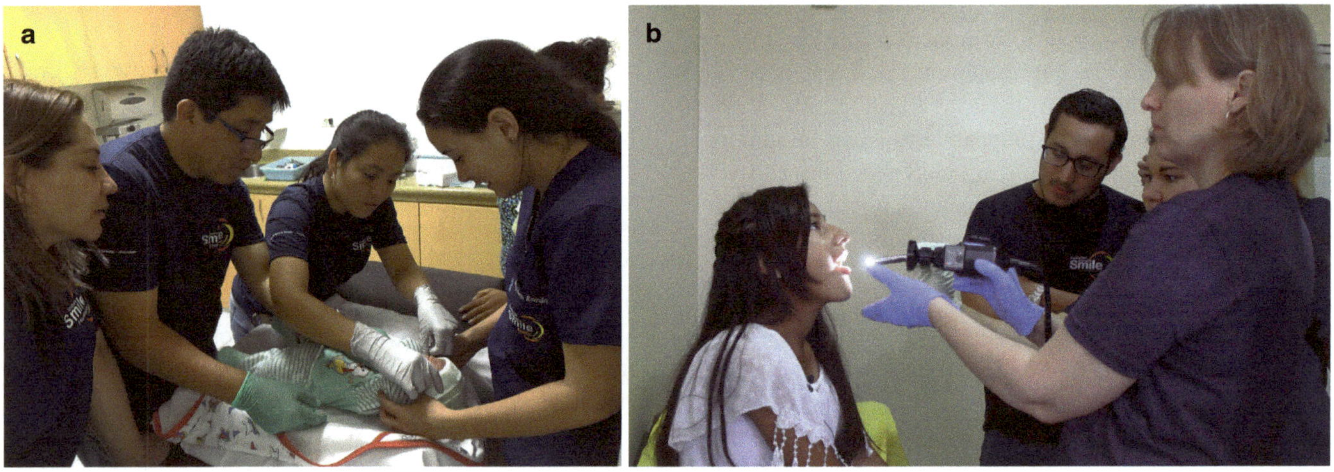


**Fig. 41.3** (**a**, **b**) Providing nasoalveolar molding (NAM) and performing nasoendoscopy at the Global Smile Foundation Cleft Center in Guayaquil, Ecuador

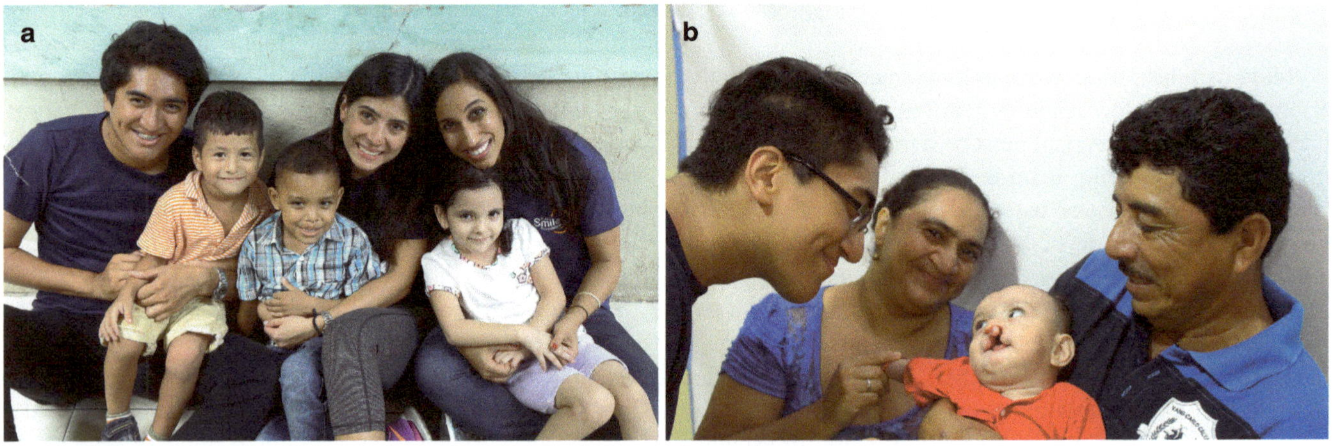


**Fig. 41.4** (**a**, **b**) Diego (left, **a**) was born with a unilateral cleft lip. He was treated by Global Smile Foundation (GSF) in infancy, and now a young adult, he is a strong advocate of GSF's vision for comprehensive cleft care throughout his community in Guayaquil, Ecuador. He helps with coordinating patient referral and follow-up and disseminating cleft awareness at a national level

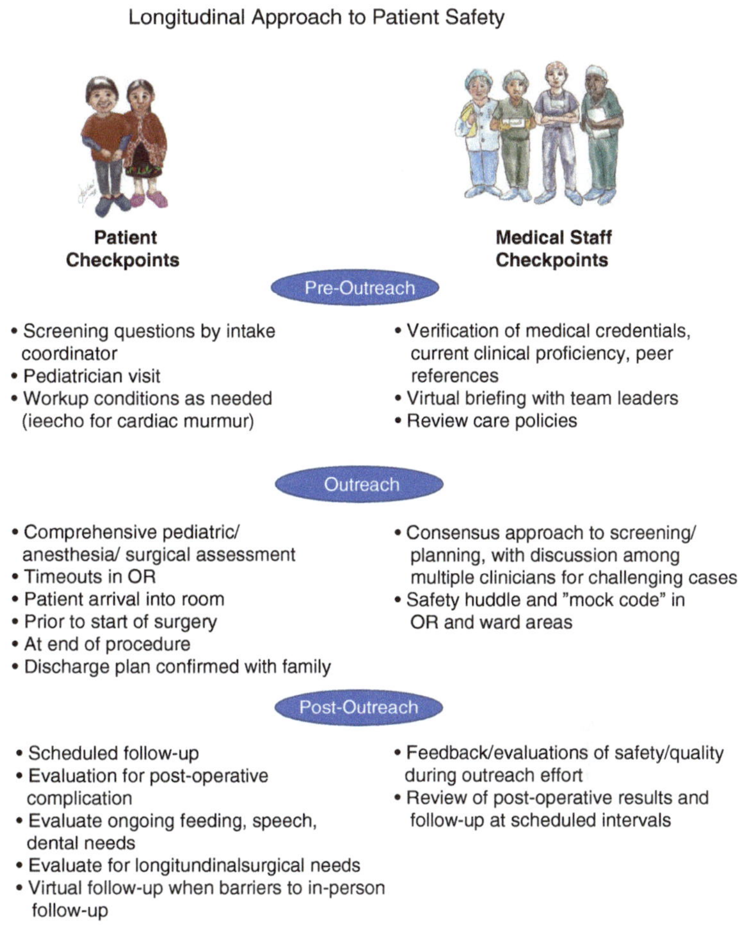


**Fig. 41.5** Longitudinal approach to patient safety. This involves both patient and medical staff checkpoints before, during, and after an outreach effort

gency response protocols have been developed which we will further elaborate on in this section [8–10]. These guidelines draw on decades of mission- and center-based cleft care by several organizations on multiple continents. An effective longitudinal approach to patient safety can be thought of as a series of both patient checkpoints and medical staff checkpoints that are carried out before, during, and after an outreach effort (Fig. 41.5).

## Credentialing

Every patient, no matter his or her circumstances, should be given access to the highest quality of care possible. All local and visiting healthcare professionals must have recognized credentials and proven experience in their fields of practice, with active licensure in their country of residency. Some host countries may request additional local credentialing. Visiting surgeons should regularly perform cleft lip and palate procedures in their own practice settings, which is defined by one organization as 50–70 cleft procedures per year. Peer references are particularly important, because they assess whether a prospective team member's character traits will contribute well to a team culture. It is the responsibility of the hosting organization to ensure that surgeons are qualified to perform cleft procedures, irrespective of their subspecialties. The consequences of a poorly performed cleft operation are devastating and should be avoided stringently. Supervising or proctoring a volunteer on their first mission experience with an organization is important to ensure technical aptitude and fit.

## Mission Preparation

Initiating a strong working relationship with key stakeholders in the community starts before the mission, laying the foundation for a successful long-term partnership and continuity of care. The multidisciplinary facets of the mission should be considered, including surgery, anesthesia, dentistry, and nursing, and their requirements addressed in coordination with local hospital leadership and coordinators [8]. Roles should be clearly defined and any potential pitfalls discussed in order to secure perioperative logistics, ancillary services, and follow-up. The availability of intensive care unit (ICU) beds and transfusion capabilities should be established. If the hospital lacks a pediatric ICU, it should at the very least be within a close distance to another healthcare facility that has intensive care capabilities.

## Emergency Response Protocols

Despite best efforts, emergencies can always happen. A clear emergency response protocol should be adopted by the cleft team and disseminated to all members. The Protocol should emphasize equipment portability, location-specific adaptability, workflow and communication, and standardization of team roles [10]. Simulations can be useful in anticipating various potential emergencies including cardiac and respiratory events, malignant hyperthermia, bleeding, loss of electricity, emergency tracheotomy, potential need for blood transfusion, and accidental needle stick exposure, among others (Fig. 41.6). The team's portable "emergency crash code" or "crash cart" suitcase outfitted with essential resuscitative items is opened and every item is reviewed. The suitcase is then placed in a designated secure location that is close to the OR, PACU, and inpatient floors and made accessible to all team members (Fig. 41.7). An on-call schedule and a reliable communication chain are established for each night and reviewed [10].

## Preoperative Screening and Case Selection

Preoperative screening, discussed in Chap. 41, can be useful in prioritizing patients for a surgical mission and enabling team members to review and prepare for potential cases in advance. Patient screening often involves the evaluation of a large number of patients (Fig. 41.8a) [8] by multiple different specialists, so a methodical process and careful coordination are important. Frequently different clinical "stations" are set up: administration, nursing (to obtain vital signs and weight), surgery, anesthesia, pediatrics, speech, dental, psychosocial care, and photography. Given the sheer number of patients and the complexity of the screening process, organi-

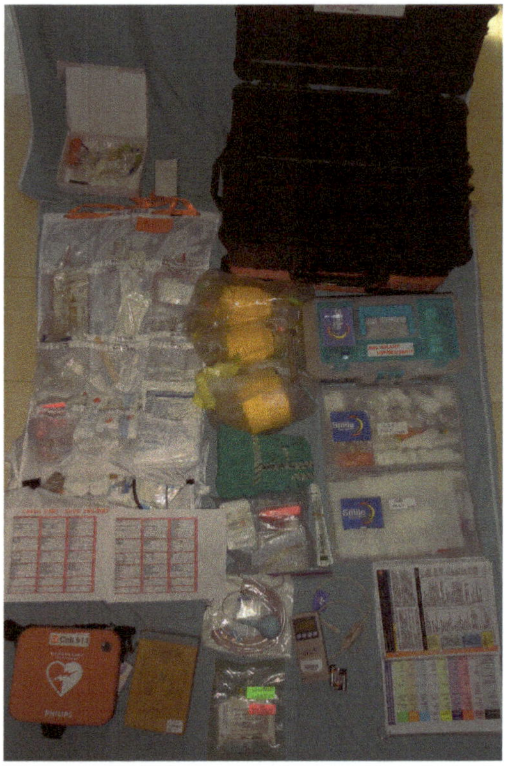

Fig. 41.7 A portable "emergency crash code" or "crash cart" suitcase outfitted with essential resuscitative items and medications should be immediately accessible to the operating room, post-anesthesia care unit, and inpatient floors and made accessible to all team members

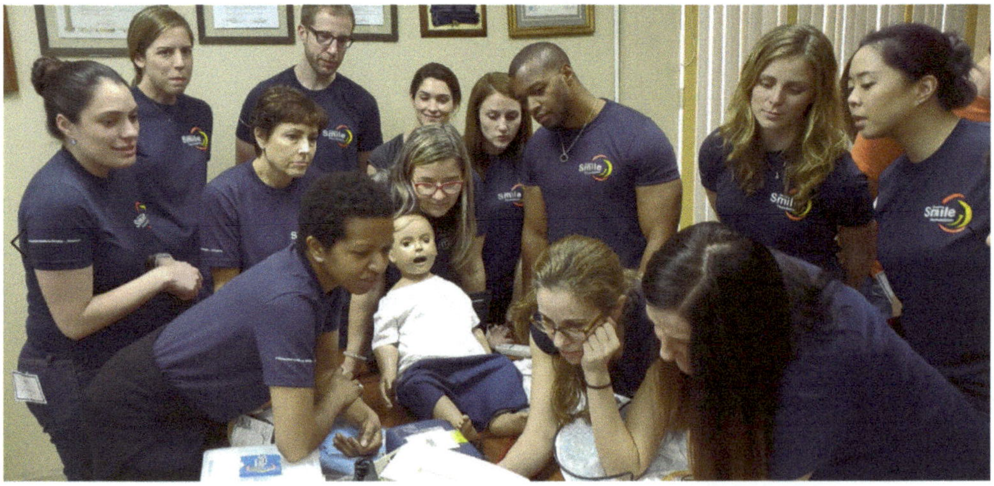

Fig. 41.6 Simulation can assist in preparation for various potential emergencies, including cardiac and respiratory events, malignant hyperthermia, bleeding, loss of electricity, emergency tracheotomy, potential need for blood transfusion, and accidental needle stick exposure, among others. Also discussed are various procedures and policies to enhance team functionality, safety, and camaraderie

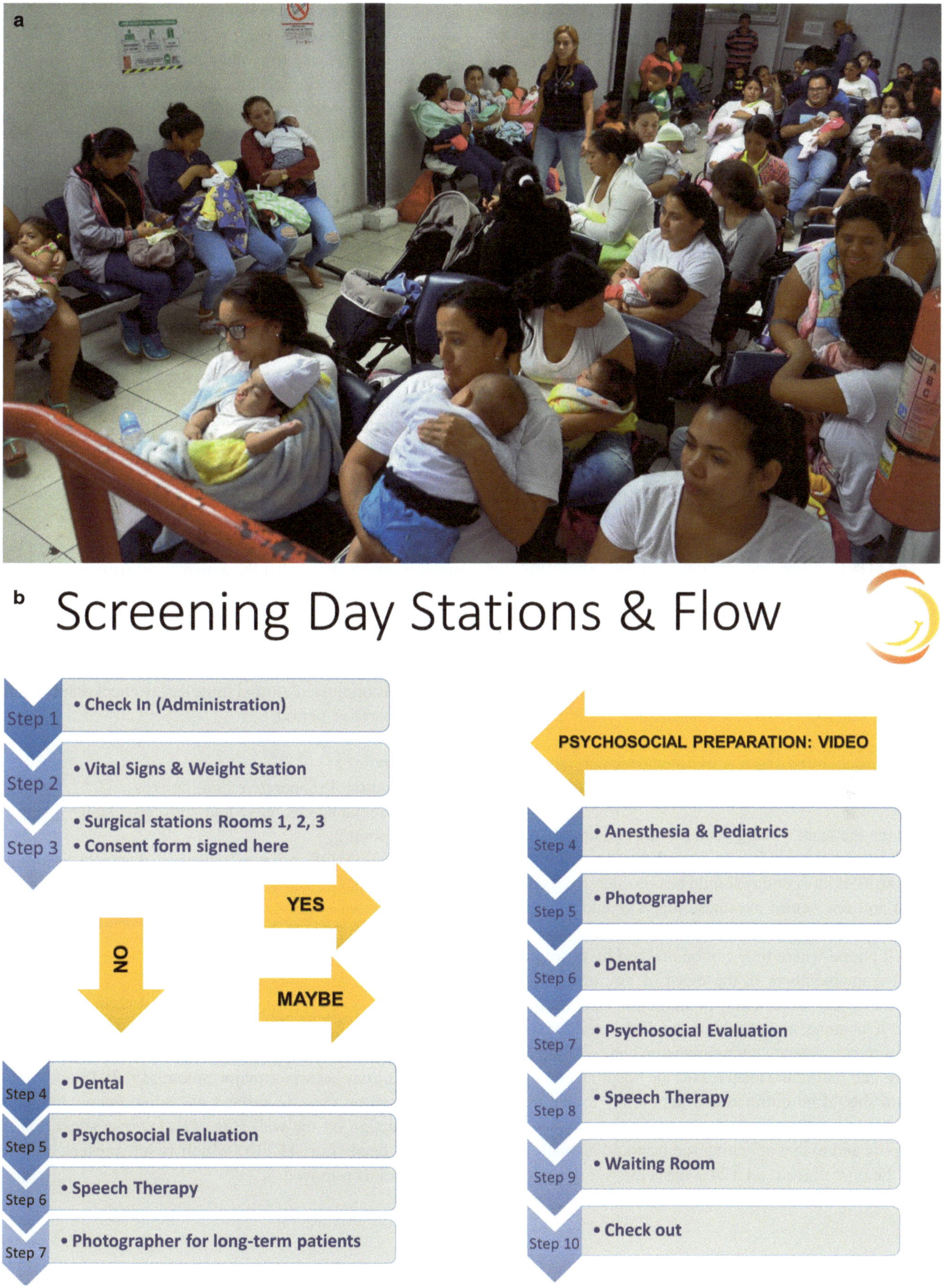


**Fig. 41.8** (**a**) Patients awaiting screening at the start of a cleft mission. (**b**) Global Smile Foundation screening day stations and flow

zation of patient flow and accurate transfer of clinical information are essential (Fig. 41.8b). Diagrammatic instructions and pamphlets or animated videos in the native language can be useful to patients and caregivers while they are waiting to be evaluated, to describe the screening and selection process and perioperative proceedings. Education is provided on causative factors for clefts, and instructions on perioperative nutrition, bottle feeding, and psychosocial support are emphasized. Bilingual translators can make the family feel at ease, reinforce the information, answer questions, and prevent any breakdown in communication.

## Perioperative Care and Safety Protocols

Before starting operative procedures, OR and PACUs are inspected by the team nurses, while the anesthesiologists and biomedical engineer confirm equipment compatibility and OR readiness and unpack equipment and supplies. When designing the schedule, younger patients are typically scheduled earlier in the day, with the exception of the first case of the week where a slightly older and lower-risk patient is selected as the checked equipment is being used for the first time [8, 11]. To allow for adequate airway monitoring, we would advise against performing palate cases within 48 hours of team departure [8, 12]. Primary cleft lip repairs or revisions for patients over the age of 12 years are done under local anesthesia with or without minor sedation. This technique can be safely and effectively performed in outreach settings by employing nerve blocks [13].

## Schedule

To manage the team's energy and morale and uphold patient safety throughout the mission, a work hour restriction of a maximum 10 hours per day should be considered. One senior surgeon and one senior anesthesiologist should together be designated as on-call physicians each night, equipped with a local cell phone where they can be reached by hospital staff or local team members in the event of any emergency. In addition, a team coordinator, pediatrician, operating room nurse, PACU nurse, and translator should be easily reachable as part of the emergency communication chain. At the end of each day, and before the team leaves the hospital, one operating room should be outfitted and kept ready to use for any potential emergent return to the operating room. Access to the hospital and to that operating room should be made available to the on-call team on a 24/7 basis [8].

## Surgical Safety Checklists

The role of surgical safety checklists in reducing mortality and morbidity is well established and has been internationally validated, with rate of death declining from 1.5% to 0.8% and the rate of inpatient complications declining from 11.0% to 7.0% [14]. Safety checklists have since become the standard of care at hospitals in the United States and multiple others around the globe [15–18]. Checklists are usually implemented as a "time out" before starting a surgical procedure. All team members should have their name clearly written on their surgical cap or identification tag and should introduce themselves at the beginning of "time out." The implementation of checklists is particularly important on international surgical outreach missions, where some team members may be working together for the first time or may be unfamiliar with assigned roles, dynamics, and the mission environment [9]. Documenting items on a checklist and listing them out loud allow team members to hold each other accountable for every item on the list.

The World Health Organization Surgical Safety Checklist (Fig. 41.9) is intended to be adapted to local contexts. In fact, much research shows that the active "contextualization" process an organization goes through to create a checklist is really important to its sustained use in the long term. A checklist adapted to cleft lip and/or palate surgery in the outreach setting has been developed by GSF (Fig. 41.10). The checklist is organized around three safety checkpoints during the perioperative period:

- Checkpoint 1:
  - Location: Preoperative holding area
  - Participants: OR nurse and anesthesia staff
- Checkpoint 2:
  - Location: OR, prior to induction of anesthesia
  - Participants: Surgeons, anesthesiologist, scrub nurse, OR nurse
- Checkpoint 3:
  - Location: OR, at the completion of the operation
  - Participants: Surgeons, anesthesiologist, scrub nurse, OR nurse

Throat packs are used frequently in cleft surgery, and a retained throat pack is a major potential risk. In addition to being listed on the safe surgery checklist, many cleft teams employ a sign on the wall (Fig. 41.11a) or a sticker on the patient's head (Fig. 41.11b) which is left present until the throat pack is removed.

## Surgical Safety Checklist

World Health Organization | Patient Safety
A World Alliance for Safer Health Care

**Before induction of anaesthesia**

(with at least nurse and anaesthetist)

**Has the patient confirmed his/her identity, site, procedure, and consent?**
- ☐ Yes

**Is the site marked?**
- ☐ Yes
- ☐ Not applicable

**Is the anaesthesia machine and medication check complete?**
- ☐ Yes

**Is the pulse oximeter on the patient and functioning?**
- ☐ Yes

**Does the patient have a:**

**Known allergy?**
- ☐ No
- ☐ Yes

**Difficult airway or aspiration risk?**
- ☐ No
- ☐ Yes, and equipment/assistance available

**Risk of >500ml blood loss (7ml/kg in children)?**
- ☐ No
- ☐ Yes, and two IVs/central access and fluids planned

**Before skin incision**

(with nurse, anaesthetist and surgeon)

- ☐ **Confirm all team members have introduced themselves by name and role.**
- ☐ **Confirm the patient's name, procedure, and where the incision will be made.**

**Has antibiotic prophylaxis been given within the last 60 minutes?**
- ☐ Yes
- ☐ Not applicable

**Anticipated Critical Events**

**To Surgeon:**
- ☐ What are the critical or non-routine steps?
- ☐ How long will the case take?
- ☐ What is the anticipated blood loss?

**To Anaesthetist:**
- ☐ Are there any patient-specific concerns?

**To Nursing Team:**
- ☐ Has sterility (including indicator results) been confirmed?
- ☐ Are there equipment issues or any concerns?

**Is essential imaging displayed?**
- ☐ Yes
- ☐ Not applicable

**Before patient leaves operating room**

(with nurse, anaesthetist and surgeon)

**Nurse Verbally Confirms:**
- ☐ The name of the procedure
- ☐ Completion of instrument, sponge and needle counts
- ☐ Specimen labelling (read specimen labels aloud, including patient name)
- ☐ Whether there are any equipment problems to be addressed

**To Surgeon, Anaesthetist and Nurse:**
- ☐ What are the key concerns for recovery and management of this patient?

This checklist is not intended to be comprehensive. Additions and modifications to fit local practice are encouraged. Revised 1 / 2009

© WHO, 2009

**Fig. 41.9** World Health Organization Surgical Safety Checklist. Reprinted with permission

## Postoperative Care

Clinical rounds should be performed twice daily at least, to evaluate all patients, monitor recovery, and manage any early signs of complications. Prior to leaving the hospital, patients and their families should be given verbal and written discharge instructions in their native language (Fig. 41.12). Postoperative care and follow-up plans should be clarified and confirmed with the local partnering medical team. During physical examination, focus should be placed on assessing the quality of the operative outcome, pain control, and any potential complications. Postoperative photographs should be taken at this time and patients given information regarding the following year's mission.

## Outcomes Evaluation, Capacity Building, and Sustainability

Meticulous team selection, mission preparation, and quality assurance through the implementation of safety checklists and emergency response protocols are the fundamental components of a culture of safety. Outcome evaluation and continuous quality control are necessary to ensure that the protocols put in place are indeed serving their purpose when properly implemented. This task is simply impossible in the absence of consistent documentation and longitudinal data collection, which are tremendous challenges for outreach teams with limited budgets and rotating staff. Electronic health records and cloud computing offer solutions for data

**Patient Surgical Safety Checklist**

**Last name:** ______________ **First name:** ______________

**Procedure:** ______________

**Surgeon:** ______________ **Anesthesia:** ______________

**Date:** ________ **Medical Record:** ______________

**TO BE COMPLETED BY PERIOP PERSON** → **TO BE COMPLETED BY OR NURSE** → **BEFORE PATIENT LEAVES ROOM**

**SIGN IN – NURSE AND ANESTHESIA**

- ❑ PATIENT IDENTIFICATION VERIFIED
- ❑ ID Band Applied
- ❑ Consent Form Complete

NPO
- ❑ LAST FOOD/MILK AT ______
- ❑ LAST WATER AT ______

DOES THE PATIENT HAVE A:

KNOWN ALLERGY?
- ❑ NO
- ❑ YES

THE CHILD IS WELL TODAY
- ❑ YES
- ❑ NO
- ❑ HCG completed (12yo or menarche)

**TIME OUT - TEAM**

- ❑ INTRODUCE SELF BY NAME AND ROLE
- ❑ INTRODUCE LOCAL TEAM
- ❑ VERBALLY CONFIRM
  - PATIENT
  - SITE
  - PROCEDURE

SURGEON VERIFIES
- ❑ WHAT ARE THE CRITICAL /UNEXPECTED STEPS
- ❑ OPERATION DURATION

ANESTHESIA VERIFIES
- ❑ ANTIBIOTICS GIVEN WITHIN 60 MINUTES OF INCISION

DIFFICULT AIRWAY/ASPIRATION RISK?
- ❑ NO
- ❑ YES, AND EQUIPMENT/ASSISTANCE AVAILABLE

RISK OF> 500 ML BLOOD LOSS(7ML/KG IN CHILDREN)?
- ❑ NO
- ❑ YES

WT______X7 =__________
- ❑ Fire Risks Reviewed

PHOTOS/ IMAGES DISPLAYED?
- ❑ YES
- ❑ NOT APPLICABLE

ANY QUESTIONS/CONCERNS FROM TEAM?

**SIGN OUT -TEAM**

- ❑ NAME OF THE PROCEDURE:
- ❑ SURGEON VERIFIES
- ❑ NURSE VERIFIES
- ❑ NEEDLES OPENED: ________
- ❑ NEEDLES ACCOUNTED FOR: ________
- ❑ INSTRUMENT COUNT FOR INVENTORY
- ❑ Blood Loss: ________
- ❑ E.T. Tube size __________

TEAM VERIFIES
- ❑ THROAT PACK REMOVED
  - o YES
  - o NOT APPLICABLE
- ❑ KEY CONCERNS FOR RECOVERY AND MANAGEMENT OF THIS PATIENT

**©Global Smile Foundation (GSF) 2020**
Last updates:May 26,2020 *'Basedon the WHO Surgical afety Checklist, URLhttp://www.who.int/patientsafety/safesurgery/en, ©WorldHealthOrganization2008Allrightsreserved.*

**Fig. 41.10** The Global Smile Foundation surgical safety checklist, which is a modification of the World Health Organization Surgical Safety Checklist, tailored to the treatment of patients with cleft lip/palate

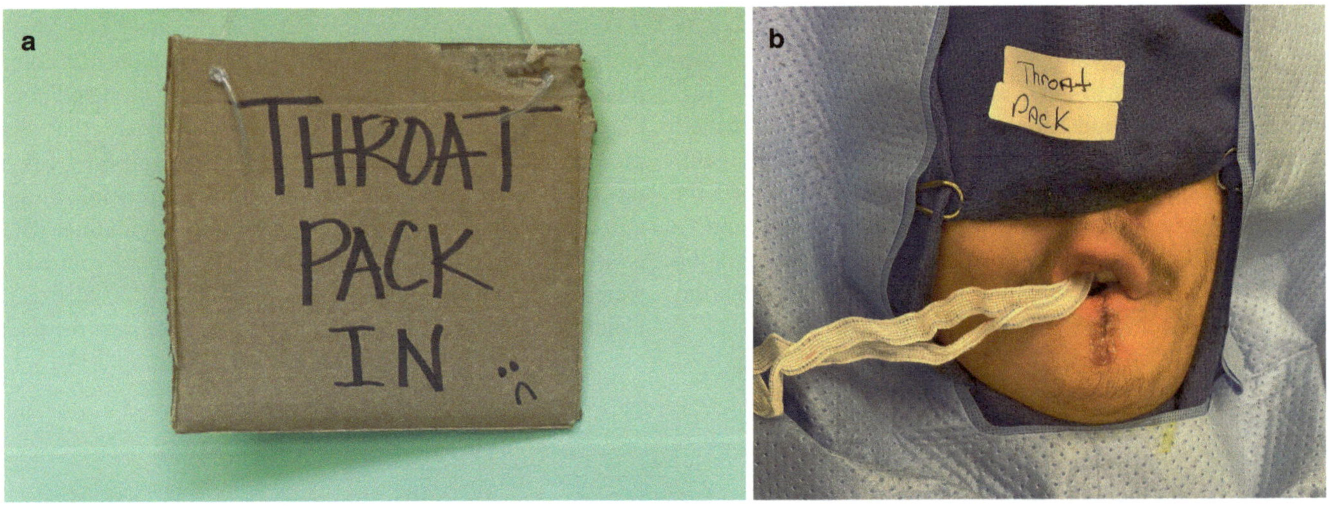


**Fig. 41.11** (**a**, **b**) "Throat pack in" sign (**a**) and sticker (**b**), which are left visible outside the patient as a reminder of the pack inside the patient

Global Smile Foundation

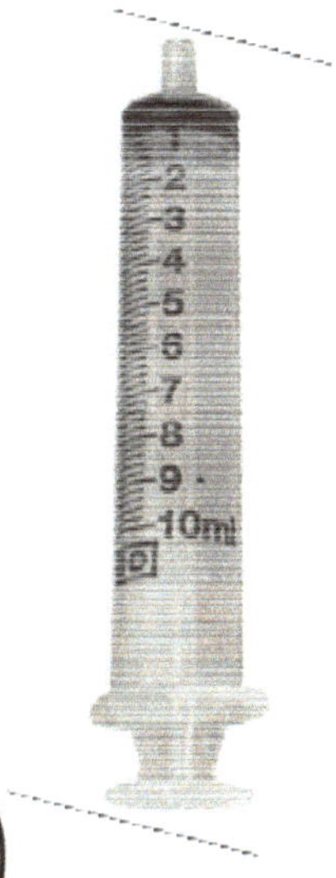


## How to Care forYour Child

**Name of Patient:** ________________________ **Allergies:**________________

**Give your child the antibiotic colored:**______________________

______________ **in the morning** **and**______________ **in the evening**

**for** _______ **days.**

**If pain medication is needed, use** ______________________ **every 4 hours (only if there is pain).**

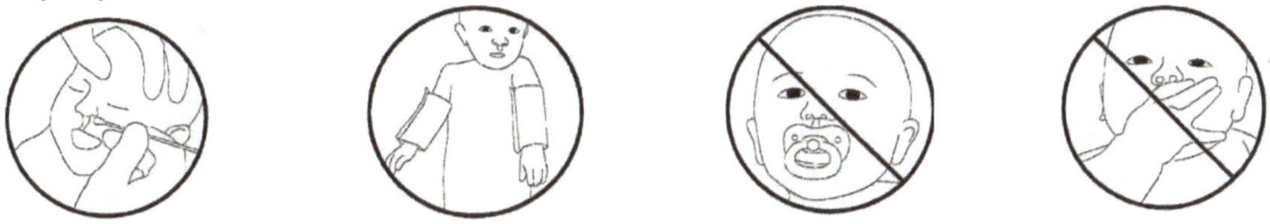

### Lip Care

- Keep lips clean and dry for 3 weeks.
- Use water to wipe your child's nose and lips
- Do not use pacifiers or bottles for 3 weeks (unless it is a specialty bottle provided by Global Smile)
- Do not allow your child to suck on anything for 3 weeks
- In 6 weeks, ___________, begin circular massage on the scar of the lip 5-6 times a day for 5-6 months

### Hands

• Do not allow your child to touch his mouth or nose for 3 weeks

• Use the braced immobilizers constantly during most of the day and night

• Allow your child to move his or her arm 3 times a day for 20 minutes. Watch your child carefully and do not allow your child to touch the mouth or nose during this time

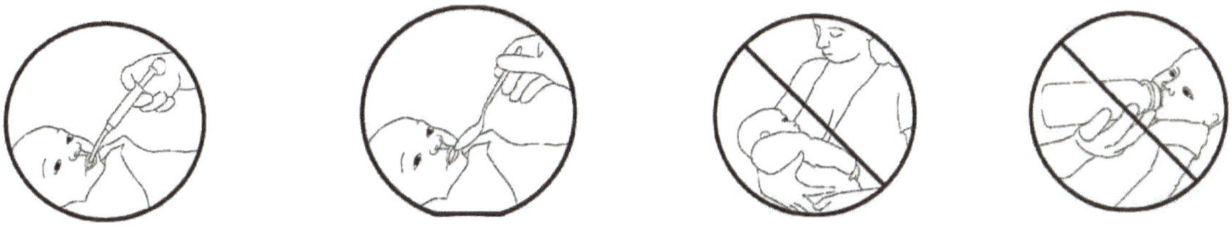

### Do Not Eat Solid Food for Two Weeks

• First day: milk, juice, soup

• For 3 weeks: milk, juice, soup, purees, creams, shakes, smoothies, yogurt.

### Feeding

• Use the syringe you are given in the hospital, a slightly inclined spoon, or a specialty bottle provided by Global Smile for 3 weeks

• Rinse your child's mouth with water after every meal

• Do not breast-feed your child for 3 weeks

### Oral Care

• Rinse your mouth with water after every meal.

• Brush your teeth gently on the outside once you are back home twice a day

• Gently wipe the tongue with a clean cloth after each meal

______________________

Return to the hospital on _____________ for the first post op check on __________________ and on _____________ for the second check with Dr. ____________________.

**** When to call for emergency ****

- **Heavy bleeding / bright red blood**
- **Difficulty breathing**
- **Unable to take food orally**

**Emergency Contact:** ______________________________________

**Parent/Guardian Signature:**__________________________________

**Date:**______________________________________________

**Fig. 41.12** Postoperative care instructions for families, utilizing pictorials storage, but the process of collecting and transferring patient information in a mission setting as part of clinical flow remains heavily dependent on paper charts for logistical and safety reasons (potential equipment failure, power outages, etc.).

Education can take many forms depending on the resources available [19]. Didactic activities during a mission can include lectures, conferences, or topical discussions among team members, local healthcare professionals and volunteers, families, or community representatives. Numerous foundations including GSF and Operation Smile have trained local surgeons by integrating them in their missions' workflow or by establishing visiting fellowships where surgeons receive training and go on to lead cleft teams in their home countries [7]. A 15-minute mini-lecture or "chalk talk" achieves three things simultaneously: it educates, it builds a sense of team, and it encourages team members to share ideas and learn from each other (Fig. 41.13).

Emerging technologies can be potentially leveraged to develop interactive educational opportunities. GSF has recently incorporated augmented reality (AR) proctoring into its cleft fellowship training model in Ecuador. Using AR software, laptop computers, and WiFi connection, GSF senior surgeons can remotely provide supervision and guidance to fellows across continental barriers during simulation-based practice including cleft repair markings and execution. Preliminary results are promising, and such technology offers innovative educational opportunities that promote graduated autonomy while delivering real-time expert feedback.

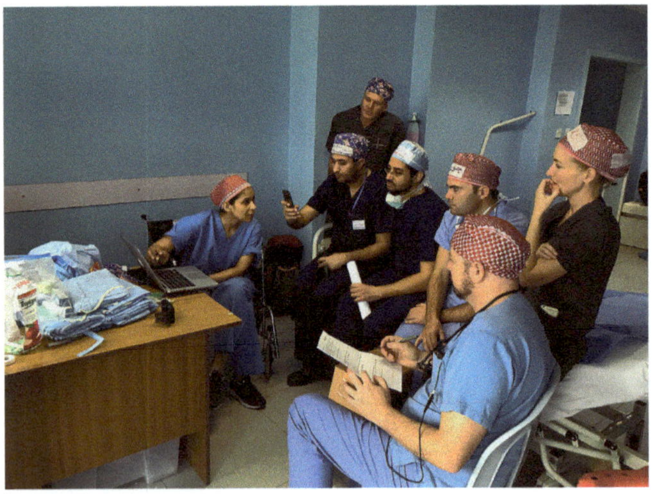

**Fig. 41.13** A cleft surgeon gives a "chalk talk" or mini-lecture on a surgical day

## Conclusion

All patients with clefts deserve the right to receive comprehensive cleft care by experienced caregivers irrespective of their socioeconomic backgrounds. Outreach programs and mission-based teams aim to address the need for such services in underserved communities throughout the world. Creating a culture of care and safety should be the guiding light for all healthcare providers treating patients with cleft lip and/or palate. Empowerment and sustainability initiatives are essential tools to support the transition from mission-based interventions to longitudinal care.

## References


1. Hunt O, Burden D, Hepper P, Johnston C. The psychosocial effects of cleft lip and palate: a systematic review. Eur J Orthod. 2005;27(3):274–85.
2. Hunt O, Burden D, Hepper P, Stevenson M, Johnston C. Self-reports of psychosocial functioning among children and young adults with cleft lip and palate. Cleft Palate Craniofac J. 2006;43(5):598–605.
3. Huijing MA, Marck KW, Combes J, et al. Facial reconstruction in the developing world: a complicated matter. Br J Oral Maxillofac Surg. 2011;49(4):292–6.
4. Fell MJ, Hoyle T, Abebe ME, et al. The impact of a single surgical intervention for patients with a cleft lip living in rural Ethiopia. J Plast Reconstr Aesthet Surg. 2014;67(9):1194–200.
5. McClenaghan F, Fell M, Martin D, Smith G, McGurk M. Surgical mission planning in the developing world. Int J Oral Maxillofac Surg. 2013;42(12):1587–91.
6. Association ACP-C. Standards of Approval for Team Care. 2016. https://acpa-cpf.org/team-care/standardscat/standards-of-approval-for-team-care/. Accessed 16 Feb 2019.
7. Jones CM, Campbell CA, Magee WP, Ayala R, Mackay DR. The expanding role of education and research in international healthcare. Ann Plast Surg. 2016;76(Suppl 3):S150–4.
8. Eberlin KR, Zaleski KL, Snyder HD. Hamdan US, medical missions for C. quality assurance guidelines for surgical outreach programs: a 20-year experience. Cleft Palate Craniofac J. 2008;45(3):246–55.
9. Patel KG, Eberlin KR, Vyas RM, Hamdan US. Use of safety measures, including the modified world health organization surgical safety checklist, during international outreach cleft missions. Cleft Palate Craniofac J. 2014;51(5):597–604.
10. Vyas RM, Eberlin KR, Hamdan US. Implementation of an emergency response protocol for overseas surgical outreach initiatives. Plast Reconstr Surg. 2013;131(4):631e–6e.
11. Tobias JD, Kim Y, Davis J. Anesthetic care in developing countries: equipment and techniques. South Med J. 2002;95(2):239–47.
12. Smoot EC 3rd, Johnson M, Graham DR, Draper GA. Operating safely in an underdeveloped country. Cleft Palate Craniofac J. 1992;29(5):444–50.
13. Eberlin KR, Vyas RM, Abi-Haidar Y, Sethna N, Hamdan US. Adult cleft lip repair under local anesthesia: an effective technique in resource-poor settings. Cleft Palate Craniofac J. 2013;50(1):59–63.

14. Haynes AB, Weiser TG, Berry WR, et al. A surgical safety checklist to reduce morbidity and mortality in a global population. N Engl J Med. 2009;360(5):491–9.
15. Semel ME, Resch S, Haynes AB, et al. Adopting a surgical safety checklist could save money and improve the quality of care in U.S. hospitals. Health Aff (Millwood). 2010;29(9):1593–9.
16. Weiser TG, Haynes AB, Dziekan G, et al. Effect of a 19-item surgical safety checklist during urgent operations in a global patient population. Ann Surg. 2010;251(5):976–80.
17. Borchard A, Schwappach DL, Barbir A, Bezzola P. A systematic review of the effectiveness, compliance, and critical factors for implementation of safety checklists in surgery. Ann Surg. 2012;256(6):925–33.
18. Fudickar A, Horle K, Wiltfang J, Bein B. The effect of the WHO surgical safety checklist on complication rate and communication. Dtsch Arztebl Int. 2012;109(42):695–701.
19. Kantar RS, Ramly EP, Almas F, et al. Sustainable cleft care through education: the first simulation-based comprehensive workshop in the Middle East and North Africa region. Cleft Palate Craniofac J. 2019;56(6):735–43.

# 42 Strengthening Surgical Systems Through Cleft Care

Eric Nagengast and William P. Magee III

## Introduction

The provision of cleft care in low-resource settings has seen massive improvements and innovation in the last half century as providers attempt to access all children while providing high-quality care. In attempts to understand the challenges to patients and practitioners, it is evident that the parts of the world with the greatest barriers to receiving and providing cleft care are also the areas with the weakest surgical health systems (Fig. 42.1) [1]. In order to provide sustainable solutions that secure safe, timely, and affordable care for all cleft patients, the surgical systems of low- and middle-income countries (LMICs) must be concomitantly strengthened. Just as cleft surgery has taken dramatic steps forward, so too has "global surgery" which seeks to improve health outcomes and equity for all people in need of surgical care [2]. By aligning the goals of cleft providers with the global surgery efforts, surgical systems can be strengthened to provide a foundation on which comprehensive cleft care can thrive.

## The Role of Surgery in a Health System

In 2008, Dr. Paul Farmer and Dr. Jim Kim declared surgery the "neglected stepchild of global health," pointing out the grave disparities in access to surgical care worldwide and the lack of prioritization of surgery in health plans [3]. Years passed without a coordinated effort to strengthen surgical care worldwide. In 2015, however, the importance of surgery was recognized on the world stage through three critical documents: The World Bank's Disease Control Priorities, Third Edition (DCP3) [4], the World Health Assembly's (WHA) Resolution 68.15 [5], and the Lancet Commission on Global Surgery's (LCOGS) "Global Surgery 2030" [6]. Long thought to be a luxury reserved for the wealthy, these three publications properly positioned surgery, in the words of Dr. Jim Kim – President of the World Bank, as an "indivisible, indispensable part of health care" [7].

DCP3 sets health priorities by using economic evaluation and global burden of disease data. The third edition is unique in that this is the first edition to contain an entire volume dedicated to surgery. The volume "Essential Surgery" identifies 44 surgical procedures (including cleft repair) that are cost-effective and implementable and treat a substantial burden of disease [4]. Universal access to these procedures could save 1.5 million lives annually. DCP3 illustrates safe surgical care is not a luxury reserved for the wealthy but rather a crucial component to any properly functioning healthcare system.

The WHA Resolution 68.15 "Strengthening Emergency and Essential Surgical Care and Anesthesia as a Component of Universal Health Coverage" called on all member states to identify and prioritize a package of essential surgical procedures [5]. Ratified unanimously, the resolution called for investments in workforce and monitoring and evaluation around essential surgery in order to integrate surgery into the primary health system.

The LCOGS estimated 5 billion people worldwide lack access to affordable, quality surgical care when needed [6]. The Commission also noted the dearth of surgical care is financially detrimental, projected to cost low- and middle-income countries (LMICs) $12.3 trillion in lost economic productivity through 2030. On the contrary, an investment of just $550 billion over this same period could scale surgical care to goal levels worldwide. As a way forward, the LCOGS proposed six metrics to monitor a surgical system and

E. Nagengast (✉)
Division of Plastic and Reconstructive Surgery, University of Southern California, Los Angeles, CA, USA
e-mail: eric.nagengast@med.usc.edu

W. P. Magee III
Division of Plastic and Reconstructive Surgery University of Southern California, Los Angeles, CA, USA

Division of Plastic and Maxillofacial Surgery, Children's Hospital Los Angeles, Los Angeles, CA, USA

Shriners Hospital for Children, Pasadena, CA, USA

© Springer Nature Switzerland AG 2021

J. W. Swanson, D. W. Low (eds.), *Global Cleft Care in Low-Resource Settings*, https://doi.org/10.1007/978-3-030-59105-2_42

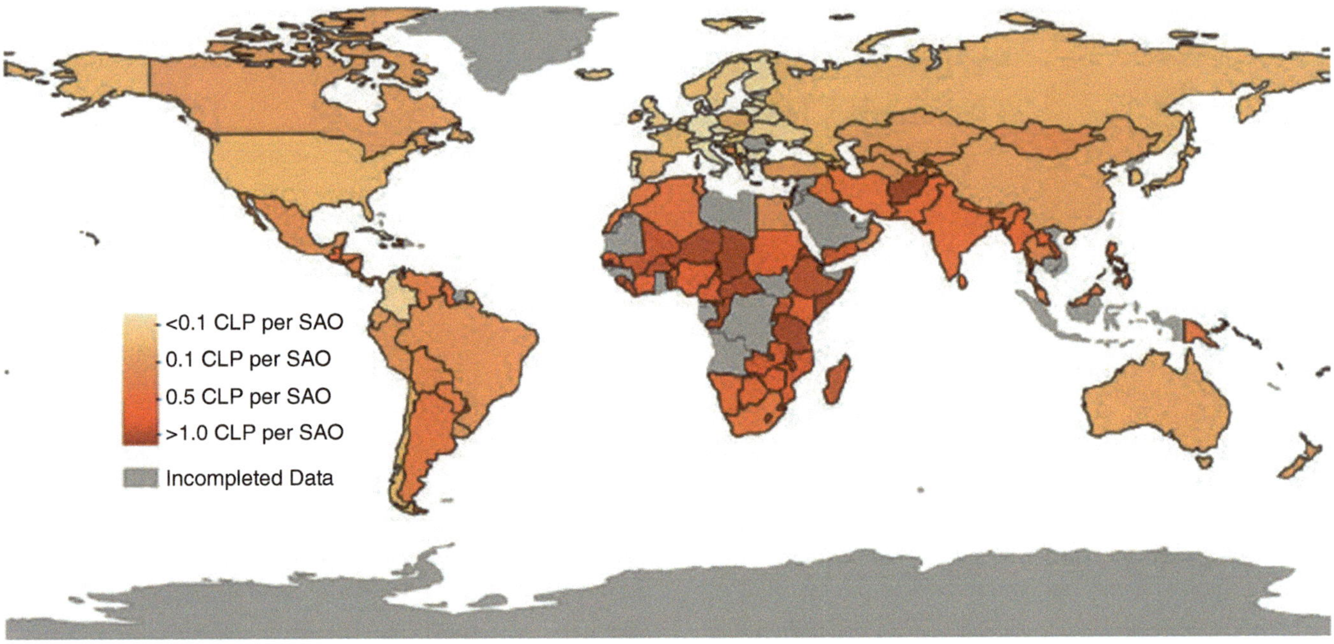


**Fig. 42.1** The estimated incidence of cleft lip and/or palate (CLP) per surgeon, anesthesiologist, and obstetrician (SAO) in each country. Darker red represents an increased ratio of newborns with CLP to members of the surgical workforce. (Reprinted by permission from Springer Nature: Springer International Publishing: Cleft Lip and Palate Treatment: A Comprehensive Guide by Massenburg et al. 2018 [1])

advised each country to create a national surgical, obstetric, and anesthesia plan (NSOAP). The NSOAP uses six key domains – service delivery, human resources, infrastructure, information management, finance, and governance (Fig. 42.2) – to outline a path to forward progress in surgical system strengthening. A number of countries have completed NSOAPs under this direction [8].

With the role of surgery recognized, the immense need defined, and a pathway forward, coordinated efforts between governments, international organizations, nongovernmental organizations (NGOs), the private sector, and care providers will be required to achieve success in the implementation of surgical system strengthening. Cleft providers and organizations have made significant contributions to the strength of current surgical systems. With a targeted effort, these providers and organizations can play a far more substantial role in strengthening surgical systems in the future.

## Strengthening of Surgical Systems Through Cleft Care

The image of a growing child with an unrepaired facial cleft is one of the most powerful examples of health disparity. Rarely seen in developed countries, this image is a reality in the poorest parts of the world [9]. These children catalyzed the birth of global initiatives in cleft and plastic surgery and drove the evolution from primarily service-based organizations to organizations with a lasting effect.

After World War II, traveling surgeons providing care in LMICs pioneered global plastic and reconstructive surgery [10–13]. At the same time, surgeons from around the world traveled to high-resource settings to receive training from select sites [14, 15]. Though small in number, pockets of reconstructive surgeons began to appear across the world. During this phase, dedicated surgeons developed notable plastic surgery hospitals including the Barsky Institute in Vietnam and Noordoff's work at Chang Gung Memorial Hospital in Taiwan [16–18]. These institutions required the surgeons to devote long periods of dedicated time spent away from their home. Many surgeons could not make such demanding commitments yet desired to use their skills to help patients with no alternative for care. In 1969, the first mission-based NGO, Interplast, was established [19].

The early surgical mission models in which medical teams travel with their supplies to a country for a short period of time in order to provide care are described as "vertical" interventions [20]. Vertical interventions address a specific health problem outside of the local health system [21]. As such, these interventions have limited effect on the local health system. Though many cleft NGOs still practice with a vertical model, many of the mission-based organizations recognized that missions alone could not match the global burden of disease [22]. Thus, groups adapted their goals to prioritize benefits for the local health systems by providing more integrated, longitudinal care [23–25]. Doing so developed more sustainable, "diagonal" programs that fortified the health system through cleft targeted interventions

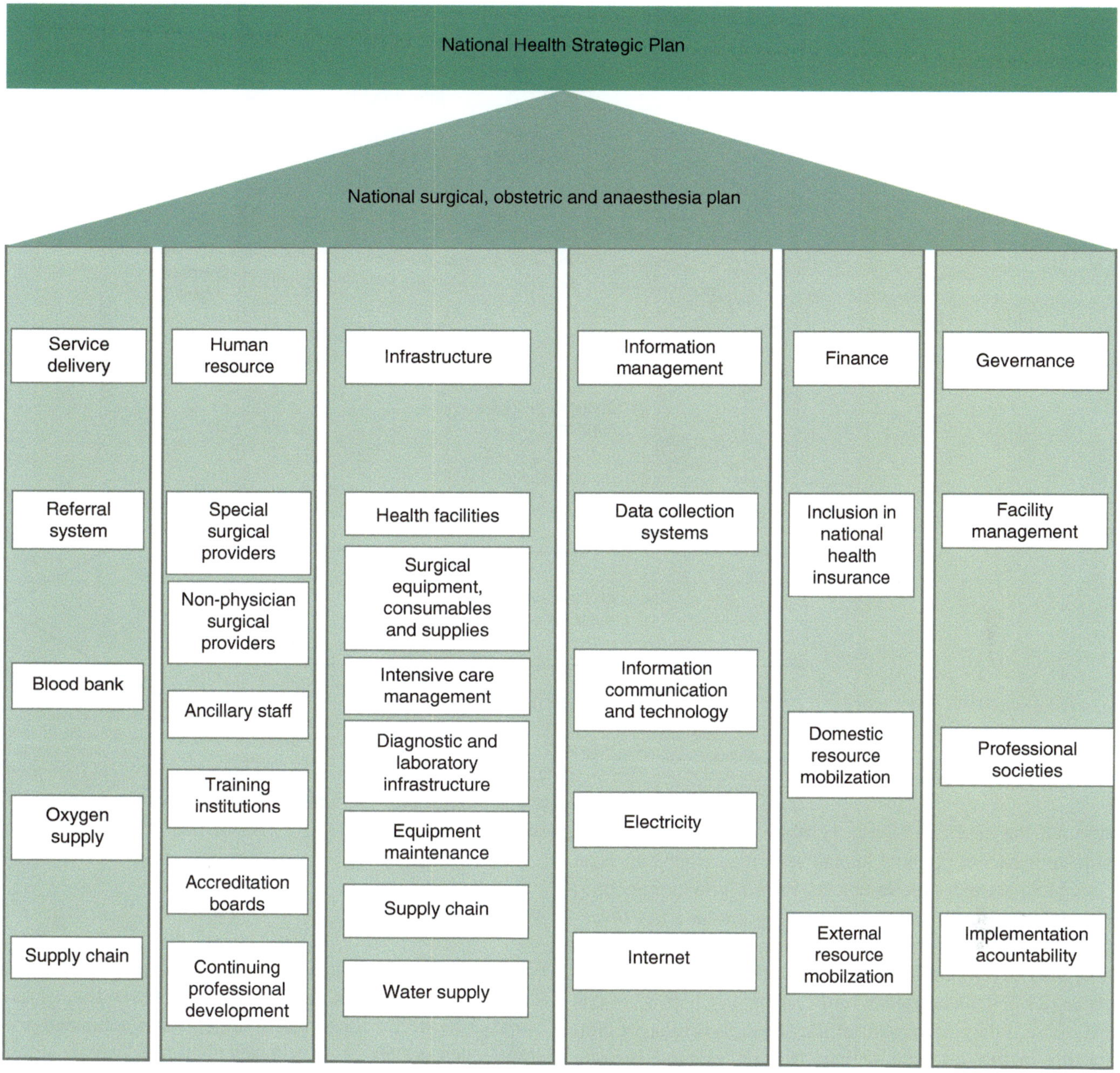


**Fig. 42.2** Modified national surgical obstetric and anesthesia plan framework from the Lancet Commission on Global Surgery [6]. (Reprinted by permission from John Wiley and Sons: British Journal of Surgery: Global surgery and the sustainable development goals by Roa et al. 2019 [57])

(Fig. 42.3) [20]. Through the diagonal approach, cleft organizations provide strength to the six domains of surgical systems: service delivery, human resources, infrastructure, information management, finance, and governance.

## Service Delivery

At the center of the mission of most of the cleft organizations is the provision of service to patients who would otherwise not receive care. Together cleft NGOs have provided care for millions of patients. Smile Train, for example, one of the largest cleft NGOs, has supported over one million cleft operations [26]. Services provided are not limited to surgery alone. Since 2011, Operation Smile has provided more than 600,000 care consultations at their comprehensive care centers across the world [27]. Service delivery requires a multitude of supporting factors that are crucial to a strong health system including supply chain management and a patient recruitment and referral system. Once these systems are in place, they can be expanded to cover more health systems and more disease processes. Acts of service are the driver that bring people together and promote the concomitant strengthening of the other surgical domains.

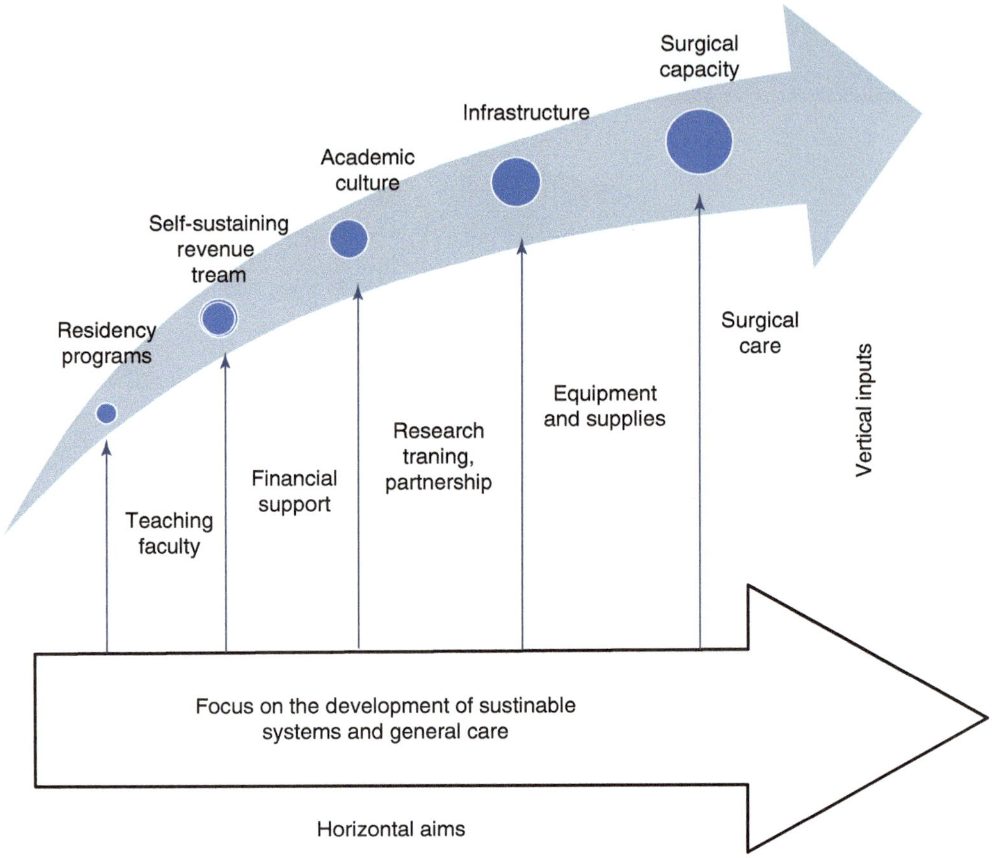


**Fig. 42.3** A diagonal approach harnesses the power of horizontal aims and vertical outputs. (Reprinted with permission from Hindawi: Plastic Surgery International: An Opportunity for Diagonal Development in Global Surgery: Cleft Lip and Palate Care in Resource-Limited Settings by Patel et al. 2012 [20])

## Human Resources

Through the service delivery platform, cleft organizations built up immense pools of human resources around surgical care. Most started with volunteers from high-income countries but later implemented training programs as a key objective [18]. Much of the training is informal, but providers have also developed formalized cleft surgeon training programs [28, 29]. Discussed in further detail in Chap. 35 of this text, these training programs utilize the high volume of cleft patients in low-resource settings to train existing surgical providers to perform cleft surgery. Organizations have also trained non-surgeons including therapists, anesthesiologists, nutritionists, medical records, biomedical technicians, nurses, community health workers, child life specialists, sterile processing, and patient coordinators [30–37]. After receiving training, many locals are hired to full-time positions contributing to a sustained health workforce [38].The globalized volunteers have not allowed for adaptations to the mission model. Local missions, utilized in Latin America and Southeast Asia, in which surgical teams from urban centers travel to rural, underserved areas, offer a practical solution for providing elective surgical care in rural areas. As seen in the aftermath of the Haitian earthquake, when natural disasters strike, the global volunteer pool can be leveraged in a similar fashion to a surgical mission to create surgical teams able to provide a number of emergency and essential surgical services [39].

## Infrastructure

Functional anesthetic and surgical equipment, as well as a safe physical space with adequate electricity and water, are essential for performing quality surgery. Self-contained programs, such as ship- or truck-based platforms, operate autonomously and are appropriate for austere environments [40]. Mission-based care subsidizes inadequacies by bringing necessary supplies and equipment. For providers to continuously provide quality care, organizations must make investments in retained infrastructure. Many organizations form partnership models in which funds go to supporting local facilities. Smile Train, for example, conducts on-site visits of partner organizations to assess the equipment necessary to operate by their standards [41]. Operation Smile invests in comprehensive care centers and operating rooms [25]. A number of organizations donate unused or reusable equipment and supplies after a mission. Much of this infrastructure and equipment is shared across surgical specialties.

## Information Management

Information management is one of the most overlooked segments of global health. The majority of low-resource settings have primitive medical record systems. This is problematic for patient safety, continuity of care, and quality improvement. Many cleft organizations provide their partner hospitals with medical record systems. One of the first cleft organizations to do so, in 2005 Operation Smile implemented an electronic record system to track patient data [9, 22]. Smile Train followed suit shortly thereafter [42]. As part of their quality standards, Smile Train requests partners to collect and share data [41]. Using the data for outcomes evaluations, cost-effectiveness analysis, and other scientific publications contributes to the local health systems and supports the need for further expansion of surgical programs [43–49].

## Finance

The many inputs needed for surgical care (providers, equipment and infrastructure, consumables) require substantial initial investments. The financial barriers to receiving care borne by patients extend far beyond the provision of surgery itself [50–52].Through media coverage and marketing campaigns, cleft NGOs have shed light on the global need for surgical care. As a testament to the attention cleft organizations have drawn to the global need for investing in surgical care, one quarter of the resources for surgery raised by NGOs comes through cleft organizations [53, 54]. Just as importantly, these funds have been spent in cost-effective ways, making the case for investing in surgery [43, 47–49, 55] (Fig. 42.4).

## Governance

Coordinated surgical systems require governance and leadership. Cleft organizations have worked with ministries of health to target priorities for providing care within local health systems. Through relationship building, cleft organizations have orchestrated public-private partnerships, NGO-NGO partnerships, and university partnerships to arrange for many of the surgical system strengthening pieces above. It is no surprise a number of the commissioners and contributors to the Lancet Commission on Global Surgery, DCP3, and the G4 alliance are cleft providers. History has taught us that team building, partnerships, and investments in local champions are necessary for large-scale success. Long-term expe-

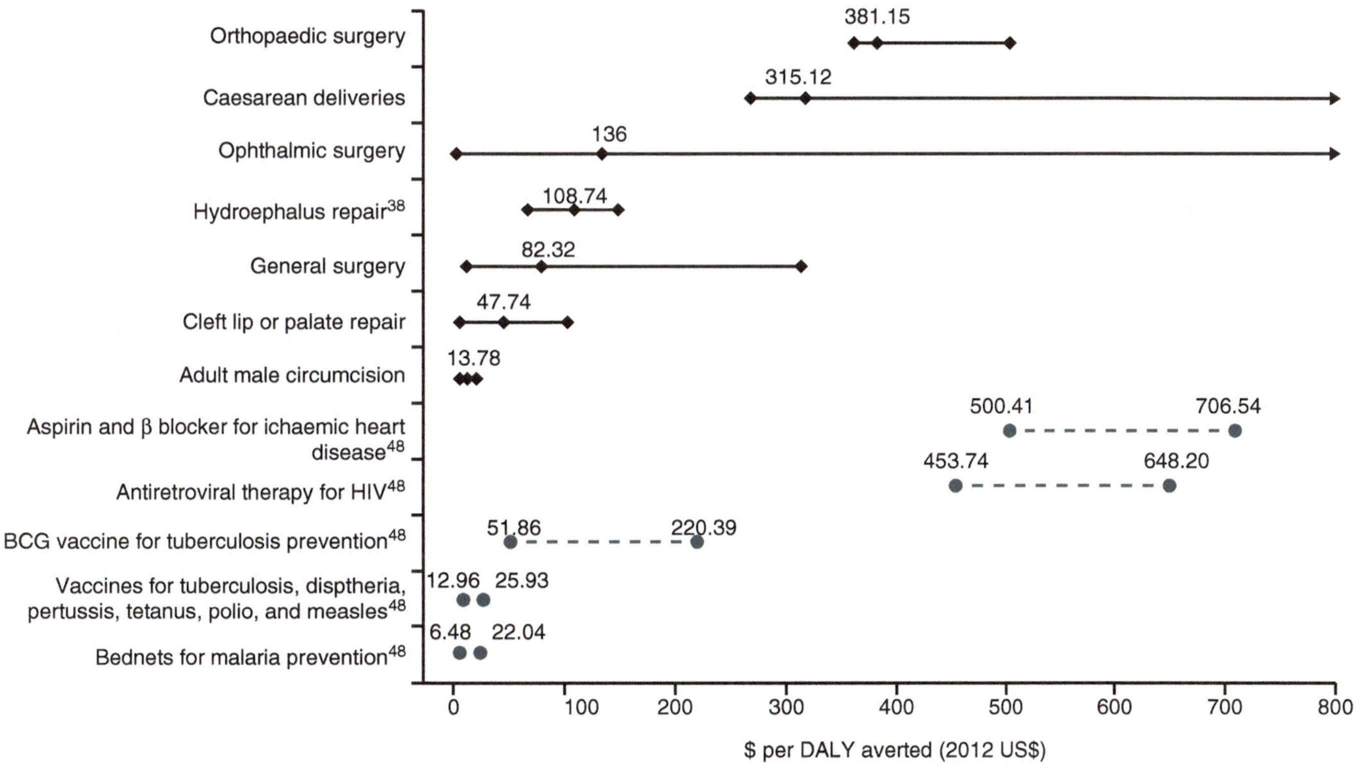


**Fig. 42.4** Surgery versus other public health interventions. Data points are medians; error bars are range. The diamonds and solid lines are for surgical interventions; circles and dashed lines are for other public health interventions. (Reprinted with permission from Elsevier: The Lancet Global Health: Cost-effectiveness of surgery and its policy implications for global health: a systematic review and analysis by Chao et al. 2014 [55])

riences in the provision of surgical care in low-resource settings are extremely valuable when orchestrating surgical efforts.

## Future Directions/Call for Action

### Overview

Adopted in 2015, the Sustainable Development Goals (SDGs) outline 17 goals necessary for ensuring peace and prosperity for all people [56]. By 2030, the SDGs aim to reduce disparity, protect the planet, and create sustainable economic growth. At least 8 of the 17 goals – including good health and well-being, gender equality, elimination of poverty, economic growth, and reducing inequalities between and among countries – will not be reached without drastic improvements in surgical systems [57]. These lofty, yet achievable goals will require partnership, leadership, and a strategic plan for universal health coverage. Cleft providers are uniquely positioned with prior experience and leadership to spearhead the strengthening of surgical systems necessary to reach universal health coverage and sustainable development.

Without cleft surgery it is estimated that the vast majority of children born with orofacial clefts in certain LMIC settings will die prematurely [58]. By 2030, a child's birthplace should not determine the health services available to him or her. Children everywhere deserve equitable access to patient-centered, comprehensive, and complete care. This means access to the same specialists and the procedures with the same level of quality. This is as true for cleft as any disease.

With these goals in mind, the traditional surgical mission model cannot be the solution for the future. Not only have surgical missions been shown to have increased rates of surgical complications compared to health system-based care [46, 59], surgical missions do not always allow for timely care, and they do not permit continuity of care [45]. Certainly, parts of our world have no alternative care or have a disease burden that vastly overwhelms the capabilities of the local health system. For these regions, surgical missions will continue to play a vital role in the provision of surgical care. But, as health systems improve, the role of the surgical mission will concomitantly fade.

The goal of all cleft providers should be investments in sustainable programs in order to transition to comprehensive models of care designed to fit the local context. In such an environment, patients have continuous access to a full spectrum of health professionals. International partnerships and NGOs will play an imperative role in the transition through coordinated efforts in service, workforce training, financing, infrastructure, information management, and governance.

Optimal cleft care, however, cannot exist within a crumbling health system nor should it. Global surgical systems need to be strengthened to provide a foundation for all surgical care. Cleft care is only a small portion of essential surgical care. Universal health coverage for essential surgery consists of three aspects: range of services covered, quality, and access to care (Fig. 42.5). While the essential surgeries

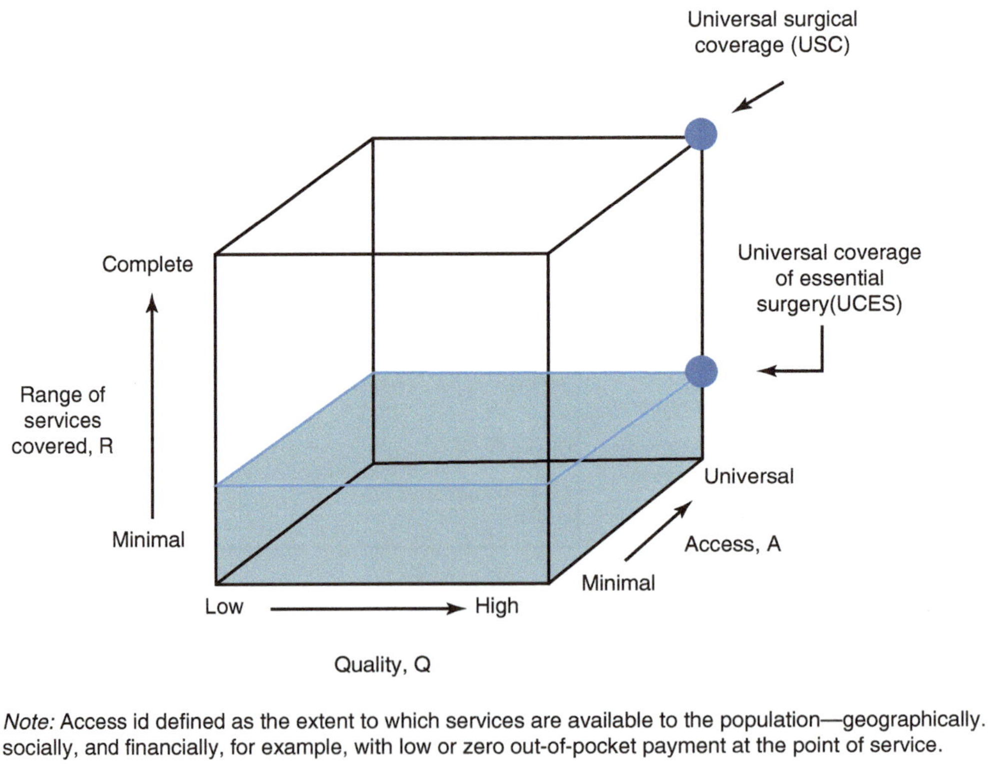


**Fig. 42.5** Dimensions of Universal Health Coverage of Essential Surgery. (Reprinted from Debas HT: Donkor P: Gawande A: Jamison DT: Kruk ME: Mock CN: 2015 *Essential Surgery: Disease Control Priorities, third edition, volume 1*. © World Bank [4])

list includes cleft care and a number of dental procedures, aside from these, cleft organizations are unlikely to greatly increase the range of surgical services offered. However, cleft providers' history of delivering high-quality care to those most in need positions them to contribute on a large scale to quality of and access to surgery.

## Quality of Care

Quality of care is defined by the WHO as "the degree to which health services for individuals and populations increase the likelihood of desired health outcomes and are consistent with current professional knowledge" [60, 61], and quality health service delivery includes seven facets: safety, equity, effectiveness, integration, people-centeredness, timeliness, and efficiency (Fig. 42.6). Poor-quality care wastes resources and causes distrust in the health system. All health systems have room to improve on quality, as a significant portion of the burden of disease worldwide is due to adverse events [62]. In fact, it is estimated that more people die within 30 days of surgery worldwide than die from HIV, malaria, and tuberculosis combined, and many of these deaths are preventable [63]. Improvements in surgical quality will greatly strengthen health systems in LMICs.

Adopting minimum standards and requirements around the provision of care can majorly impact safety, equity, and effectiveness of care [60]. Implementation of the WHO Surgical Safety Checklist significantly decreased surgical complications and mortality in LMICs as well as high-income countries [64]. Such standards improve the quality of surgery regardless of the procedure or specialty. For many cleft organizations, safety standards already exist. Therefore, cleft providers should work with ministries of health and other local stakeholders to develop and implement standards in all countries in which they work. Cleft organizations should also train and supervise local healthcare providers on the standards of care. To incentivize the adoption and implementation of standards of care, organizations may offer hospitals or surgical centers a form of accreditation when they achieve the standards.

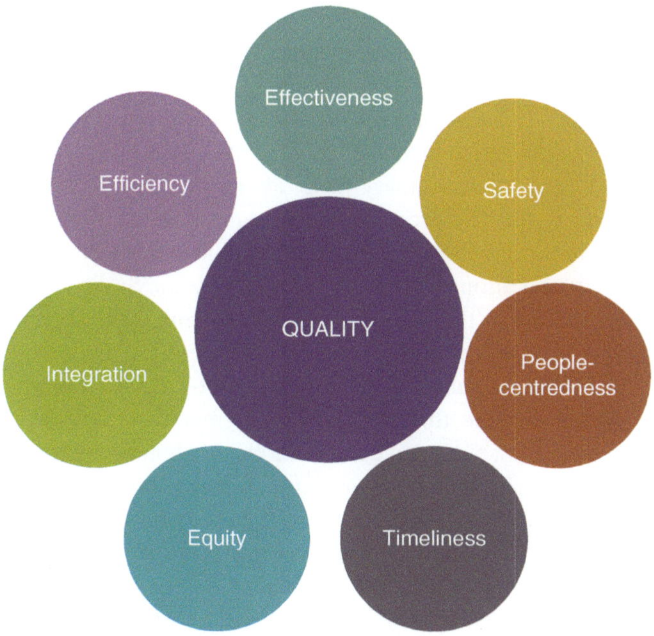


**Fig. 42.6** Elements of health care quality. (Reprinted from Delivering Quality Health Services: A Global Imperative, World Health Organization Copyright (2018) [60])

Few surgical conditions are treated as longitudinally as a facial cleft. Prior experience in multidisciplinary, comprehensive care puts cleft organizations in a unique position to improve integration, effectiveness, timeliness, efficiency, and people-centeredness of health systems. Cleft organizations should work to train ancillary providers such as nutritionists, therapists, and community health workers. Such roles transcend surgical specialty and drive many aspects of quality of care. Cleft providers can also work with ministries of health and other surgical specialties to discern the most effective way to integrate multidisciplinary care teams into the surgical system.

In order to quantify changes in quality of care, improvements must be made in monitoring and evaluation. Too little is currently invested in information systems, especially in LMICs where less than 1% of health expenditures is directed toward data management [65]. Cleft providers should strive for integrated information management systems that allow for longitudinal tracking across specialties. These systems should be shared with and integrated into the local health systems. At minimum, all surgical providers should be collecting data in line with the surgical metrics of the Lancet Commission on Global Surgery [6]. But, to best drive quality improvement, data must also be collected and analyzed on processes and outcomes. Complete and accurate collection of data should be rewarded regardless of the findings. It is imperative that negative outcomes and adverse events not be punished but instead used to impact change and improve quality of care. Providers with sophisticated collection and usage of data will be better positioned to drive quality improvements and improve access to surgical care.

## Access to Care

Access to care is categorized by acceptability or willingness to seek care, physical access, and financial access [66]. All three branches of access to care must be addressed concomitantly to maximize usage of care. Cleft patients, long recognized as vulnerable, have generated much focus to mitigate barriers across all three domains; many of these insights can be applied more broadly across surgical conditions.

If patients in need are unwilling to seek care, the health system is not serving the community appropriately. People are more likely to use a system when they expect a good outcome; improvements in quality will thus improve acceptability. Patient recruitment is also important. Community health workers are proven to be a cost-effective way of accessing and educating patients [67]. Training community health workers to recognize common surgical diseases and guide patients to surgical care will improve overall acceptability.

Using patient, provider, and hospital data, strategic programs should be deployed in line with the local NSOAP and the needs of the health system to improve physical access to surgery. Future efforts should focus on training providers, infrastructure investment, and supply chain management to ensure quality essential equipment and medicines. The most important of these is likely the training of providers as human resources may overcome the shortfalls in infrastructure and equipment, but the opposite is not true. The greatest strength of cleft organizations is the enormous volunteer pool. These volunteers are used to fill gaps in service delivery, but they should also be leveraged as global educators. Cleft organizations have shown promise in training surgeons to perform cleft surgery [28], but there is also a dire need for nonsurgical training, including anesthetists, therapists, nutritionists, nursing, community health workers, biomedical technicians, and more. Through synergistic partnerships with local universities, innovation in education can be achieved by producing programs that effectively utilize the global volunteer pool as formal educators.

Cleft organizations have set up operating rooms in the most isolated regions of the world. Building off of this experience, efforts should be directed to create lasting and sustainable infrastructure in areas of need. Locations in which any surgical NGOs work should be equipped to function with essential equipment and infrastructure to carry out safe surgery year long.

Access to surgery in much of the world is most limited by cost. Worldwide surgical services are grossly underfunded, and a massive increase in investment is needed to reach universal health coverage. Cleft organizations have been extremely successful in raising funds for surgical efforts [53], largely from private donors. If large-scale investments in surgical systems are to be made, new sources of funding must be secured. Since 2015, surgery has become recognized as an important part of a health system, and more sophisticated donors are entering the space. Targeting and marketing programs toward the strengthening of surgical systems will be necessary to gain support from formalized global health funds such as the Gates Foundation, USAID, or the Department for International Development (DFID). Still, more partners are needed. Many of the world's largest corporations are increasing philanthropic campaigns. Corporate philanthropic involvement will not only increase funding for surgery but may also bring specialized expertise valuable for global surgical efforts and innovation. Organizations that collect and utilize data well and are able to show impact in surgical system strengthening will be best positioned to secure these new sources of capital.

**Solutions from the Field:** ***Surgery for the People*** **in Nicaragua**

In Nicaragua, a collaboration between the Ministry of Health (MoH) and Operation Smile has sought to expand a partnership focused on cleft surgery to broader surgical care improvement in rural district hospitals. Since 1994, Operation Smile Nicaragua's model has evolved from international missions to a primarily local volunteer base conducting local missions to, more recently, a comprehensive cleft center. Much of this work has been in close collaboration with the Nicaraguan MoH including shared cleft patient referral and registry processes, shared clinicians, and surgical care in public hospitals. The Nicaraguan government announced its prioritization of access to surgery at the 2015 UN General Assembly, creating a political environment conducive to expansion of services in the field. Operation Smile sought to train all 1200 perioperative physicians, nurses, and technicians in Nicaragua in resuscitation – basic and advanced life support, including pediatric advanced life support – and succeeded in reaching more than 90% of eligible staff in 2016.

In 2017, the *Surgery for the People* pilot program was launched to increase access to and impact of surgical care at two primary hospitals in rural Las Minas, Nicaragua. The program has brought a "surgical ecosystem perspective" to these district hospitals through a collaboration with the MoH and Operation Smile and supported by the UBS Optimus Foundation. Las Minas is well known to the Operation Smile staff through cleft patient outreach: its population of 250,000 needs to travel more than 8–12 hours to reach the nearest regional hospital, and current surgical volume per population is at 20% of the minimum goal volume based on LCOGS thresholds. There are numerous critical inputs to an optimally functioning surgical "ecosystem" – often categorized as the "4 Ss": staff, space, stuff, and systems. Safe surgery requires that all 4 Ss be present at the same time – the absence of one, for instance, a functioning autoclave or clean water, can be rate limiting. The 4 Ss represent the "supply side" of the equation. Often overlooked is the "demand side" – the patient – who, in such environments, often faces substantial and complex barriers to care. The program's patient-centric view reveals critical surgical ecosystem components that transcend the operating room. A functioning surgical ecosystem includes components such as community health workers to identify and follow-up patients and a biomedical technician program to rehabilitate essential equipment.

The program has built and upgraded operating rooms, implemented appropriate equipment such as the Arbutus orthopedic drill and Gradian Universal Anesthesia Machine, and brought new systems through collaborations with partners such as the Global Initiative for Children's Surgery, Panamerican Trauma Society, and Lifebox. Importantly, students and faculty of the local Las Minas University have provided critical workforce and talent and through internships have developed skills in research. These local investments fit with the core mission of building durable capacity, which may in the future help alleviate ongoing challenges such as anesthesia provider migration. The program legacy will hopefully surpass surgery: once a hospital can more effectively deliver surgery, it can more appropriately treat a full spectrum of disease processes. Preliminary findings show a 20–40% increase in surgical volume as well as improved patient safety and satisfaction, but certain challenges such as anesthesia workforce constraints persist.

## Conclusion

Surgical systems require more infrastructure and human resources than most of medical care, which until recently has left surgery largely forgotten in global health. In order to reduce the global disparity and secure the economic prosperity targeted by the SDGs, substantial strides must be taken toward universal health coverage for surgical care. This monumental undertaking will require cooperation and partnerships between NGOs, governments, donors, corporations, and healthcare providers. Cleft organizations have substantially contributed to surgical systems of LMICs through service delivery, cultivating relationships, and building local and international leaders. The past experiences of cleft providers should be a foundation and a catalyst for the future surgical system strengthening needed to ensure a sustainable and prosperous future for all people. By focusing on improving quality of and access to surgical care, cleft providers can align their goals with global surgery efforts to strengthen surgical systems building a framework in which comprehensive cleft care can thrive.

## References


1. Massenburg BB, Riesel JN, Hughes CD, Meara JG. Global cleft lip and palate care: a brief review. In: Alonso N, Raposo-Amaral CE, editors. Cleft lip and palate treatment: a comprehensive guide. Cham: Springer International Publishing; 2018. p. 15–23.
2. Dare AJ, Grimes CE, Gillies R, Greenberg SL, Hagander L, Meara JG, et al. Global surgery: defining an emerging global health field. Lancet (London, England). 2014;384(9961):2245–7. https://doi.org/10.1016/s0140-6736(14)60237-3.
3. Farmer PE, Kim JY. Surgery and global health: a view from beyond the OR. World J Surg. 2008;32(4):533–6. https://doi.org/10.1007/s00268-008-9525-9.
4. Debas HT, Donkor P, Gawande A, Jamison DT, Kruk ME, Mock CN. Essential surgery: disease control priorities, vol. 1. 3rd ed. Washington, D.C.: World Bank; 2015.
5. Sixty-Eighth World Health Assembly. WHA Resolution 68·15 – Strengthening Emergency and Essential Surgical Care and Anaesthesia as a Component of Universal Health Coverage. 2015.
6. Meara JG, Leather AJ, Hagander L, Alkire BC, Alonso N, Ameh EA, et al. Global surgery 2030: evidence and solutions for achieving health, welfare, and economic development. Lancet (London, England). 2015;386(9993):569–624. https://doi.org/10.1016/s0140-6736(15)60160-x.
7. The World Bank. Transcript of recorded video remarks by Jim Yong Kim, President of the World Bank Group, to the Lancet Commission on Global Surgery, January 17, 2014. 2014. http://www.globalsurgery.info/wp-content/uploads/2014/01/Jim-Kim-Global-Surgery-Transcribed.pdf.
8. Citron I, Jumbam D, Dahm J, Mukhopadhyay S, Nyberger K, Iverson K, et al. Towards equitable surgical systems: development and outcomes of a national surgical, obstetric and anaesthesia plan in Tanzania. BMJ Glob Health. 2019;4(2):e001282. https://doi.org/10.1136/bmjgh-2018-001282.
9. McQueen KA, Magee W, Crabtree T, Romano C, Burkle FM Jr. Application of outcome measures in international humanitarian aid: comparing indices through retrospective analysis of corrective surgical care cases. Prehosp Disaster Med. 2009;24(1):39–46.
10. Hughes CD, Alkire B, Martin C, Semer N, Meara JG. American plastic surgery and global health: a brief history. Ann Plast Surg. 2012;68(2):222–5. https://doi.org/10.1097/SAP.0b013e318209a5e8.
11. Adenwalla HS, Narayanan PV, Rajshree CJ. The history and evolution of cleft surgery in India. Indian J Plast Surg. 2005;38(2):188–91. https://doi.org/10.4103/0970-0358.19798.
12. Stark RB. The export of plastic surgical training programs to emerging countries. Plast Reconstr Surg. 1967;39(6):541–8.
13. Rees TD, Raassen T, Wachira J, Mustafa O, Adams-Ray B. The flying doctors of east Africa. Bull Am Coll Surg. 1994;79(10):12–20.
14. Rautio J, Somer M, Pettay M, Klockars T, Elfving-Little U, Holtta E, et al. Treatment of cleft lip and palate in Finland. Duodecim; laaketieteellinen aikakauskirja. 2010;126(11):1286–94.
15. Saman M. In memoriam: Fernando Ortiz Monasterio, MD (1923–2012). JAMA Facial Plast Surg. 2014;16(1):69–70. https://doi.org/10.1001/jamafacial.2013.1321.
16. Barsky AJ. Establishing a plastic surgical unit in South Vietnam. Plast Reconstr Surg. 1970;45(5):431–4.
17. Snyder P. Remembering M. Samuel Noordhoff MD, 1927–2018, whose impact was felt worldwide. American Society of Plastic Surgeons. 2018. https://www.plasticsurgery.org/for-medical-professionals/resources-and-education/publications/psn-extra/news/remembering-m-samuel-noordhoff-md-1927-2018-whose-impact-was-felt-worldwide. Accessed 10 Mar 2019.
18. Goh RC, Wang R, Chen PK, Lo LJ, Chen YR. Strategies for achieving long-term effective outcome in cleft missions: the

Noordhoff Craniofacial Foundation and Chang Gung Memorial Hospital. J Craniofac Surg. 2009;20(Suppl 2):1657–60. https://doi.org/10.1097/SCS.0b013e3181b2d5fb.
19. Laub DR. Humanitarianism in plastic surgery. Ann Plast Surg. 1981;7(2):99–101.
20. Patel PB, Hoyler M, Maine R, Hughes CD, Hagander L, Meara JG. An opportunity for diagonal development in global surgery: cleft lip and palate care in resource-limited settings. Plast Surg Int. 2012;2012:892437. https://doi.org/10.1155/2012/892437.
21. Msuya J. Horizontal and vertical delivery of health services : what are the trade offs. Washington, D.C.: World Bank; 2003. http://documents.worldbank.org/curated/en/914491468761944686/Horizontal-and-vertical-delivery-of-health-services-what-are-the-trade-offs.
22. Patel PS, Chung KY, Kasrai L. Innovate global plastic and reconstructive surgery: cleft lip and palate charity database. J Craniofac Surg. 2018;29(4):937–42. https://doi.org/10.1097/scs.0000000000004374.
23. Roldan JC, Pape HD, Koch H, Koller M. Ten-year cleft surgery in Nepal: achievements and lessons learned for better cleft care abroad. Plast Reconstr Surg Glob Open. 2016;4(5):e711. https://doi.org/10.1097/gox.0000000000000702.
24. Jones CM, Campbell CA, Magee WP, Ayala R, Mackay DR. The expanding role of education and research in international healthcare. Ann Plast Surg. 2016;76(Suppl 3):S150–4. https://doi.org/10.1097/sap.0000000000000721.
25. Magee WP, Raimondi HM, Beers M, Koech MC. Effectiveness of international surgical program model to build local sustainability. Plast Surg Int. 2012;2012:185725. https://doi.org/10.1155/2012/185725.
26. Smile Train. 2019.
27. Ruben Ayala CMOOS. Re: number of surgeries performed. electronic mail ed2019.
28. McCullough M, Campbell A, Siu A, Durnwald L, Kumar S, Magee WP 3rd, et al. Competency-based education in low resource settings: development of a novel surgical training program. World J Surg. 2018;42(3):646–51. https://doi.org/10.1007/s00268-017-4205-2.
29. Nagengast ES, Campbell A, Restrepo C, Munabi NCO, McCullough M, Deshpande G, et al. Reverse innovation in surgical education: subspecialty training in a low-resource setting. 2019.
30. Fast O, Fast C, Fast D, Veltjens S, Salami Z, White MC. Limited sterile processing capabilities for safe surgery in low-income and middle-income countries: experience in the republic of Congo, Madagascar and Benin. BMJ Glob Health. 2017;2(Suppl 4):e000428. https://doi.org/10.1136/bmjgh-2017-000428.
31. White MC, Peterschmidt J, Callahan J, Fitzgerald JE, Close KL. Interval follow up of a 4-day pilot program to implement the WHO surgical safety checklist at a Congolese hospital. Glob Health. 2017;13(1):42. https://doi.org/10.1186/s12992-017-0266-0.
32. White M, Close K. Lasting impact: insights from a surgical mission-based mentoring training programme in the republic of Congo. BMJ Glob Health. 2016;1(3):e000102. https://doi.org/10.1136/bmjgh-2016-000102.
33. Mercy Ships. Mentoring. https://www.mercyships.org/surgeries-more/mentoring/. Accessed 10 Mar 2019.
34. Operation Smile. Saving lives through education 2019. https://www.operationsmile.org/saving-lives-through-education. Accessed 10 Mar 2019.
35. O'Brien L, Hardman A. Developing hand therapy skills in Bangladesh: experiences of Australian volunteers. J Hand Ther. 2014;27(1):30–7. https://doi.org/10.1016/j.jht.2013.09.006.
36. Silinzieds A, Simmons L, Edward KL, Mills C. Nurse education in developing countries–Australian plastics and microsurgical nurses in Nepal. Plastic Surg Nurs. 2012;32(4):148–55. https://doi.org/10.1097/PSN.0b013e3182728267.
37. Campbell A, Restrepo C, Mackay D, Sherman R, Varma A, Ayala R, et al. Scalable, sustainable cost-effective surgical care: a model for safety and quality in the developing world, part III: impact and sustainability. J Craniofac Surg. 2014;25(5):1685–9. https://doi.org/10.1097/scs.0000000000001207.
38. Nagengast ES, Caterson EJ, Magee WP Jr, Hatcher K, Ramos MS, Campbell A. Providing more than health care: the dynamics of humanitarian surgery efforts on the local microeconomy. J Craniofac Surg. 2014;25(5):1622–5. https://doi.org/10.1097/scs.0000000000001133.
39. Operation Smile. Haiti. 2019. https://www.operationsmile.org/content/haiti. Accessed 14 Mar 2019.
40. Mercy Ships. Change Lives. Restore Joy. 2019. https://www.mercyships.org.
41. Braun TL, Louis MR, Dickey RM, Buchanan EP. A sustainable and scalable approach to the provision of cleft care: a focus on safety and quality. Plast Reconstr Surg. 2018;142(2):463–9. https://doi.org/10.1097/prs.0000000000004580.
42. Patil SB, Kale SM, Khare N, Math M, Jaiswal S, Jain A. Changing patterns in demography of cleft lip-cleft palate deformities in a developing country: the Smile Train effect–what lies ahead? Plast Reconstr Surg. 2011;127(1):327–32. https://doi.org/10.1097/PRS.0b013e3181f95b9c.
43. Hackenberg B, Ramos MS, Campbell A, Resch S, Finlayson SR, Sarma H, et al. Measuring and comparing the cost-effectiveness of surgical care delivery in low-resource settings: cleft lip and palate as a model. J Craniofac Surg. 2015;26(4):1121–5. https://doi.org/10.1097/scs.0000000000001829.
44. Hamze H, Mengiste A, Carter J. The impact and cost-effectiveness of the Amref Health Africa-Smile train cleft lip and palate surgical repair programme in eastern and Central Africa. Pan Afr Med J. 2017;28:35. https://doi.org/10.11604/pamj.2017.28.35.10344.
45. Bermudez L, Carter V, Magee W Jr, Sherman R, Ayala R. Surgical outcomes auditing systems in humanitarian organizations. World J Surg. 2010;34(3):403–10. https://doi.org/10.1007/s00268-009-0253-6.
46. Maine RG, Hoffman WY, Palacios-Martinez JH, Corlew DS, Gregory GA. Comparison of fistula rates after palatoplasty for international and local surgeons on surgical missions in Ecuador with rates at a craniofacial center in the United States. Plast Reconstr Surg. 2012;129(2):319e–26e. https://doi.org/10.1097/PRS.0b013e31823aea7e.
47. Corlew DS, Alkire BC, Poenaru D, Meara JG, Shrime MG. Economic valuation of the impact of a large surgical charity using the value of lost welfare approach. BMJ Glob Health. 2016;1(4):e000059. https://doi.org/10.1136/bmjgh-2016-000059.
48. Poenaru D, Lin D, Corlew S. Economic valuation of the global burden of cleft disease averted by a large cleft charity. World J Surg. 2016;40(5):1053–9. https://doi.org/10.1007/s00268-015-3367-z.
49. Magee WP Jr, Vander Burg R, Hatcher KW. Cleft lip and palate as a cost-effective health care treatment in the developing world. World J Surg. 2010;34(3):420–7. https://doi.org/10.1007/s00268-009-0333-7.
50. Shrime MG, Hamer M, Mukhopadhyay S, Kunz LM, Claus NH, Randall K, et al. Effect of removing the barrier of transportation costs on surgical utilisation in Guinea, Madagascar and the republic of Congo. BMJ Glob Health. 2017;2(Suppl 4):e000434. https://doi.org/10.1136/bmjgh-2017-000434.
51. Yao CA, Swanson J, Chanson D, Taro TB, Gura B, Figueiredo JC, et al. Barriers to reconstructive surgery in low- and middle-income countries: a cross-sectional study of 453 cleft lip and cleft palate patients in Vietnam. Plast Reconstr Surg. 2016;138(5):887e–95e. https://doi.org/10.1097/prs.0000000000002656.
52. Swanson JW, Yao CA, Auslander A, Wipfli H, Nguyen TH, Hatcher K, et al. Patient barriers to accessing surgical cleft care in Vietnam:

a multi-site, cross-sectional outcomes study. World J Surg. 2017;41(6):1435–46. https://doi.org/10.1007/s00268-017-3896-8.
53. Gutnik L, Yamey G, Riviello R, Meara JG, Dare AJ, Shrime MG. Financial contributions to global surgery: an analysis of 160 international charitable organizations. Springerplus. 2016;5(1):1558. https://doi.org/10.1186/s40064-016-3046-z.
54. Gutnik L, Dieleman J, Dare AJ, Ramos MS, Riviello R, Meara JG, et al. Funding allocation to surgery in low and middle-income countries: a retrospective analysis of contributions from the USA. BMJ Open. 2015;5(11):e008780. https://doi.org/10.1136/bmjopen-2015-008780.
55. Chao TE, Sharma K, Mandigo M, Hagander L, Resch SC, Weiser TG, et al. Cost-effectiveness of surgery and its policy implications for global health: a systematic review and analysis. Lancet Glob Health. 2014;2(6):e334–45. https://doi.org/10.1016/s2214-109x(14)70213-x.
56. United Nations. Sustainable Development Goals. 2015. https://www.un.org/sustainabledevelopment/. Accessed 21 Feb 2019.
57. Roa L, Jumbam DT, Makasa E, Meara JG. Global surgery and the sustainable development goals. Br J Surg. 2019;106(2):e44–52. https://doi.org/10.1002/bjs.11044.
58. Mossey PA, Modell B. Epidemiology of oral clefts 2012: an international perspective. Front Oral Biol. 2012;16:1–18. https://doi.org/10.1159/000337464.
59. Rossell-Perry P, Segura E, Salas-Bustinza L, Cotrina-Rabanal O. Comparison of two models of surgical care for patients with cleft lip and palate in resource-challenged settings. World J Surg. 2015;39(1):47–53. https://doi.org/10.1007/s00268-013-2395-9.
60. World Health Organization, World Bank Group, OECD. Delivering quality health services: a global imperative. 2018.
61. Institute of Medicine. Crossing the quality chasm: a new health system for the 21st century. Washington, D.C.: The National Academies Press; 2001.
62. Slawomirski L, Auraaen A, Klazinga NS. The economics of patient safety. 2017. https://doi.org/10.1787/5a9858cd-en.
63. Nepogodiev D, Martin J, Biccard B, Makupe A, Bhangu A. Global burden of postoperative death. Lancet (London, England). 2019;393(10170):401. https://doi.org/10.1016/s0140-6736(18)33139-8.
64. Haynes AB, Weiser TG, Berry WR, Lipsitz SR, Breizat AH, Dellinger EP, et al. A surgical safety checklist to reduce morbidity and mortality in a global population. N Engl J Med. 2009;360(5):491–9. https://doi.org/10.1056/NEJMsa0810119.
65. Management of patient information: trends and challenges in member states: based on the findings of the second global survey on eHealth [database on the internet]. World Health Organization. 2012. Available from: http://www.who.int/iris/handle/10665/76794. Accessed.
66. Evans DB, Hsu J, Boerma T. Universal health coverage and universal access. Bull World Health Organ. 2013;91(8):546–a. https://doi.org/10.2471/blt.13.125450.
67. World Health Organization. WHO guideline on health policy and system support to optimize community health worker programmes. Geneva: World Health Organization; 2018.

# Afterword: The Wonder of the Smile

Mohamed El-Shazly

Faces are the doors to ourselves. They sense and interpret the outside world, express how we feel to those around us, and thus both comprise and influence our many interactions. The smile is among our most communicative facial actions; a cleft lip a forbidding deformity which hides this most sensible expression. Reconstructing a cleft lip is at its heart the reconstruction of a smile. Consequently, we—as surgeons and others working in this field—work in large degree to recreate this important social element.

The smile mechanism implicates sophisticated anatomical, psychological, and biochemical pathways, which we are just beginning to understand. A smile is thought to involve 17 of the 43 facial muscles. (A frown uses all 43.) Yet unlike a frown, there are many permutations to a smile. In fact, there are smile gradations, ranging from the Grade 1 "Mona Lisa" smile to the Grade 4 "full denture" variety. One group of facial muscles can present a specific look, while multiple muscle groups can simultaneously contract to present another look. In fact, the Facial Action Coding System developed by psychologist Paul Ekman assigns each of the 43 facial distinctive facial muscles a number, called an "action unit." Facial expressions of emotion can be cataloged, much like music into notes on a score.

Unlike the counteraction of biceps and triceps on the elbow, the muscles of facial expression are not opposed in manifesting happiness or anger, creating smile or frown. The contraction-relaxation mode of these muscles presents a special type of expression; the interwoven attachments of muscle to fascia to the dermis of our facial skin can create patterns that are complex.

Some critical questions arise: When do the facial muscles move? Is this voluntary or spontaneous, emotional or non-emotional? A spontaneous smile circuit with only a direct cortical pathway produces what are known as "real" or "emotional" smiles. A voluntary smile circuit with direct and indirect pathways would, in contrary, lead to the fake or the social smile. Yet smiles are so connected to our afferent senses that we smile when we are seeing what we like, listening to funny or nice words, touching lovely persons, smelling beautiful odor, or tasting a favorable food. Further, a "sixth sense" of perception may be responsible for us smiling when we expect happy things. Is a smile when sleeping due to the emotion from a dream, or involuntary? Apparently, we smile with, without, before or after any of the known senses. It works as a common factor in our daily life.

And, finally, what moves these muscles? The answer may reveal struggle between happiness and stress hormones; endorphins versus cortisol. At least 20 types of endorphins have been demonstrated as neurotransmitters. And although they are all released when a smile flashes across the face, no one actually knows if the smile released the endorphins or the endorphins caused the smile! What is clear, however, is that the degree of the smile – it's grade – is absolutely correlated to the amount of endorphins released. The cortisol, as the stress hormone, takes more time to penetrate the face because its release is a multi-step process involving two additional hormones; adrenaline and nor-adrenaline. Voluntarily hiding a smile is often hard to do and occurs after the fact. Even attempting to counteract the smiling muscles cannot disguise the ocular muscles that often accompany the full, emotional smile.

While we may only imperfectly understand the psychological and biochemical processes that create a smile, we can agree on its centrality as a human emotion for good. A mended smile enables a child to be whole, and allows them this most important faculty of expressing who they are. Think about it and whatever it is, go and fix it on the faces in need.

M. El-Shazly
Professor of Plastic Surgery, Assiut University, Regional Director MENA – Operation Smile, Asyut, Egypt

© Springer Nature Switzerland AG 2021

J. W. Swanson, D. W. Low (eds.), *Global Cleft Care in Low-Resource Settings*, https://doi.org/10.1007/978-3-030-59105-2

# Index



© Springer Nature Switzerland AG 2021
J. W. Swanson, D. W. Low (eds.), *Global Cleft Care in Low-Resource Settings*, https://doi.org/10.1007/978-3-030-59105-2

FSC
www.fsc.org
MIX
Papier | Fördert gute Waldnutzung
FSC® C083411

Kolibri 360 GmbH
Ferdinand-Jühlke-Straße 7
99095 Erfurt, Deutschland
produktsicherheit@kolibri360.de